The 20th Anniversary of Pharmaceuticals—Multi-Targeted Natural Products as Therapeutics

The 20th Anniversary of Pharmaceuticals—Multi-Targeted Natural Products as Therapeutics

Guest Editors

Elena Y. Enioutina
Kathleen M. Job
Catherine M. Sherwin

MDPI

Basel • Beijing • Wuhan • Barcelona • Belgrade • Novi Sad • Cluj • Manchester

Guest Editors
Elena Y. Enioutina
Pediatrics
University od Utah
Salt Lake City
United States

Kathleen M. Job
Pediatrics
University of Utah
Salt Lake City
United States

Catherine M. Sherwin
Internal Medicine
The University of
Western Australia
Perth
Australia

Editorial Office
MDPI AG
Grosspeteranlage 5
4052 Basel, Switzerland

This is a reprint of the Special Issue, published open access by the journal *Pharmaceuticals* (ISSN 1424-8247), freely accessible at: https://www.mdpi.com/journal/pharmaceuticals/special_issues/93CN46HT0Q.

For citation purposes, cite each article independently as indicated on the article page online and as indicated below:

Lastname, A.A.; Lastname, B.B. Article Title. *Journal Name* **Year**, *Volume Number*, Page Range.

ISBN 978-3-7258-3774-8 (Hbk)
ISBN 978-3-7258-3773-1 (PDF)
https://doi.org/10.3390/books978-3-7258-3773-1

Contents

Preface

Preparations from medicinal herbs or marine products may contain hundreds, if not thousands, of bioactive molecules. These molecules target the functions of different organs and systems and potentiate the activities of other bioactive molecules present in the formulation. Therefore, therapeutics prepared from natural products may be of special interest to healthcare professionals, enabling them to successfully treat multifactorial diseases.

This Special Issue summarizes the latest research findings on identifying natural products targeting multiple pathways and body functions that can successfully treat multifactorial diseases. Research articles presented in this issue may be of great interest to pharmacologists, pharmacists, and physicians interested in the complementary treatment of disease.

The Guest Editors would like to thank all contributors to the issue and the Assistant Editor, Ms. Kate Zhou.

Elena Y. Enioutina, Kathleen M. Job, and Catherine M. Sherwin
Guest Editors

pharmaceuticals

Editorial

The Special Issue "The 20th Anniversary of Pharmaceuticals—Multi-Targeted Natural Products as Therapeutics" Editorial—Multi-Targeted Therapeutics from Natural Sources: What Do We Know?

Elena Y. Enioutina [1,*], Katheleen M. Job [1] and Catherine M. Sherwin [2]

1 The Division of Clinical Pharmacology, Pediatrics, The Spencer Fox Eccles School of Medicine, Salt Lake City, UT 84108, USA; kate.job@hsc.utah.edu
2 Internal Medicine, UWA Medical School, The University of Western Australia, Perth, WA 6009, Australia; catherine.sherwin85@gmail.com
* Correspondence: elena.enioutina@hsc.utah.edu

Received: 31 January 2025
Revised: 14 March 2025
Accepted: 14 March 2025
Published: 21 March 2025

Citation: Enioutina, E.Y.; Job, K.M.; Sherwin, C.M. The Special Issue "The 20th Anniversary of Pharmaceuticals—Multi-Targeted Natural Products as Therapeutics" Editorial—Multi-Targeted Therapeutics from Natural Sources: What Do We Know? *Pharmaceuticals* **2025**, *18*, 442. https://doi.org/10.3390/ph18040442

Herbal and marine products in the form of extracts, infusions, and decoctions have been used for centuries in folk and traditional medicine. Preparations typically contain multiple biologically active compounds. The World Health Organization (WHO) estimated that about 65% of consumers worldwide use natural remedies containing bioactive molecules to treat various diseases [1]. Most single-molecule drugs of natural origin were developed in the middle of the 20th century through the active screening of natural products for bioactive molecules [2]. Examples include artemisinin, cyclosporine, taxol, doxorubicin, and many others. However, at the beginning of the 21st century, we saw a decline in the number of "natural drugs" introduced to the market. A limiting factor could be explained by the pharmaceutical industry blockbuster model, implying the development of few drugs that make a bulk profit (e.g., USD 1 billion in sales for a drug per year [2]). Another reason for this decline could be the introduction of the high-throughput screening of synthetic libraries. A limitation to the large-scale production of "natural drugs" is the availability of herbal or marine sources for their production. However, the research community has expressed great interest in investigating new therapeutics from natural sources. The Special Issue "The 20th Anniversary of Pharmaceuticals—Multi-Targeted Natural Products as Therapeutics" has had great success, with 25 articles published. These comprise eight review articles and seventeen research articles. This Special Issue aimed to summarize and examine the latest research findings in identifying natural products targeting multiple pathways and body functions that can successfully treat multifactorial diseases. The Guest Editors are thankful for all contributors.

The results of the analysis of studies published in this Special Issue showed that many bioactive compounds in natural products affect various body functions or target multiple pathways. A combination of bioactive molecules in an extract or decoctions usually affects various body functions. Interestingly, some molecules belonging to the same chemical class may target different pathways, often resulting in potential therapeutic effects [Contributions 1–3]. Torres-Sanchez A. et al., for example, reported that pentacyclic triterpenes stimulate human lung carcinoma cell apoptosis, S-phase and G2/M-phase cycle arrest, and the downregulation of MAPK/PI3K and STAT3 gene expression [Contribution 1]. Lung cancers are some of the most common malignancies worldwide, with a poor survival rate [3]. Multiple new treatment strategies have been proposed, from nanoparticle drug delivery to malignant cells and minimally invasive photothermal therapy to the molecular targeting of pathways and receptors involved in malignant cell expansion. The addition of pentacyclic triterpenes as an adjuvant therapy to already existing treatment regimens could significantly improve the survival rate and life satisfaction of treated patients.

Some articles in this Special Issue also focused on the effects of bioactive molecules on immune system functions [Contributions 4–8] [4]. Over the past decade, numerous publications have demonstrated the immunomodulatory activities of traditional medicine preparations and their biologically active components [5–9]. For example, the immunomodulatory properties of ginsenosides isolated from *Panax notoginseng* were found to depend on the ginsenosides' structure and can demonstrate immunosuppressive or immunostimulatory properties [6]. Glycoprotein isolated from *Dioscorea batatas* Decne activated macrophages through the TLR-4 receptor and stimulated nuclear factor-κB (NF-kB), c-Jun N-terminal kinase, and several other pathways, resulting in the production of IL-1β, IL-6, and TNF-α [10]. The bark of *Dioscorea batatas* Decne demonstrated anti-inflammatory activity by inhibiting inducible nitric oxide synthase (iNOS) and Cyclooxygenase-2 (COX-2) expression in LPS-activated RAW264.7 cells via the suppression of NF-κB p65 subunit nuclear translocation [11]. Catechins from green tea modulated the activity of T cells [12]. Gasmi A. et al. reviewed the immunomodulatory properties of polyphenols, terpenoids, β-glucans, and vitamins [Contribution 4, 29 citations as of 30 January 2025]. Beta-glucans activate phagocytic cells (e.g., neutrophils, monocytes, and macrophages), antigen-presenting dendritic cells, Natural Killer (NK) cells through scavenger receptors, Dectin-1, complement receptor 3, and Toll-Like Receptors (TLRs) 2/6 [13,14]. Additionally, β -glucans demonstrate anti-angiogenic properties, which, combined with activated cytotoxic NK cells, may reduce tumor proliferation and metastasis development [14]. Glucans, as natural polysaccharides, could also be valuable as drug-delivery vessels. The data presented in Contribution 6 indicated that cannabidiol extract (CBD) reduces IL-5 and IL-13, which are key cytokines involved in asthma development. An animal model of asthma showed that CBD treatment reduced the levels of IgE and asthma-associated cytokines alongside lung infiltration by immune cells.

Medicinal herbs or their bioactive compounds often simultaneously display immunomodulatory and antimicrobial activity, which can be particularly advantageous in this era of multidrug-resistant bacteria [15]. Herbal extracts often show a broad spectrum of antimicrobial activities against bacteria, viruses, and fungi. Wang et al. investigated the mechanisms behind the antimicrobial activity of walnut green husk extracts against *Staphylococcus aureus*, *Bacillus subtilis*, and *Escherichia coli* [16]. The authors determined that the extracts stimulated intracellular ions and alkaline phosphatase leakage from bacteria, reduced ATPase activity, and upregulated pathways associated with RNA degradation and oxidative phosphorylation. The data presented by Fernandes M. et al. showed that sliver nanoparticles synthesized with the help of extracts from brown algae (*Cystoseira baccata* and *Cystoseira tamariscifolia*) had strong bactericidal or bacteriostatic effects against *Pseudomonas aeruginosa* and *Escherichia coli* [17]. The authors of Contributions 9–12 also focused on the antimicrobial activities of several natural products and their bioactive compounds. The *Kielmeyera membranacea* extract and biflavonoid podocarpus flavone A from *Kielmeyera membranacea* demonstrated anti-*Mycobacterium marinum* activity in vitro and in infected zebrafish [Contribution 12]. Treatment with podocarpus flavone A stimulated the expression of IL-12 and TNF-α cytokines in fish larvae after 5 days of infection. This contribution is especially important due to the growing number of cases of multi-drug-resistant tuberculosis. Hamdi A. et al. screened and ADME-profiled essential oils isolated from *Citrus limon* L. and *Citrus paradisi* L. for their antimicrobial and anti-coagulate activity [Contribution 10]. The essential oils showed bactericidal activity against Gram-positive and Gram-negative bacteria and fungicidal activity against Candida species.

Hepatoprotective and liver function-improving activities are most often associated with silymarin isolated from milk thistle [18,19]. Recently, more studies have investigated the effects of other medicinal herbs on liver functions [20–22]. Contributions 13–15 describe the hepatoprotective, anti-lipidemic, anti-glycemic, choleretic, and hepato-regenerative activities of extracts from *Cichorium intybus*, *Hypericum perforatum*, and polyherbal extract from Cassia *auriculata* leaf, *Centella asiatica* leaf, and *Zingiber officinale* rhizome. The data presented in these articles clearly demonstrated that these extracts regulate glucose and lipid metabolism, protect the liver from xenobiotic injury, and may accelerate liver regeneration.

In conclusion, it appears that there is considerable interest in investigating the effects of purified extracts prepared from natural products or bioactive molecules from these extracts. The PubMed search for natural products and therapeutics displayed 33,703 articles, including 7548 reviews published in 2023–2024, suggesting that researchers have expressed considerable interest in investigating new properties of natural products and summarizing knowledge from previous research. The ability of bioactive molecules to affect multiple signaling pathways and improve several body functions has the potential to decrease the use of multiple drugs for the treatment of different conditions. Additionally, such natural drugs can be used as adjuvant therapies along with conventional regimens to provide positive therapeutic outcomes.

Acknowledgments: The Guest Editors are thankful to all contributors to the Special Issue.

Conflicts of Interest: The author declares no conflicts of interest.

List of Contributions

1. Torres-Sanchez, A.; Torres, G.; Estrada, S.; Perez, D.; Garcia, C.; Milian, M.; Velazquez, E.; Molina, V.; Delgado, Y. Unraveling the Impact of Six Pentacyclic Triterpenes Regulating Metabolic Pathways on Lung Carcinoma Cells. *Pharmaceuticals* **2024**, *17*, 694. https://doi.org/10.3390/ph17060694.
2. Pessoa, R.T.; Santos da Silva, L.Y.; Alcântara, I.S.; Silva, T.M.; Silva, E.d.S.; da Costa, R.H.S.; da Silva, A.B.; Ribeiro-Filho, J.; Pereira Bezerra Martins, A.O.B.; Coutinho, H.D.M.; et al. Antinociceptive Potential of *Ximenia americana* L. Bark Extract and Caffeic Acid: Insights into Pain Modulation Pathways. *Pharmaceuticals* **2024**, *17*, 1671. https://doi.org/10.3390/ph17121671.
3. Kumbukgahadeniya, P.; Baek, E.-B.; Hong, E.-J.; Song, J.-Y.; Kwak, Y.-G.; Jang, M.-R.; Ji, H.-S.; Kwun, H.-J. Prunella vulgaris Extract Ameliorates Testosterone-Induced Benign Prostatic Hyperplasia by Regulating Androgen Levels, Cell Proliferation, and Apoptosis. *Pharmaceuticals* **2024**, *17*, 1516. https://doi.org/10.3390/ph17111516.
4. Gasmi, A.; Shanaida, M.; Oleshchuk, O.; Semenova, Y.; Mujawdiya, P.K.; Ivankiv, Y.; Pokryshko, O.; Noor, S.; Piscopo, S.; Adamiv, S.; et al. Natural Ingredients to Improve Immunity. *Pharmaceuticals* **2023**, *16*, 528. https://doi.org/10.3390/ph16040528.
5. Dontje, A.E.W.K.; Schuiling-Veninga, C.C.M.; van Hunsel, F.P.A.M.; Ekhart, C.; Demirci, F.; Woerdenbag, H.J. The Therapeutic Potential of Essential Oils in Managing Inflammatory Skin Conditions: A Scoping Review. *Pharmaceuticals* **2024**, *17*, 571. https://doi.org/10.3390/ph17050571.
6. Aswad, M.; Pechkovsky, A.; Ghanayiem, N.; Hamza, H.; Dotan, Y.; Louria-Hayon, I. High-CBD Extract (CBD-X) in Asthma Management: Reducing Th2-Driven Cytokine Secretion and Neutrophil/Eosinophil Activity. *Pharmaceuticals* **2024**, *17*, 1382. https://doi.org/10.3390/ph17101382.
7. Shin, J.; Kim, D.-U.; Bae, G.-S.; Han, J.-Y.; Lim, D.-W.; Lee, Y.-M.; Kim, E.; Kwon, E.; Han, D.; Kim, S. Antidepressant-like Effects of *Cannabis sativa* L. Extract in an Lipopolysaccharide Model: Modulation of Mast Cell Activation in Deep Cervical Lymph Nodes and Dura Mater. *Pharmaceuticals* **2024**, *17*, 1409. https://doi.org/10.3390/ph17101409.
8. Machado, I.D.; Borges, P.P.; Giacomozzi, L.J.A.; Benvenutti, L.; Santin, J.R.; dos Santos, S.C.; Rau, M.; Begnini, I.M.; Rebelo, R.A.; Coutinho, H.D.M.; et al. Vernonanthura tweediana (Baker) H. Rob. (Asteraceae), an Ordinary Bush or an Anti-Inflammatory and Immunomodulator Aromatic Species? *Pharmaceuticals* **2024**, *17*, 1492. https://doi.org/10.3390/ph17111492.

9. Veldman, L.B.M.; Belt-Van Zoen, E.; Baars, E.W. Mechanistic Evidence of *Andrographis paniculata* (Burm. f.) Wall. ex Nees, *Pelargonium sidoides* DC., *Echinacea* Species and a Combination of *Hedera helix* L., *Primula veris* L./*Primula elatior* L. and *Thymus vulgaris* L./*Thymus zygis* L. in the Treatment of Acute, Uncomplicated Respiratory Tract Infections: A Systematic Literature Review and Expert Interviews. *Pharmaceuticals* **2023**, *16*, 1206. https://doi.org/10.3390/ph16091206.
10. Hamdi, A.; Horchani, M.; Jannet, H.B.; Snoussi, M.; Noumi, E.; Bouali, N.; Kadri, A.; Polito, F.; De Feo, V.; Edziri, H. In Vitro Screening of Antimicrobial and Anti-Coagulant Activities, ADME Profiling, and Molecular Docking Study of *Citrus limon* L. and *Citrus paradisi* L. Cold-Pressed Volatile Oils. *Pharmaceuticals* **2023**, *16*, 1669. https://doi.org/10.3390/ph16121669.
11. Reyna-Urrutia, V.A.; Robles-Zepeda, R.E.; Estevez, M.; Gonzalez-Reyna, M.A.; Alonso-Martínez, G.V.; Cáñez-Orozco, J.R.; López-Romero, J.C.; Torres-Moreno, H. Microparticles Loaded with *Bursera microphylla* A. Gray Fruit Extract with Anti-Inflammatory and Antimicrobial Activity. *Pharmaceuticals* **2024**, *17*, 1565. https://doi.org/10.3390/ph17121565.
12. Araujo, M.H.d.; Muñoz Sánchez, S.; Simão, T.L.B.V.; Nowik, N.; Antunes, S.S.; Pinto, S.C.; Sorze, D.; Boldrin, F.; Manganelli, R.; Correia Romeiro, N.; et al. Exploring the Antimycobacterial Potential of Podocarpusflavone A from *Kielmeyera membranacea*: In Vitro and In Vivo Insights. *Pharmaceuticals* **2024**, *17*, 1560. https://doi.org/10.3390/ph17121560.
13. Krepkova, L.V.; Babenko, A.N.; Lemyaseva, S.V.; Saybel, O.L.; Sherwin, C.M.; Enioutina, E.Y. Modulation of Hepatic Functions by Chicory (*Cichorium intybus* L.) Extract: Preclinical Study in Rats. *Pharmaceuticals* **2023**, *16*, 1471. https://doi.org/10.3390/ph16101471.
14. Alhamhoom, Y.; Ahmed, S.S.; M., R.K.; Salahuddin, M.; D. R., B.; Ahmed, M.M.; Farhana, S.A.; Rahamathulla, M. Synergistic Antihyperglycemic and Antihyperlipidemic Effect of Polyherbal and Allopolyherbal Formulation. *Pharmaceuticals* **2023**, *16*, 1368. https://doi.org/10.3390/ph16101368.
15. Mohagheghzadeh, A.; Badr, P.; Mohagheghzadeh, A.; Hemmati, S. *Hypericum perforatum* L. and the Underlying Molecular Mechanisms for Its Choleretic, Cholagogue, and Regenerative Properties. *Pharmaceuticals* **2023**, *16*, 887. https://doi.org/10.3390/ph16060887.

References

1. Chopra, B.; Dhingra, A.K. Natural products: A lead for drug discovery and development. *Phytother. Res.* **2021**, *35*, 4660–4702. [CrossRef]
2. Li, J.W.; Vederas, J.C. Drug discovery and natural products: End of an era or an endless frontier? *Science* **2009**, *325*, 161–165. [CrossRef] [PubMed]
3. Li, Y.; Yan, B.; He, S. Advances and challenges in the treatment of lung cancer. *Biomed. Pharmacother.* **2023**, *169*, 115891. [CrossRef]
4. Lin, H.; Han, R.; Wu, W. Glucans and applications in drug delivery. *Carbohydr. Polym.* **2024**, *332*, 121904. [CrossRef] [PubMed]
5. Wang, K.; Yin, J.; Chen, J.; Ma, J.; Si, H.; Xia, D. Inhibition of inflammation by berberine: Molecular mechanism and network pharmacology analysis. *Phytomedicine* **2024**, *128*, 155258. [CrossRef]
6. Yang, C.; Qu, L.; Wang, R.; Wang, F.; Yang, Z.; Xiao, F. Multi-layered effects of Panax notoginseng on immune system. *Pharmacol. Res.* **2024**, *204*, 107203. [CrossRef] [PubMed]
7. Zhang, M.; Wu, X.; Gao, H.; Zhang, L.; Li, Y.; Li, M.; Zhao, C.; Wei, P.; Ou, L. Chinese Herbal Medicine for Irritable Bowel Syndrome: A Perspective of Local Immune Actions. *Am. J. Chin. Med.* **2024**, *52*, 2079–2106. [CrossRef]
8. Shen, M.; Li, Z.; Wang, J.; Xiang, H.; Xie, Q. Traditional Chinese herbal medicine: Harnessing dendritic cells for anti-tumor benefits. *Front. Immunol.* **2024**, *15*, 1408474. [CrossRef]
9. Mok, H.L.; Cheng, K.W.; Xu, Y.; Huang, C.; Lyu, C.; Xu, J.; Hu, D.; Zhu, L.; Lin, C.; Tan, H.Y.; et al. Modified Zhenwu Decoction suppresses chronic colitis via targeting macrophage CCR2/Fyn/p38 MAPK signaling axis. *Phytomedicine* **2024**, *129*, 155694. [CrossRef]
10. Huong, P.T.; Jeon, Y.J. Macrophage activation by glycoprotein isolated from Dioscorea batatas. *Toxicol. Res.* **2011**, *27*, 167–172. [CrossRef]
11. Jin, M.; Suh, S.J.; Yang, J.H.; Lu, Y.; Kim, S.J.; Kwon, S.; Jo, T.H.; Kim, J.W.; Park, Y.I.; Ahn, G.W.; et al. Anti-inflammatory activity of bark of Dioscorea batatas DECNE through the inhibition of iNOS and COX-2 expressions in RAW264.7 cells via NF-κB and ERK1/2 inactivation. *Food Chem. Toxicol.* **2010**, *48*, 3073–3079. [CrossRef] [PubMed]
12. Alhazmi, H.A.; Najmi, A.; Javed, S.A.; Sultana, S.; Al Bratty, M.; Makeen, H.A.; Meraya, A.M.; Ahsan, W.; Mohan, S.; Taha, M.M.E.; et al. Medicinal Plants and Isolated Molecules Demonstrating Immunomodulation Activity as Potential Alternative Therapies for Viral Diseases Including COVID-19. *Front. Immunol.* **2021**, *12*, 637553. [CrossRef]

13. Chan, G.C.; Chan, W.K.; Sze, D.M. The effects of beta-glucan on human immune and cancer cells. *J. Hematol. Oncol.* **2009**, *2*, 25. [CrossRef] [PubMed]
14. Akramiene, D.; Kondrotas, A.; Didziapetriene, J.; Kevelaitis, E. Effects of beta-glucans on the immune system. *Medicina (Kaunas)* **2007**, *43*, 597–606.
15. Enioutina, E.Y.; Teng, L.; Fateeva, T.V.; Brown, J.C.S.; Job, K.M.; Bortnikova, V.V.; Krepkova, L.V.; Gubarev, M.I.; Sherwin, C.M.T. Phytotherapy as an alternative to conventional antimicrobials: Combating microbial resistance. *Expert. Rev. Clin. Pharmacol.* **2017**, *10*, 1203–1214. [CrossRef]
16. Wang, L.; Li, W.; Li, X.; Liu, J.; Chen, Y. Antimicrobial Activity and Mechanisms of Walnut Green Husk Extract. *Molecules* **2023**, *28*, 7981. [CrossRef]
17. Fernandes, M.; González-Ballesteros, N.; da Costa, A.; Machado, R.; Gomes, A.C.; Rodríguez-Argüelles, M.C. Antimicrobial and anti-biofilm activity of silver nanoparticles biosynthesized with Cystoseira algae extracts. *J Biol Inorg Chem* **2023**, *28*, 439–450. [CrossRef]
18. Federico, A.; Dallio, M.; Loguercio, C. Silymarin/Silybin and Chronic Liver Disease: A Marriage of Many Years. *Molecules* **2017**, *22*, 191. [CrossRef] [PubMed]
19. Mohammadi, S.; Ashtary-Larky, D.; Asbaghi, O.; Farrokhi, V.; Jadidi, Y.; Mofidi, F.; Mohammadian, M.; Afrisham, R. Effects of silymarin supplementation on liver and kidney functions: A systematic review and dose-response meta-analysis. *Phytother. Res.* **2024**, *38*, 2572–2593. [CrossRef]
20. Li, J.; Guo, H.; Dong, Y.; Yuan, S.; Wei, X.; Zhang, Y.; Dong, L.; Wang, F.; Bai, T.; Yang, Y. Polysaccharides from Chinese herbal medicine: A review on the hepatoprotective and molecular mechanism. *Chin. J. Nat. Med.* **2024**, *22*, 4–14. [CrossRef]
21. Islam Shawon, S.; Nargis Reyda, R.; Qais, N. Medicinal herbs and their metabolites with biological potential to protect and combat liver toxicity and its disorders: A review. *Heliyon* **2024**, *10*, e25340. [CrossRef] [PubMed]
22. Nasir, F.; Itrat, M.; Khan, F. Evidence-Based Unani Pharmacotherapeutics for the Treatment of Non-Alcoholic Fatty Liver Disease: A Mechanistic Review. *Altern. Ther. Health Med.* **2024**, *30*, 32–42. [PubMed]

pharmaceuticals

Article

Antinociceptive Potential of *Ximenia americana* L. Bark Extract and Caffeic Acid: Insights into Pain Modulation Pathways

Renata Torres Pessoa [1], Lucas Yure Santos da Silva [1], Isabel Sousa Alcântara [1], Tarcísio Mendes Silva [1], Eduardo dos Santos Silva [1], Roger Henrique Sousa da Costa [1], Aparecida Barros da Silva [1], Jaime Ribeiro-Filho [1,2], Anita Oliveira Brito Pereira Bezerra Martins [1], Henrique Douglas Melo Coutinho [3], Jean Carlos Pereira Sousa [4], Andréa Rodrigues Chaves [4], Ricardo Neves Marreto [5] and Irwin Rose Alencar de Menezes [1,*]

1 Laboratory of Pharmacology and Molecular Chemistry, Department of Chemical Biology, Regional University of Cariri (URCA), Rua Coronel Antônio Luis 1161, Pimenta, Crato 63105-000, Ceará, Brazil; renata.pessoa@urca.br (R.T.P.); lucas.yure@urca.br (L.Y.S.d.S.); isabel.alcantara@urca.br (I.S.A.); tarcisio.mendes@urca.br (T.M.S.); eduardodos.santos@urca.br (E.d.S.S.); rogerhenrique8@hotmail.com (R.H.S.d.C.); aparecida.barros@urca.br (A.B.d.S.); jaime.ribeiro@fiocruz.br (J.R.-F.); anita.oliveira@urca.br (A.O.B.P.B.M.)

2 Oswaldo Cruz Foundation (FIOCRUZ), Fiocruz Ceará, R. São José, S/N—Precabura, Eusébio 61773-270, Ceará, Brazil

3 Laboratory of Microbiology and Molecular Biology, Department of Biological Chemistry, Regional University of Cariri (URCA), Crato 63105-000, Ceará, Brazil; hdmcoutinho@gmail.com

4 Institute of Chemistry, Federal University of Goiás, Goiânia 74001-970, Goiás, Brazil; jeanpsousa01@gmail.com (J.C.P.S.); andrea_chaves@ufg.br (A.R.C.)

5 Faculty of Pharmacy, Federal University of Goiás, Goiânia 74605-170, Goiás, Brazil; ricardomarreto@ufg.br

* Correspondence: irwin.alencar@urca.br

Citation: Pessoa, R.T.; Santos da Silva, L.Y.; Alcântara, I.S.; Silva, T.M.; Silva, E.d.S.; da Costa, R.H.S.; da Silva, A.B.; Ribeiro-Filho, J.; Pereira Bezerra Martins, A.O.B.; Coutinho, H.D.M.; et al. Antinociceptive Potential of *Ximenia americana* L. Bark Extract and Caffeic Acid: Insights into Pain Modulation Pathways. *Pharmaceuticals* **2024**, *17*, 1671. https://doi.org/10.3390/ph17121671

Academic Editors: Catherine Sherwin, Elena Y. Enioutina and Kathleen M. Job

Received: 6 November 2024
Revised: 28 November 2024
Accepted: 7 December 2024
Published: 11 December 2024

Abstract: Background/Objectives: This study evaluated the antinociceptive effect of the *Ximenia americana* L. bark extract (HEXA) and its primary component, caffeic acid (CA), through in vivo assays. **Methods**: The antinociceptive properties were assessed using abdominal writhing, hot plate, and Von Frey tests. Additionally, the study investigated the modulation of various pain signaling pathways using a pharmacological approach. **Results:** The results demonstrated that all doses of the HEXA significantly increased latency in the hot plate test, decreased the number of abdominal contortions, reduced hyperalgesia in the Von Frey test, and reduced both phases of the formalin test. Caffeic acid reduced licking time in the first phase of the formalin test at all doses, with the highest dose showing significant effects in the second phase. The HEXA potentially modulated α_2-adrenergic (52.99%), nitric oxide (57.77%), glutamatergic (33.66%), vanilloid (39.84%), cyclic guanosine monophosphate (56.11%), and K^+ATP channel-dependent pathways (38.70%). Conversely, CA influenced the opioid, glutamatergic (53.60%), and vanilloid (34.42%) pathways while inhibiting nitric oxide (52.99%) and cyclic guanosine monophosphate (38.98%). **Conclusions:** HEXA and CA exhibit significant antinociceptive effects due to their potential interference in multiple pain signaling pathways. While the molecular targets remain to be fully investigated, HEXA and CA demonstrate significant potential for the development of new analgesic drugs.

Keywords: natural compounds; HPLC; nociception; anti-inflammatory; mechanism of action; pain

1. Introduction

Pain is a sensory and emotional experience that signals actual or potential harm to the body, thus providing an essential protective function against threats to the organism's health [1]. Pain can be classified based on duration as acute, subchronic, or chronic [2] and based on the origin of the signaling stimulus as neuropathic or inflammatory [1].

Acute pain is immediate and prevents damage and protects injured tissue [2]. On the other hand, chronic pain lasts more than ten days. This issue is a major global health concern that impacts people in physical, economic, emotional, and social ways [3,4]. In both cases, the pain usually requires management, which is mainly performed with the use of analgesic drugs.

Nonsteroidal anti-inflammatory drugs (NSAIDs) are the most used drugs in the treatment of acute, moderate, or chronic pain [5]. Their mechanism of action involves the peripheral and central inhibition of the cyclooxygenase enzymes (COX-1 and COX-2), which inhibits the production of lipid mediators such as prostaglandins, thromboxanes, and leukotrienes [6]. However, the long-term use of NSAIDs is associated with severe adverse effects, including nausea, dyspepsia, abdominal pain, skin reactions, and nephropathy, among others [7]. In addition, NSAIDs present significant therapeutic limitations, so in many cases, the use of opioid analgesics is necessary. However, these drugs pose even more significant risks for patients. Therefore, research targeting new therapeutic alternatives with fewer adverse effects can significantly improve the pharmacological management of pain disorders [8].

In this context, medicinal plants are an ancient source of therapeutic resources in treating various diseases [9]. The pharmacological properties associated with the traditional use of medicinal species are due to the presence of bioactive compounds, indicating that medicinal plants are sources of new molecules with therapeutic potential [10] and, as such, may help develop new drugs to treat pain [11]. Historically, bark is a common ingredient that has been utilized for centuries in traditional medicine for the treatment of various diseases. This part of the plant contains different active compounds, such as tannins, salicylates, flavonoids, and alkaloids, contributing to its analgesic effects [12,13].

Ximenia americana L. is popularly known in Brazil as wild plum, *"ambuí"*, thorn plum, and Brazilian sandalwood [14,15]. Previous research has demonstrated that *X. americana* has antioxidant [16], gastroprotective [17], antiparasitic [18], wound healing [19], antiedematogenic [20], and antinociceptive [21] biological properties. Phytochemical studies have identified caffeic acid (CA) as a major constituent in *X. americana* [18,22,23]. Also known as 3,4-hydroxycinnamic acid, this compound is usually found in numerous fruits and vegetables, such as prunes, artichokes, eggplant, and grapes [24]. Research in pharmacology has uncovered a range of biological activities associated with CA, such as neuroprotective [25], antimicrobial [26], anticancer [27], anti-inflammatory [28], antinociception [29], and antiviral [30] activities.

Considering the ethnopharmacological evidence of *X. americana* as a promising medicinal plant, this study aimed to investigate the antinociceptive effect of *X. americana* L. bark extract (HEXA) and its main constituent, caffeic acid (CA), in animal models, to understand how these compounds can act in modulating pain induced by different stimuli.

2. Results

In our previous paper, we demonstrated the predominance of polyphenols in the hydroethanolic bark extract of *X. Americana* through HPLC analysis, where nine compounds were identified. Upon the new chemical approach by UPLC-MS/MS, caffeic acid and quercetin were confirmed as the major constituents (Figure S1 in Supplementary Material).

The ESI-MS analysis revealed the MS/MS pattern for CA dominating the loss of a water molecule (18 Da), characterizing the fragment of m/z 161.05 ($[M\text{-}H_2O]^-$) and sequentially the decarboxylation of CO_2 (44 Da), which can be explained by the Diels–Alder rearrangement reaction allowing the visualization of the fragment of m/z 135.05 ($[M\text{-}CO_2]^-$), as identified by [31] (Figure S1A,B) in the Supplementary Material. The Molecular Networking tool with gold classification was successfully applied to correlate the fragmentation spectrum of caffeic acid and other compounds of the extract of *X. americana* L. (Table S1; see Supplementary Material) with the GNPS spectral library, allowing the confirmation of its molecular identity.

2.1. HEXA Failed in Inducing Central Nervous System Effects in Mice

The treatment with HEXA (200 mg/kg) did not alter the animals' motor coordination compared to the negative control group in the rotarod test. In addition, the number of falls and the time the treated animals spent on the bar was similar to the negative control group. Concerning the open-field test, the treatment with HEXA (200 mg/kg) did not affect behavioral parameters such as rearing (lifting) and grooming (self-cleaning), nor did it alter the number of crossings. Together, these results suggest that HEXA has no evident central nervous system activity.

2.2. HEXA Has Antinociceptive Activity In Vivo: Central and Peripheral Effects

The administration of acetic acid induces abdominal writhing in untreated mice. treatments with HEXA at doses of 50, 100, and 200 mg/kg caused a significant reduction in the amount of abdominal writhing by 84.99%, 87.99%, and 89.49% ($p < 0.0001$), respectively, compared to the untreated group (Figure 1A).

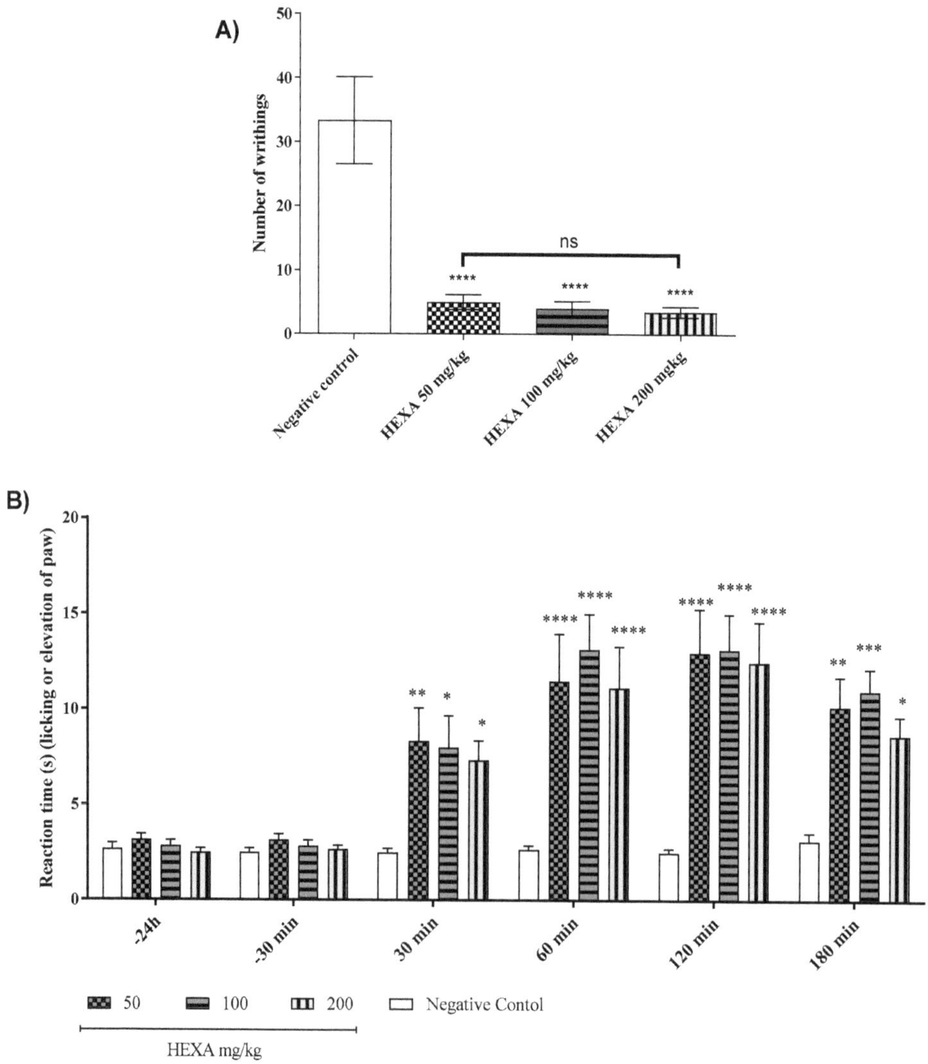

Figure 1. *Cont.*

C)

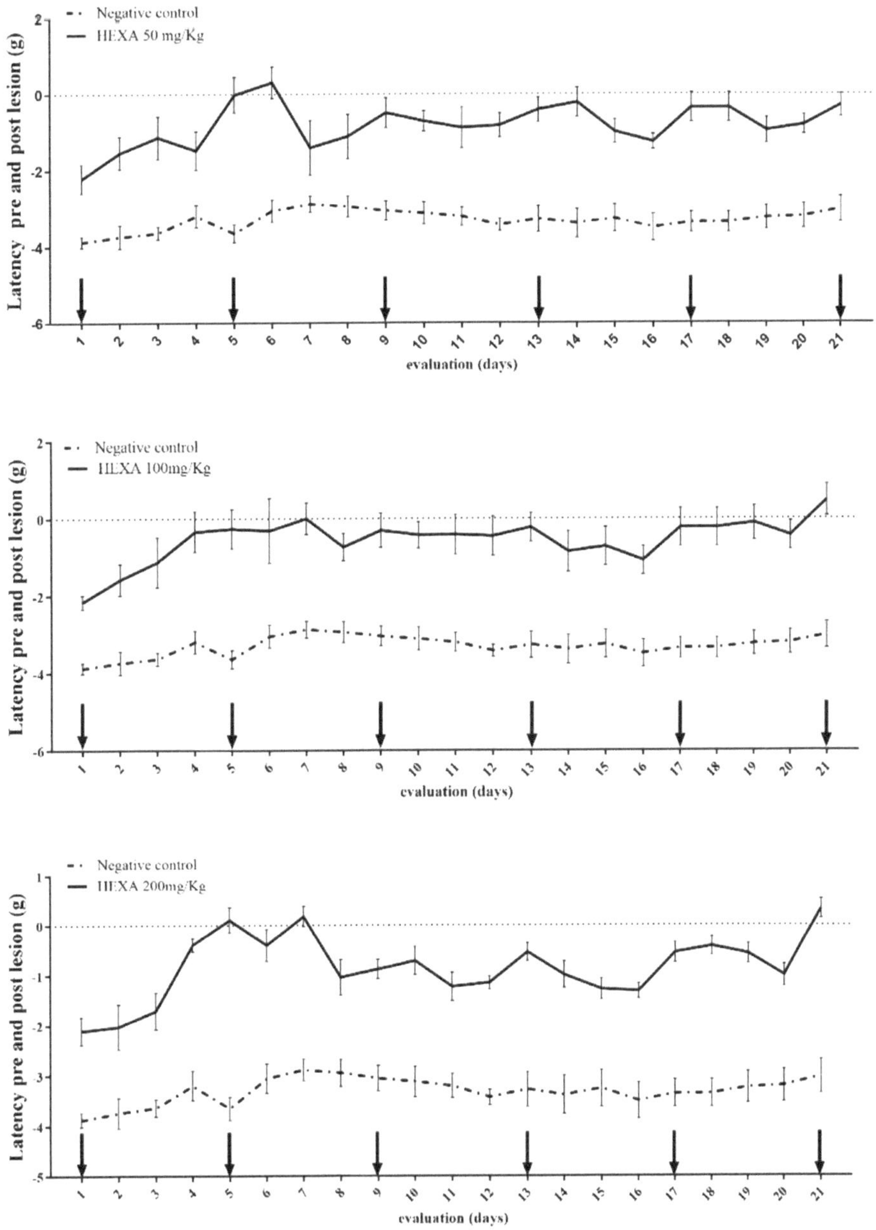

Figure 1. Antinociceptive effect of HEXA (50, 100, and 200 mg/kg) by acetic acid-induced abdominal writhing test (**A**); the hot plate test (**B**) and the hypernociception measure by Von Frey test induced by CFA (**C**). The arrow indicates the treatment day. One-way ANOVA followed by Tukey's test. (* $p < 0.05$; ** $p < 0.01$; *** $p < 0.001$; **** $p < 0.0001$; ns = not significant when compared to the negative control group) for the acetic acid-induced abdominal writhing test. Two-way ANOVA followed by Tukey's test (* $p < 0.05$; ** $p < 0.01$; *** $p < 0.001$; **** $p < 0.0001$ when compared to the negative control group) for hot plate and hypernociception induced by CFA assay.

In the hot plate model, treatments with HEXA at doses of 50, 100, and 200 mg/kg significantly increased the time the animals remained on the hot plate by 69.17%, 68.13%, and 71.98%, ($p < 0.0001$), respectively, when compared to the negative control group. A time-point analysis revealed that the lowest dose (50 mg/kg) increased the latency by 66.67%, 56.89%, 48%, and 67.89% at 30, 60, 120, and 180 min. ($p < 0.0001$). In these respective time points, the dose of 100 mg/kg increased the permanence by 68%, 50.62%, 47.32%, and 65.27%, while the dose of 200 mg/kg increased the permanence of the animals by 70.67%, 58.12%, 50%, and 72.63% ($p < 0.0001$) (Figure 1B) (F (15, 120) = 2951).

The treatments with HEXA at 50, 100, and 200 mg/kg significantly increased the pain threshold by 75.30%, 83.32%, and 74.52%, respectively, thus demonstrating the antinociceptive activity of HEXA in this model when compared to the negative control group. Regarding the time intervals, treatment with HEXA at a dose of 50 mg/kg increased the pain threshold by 42.83% (day 01), 58.83% (day 02), 69.01% (day 03), 54% (day 04), 99.39% (day 05), 90% (day 06), 51.44% (day 07), 62.43% (day 08), 84% (day 09), 77.22% (day 10), 72.49% (day 11), 76.05% (day 12), 87.46% (day 13), 93.44% (day 14), 69.67% (day 15), 64.18% (day 16), 89.42% (day 17), 89.42% (day 18), 70.50% (day 19), 74.70% (day 20), and 89.89% (day 21) ($p < 0.0001$) when compared to the negative control group (Figure 1C).

On the other hand, treatment with HEXA at a dose of 100 mg/kg increased the threshold by 44.41% (day 01), 57.95% (day 02), 69.17% (day 03), 89.24% (day 04), 92.85% (day 05), 89.64% (day 06), 99.80% (day 07), 74.90% (day 08), 89.82% (day 09), 86.30% (day 10), 87.02% (day 11), 86.57% (day 12), 99.99% (day 13), 74.75% (day 14), 77.68% (day 15), 68.94% (day 16), 93.06% (day 17), 93.06% (day 18), 96.40% (day 19), 86.31% (day 20), and 84.37% (day 21) ($p < 0.0001$), respectively, when compared to the negative control group (Figure 1C).

Finally, treatment with HEXA at a dose of 200 mg/kg increased the threshold by 45.70% (day 01), 45.92% (day 02), 53.12% (day 03), 87.85% (day 04), 97.11% (day 05), 87.09% (day 06), 93.83% (day 07), 64.70% (day 08), 71.28% (day 09), 77.22% (day 10), 61.66% (day 11), 66.50% (day 12), 99.98% (day 13), 70.66% (day 14), 60.81% (day 15), 96.24% (day 16), 83.64% (day 17), 83.64% (day 18), 99.98% (day 19), 68.62% (day 20), and 89.15% (day 21) ($p < 0.0001$), respectively, when compared to the negative control group (Figure 1C).

2.3. Formalin-Induced Nociception Test of HEXA and CA

Animals treated with HEXA showed a significant reduction in paw-licking time in the first phase and the second phase compared to the negative control group. In the first phase (Figure 2A), treatment with doses of 50, 100, and 200 mg/kg caused a reduction of 77.63%, 59.37%, and 58.44% ($p < 0.001$, F = 0.114), respectively, while in the second phase (Figure 2B), the same doses caused reductions of 56.74%, 69.43, and 54.02% ($p < 0.0001$, F = 15.08), respectively, compared to the control group. On the other hand, treatment with CA at doses of 0.8 and 1.8 mg/kg reduced paw-licking time by 36.40% and 22.17% ($p < 0.0001$, F = 46.26), respectively, in the first phase (Figure 2C). However, only the 1.8 mg/kg dose reduced licking time significantly by 47.97% ($p < 0.0001$, F = 23.55) in the second phase (Figure 2D) when compared to the control group.

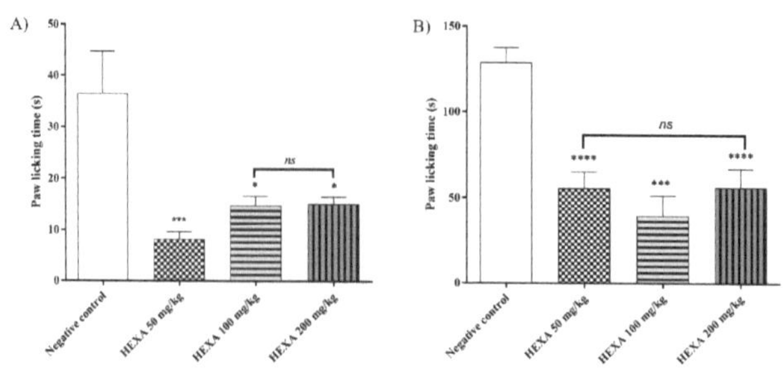

Figure 2. *Cont.*

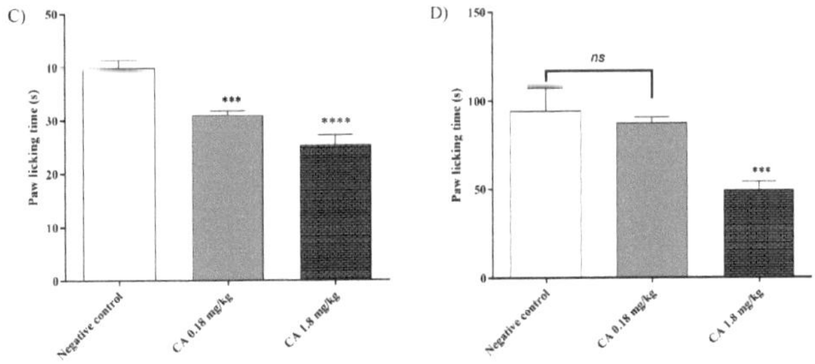

Figure 2. Evaluation of the antinociceptive effect of HEXA (50, 100, and 200 mg/kg) and CA (0.18 and 1.8 mg/kg) on the neurogenic phase (phase 1—(**A**,**C**)) and inflammatory phase (phase 2—(**B**,**D**)) against formalin-induced pain in mice. These values represent the arithmetic mean ± SE (Standard Error of the Mean) (n = 6/group). One-way ANOVA followed by Tukey's test. (* $p < 0.05$; *** $p < 0.001$; **** $p < 0.0001$; ns = not significant when compared to the negative control group).

2.4. Analysis of Signaling Pathways Underlying the Analgesic Effect of HEXA and CA

2.4.1. Vanilloid System

The administration of HEXA (100 mg/kg), CA (1.8 mg/kg), and ruthenium red (a non-selective antagonist of transient potential receptors -TRP) significantly reduced paw-licking time by 39.84%, 34.42%, and 99.77% ($p < 0.0001$, F = 131.5), respectively, in animals challenged with capsaicin, a TRPV1 receptor agonist, when compared to the negative control group (Figure 3A). However, while the antagonist fully inhibited the nociceptive response, the natural products caused partial inhibition.

2.4.2. Glutamatergic Pathway

The treatment with HEXA (100 mg/kg), CA (1.8 mg/kg), and ascorbic acid reduced the licking time by 33.66%, 53.60%, and 68.44% ($p < 0.0001$, F = 12.71) respectively, after intraplantar injection of glutamate, compared to challenged and non-treated animals. These results demonstrate the potential participation of the glutamatergic pathway in the antinociceptive effect of the compounds (Figure 3B).

2.4.3. Opioid Pathway

The administration of HEXA (100 mg/kg), CA (1.8 mg/kg), and morphine significantly reduced nociception time by 57.28%, 51.21%, and 94.20%, ($p < 0.0001$, F = 26.36), respectively, when compared to the negative control group (Figure 3C). Notably, the magnitude of inhibition was significantly higher in the morphine group. When the animals received pretreatment with naloxone, the antinociceptive effect of HEXA and CA was reversed, suggesting that both treatments could modulate nociception by interfering with the opioid system.

2.4.4. L-Arginine/Nitric Oxide/cGMP Pathway

Swiss mice treated with HEXA (100 mg/kg), CA (1.8 mg/kg), and L-NOARG had nociception time significantly reduced by 57.77%, 52.99%, and 51.68%, ($p < 0.0001$, F = 36.14), respectively, in comparison with the negative control group. The pretreatment with L-arginine was found to reverse the analgesic effect of HEXA and CA, suggesting an interference of HEXA and CA on the NO signaling pathway (Figure 3D).

2.4.5. Cyclic Guanosine Monophosphate (cGMP) Pathway

The treatment with HEXA (100 mg/kg), CA (1.8 mg/kg), and methylene blue reduced the animals' licking time by 56.11%, 38.98%, and 98.8% ($p < 0.0001$, F = 17.14) respectively, when compared to untreated animals. However, pretreatment with methylene blue did not affect the analgesic effect of HEXA and CA (Figure 3E). Nevertheless, the participation of this pathway in the mechanisms underlying the antinociceptive effect of the compounds cannot be ruled out.

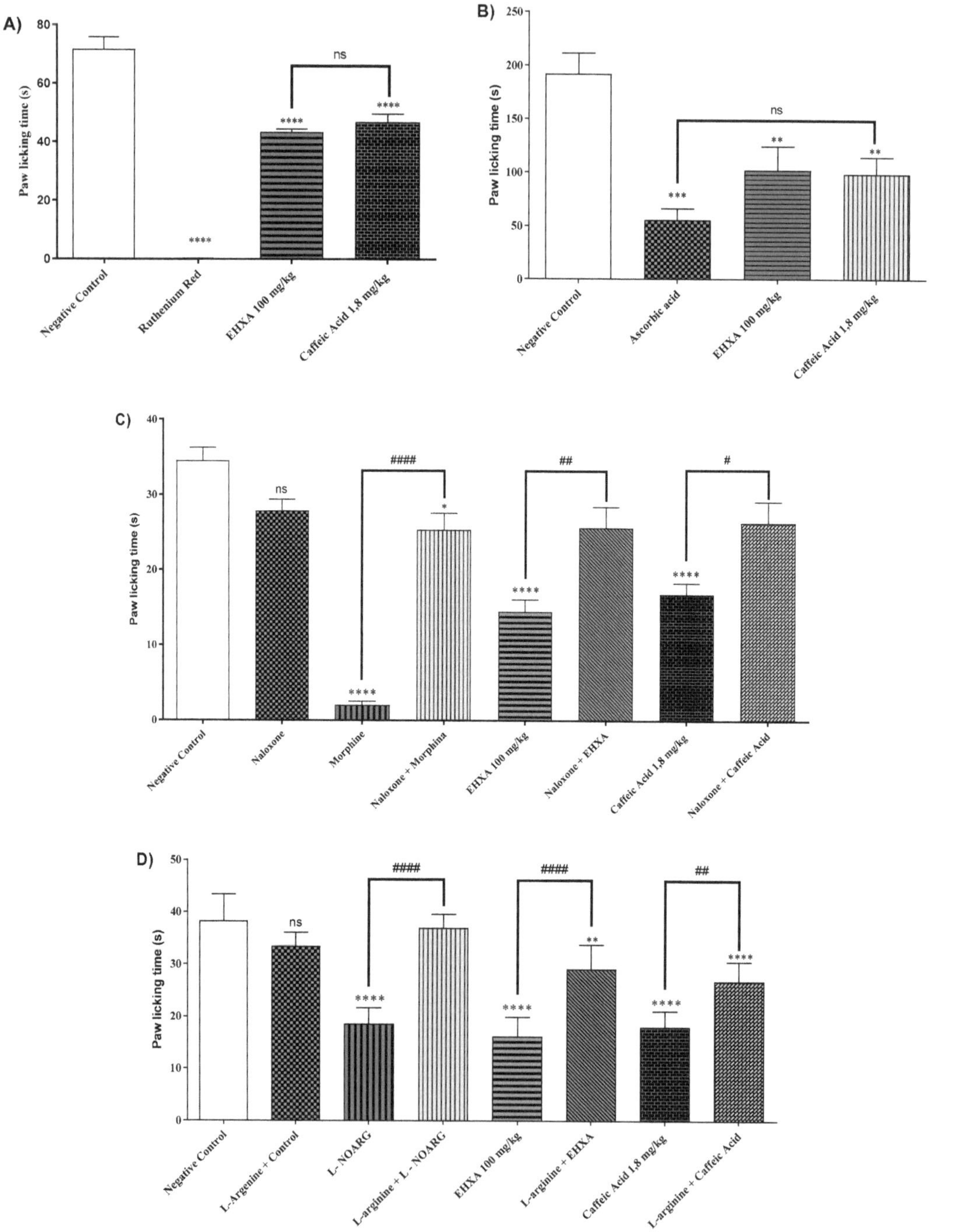

Figure 3. *Cont.*

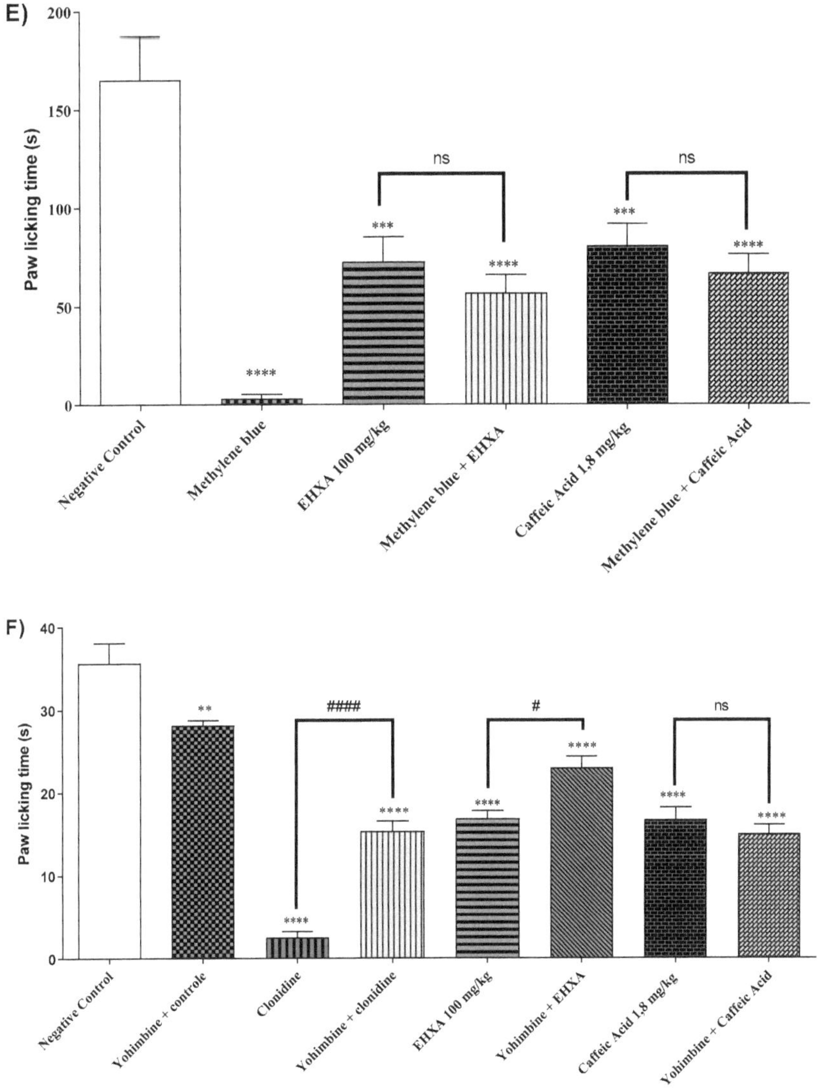

Figure 3. *Cont.*

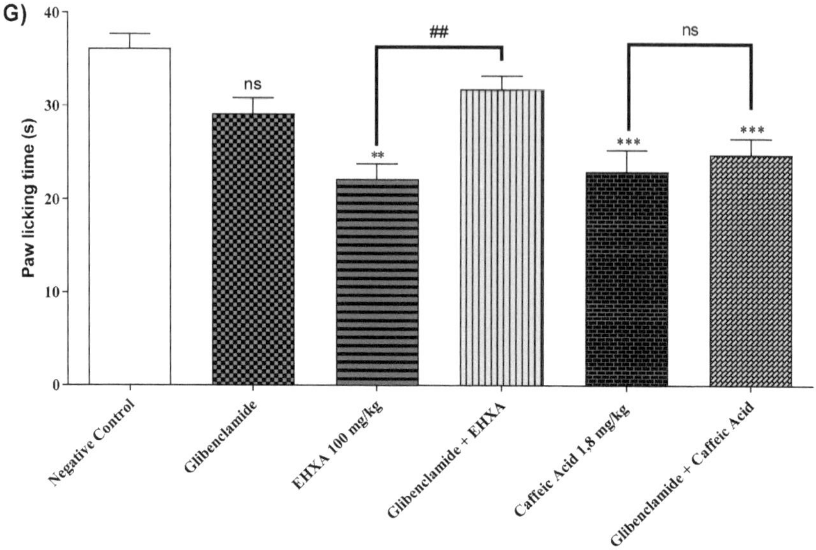

Figure 3. Signaling pathways underlying the antinociceptive response of HEXA (100 mg/kg) and CA (1.8 mg/kg) in the antinociceptive response: (**A**) vanilloid; (**B**) glutamatergic; (**C**) opioid; (**D**) L-Arginine/Nitric Oxide/cGMP; (**E**) cyclic guanosine monophosphate. (**F**) Participation of α2-adrenergic receptors; (**G**) K+ATP channels against formalin-induced pain in mice. Values present the mean ± SE (Standard Error of the Mean) (n = 6/group). One-way (ANOVA) followed by the Tukey test (* $p < 0.05$; ** $p < 0.01$; *** $p < 0.001$; **** $p < 0.0001$ when compared to the negative control group; # $p < 0.05$; ## $p < 0.01$; #### $p < 0.0001$ when comparing agonist vs. antagonist + agonist or HEXA alone vs. antagonist + HEXA group; ns = not significant).

2.4.6. Involvement of the α_2-Adrenergic Receptor

The groups of mice treated with HEXA (100 mg/kg), CA (1.8 mg/kg), and clonidine (α_2 receptor agonist) had nociception time significantly reduced by 52.99%, 53.27%, and 92.99%, ($p < 0.0001$, F = 54.83), respectively, in comparison with the negative control group. The pretreatment with yohimbine (α_2 receptor antagonist) was found to reverse the analgesic effect of HEXA and CA, suggesting that these products interfere with α_2-adrenergic receptor signaling (Figure 3F).

2.4.7. K+ATP Channel-Dependent Signaling

When treated with HEXA at a dose of 100 mg/kg and CA at a dose of 1.8 mg/kg, the animals showed a decrease in paw-licking time by 38.70% and 36.41% ($p < 0.0001$, F = 10.04) respectively, compared to the control group. In the HEXA group, and when the animals received pretreatment with glibenclamide, the pain-relieving effect was reversed. However, this effect was not observed in the combined treatment with glibenclamide and CA (see Figure 3G), suggesting that HEXA components could partially act on K+ATP channels. However, this effect was not observed in the combined treatment with glibenclamide and CA (Figure 3G).

2.4.8. Cholinergic Pathway

The treatment with HEXA (100 mg/kg), CA (1.8 mg/kg), and acetylcholine reduced nociception time by 53.33%, 39.55%, and 62.67% ($p < 0.0001$, F = 17.15), respectively, when compared to the control group. When the animals in the HEXA and CA groups received pretreatment with atropine, the antinociceptive effect was not affected, indicating that there is no clear relationship between this mechanism and the analgesic effect of the natural products investigated in this study (Figure 4A).

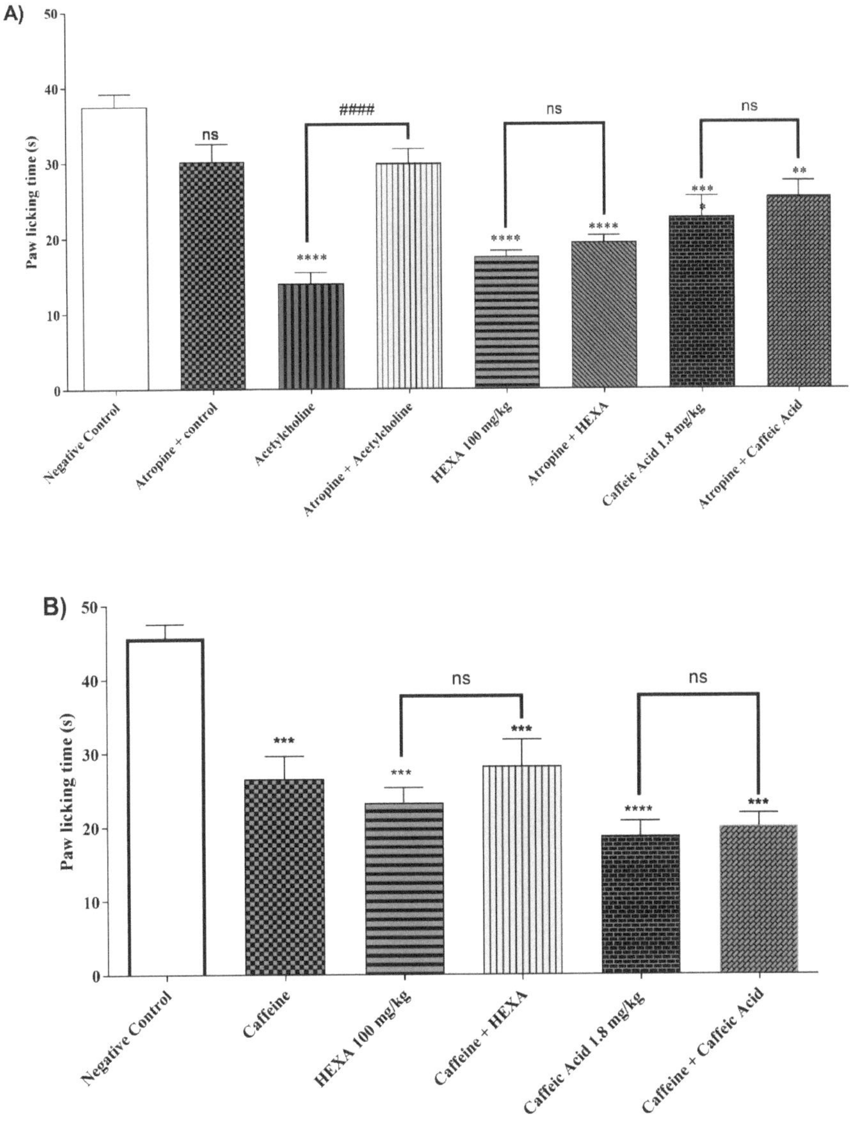

Figure 4. *Cont.*

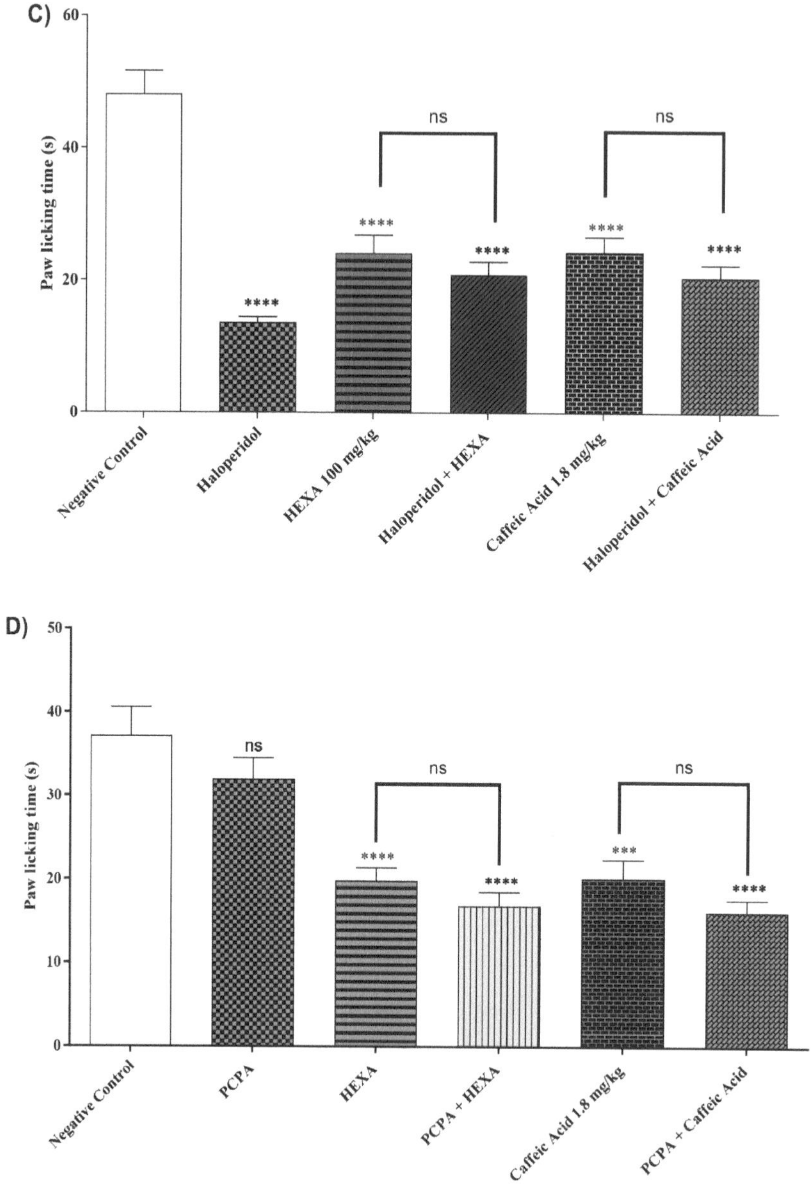

Figure 4. Participation of (**A**) cholinergic, (**B**) adenosinergic, (**C**) dopaminergic pathway, and (**D**) serotonergic system for the antinociceptive response of HEXA (100 mg/kg) and CA (1.8 mg/kg) against formalin-induced pain in mice. The values present the mean ± SE (Standard Error of the Mean) (n = 6/group). One-way (ANOVA) followed by the Tukey test (* $p < 0.05$; ** $p < 0.01$, *** $p < 0.001$; **** $p < 0.0001$ when compared to the negative control group; #### $p < 0.0001$ when comparing agonist vs. agonist + antagonist; ns = not significant).

2.4.9. Adenosinergic Pathway

The treatment with HEXA (100 mg/kg) and CA (1.8 mg/kg) significantly reduced the animals' licking time by 49.27% and 59.12% ($p < 0.0001$, F = 15.37), respectively, after intraplantar formalin injection compared to the control group. However, there was no statistical difference when the animals in the HEXA and CA groups received pretreatment with caffeine, a non-specific inhibitor of the pathway (see Figure 4B).

2.4.10. Dopaminergic System

The treatment with HEXA (100 mg/kg) and CA (1.8 mg/kg) significantly reduced by 41.87% and 49.49%, ($p < 0.0001$, F = 23.70), respectively, the animals' licking time after when compared to the negative control group. However, no statistical difference was observed when the animals of the HEXA and CA groups received pretreatment with haloperidol, thus suggesting that none of these substances inhibit the adenosinergic signaling pathway (Figure 4C).

2.4.11. Involvement of the Serotonergic System

After receiving HEXA (100 mg/kg) and CA (1.8 mg/kg) treatments, the animals showed a 46.65% and 45.73% ($p < 0.0001$, F = 15.33) reduction in licking time compared to the control group. Additionally, when the HEXA and CA groups were given a pretreatment of PCPA, the antinociceptive effect was sustained, indicating that both HEXA and CA do not affect the serotonergic signaling pathway (Figure 4D).

3. Discussion

This study contributes new insights into the potential mechanisms of action underlying the antinociceptive effect of *Ximenia americana* L. bark extract (HEXA) and its major constituent caffeic acid (CA). In this context, significant reductions in pain responses were demonstrated through different assessment tests such as formalin, acetic acid, hot plate, and complete Freund's adjuvant as well as through the pharmacological modulation of pain signaling pathways that to date have not been previously reported in the literature. Previous studies have shown that HEXA has clinical safety by presenting low toxicity (LD_{50} > 2000 mg/kg), as well as caffeic acid (LD_{50} = 4850 mg/kg) [32,33].

In our previously published data, our research group demonstrated that the extract of *Ximenia americana* L. used in this study (HEXA) has a unique chemical profile. It is characterized by the presence of alkaloids, steroids, saponins, glycosides, cyanogenic glycosides, anthraquinone, and, principally, flavonoids, terpenoids, and tannin derivatives. The quantitative analysis by HPLC revealed rutin, gallic acid, quercetin, catechin, kaempferol, chlorogenic acid, ellagic acid, caffeic acid, and quercitrin as the main compounds [18,22,23,34]. The literature's comprehensive chemical profile, combined with the isolation of several other compounds from this species, including sambunigrin, gallic acid, catechin, and different stereoisomers of (epi)catechin, gallotannins quercetin, quercetin-3-O-β-xylopyranoside, quercetin-3-O-(6″-galloyl)-β-glucopyranoside quercitrin, avicularin, β-glucogalin, 1,6-digalloyl-β-glucopyranose, and kaempferol-3-O-(6″-galloyl)-β-glucopyranoside [16,35–39], underscores its potential for drug discovery, providing a solid foundation for further research in pharmacology.

Previous research by Coutinho et al. (2009) demonstrated that quercitrin presents anti-inflammatory effects, while epicatechin isolated from ethanolic extracts of *X. americana* bark [40,41] and flavonoid-rich fractions obtained from the roots of this species showed antinociceptive activity and antioxidant potential [42]. In addition, caffeic acid has previously been shown to have biological activities such as antimicrobial [26], anticancer [43], muscle relaxant [44], antioxidant [45], gastroprotective, and antinociceptive activities. Corroborating with our results, the literature shows evidence that this antinociceptive effect is dose-dependent and may be mediated by nitric oxide [46] through the downregulation of NF-κB, α_2-adrenergic and opioidergic receptors [29], but it does not involve serotonergic pathways.

Thus, the antinociceptive activity of the HEXA can be justified by the presence of bioactive compounds with proven pharmacological properties. Our studies demonstrated the therapeutic potential of various formulations obtained from different parts of *X. americana*.

For instance, an extract from the stem of this species showed topical anti-inflammatory potential in ear edema models [22], while the ethanol extract showed anticonvulsant activity in models of acute inflammation [47]. Moreover, the total polysaccharides obtained from *X. americana* showed anti-inflammatory and antinociceptive action in a model of acute pancreatitis. It was demonstrated that their pharmacological actions might occur through type 2 cannabinoid receptors [48].

Regarding the biological activities investigated in the present study, it was observed through the open-field and rotarod tests that HEXA, at the highest dose evaluated in the present study, did not promote central nervous system activity, suggesting that the antinociceptive effects observed in this study do not occur due to a change in behavioral parameters such as incoordination from either stimulant or depressant, evaluated in the rotarod and open-field models. The study found that HEXA, when orally administered at doses of 50, 100, and 200 mg/kg, demonstrated an antinociceptive effect by reducing nociception in mice models challenged with acetic acid and formalin, as evidenced by decreased abdominal writhing and paw licking. The results of the study showed that HEXA significantly reduced the amount of writhing, indicating a possible peripheral analgesic effect by inhibiting the release of these mediators.

Regarding the formalin test, treatment with HEXA and CA significantly reduced nociception in both the first and second phases of the test, suggesting a possible inhibition of cell activation and mediator release. Zhen et al. (2015) demonstrated that an extract obtained from *X. caffra*, chemically characterized by the presence of phenolic compounds also identified in *X. americana*, including gallic acid, catechin, quercetin, and kaempferol and its derivatives, showed antioxidant, antiproliferative, and anti-inflammatory potential, reinforcing the potential action of the extract on the inflammatory component of the nociceptive response [49]. In the hot plate test, the HEXA significantly increased the time the animals remained on the plate, which suggests the intriguing possibility that the extract may also act at a supraspinal level.

Complete Freund's adjuvant (CFA) is commonly used in chronic in vivo models. It triggers an inflammatory process that lowers nociceptive thresholds, leading to the development of allodynia and hyperalgesia in inflamed limbs. This compound induces an inflammatory response involving mediators such as histamine, serotonin, cytokines, glutamate, and prostaglandins [50,51], resulting in edema and persistent mechanical hyperalgesia in chronic models [52], as well as causing long-lasting mechanical allodynia in mice [53]. The latest findings demonstrate that HEXA significantly reduces allodynia and hyperalgesia, supporting the idea that this extract might inhibit the release of nociceptive process mediators, as previously suggested in this study. A study by Gamato et al. (2011) revealed that caffeic acid was more potent than its derivative rosmarinic acid in nociception models, with the 10 mg/kg dose showing the most significant antinociceptive potential [54].

The extract of *X. americana* stem significantly reduced the chronic inflammatory process in a tendinitis model [55]. The study conducted by Da Palma et al. (2020) demonstrated that hydroalcoholic extracts obtained from the leaves and bark of *X. americana* presented wound-healing effects in acute, subchronic, and chronic stages of injury in mice. Thus, the therapeutic potential of this species in treating acute pain in both the acute and chronic phases is suggested. Given these results, the present study aimed to investigate the potential signaling pathways underlying the analgesic effects of HEXA and its major constituent caffeic acid. For this purpose, we chose signaling pathways that are critically involved in the painful process, including the opioid, cholinergic, α2-adrenergic, adenosinergic, dopaminergic, glutamatergic, vanilloid, and serotoninergic pathways as well as those mediated by cyclic guanosine monophosphate, nitric oxide, and K+ATP channels.

The opioid signaling pathway involves G protein-coupled receptors (Gi/0 subfamily), whose activation inhibits the enzyme adenylate cyclase, leading to the degradation of cyclic adenosine monophosphate (cAMP) and blocking downstream events mediated by protein kinase A (PKA) [56]. Moreover, through this signaling pathway, opioid agonists open potassium channels and inhibit the opening of voltage-gated calcium channels [57], reducing the activity of nociceptor neurons and the release of neurotransmitters [56]. The results obtained in this study indicate that HEXA and CA can interfere with the opioid signaling pathway, which corroborates the results obtained in the hot plate assay.

Nitric oxide (NO) indirectly mediates the inflammatory process, contributing to vascular and cellular events. Since this mediator is produced from L-arginine under the action of NO-synthase (NOS), the inhibition of this synthesis pathway is associated with the inhibition of the pain process [58,59]. L-NOArg, an L-arginine analog, competitively inhibits NOS, blocking thus nitric oxide synthesis [60]. The present study showed that both HEXA and CA affect NO-mediated pain, corroborating the study by Kolgazi et al. (2021), who suggested that the gastroprotective potential of caffeic acid depends on the modulation of the nitric oxide pathway by regulation of NF-κB through NIK/IKK and c-Src/ERK signaling pathways [61].

The vanilloid receptor pathway or transient receptor potential vanilloid type 1 (TRPV1) is sensitive to a variety of harmful stimuli, such as temperatures elevated to ±42 °C, lipid mediators, and vanilloid compounds such as capsaicin and resiniferatoxin [62,63]. The activation of these receptors results in neuron depolarization, leading to the release of multiple neuropeptides [64]. Ruthenium red, a non-selective antagonist of vanilloid receptors, is used to evaluate the potential interaction of substances with vanilloid receptors [65]. Glutamate induces a nociceptive response by activating glutamatergic receptors at supraspinal, spinal, and peripheral sites [66]. This neurotransmitter activates AMPA (α-amino-3-hydroxy-5-methyl-4-isoxazole propionic acid) and NMDA (N-Methyl-D-Aspartic acid) receptors, thus allowing the passage of Na^+ and Ca^{2+}, facilitating the action potential and subsequent nociceptive responses [67].

Such inhibition also results in the availability of cGMP, providing peripheral antinociception through the opening of ATP-sensitive K^+ channels [68]. On the other hand, the administration of methylene blue causes the activation of the guanylate cyclase enzyme, which catalyzes cGMP production [69]. In the present study, it was evidenced that both HEXA and CA act synergistically. The analgesic pathway mediated by α_2 receptors involves Gi-mediated inhibition of presynaptic Ca^{2+} channels, preventing glutamate (excitatory neurotransmitter) from being released from primary afferent fibers [70]. Simultaneously, the opening of K^+ channels results in hyperpolarization, causing a decrease in the excitability of postsynaptic cells [71]. Agonists of these receptors have analgesic properties involving peripheral and central mechanisms [72]. In this study, the evaluation of HEXA in this pathway indicates that the antinociceptive effect of this extract can involve the participation of these receptors.

K+ATP channels are directly involved in cell hyperpolarization, consecutively decreasing intracellular concentrations of Ca^{2+} and reducing the release of neurotransmitters, thus inhibiting nociception. Experimentally, the administration of glibenclamide blocks these channels [73]. From the results obtained in the study, it is reasonable to hypothesize that the action of HEXA affects the activation of potassium channels, contributing to the observed analgesic effect.

The findings of this study indicate that HEXA exhibits antinociceptive effects both centrally and peripherally. These effects may be attributed to its ability to suppress the release of inflammatory mediators or regulate their interaction with receptors involved in pain perception. This research revealed that the components of the extract of *X. americana* can influence multiple pain pathways with the modulation of α2-adrenergic, nitric oxide, glutamatergic, vanilloid, cyclic guanosine monophosphate, and K+ATP channel-dependent pathways. On the other hand, caffeic acid specifically influences the opioid, glutamatergic, and vanilloid pathways by inhibiting nitric oxide and cyclic guanosine monophosphate.

4. Materials and Methods

4.1. Drugs, Reagents, and Doses

The substances used in this study were obtained from Sigma-Aldrich. The other substances used in the tests were the following: formalin (PubChem CID = 712), morphine (5 mg/kg; s.c.) (PubChem CID = 5288826), L-NOARG ((PubChem CID = 440005), ruthenium red (PubChem CID = 117587625), capsaicin (PubChem CID = 1548943), glutamate (PubChem CID = 23689119), methylene blue (PubChem CID = 6099), clonidine (PubChem CID = 20179), yohimbine (PubChem CID = 6169), glibenclamide (PubChem CID = 3488), acetylcholine (PubChem CID = 6060), atropine (PubChem CID = 174174), caffeine (PubChem CID = 2519), and p-chlorophenyl alanine (PubChem CID = 46520). Methanol, acetonitrile (LiChrosolv®, ≥99.9%), and ammonium hydroxide (NH4OH) were purchased from Sigma-Aldrich (St. Louis, MO, USA).

HEXA was obtained as previously described by da Silva et al. (2018) [20] and administered at 50, 100, and 200 mg/kg orally. Caffeic acid (PubChem CID = 689043) was administered at 0.18 mg/kg and 1.8 mg/kg.

4.2. *Chemical Profile by Electrospray Ionization–Mass Spectrometry (ESI-MS) Analysis*

In the previous work, Silva et al. (2018), we determined the chemical profile of HEXA compounds, identifying 21 compounds using HPLC-DAD. However, in the current study, the analysis focuses specifically on the compound caffeic acid. For this purpose, electrospray ionization–mass spectrometry (ESI-MS) analysis was utilized.

The sample was prepared by dissolving the dried extract in 1 mL of a methanol/acetonitrile mixture (2:1, *v:v*) containing 10 µL of ammonium hydroxide. The ESI-MS analyses were performed on a high-resolution Quadrupole-Orbitrap hybrid mass spectrometer (Q-Exactive, Thermo Scientific, Waltham, MA, USA). The ESI source conditions were set as follows: negative ionization mode, spray voltage of 3.2 kV, capillary temperature of 320 °C, S-Lens RF level at 45 V, sheath gas flow rate at 8 L min^{-1}, and auxiliary gas flow rate at 5 L.min^{-1}, and for MSMS, a collision energy of 15 eV was used.

Compound Annotation

The mass spectrometer data files were converted from (.raw) to (.mzML) format using MSconvert software v.3 (ProteoWizard, Palo Alto, CA, USA) and processed using the online platform (https://gnps.ucsd.edu/ProteoSAFe/static/gnps-splash.jsp, accessed on 10 July 2024) to retrieve compound information. Molecular annotations were based on the comparison of experimental MS/MS spectra with the GNPS spectral library using tools such as Molecular Networking [74].

4.3. *Animals*

The animals used were Swiss mice (*Mus musculus*) of both sexes weighing 20–30 g and housed in polypropylene cages (410 × 282 × 150 mm; n = 6) at 24 ± 2 °C with a 12 h light/dark cycle, with free access to water and specific chow (Labina, Presence®). Mice were fasted from solids for 6–8 h before experiments.

4.4. *Ethical Information*

The study adhered to guidelines from CONCEA, U.K. Animals (Scientific Procedures) Act, 1986, EU Directive 2010/63/EU, and NIH guidelines. Protocols were approved by the Ethics Committee on Animal Use of URCA (approval number 180/2020.2).

4.5. *Evaluation of the Effects of HEXA on the Central Nervous System*

4.5.1. Rotarod Performance Test

Mice (n = 3/group) were treated with water (10 mL/kg; p.o.) or HEXA (200 mg/kg; p.o.). After 1 h, the number of falls and time on the rotating rod were recorded [75].

4.5.2. Open-Field Test

Mice (n = 3/group) were treated with water (10 mL/kg; p.o.) or HEXA (200 mg/kg; p.o.). After 1 h, the number of fields explored in a 30 cm^2 open field was observed for 5 min [76].

4.6. Screening for the Antinociceptive Effect

The antinociceptive effect was assessed using acetic acid-induced writhing, formalin, hot plate, and Von Frey tests. Mice were divided into groups (n = 6) and treated with water (10 mL/kg; p.o.) or HEXA (50, 100, or 200 mg/kg; p.o.) [77]. The experimental timeline is shown in Figure 1.

4.6.1. Acetic Acid-Induced Abdominal Contortions

Mice (n = 6/group) were treated with water (10 mL/kg; p.o.) or HEXA (50, 100, or 200 mg/kg; p.o.) 1 h before 0.6% acetic acid (i.p.). The amount of writhing was recorded for 30 min [76,78].

4.6.2. The Formalin Test

Mice (n = 6/group) were treated with water (10 mL/kg; p.o.), HEXA (50, 100, or 200 mg/kg; p.o.), or CA (0.18, 1.8 mg/kg). After 1 h, 2.5% formalin (20 μL) was administered, and the nociceptive response was observed at 0–5 min and 15–30 min post injection [79].

4.7. Evaluation of Central and Peripheral Antinociceptive Responses

4.7.1. Hot Plate Test

Mice (n = 6/group) were treated with water (10 mL/kg; p.o.) or HEXA (50, 100, or 200 mg/kg; p.o.). Latency time was recorded at various intervals up to 180 min post treatment [76,80].

4.7.2. Mechanical Pressure Hypernociception (Von Frey Test)

Mice (n = 6/group) were subjected to mechanical stimulation in the right paw at 24 h and 30 min (basal measure) before the test. After 30 min, the animals received an injection (20 μL/paw) of complete Freund's adjuvant (CFA) (1 mg/mL) in the right hind paw. The animals were treated with water (10 mL/kg; p.o.) or HEXA (50, 100, or 200 mg/kg, p.o.). Subsequently, treatments were carried out on the 5th, 9th, 13th, 17th, and 21st days after induction. The test was performed using the Von Frey apparatus. Briefly, the animals were placed individually in glass boxes (12 × 20 × 20 cm) supported on an elevated surface and covered with a wire mesh. After 1 h of acclimatization, the stimulus was applied with a rod with a constant force on the plantar surface of the right hind paw (to assess hypernociception to the lesion in injured mice) using the Von Frey filament resistance apparatus for 21 consecutive days. The force in (g) was determined by removing the paw from the filament. The force was applied six times, and the average of the three most similar values was considered [81,82].

4.8. Investigation of the Signaling Pathways Associated with the Analgesic Effect of HEXA and AC

The effect of HEXA (100 mg/kg; b.w.) or CA (1.8 mg/kg; b.w.) on pain signaling pathways was evaluated using the formalin assay through the pharmacological signaling pathways, including opioid receptor, nitric oxide, vanilloid, glutamatergic, cyclic guanosine monophosphate pathway, adrenergic α-2, K+ATP channels, cholinergic, adenosinergic, dopaminergic, and the serotonergic pathways.

In the formalin model, mice (n = 6) were pretreated with HEXA (100 mg/kg; p.o.), CA (1.8 mg/kg; p.o.), or, according to the signaling pathway: opioid—morphine (agonist—5 mg/kg; s.c.) and naloxone (antagonist—4 mg/kg; i.p.) [83]; nitric oxide—L-NOARG (nitric oxide synthase (NOS) inhibitor—75 mg/kg; i.p.) and L-arginine (NOS substrate—600 mg/kg; i.p.) [84,85]; vanilloid—ruthenium red (non-selective TRP antagonist—3 mg/kg; i.p.) and capsaicin (TRPV1 receptor agonist—5.2 nmol/paw) [66]; glutamatergic—ascorbic acid (100 mg/kg; i.p.) and buffered glutamate (20 μmol/paw) [86–89]; cGMP—methylene blue (guanylate cyclase inhibitor—20 mg/kg; i.p.) [66]; α_2-adrenergic—clonidine (agonist—0.1 mg/kg; i.p.) and yohimbine (antagonist—0.15 mg/kg; i.p.) [90]; K+ATP channels—glibenclamide (K+ATP channel blocker—3 mg/kg; i.p.) [66,91]; cholinergic—acetylcholine (agonist—1 mg/kg; i.p.) and atropine (antagonist—1 mg/kg; i.p.) [85]; adenosinergic—caffeine (10 mg/kg; i.p.) [92]; dopaminergic—haloperidol (non-selective dopamine receptor antagonist—0.2 mg/kg; i.p.) [93,94]; and serotoninergic—p-chlorophenyl alanine (PCPA) (serotonin receptor antagonist—100 mg/kg; i.p.) [95,96].

4.9. Statistical Analysis

The values were expressed as mean ± SEM. Data were analyzed by one-way ANOVA followed by Tukey's test or two-way ANOVA followed by Dunnett's or Tukey's post hoc, using the GraphPad Software version 6.1. p-values < 0.05 were considered significant.

5. Conclusions

In conclusion, HEXA and CA have significant antinociceptive effects in the absence of evident central nervous system (CNS) toxicity in mice and, as such, have the potential to be used in the development of new analgesic drugs. The present results bring new insights into the antinociceptive effects of HEXA and CA as well as the main mechanisms underlying their effects in pain management, shedding light on the search for new therapeutic alternatives.

Supplementary Materials: The following supporting information can be downloaded at: https://www.mdpi.com/article/10.3390/ph17121671/s1, Figure S1: Chromatogram of ESI-MS scanning by UPLC-MS; Table S1: Results of compound annotation in the hydroethanolic extract of *X. americana* L. through molecular network analysis.

Author Contributions: Conceptualization and resources, R.T.P.; methodology and resources, L.Y.S.d.S. and I.S.A.; validation and formal analysis, T.M.S.; investigation and data curation, E.d.S.S.; formal analysis and visualization, R.H.S.d.C.; investigation and visualization, A.B.d.S.; writing—original draft and supervision, J.R.-F.; methodology and writing—original draft, A.O.B.P.B.M.; writing—review and editing and. visualization, H.D.M.C.; methodology and validation, J.C.P.S.; methodology and investigation, A.R.C.; methodology and validation, R.N.M.; project administration and writing—review and editing, I.R.A.d.M. All authors have read and agreed to the published version of the manuscript.

Funding: Acknowledges financial support from CNPq-PQ (Grant 303438/2021-5) and FUNCAP-UNIVERSAL (Grant 404780/2021-0) and CNPq (Grant 406522/2021-9-1).

Institutional Review Board Statement: The animal study protocol was approved by the Institutional Ethics Committee on Animal Use of Regional University of Cariri—URCA (approval number 180/2020.2).

Informed Consent Statement: Not applicable.

Data Availability Statement: Data is contained within the article or Supplementary Material.

Acknowledgments: The authors would like to thank the financial support provided by Coordination for the Improvement of Higher Education Personnel—Brazil (CAPES); Cearense Foundation to Support Scientific and Technological Development (FUNCAP)—finance code BPI; National Council for Scientific and Technological Development (CNPq)—finance code 304291/2017-0; and Financier of Studies and Projects—Brasil (FINEP). This article is a contribution of the National Institute of Science and Technology—Ethnobiology, Bioprospecting, and Nature Conservation/CNPq/FACEPE and Excitotoxicity and Neuroprotection (INCT-EN); National Institute of Science and Technology of the Health Economic–Industrial Complex (iCEIS); and National Institute of Science and Technology in Analytical Chemistry of Food: Food Safety and Characterization of Functional Foods (INCT-ALIM) for the support offered to carry out this work.

Conflicts of Interest: The authors declare that they have no known competing financial interests or personal relationships that could have appeared to influence the work reported in this paper.

References

1. Baral, P.; Udit, S.; Chiu, I.M. Pain and Immunity: Implications for Host Defence. *Nat. Rev. Immunol.* **2019**, *19*, 433–447. [CrossRef] [PubMed]

2. Matsuda, M.; Huh, Y.; Ji, R.R. Roles of Inflammation, Neurogenic Inflammation, and Neuroinflammation in Pain. *J. Anesth.* **2019**, *33*, 131–139. [CrossRef] [PubMed]
3. Arthur, J.; Bruera, E. Balancing Opioid Analgesia with the Risk of Nonmedical Opioid Use in Patients with Cancer. *Nat. Rev. Clin. Oncol.* **2019**, *16*, 213–226. [CrossRef] [PubMed]
4. Cohen, S.P.; Vase, L.; Hooten, W.M. Chronic Pain: An Update on Burden, Best Practices, and New Advances. *Lancet* **2021**, *397*, 2082–2097. [CrossRef] [PubMed]
5. Day, R.O.; Graham, G.G. Non-Steroidal Anti-Inflammatory Drugs (NSAIDs). *BMJ* **2013**, *346*, f3195. [CrossRef]
6. Lima, C.P.; Silva, H.R.D.O.; Pogian, V.B.; Santos, V.G. Pharmaceutical Evaluation of the Risks of the Use of Non-Steroid Anti-Inflammatories. *Unisanta Health Sci.* **2020**, *4*, 1–20.
7. Silva, L.A.; Gerica, O.; Al, H. Review on Non-Steroid Antiinflammatory: Acetylsalicylic Acid. *Rev. Iniciaç. Cient. Ext.* **2018**, *1*, 169–174.
8. Mohammad, F.; Hasan, E.; Wedad, A.; Mohamed, E.G. Natural Antioxidant Flavonoids in Formalin-Induced Mice Paw Inflammation; Inhibition of Mitochondrial Sorbitol Dehydrogenase Activity. *J. Biochem. Mol. Toxicol.* **2017**, *31*, e21896. [CrossRef]
9. Mussin, J.; Giusiano, G. Ethno–Phytopharmacology: Product Validation Process Based on Traditional Knowledge of Medicinal Plants. In *Agricultural, Forestry and Bioindustry Biotechnology and Biodiscovery*; Springer: Berlin/Heidelberg, Germany, 2020; pp. 331–353.
10. Ribeiro, D.A.; de Oliveira, L.G.S.; de Macêdo, D.G.; de Menezes, I.R.A.; da Costa, J.G.M.; da Silva, M.A.P.; Lacerda, S.R.; de Almeida Souza, M.M. Promising Medicinal Plants for Bioprospection in a Cerrado Area of Chapada Do Araripe, Northeastern Brazil. *J. Ethnopharmacol.* **2014**, *155*, 1522–1533. [CrossRef]
11. Sreekeesoon, D.P.; Mahomoodally, M.F. Ethnopharmacological Analysis of Medicinal Plants and Animals Used in the Treatment and Management of Pain in Mauritius. *J. Ethnopharmacol.* **2014**, *157*, 181–200. [CrossRef]
12. Da Silva-Leite, K.E.S.; Assreuy, A.M.S.; Mendonça, L.F.; Damasceno, L.E.A.; De Queiroz, M.G.R.; Mourão, P.A.S.; Pires, A.F.; Pereira, M.G. Polysaccharide Rich Fractions from Barks of *Ximenia americana* Inhibit Peripheral Inflammatory Nociception in Mice Antinociceptive Effect of *Ximenia americana* Polysaccharide Rich Fractions. *Rev. Bras. Farmacogn.* **2017**, *27*, 339–345. [CrossRef]
13. Jahromi, B.; Pirvulescu, I.; Candido, K.D.; Knezevic, N.N. Herbal Medicine for Pain Management: Efficacy and Drug Interactions. *Pharmaceutics* **2021**, *13*, 251. [CrossRef] [PubMed]
14. Da Silva, G.G.; De Souza, P.A.; De Morais, P.L.D.; Dos Santos, E.C.; Moura, R.D.; Menezes, J.B. Caracterização Do Fruto de Ameixa Silvestre (*Ximenia americana* L.). *Rev. Bras. Frutic.* **2008**, *30*, 311–314. [CrossRef]
15. Shettar, A.K.; Sateesh, M.K.; Kaliwal, B.B.; Vedamurthy, A.B. In Vitro Antidiabetic Activities and GC-MS Phytochemical Analysis of *Ximenia americana* Extracts. *S. Afr. J. Bot.* **2017**, *111*, 202–211. [CrossRef]
16. Almeida, M.L.B.; Freitas, W.E.D.S.; De Morais, P.L.D.; Sarmento, J.D.A.; Alves, R.E. Bioactive Compounds and Antioxidant Potential Fruit of *Ximenia americana* L. *Food Chem.* **2016**, *192*, 1078–1082. [CrossRef]
17. Aragão, T.P.; dos Prazeres, L.D.K.T.; Brito, S.A.; Neto, P.J.R.; Rolim, L.A.; da Silva Almeida, J.R.G.; Caldas, G.F.R.; Wanderley, A.G. alves Contribution of Secondary Metabolites to the Gastroprotective Effect of Aqueous Extract of *Ximenia americana* L. (Olacaceae) Stem Bark in Rats. *Molecules* **2018**, *23*, 112. [CrossRef]
18. de Menezes, I.R.A.; da Costa, R.H.S.; Augusti Boligon, A.; Rolón, M.; Coronel, C.; Vega, C.; Melo Coutinho, H.D.; da Costa, M.S.; Tintino, S.R.; Silva Pereira, R.L.; et al. *Ximenia americana* L. Enhances the Antibiotic Activity and Inhibit the Development of Kinetoplastid Parasites. *Comp. Immunol. Microbiol. Infect. Dis.* **2019**, *64*, 40–46. [CrossRef]
19. Da Palma, A.F.M.; Marques, L.K.M.; Carneiro, R.D.S.; Carvalho, G.F.S.; Ferreira, D.C.L.; Sant'Ana, A.E.G.; Maia Filho, A.L.M.; Marques, R.B.; Alves, W.D.S.; Uchôa, V.T.; et al. Evaluation of Hydroalcoholic Extracts of Stem and Leaves of *Ximenia americana* L. In the Healing of Excisional Acute Wounds in Mice. *Rev. Virtual Quim.* **2020**, *12*, 37–50. [CrossRef]
20. da Silva, B.A.F.; da Costa, R.H.S.; Fernandes, C.N.; Leite, L.H.I.; Ribeiro-Filho, J.; Garcia, T.R.; Coutinho, H.D.M.; Wanderley, A.G.; de Menezes, I.R.A. HPLC Profile and Antiedematogenic Activity of *Ximenia americana* L. (Olacaceae) in Mice Models of Skin Inflammation. *Food Chem. Toxicol.* **2018**, *119*, 199–205. [CrossRef]
21. Soro, T.Y.; Zahoui, O.S.; Nene-bi, A.S. Analgesic Activity of the Fractions of the Aqueous Extract of *Ximenia americana* (Linné) (Olacaceae). *Int. J. Pharmacol. Toxicol.* **2016**, *4*, 1. [CrossRef]
22. Kefelegn, G.A.; Desta, B. *Ximenia americana*: Economic importance, medicinal value, and current status in Ethiopia. *Sci. World J.* **2021**, *1*, 8880021. [CrossRef] [PubMed]
23. da Costa, R.H.S.; Martins, A.O.B.P.B.; de Oliveira, M.R.C.; Alcântara, I.S.; Ferreira, F.F.; dos Santos, F.F.C.; de Araújo Delmondes, G.; da Cunha, F.A.B.; Coutinho, H.D.M.; de Menezes, I.R.A. Acaricide Activity of the *Ximenia americana* L. (Olacaceae) Stem Bark Hydroethanolic Extract against Rhipicephalus (Boophilus) Microplus. *Biologia* **2022**, *77*, 1667–1674. [CrossRef]
24. Cizmarova, B.; Hubkova, B.; Bolerazska, B.; Marekova, M.; Birkova, A. Caffeic Acid: A Brief Overview of Its Presence, Metabolism, and Bioactivity. *Bioact. Compd. Health Dis.* **2020**, *3*, 74–81. [CrossRef]
25. Alam, M.; Ahmed, S.; Elasbali, A.M.; Adnan, M.; Alam, S.; Hassan, M.I.; Pasupuleti, V.R. Therapeutic Implications of Caffeic Acid in Cancer and Neurological Diseases. *Front. Oncol.* **2022**, *12*, 860508. [CrossRef] [PubMed]
26. Khan, F.; Bamunuarachchi, N.I.; Tabassum, N.; Kim, Y.M. Caffeic Acid and Its Derivatives: Antimicrobial Drugs toward Microbial Pathogens. *J. Agric. Food Chem.* **2021**, *69*, 2979–3004. [CrossRef]

27. Nasr Bouzaiene, N.; Kilani Jaziri, S.; Kovacic, H.; Chekir-Ghedira, L.; Ghedira, K.; Luis, J. The Effects of Caffeic, Coumaric and Ferulic Acids on Proliferation, Superoxide Production, Adhesion and Migration of Human Tumor Cells in Vitro. *Eur. J. Pharmacol.* **2015**, *766*, 99–105. [CrossRef]
28. Zielińska, D.; Zieliński, H.; Laparra-Llopis, J.M.; Szawara-Nowak, D.; Honke, J.; Giménez-Bastida, J.A. Caffeic Acid Modulates Processes Associated with Intestinal Inflammation. *Nutrients* **2021**, *13*, 554. [CrossRef]
29. Park, S.H.; Sim, Y.B.; Kim, S.M.; Lee, J.K.; Jung, J.S.; Suh, H.W. The Effect of Caffeic Acid on the Antinociception and Mechanisms in Mouse. *J. Appl. Biol. Chem.* **2011**, *54*, 177–182. [CrossRef]
30. Crevar-Sakač, M.; Vujić, Z.; Kotur-Stevuljević, J.; Ivanišević, J.; Jelić-Ivanović, Z.; Milenković, M.; Markelić, M.; Vujčić, Z. Uticaj Atorvastatina i Tinkture Lista Artičoke Na Oksidativni Stres Kod Pacova Sa Hiperholesterolemijom. *Vojnosanit. Pregl.* **2016**, *73*, 178–187. [CrossRef]
31. Wu, Z.-J.; Ma, X.-L.; Fang, D.-M.; Qi, H.-Y.; Ren, W.-J.; Zhang, G.-L. Analysis of Caffeic Acid Derivatives from *Osmanthus Yunnanensis* Using Electrospray Ionization Quadrupole Time-of-Flight Mass Spectrometry. *Eur. J. Mass Spectrom.* **2009**, *15*, 415–429. [CrossRef]
32. Pessoa, R.T.; Alcântara, I.S.; da Silva, L.Y.S.; da Costa, R.H.S.; Silva, T.M.; de Morais Oliveira-Tintino, C.D.; Ramos, A.G.B.; de Oliveira, M.R.C.; Martins, A.O.B.P.B.; de Lacerda, B.C.G.V.; et al. *Ximenia americana* L.: Chemical Characterization and Gastroprotective Effect. *Analytica* **2023**, *4*, 141–158. [CrossRef]
33. Liu, Y.; Qiu, S.; Wang, L.; Zhang, N.; Shi, Y.; Zhou, H.; Liu, X.; Shao, L.; Liu, X.; Chen, J.; et al. Reproductive and Developmental Toxicity Study of Caffeic Acid in Mice. *Food Chem. Toxicol.* **2019**, *123*, 106–112. [CrossRef] [PubMed]
34. Brandão, D.O.; Fernandes, F.H.A.; Júnior, F.J.L.R.; Silva, P.C.D.; Santana, C.P.; De Medeiros, F.D.; Véras, G.; Medeiros, A.C.D. Validation of UPLC Method for Determination of Gallic Acid from *Ximenia americana* L. *Planta Med.* **2014**, *80*, P2O60. [CrossRef]
35. de Araújo, M.R.S.; da Costa Assunção, J.C.; Dantas, I.N.F.; Costa-Lotufo, L.V.; Monte, F.J.Q. Chemical Constituents of *Ximenia americana*. *Nat. Prod. Commun.* **2008**, *3*, 1934578X0800300605. [CrossRef]
36. Le, N.H.T.; Malterud, K.E.; Diallo, D.; Paulsen, B.S.; Nergård, C.S.; Wangensteen, H. Bioactive Polyphenols in *Ximenia americana* and the Traditional Use among Malian Healers. *J. Ethnopharmacol.* **2012**, *139*, 858–862. [CrossRef]
37. Queiroz Monte, F.J.; de Lemos, T.L.G.; de Arajo, M.R.S.; Sousa Gomes, E. de *Ximenia americana*: Chemistry, Pharmacology and Biological Properties, a Review. *Phytochem.—A Glob. Perspect. Their Role Nutr. Health* **2012**, *1*, 429–450. [CrossRef]
38. Siddaiah, M.; Jayavcera, K.N.; Mallikarjuna, R.P.; Ravindra, R.K.; Yasodha, K.Y.; Narender, R.G. Phytochemical Screening and Analgesic Activity of Methanolic Extract of *Ximenia americana*. *J. Pharm. Chem.* **2009**, *3*, 23–25.
39. Hemamalini, K.; Srikanth, A.; Sunny, G.; Praneethkumar, H. Phytochemical Screening and Analgesic Activity of Methanolic Extract of *Ximenia americana*. *J. Curr. Pharma Res.* **2011**, *1*, 153.
40. Coutinho, M.A.S.; Muzitano, M.F.; Costa, S.S. Flavonoids: Potential Therapeutic Agents for the Inflammatory Process. *Rev. Virtual Quím.* **2009**, *1*, 241–256. [CrossRef]
41. Dias, T.L.M.F.; Melo, G.M.A.; Da Silva, Y.K.C.; Queiroz, A.C.; Goulart, H.F.; Alexandre-Moreira, M.S.; Santana, A.E.G.; Uchôa, V.T. Antinociceptive and Anti-Inflammatory Activities of the Ethanolic Extract, of Fractions and of Epicatechin Isolated from the Stem Bark of *Ximenia americana* L. (Oleacaceae). *Rev. Virtual Quim.* **2018**, *10*, 86–101. [CrossRef]
42. Kiessoun, K.; Ouattara, N.; Arsène, M.; Souza, A.; Sytar, O.; Brestic, M.; Mamoudou, D.H. Anti-Nociceptive and Anti-Inflammatory Properties of Polyphenol-Rich Fractions of Roots from *Ximenia americana* L., (Olacaceae), in Experimental Mice. *Int. J. Pharm. Pharm. Res.* **2018**, *12*, 281–297.
43. Matejczyk, M.; Świsłocka, R.; Golonko, A.; Lewandowski, W.; Hawrylik, E. Cytotoxic, Genotoxic and Antimicrobial Activity of Caffeic and Rosmarinic Acids and Their Lithium, Sodium and Potassium Salts as Potential Anticancer Compounds. *Adv. Med. Sci.* **2018**, *63*, 14–21. [CrossRef] [PubMed]
44. de Alencar Silva, A.; Pereira-de-Morais, L.; Rodrigues da Silva, R.E.; de Menezes Dantas, D.; Brito Milfont, C.G.; Gomes, M.F.; Araújo, I.M.; Kerntopf, M.R.; Alencar de Menezes, I.R.; Barbosa, R. Pharmacological Screening of the Phenolic Compound Caffeic Acid Using Rat Aorta, Uterus and Ileum Smooth Muscle. *Chem. Biol. Interact.* **2020**, *332*, 109269. [CrossRef] [PubMed]
45. Amorati, R.; Pedulli, G.F.; Cabrini, L.; Zambonin, L.; Landi, L. Solvent and PH Effects on the Antioxidant Activity of Caffeic and Other Phenolic Acids. *J. Agric. Food Chem.* **2006**, *54*, 2932–2937. [CrossRef] [PubMed]
46. Kolgazi, M.; Cilingir, S.; Yilmaz, O.; Gemici, M.; Yazar, H.; Ozer, S.; Acikel-Elmas, M.; Arbak, S.; Suyen, G.G. Caffeic Acid Attenuates Gastric Mucosal Damage Induced by Ethanol in Rats via Nitric Oxide Modulation. *Chem. Biol. Interact.* **2021**, *334*, 109351. [CrossRef]
47. Quintans-Júnior, L.J.; De Almeida, R.N.; Falcão, A.C.G.M.; de Fátima Agra, M.; De Sousa, M.d.F.V.; Barbosa-Filho, J.M. Avaliação Da Atividade Anticonvulsivante de Plantas Do Nordeste Brasileiro. *Acta Farm. Bonaer.* **2002**, *21*, 179–184.
48. da Silva-Leite, K.E.S.; Girão, D.K.F.B.; de Freitas Pires, A.; Assreuy, A.M.S.; de Moraes, P.A.F.; Cunha, A.P.; Ricardo, N.M.P.S.; Criddle, D.N.; de Souza, M.H.L.P.; Pereira, M.G.; et al. *Ximenia americana* Heteropolysaccharides Ameliorate Inflammation and Visceral Hypernociception in Murine Caerulein-Induced Acute Pancreatitis: Involvement of CB2 Receptors. *Biomed. Pharmacother.* **2018**, *106*, 1317–1324. [CrossRef]
49. Zhen, J.; Guo, Y.; Villani, T.; Carr, S.; Brendler, T.; Mumbengegwi, D.R.; Kong, A.N.T.; Simon, J.E.; Wu, Q. Phytochemical Analysis and Anti-Inflammatory Activity of the Extracts of the African Medicinal Plant Ximenia Caffra. *J. Anal. Methods Chem.* **2015**, *2015*, 948262. [CrossRef]

50. Ferreira, J.; Campos, M.M.; Pesquero, J.B.; Araújo, R.C.; Bader, M.; Calixto, J.B. Evidence for the Participation of Kinins in Freund's Adjuvant Induced Inflammatory and Nociceptive Responses in Kinin B1 and B2 Receptor Knockout Mice. *Neuropharmacology* **2001**, *41*, 1006–1012. [CrossRef]
51. Billiau, A.; Matthys, P. Modes of Action of Freund's Adjuvants in Experimental Models of Autoimmune Diseases. *J. Leukoc. Biol.* **2001**, *70*, 849–860. [CrossRef]
52. Dutra, R.C.; Campos, M.M.; Santos, A.R.S.; Calixto, J.B. Medicinal Plants in Brazil: Pharmacological Studies, Drug Discovery, Challenges and Perspectives. *Pharmacol. Res.* **2016**, *112*, 4–29. [CrossRef] [PubMed]
53. Sandkühler, J. Models and Mechanisms of Hyperalgesia and Allodynia. *Physiol. Rev.* **2009**, *89*, 707–758. [CrossRef] [PubMed]
54. Gamaro, G.D.; Suyenaga, E.; Borsoi, M.; Lermen, J.; Pereira, P.; Ardenghi, P. Effect of Rosmarinic and Caffeic Acids on Inflammatory and Nociception Process in Rats. *ISRN Pharmacol.* **2011**, *2011*, 451682. [CrossRef] [PubMed]
55. Leal, S.S.; Uchôa, V.T.; Figuerêdo-Silva, J.; Soares, R.B.; Mota, D.M.; De Alencar, R.C.; Filho, A.L.M.M.; Sant'Ana, A.E.G.; Beltrame Junior, M. Eficácia Da Fonoforese Com *Ximenia americana* L. Na Inflamação de Tendão de Ratos. *Rev. Bras. Med. Esporte* **2016**, *22*, 355–360. [CrossRef]
56. Dhawan, B.N.; Cesselin, F.; Raghubir, R.; Reisine, T.; Bradley, P.B.; Portoghese, P.S.; Hamon, M. International Union of Pharmacology. XII. Classification of Opioid Receptors. *Pharmacol. Rev.* **1996**, *48*, 567–592.
57. Stein, C.; Hassan, A.H.S.; Lehrberger, K.; Stein, C.; Giefing, J.; Yassouridis, A. Local Analgesic Effect of Endogenous Opioid Peptides. *Lancet* **1993**, *342*, 321–324. [CrossRef]
58. Jin, W.Y.; Liu, Z.; Liu, D.; Yu, L.C. Antinociceptive Effects of Galanin in the Central Nucleus of Amygdala of Rats, an Involvement of Opioid Receptors. *Brain Res.* **2010**, *1320*, 16–21. [CrossRef]
59. Shih, C.C.; Hwang, H.R.; Chang, C.I.; Su, H.M.; Chen, P.C.; Kuo, H.M.; Li, P.J.; Wang, H.M.D.; Tsui, K.H.; Lin, Y.C.; et al. Anti-Inflammatory and Antinociceptive Effects of Ethyl Acetate Fraction of an Edible Red Macroalgae Sarcodia Ceylanica. *Int. J. Mol. Sci.* **2017**, *18*, 2437. [CrossRef]
60. Iacopucci, A.P.; Mello, R.O.; Barbosa-Silva, R.; Melo-Thomas, L. L-NOARG-Induced Catalepsy Can Be Influenced by Glutamatergic Neurotransmission Mediated by NMDA Receptors in the Inferior Colliculus. *Behav. Brain Res.* **2012**, *234*, 149–154. [CrossRef]
61. Kim, S.R.; Jung, Y.R.; Kim, D.H.; An, H.J.; Kim, M.K.; Kim, N.D.; Chung, H.Y. Caffeic Acid Regulates LPS-Induced NF-KB Activation through NIK/IKK and c-Src/ERK Signaling Pathways in Endothelial Cells. *Arch. Pharm. Res.* **2014**, *37*, 539–547. [CrossRef]
62. Tominaga, M.; Caterina, M.J.; Malmberg, A.B.; Rosen, T.A.; Gilbert, H.; Skinner, K.; Raumann, B.E.; Basbaum, A.I.; Julius, D. The Cloned Capsaicin Receptor Integrates Multiple Pain-Producing Stimuli. *Neuron* **1998**, *21*, 531–543. [CrossRef] [PubMed]
63. Devesa, I.; Planells-Cases, R.; Fernández-Ballester, G.; González-Ros, J.M.; Ferrer-Montiel, A.; Fernández-Carvajal, A. Role of the Transient Receptor Potential Vanilloid 1 in Inflammation and Sepsis. *J. Inflamm. Res.* **2011**, *4*, 67–81. [CrossRef] [PubMed]
64. Gamse, R.; Holzer, P.; Lembeck, F. Indirect Evidence for Presynaptic Location of Opiate Receptors on Chemosensitive Primary Sensory Neurones. *Naunyn-Schmiedeberg's Arch. Pharmacol.* **1979**, *308*, 281–285. [CrossRef] [PubMed]
65. Maia, J.L.; Lima-Júnior, R.C.P.; Melo, C.M.; David, J.P.; David, J.M.; Campos, A.R.; Santos, F.A.; Rao, V.S.N. Oleanolic Acid, a Pentacyclic Triterpene Attenuates Capsaicin-Induced Nociception in Mice: Possible Mechanisms. *Pharmacol. Res.* **2006**, *54*, 282–286. [CrossRef] [PubMed]
66. Beirith, A.; Santos, A.R.S.; Calixto, J.B. Mechanisms Underlying the Nociception and Paw Oedema Caused by Injection of Glutamate into the Mouse Paw. *Brain Res.* **2002**, *924*, 219–228. [CrossRef]
67. Vorobeychik, Y.; Willoughby, C.D.; Mao, J. NMDA Receptor Antagonists in the Treatment of Pain. In *Comprehensive Treatment of Chronic Pain by Medical, Interventional, and Integrative Approaches*; Springer: New York, NY, USA, 2013; pp. 61–67.
68. Soares, A.C.; Leite, R.; Tatsuo, M.A.K.F.; Duarte, I.D.G. Activation of ATP-Sensitive K+ Channels: Mechanism of Peripheral Antinociceptive Action of the Nitric Oxide Donor, Sodium Nitroprusside. *Eur. J. Pharmacol.* **2000**, *400*, 67–71. [CrossRef]
69. Garthwaite, J. Glutamate, Nitric Oxide and Cell-Cell Signalling in the Nervous System. *Trends Neurosci.* **1991**, *14*, 60–67. [CrossRef]
70. Kimura, M.; Saito, S.; Obata, H. Dexmedetomidine Decreases Hyperalgesia in Neuropathic Pain by Increasing Acetylcholine in the Spinal Cord. *Neurosci. Lett.* **2012**, *529*, 70–74. [CrossRef]
71. Obata, H. Analgesic Mechanisms of Antidepressants for Neuropathic Pain. *Int. J. Mol. Sci.* **2017**, *18*, 2483. [CrossRef]
72. Chan, A.K.M.; Cheung, C.W.; Chong, Y.K. Alpha-2 Agonists in Acute Pain Management. *Expert Opin. Pharmacother.* **2010**, *11*, 2849–2868. [CrossRef]
73. Lopes, L.D.S.; Marques, R.B.; Fernandes, H.B.; Pereira, S.D.S.; Ayres, M.C.C.; Chaves, M.H.; Almeida, F.R.C. Mechanisms of the Antinociceptive Action of (-) Epicatechin Obtained from the Hydroalcoholic Fraction of Combretum Leprosum Mart & Eic in Rodents. *J. Biomed. Sci.* **2012**, *19*, 2–7. [CrossRef]
74. Wang, M.; Carver, J.J.; Phelan, V.V.; Sanchez, L.M.; Garg, N.; Peng, Y.; Nguyen, D.D.; Watrous, J.; Kapono, C.A.; Luzzatto-Knaan, T.; et al. Sharing and Community Curation of Mass Spectrometry Data with GNPS. *Nat. Biotechnol.* **2016**, *34*, 828. [CrossRef] [PubMed]
75. Dunham, N.W.; Miya, T.S. A Note on a Simple Apparatus for Detecting Neurological Deficit in Rats and Mice. *J. Am. Pharm. Assoc.* **1957**, *46*, 208–209. [CrossRef] [PubMed]
76. Lapa, A.J.J.; Souccar, C.; Lima-Landman, M.T.R.; Castro, M.S.D.A.; Lima, T.C.M. *Pharmacological Activity Evaluation Methods of Medicinal Plants*; Sociedade Brasileira de Plantas Medicinais: São Paulo, Brasil, 2008.

77. Gaichu, D.M.; Mawia, A.M.; Gitonga, G.M.; Ngugi, M.P.; Mburu, D.N. Phytochemical screening and antipyretic activities of dichloromethane-methanolic leaf and stem bark extracts of *Ximenia americana* in rat models. *J. Herbmed Pharmacol.* **2017**, *6*, 3–107.
78. Koster, R.; Anderson, M.; De Beer, E.J. Acetic Acid for Analgesic Screening. *Fed. Proc.* **1959**, *18*, 412–417.
79. Tjølsen, A.; Berge, O.-G.; Hunskaar, S.; Rosland, J.H.; Hole, K. The Formalin Test: An Evaluation of the Method. *Pain* **1992**, *51*, 5–17. [CrossRef]
80. Bannon, A.; Malmberg, A. Models of Nociception: Hot-Plate, Tail-Flick, and Formalin Tests in Rodents. *Curr. Protoc. Neurosci.* **2007**, *41*, 8–9. [CrossRef]
81. Martinov, T.; Mack, M.; Sykes, A.; Chatterjea, D. Measuring Changes in Tactile Sensitivity in the Hind Paw of Mice Using an Electronic von Frey Apparatus. *J. Vis. Exp.* **2013**, *82*, e51212. [CrossRef]
82. Tena, B.; Escobar, B.; Arguis, M.J.; Cantero, C.; Rios, J.; Gomar, C. Reproducibility of Electronic von Frey and von Frey Monofilaments Testing. *Clin. J. Pain* **2012**, *28*, 318–323. [CrossRef]
83. Stevenson, G.W.; Bilsky, E.J.; Negus, S.S. Targeting Pain-Suppressed Behaviors in Preclinical Assays of Pain and Analgesia: Effects of Morphine on Acetic Acid-Suppressed Feeding in C57BL/6J Mice. *J. Pain* **2006**, *7*, 408–416. [CrossRef]
84. Miller, E.C.; Swanson, A.B.; Phillips, D.H.; Fletcher, T.L.; Liem, A.; Miller, J.A. Structure-Activity Studies of the Carcinogenicities in the Mouse and Rat of Some Naturally Occurring and Synthetic Alkenylbenzene Derivatives Related to Safrole and Estragole. *Cancer Res.* **1983**, *43*, 1124–1134. [PubMed]
85. Schechtmann, G.; Song, Z.; Ultenius, C.; Meyerson, B.A.; Linderoth, B. Cholinergic Mechanisms Involved in the Pain Relieving Effect of Spinal Cord Stimulation in a Model of Neuropathy. *Pain* **2008**, *139*, 136–145. [CrossRef] [PubMed]
86. Lam, D.K.; Sessle, B.J.; Cairns, B.E.; Hu, J.W. Neural Mechanisms of Temporomandibular Joint and Masticatory Muscle Pain: A Possible Role for Peripheral Glutamate Receptor Mechanisms. *Pain Res. Manag.* **2005**, *10*, 145–152. [CrossRef] [PubMed]
87. Li, P.; Zhuo, M. Silent Glutamatergic Synapses and Nociception in Mammalian Spinal Cord. *Nature* **1998**, *393*, 695–698. [CrossRef] [PubMed]
88. Majewska, M.D.; Bell, J.A.; London, E.D. Regulation of the NMDA Receptor by Redox Phenomena: Inhibitory Role of Ascorbate. *Brain Res.* **1990**, *537*, 328–332. [CrossRef] [PubMed]
89. Zeraati, F.; Araghchian, M.; Farjoo, M.H. Ascorbic Acid Interaction With Analgesic Effect of Morphine and Tramadol in Mice. *Anesthesiol. Pain Med.* **2014**, *4*, e19529. [CrossRef]
90. Santos, A.R.S.; Gadotti, V.M.; Oliveira, G.L.; Tibola, D.; Paszcuk, A.F.; Neto, A.; Spindola, H.M.; Souza, M.M.; Rodrigues, A.L.S.; Calixto, J.B. Mechanisms Involved in the Antinociception Caused by Agmatine in Mice. *Neuropharmacology* **2005**, *48*, 1021–1034. [CrossRef]
91. Ocaña, M.; Cendán, C.M.; Cobos, E.J.; Entrena, J.M.; Baeyens, J.M. Potassium Channels and Pain: Present Realities and Future Opportunities. *Eur. J. Pharmacol.* **2004**, *500*, 203–219. [CrossRef]
92. Ferré, S.; Diamond, I.; Goldberg, S.R.; Yao, L.; Hourani, S.M.O.; Huang, Z.L.; Urade, Y.; Kitchen, I. Adenosine A2A Receptors in Ventral Striatum, Hypothalamus and Nociceptive Circuitry. *Prog. Neurobiol.* **2007**, *83*, 332–347. [CrossRef]
93. Finan, P.H.; Smith, M.T. The Comorbidity of Insomnia, Chronic Pain, and Depression: Dopamine as a Putative Mechanism. *Sleep Med. Rev.* **2013**, *17*, 173–183. [CrossRef]
94. Wood, P.B. Mesolimbic Dopaminergic Mechanisms and Pain Control. *Pain* **2006**, *120*, 230–234. [CrossRef] [PubMed]
95. Maleki, N.; Nayebi, A.M.; Garjani, A. Effects of Central and Peripheral Depletion of Serotonergic System on Carrageenan-Induced Paw Oedema. *Int. Immunopharmacol.* **2005**, *5*, 1723–1730. [CrossRef] [PubMed]
96. Suzuki, R.; Rygh, L.J.; Dickenson, A.H. Bad News from the Brain: Descending 5-HT Pathways That Control Spinal Pain Processing. *Trends Pharmacol. Sci.* **2004**, *25*, 613–617. [CrossRef] [PubMed]

pharmaceuticals

MDPI

Article

Exploring the Antimycobacterial Potential of Podocarpusflavone A from *Kielmeyera membranacea*: In Vitro and In Vivo Insights

Marlon Heggdorne de Araujo [1,2], Salomé Muñoz Sánchez [2], Thatiana Lopes Biá Ventura Simão [3], Natalia Nowik [2], Stella Schuenck Antunes [1,4], Shaft Corrêa Pinto [1], Davide Sorze [5], Francesca Boldrin [5], Riccardo Manganelli [5], Nelilma Correia Romeiro [4], Elena B. Lasunskaia [3], Fons J. Verbeek [6], Herman P. Spaink [2] and Michelle Frazão Muzitano [1,*]

1 Laboratório de Produtos Bioativos (LPBio), Instituto de Ciências Farmacêuticas, Universidade Federal do Rio de Janeiro, Campus Macaé, Macaé 27930-560, RJ, Brazil; marlon.heggdorne@gmail.com (M.H.d.A.); stellantunes@yahoo.com.br (S.S.A.); shaftcp@yahoo.com.br (S.C.P.)

2 Department of Animal Sciences and Health, Institute of Biology (IBL), Leiden University, 2333 BE Leiden, The Netherlands; s.munoz.sanchez@biology.leidenuniv.nl (S.M.S.); h.p.spaink@biology.leidenuniv.nl (H.P.S.)

3 Laboratório de Biologia do Reconhecer (LBR), Centro de Biociências e Biotecnologia, Universidade Estadual do Norte Fluminense Darcy Ribeiro, Campos dos Goytacazes 28013-602, RJ, Brazil; thativentura@yahoo.com.br (T.L.B.V.S.); elena@uenf.br (E.B.L.)

4 Laboratório Integrado de Computação Científica (LICC), Universidade Federal do Rio de Janeiro, Campus Macaé, Macaé 27930-560, RJ, Brazil; nelilmaromeiro@gmail.com

5 Department of Molecular Medicine, University of Padova, 35121 Padova, Italy; davide.sorze@studenti.unipd.it (D.S.); francesca.boldrin@unipd.it (F.B.); riccardo.manganelli@unipd.it (R.M.)

6 Leiden Institute of Advanced Computer Science, Leiden University, 2333 CA Leiden, The Netherlands; f.j.verbeek@liacs.leidenuniv.nl

* Correspondence: mfmuzitano@macae.ufrj.br or mfmuzitano@gmail.com; Tel.: +55-22-2141-4029

Citation: Araujo, M.H.d.; Muñoz Sánchez, S.; Simão, T.L.B.V.; Nowik, N.; Antunes, S.S.; Pinto, S.C.; Sorze, D.; Boldrin, F.; Manganelli, R.; Correia Romeiro, N.; et al. Exploring the Antimycobacterial Potential of Podocarpusflavone A from *Kielmeyera membranacea*: In Vitro and In Vivo Insights. *Pharmaceuticals* **2024**, *17*, 1560. https://doi.org/10.3390/ph17121560

Academic Editors: Catherine Sherwin, Elena Y. Enioutina and Kathleen M. Job

Received: 26 September 2024
Revised: 13 November 2024
Accepted: 15 November 2024
Published: 21 November 2024

Abstract: Background/Objectives: Tuberculosis (TB) is one of the leading infectious causes of death worldwide, highlighting the importance of identifying new anti-TB agents. In previous research, our team identified antimycobacterial activity in *Kielmeyera membranacea* leaf extract; therefore, this study aims to conduct further exploration of its potential. **Methods**: Classical chromatography was applied for fractionation and spectrometric techniques were utilized for chemical characterization. For in vitro tests, samples were assessed against *Mycobacterium tuberculosis* and *Mycobacterium marinum*. The toxicity and efficacy of active samples were evaluated in vivo using different zebrafish models. Chemogenomics studies were applied to predict the isolated active compound's potential mode of action. **Results**: We performed fractionation of *K. membranacea* ethanolic extract (EE) and then its dichloromethane fraction (DCM), and the biflavonoid podocarpusflavone A (PCFA) was isolated and identified as a promising active compound. The EE and PCFA were found to be non-toxic to zebrafish larvae and were able to inhibit *M. tuberculosis* growth extracellularly. Additionally, PCFA demonstrated antimycobacterial activity within infected macrophages, especially when combined with isoniazid. In addition, the EE, DCM, and PCFA have shown the ability to inhibit *M. marinum's* growth during in vivo zebrafish larvae yolk infection. Notably, PCFA also effectively countered systemic infection established through the caudal vein, showing a similar inhibitory activity profile to rifampicin, both at 32 μM. A reduction in the transcriptional levels of pro-inflammatory cytokines confirmed the infection resolution. The protein tyrosine phosphatase B (PtpB) of *M. tuberculosis*, which inhibits the macrophage immune response, was predicted as a theoretical target of PCFA. This finding is in agreement with the higher activity observed for PCFA intracellularly and in vivo on zebrafish, compared with the direct action in *M. tuberculosis*. **Conclusions**: Here, we describe the discovery of PCFA as an intracellular inhibitor of *M. tuberculosis* and provide evidence of its in vivo efficacy and safety, encouraging its further development as a combination drug in novel therapeutic regimens for TB.

Keywords: biflavone; podocarpusflavone A; zebrafish; tuberculosis; *Kielmeyera*; cytokines; toxicity

1. Introduction

Tuberculosis (TB) is an infectious disease that affects the lungs and is caused by *Mycobacterium tuberculosis*. Globally, in 2023, an estimated 10.8 million people fell ill with TB, resulting in 1.25 million deaths [1]. Additionally, drug-resistant TB remains a significant public health threat. From 2018 to 2023, over 8.2 million people worldwide enrolled in treatment for multidrug-resistant or rifampicin-resistant TB (MDR/RR-TB). In 2023 alone, 188,666 cases were identified, including 159,684 cases of MDR/RR-TB and 28,982 cases of pre-extensive drug-resistant (pre-XDR) TB or extensively drug-resistant TB (XDR-TB). Current data indicate a treatment success rate for RR-TB between 50 and 75%, emphasizing the critical need to study new, effective, and safe anti-TB drugs [1].

Natural products are part of an essential strategy for the development of new drugs for the treatment of TB [2,3]. In this scenario, the coastal ecosystem of the restinga, which belongs to the Atlantic Forest biome, is a recognized biodiversity hotspot. Its extreme environmental conditions can lead to diverse production of secondary metabolites. Among the plants that occur in restingas, *Kielmeyera* species (*Calophyllaceae*) can be highlighted for their antimicrobial potential against bacteria [4–6] and fungi [7], in addition to their antiglycation [8], anticancer [9], and anxiolytic [10] activities. Regarding their chemical composition, procyanidins [8], coumarins [9], xanthones [5], long-chain fatty acid compounds [11], and sesquiterpenes [6] have been described. However, there is limited research on *K. membranacea* Casar., with published information mainly addressing its botanical and ecological characteristics [12], except for a prior screening study conducted by our research group, which identified the in vitro antimycobacterial activity of *Kielmeyera membranacea* [13]. In this previous study, different plant species collected at the Jurubatiba National Park, a protected restinga area in the Northeast of Rio de Janeiro (Brazil), were evaluated against *Mycobacterium bovis* BCG. *Kielmeyera membranacea* was among the most active species, especially its dichloromethane fraction, which inhibited the extracellular growth of *M. bovis* BCG and *M. tuberculosis* H37Rv strains [13]. Therefore, considering the urgent need for new anti-TB compounds, the present study aimed to investigate the *Kielmeyera membranacea* extract, fraction, and isolated compound, including in vitro and in vivo experiments.

Studies of anti-TB activity with bioactive natural products using in vivo models are still scarce, both due to the difficulty in simulating the human pathology using animal models and because in vivo experiments require a more significant amount of samples to treat the groups of animals. In this context, the zebrafish (*Danio rerio*) model uses compounds economically while maintaining the experimental complexity of in vivo models [14]. *Mycobacterium marinum* is a natural pathogen of zebrafish and can cause granulomatous lesions with host tissue necrosis [15], being genetically related to the *M. tuberculosis* complex. In zebrafish, it causes a disease that resembles TB in humans [16], allowing investigators to quickly assess the inhibitory effects of natural products on mycobacterial growth [16,17] and also to evaluate toxic effects during larval development [18].

In view of the importance of conducting research to find new anti-TB compounds, the present study focused on evaluating the antimycobacterial activity of podocarpusflavone A, isolated from *Kielmeyera membranacea,* in vitro and in vivo through the *M. marinum*-infected zebrafish larval model. In addition, the antimycobacterial activity and the toxicological profile of the ethanol extract (EE) of *Kielmeyera membranacea* were investigated in vivo. Therefore, this original study provides important and robust data regarding the in vitro and in vivo antimycobacterial activity of podocarpusflavone A for the first time; in addition, it contributes to the knowledge about the species *Kielmeyera membranacea.*

2. Results and Discussion

2.1. Chemical Study of Kielmeyera Membranacea

Kielmeyera membranacea is a promising species with great antimycobacterial activity. In our earlier study, we found that the dichloromethane fraction (DCM) derived from the ethanol extract (EE) of *K. membranaceae* can inhibit both the avirulent *M. bovis* BCG and the virulent *M. tuberculosis* H37Rv strain. For this reason, the dichloromethane fraction was fractionated, and this process yielded six subfractions (F1–6), with the last two presenting the most promising antimycobacterial activity (Section 2.2). Therefore, F5 and F6 were analyzed by UPLC-MS/MS, and the compounds were identified based on their MS_n data and by comparison with MS databases and the literature (Figure 1A–D).

In the F5 chromatogram, only one peak was observed with t_R 12.72 min and a protonated molecule of m/z 553 $[M+H]^+$, corresponding to $C_{31}H_{20}O_{10}$ (Figure 1A,B). In the F6 chromatogram, two peaks were observed, the first with t_R 11.31 min and a protonated molecule of m/z 539 $[M+H]^+$, corresponding to $C_{30}H_{18}O_{10}$ (Figure 1C,D), probably corresponding to amentoflavone. The second peak with t_R 12.76 min was identified as the same flavonoid of F5 after comparing UV spectra and the MS fragmentation patterns. The compound isolated in F5 was further characterized by NMR spectroscopy as the biflavone podocarpusflavone A (PCFA) (Figure 1E), in accordance with the literature [19]. ^{1}H and ^{13}C NMR spectra are presented in the Supplementary Material Figure S1.

Podocarpusflavone A: ^{1}H NMR (DMSO-d_6, 500 MHz) δ 6.82 (s, H-3), 6.17 (*d, J* 1.8 Hz, H-6), 6.41 (*d, J* 1.8 Hz, H-8), 8.04 (*d, J* 2.2 Hz, H-2′), 7.11 (*d, J* 8.6 Hz, H-5′), 7.99 (*dd, J* 2.2; 8.6 Hz, H-6′), 6.88 (*s*, H-3″), 6.35 (*s*, H-6″), 7.70 (*br d, J* 8.9 Hz, H-2‴ and H-6‴), 6.89 (*br d, J* 8.9 Hz, H-3‴ and H-5‴), 3.73 (*s*, 4‴-OCH3), 12.89 (*s*, 5-OH), 13.09 (*s*, 5″-OH); ^{13}C *NMR (DMSO-d_6*, 125 MHz) δ 164.0 (C-2), 102.1 (C-3), 181.8 (C-4), 161.5 (C-5), 98.8 (C-6), 164.1 (C-7), 94.0 (C-8), 157.4 (C-9), 103.7 (C-10), 120.5 (C-1′), 131.4 (C-2′), 120.6 (C-3′), 160.6 (C-4′), 116.7 (C-5′), 127.7 (C-6′), 164.0 (C-2″), 103.3 (C-3″), 182.1 (C-4″), 160.6 (C-5″), 99.2 (C-6″), 163.1 (C-7″), 104.5 (C-8″), 154.6 (C-9″), 103.4 (C-10″), 123.1 (C-1‴), 128.1 (C-2‴), 114.5 (C-3‴), 162.2 (C-4‴), 114.5 (C-5‴), 128.1 (C-6‴), 55.5 (4‴-OCH_3); ESI-MS m/z 553.37 [M+]+ (calculated for $C_{31}H_{20}O_{10}$, 552.45).

PCFA, also known as 4‴*O*-methylamentoflavone, is a dimer of apigenin and acacetin (4′-methyl ether derivative of apigenin) and has a C3′→C8″ interflavonoid linkage. Although PCFA has been described for some plant species belonging to the genera *Podocarpus* (Podocarpaceae) [20], *Garcinia* (Clusiaceae) [21], and *Juniperus* (Cupressaceae) [22], for the genus *Kielmeyera* there is only one report for *Kielmeyera variabilis* [19] and no reports of *K. membranacea*. Moreover, PCFA has exhibited anticancer [20,23], antileishmanial [24], antiviral [25,26], and antioxidant [19] activities. It can also inhibit NO production in LPS-stimulated macrophages [27] and NADPH oxidase and ROS production in stimulated human neutrophils [28].

2.2. Antimycobacterial Activity on Extracellular Bacteria and in Infected Human Macrophages

Aiming to select the best conditions for in vivo experiments, the minimum inhibitory concentration (MIC) of PCFA was evaluated in the *M. marinum* Wasabi strain. PCFA (F5) showed a MIC_{50} value of 34.38 ± 1.88 μM (equivalent to 18.99 ± 1.03 μg/mL) and was more active than the EE and DCM samples (MIC_{50} of 91.82 ± 1.62 and 125.1 ± 4.34 μg/mL, respectively) (Figure 2). The other fractions, F1-4 and F6, showed low inhibition of mycobacterial growth (Figure 2 and Supplementary Material Figure S2 for F1–4). PCFA has also been demonstrated to be effective against *M. marinum* E11 mCherry strain, *M. tuberculosis* strains H37Rv and M299 (hypervirulent), with MIC_{50} 34.83 ± 1.56, 87.38 ± 1.08 and 99.61 ± 1.03 μM, respectively, suggesting that PCFA is partially responsible for the activity of the DCM (Figure 3).

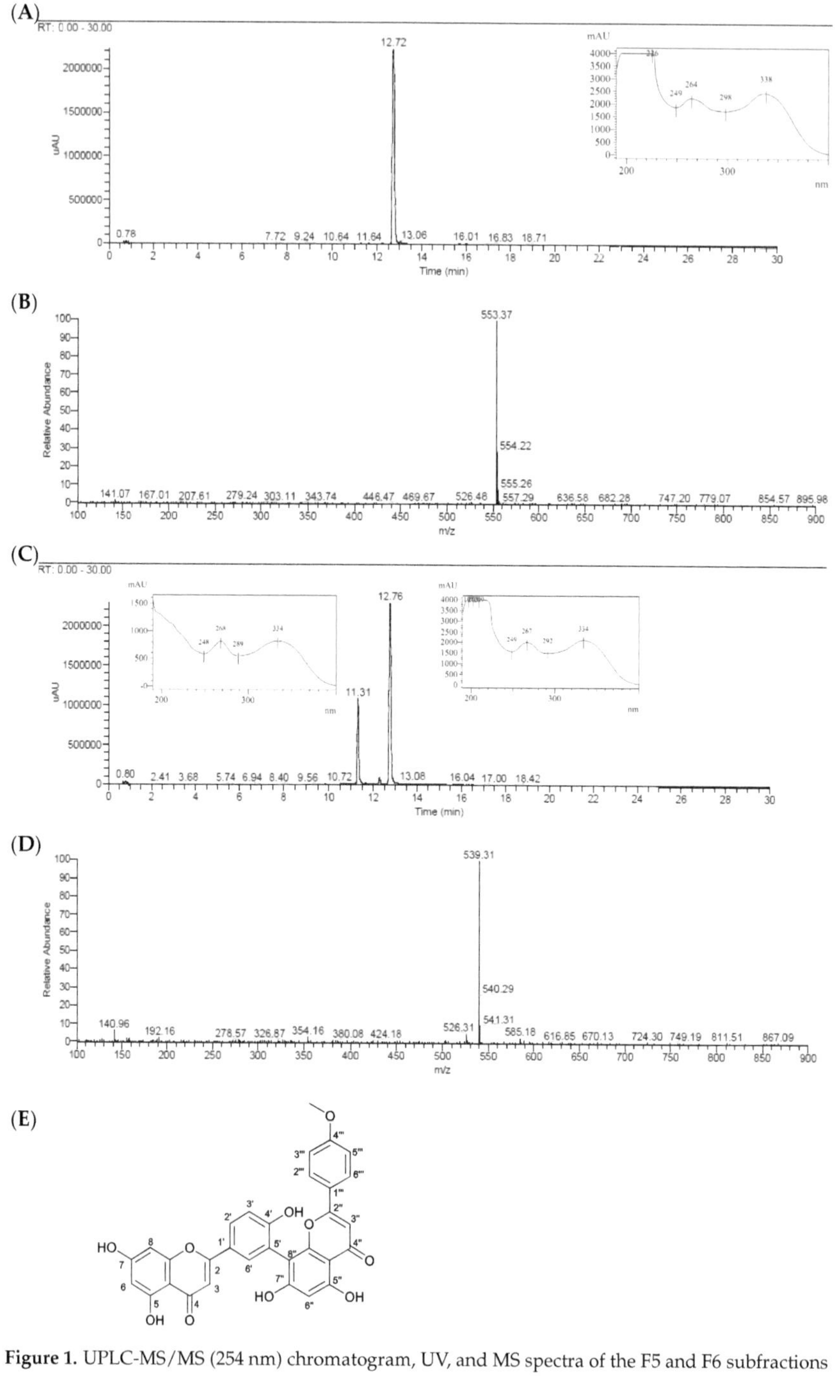

Figure 1. UPLC-MS/MS (254 nm) chromatogram, UV, and MS spectra of the F5 and F6 subfractions purified from dichloromethane fraction (DCM) of *Kielmeyera membranacea*. (**A**) F5 chromatogram and UV spectrum of the peak with t_R 12.72 min (podocarpusflavone A—PCFA). (**B**) F5 mass spectrum of the peak with t_R 12.72 min. (**C**) F6 chromatogram and UV spectra of the peak with t_R 11.31 and 12.76 min. (**D**) F6 mass spectrum of the peak with t_R 11.31 min. (**E**) PCFA structure.

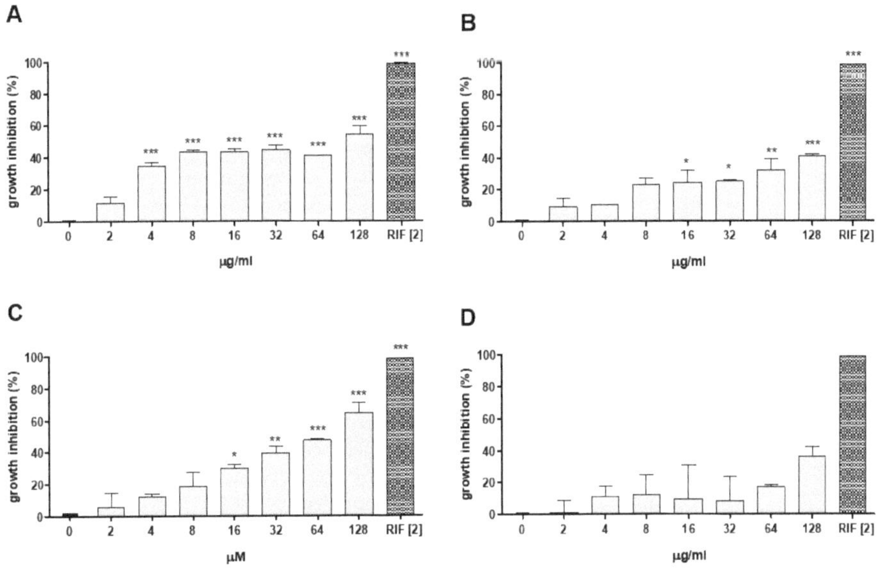

Figure 2. Growth inhibition of *Mycobacterium marinum* Wasabi by *Kielmeyera membranacea*. (**A**) ethanolic extract (EE); (**B**) dichloromethane fraction (DCM); (**C**) podocarpusflavone A (PCFA; F5); and (**D**) F6. Microplate assay with green-fluorescent bacteria after 5 days of incubation. Fluorescence reading was performed using excitation at 493 nm and emission at 509 nm. *M. marinum* treated with rifampicin (RIF) at a concentration of 2 µg/mL was used as a positive control, and untreated *M. marinum* was used as a negative control. *** $p < 0.001$, ** $p < 0.01$, and * $p < 0.05$ when compared to the untreated group (0).

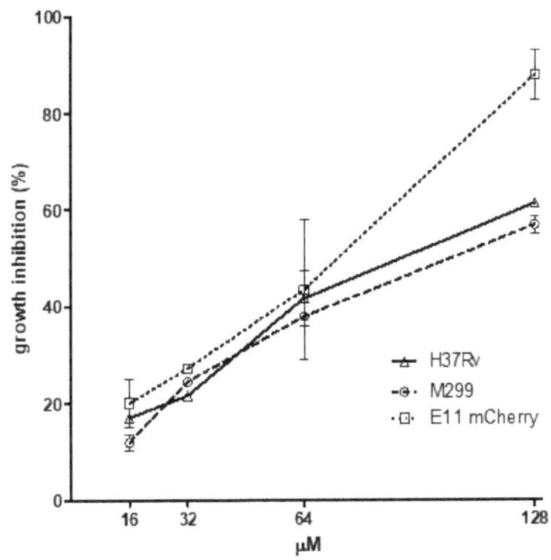

Figure 3. Growth inhibition of *Mycobacterium* strains by podocarpusflavone A (PCFA). Microplate assay after 5 days of incubation in the presence of PCFA (16–128 µM). Growth of *Mycobacterium tuberculosis* strains H37Rv and M299 was evaluated by the MTT test. The growth of *M. marinum* E11 mCherry red-fluorescent bacteria was assessed by measuring bacterial fluorescence (excitation at 588 nm and emission at 610 nm). The untreated *Mycobacterium* strains were used as a negative control, and rifampicin (RIF) was used as a positive control, with MIC values for each of the strains equal to 0.3 µg/mL for M299; 1 µg/mL for H37Rv and 4 µg/mL for E11 mCherry, respectively.

The ability of PCFA, or isoniazid either on its own or in combination therapy with (INH), to inhibit the intracellular growth of mycobacteria was tested in THP-1-derived macrophages infected with *M. tuberculosis* H37Rv strain (Figure 4). This in vitro-infected macrophage model allows researchers to mimic the environment typically encountered by mycobacteria during infection [29]. The results demonstrated that PCFA alone at 64 and 128 μM was able to reduce bacterial growth when compared to untreated bacteria, as well as when compared to INH 0.5× MIC (0.032 μg/mL) at days 2 and 4 (Figure 4A). PCFA also reduced mycobacterial growth in combination with INH: INH 0.5× MIC + PCFA 64 μM was more efficient than INH 0.5× MIC alone. Likewise, INH 1× MIC + PCFA 32 μM and INH 1× MIC + PCFA 64 μM were more efficient than INH 1× MIC alone (0.063 μg/mL) (Figure 4B). Interestingly, the inhibitory effect was increased with the combined INH 1× MIC+ PCFA 64 μM, resulting in statistical significance on days 2, 4, and 7 (Figure 4B). Moreover, on days 4 and 7, the observed effect for the combination INH 1× MIC + PCFA 64 μM (Figure 4B) was higher than the sum of the single effects of INH 1× and PCFA 64 μM (Figure 4A). No significant toxicity was observed for PCFA on non-infected THP-1 macrophage culture, while it exhibited selectivity against the *M. tuberculosis* H37Rv strain. These findings indicate that further studies should be conducted to better characterize PCFA as a combination drug regarding novel combination regimens for TB treatment. In these multidrug regimens, a companion drug is used to prevent treatment failure due to acquired resistance to the core drugs. Some also help to reduce the risk of relapse [30].

INH is an essential first-line anti-TB drug with a well-described mechanism of action. In general, after activation by catalase-peroxidase (KatG), INH leads to the inhibition of enoyl acyl transporter reductase (InhA), which is involved in the biosynthesis of mycolic acids, essential constituents of the bacterial cell wall [31]. In this context, the mode of action of PCFA remains to be studied, and its prediction has been described in Section 2.5. However, the higher inhibitory effect of PCFA and INH together, when compared to the sum of their single effects, suggests that PCFA may act synergistically with INH.

2.3. *In Vivo Toxicological Analysis*

To determine the possible toxicity of the *Kielmeyera membranacea* samples in an in vivo model, zebrafish embryos were treated with EE, DCM (4–128 μg/mL), and PCFA (4–128 μM), and the embryos' survival was examined by counting viable and dead larvae (Figure 5A–C). As can be seen in Figure 5, groups treated with EE (4, 8, 16, 32, 64, 128 μg/mL) showed no mortality (0%) at 2 h post-fertilization (hpf) (Figure 5A). These results should provide encouragement for researchers to conduct other pharmacological studies with *K. membranacea*, considering the good toxicological profile observed in vivo by the well-accepted fish embryo toxicity test (FET) with zebrafish (*Danio rerio*) [32]. PCFA showed no significant differences in embryo mortality compared to the control group (CTL) (Figure 5C). The group treated with valproic acid (VPA—15 μM), a zebrafish larvae control toxic drug, showed a high mortality rate (90%) (Figure 5A–C). The solvent used, DMSO (0.1% *v*/*v*), resulted in no fatalities (0% mortality rate at 2, 24, and 48 hpf).

Based on the antimycobacterial and toxicological results, a 32 μM dose was tested for in vivo efficacy against *M. marinum* infection. This dose did not result in any gross morphological change to embryonic development and was near the MIC_{50} of PCFA.

2.4. *In Vivo Antimycobacterial Activity of Kielmeyera Membranacea Extract, Fraction, and Podocarpusflavone A Tested in the Zebrafish Mycobacterium marinum Infection Model*

Initially, the antibacterial efficacy of the EE, DCM, and PCFA was assessed by monitoring the fluorescence intensity correlating with bacterial burden present either in the total body or only in the tail region of 5-day-old zebrafish larvae using COPAS analysis after yolk infection (Figure 6A,B). Larvae treated with the EE showed a reduction in the bacterial burden after 24 and 48 h. It is important to mention that, after 24 h, the EE and DCM showed similar in vivo activity despite the slightly higher in vitro extracellular antimycobacterial activity observed for the EE (Figure 2). The DCM was not evaluated at 48 h due to its toxicity. PCFA showed an inhibition trend after 24 h. However, after 48 h, it caused a statistically significant decrease in the bacterial burden, suggesting a time-dependent effect. Regarding macrophage fluorescence, it can be seen that PCFA significantly enhanced it after *M. marinum* infection at 24 and 48 h, which can be correlated with a high migration pattern associated with the infection site (Figure 6C,D).

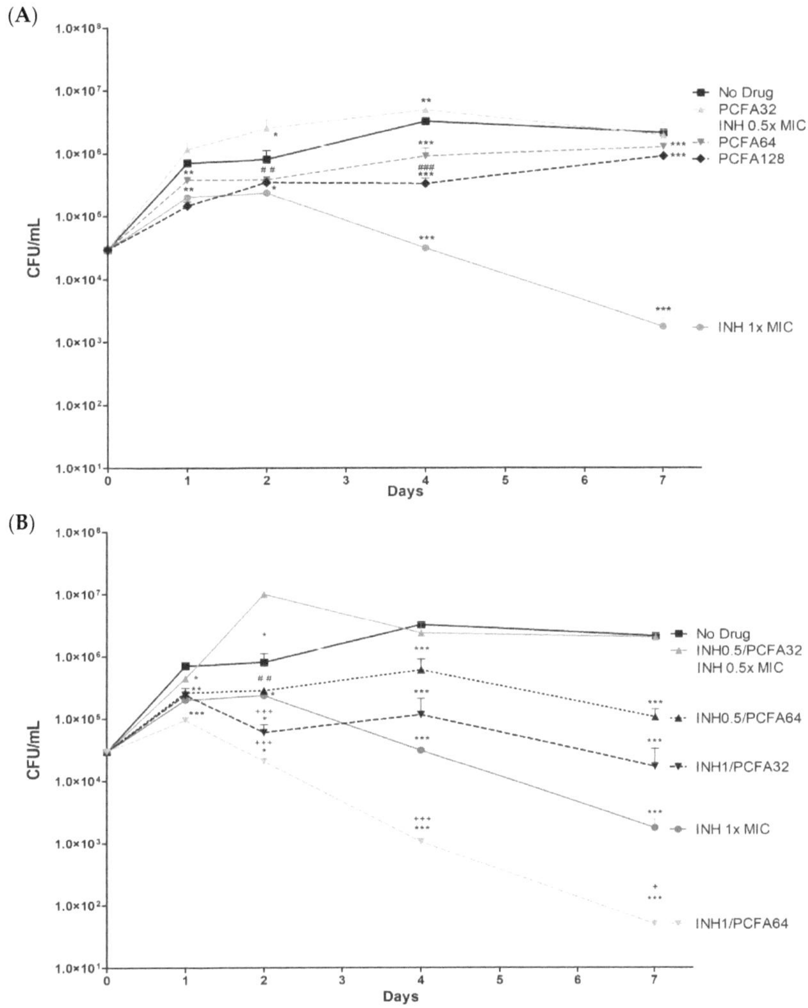

Figure 4. Effect of podocarpusflavone A (PCFA), isoniazid (INH), and INH-PCFA combinations on *Mycobacterium tuberculosis* H37Rv strain growth in THP-1-derived macrophages. (**A**) THP-1 macrophages were infected and treated with PCFA at 32, 64, and 128 μM and INH at 0.5× MIC (0.032 μg/mL) and 1× MIC (0.063 μg/mL). (**B**) THP-1 macrophages infected and treated with combinations of INH-PCFA. The intracellular viability of the bacteria was determined by CFU counting. Values were reported as mean ± error. The mean value of each group was significantly different from the mean value of the controls, as indicated in the graph after the two-way ANOVA analysis. *** $p < 0.001$, ** $p < 0.01$, and * $p < 0.05$ compared to no drug. ### $p < 0.001$ and ## $p < 0.01$ compared to INH 0.5× MIC. +++ $p < 0.001$ and + $p < 0.05$ compared to INH 1× MIC.

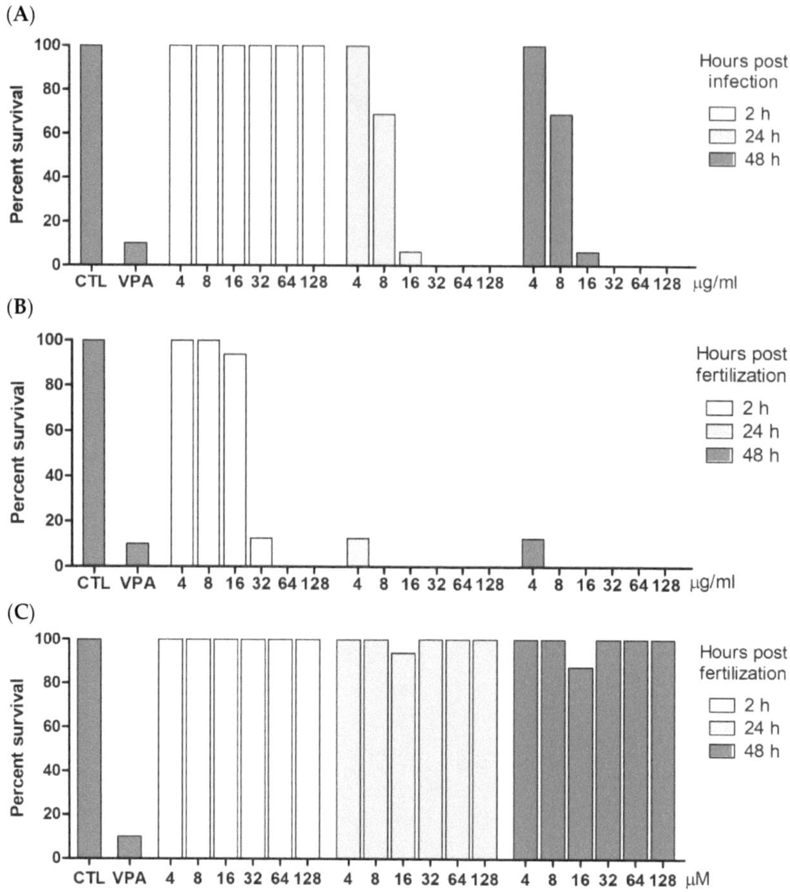

Figure 5. Viability of zebrafish larvae treated with *Kielmeyera membranacea* samples. The wild-type zebrafish larvae were treated with ethanolic extract (EE) (**A**), dichloromethane fraction (DCM) (**B**), and PCFA (**C**) for 2, 24, and 48 hpf, and viability was evaluated by microscopy-based morphological analysis. CTL (negative control, dilution water) and VPA (positive control, valproic acid—15 µM).

At the final step of the in vivo study, larvae infected through the caudal vein by *M. marinum* microinjection were treated with PCFA at 32 µM for 5 days and refreshed every second day. Quantification of the systemic bacterial burden of *M. marinum*, through fluorescence imaging with repeated measurements of each larva, showed a statistically significant decrease at day 5 post-infection. Compared with the infected and untreated larvae at 5 dpi, there were fewer total infection foci and the areas of infection were smaller, clearly demonstrating the potential of PCFA to reduce (81.93 ± 8.76%) the bacterial burden in a biologically relevant setting (Figure 7). A similar effect was observed with rifampicin at the same concentration, 32 µM.

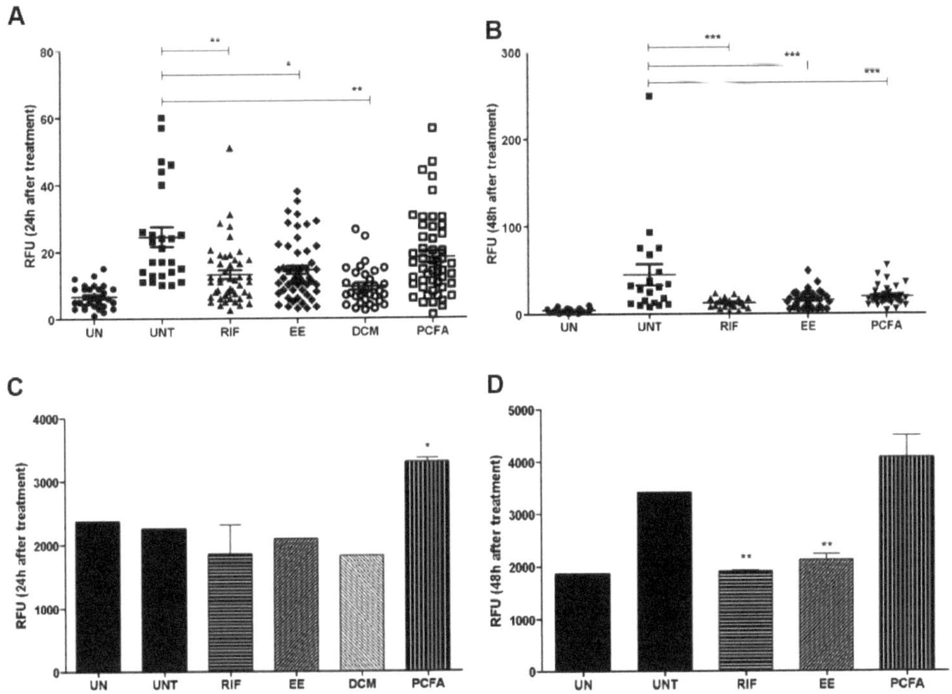

Figure 6. Effect of treatment with the ethanolic extract (EE), dichloromethane fraction (DCM) (32 μg/mL), and podocarpusflavone A (PCFA) (32 μM) on mycobacterial growth (mCherry E11) in 4- and 5-day-old Tg(mpeg1:eGFP)gl22 larvae after yolk sac injection of *Mycobacterium marinum*. (**A**) Red-fluorescent mycobacteria measured by COPAS analysis after 24 h, and (**B**) 48 h. (**C**) Green-fluorescent macrophages were measured by COPAS analysis after 24 h and (**D**) 48 h. UN: uninfected; UNT: untreated; RIF: rifampicin. *** $p < 0.001$ ** $p < 0.01$ and * $p < 0.05$ when compared to the infected and untreated group (UNT).

2.5. Podocarpusflavone: A Mode of Action Study

Chemogenomics studies were used to predict the potential mode of action of PCFA in *M. tuberculosis*. Protein tyrosine phosphatase B (PtpB), one of the virulence factors secreted into the host cell by *M. tuberculosis*, was predicted as the target responsible for the antimycobacterial activity of PCFA. Meaningful interactions for enzyme inhibition were observed via visual inspection (Figure 8). For instance, the molecule interacts with hydrogen bonds with residues Arg166 and Asp165 and achieves hydrophobic/aromatic interactions with the side chain of Phe161 with a geometry like the π stacking proposed for the polyphenol compound kuwanol E [33,34]. Besides kuwanol E, few PtpB inhibitors have been reported in the literature, as reviewed by Kuban-Jankowska [35]. Using Protein BLAST alignment protein sequence (http://blast.ncbi.nlm.nih.gov/Blast.cgi) accessed on 18 August 2023, we found that *M. tuberculosis* PtpB is 78% identical in the amino acid sequence and 84% identical in the catalytic domain in comparison to *M. marinum* PtpB (Figure 9).

Notably, PtpB prevents infected macrophage apoptosis by activating Akt and blocking caspase 3 activity [36]. Recently, it has been shown that PtpB inhibits gasdermin D (GSDMD)-dependent pyroptosis to promote *M. tuberculosis* intracellular survival in macrophages [37]. In addition, PtpB attenuates host immune defenses by interfering with signal transduction pathways in macrophages and, therefore, is a promising target for new anti-TB drug development [33,34,38]. Specifically, PtpB blocks the IFN-γ stimulated IL-6 production by downregulating ERK 1/2 and p38 activity [39]. IL-6 plays an important role in fighting *M. tuberculosis* infection, upregulating microbicidal activity in macrophages and initiating the systemic immune response [40]; its suppression contributes to *M. tuberculosis* intracellular survival. Consequently, the genetic inactivation of PtpB in *M. tuberculosis* accelerated mycobacterial cell death in activated macrophages and in the guinea pig model [39,41].

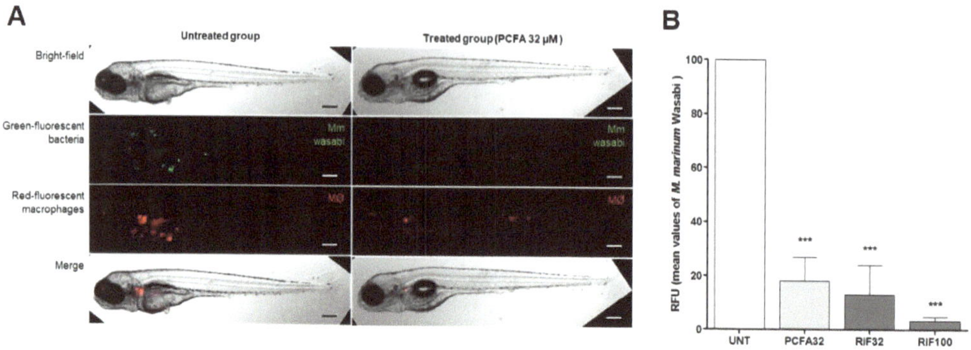

Figure 7. Caudal vein injection of *Mycobacterium marinum* and effect of treatment on infected larvae. Fluorescence microscopy images of fluorescent zebrafish and *M. marinum*. (**A**) Transgenic zebrafish larva with red fluorescent macrophages Tg(mpeg1:mCherry)gl23 infected with green fluorescent *M. marinum* (Wasabi), untreated or treated with PCFA (podocarpusflavone A) at 32 µM after 3 days. (**B**) Mean values of relative fluorescence units of green-fluorescent bacteria after 3 days with PCFA (32 µM) and rifampicin (RIF) (32 and 100 µM) treatment. Scale bar: 250 µm. *** $p < 0.001$ compared to the infected and untreated group (UNT).

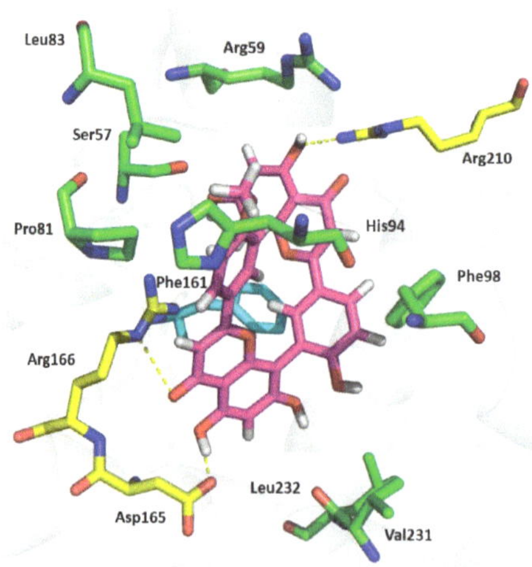

Figure 8. Molecular docking of podocarpusflavone A (PCFA) and PtpB of *Mycobacterium tuberculosis*. The carbon atoms of the molecule are colored pink at the ATP-binding site of PtpB. The amino acid residues in green show the interactions between van der Waals forces, the residues depicted in yellow are those involved in hydrogen bonding, π-π stacking is indicated in light blue, oxygen atoms are shown in red, and nitrogen atoms are shown in dark blue. Yellow dashed lines indicate hydrogen bonding. Picture made with Pymol, version 0.99.

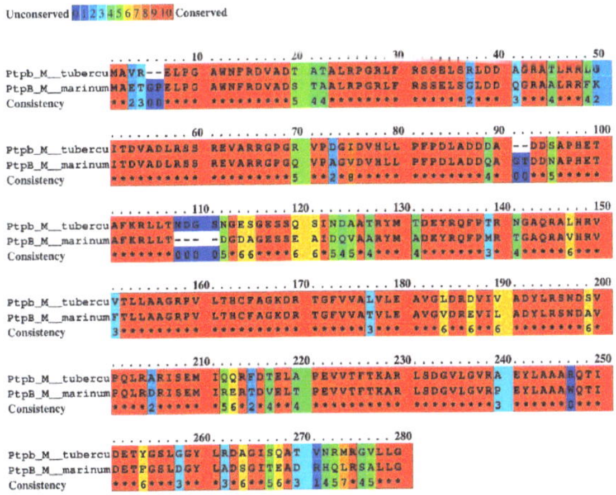

Figure 9. Amino acid sequence alignment of PtpB of *Mycobacterium tuberculosis* and *M. marinum*, * refers to the same amino acid residues in protein alignment, showing the consistency of the results. Image from the server Praline (https://www.ibi.vu.nl/programs/pralinewww/) accessed on 29 October 2024.

The prediction of PtpB as the target of PCFA concurs with the experimental results, considering that the observed activity of PCFA is promising, mainly with regard to macrophage and zebrafish infection. These results showed the importance of the reversion (or at least partial reversion) of the immune response inhibition modulated by PtpB. The combination of a PtpB inhibitor, which reduces *M. tuberculosis'* ability to evade immune responses, with a bactericidal antitubercular agent representing a highly promising strategy for TB treatment [35]. In this context, the activity observed using the combination of INH and PCFA (Figure 4) further corroborates this concept. Notably, no intrinsic roles have been identified between PtpB and the INH-related enzymes InhA and KatG.

2.6. Expression of Cytokines and Macrophage Markers in Zebrafish Infected with *Mycobacterium marinum*

Given that the in silico study predicted a potential interaction between PCFA and PtpB, which may be linked to the immune response, we evaluated the expression of cytokines. For this purpose, mRNA was obtained from the infected zebrafish larvae cells to characterize the profile of the host's immune response in the acute phase of infection with mycobacteria. This was achieved through quantification of the relative expression of mRNAs responsible for encoding important antimycobacterial defense mediators by real-time qPCR. After 5 days of infection with *M. marinum*, the relative expression of mRNA of IL-10, IL-6, IL-12, TNF-α, and the chemokine receptor CXCR3 was measured in whole fish.

Consistent with the established role of inflammatory mediators in host defense against mycobacterial infection [42–45], the pro-inflammatory cytokines IL-12 and TNF-α expression were upregulated on day 5 post-infection in zebrafish larvae. After being treated with PCFA or rifampicin for 72 h, infected zebrafish larvae exhibited reduced transcriptional levels of the pro-inflammatory cytokines IL-12 and TNF-α, presumably indicating the resolution of the infection (Figure 10). In contrast, no statistically significant difference was observed for IL-6 between infected and non-infected controls. It is known that mycobacteria can modulate host IL-6 production, facilitating disease progression [40]. However, after PCFA treatment, a statistically significant increase was observed in the IL-6 mRNA level (Figure 10), which could be attributed to the inhibition of PtpB by PCFA, as predicted in silico, since PtpB blocks IL-6 production [39].

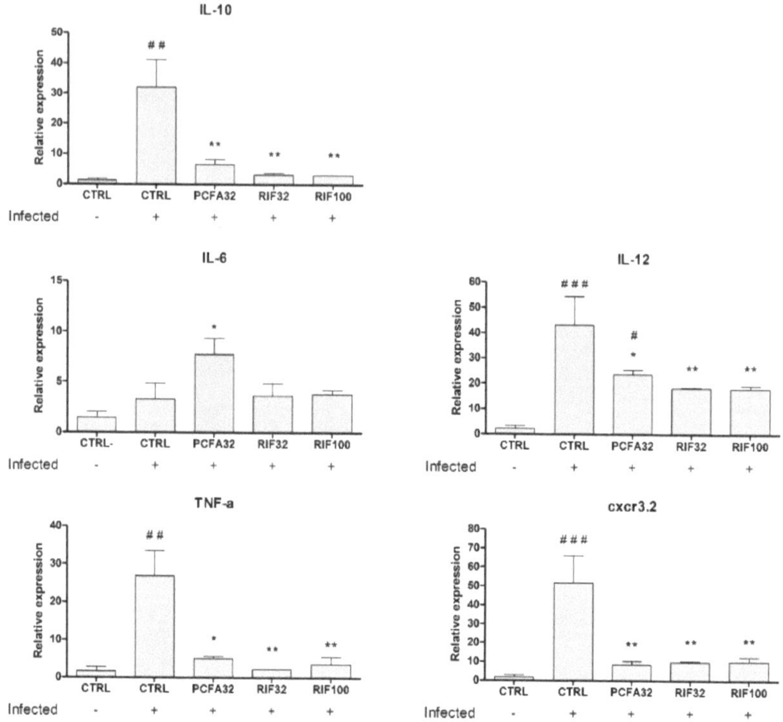

Figure 10. Expression levels of cytokines and macrophage markers in zebrafish larvae infected with *Mycobacterium marinum* determined by RT-qPCR. The Tg(mpeg1:mCherry)gl23 zebrafish larvae, infected (+) or non-infected (−) with *M. marinum*, were treated with podocarpusflavone A at 32 μM (PCFA32), rifampicin at 32 or 100 μM (RIF32 and RIF100) or were left untreated (CTRL) for 5 days, and relative expression of mRNA was measured for IL-12, IL-6, TNF-α, IL-10, and CXCR3.2. The expression of each target gene was related to the expression of the housekeeping ppial gene. The data were expressed as the mean ± SEM. * $p < 0.05$ and ** $p < 0.01$ compared to the CTRL infected group and # $p < 0.05$, ## $p < 0.01$ and ### $p < 0.001$ as compared to the CTRL non-infected group.

IL-10, the only anti-inflammatory cytokine evaluated in the present study, weakens the immune defense against *M. marinum* in infected zebrafish. Therefore, its levels are enhanced after infection as a mycobacterial survival immunomodulatory mechanism [46]. However, the treatment with PCFA or rifampicin reduced its levels due to infection control.

Macrophages are the primary cells of the host's innate immune defense that interact with mycobacteria, and are stimulated to produce a variety of inflammatory mediators, like those described above: IL-6, IL-12, and TNF-α. Moreover, macrophages play a pivotal role in mycobacterial infections because they are motile and phagocytic cells while being a constituent cell type of the characteristic granulomas [47]. At the transcriptional level, infection in zebrafish triggers the expression of cxcr3.2 in macrophages, enhancing bacterial containment by increasing macrophage motility. This, in turn, facilitates macrophage-mediated bacterial dissemination and leads to a higher number of granulomas. Also, notably, cxcr3.2 is a functional homolog of human CXCR3 [48,49]. As shown in Figure 10, the cxcr3.2 level was enhanced due to the infection, and the treatment with PCFA and rifampicin attenuated its level; this can be directly associated with the infection resolution.

3. Materials and Methods

3.1. Reagents

Middlebrook 7H9 mycobacterial media was obtained from Difco (Detroit, MI, USA), while ADC supplements were sourced from BD Biosciences (Sparks, MD, USA). Rifampicin and MTT (3-(4,5-dimethylthiazol-2-yl)-2,5-diphenyltetrazolium bromide) were acquired from Sigma-Aldrich (St. Louis, MO, USA). Samples were dissolved in dimethyl sulfoxide (DMSO, Sigma Aldrich), whereas other reagents used for cell culture were dissolved in sterile phosphate-buffered saline (PBS) and sterilized by filtration.

3.2. General Experimental Procedures

^1H and ^{13}C NMR spectra of F5 (podocarpusflavone A) were obtained from 500 and 125 MHz, respectively, on a Varian MERCURY-VX 500 MHz. Size exclusion chromatography was performed on Sephadex LH-20. Eluates were monitored by thin-layer chromatography (TLC) on silica 60 F254 using chloroform–methanol (6:1), visualized under UV light, and revealed with phosphoric vanillin under heating. The fractions were analyzed by HPLC-DAD on a Shimadzu SCL-10A with Diode Array Detector SPD-M10A with absorptions measured from 200 to 600 nm.

3.3. Plant Material

Extract and fractions from leaves of previously obtained *Kielmeyera membranacea* Casar. (Calophyllaceae) [13] were used for the development of this research. Briefly, *K. membranacea* leaves were collected at Carapebus, Rio de Janeiro, Brazil. The plant material was identified by a botanist, Prof. Dr. Tatiana U. P. Konno, and a voucher specimen was deposited in the herbarium of UFRJ-RJ (RFA 38752). The leaves were then air-dried at room temperature, ground into a fine powder, and extracted through maceration with ethanol until fully exhausted. The crude extract (EE), obtained by rotary evaporation at 45 °C, was dissolved in H_2O: MeOH (1:9), and fractions were obtained sequentially by liquid–liquid partition. Firstly, hexane was obtained, then, after MeOH removal, dichloromethane was obtained, resulting in the dichloromethane fraction (DCM). This research adhered to all applicable federal guidelines and institutional policies regarding the use of botanical material for research purposes (SISBIO/ICMBio No 62.455-11; SISGEN/MMA No: AAA989F).

3.4. Isolation and Characterization of Podocarpusflavone A

An aliquot of 1888 mg of the dichloromethane fraction was chromatographed on a Sephadex LH-20 gel column (GE Healthcare, Chicago, IL, USA) (60 × 5.5 cm; methanol), yielding 6 subfractions. After thin-layer chromatography (TLC) analysis, subfraction 5 (F5) was identified as an isolated compound 1 (101.9 mg). Compound 1 was identified as the biflavone podocarpusflavone A based on MS data (UPLC-MS/MS analysis), m/z 553.37 [M+H]+, and NMR spectroscopic data, in accordance with previous reports from the literature [20].

3.5. UPLC-MS/MS Analysis

The analysis of the subfractions obtained from the dichloromethane fraction was performed using a Dionex Focused Ultimate 3000 equipped with a DAD detector coupled with an LCQ Fleet Ion Trap Mass Spectrometer ThermoFisher Scientific (Waltham, MA, USA). The chromatographic conditions were an Ascentis® Express C18 column (100 mm × 4.6 mm; 1.7 µm particle size) Supelco® (Bellefonte, PA, USA) maintained at 25 °C, flow rate 0.2 mL/min, injection volume of 5 µL. The eluents were H_2O (0.01% H_3PO_4) (A) and acetonitrile (ACN, B). The mobile phase elution was performed in the following gradient mode: 0–15 min, A–B (90:10→10:90); 15–20 min, A–B (10:90→0:100); 20–35 min, A–B (0:100→0:100); 35–37 min, A–B (0:100→90:10); 37–40 min, A–B (90:10→90:10), and 40 min as total time analysis. The mass spectrometry parameters were as follows: capillary voltage of 36 V, nebulization 5.5 Bar, drying gas flow of 10 L/min, drying temperature of 250 °C, and collision energy of 35 eV. Signal acquisition was performed in positive ion mode at m/z between 100 and 900 and MS2 of the base peak ions. The results were processed using XCalibur software ThermoFisher Scientific Version 2.0 (Waltham, MA, USA).

3.6. Bacterial Strain Preparation

The bacterial strains *Mycobacterium tuberculosis* H37Rv (a low virulent laboratory strain, ATCC 27294) and Beijing M299 (a highly virulent strain isolated from TB patient in Mozambique) were used for in vitro tests. Mycobacterial strains were cultured at 37 °C in Middlebrook 7H9 supplemented with 0.5% glycerol, 0.05% Tween-80, and 10% acid-albumin-dextrose-catalase (ADC). The bacterial strains *M. marinum* E11, expressing mCherry fluorescent protein and *M. marinum* Wasabi, expressing green fluorescent protein [49] were used for in vitro and in vivo tests inducing an infection by yolk or caudal vein in zebrafish embryos, respectively. Briefly, a colony of *M. marinum* was picked from 7H10 supplemented with 10% oleic acid-albumin-dextrose-catalase (OADC), and the colony was suspended in 7H9 supplemented with 10% ADC and cultured overnight at 28 °C. After 24 h, the OD at 600 nm (OD600) was measured (Eppendorf Biophotometer 6131, Eppendorf, Hamburg, Germany). Bacteria in the logarithmic growth phase were harvested and washed three times with sterile PBS. The inoculum was resuspended to a target concentration of 200 colony-forming units CFU/ηL in 2% polyvinylpyrrolidone-40 solution (PVP40) for both in vitro and in vivo infection tests [50].

3.7. In Vitro Antimycobacterial Activity

During the mid-logarithmic growth phase, bacterial suspensions were plated in a 96-well microplate at 1×10^6 CFU/well. The samples were added at 128, 64, 32, and 16 μg/mL or μM (for PCFA), along with rifampicin at concentrations ranging from 0.0032 to 4 μg/mL. The plates were sealed and incubated at 32 °C or 37 °C for *M. marinum* and *M. tuberculosis*, respectively, and 5% CO_2 for 5 days. After these periods, the *M. tuberculosis* cultures were incubated for 3 h with MTT solution (5 mg/mL) and then treated with lysis buffer (20% w/v SDS/50% dimethylformamide—DMF in distilled water, pH 4.7) for 18 h. The optical density was measured at 570 nm [51]. The *M. marinum* fluorescent cultures were analyzed by fluorescence using 588 nm excitation and 610 nm emission for the E11 strain, and 493 nm excitation and 509 nm emission for the Wasabi strain. Mycobacteria treated and untreated with rifampicin were used as positive and negative controls, respectively.

3.8. Cytotoxicity and Infection of Macrophages

THP-1 macrophage cells were cultured and differentiated into macrophages with 50 ng/mL phorbol 12-myristate 13-acetate (PMA; Sigma-Aldrich). After 24 h, PMA was removed, and cells were treated with the samples. After 24, 48, 72, and 144 h, cell viability was measured using MTT. Then, to evaluate the sample's intracellular antimycobacterial activity, following differentiation, the cells were infected with *M. tuberculosis* H37Rv strain at a multiplicity of infection (MOI) of 1:10. After 3 h of infection, extracellular bacteria were further removed by washing with warm PBS. Fresh medium with different treatments was added (isolated compound at 32, 64, and 128 μM, isoniazid (INH) at 0.5× and 1× MIC, 0.063 μg/mL, and their combinations). Macrophages were lysed at 0 h and 1, 2, 4, and 7 days after infection, plated on 7H10 agar plates, and incubated at 37 °C to determine total CFU after 10–14 days [52,53].

3.9. Zebrafish Husbandry

Zebrafish were maintained and handled in accordance with international consensus protocols [54]. The design and execution of all experiments complied with European regulations, in which zebrafish embryos and larvae were not considered experimental animals throughout our experiments (0–5 days post-fertilization [dpf]). Adult wild-type, Tg(mpeg1:eGFP)gl22 and Tg(mpeg1:mCherry)gl23 zebrafish were kept in glass aquaria (max 6 L^{-1}, volume 10 L, 120 × 220 × 490 mm; Fleuren & Nooijen BV, Nederweert, The Netherlands) with circulating water (27.7 °C ± 0.1 on a 14 h/10 h light/dark cycle, lights on at 08:00). Artemia or Gemma Micro/Diamond (Skretting, Nutreco NV, Amersfoort, The Netherlands) were used for adult zebrafish feeding, and the water quality was monitored with a JUMO ACQUIS. For breeding, the zebrafish were kept overnight, and in the morning, the dividers between males and females were removed to collect fertilized eggs. Eggs, embryos, and larvae were kept in E3 medium (60 μg/mL^{-1} Instant Ocean Sea Salts [Sera, Heinsberg, Germany] in demineralized water, daily refreshed) at 28 °C.

3.10. *Toxic Effect on Zebrafish Larvae*

The wild-type zebrafish were maintained and handled, and the eggs were prepared as described in the previous section. The tests were performed in accordance with the fish embryo toxicity guide [55] and the scheme proposed by Lammer [32]. Ten wells of a 24-well plate were assigned to each sample concentration of treatment and negative and positive controls. A fertilized egg was added to each well with 2 mL of fish water solution. The plates were incubated at 28 °C, and the toxic effect was evaluated by analyzing the morphological patterns of zebrafish development recorded at 2, 24, and 48 h post-fertilization (hpf).

3.11. *Inhibition of Mycobacterium marinum Growth by Yolk Infection*

The Tg(mpeg1:eGFP)gl22 zebrafish embryos at 2 to 4 hpf were anesthetized with 0.02% (*w*/*v*) of ethyl 3-aminobenzoate (tricaine) buffer 10 min before injection and injected with 1 nL of 50 CFU/nL *M. marinum* E11 mCherry strain using the microinjection system (Femto-Jet, Eppendorf, Hamburg, Germany). The Petri plates (92 × 16 mm) with 50 embryos were incubated at 28 °C. After 3 days, infected larvae were analyzed using COPAS™ (Complex Object Parametric Analyzer and Sorter) to check the established infection. Waterborne treatment with compounds commenced, and larvae were kept in E3 medium with compounds during the entire treatment at 28 °C. COPAS analysis and imaging were performed at 24 and 48 h post-treatment.

3.12. *Inhibition of Mycobacterium marinum Growth by Caudal Vein Infection*

The Tg(mpeg1:mCherry)gl23 zebrafish embryos were dechorionated manually at 24 hpf. Embryos of 30 hpf were anesthetized with 0.02% (*w*/*v*) of tricaine buffer 10 min prior and injected with 1 nL of 200 CFU/nL *M. marinum* Wasabi strain into the caudal vein at the blood island [41]. After injection, the larvae were kept at 28 °C overnight to check the establishment of the infection. Then, the embryos were transferred to 24-well plates (Greiner Bio-One) with compound solutions at 32 μM in an E3 medium. The waterborne treatment with compounds was refreshed every 48 h. For the duration of treatment, larvae were kept at 28 °C in an E3 medium with compounds until imaging or sampling took place. Quantification of the bacterial burden within individual larvae was analyzed through fluorescence imaging at 3 days post-treatment (dpt) and 4 days post-infection (dpi) to assess individual early bactericidal responses. The group size was designed at $n = 20$, and rifampicin at 32 and 100 μM was used as a positive control.

3.13. *RNA Isolation, cDNA Synthesis, and RT-qPCR*

Pools of twenty Tg(mpeg1:mCherry)gl23 larvae were homogenized in 1 mL of TRIzol reagent (Life Technologies, Carlsbad, CA, USA). Subsequently, total RNA was extracted and purified using RNeasy MinElute Cleanup Kit (Qiagen, Hilden, Germany), according to the manufacturer's instructions. cDNAs were synthesized from 200 ng total RNAs, and qPCR was performed by using the iScript™ cDNA Synthesis Kit (Bio-Rad, Hercules, CA, USA) and iQ™ SYBR Green Supermix (Bio-Rad), according to the manufacturer's protocols. RT-qPCR was conducted using the MyiQ Single-Color Real-Time PCR Detection System (Bio-Rad). The cycling started with a 3 min 95 °C pre-denaturation, followed by 40 cycles of 15 s 95 °C denaturation, 30 s annealing at 60 °C, and elongation for 30 s at 72 °C, with 0.5 °C increments every 10 s. For every sample, the threshold cycle (Ct) value was determined from the Ct value of a non-infected control sample, and the fold change of gene expression was calculated and normalized against the expression of the housekeeping gene ppial. The results were analyzed using the ΔΔCt method [56].

3.14. Statistical Analysis

GraphPad Prism 5.0 and 10 were used for statistical analysis. One-way analysis of variance (ANOVA) with Tukey's post-test or two-way analysis of variance (ANOVA) were used to evaluate paired replicates. The *p*-values of less than 0.05 were considered significant. IC_{50}, MIC_{50}, and CC_{50} values were calculated by non-linear regression analysis of log[concentration]/inhibition curves by GraphPad Prism 5 Software applying a sigmoidal dose–response variable slope curve fitting using the different percentage obtained for each corresponding concentration in triplicate and were expressed as means with corresponding 95% confidence intervals.

3.15. In Silico Prediction of Podocarpusflavone A Mode of Action (MOA)

The active compound PCFA was drawn in ChemAxon's MarvinSketch v. 6.2.1, saved in sdf format and then standardized with ChemAxon's Standardizer v. 6.2.1. After this step, the compound was saved in Excel in the smiles molecular format. The smiles notation was then saved in csv format, and the biological targets were predicted using the command "python predict_binary.py input.csv 30 0.5" using Pidgin chemogenomics software v. 2 [57,58].

3.16. Molecular Docking Studies

GOLD v. 5.535 was applied to conduct the molecular docking studies using chain A of the 3D structure of the *M. tuberculosis* target protein tyrosine phosphatase B (PtpB), PDB code 2OZ5 [33], obtained by X-ray diffraction with 2 Å of resolution in a complex with its inhibitor (oxalylamino-methylene)-thiophene sulfonamide (OMTS). The protonation states of charged residues from podocarpusflavone A were defined at pH 7.4 using PROPKA 3.0 available on the PDB2PQR server [59]. Before docking studies, redocking of the inhibitor OMTS was performed with GOLD v.5.535, using ChemPLP, GoldScore, and ChemScore scoring functions, with search radii of 10, 15, and 20 Å, respectively, using the carbon atom #1130 belonging to Phe161 as a reference. After redocking, the best function and radius were chosen for the lowest value of Root Mean Square Deviation (RMSD) between the inhibitor (OMTS) removed from the crystal and the top pose obtained by the redocking methodology. Hermes software, available in Gold Suite (GOLD v. 5.535), was used to calculate the RMSD values. The 3D structure of podocarpusflavone A was constructed in Spartan'10 (Wavefunction Inc., Irvine, CA, USA), and the prediction of the molecular ionization states in the physiological pH was carried out with ChemAxon's MarvinView, version 6.2.1 (http://www.chemaxon.com) accessed on 9 August 2023. Finally, the compound was energy-optimized in Spartan'10 using the B3LYP/6-31G * density functional method [60]. Analysis of the interactions between podocarpusflavone A and PtpB was performed in Pymol v. 0.99 (The PyMOL Molecular Graphics System, Schrodinger, LLC, New York, NY, USA) and Discovery Studio v. 16.1.0 (BIOVIA, Discovery Studio Visualizer, 2015).

4. Conclusions

Our study demonstrated the promising in vivo antimycobacterial activity of the *Kielmeyera membranacea* extract, displaying a favorable in vivo toxicological profile. We isolated and characterized podocarpusflavone A (PCFA) as an active compound in this extract. Intracellularly, PCFA reduced *Mycobacterium tuberculosis* H37Rv strain growth, particularly when combined with isoniazid. In addition, PCFA was active in two in vivo zebrafish larvae *M. marinum* infection models, which was a stimulating finding. Specifically, when the systemic infection was established by bacterial microinjection via the caudal vein, the efficacy of PCFA was comparable to that of rifampicin at 32 μM. In silico predictions further suggest that PCFA interacts with mycobacterial protein tyrosine phosphatase (PtpB), potentially blocking *M. tuberculosis*'s key immune evasion mechanism. This finding corroborates the positive modulation of IL-6 in vivo and the enhanced intracellular in vitro and in vivo antimycobacterial activity observed for PCFA. In short, our findings support further mammalian studies to explore the anti TB potential of PCFA.

Supplementary Materials: The following supporting information can be downloaded at https://www.mdpi.com/article/10.3390/ph17121560/s1, Figure S1. NMR spectra of the biflavone podocarpusflavone A (PCFA); Figure S2. Growth inhibition of Mycobacterium marinum Wasabi by subfractions of dichloromethane fraction from Kielmeyera membranacea.

Author Contributions: Conceptualization, M.F.M. and M.H.d.A.; methodology, M.F.M., E.B.L., F.J.V., H.P.S., N.C.R., R.M., F.B., S.C.P. and M.H.d.A.; formal analysis, M.H.d.A.; investigation, M.H.d.A., N.N., S.M.S., D.S., F.B., T.L.B.V.S., S.C.P. and S.S.A.; resources, M.H.d.A., F.J.V., H.P.S. and M.F.M.; data curation, M.H.d.A. and M.F.M.; writing—original draft preparation, M.H.d.A., S.S.A. and M.F.M.; writing—review and editing, M.H.d.A., S.S.A., N.C.R., S.M.S., D.S., F.B., E.B.L., F.J.V., H.P.S., R.M. and M.F.M.; supervision, F.J.V., H.P.S., N.C.R., R.M. and M.F.M.; project administration, M.F.M.; funding acquisition, M.H.d.A., M.F.M., N.C.R., R.M. and H.P.S. All authors have read and agreed to the published version of the manuscript.

Funding: This study was funded by Fundação de Amparo à Pesquisa do Estado do Rio de Janeiro (FAPERJ), Brazil (Project No. 201.136/2022 and 211.560/2021), Conselho Nacional de Desenvolvimento Científico e Tecnológico (CNPq), Brazil (Project No. 403236/2023) and the Coordenação de Aperfeiçoamento de Pessoal de Nível Superior (CAPES), Brazil (Project No. 88881.312022/2018 and 001). RM is supported by EU funding within the MUR PNRR Extended Partnership Initiative on Emerging Infectious Diseases (Project No. PE00000007, INF-ACT).

Institutional Review Board Statement: Not applicable.

Informed Consent Statement: Not applicable.

Data Availability Statement: Data are contained within the article and Supplementary Materials.

Conflicts of Interest: The authors declare no conflicts of interest.

References

1. WHO, World Health Organization. Global Tuberculosis Report. 2024. Available online: https://www.who.int/publications/i/item/9789240101531 (accessed on 5 November 2024).
2. Dong, M.; Pfeiffer, B.; Altmann, K.H. Recent developments in natural product-based drug discovery for tuberculosis. *Drug Discov. Today* **2017**, *22*, 585–591. [CrossRef] [PubMed]
3. Sharifi-Rad, M.; Lankatillake, C.; Dias, D.A.; Docea, A.O.; Mahomoodally, M.F.; Lobine, D.; Chazot, P.L.; Kurt, B.; Boyunegmez, T.T.; Catarina, M.A.; et al. Impact of Natural Compounds on Neurodegenerative Disorders: From Preclinical to Pharmacotherapeutics. *J. Clin. Med.* **2020**, *9*, 1061. [CrossRef] [PubMed]
4. Sousa, Z.L.; de Oliveira, F.F.; da Conceição, A.O.; Silva, L.A.; Rossi, M.H.; Santos, J.D.S.; Andrioli, J.L. Biological activities of extracts from *Chenopodium ambrosioides* Lineu and *Kielmeyera neglecta* Saddi. *Ann. Clin. Microbiol. Antimicrob.* **2012**, *11*, 20. [CrossRef] [PubMed]
5. Coqueiro, A.; Choi, Y.H.; Verpoorte, R.; Gupta, K.B.; De Mieri, M.; Hamburger, M.; Young, M.C.; Stapleton, P.; Gibbons, S.; Bolzani, V.d.S. Antistaphylococcal Prenylated Acylphoroglucinol and Xanthones from Kielmeyera variabilis. *J. Nat. Prod.* **2016**, *79*, 470–476. [CrossRef] [PubMed]
6. Martins, C.d.M.; do Nascimento, E.A.; de Morais, S.A.; de Oliveira, A.; Chang, R.; Cunha, L.C.; Martins, M.M.; Martins, C.H.; Moraes, T.D.S.; Rodrigues, P.V.; et al. Chemical Constituents and Evaluation of Antimicrobial and Cytotoxic Activities of *Kielmeyera coriacea* Mart. & Zucc. Essential Oils. *Evid. Based Complement. Altern. Med.* **2015**, *2015*, 842047.
7. Cortez, D.A.G.; Young, M.C.M.; Marston, A.; Wolfender, J.L.; Hostettmann, K. Xanthones, triterpenes and a biphenyl from *Kielmeyera coriacea*. *Phytochemistry* **1998**, *47*, 1367–1374. [CrossRef]
8. Justino, A.B.; Santana, E.C.; Franco, R.R.; Queiroz, J.S.; Silva, H.C.G.; de Lima, J.P.J.; Saraiva, A.L.; Martins, M.M.; Lemos de Morais, S.A.; de Oliveira, A.; et al. Antioxidant compounds of *Kielmeyera coriacea* Mart. with α-amylase, lipase and advanced glycation end-product inhibitory activities. *J. Pharm. Biomed. Anal.* **2021**, *206*, 114387. [CrossRef]
9. Boness, H.V.M.; Santos, N.A.S.; Costa, I.B.; Queiroz, C.K.L.; Marques, E.J.; El-Bachá, R.S.; Cruz, F.G. Prenylated 4-phenylcoumarins and 4-alkylcoumarins from *Kielmeyera argentea* and their cytotoxic activity. *Fitoterapia* **2021**, *149*, 104836. [CrossRef]
10. Biesdorf, C.; Cortez, D.A.; Audi, E.A. Assessment of anxiolytic and panicolytic effects of dichloromethane fraction from stems of *Kielmeyera coriacea*. *Phytomedicine* **2012**, *19*, 374–377. [CrossRef]

11. Figueiredo, C.R.; Matsuo, A.L.; Massaoka, M.H.; Girola, N.; Azevedo, R.A.; Rabaça, A.N.; Farias, C.F.; Pereira, F.V.; Matias, N.S.; Silva, L.P.; et al. Antitumor activity of *kielmeyera coriacea* leaf constituents in experimental melanoma, tested in vitro and in vivo in syngeneic mice. *Adv. Pharm. Bull.* **2014**, *4*, 429–436.
12. Correia, M.C.R.; Lima, H.A.d.; Silva, R.C.P.D. Caracterização dos frutos, sementes e plântulas de espécies de Clusiaceae das restingas do Rio de Janeiro. *Rodriguésia* **2013**, *64*, 61–73. [CrossRef]
13. Araujo, M.H.; Simão, T.L.B.V.; Konno, T.U.P.; Guimarães, D.O.; Leal, I.C.R.; Lasunskaia, E.; Muzitano, F.M. Anti-mycobacterial and anti-inflammatory activity of Restinga plants: A dual approach in searching for new drugs to treat severe tuberculosis. *Rodriguesia* **2021**, *72*, e01152019. [CrossRef]
14. Ali, S.; Champagne, D.L.; Spaink, H.P.; Richardson, M.K. Zebrafish embryos and larvae: A new generation of disease models and drug screens. *Birth Defects Res. C. Embryo Today* **2011**, *93*, 115–133. [CrossRef] [PubMed]
15. Torraca, V.; Masud, S.; Spaink, H.P.; Meijer, A.H. Macrophage-pathogen interactions in infectious diseases: New therapeutic insights from the zebrafish host model. *Dis. Mod. Mech.* **2014**, *7*, 785–797. [CrossRef] [PubMed]
16. Takaki, K.; Davis, J.M.; Winglee, K.; Ramakrishnan, L. Evaluation of the pathogenesis and treatment of *Mycobacterium marinum* infection in zebrafish. *Nat. Prot.* **2013**, *8*, 1114–1124. [CrossRef]
17. Takaki, K.; Cosma, C.L.; Troll, M.A.; Ramakrishnan, L. An in vivo platform for rapid high-throughput antitubercular drug discovery. *Cell Rep.* **2012**, *26*, 175–184. [CrossRef]
18. Feitosa, N.M.; Richardson, R.; Bloch, W.; Hammerschmidt, M. Basement Membrane Diseases in Zebrafish. In: Detrich, H.W., Westerfield, M., Zon, L.I. (Org.). Methods in Cell Biology: The Zebrafish, Disease Models and Chemical Screens. *Elsevier Corp.* **2011**, *105*, 191–222.
19. Coqueiro, A.; Regasini, L.O.; Skrzek, S.C.G.; Queiroz, M.M.F.; Silva, D.H.S.; Bolzani, V.d.S. Free Radical Scavenging Activity of Kielmeyera variabilis (Clusiaceae). *Molecules* **2013**, *18*, 2376–2385. [CrossRef]
20. Yeh, P.H.; Shieh, Y.D.; Hsu, L.C.; Kuo, L.M.; Lin, J.H.; Liaw, C.C.; Kuo, Y.H. Naturally Occurring Cytotoxic [3′→8″]-Biflavonoids from Podocarpus nakaii. *J. Trad. Complem. Med.* **2012**, *2*, 220–226. [CrossRef]
21. Yu, S.; Yan, H.; Zhang, L.; Shan, M.; Chen, P.; Ding, A.; Li, S.F. A Review on the Phytochemistry, Pharmacology, and Pharmacokinetics of Amentoflavone, a Naturally-Occurring Biflavonoid. *Molecules* **2017**, *22*, 299. [CrossRef]
22. Lim, D.J.; Song, J.S.; Lee, B.H.; Son, Y.K.; Kim, Y. Qualitative and Quantitative Analysis of the Major Bioactive Components of *Juniperus chinensis* L. Using LC-QTOF-MS and LC-MS/MS and Investigation of Antibacterial Activity against Pathogenic Bacteria. *Molecules* **2023**, *28*, 3937. [CrossRef] [PubMed]
23. Meng, H.; Pang, Y.; Liu, G.; Luo, Z.; Tan, H.; Liu, X. Podocarpusflavone A inhibits cell growth of skin cutaneous melanoma by suppressing STAT3 signaling. *J. Dermatol. Sci.* **2020**, *100*, 201–208. [CrossRef] [PubMed]
24. Camacho, M.R.; Mata, R.; Castaneda, P.; Kirby, G.C.; Warhurst, D.C.; Croft, S.L.; Phillipson, J.D. Bioactive compounds from Celaenodendron mexicanum. *Planta Med.* **2000**, *66*, 463–468. [CrossRef] [PubMed]
25. Coulerie, P.; Eydoux, C.; Hnawia, E.; Stuhl, L.; Maciuk, A.; Lebouvier, N.; Canard, B.; Figadère, B.; Guillemot, J.C.; Nour, M. Biflavonoids of Dacrydium balansae with potent inhibitory activity on dengue 2 NS5 polymerase. *Planta Med.* **2012**, *78*, 672–677. [CrossRef] [PubMed]
26. Sharma, M.; Mahto, J.K.; Dhaka, P.; Neetu, N.; Tomar, S.; Kumar, P. MD simulation and MM/PBSA identifies phytochemicals as bifunctional inhibitors of SARS-CoV-2. *J. Biomol. Struct. Dyn.* **2022**, *40*, 12048–12061. [CrossRef]
27. Trang, D.T.; Huyen, L.T.; Nhiem, N.X.; Quang, T.H.; Hang, D.T.T.; Yen, P.H.; Tai, B.H.; Anha, H.L.T.; Binh, N.Q.; Van Minh, C.; et al. Tirucallane glycoside from the leaves of *Antidesma bunius* and inhibitory NO production in BV2 cells and RAW264.7 macrophages. *Nat. Prod. Commun.* **2016**, *11*, 935–937. [CrossRef]
28. Saroni Arwa, P.; Zeraik, M.L.; Ximenes, V.F.; da Fonseca, L.M.; Bolzani, V.d.S.; Siqueira Silva, D.H. Redox-active biflavonoids from *Garcinia brasiliensis* as inhibitors of neutrophil oxidative burst and human erythrocyte membrane damage. *J. Ethnopharmacol.* **2015**, *4*, 410–418. [CrossRef]
29. Marrapu, V.K.; Chaturvedi, V.; Singh, S.; Singh, S.; Sinha, S.; Bhandari, K. Novel aryloxy azolyl chalcones with potent activity against *Mycobacterium tuberculosis* H37Rv. *Eur. J. Med. Chem.* **2011**, *46*, 4302–4310. [CrossRef]
30. Van Deun, A.; Decroo, T.; Piubello, A.; de Jong, B.C.; Lynen, L.; Rieder, H.L. Principles for constructing a tuberculosis treatment regimen: The role and definition of core and companion drugs. *Int. J. Tuberc. Lung Dis.* **2018**, *22*, 239–245. [CrossRef]
31. Sankar, J.; Chauhan, A.; Singh, R.; Mahajan, D. Isoniazid-historical development, metabolism associated toxicity and a perspective on its pharmacological improvement. *Front. Pharmacol.* **2024**, *15*, 1441147. [CrossRef]
32. Lammer, E.; Carr, G.J.; Wendler, K.; Rawlings, J.M.; Belanger, S.E.; Braunbeck, T. Is the fish embryo toxicity test (FET) with the zebrafish (*Danio rerio*) a potential alternative for the fish acute toxicity test? *Comp. Biochem. Physiol. Part. C* **2009**, *149*, 196–209. [CrossRef] [PubMed]
33. Grundner, C.; Perrin, D.; Van Huijsduijnen, R.H.; Swinnen, D.; Gonzalez, J.; Gee, C.L.; Wells, T.N.; Alber, T. Structural basis for selective inhibition of *Mycobacterium tuberculosis* protein tyrosine phosphatase PtpB. *Structure* **2007**, *15*, 499–509. [CrossRef] [PubMed]

34. Mascarello, A.; Mori, M.; Chiaradia-Delatorre, L.D.; Menegatti, A.C.L.; Monache, F.D.; Ferrari, F.; Yunes, R.A.; Nunes, R.J.; Terenzi, H.; Botta, B.; et al. Discovery of *Mycobacterium tuberculosis* protein tyrosine phosphatase B (PtpB) inhibitors from natural products. *PLoS ONE* **2013**, *8*, e77081. [CrossRef] [PubMed]
35. Kuban-Jankowska, A.; Kostrzewa, T.; Gorska-Ponikowska, M. Bacterial protein tyrosine phosphatases as possible targets for antimicrobial therapies in response to antibiotic resistance. *Antioxidants* **2022**, *11*, 2397. [CrossRef]
36. Wong, D.; Chao, J.D.; Av-Gay, Y. *Mycobacterium tuberculosis*-secreted phosphatases: From pathogenesis to targets for TB drug development. *Trends Microbiol.* **2013**, *21*, 100–109. [CrossRef]
37. Chai, Q.; Yu, S.; Zhong, Y.; Lu, Z.; Qiu, C.; Yu, Y.; Zhang, X.; Zhang, Y.; Lei, Z.; Qiang, L.; et al. A bacterial phospholipid phosphatase inhibits host pyroptosis by hijacking ubiquitin. *Science* **2022**, *378*, eabq0132. [CrossRef]
38. Morrell, T.E.; Rafalska-Metcalf, I.U.; Yang, H.; Chu, J. Compound molecular logic in accessing the active site of *Mycobacterium tuberculosis* protein tyrosine phosphatase B. *J. Am. Chem. Soc.* **2018**, *140*, 14747–14752. [CrossRef]
39. Zhou, B.; He, Y.; Zhang, X.; Xu, J.; Luo, Y.; Wang, Y.; Franzblau, S.G.; Yang, Z.; Chan, R.J.; Liu, Y.; et al. Targeting *Mycobacterium* protein tyrosine phosphatase B for antituberculosis agents. *Proc. Natl. Acad. Sci. USA* **2010**, *107*, 4573–4578. [CrossRef]
40. Boni, F.G.; Hamdi, I.; Koundi, L.M.; Shrestha, K.; Xie, J. Cytokine storm in tuberculosis and IL-6 involvement. *Infect. Genet. Evol.* **2022**, *97*, 105166. [CrossRef]
41. Washburn, A.; Abdeen, S.; Ovechkina, Y.; Ray, A.M.; Stevens, M.; Chitre, S.; Sivinski, J.; Park, Y.; Johnson, J.; Hoang, Q.Q.; et al. Dual-targeting GroEL/ES chaperonin and protein tyrosine phosphatase B (PtpB) inhibitors: A polypharmacology strategy for treating *Mycobacterium tuberculosis* infections. *Bioorganic Med. Chem. Lett.* **2019**, *29*, 1665–1672. [CrossRef]
42. Clay, H.; Volkman, H.E.; Ramakrishnan, L. Tumor necrosis factor signaling mediates resistance to mycobacteria by inhibiting bacterial growth and macrophage death. *Immunity* **2008**, *29*, 283–294. [CrossRef] [PubMed]
43. Holt, A.; Mitra, S.; van der Sar, A.M.; Alnabulsi, A.; Secombes, C.J.; Bird, S. Discovery of zebrafish (*Danio rerio*) interleukin-23 alpha (IL-23α) chain, a subunit important for the formation of IL-23, a cytokine involved in the development of Th17 cells and inflammation. *Mol. Immunol.* **2011**, *48*, 981–991. [CrossRef] [PubMed]
44. Vemula, M.H.; Medisetti, R.; Ganji, R.; Jakkala, K.; Sankati, S.; Chatti, K.; Banerjee, S. *Mycobacterium tuberculosis* Zinc Metalloprotease-1 Assists Mycobacterial Dissemination in Zebrafish. *Front. Microbiol.* **2016**, *29*, 1347. [CrossRef] [PubMed]
45. Roca, F.J.; Whitworth, L.J.; Redmond, S.; Jones, A.A.; Ramakrishnan, L. TNF Induces Pathogenic Programmed Macrophage Necrosis in Tuberculosis through a Mitochondrial-Lysosomal-Endoplasmic Reticulum Circuit. *Cell* **2019**, *178*, 1344–1361.e11. [CrossRef] [PubMed]
46. Harjula, S.E.; Ojanen, M.J.T.; Taavitsainen, S.; Nykter, M.; Rämet, M. Interleukin 10 mutant zebrafish have an enhanced interferon-gamma response and improved survival against a *Mycobacterium marinum* infection. *Sci. Rep.* **2018**, *8*, 10360. [CrossRef]
47. Meijer, A.H. Protection and pathology in TB: Learning from the zebrafish model. *Semin. Immunopathol.* **2016**, *38*, 261–273. [CrossRef]
48. Torraca, V.; Cui, C.; Boland, R.; Bebelman, J.P.; Van der Sar, A.M.; Smit, M.J.; Siderius, M.; Spaink, H.P.; Meijer, A.H. The CXCR3-CXCL11 signaling axis mediates macrophage recruitment and dissemination of mycobacterial infection. *Dis. Mod. Mech.* **2015**, *8*, 253–269. [CrossRef]
49. Varela, M.; Meijer, A.H. A fresh look at mycobacterial pathogenicity with the zebrafish host model. *Mol. Microbiol.* **2022**, *117*, 661–669. [CrossRef]
50. Aubry, A.; Jarlier, V.; Escolano, S.; Truffot-Pernot, C.; Cambau, E. Antibiotic susceptibility pattern of Mycobacterium marinum. *Antimicrob. Agents Chemother.* **2000**, *44*, 3133–3136. [CrossRef]
51. Gomez-Flores, R.; Gupta, S.; Tamez-Guerra, R.; Mehta, R.T. Determination of MICs for *Mycobacterium avium-M. Intracellular* complex in liquid medium by a colorimetric method. *J. Clin. Microbiol.* **1995**, *33*, 1842–1846. [CrossRef]
52. Manganelli, R.; Voskuil, M.I.; Schoolnik, G.K.; Smith, I. The Mycobacterium tuberculosis ECF sigma factor sE: Role in global gene expression and survival in macrophages. *Mol. Microbiol.* **2001**, *41*, 423–437. [CrossRef] [PubMed]
53. Boldrin, F.; Anso, I.; Alebouyeh, S.; Sevilla, I.A.; Geijo, M.; Garrido, J.M.; Marina, A.; Cioetto Mazzabò, L.; Segafreddo, G.; Guerin, M.E.; et al. The Phosphatidyl-myo-Inositol Dimannoside Acyltransferase PatA Is Essential for *Mycobacterium tuberculosis* Growth In Vitro and In Vivo. *J. Bacteriol.* **2021**, *203*, e00439-e20. [CrossRef] [PubMed]
54. Westerfield, M. *The Zebrafish Book: A Guide for the Laboratory Use of Zebrafish (Danio Rerio)*, 4th ed.; University Oregon Press: Eugene, OR, USA, 2000.
55. OECD. Test No. 236: Fish Embryo Acute Toxicity (FET) Test. In *OECD Guidelines for the Testing of Chemicals, Section 2*; OECD iLibrary: Ithaca, NY, USA, 2013; pp. 1–22.
56. Livak, K.J.; Schmittgen, T.D. Analysis of relative gene expression data using real-time quantitative PCR and the 2 (-Delta Delta C(T)) Method. *Methods* **2001**, *25*, 402–408. [CrossRef] [PubMed]
57. Mervin, L.H.; Afzal, A.M.; Drakakis, G.; Lewis, R.; Engkvist, O.; Bender, A. Target prediction utilizing negative bioactivity data covering large chemical space. *J. Cheminformatics* **2015**, *7*, 51. [CrossRef]
58. Mervin, L.H.; Bulusu, K.C.; Kalash, L.; Afzal, A.M.; Svensson, F.; Firth, M.A.; Barrett, I.; Engkvist, O.; Bender, A. Orthologue chemical space and its influence on target prediction. *Bioinformatics* **2018**, *34*, 72–79. [CrossRef]

59. Todd, J.D.; Jens, E.N.; McCammon, J.A.; Baker, N.A. PDB2PQR: An automated pipeline for the setup of Poisson–Boltzmann electrostatics calculations. *Nucleic Acids Res.* **2004**, *32*, W665–W667.
60. Hehre, W.J. *A Guide to Molecular Mechanics and Quantum Chemical Calculations*; Wavefunction, Inc.: Irvine, CA, USA, 2003.

pharmaceuticals

MDPI

Article

Microparticles Loaded with *Bursera microphylla* A. Gray Fruit Extract with Anti-Inflammatory and Antimicrobial Activity

Víctor Alonso Reyna-Urrutia [1], Ramón Enrique Robles-Zepeda [2], Miriam Estevez [3], Marlen Alexis Gonzalez-Reyna [3], Grecia Vianney Alonso-Martínez [1], Juan Ramón Cáñez-Orozco [2], Julio César López-Romero [1,*] and Heriberto Torres-Moreno [1,*]

1 Department of Chemical Biological and Agricultural Sciences, University of Sonora, Avenida University and Irigoyen, Caborca 83600, Sonora, Mexico; alonso.reyna@unison.mx (V.A.R.-U.); a220219607@unison.mx (G.V.A.-M.)

2 Department of Chemical Biological Sciences, University of Sonora, Blvd. Luis Encinas y Rosales, Hermosillo 83000, Sonora, Mexico; robles.zepeda@unison.mx (R.E.R.-Z.); a210218361@unison.mx (J.R.C.-O.)

3 Center for Applied Physics and Advacend Technologya, National Autonomous University of Mexico, Juriquilla Campus, Juriquilla 76230, Queretaro, Mexico; miries@fata.unam.mx (M.E.); marlenreyna@gmail.com (M.A.G.-R.)

* Correspondence: julio.lopez@unison.mx (J.C.L.-R.); heriberto.torres@unison.mx (H.T.-M.); Tel.: +52-668-119-3447 (J.C.L.-R.); +52-662-307-6838 (H.T.-M.)

Abstract: Background: *Bursera microphylla* (B) A. Gray, a plant native to northwest Mexico, has long been utilized in traditional medicine for its anti-inflammatory effects. Previous studies have highlighted the bioactivity of *B. microphylla* fruit extract. Chitosan (Cs), a biopolymer known for its favorable physicochemical properties, has proven effective in encapsulating bioactive compounds. This study aimed to synthesize and characterize Cs-based microparticles containing *B. microphylla* fruit extract and evaluate their in vitro anti-inflammatory activity. **Methods:** Cs-based three-dimensional hydrogels were synthesized using physical cross-linking with ammonium hydroxide, incorporating *B. microphylla* fruit extract. The hydrogels were freeze-dried and mechanically ground into microparticles. The physicochemical properties of the microencapsulates were analyzed through scanning electron microscopy (SEM), optical microscopy (OM), Fourier transform infrared spectroscopy (FTIR), thermogravimetric analysis (TGA), and moisture absorption tests. Anti-inflammatory activity was assessed by measuring nitric oxide (NO) reduction in LPS-activated RAW 264.7 cells. Antimicrobial activity was evaluated against *Staphylococcus aureus*. **Results:** SEM and OM analyses revealed irregular morphologies with rounded protuberances, with particle sizes ranging from 135 to 180 µm. FTIR spectra indicated that no new chemical bonds were formed, preserving the integrity of the original compounds. TGA confirmed that the encapsulated extract was heat-protected. The moisture absorption test indicated the microparticles' hydrophilic nature. In vitro, the microencapsulated extract reduced NO production by 46%, compared to 32% for the non-encapsulated extract. The microencapsulated extract was effective in reducing the microbial load of *S. aureus* between 15–24%. **Conclusions:** Cs-based microencapsulates containing *B. microphylla* fruit extract exhibited no chemical interactions during synthesis and demonstrated significant anti-inflammatory and antimicrobial activity. These results suggest that the Cs-based system is a promising candidate for managing inflammatory conditions.

Keywords: *Bursera microphylla*; chitosan; microparticles; encapsulation and bioactivity

Citation: Reyna-Urrutia, V.A.; Robles-Zepeda, R.E.; Estevez, M.; Gonzalez-Reyna, M.A.; Alonso-Martínez, G.V.; Cáñez-Orozco, J.R.; López-Romero, J.C.; Torres-Moreno, H. Microparticles Loaded with *Bursera microphylla* A. Gray Fruit Extract with Anti-Inflammatory and Antimicrobial Activity. *Pharmaceuticals* **2024**, *17*, 1565. https://doi.org/10.3390/ph17121565

Academic Editor: Silviya Petrova Zustiak

Received: 1 November 2024
Revised: 15 November 2024
Accepted: 18 November 2024
Published: 21 November 2024

1. Introduction

The multiplication of inflammation-related diseases has considerably increased the rate of prescription of non-steroidal anti-inflammatory drugs (NSAIDs) and corticosteroids [1,2]. Due to their effectiveness in reducing pain and inflammation, NSAIDs and corticosteroids are among the most used treatments for these conditions. However, the prolonged and excessive use of these drugs is related to a wide range of side effects, with gastrointestinal and cardiovascular complications being the most common [3,4]. For this reason, it is necessary to develop more effective anti-inflammatory agents with a better safety profile [5,6].

On the other hand, bacterial infections have become a severe public health challenge worldwide [7]. In this way, it is estimated that bacterial infections generated by antibiotic-resistant strains will constitute the greatest cause of death in the world in 2050 [8]. The resistance phenomenon makes traditional antibiotic treatments ineffective, causing infectious processes that are more difficult to treat. *S. aureus* is one of the most important microorganisms in the clinical area because it is one of the most common pathogens isolated in infectious processes [9]. In turn, it is important to mention that the World Health Organization (WHO) considers this pathogen a high-priority microorganism due to its high resistance characteristics to antibiotics [10]. For this reason, it is necessary to find new pharmacological strategies that can effectively treat bacterial infections.

In this sense, pharmaceutical engineering has opted to develop encapsulating systems from synthetic or natural polymers such as chitosan (Cs). This biomaterial is a polysaccharide industrially obtained from the alkaline deacetylation of crustacean chitin (exoskeleton of shrimp and crab) [11]. Cs is a non-toxic biopolymer with many biomedical applications (hemostatic, antimicrobial, cytocompatibility, biocompatibility, etc.). The Food and Drug Administration (FDA) considers this biopolymer as GRAS (Generally Recognized as Safe) with commercial availability at a low cost [12,13]. The cationic nature of Cs in acidic conditions favors the development of materials with different geometries, such as nano/microparticles, emulsions, fibers, hydrogels, films, and membranes. Cs, in its various forms, has been widely used as a matrix for the encapsulation of extracts, essential oils, and bioactive compounds [13–15]. Ionic gelation is one of the most promising encapsulation techniques since no chemical agents are used as cross-linking agents, and the biocompatibility of the polymeric matrix is not affected [15,16]. By enhancing the availability of the amino group in the Cs molecule, which is responsible for its bioactive properties and serves as the functional group used during chemical cross-linking, it becomes possible to obtain materials with unexplored stability and bioactivity [17]. In this way, by using ammonium hydroxide, physical bonds are generated that prevent cross-linking with the functional group, leaving the amino group free to be utilized for its bioactive properties. The materials are then lyophilized for preservation. For this reason, chitosan can serve as an encapsulating vehicle for the active compounds of medicinal plants.

Bursera microphylla A. Gray (*Burseraceae*) commonly named "torote", "white torote", "copal" or "elephant tree", is a medicinal plant native to the desert region of northern Mexico and the southwestern United States, which covers the vast majority of the area geography of the Sonora Desert [18,19]. In traditional Mexican medicine, the Seri ethnic group makes use of the bark, fruits, and leaves of the plant to treat various disorders such as wound healing, sore throat, and headache. Currently, the preparation of tinctures based on *B. microphylla* has been reported as a remedy to control gum sores and teeth with abscesses. Stems and leaves of *B. microphylla* have also been used for the treatment of pain when urinating and as an anti-inflammatory [19,20].

In vitro studies demonstrate that *B. microphylla* fruit extracts inhibit the production of inflammatory mediators such as NO and TNF-α in RAW 264.7 cells activated with bacterial LPS [21,22]. However, no microsystem has been developed to encapsulate *B. microphylla* extract for therapeutic purposes. Due to the bioactive properties of *B. microphylla* extracts, the objective of this research was to synthesize and characterize a Cs-encapsulating polymeric system that maintains or enhances the properties of the extract. The function of these Cs microsystems is to potentiate the bioactivity of the extract by controlling its release, improving its bioavailability, and the absorption of bioactive compounds through the epithelial layers. This is reflected in the use of a smaller number of doses during therapy, which impacts the reduction in treatment costs. Furthermore, these microsystems reduce problems of physical or chemical instability of bioactive compounds by protecting them from unfavorable environmental conditions, reducing their volatilization and/or degradation [23]. The potential of these microparticles could be particularly relevant in treating chronic inflammatory conditions such as inflammatory bowel disease, which are areas of significant interest in pharmaceutical research.

2. Results and Discussion

2.1. Physicochemical Characterization of Microparticles

2.1.1. Microparticle Morphology

The morphological characteristics of the microparticles (Cs, CsB-0.5 and CsB-1.0) are shown in Figure 1. By OM and SEM, it was observed that these materials presented a heterogeneous morphology with irregularities.

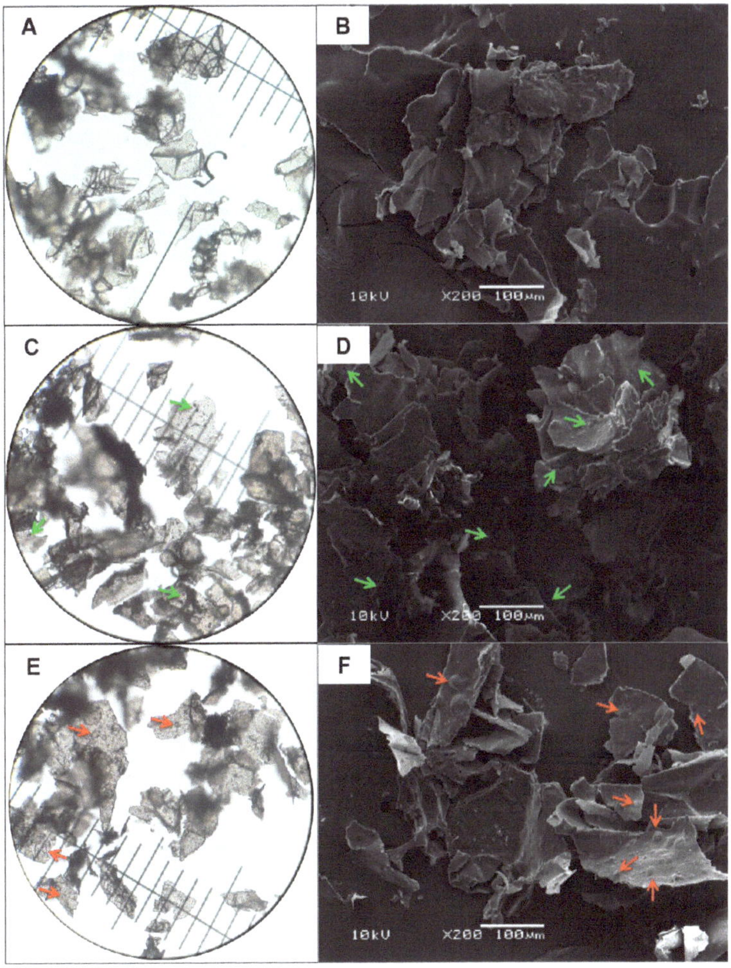

Figure 1. SEM micrographs (**right** column) at 200× and OM micrographs (**left** column) of microparticles. (**A**,**B**) Cs, (**C**,**D**) CsB-0.5 and (**E**,**F**) CsB-1.0. Cs: chitosan, CsB-0.5: chitosan-0.5% *Bursera microphylla* extract and CsB-1.0: chitosan-0.5% *Bursera microphylla* extract. Green and red arrows indicate *B. microphylla* extract present in the microparticles. (**A**,**C**,**E**; **left** column): 10 µm scale on the ruler.

In CsB-0.5 (Figure 1C,D) marked with green arrows, round bodies can be observed in the walls that make up the three-dimensional network of the encapsulating microsystem.

These findings were more evident in CsB-1.0 (Figure 1E,F), where larger rounded bodies were observed. In the microparticles loaded with 0.5% extract, it was possible to observe larger round bodies within the polymeric matrix; these changes were more evident in the 1.0% formulation (see red arrows). These findings suggest the presence of the extract in the walls that make up the three-dimensional network of the encapsulating microsystem (see red arrows). These findings indicate that the formation of round bodies could be associated with the incorporation of the extract into the encapsulating matrix.

2.1.2. Microparticle Size Distribution and Specific Surface Area

Analysis of the size of the Cs microparticles showed a bimodal distribution, where the most abundant particle size frequencies were 135 μm and 270 μm (Figure 2). In contrast, microparticles loaded with *B. microphylla* fruit extract showed a single particle size distribution. CsB-0.5 microparticles presented a skewed distribution to the right with a predominant particle size frequency of 135 μm and 180 μm. Meanwhile, CsB-1.0 shows a slightly unimodal distribution skewed to the right, with a higher frequency of 180 microns. Although the microparticles presented non-uniform distributions, in all cases the most predominant distribution frequencies exceeded 50%.

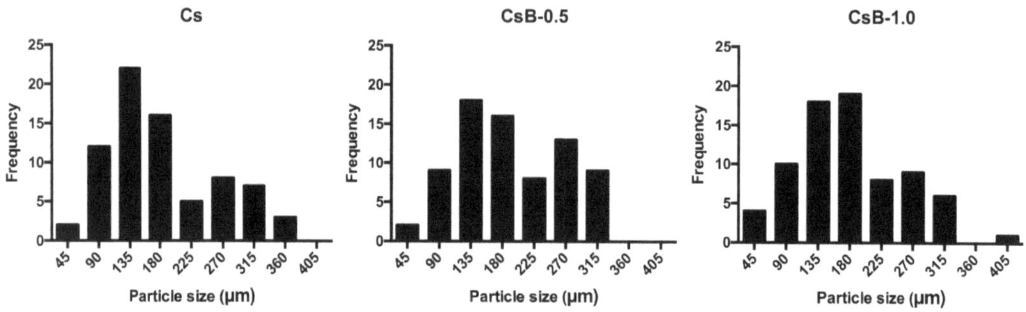

Figure 2. Particle size distribution of the microencapsulation of Cs, CsB-0.5 and CsB-1.0 of *B. microphylla*. Cs: chitosan microparticles; B: *B. microphylla* extract; CsB-0.5: chitosan microparticles loaded with 0.5% of *B. microphylla* extract; and CsB-1.0: chitosan microparticles loaded with 1.0% of *B. microphylla* extract.

The specific surface area (SSA) of the encapsulating systems is shown in Table 1. The SSA value was 110.5% higher for CsB-0.5 concerning Cs. Similarly, the SSA of CsB-0.5 was 45% higher compared to CsB-1. The higher SSA of CsB-0.5 could be related to the formation of small protuberances on the walls of the microparticles. On the other hand, the increase in the concentration of extract in CsB-1 produces larger protuberances, which causes the SSA to reduce. These treatments show behaviors with promising values that will benefit the bioactivity, contact area, and bioavailability of the extract incorporated into the designed microparticles. However, the SSA values of the microparticles with the *B. microphylla* extract are higher than those reported for other microencapsulations in which the major component is Cs as an encapsulating matrix or transport vehicle of a principle/drug. These values could indicate the bioavailability of our encapsulating systems, which acquire a high free contact area that may be required when coming into contact with physiological fluids, and the extract found in the three-dimensional structure of the particulate materials can be released to present adequate bioactivity [24–27]. Moreover, enhancing the bioavailability through controlled release mechanisms is crucial in developing more efficient drug delivery systems, potentially reducing dosage frequency and improving patient ease of treatment.

Table 1. Specific surface area (SSA) of encapsulating materials with chitosan as polymer matrix.

Composition	SSA (m^2/g)	Reference
Cs	05.753	This work
CsB-0.5	12.111	This work
CsB-1.0	03.220	This work
Cs-ethylene glycol diglycidyl ether	00.620	[28]
Cs-sodium lauryl sulphate	00.670	[29]
Cs	01.200	[30]
Carboxymethyl-Cs	00.490	[31]
Tin (IV)-Cs	0.3020	[32]
Polyvinyl alcohol-Cs	01.948	[33]
Polyethylene glycol-Cs	02.679	[33]
Aliquant 336-Cs	02.430	[34]

Cs: chitosan; B: *B. microphylla* extract.

2.1.3. Structure for the Fourier Transform Infrared Spectroscopy (FTIR)

Figure 3 presents the FTIR spectra of the microencapsulation. All spectra were similar, showing the characteristic absorption bands of Cs. In the wavenumber range of 3500 to 3300 cm^{-1}, a relatively broad and intense band was observed, corresponding to the stretching vibrations of the O-H and N-H bonds. Peaks were also detected at 2923 and 2880 cm^{-1}, associated with methylene groups, band at 1653 cm^{-1}, which is associated with the C=O stretch of amide I and, at 1580 cm^{-1}, related to the deformation of amide II [35–37] and, finally, in the range of 1200 to 500 cm^{-1}, characteristic signals of the saccharide structure [38].

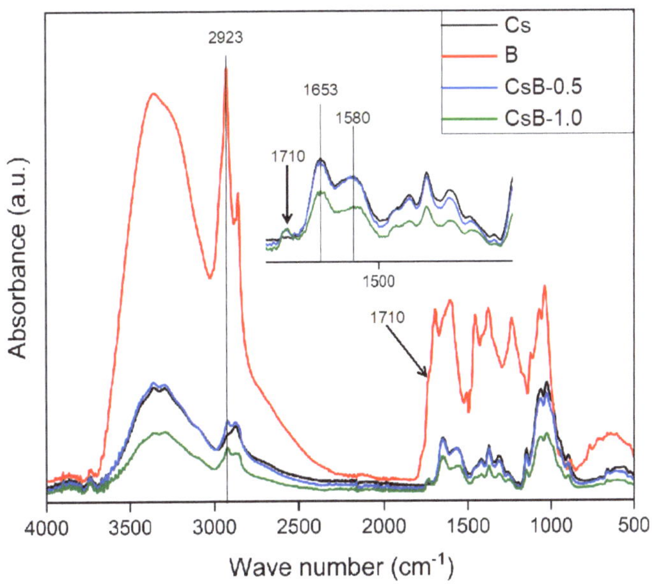

Figure 3. FTIR spectra of microencapsulation. Cs: chitosan microparticles; B: *B. microphylla* extract; CsB-0.5: chitosan microparticles loaded with 0.5% of *B. microphylla* extract; and CsB-1.0: chitosan microparticles loaded with 1.0% of *B. microphylla* extract.

The microparticles loaded with *B. microphylla* extract (CsB-0.5 and CsB-1.0) showed a signal at 1710 cm^{-1} corresponding to the stretching vibration of C=O, characteristic of the aldehydes and ketones groups. Another signal with greater intensity that could be associated with the presence of the extract components in the microparticles was observed at 2923 cm^{-1} [39]. Comparative analysis of the rest of the FTIR signals shows that the extract-loaded microparticles and the unloaded microparticles present similar signal patterns, indicating that there is no presence of new functional groups in the loaded materials. The above confirms the absence of chemical interactions between Cs and the *B. microphylla* extract, suggesting that the components of the extract do not change in their chemical structure during the microparticle synthesis process, so the activity of the extract is not affected. When there is an interaction between the extract and chitosan, they make use of the free amino group of the chitosan polymer chains and this will stimulate a slow release caused by a degradation mechanism. On the other hand, if there is no interaction with the extract in which the encapsulation mechanism is entrapped in the chitosan polymer chains, a pH-triggered release is encouraged, dependent on the protonation/deprotonation of the chitosan amine groups after diffusion of the extract from the microparticle matrix [40].

2.1.4. Thermogravimetric Analysis (TGA)

The thermogravimetric analysis (Figure 4) compares the thermal stability of the microparticles with *B. microphylla* fruit extract. The extract showed a mass loss of ≈60% between 50–100 °C, with a maximum peak observed at 78 °C (see red arrow). On the other hand, for microparticles (Cs, CsB-0.5, and CsB-1.0), a mass loss of ≈6% was observed at ≈100 °C due to the loss of water molecules. The second mass loss for the microparticles occurred at 303 °C (see blue arrow), as a result of the degradation of the saccharides of the Cs molecule [41–43]. Similar behavior was observed in the microparticle loaded with *B. microphylla* extract (CsB-0.5% and CsB-1.0%), where the Cs matrix conferred thermal stability to the extract encapsulated in the walls of the polymeric matrix, helping to protect the extract from decomposition or degradation at high temperatures.

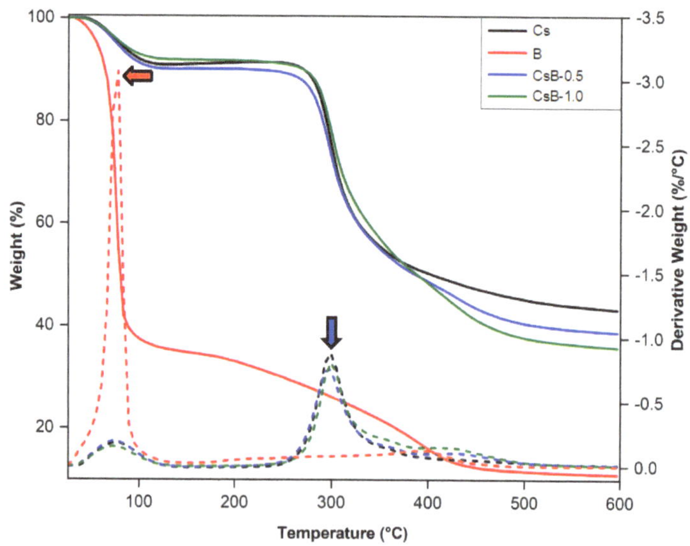

Figure 4. Thermogravimetric analysis of the synthesized microparticles. Cs: chitosan microparticles; B: *B. microphylla* extract; CsB-0.5: chitosan microparticles loaded with 0.5% of *B. microphylla* extract; and CsB-1.0: chitosan microparticles loaded with 1.0% of *B. microphylla* extract. Red arrow: Maximum loss of *B. microphylla* extract; Blue arrow: Maximum loss of Cs end Cs with *B. microphylla* extract. Dashed lines represent the derivative of the mass loss of the treatments.

2.1.5. Moisture Absorption

Moisture absorption analysis showed microparticles (Cs, CsB-0.5, and CsB-1.0) presented maximum moisture absorption of 20–22% at 40 ± 1% R.H. On the other hand, the maximum moisture absorption for all microparticles was found between 37–40% at

80 ± 1% R.H. (Figure 5). The behaviors were with values similar to those reported in the literature where Cs is the majority polymeric matrix of the material, achieving an equilibrium moisture absorption of 41% at high R.H. values [44]. These results demonstrate that microparticles have a hydrophilic character when exposed to high relative humidity. This property of the materials can be beneficial in terms of exposure to physiological fluids since when in contact with these systems, it causes a release of the extracts encapsulated in the polymeric matrix. It should also be mentioned that the hydrophilic character of the Cs matrix is conferred to the free amino group of the Chitosan polymeric chain, confirming the null chemical interaction between *B. microphylla* extracts and the Cs structural chain [45].

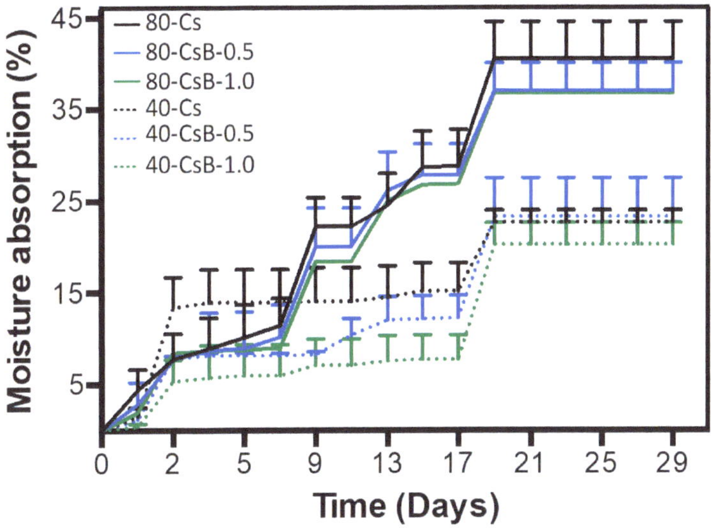

Figure 5. Moisture absorption of microparticles at a relative humidity of 40 ± 1% and 80 ± 1%. Values of n = 3 ± SD are shown. Cs: chitosan microparticles; B: *B. microphylla* extract; CsB-0.5: chitosan microparticles loaded with 0.5% of *B. microphylla* extract; and CsB-1.0: chitosan microparticles loaded with 1.0% of *B. microphylla* extract.

2.2. Bioactive Characterization of Microparticles

2.2.1. Cytotoxic Effect

Assessing the anti-inflammatory effect in cell models must be accompanied by determining the cytotoxic effect of the treatments, to guarantee that the effect is associated with the inhibition of the inflammation and not by the induction of cell death [46]. The results (Figure 6) showed that in general, microparticles did not show cytotoxic effects on RAW 264.7 cells. Except at (200 µg/mL) Cs, CsB-0.5 and CsB-1 reduced the cell viability by 87, 86 and 84%, respectively. These results are consistent with those reported by Torres-Moreno et al. (2022) for extracts of stems, fruits, and leaves of *B. microphylla*, where viability was at 90% in the different extract concentrations assessed in said research [21]. While the encapsulation of *B. microphylla* extract within chitosan microparticles shows promise, potential side effects such as immunogenicity or allergic reactions must be thoroughly evaluated in future studies to ensure patient safety. It should be mentioned that the cytotoxic effect of the investigation with the pure extract showed higher cytotoxic activity compared to the microencapsulation of the extract in the Cs matrix.

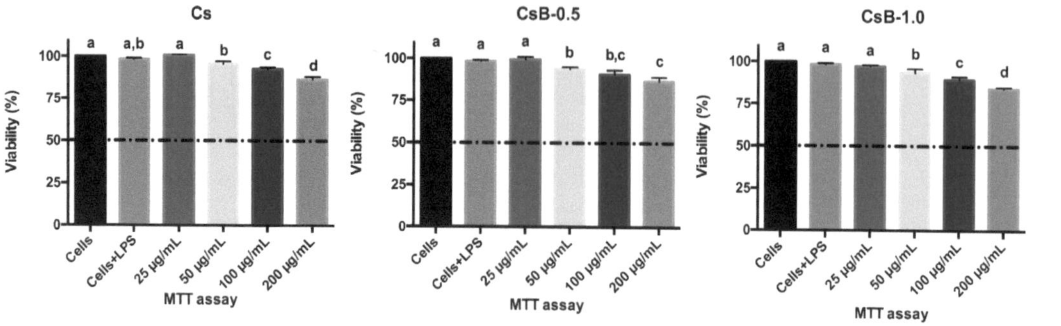

Figure 6. Cytotoxic effect of microparticles on RAW 264.7. Bars with different letters a–d indicate statistically significant differences ($p < 0.05$). All values represent the mean ± standard deviation of three independent experiments (±SD, $n = 3$). LPS = Lipopolysaccharide. Cs: chitosan microparticles; B: *B. microphylla* extract; CsB-0.5: chitosan microparticles loaded with 0.5% of *B. microphylla* extract; and CsB-1.0: chitosan microparticles loaded with 1.0% of *B. microphylla* extract.

2.2.2. Effect on the Nitric Oxide (NO) Production

Figure 7 shows the anti-inflammatory activity of the Cs encapsulating systems. The ability of these particulate materials to reduce NO production in RAW 264.7 macrophages activated with LPS was evaluated. The results show that stimulation of macrophages with LPS leads to a 3.2-fold increase in NO production compared to the basal level shown with untreated cells. In the cells treated with CsB-0.5 and CsB-1.0 (200 µg/mL), the NO levels were reduced by 39.4 and 46.0%, respectively. This effect was greater than that shown by the unloaded Cs microparticles, where at the maximum concentration tested (200 µg/mL), a reduction in NO production of 32% was observed. These effects are relatively lower compared to the observed for the extract because the microparticles contain 0.5% and 1% of the extract. Therefore, these findings suggest that the *B. microphylla* extract can be used more efficiently by incorporating it into the Cs matrix. [47]. This NO reduction effect is highly significant, as NO is a pro-inflammatory mediator involved in the development of various diseases of major concern to the healthcare sector, including diabetes, cardiovascular diseases, arthritis, allergies, and cancer, among others. This reduction could have broad functional applications in counteracting these conditions [48,49]. Similarly, it is relevant that it was possible to raise the IC_{50} of the *B. microphila* extract with values in its different seasonalities <200 µg/mL to values >200 µg/mL shown in the CsB-0.5% Ex encapsulant system [21]. The above is of great advantage since a smaller amount of encapsulated extract would be used in the microparticle to achieve the effectiveness of the extract. This increases the functionality of the extract combined with Cs to obtain microparticles loaded with the *B. microphylla* extract in a polymeric matrix with a synergistic behavior in its bioactivity.

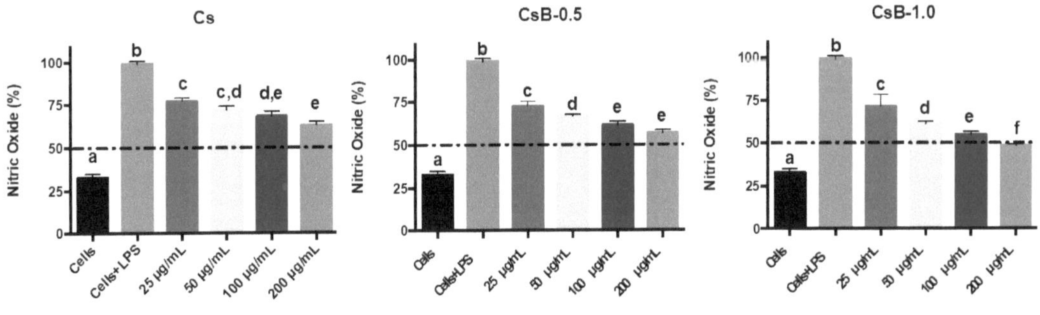

Figure 7. Effect of encapsulating systems of *B. microphylla* extracts of fruits on the production of NO in RAW 264.7-activated with LPS. Bars with different letters a–f indicate statistical differences ($p < 0.05$). All values represent the mean ± standard deviation of three independent experiments (±SD, $n = 3$). LPS = Lipopolysaccharide. Cs: chitosan microparticles; B: *B. microphylla* extract; CsB-0.5: chitosan microparticles loaded with 0.5% of *B. microphylla* extract; and CsB-1.0: chitosan microparticles loaded with 1.0% of *B. microphylla* extract.

2.2.3. Antimicrobial Evaluation

Results obtained in the antimicrobial evaluation of microparticles loaded with *B. microphylla* extract are presented in Figure 8. Results show that microparticles loaded with *B. microphylla* extract significantly reduce the microbial load in both treatments, with the CsB-1.0 treatment being the most effective, reducing 24% of the logarithmic count, followed by CsB-0.5 treatment, decreasing 15% of the logarithmic count. The results suggest that microparticles can release the extracts and their chemical compounds and interact with *S. aureus*, causing bacterial cell damage. The results presented in this study showed novel and original information because this is the first study that reports the antimicrobial activity of *B. microphylla*. Additionally, it is important to highlight that *S. aureus* is one of the most important Gram-positive bacteria in the health area because it is one of the main pathogens acquired and transmitted at clinical and community levels and also develops the ability to tolerate the effect of antimicrobial therapies [9]. The antimicrobial effect of *B. microphylla* can be associated with the presence of chemical compounds. Previous studies of our research group have demonstrated that *B. microphylla* fruit extract showed phenolic compounds such as flavonoids, phenolic acids, and lignans [21,22]. In this way, phenolic compounds have demonstrated a potent antimicrobial effect against *S. aureus*. The antimicrobial mode of action of phenolic compounds is related to their capacity to interact with bacterial enzymes and toxins, cell walls, and bacterial membranes, interfere with metabolic pathways, induce DNA fragmentation, and suppress virulence genes [50–52]. Based on the above, the results offered an important basis for future studies in which the concentration of *B. microphylla* extract in the microparticles can be increased to improve the antimicrobial effect. In addition, it seems feasible to carry out antimicrobial evaluations in other bacterial strains, such as antibiotic-resistant clinical isolates. The above is performed to use these polymeric matrices as possible alternatives for the development of pharmacological therapies.

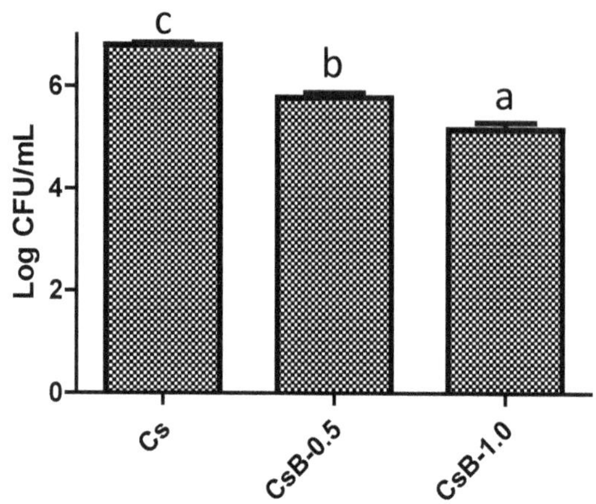

Figure 8. Antimicrobial activity of microparticles loaded with *B. microphylla* A. Gray fruit extract against *S. aureus*. Bars with different letters a–c indicate statistical differences ($p < 0.05$). All values represent the mean ± standard deviation of three independent experiments (±SD, $n = 3$). Cs: chitosan microparticles; B: *B. microphylla* extract; CsB-0.5: chitosan microparticles loaded with 0.5% of *B. microphylla* extract; and CsB-1.0: chitosan microparticles loaded with 1.0% of *B. microphylla* extract.

3. Materials and Methods

3.1. Materials

Chitosan (Cs) with catalog No. 448877 was used to prepare the microparticles. Ethyl alcohol (EA, 94.9–96%, No. 493538) was used to obtain the plant extract of *Bursera microphylla*. Ammonium hydroxide (AH, 28% NH_3 in H_2O, ≥99.99% trace metals basis, No. 338818) and glacial acetic acid (AA, ≥99.5% purity No. 33209) were used to make the hydrogels. Magnesium nitrate hexahydrate (MNH, 99%, No. 237175) and sodium sulfate decahydrate (SSD, 99%, No. 403008) were used to measure relative humidity absorption. Griess reagent (catalog No. G4410), MTT (catalog No. 88417), and isopropanol (catalog No. 563935) were used in the in vitro assays. All solvents and reagents were purchased from Sigma-Aldrich (Toluca, Mexico).

3.2. Plant Material and Extract Elaboration

Bursera microphylla specimens were collected in the State of Sonora of Mexico in the "Puerto Lobos" area (30.177211, −112.664644) of the municipality of Caborca during the spring (30 April 2023). The collected fruits were weighed and placed in a flask with ethanol (1:10 *w/v*) at 25 °C for 10 days with daily manual shaking. The extracts were filtered and evaporated in an IKA rotary evaporator model RV-10B-S99 of 125 rpm, heating to 50 °C. Once the ethanolic extracts were obtained, they were dried and stored at 4 °C until use.

3.3. Obtaining Microparticles

Different solutions were prepared for the synthesis of microencapsulation with/without *Bursera microphylla* extract: (1) Cs solution at 2% (*w/w*) was prepared, dissolving in 0.3 M glacial acetic acid at room temperature then stirred until completely dissolved [53]. (2) Cs solutions were prepared with 0.5–1.0% *B. microphylla* extract, CsB-0.5 (99.5/0.5) and CsB-1.0 (99/01), ratio (*w/w*), respectively. Where the extract was mixed in the Cs solution for 30 min [54].

Aliquots of the polymer suspensions were made in 10 mL beakers and placed inside a hermetically closed chamber, containing 100 mL of ammonium hydroxide. Physical cross-linking (gelation) was induced by ammonia diffusion for 24 h [55]. Subsequently, the hydrogels were washed with distilled water to eliminate ammonium acetate (CH_3COONH_4), and the rest of the ammonium hydroxide (NH_4OH) remained in the hydrogels until a pH of 7 was reached. Afterward, the hydrogels were placed in a refrigerator at a temperature of −26 °C for 24 h to later be introduced into a freeze dryer (SCIENTZ-10N LYOPHILIZER, Kansas City, MO, USA) for 24 h at 58 °C and pressure of 1 Pa [17]. Once the hydrogels were obtained, they were mechanically crushed for 5 min to obtain the microparticulate materials.

3.4. *Physicochemical Characterization of Microparticles*

3.4.1. Scanning Electron Microscope (SEM) and Optical Microscopy (OM)

The surface morphology and size of the microparticles were analyzed by scanning electron microscope (SEM) and optical microscopy (OM). For SEM, Hitachi SU8230 equipment at 10 kV was used. The samples were mounted on aluminum tape and coated with gold, using Desk II high vacuum model LLC equipment. For OM, a LABOMED Model CX, Lamp 12 V 20 W device from Labo America, Inc., Fullerton, CA, USA was used. An OEM model objective micrometer was used to measure the apparent length of the microparticles.

3.4.2. Specific Surface Area (SSA)

Surface specific area (SSA) is a property of solids defined as the total surface area of a material per unit of mass, this physical value is crucial in the characterization of pharmaceutical powders since it can provide information about their bioactive properties [56–58]. The analysis of SSA of the microparticles was carried out by nitrogen adsorption at 77 K to determine the specific surface area of the scaffolds, using Quentachome NOVA 2200e instruments Boynton Beach, FL, USA. The samples were previously degassed for 24 h, at 90 °C, to eliminate air and humidity present in the samples. The Brunauer–Emmett–Teller (BET) model was used to calculate the specific surface area of the materials obtained [59].

3.4.3. Fourier Transform Infrared Spectroscopy (FTIR)

Fourier Transform Infrared Spectroscopy (FTIR) is used to monitor encapsulation processes since it allows analyzing the possible chemical bonds established between the encapsulating polymer and the active ingredient [60–62]. The spectra of analysis of the microparticles were obtained using a Perkin Elmer Spectrum Two FTIR spectrometer Fremont, CA, USA. A spectrum was analyzed in the wavenumber range of 4000–650 cm^{-1} with a resolution of 4 cm^{-1} and a ratio of 100 scans.

3.4.4. Thermalgravimetric Analysis (TGA)

Thermogravimetric Analysis (TGA) helps to understand the thermal decomposition and the stability of formulations at high temperatures [63,64]. The thermogravimetric analysis of the microparticles was carried out in a Mettler Toledo TGA/DSC 2+ thermal analyzer (Greifensee, Switzerland), with a nitrogen atmosphere. Microparticles were measured between 25 and 600 °C with a heating ramp of 10°/min.

3.4.5. Moisture Absorption

The analysis of the effect of humidity on formulation prototypes helps to understand their behavior in demanding environmental conditions. Humidity absorption is a gravimetric method that monitors the change in the humidity content of a polymer over time [65]. Its behavior also tells us if the material is hydrophilic or hydrophobic [66]. To perform the analysis, the freeze-drying process microparticles were stored under two relative humidity percentages (RH): 40 ± 1% and 80 ± 1%, using magnesium nitrate hexahydrate (Mg $(NO_3)_2 \cdot 6H_2O$) and sodium sulfate decahydrate ($Na_2SO_4 \cdot 10H_2O$), respectively. The mass of each of the samples was taken at the beginning of the study until equilibrium was reached. The percentage of moisture absorption (M. A.) is given by Equation (1):

$$A(t) = \left(\frac{mt - m0}{m0}\right) \times 100 \quad (1)$$

where $m0$ is the mass of the sample at the beginning of the exposure to moisture and mt is the mass of the sample after a time t in days. The mean and standard deviation are obtained in triplicate for each microparticle.

3.5. *In Vitro Analysis of Microparticles*

3.5.1. Sample Sterilization

The samples were sterilized by exposure to UV radiation for 20 min using a laminar flow hood (Labconco®, Class II type A2, Kansas City, MO, USA).

3.5.2. Cell Culture

Macrophages transformed by Abelson leukemia virus (RAW 264.7) were provided by Dr. Emil A. Unanue from the Department of Pathology and Immunology, Washington University, St. Louis, MO. USA. The RAW 264.7 cell line (Abelson leukemia virus-induced murine macrophages) was cultured in DMEM (Dulbecco's modified Eagle's medium) supplemented with 5% heat-inactivated fetal bovine serum and penicillin (100 U/mL) in 25 cm^2 culture plates. Incubation was performed in an Isotherm incubator under the following conditions: 5% CO_2, 37 °C and 95% relative humidity (Thermo Fisher Scientific, Waltham, MA, USA).

3.5.3. Cytotoxic Effect

After RAW 264.7 cells reached 80% of confluence, they were detached by enzymatic digestion with 3 mL of trypsin and collected in DMEM. Subsequently, the cells were centrifuged (Beckman Coulter® Allegra X-15R with SX4750 rotor, Brea, CA, USA) for 7 min at 1700 rpm and 4 °C. The supernatant was discarded, and the cell pellet was re-suspended with DMEM. A RAW 264.7 cell suspension with 500,000 cells/mL (cell viability > 90%) was placed in a 96-well plate (Costar, Corning, NY, USA) and incubated for 24 h. Subsequently, the cells were treated with the microparticles 0–200 µg/mL and 1 µg/mL of LPS (lipopolysaccharide) for 24 h by the indirect method (the microparticles were placed in a pH 5 buffer for 4 h and then 100 µL of the supernatant was taken to treat the cells). Then, 5 mg/mL of MTT (3-(4,5-dimethylthiazol-2-yl)-2,5-diphenyltetrazolium bromide) was added to lead to incubation for 4 h. Finally, the formazan crystals were resuspended with isopropanol and read at an absorbance at 570–630 nm in a model iMARK BIO-RAD® (Gurgaon, India) microplate reader. Concentrations of the extracts tested where 90% or more cell viability was present are considered non-cytotoxic [67].

3.5.4. Quantification of Nitric Oxide (NO) Production

The level of NO production will be analyzed in the supernatant of LPS-activated RAW 264.7 cells using Griess reagent. The cell suspension (50,000 cells/mL) was seeded in a 96-well plate (Costar, Corning, NY, USA) and incubated for 24 h. Subsequently, the cells are stimulated or not with LPS (1 µg/mL) in the presence or absence of the microparticles. Subsequently, 100 µL of the supernatant is mixed with an equal volume of Griess reagent and the reaction is subsequently incubated for 10 min at room temperature. Finally, the absorbance is read at 540 nm in a microplate reader (iMARK BIO-RAD® microplate reader). A nitrite standard curve is used to determine NO levels. IC_{50} values (concentration required to inhibit 50% of NO production) are calculated using linear regression [67].

3.5.5. Antimicrobial Activity

Antimicrobial evaluation of microparticles loaded with *B. microphylla* A. Gray fruit extract was performed using the method described by CLSI. Overnight culture bacteria (37 °C) was adjusted at 0.5 McFarland (1×10^8 CFU/mL). Afterward, 0.1 mL of the bacterial suspension was mixed with 9.9 mL of Mueller Hinton broth reaching a concentration of 1×10^6 CFU/mL. Subsequently, microparticles loaded with *B. microphylla* extract were mixed with Mueller Hinton broth. A 1:1 proportion of bacterial inoculum and microparticles was combined and incubated for 24 h at 37 °C. Microparticles without *B. microphylla* extract was used as a control. After, 50 µL of each treatment was combined with saline solution (0.85% *w/v*) in a proportion 1:10, performing serial dilution. Each dilution (10 µL) was plated on plate count agar. The plates were incubated for 24 h at 37 °C. Finally, the results were reported as CFU/mL after the colony's enumeration.

3.6. Statistical Analysis

Data were expressed as mean ± standard deviation. Statistical analysis was performed via a one-way analysis of variance (ANOVA) followed by a Tukey's test in the GraphPad PRISM® version 6.0c program, Boston, MA, USA. A value of $p < 0.05$ was considered statistically significant.

4. Conclusions

In this research, it was possible to synthesize Cs microparticles loaded with *B. microphylla* fruit extract with anti-inflammatory and antimicrobial effects. The clinical implications of these findings suggest that chitosan-based microparticles could serve as a safer alternative to traditional NSAIDs, reducing the risk of gastrointestinal and cardiovascular side effects associated with prolonged use and could be an alternative for the treatment of infections caused by *S. aureus*.

More studies are needed to assess the anti-inflammatory effect in vivo models to continue profiling the CsB-0.5 end CsB-1.0 encapsulating system of *B. microphylla*, as a pharmaceutical candidate for the treatment and control of inflammation and infections caused by *S. aureus*.

Future Prospects

Future studies will focus on preclinical evaluations in animal models to further assess the efficacy and safety profile of these microparticles, paving the way for clinical trials.

The scalability of the production process for these chitosan-based microparticles is another critical consideration. Future work will focus on optimizing the synthesis process to ensure cost-effectiveness and reproducibility at an industrial scale.

While chitosan is a well-known biopolymer, exploring the combination with other natural polymers such as alginate or gelatin could further enhance the stability and bioactivity of the encapsulated compounds.

Author Contributions: Conceptualization, investigation, resources, and supervision, V.A.R.-U., J.C.L.-R. and H.T.-M.; investigation, methodology, and validation, V.A.R.-U., R.E.R.-Z., M.E., M.A.G.-R., G.V.A.-M., J.R.C.-O., J.C.L.-R. and H.T.-M.; data curation and validation, V.A.R.-U., R.E.R.-Z., J.C.L.-R. and H.T.-M.; writing of the original draft, V.A.R.-U.; writing, review, and editing, J.C.L.-R. and H.T.-M. All authors have read and agreed to the published version of the manuscript.

Funding: This research is funded by the CONAHCYT project CBF-2023-2024-3824.

Institutional Review Board Statement: Not applicable.

Informed Consent Statement: Not applicable.

Data Availability Statement: The raw data supporting the conclusions of this article will be made available by the authors on request.

Acknowledgments: Víctor Reyna-Urrutia thanks CONAHCYT for his postdoctoral fellowship. He also thanks the University of Sonora, Caborca Campus, for providing the facilities to carry out the research. We thank Rita Sulub-Sulub for her support of her in the TGA tests. The authors thank Daniella E. Pacheco Catalana and José Martín Baas López for the BET analysis measurements (CONAHCYT N° 254667, Consolidation of the Southeast Renewable Energy Laboratory, LENERSE).

Conflicts of Interest: The authors declare no conflicts of interest.

References

1. Kaur, B.; Singh, P. Inflammation: Biochemistry, Cellular Targets, Anti-Inflammatory Agents and Challenges with Special Emphasis on Cyclooxygenase-2. *Bioorg. Chem.* **2022**, *121*, 105663. [CrossRef]

2. Ishitsuka, Y.; Kondo, Y.; Kadowaki, D. Toxicological Property of Acetaminophen: The Dark Side of a Safe Antipyretic/Analgesic Drug? *Biol. Pharm. Bull.* **2020**, *43*, 195–206. [CrossRef]
3. Sohail, R.; Mathew, M.; Patel, K.K.; Reddy, S.A.; Haider, Z.; Naria, M.; Habib, A.; Abdin, Z.U.; Razzaq Chaudhry, W.; Akbar, A. Effects of Non-Steroidal Anti-Inflammatory Drugs (NSAIDs) and Gastroprotective NSAIDs on the Gastrointestinal Tract: A Narrative Review. *Cureus* **2023**, *14*, e37080. [CrossRef]
4. Ghosh, R.; Alajbegovic, A.; Gomes, A.V. NSAIDs and Cardiovascular Diseases: Role of Reactive Oxygen Species. *Oxid. Med. Cell. Longev.* **2015**, *2015*, 536962. [CrossRef]
5. Mohi-ud-din, R.; Chawla, A.; Sharma, P.; Mir, P.A.; Potoo, F.H.; Reiner, Ž.; Reiner, I.; Ateşşahin, D.A.; Sharifi-Rad, J.; Mir, R.H.; et al. Repurposing Approved Non-Oncology Drugs for Cancer Therapy: A Comprehensive Review of Mechanisms, Efficacy, and Clinical Prospects. *Eur. J. Med. Res.* **2023**, *28*, 345. [CrossRef]
6. Godman, B.; McCabe, H.; D Leong, T.; Mueller, D.; Martin, A.P.; Hoxha, I.; Mwita, J.C.; Rwegerera, G.M.; Massele, A.; Costa, J.; et al. Fixed Dose Drug Combinations—Are They Pharmacoeconomically Sound? Findings and Implications Especially for Lower- and Middle-Income Countries. *Expert Rev. Pharmacoecon. Outcomes Res.* **2020**, *20*, 1–26. [CrossRef]
7. Li, Y.; Xia, X.; Hou, W.; Lv, H.; Liu, J.; Li, X. How Effective Are Metal Nanotherapeutic Platforms Against Bacterial Infections? A Comprehensive Review of Literature. *Int. J. Nanomed.* **2023**, *18*, 1109–1128. [CrossRef] [PubMed]
8. Naghavi, M.; Vollset, S.E.; Ikuta, K.S.; Swetschinski, L.R.; Gray, A.P.; Wool, E.E.; Robles Aguilar, G.; Mestrovic, T.; Smith, G.; Han, C.; et al. Global Burden of Bacterial Antimicrobial Resistance 1990–2021: A Systematic Analysis with Forecasts to 2050. *Lancet* **2024**, *404*, 1199–1226. [CrossRef] [PubMed]
9. Tălăpan, D.; Sandu, A.-M.; Rafila, A. Antimicrobial Resistance of Staphylococcus Aureus Isolated between 2017 and 2022 from Infections at a Tertiary Care Hospital in Romania. *Antibiotics* **2023**, *12*, 974. [CrossRef] [PubMed]
10. Mancuso, G.; Midiri, A.; Gerace, E.; Biondo, C. Bacterial Antibiotic Resistance: The Most Critical Pathogens. *Pathogens* **2021**, *10*, 1310. [CrossRef] [PubMed]
11. Cocoletzi, H.H.; Almanza, E.Á.; Agustin, O.F.; Nava, E.L.V.; Cassellis, E.R. Obtaining and Characterizing Chitosan from Shrimp Exoskeletons. *Surfaces and Void* **2009**, *22*, 57–60. Available online: https://www.researchgate.net/publication/260992204_Obtencion_y_caracterizacion_de_quitosano_a_partir_de_exoesqueletos_de_camaron (accessed on 31 October 2024).
12. Huang, Y.; Onyeri, S.; Siewe, M.; Moshfeghian, A.; Madihally, S.V. In Vitro Characterization of Chitosan-Gelatin Scaffolds for Tissue Engineering. *Biomaterials* **2005**, *26*, 7616–7627. [CrossRef]
13. Kumar, A.; Kumar, A. *Chitosan as a Biomedical Material: Properties and Applications*; Nova Science Publishers: Hauppauge, NY, USA, 2017; pp. 139–154.
14. Kumar, S.; Ye, F.; Dobretsov, S.; Dutta, J. Chitosan Nanocomposite Coatings for Food, Paints, and Water Treatment Applications. *Appl. Sci.* **2019**, *9*, 2409. [CrossRef]
15. Detsi, A.; Kavetsou, E.; Kostopoulou, I.; Pitterou, I.; Pontillo, A.R.N.; Tzani, A.; Christodoulou, P.; Siliachli, A.; Zoumpoulakis, P. Nanosystems for the Encapsulation of Natural Products: The Case of Chitosan Biopolymer as a Matrix. *Pharmaceutics* **2020**, *12*, 669. [CrossRef] [PubMed]
16. Roy, S.G.; Shirsat, N.S.; Mishra, A.C.; Waghulde, S.O.; Kale, M.K. A Review on Chitosan Nanoparticles Applications in Drug Delivery. *J. Pharmacogn. Phytochem.* **2018**, *7*, 1–4. [CrossRef]
17. Reyna-Urrutia, V.A.; Mata-Haro, V.; Cauich-Rodriguez, J.V.; Herrera-Kao, W.A.; Cervantes-Uc, J.M. Effect of Two Crosslinking Methods on the Physicochemical and Biological Properties of the Collagen-Chitosan Scaffolds. *Eur. Polym. J.* **2019**, *117*, 424–433. [CrossRef]
18. Bianchi, E.; Caldwell, M.E.; Cole, J.R. Antitumor Agents from *Bursera microphylla* (*Burseraceae*) I. Isolation and Characterization of Deoxypodophyllotoxin. *J. Pharm. Sci.* **1968**, *57*, 696–697. [CrossRef]
19. Gigliarelli, G.; Zadra, C.; Cossignani, L.; Robles Zepeda, R.E.; Rascón-Valenzuela, L.A.; Velázquez-Contreras, C.A.; Marcotullio, M.C. Two New Lignans from the Resin of *Bursera microphylla* A. Gray and Their Cytotoxic Activity. *Nat. Prod. Res.* **2018**, *32*, 2646–2651. [CrossRef] [PubMed]
20. Adorisio, S.; Fierabracci, A.; Gigliarelli, G.; Muscari, I.; Cannarile, L.; Liberati, A.M.; Marcotullio, M.C.; Riccardi, C.; Curini, M.; Robles Zepeda, R.E.; et al. The Hexane Fraction of *Bursera microphylla* A Gray Induces p21-Mediated Antiproliferative and Proapoptotic Effects in Human Cancer–Derived Cell Lines. *Integr. Cancer Ther.* **2017**, *16*, 426–435. [CrossRef] [PubMed]
21. Torres-Moreno, H.; López-Romero, J.C.; Vidal-Gutiérrez, M.; Rodríguez-Martínez, K.L.; Robles-Zepeda, R.E.; Vilegas, W.; Velarde-Rodríguez, G.M. Seasonality Impact on the Anti-Inflammatory, Antiproliferative Potential and the Lignan Composition of *Bursera microphylla*. *Ind. Crops Prod.* **2022**, *184*, 115095. [CrossRef]
22. Vidal Gutiérrez, M.; Torres Moreno, H.; Velázquez Contreras, C.A.; Rascón Valenzuela, L.A.; Robles Zepeda, R.E. Actividad Antioxidante Y Antiproliferativa de Seis Plantas Medicinales Del Noroeste de México. *Biotecnia* **2020**, *22*, 40–45. [CrossRef]
23. Marisa Ribeiro, A.; Estevinho, B.N.; Rocha, F. Microencapsulation of Polyphenols—The Specific Case of the Microencapsulation of Sambucus Nigra L. Extracts—A Review. *Trends Food Sci. Technol.* **2020**, *105*, 454–467. [CrossRef]
24. Kravanja, G.; Primožič, M.; Knez, Ž.; Leitgeb, M. Chitosan-Based (Nano)Materials for Novel Biomedical Applications. *Molecules* **2019**, *24*, 1960. [CrossRef] [PubMed]
25. Tamilarasi, G.P.; Krishnan, M.; Sabarees, G.; Gouthaman, S.; Alagarsamy, V.; Solomon, V.R. Emerging Trends in Curcumin Embedded Electrospun Nanofibers for Impaired Diabetic Wound Healing. *Appl. Nano* **2022**, *3*, 202–232. [CrossRef]

26. Pateiro, M.; Gómez, B.; Munekata, P.E.S.; Barba, F.J.; Putnik, P.; Kovačević, D.B.; Lorenzo, J.M. Nanoencapsulation of Promising Bioactive Compounds to Improve Their Absorption, Stability, Functionality and the Appearance of the Final Food Products. *Molecules* **2021**, *26*, 1547. [CrossRef] [PubMed]
27. Min, J.B.; Kim, E.S.; Lee, J.-S.; Lee, H.G. Preparation, Characterization, and Cellular Uptake of Resveratrol-Loaded Trimethyl Chitosan Nanoparticles. *Food Sci. Biotechnol.* **2017**, *27*, 441–450. [CrossRef]
28. Azlan, K.; Wan Saime, W.N.; Lai Ken, L. Chitosan and Chemically Modified Chitosan Beads for Acid Dyes Sorption. *J. Environ. Sci.* **2009**, *21*, 296–302. [CrossRef] [PubMed]
29. Piyamongkala, K.; Mekasut, L.; Pongstabodee, S. Cutting Fluid Effluent Removal by Adsorption on Chitosan and Sds-Modified Chitosan. *Macromol. Res.* **2008**, *16*, 492–502. [CrossRef]
30. Pivarčiová, L.; Rosskopfová, O.; Galamboš, M.; Rajec, P.; Hudec, P. Sorption of Pertechnetate Anions on Chitosan. *J. Radioanal. Nucl. Chem.* **2016**, *308*, 93–98. [CrossRef]
31. Luo, W.; Bai, Z.; Zhu, Y. Fast Removal of Co(II) from Aqueous Solution Using Porous Carboxymethyl Chitosan Beads and Its Adsorption Mechanism. *RSC Adv.* **2018**, *8*, 13370–13387. [CrossRef]
32. Shekhawat, A.; Kahu, S.; Saravanan, D.; Jugade, R. Tin(IV) Cross-Linked Chitosan for the Removal of As(III). *Carbohydr. Polym.* **2017**, *172*, 205–212. [CrossRef]
33. Rajeswari, A.; Amalraj, A.; Pius, A. Adsorption Studies for the Removal of Nitrate Using chitosan/PEG and chitosan/PVA Polymer Composites. *J. Water Process Eng.* **2016**, *9*, 123–134. [CrossRef]
34. Cui, H.; Chen, J.; Yang, H.; Wang, W.; Liu, Y.; Zou, D.; Liu, W.; Men, G. Preparation and Application of Aliquat 336 Functionalized Chitosan Adsorbent for the Removal of Pb(II). *Chem. Eng. J.* **2013**, *232*, 372–379. [CrossRef]
35. Santos-López, G.; Argüelles-Monal, W.; Carvajal-Millan, E.; López-Franco, Y.L.; Recillas-Mota, M.T.; Lizardi-Mendoza, J. Aerogels from Chitosan Solutions in Ionic Liquids. *Polymers* **2017**, *9*, 722. [CrossRef]
36. Malheiro, V.N.; Caridade, S.G.; Alves, N.M.; Mano, J.F. New Poly(ε-Caprolactone)/chitosan Blend Fibers for Tissue Engineering Applications. *Acta Biomater.* **2010**, *6*, 418–428. [CrossRef]
37. Thein-Han, W.W.; Kitiyanant, Y.; Misra, R.D.K. Chitosan as Scaffold Matrix for Tissue Engineering. *Mater. Sci. Technol.* **2013**, *24*, 1062–1075. [CrossRef]
38. Bolaina-Lorenzo, E.; Martinez-Ramos, C.; Monleón-Pradas, M.; Herrera-Kao, W.; Cauich-Rodriguez, J.V.; Cervantes-Uc, J.M. Electrospun Polycaprolactone/chitosan Scaffolds for Nerve Tissue Engineering: Physicochemical Characterization and Schwann Cell Biocompatibility. *Biomed. Mater.* **2017**, *12*, 015008. [CrossRef] [PubMed]
39. Ellerbrock, R.H.; Gerke, H.H. FTIR Spectral Band Shifts Explained by OM–cation Interactions. *J. Plant Nutr. Soil Sci.* **2021**, *184*, 388–397. [CrossRef]
40. Antunes, J.C.; Domingues, J.M.; Miranda, C.S.; Silva, A.F.G.; Homem, N.C.; Amorim, M.T.P.; Felgueiras, H.P. Bioactivity of Chitosan-Based Particles Loaded with Plant-Derived Extracts for Biomedical Applications: Emphasis on Antimicrobial Fiber-Based Systems. *Mar. Drugs* **2021**, *19*, 359. [CrossRef] [PubMed]
41. Reyna-Urrutia, V.A.; Estevez, M.; González-González, A.M.; Rosales-Ibáñez, R. 3D Scaffolds of Caprolactone/chitosan/polyvinyl Alcohol/hydroxyapatite Stabilized by Physical Bonds Seeded with Swine Dental Pulp Stem Cell for Bone Tissue Engineering. *J. Mater. Sci. Mater. Med.* **2022**, *33*, 81. [CrossRef] [PubMed]
42. Kaya, M.; Baran, T.; Mentes, A.; Asaroglu, M.; Sezen, G.; Tozak, K.O. Extraction and Characterization of A-Chitin and Chitosan from Six Different Aquatic Invertebrates. *Food Biophys.* **2014**, *9*, 145–157. [CrossRef]
43. Ferfera-Harrar, H.; Dairi, N. Green Nanocomposite Films Based on Cellulose Acetate and Biopolymer-Modified Nanoclays: Studies on Morphology and Properties. *Iran. Polym. J.* **2014**, *23*, 917–931. [CrossRef]
44. Reyna-Urrutia, V.A.; Rosales-Ibáñez, R.; González-González, A.M.; Estevez, M.; Rodríguez-Martínez, J.J.; González-Reyna, M. Biological Activity of a Chitosan-Carboxymethylcellulose-Zinc Oxide and Calcium Carbonate in 3D Scaffolds Stabilized by Physical Links for Bone Tissue Engineering. *J. Biomater. Appl.* **2023**, *37*, 1776–1788. [CrossRef] [PubMed]
45. Lee, D.W.; Lim, C.; Israelachvili, J.N.; Hwang, D.S. Strong Adhesion and Cohesion of Chitosan in Aqueous Solutions. *Langmuir* **2013**, *29*, 14222–14229. [CrossRef]
46. Araújo, L.C.C.; Aguiar, J.S.; Napoleão, T.H.; Mota, F.V.B.; Barros, A.L.S.; Moura, M.C.; Coriolano, M.C.; Coelho, L.C.B.B.; Silva, T.G.; Paiva, P.M.G. Evaluation of Cytotoxic and Anti-Inflammatory Activities of Extracts and Lectins from Moringa Oleifera Seeds. *PLoS ONE* **2013**, *8*, e81973. [CrossRef]
47. Vidal-Gutiérrez, M.; Robles-Zepeda, R.E.; Vilegas, W.; Gonzalez-Aguilar, G.A.; Torres-Moreno, H.; López-Romero, J.C. Phenolic Composition and Antioxidant Activity of *Bursera Microphylla* A. Gray. *Ind. Crops Prod.* **2020**, *152*, 112412. [CrossRef]
48. Kany, S.; Vollrath, J.T.; Relja, B. Cytokines in Inflammatory Disease. *Int. J. Mol. Sci.* **2019**, *20*, 6008. [CrossRef]
49. Pahwa, R.; Goyal, A.; Jialal, I. Chronic inflammation. In *StatPearls [Internet]*; LLCStatPearls Publishing: Treasure Island, FL, USA, 2023. [PubMed]
50. Miklasińska-Majdanik, M.; Kępa, M.; Wojtyczka, R.D.; Idzik, D.; Wąsik, T.J. Phenolic Compounds Diminish Antibiotic Resistance of Staphylococcus Aureus Clinical Strains. *Int. J. Environ. Res. Public Health* **2018**, *15*, 2321. [CrossRef] [PubMed]
51. Ecevit, K.; Barros, A.A.; Silva, J.M.; Reis, R.L. Preventing Microbial Infections with Natural Phenolic Compounds. *Futur. Pharmacol.* **2022**, *2*, 460–498. [CrossRef]
52. Chen, X.; Lan, W.; Xie, J. Natural Phenolic Compounds: Antimicrobial Properties, Antimicrobial Mechanisms, and Potential Utilization in the Preservation of Aquatic Products. *Food Chem.* **2024**, *440*, 138198. [CrossRef] [PubMed]

53. Cheng, J.; Zhu, H.; Huang, J.; Zhao, J.; Yan, B.; Ma, S.; Zhang, H.; Fan, D. The Physicochemical Properties of Chitosan Prepared by Microwave Heating. *Food Sci. Nutr.* **2020**, *8*, 1987–1994. [CrossRef] [PubMed]
54. Yuan, G.; Lv, H.; Yang, B.; Chen, X.; Sun, H. Physical Properties, Antioxidant and Antimicrobial Activity of Chitosan Films Containing Carvacrol and Pomegranate Peel Extract. *Molecules* **2015**, *20*, 11034–11045. [CrossRef] [PubMed]
55. Montembault, A.; Viton, C.; Domard, A.; Genevrier, L.; Goa, D.; Moulins, Z.I.L.T. Rheometric Study of the Gelation of Chitosan in Aqueous Solution without Cross-Linking Agent. *Biomacromolecules* **2005**, *6*, 653–662. [CrossRef] [PubMed]
56. Vecstaudža, J. *Amorphous Calcium Phosphate Biomaterials with High Specific Surface Area*; Riga Technical University: Latvia, Riga, 2021. [CrossRef]
57. Trzaskowska, M.; Vivcharenko, V.; Przekora, A. The Impact of Hydroxyapatite Sintering Temperature on Its Microstructural, Mechanical, and Biological Properties. *Int. J. Mol. Sci.* **2023**, *24*, 5083. [CrossRef]
58. Ghasemi-Mobarakeh, L.; Kolahreez, D.; Ramakrishna, S.; Williams, D. Key Terminology in Biomaterials and Biocompatibility. *Curr. Opin. Biomed. Eng.* **2019**, *10*, 45–50. [CrossRef]
59. Robitzer, M.; David, L.; Rochas, C.; Di Renzo, F.; Quignard, F. Supercritically-Dried Alginate Aerogels Retain the Fibrillar Structure of the Hydrogels. *Macromol. Symp.* **2008**, *273*, 80–84. [CrossRef]
60. Stefan, M.; Vlaicu, I.D.; Nistor, L.C.; Ghica, D.; Nistor, S.V. Origin and Chemical Composition of the Amorphous Material from the Intergrain Pores of Self-Assembled Cubic ZnS:Mn Nanocrystals. *Appl. Surf. Sci.* **2017**, *426*, 342–350. [CrossRef]
61. Basiuk, V.A. Quantum Chemical Calculations of Infrared Spectra for the Identification of Unknown Compounds by GC/FTIR/MS in Exobiological Simulation Experiments. *Adv. Sp. Res.* **2001**, *27*, 255–260. [CrossRef]
62. Kowalczuk, D.; Pitucha, M. Application of FTIR Method for the Assessment of Immobilization of Active Substances in the Matrix of Biomedical Materials. *Materials* **2019**, *12*, 2972. [CrossRef]
63. Olatunji, O.O.; Akinlabi, S.A.; Mashinini, M.P.; Fatoba, S.O.; Ajayi, O.O. Thermo-Gravimetric Characterization of Biomass Properties: A Review. *IOP Conf. Ser. Mater. Sci. Eng.* **2018**, *423*, 12175. [CrossRef]
64. Liu, S.; Yu, D.; Chen, Y.; Shi, R.; Zhou, F.; Mu, T. High-Resolution Thermogravimetric Analysis Is Required for Evaluating the Thermal Stability of Deep Eutectic Solvents. *Ind. Eng. Chem. Res.* **2022**, *61*, 14347–14354. [CrossRef]
65. Krauklis, A.E.; Karl, C.W.; Rocha, I.B.C.M.; Burlakovs, J.; Ozola-Davidane, R.; Gagani, A.I.; Starkova, O. Modelling of Environmental Ageing of Polymers and Polymer Composites—Modular and Multiscale Methods. *Polymers* **2022**, *14*, 216. [CrossRef]
66. Lee, P.-C.; Kang, D.; Oh, J.T.; Seo, J.Y.; Shin, D.; Jung, J.-U.; Ko, Y.K.; Ha, J.U.; Kim, M.-G. Reducing Moisture Absorption in Polypropylene Nanocomposites for Automotive Headlamps Using Hydrophobicity-Modified Graphene/Montmorillonite. *Nanomaterials* **2023**, *13*, 1439. [CrossRef] [PubMed]
67. Torres-Moreno, H.; López-Romero, J.C.; Vázquez-Solorio, J.Y.; Velázquez-Contreras, C.A.; Garibay-Escobar, A.; Díaz-López, R.; Robles-Zepeda, R.E. Antioxidant, Anti-Inflammatory and Antiproliferative Properties of Ibervillea Sonorae. *S. Afr. J. Bot.* **2019**, *125*, 207–213. [CrossRef]

pharmaceuticals

Article

Prunella vulgaris Extract Ameliorates Testosterone-Induced Benign Prostatic Hyperplasia by Regulating Androgen Levels, Cell Proliferation, and Apoptosis

Poornima Kumbukgahadeniya [1], Eun-Bok Baek [1], Eun-Ju Hong [1], Jun-Yeop Song [1], Youn-Gil Kwak [2], Mi-Ran Jang [2], Hyo-Seong Ji [2] and Hyo-Jung Kwun [1,*]

1 Department of Veterinary Pathology, College of Veterinary Medicine, Chungnam National University, Daejeon 34134, Republic of Korea; poornima.lakshini93@gmail.com (P.K.); baekeunbok@hanmail.net (E.-B.B.); bioeun59@naver.com (E.-J.H.); qldqld0610@gmail.com (J.-Y.S.)

2 Huons Foodience Co., Ltd., 19, Insam Gwangjang ro, Geumsan eup, Geumsan gun 32724, Republic of Korea; kyg@huonsfoodience.com (Y.-G.K.); rose86mr@huonsfoodience.com (M.-R.J.); hsji@huonsfoodience.com (H.-S.J.)

* Correspondence: hyojung@cnu.ac.kr; Tel.: +82-42-821-7403

Abstract: Background/Objectives: Benign prostatic hyperplasia (BPH) is a prevalent urological condition affecting elderly men. *Prunella vulgaris* L. (PV), a perennial herbaceous plant native to Europe and Asia, has anti-inflammatory, antioxidant, and antimicrobial effects. In this study, we determined the effect of PV extract on the development of BPH. Methods: Rats were treated via a daily hypodermic injection of testosterone propionate (TP; 3 mg/kg) for 4 weeks. Groups of BPH rats were treated with or without PV (60 or 80 mg/kg) by oral gavage. Results: In BPH model rats, PV considerably reduced their relative prostate weight and serum concentrations of dihydrotestosterone (DHT) and testosterone. The TP-induced increases in epithelial thickness in the prostate, proliferating cell nuclear antigen (PCNA) expression, and cyclin D1 expression were remarkably reduced, whereas terminal deoxynucleotidyl transferase dUTP nick-end labeling (TUNEL)-positive cells and cleaved caspase-3 levels were increased, in PV-treated rats compared to BPH rats. The mRNA expression levels of growth factors, such as transforming growth factor-β (TGF-β), fibroblast growth factor (FGF), and insulin-like growth factor (IGF-2), were significantly reduced in PV-treated rats. Mechanistically, the TP-induced activation of c-Jun N-terminal kinase (JNK) was reduced by PV administration. Conclusions: These results designate that PV effectively ameliorates the development of testosterone-induced BPH through anti-androgenic, anti-proliferative, and pro-apoptotic activities, suggesting that it could be a potential therapeutic substance for BPH.

Keywords: benign prostatic hyperplasia; *Prunella vulgaris* L.; proliferation; apoptosis; growth factors

Citation: Kumbukgahadeniya, P.; Baek, E.-B.; Hong, E.-J.; Song, J.-Y.; Kwak, Y.-G.; Jang, M.-R.; Ji, H.-S.; Kwun, H.-J. *Prunella vulgaris* Extract Ameliorates Testosterone-Induced Benign Prostatic Hyperplasia by Regulating Androgen Levels, Cell Proliferation, and Apoptosis. *Pharmaceuticals* **2024**, *17*, 1516. https://doi.org/10.3390/ph17111516

Academic Editors: Elena Y. Enioutina, Kathleen M. Job and Catherine Sherwin

Received: 28 October 2024
Revised: 8 November 2024
Accepted: 9 November 2024
Published: 11 November 2024

1. Introduction

Benign prostatic hyperplasia (BPH) is a prevalent urological condition affecting elderly men, with an estimated prevalence of 8% at 40, 50% at 60, and 80% at 90 years of age [1]. BPH involves non-malignant, hyperplastic, and progressive histopathological changes in the prostate's transitional zone; this causes prostatic nodule formation, inflammation, fibrosis, and alterations in smooth muscle function, leading to urethral blockage and lower urinary tract symptoms (LUTS) [2,3]. The exact molecular mechanism underlying BPH remains uncertain, but the increased cell count may be due to impaired programmed cell death and epithelial and stromal cell proliferation [4]. The normal development and functions of the prostate depend on the reduction of testosterone to dihydrotestosterone (DHT), which interacts with androgen receptors (ARs) to promote protein synthesis and prostate cell proliferation [5–7]. As males age, testosterone levels decline; BPH patients, however, experience increased DHT secretion and a consequent enlargement of prostate volume [8,9]. Several studies have identified growth factors involved in BPH, including transforming growth factor beta (TGF-β) family members, fibroblast growth factor (FGF), and insulin-like growth factor type (IGF) [10,11]. These growth factors regulate the signaling among epithelial cells and stroma in the prostate gland to regulate cellular proliferation and apoptosis [12].

Treatment options for symptomatic BPH include lifestyle changes and/or medical, device-based, or surgical therapies [13–15]. The drugs utilized, which may be used alone or in combination, include 5-alpha-reductase antagonists (5-ARIs), alpha-adrenergic antagonists (α1-blockers), and phosphodiesterase-5 enzyme antagonists. The most used medications are 5-ARIs, α1-blockers, and cocktails of the two combined (tamsulosin and dutasteride) [16–18]. However, these medications have potential adverse effects such as a decreased libido, erectile dysfunction, gynecomastia, depression and anxiety, and an increased risk of high-grade prostate cancer, etc. [19]. Due to these side effects, the therapeutic application of plant extracts, called phytotherapy, has become an alternative approach for managing BPH [20]. Phyto therapeutic agents are common in Europe, and their use is increasing in Western populations [20].

Prunella vulgaris L. (PV) is a perennial herbaceous plant that is native to Europe and Asia and grows in temperate regions worldwide, including Korea [21]. PV has long been used as a therapeutic agent in conventional medicine, such as in treating thyroid dysfunction, pulmonary tuberculosis, mastitis, arterial hypertension, and infectious hepatitis [22,23]. PV can also be used in patients with goiter, dermatitis, and dermal allergy. It shows anti-allergic, antioxidant, antimicrobial, and anti-inflammatory activities [23,24]. While PV extract is generally considered safe, it is important to be aware of potential side effects such as gastrointestinal discomfort and allergic reactions [25]. PV's main components include phenolic acids, mono- and sesquiterpenoids, higher fatty acids, pentacyclic triterpenes, flavonoids, vitamins, polysaccharides, nitrogen-containing compounds, and tannins. The bioactive components of PV include caffeic acid, rosmarinic acids, oleanolic acid (OA), and ursolic acid (UA) [21,23,24]. Rosmarinic acid, a combination ester of lactic and caffeic acid, is an effective natural antioxidant against free radical pathologies, such as atherosclerosis, radiation sickness, and cancer [23,24]. It binds oxygen free radicals and inhibits UVA-modulated protein expression [24]. OA and UA are classified as pentacyclic triterpenoids and have been extensively studied in vitro and in vivo for their biological activities [26].

While there is no specific research directly linking PV extract to BPH treatment, its potential anti-inflammatory, antiproliferative, and antioxidant properties could be beneficial. These properties may help to reduce prostate inflammation and oxidative stress, which are often associated with BPH [27]. Previous studies highlighted that PV extract can induce cancer cell apoptosis, inhibit angiogenesis, and suppress tumor cell migration and invasion, and PV-containing herbal mixtures can remodel the tumor immune microenvironment by increasing anti-tumor immune cells and suppressing immune-suppressive cells [25,28]. This can enhance the effectiveness of cancer immunotherapy. Based on this literature, it can be concluded that PV is a potential candidate in treatments for BPH. Here, we utilized a testosterone-induced rat BPH model to determine the medicinal effects of PV against BPH and their fundamental molecular mechanism(s).

2. Results

2.1. HPLC Analysis of PV Extract

The triterpenoids in PV extract were identified using HPLC analysis. OA and UA were determined by comparing the retention times of peaks in the crude extract to those of known standards and were detected in significant amounts (2.03 ± 0.01 and 7.03 ± 0.03 mg/g of extract) (Figure 1). The results showed that OA and UA are major compounds of PV extract.

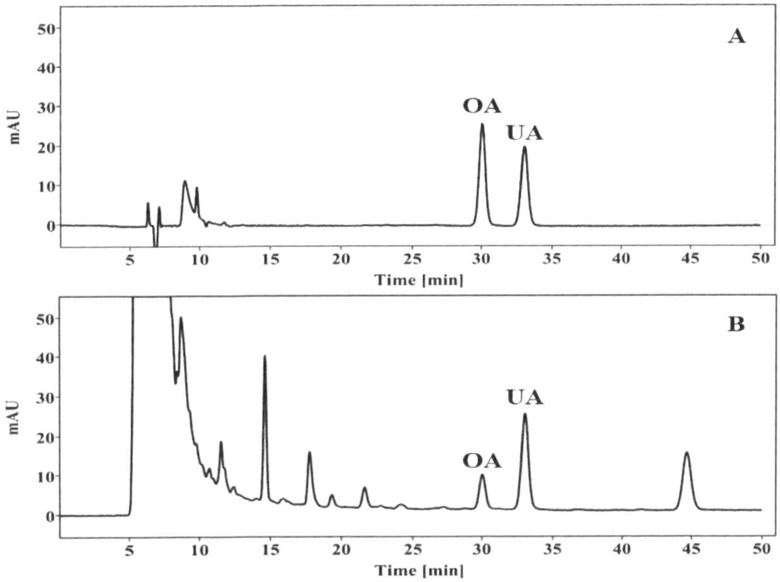

Figure 1. Chromatogram of triterpenoids in PV extract. (**A**) Standard and (**B**) PV extract detected at 210 nm.

2.2. *PV Extract Reduces Prostate Relative Weight in Rat BPH Model*

Prostate relative weights were increased in the BPH group (0.346 ± 0.075%) compared to the NC group (0.185 ± 0.031%). Compared to the BPH group, significantly lower prostate weights were seen in groups treated with finasteride (0.292 ± 0.059%), PV at 60 mg/kg (0.289 ± 0.064%), and PV at 80 mg/kg (0.287 ± 0.053%) (Table 1). The percent inhibition of prostate gland growth in the finasteride (BPH + FIN) and PV (BPH + PV60, BPH + PV80) groups were 66.49%, 35.87%, and 36.64%, respectively (Table 1). There was no statistically significant variation in the body mass of the rats across the different experimental groups.

Table 1. Effect of PV extract on prostatic relative weight and inhibition of growth percent.

Group	Treatment	Body Weight (g)	Relative Prostate Weight (%)	Inhibition of Growth (%)
NC	Corn oil + PBS	431.1 ± 19.3	0.185 ± 0.031	-
BPH	TP + PBS	393.2 ± 14.5	0.346 ± 0.075 ##	-
BPH + FIN	TP + finasteride	450.3 ± 24.6	0.292 ± 0.059 *	66.49
BPH + PV60	TP + PV 60 mg/kg	406.7 ± 22.2	0.289 ± 0.064 *	35.87
BPH + PV80	TP + PV80 mg/kg	454.1 ± 24.2	0.287 ± 0.053 *	36.64

NC, PBS- and corn oil-dispensed rats; BPH, PBS- and testosterone-dispensed rats; BPH + FIN, testosterone- and finasteride-dispensed rats; BPH + PV60, testosterone- and PV 60 mg/kg-dispensed rats; BPH + PV80, testosterone- and PV 80 mg/kg-dispensed rats. Representation of results as average ± SD. Comparison ## $p < 0.01$ with the NC group; comparison * $p < 0.05$ with the BPH group.

2.3. *PV Extract Downregulates the Serum Levels of DHT and Testosterone in a Rat BPH Model*

The BPH group exhibited significant increases in serum levels of DHT and testosterone in comparison to the NC cohort, and those levels were significantly lower in the finasteride- and PV-treated cohort than in the BPH cohort (Figure 2).

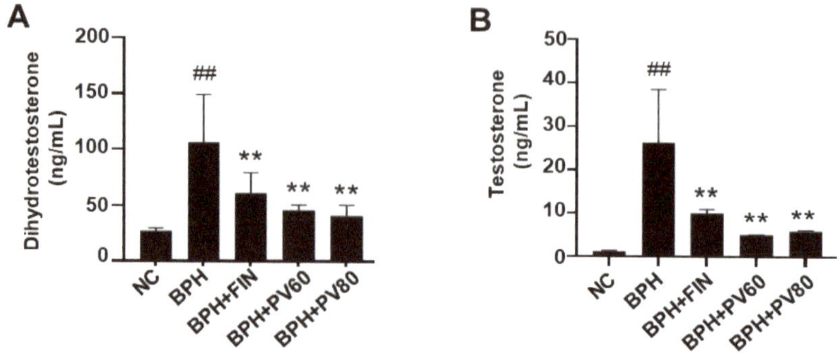

Figure 2. Effects of PV extract on serum levels of dihydrotestosterone and testosterone. (**A**) Serum level of dihydrotestosterone. (**B**) Serum level of testosterone. NC, PBS- and corn oil-dispensed rats; BPH, PBS- and testosterone-dispensed rats; BPH + FIN, testosterone- and finasteride-dispensed rats; BPH + PV60, testosterone- and PV 60 mg/kg-dispensed rats; BPH + PV80, testosterone- and PV 80 mg/kg-dispensed rats. Representation of results as average ± SD. Comparison ## $p < 0.01$ with the NC group; comparison ** $p < 0.01$ with the BPH group.

2.4. PV Extract Reduces the Epithelium Thickness of the Prostate Gland in a Rat BPH Model

The prostate glands of the NC group showed no histological change, whereas the BPH group exhibited increases in epithelial hyperplasia and glandular epithelial thickness (Figure 3). Treatment with finasteride and PV extract significantly reduced the thickness of the prostatic epithelium in comparison to that seen in the BPH group (Figure 3).

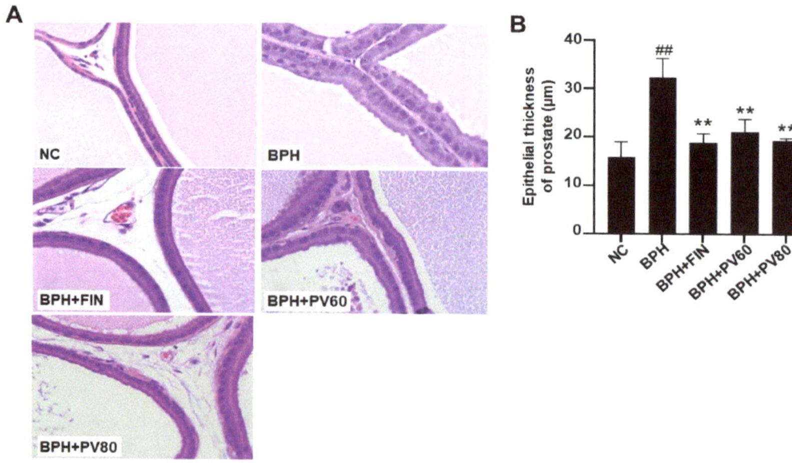

Figure 3. Effects of PV extract on the epithelium thickness of the prostate gland in a rat BPH model. (**A**) Representative images of hematoxylin and eosin (H&E)-stained prostate tissues (magnification, ×400). (**B**) The epithelial thickness of the prostate gland. NC, PBS- and corn oil-dispensed rats; BPH, PBS- and testosterone-dispensed rats; BPH + FIN, testosterone- and finasteride-dispensed rats; BPH + PV60, testosterone- and PV 60 mg/kg-dispensed rats; BPH + PV80, testosterone- and PV 80 mg/kg-dispensed rats. Representation of results as average ± SD. Comparison ## $p < 0.01$ with the NC group; comparison ** $p < 0.01$ with the BPH group.

2.5. PV Extract Suppresses the Proliferation of Prostate Cells in a Rat BPH Model

Immunohistochemical staining showed that the count of proliferating cell nuclear antigen (PCNA)-positive cells was significantly increased in the BPH cohort compared to the NC cohort (Figure 4A,B), whereas the numbers in the finasteride and PV cohorts were considerably less than that in the BPH group (Figure 4A,B). Western blot analysis showed that cyclin D1 expression was significantly upregulated in the BPH group compared to NC, but this change was alleviated in the groups of finasteride and PV (Figure 4C).

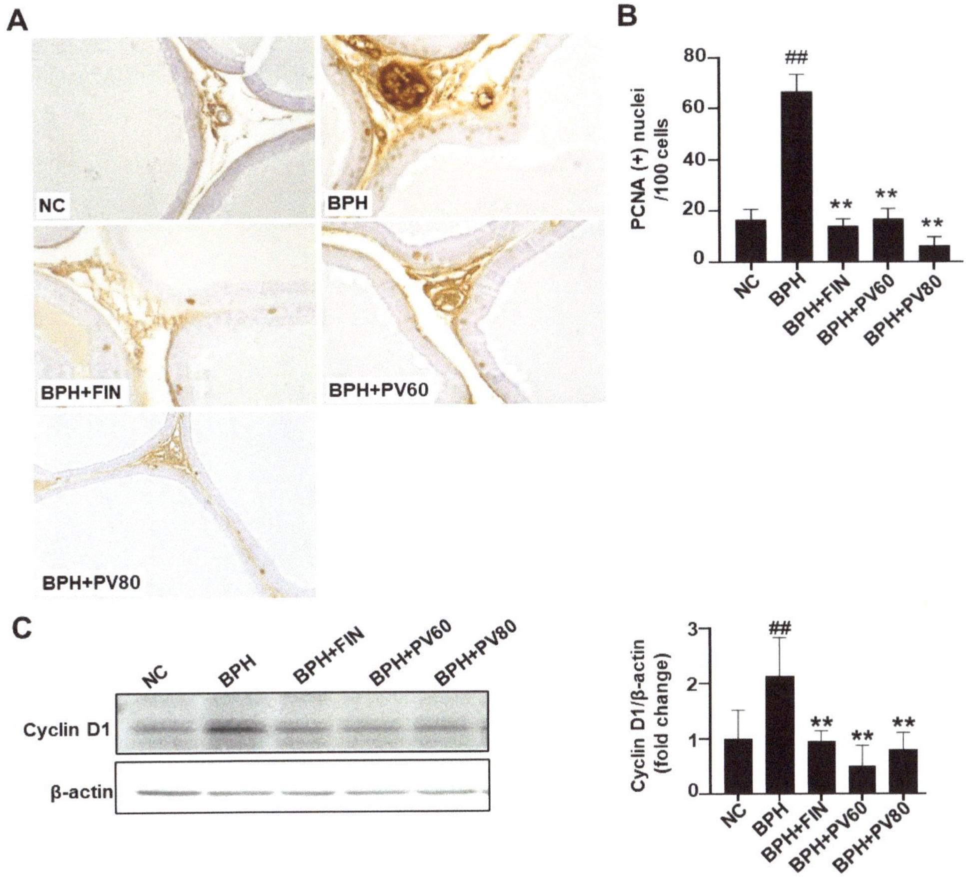

Figure 4. Effects of PV extract on prostate cell proliferation in a rat BPH model. (**A**) Respective images showing immunohistochemical analysis of targeting proliferative cell nuclear antigen (PCNA, magnification, ×400). (**B**) Quantitative analysis of PCNA-positive cells. (**C**) Expression of cyclin D1. NC, PBS- and corn oil-dispensed rats; BPH, PBS- and testosterone-dispensed rats; BPH + FIN, testosterone- and finasteride-dispensed rats; BPH + PV60, testosterone- and PV 60 mg/kg-dispensed rats; BPH + PV80, testosterone- and PV 80 mg/kg-dispensed rats. Representation of results as average ± SD. Comparison ## $p < 0.01$ with the NC group; comparison ** $p < 0.01$ with the BPH group.

2.6. PV Extract Elevates Apoptosis of Prostatic Cells in Rat BPH Model

Compared with the NC batch, the count of terminal deoxynucleotidyl transferase dUTP nick-end labeling (TUNEL)-positive cells was reduced in the BPH cohort. However, the TUNEL-positive cell count was remarkably enhanced in the finasteride and PV groups relative to the BPH group (Figure 5A,B). Western blot analysis showed that the expression level of cleaved caspase-3 was upregulated in the PV groups compared to the BPH group (Figure 5C).

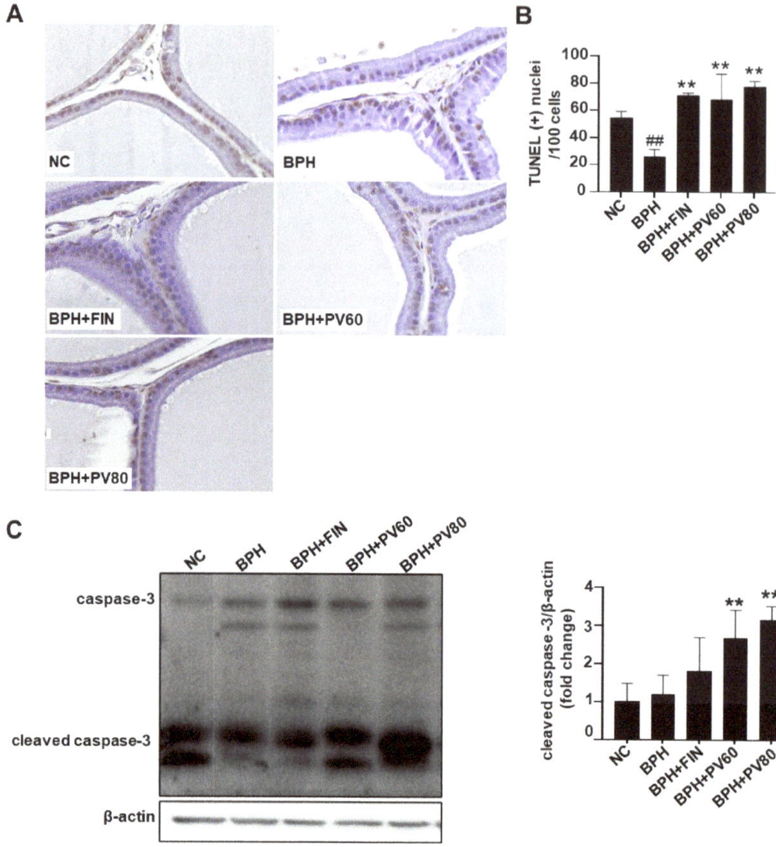

Figure 5. Effects of PV extract on the apoptosis of prostate cells in a rat BPH model. (**A**) Terminal deoxynucleotidyl transferase dUTP nick-end labeling (TUNEL) staining (magnification, ×400). (**B**) As a percentage, the count of TUNEL-positive cells. (**C**) Cleaved caspase-3 expression in prostate tissue. NC, PBS- and corn oil- dispensed rats; BPH, PBS- and testosterone-dispensed rats; BPH + FIN, testosterone- and finasteride-dispensed rats; BPH + PV60, testosterone- and PV 60 mg/kg-dispensed rats; BPH + PV80, testosterone- and PV 80 mg/kg-dispensed rats. Representation of results as average ± SD. Comparison ## $p < 0.01$ with the NC group; comparison ** $p < 0.01$ with the BPH group.

2.7. PV Extract Decreases the Expression Levels of Growth Factors in a Rat BPH Model

The mRNA expression levels of IGF-2, TGF-β, and FGF in the BPH cohort were increased compared to those in the NC cohort; nevertheless, the finasteride and PV groups showed significant reductions in the expression levels of IGF-2, TGF-β, and FGF compared to those in the BPH cohort (Figure 6).

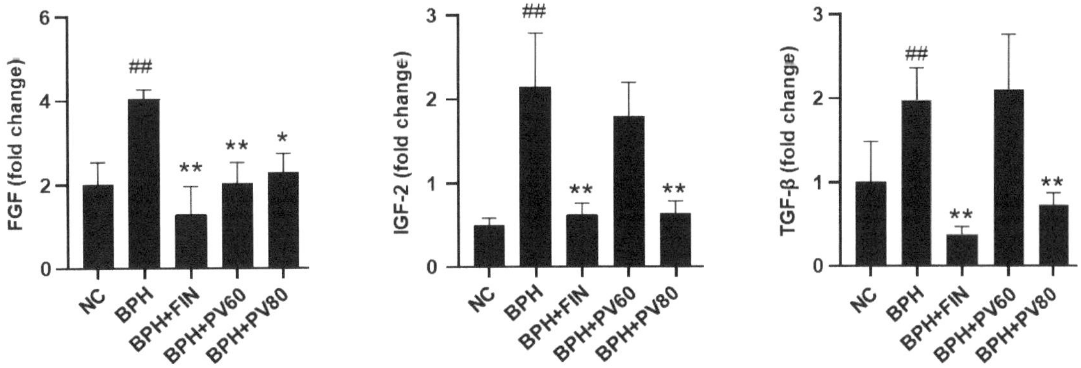

Figure 6. Effects of PV extract on growth factor expression levels in a rat BPH model. The prostatic mRNA levels of FGF, IGF-2, and TGF-β. NC, PBS- and corn oil-dispensed rats; BPH, PBS- and testosterone-dispensed rats; BPH + FIN, testosterone- and finasteride-dispensed rats; BPH + PV60, testosterone- and PV 60 mg/kg-dispensed rats; BPH + PV80, testosterone- and PV 80 mg/kg-dispensed rats. Representation of results as average ± SD. Comparison ## $p < 0.01$ with the NC group; comparison * $p < 0.05$ and ** $p < 0.01$ with the BPH group.

2.8. PV Extract Reduces JNK Activation in a Rat BPH Model

The phosphorylation of c-Jun N-terminal kinase (JNK) (indicating its activation) was elevated in the BPH group compared with the NC group but reduced in the finasteride and PV groups compared to the BPH group (Figure 7).

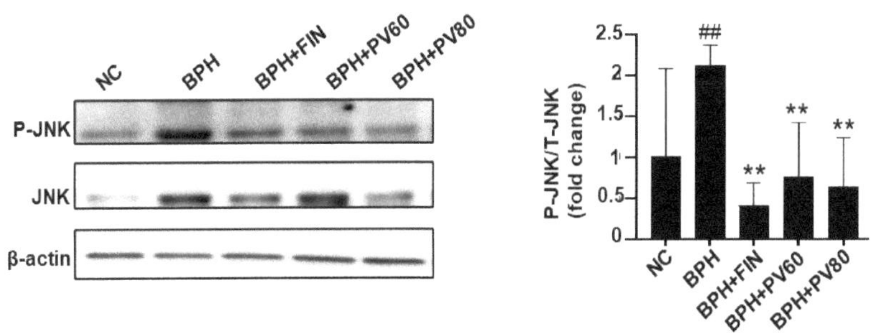

Figure 7. Effects of PV extract on JNK activation in a rat BPH model. Western blot analysis of total JNK (T-JNK) and phosphorylated JNK (P-JNK) expression. NC, PBS- and corn oil-dispensed rats; BPH, PBS- and testosterone-dispensed rats; BPH + FIN, testosterone- and finasteride-dispensed rats; BPH + PV60, testosterone- and PV 60 mg/kg-dispensed rats; BPH + PV80, testosterone- and PV 80 mg/kg-dispensed rats. Representation of results as average ± SD. Comparison ## $p < 0.01$ with the NC group; comparison ** $p < 0.01$ with the BPH group.

3. Discussion

BPH is a degenerative disorder characterized by prostatic hypertrophy with LUTS [2]. Our current study focused on whether PV extract exhibits protective effects in testosterone-induced BPH model rats. Our analytic results revealed that PV extract attenuates the testosterone-mediated elevations in relative prostate weight, serum testosterone, and serum DHT in BPH model rats. The administration of PV extract also markedly reduced testosterone-induced increases in prostatic glandular epithelial cells and growth factor expression and activated apoptotic signaling pathways in BPH model rats. These findings suggest that PV extract inhibits the advancement of testosterone-induced BPH.

Testicular androgens, such as testosterone and DHT, are essential for prostate development [29,30]. DHT is predominantly generated by 5α-reductase (5αR) from testosterone; it binds androgen receptors with high affinity, and the DHT–androgen receptor complex initiates the transcription and ultimately regulates the cell cycle, cell growth, and differentiation of prostate stromal and epithelial cells to promote enlargement of the prostate and BPH pathogenesis [29]. Finasteride is a 4-azasteroid antagonist of 5αR [31] that functions by forming a stable complex with, and thereby selectively inhibiting, the enzyme 5αR [30] to obstruct the peripheral transformation of testosterone into DHT. This substantially reduces the tissue and serum concentrations of DHT, leading to a concomitant decrease in prostatic size [32]. Despite these beneficial actions, however, finasteride is associated with significant adverse effects. This has prompted researchers to explore alternative therapeutic agents that may be utilized to manage BPH while minimizing side effects [33]. Here, we show that BPH model rats exhibit increases in serum levels of testosterone and DHT, but this is ameliorated by treatment with PV extract.

One of the most well-known causes of BPH is an imbalance between cell proliferation and death [34,35]. In the cellular proliferation process, PCNA critically contributes to DNA replication and repair, while nuclear cyclin D1 regulates cell cycle progression [36,37]. Our present results revealed that PV treatment attenuated the relative protein expression level of cyclin D1 in the BPH model and significantly decreased the numbers of PCNA-positive nuclei on immunohistochemical analysis, in comparison to these parameters in the BPH group. Regarding apoptosis, we examined the level of cleaved caspase 3, which is an important tumor gene and apoptotic protein [10,12], and found that cleaved caspase 3 was downregulated in the BPH cohort, and this outcome was ameliorated in the finasteride- and PV-treated categories. This suggests that both treatments are inducing apoptosis in prostate cells. The fact that the NC and BPH groups show similar levels of cleaved caspase-3 indicates that BPH itself may not significantly alter the apoptotic rate in prostate cells. However, both finasteride and PV extract seem to enhance apoptosis. According to the antiproliferative results, finasteride and PV extract primarily induce apoptosis, while significantly affecting cell proliferation; this could be beneficial in reducing prostate enlargement. However, with regards to the apoptotic effect of PV, previous studies demonstrated that PV extract induced apoptosis by upregulating the expression of cleaved caspase-3, along with other apoptotic markers like Bax [38]. While the results presented in Figure 5C suggest that PV extract can induce apoptosis in prostate cells, further investigation is needed to determine the optimal balance between cell proliferation and apoptosis to achieve effective BPH treatment. The numbers of TUNEL-positive cells were also increased in the PV- and finasteride-administrated categories, relative to the BPH cohort. We herein identified UA as a major compound of PV extract. A previous study showed that UA is nontoxic against healthy cells but exhibits apoptotic effects against cervical, breast, and colorectal cancer cells [26]. Here, we provide evidence that PV extract attenuates cell proliferation and increases apoptosis in testosterone-induced BPH model rats.

Growth factors, particularly members of the FGF, IGF, and TGF-β families, are crucial for the development and progression of BPH [39,40]. FGF has been identified in BPH stromal cells and prostate cancer epithelial cells, where it plays significant roles in tumor growth, cellular proliferation, and prostatic growth [41]. Previous studies examining the relevant roles of growth factors (e.g., IGFs) have suggested that they may contribute to the development of BPH through androgen-independent mechanisms [42,43]. High IGF-1 blood levels have been associated with prostatic malignancy [44], while IGF-2 reportedly promotes cellular proliferation and growth in the prostate gland [45]. T lymphocyte-secreted TGF-β plays important roles in regulating the proliferation and differentiation of the prostate stroma [39,46]. Previous studies showed that sulfated polysaccharide extracted from PV attenuates the expression of FGF on endothelial cells [47] and that PV can downregulate TGF-β expression in models of renal injury and extrinsic aging [48]. Here, we report that the levels of FGF, IGF-2, and TGF-β are significantly higher in the prostates of BPH rats compared to those of the NC group, and these differences are notably rescued in the PV group compared to the BPH group. Our present findings suggest that PV may potentially alleviate BPH by influencing growth factor responses to regulate cellular proliferation and prostatic growth.

The MAPK family member, JNK, is activated by phosphorylation and acts as a vital serine/threonine protein kinase for normal cell proliferation and development [49]. Some studies have suggested that JNK is regulated in the enlarged prostate and/or during the proliferation of prostate stromal cells [50], while others found that an interaction with AR triggers JNK phosphorylation and downstream signaling to facilitate cell cycle progression in BPH and prostate cancer [51]. Testosterone and DHT are reported to rapidly and transiently activate MAPK in cultured hippocampal neurons, as evidenced by the phosphorylation of JNK [52]. The JNK signaling pathway is critical for FGF-induced epithelial cell proliferation [53] and IGF and TGF-β induced cellular proliferation [54], all of which are important for the development of BPH. Previous reports found that PV extract can attenuate phospho-JNK levels in various cell types, including INS-1 cells and normal human dermal fibroblasts [55]. Here, we show that the phosphorylation of JNK is increased in the prostate tissues of BPH rats, and this change is significantly ameliorated by PV extract.

In our study, we tested multiple concentrations of PV extract against BPH rats. The highest concentration, 80 mg/kg, achieved effective results in many parts of the study. While increasing the dosage of PV above 80 mg/kg might seem like a straightforward approach to enhance its effectiveness, it is important to consider the potential risks and limitations associated with higher doses, such as increased toxicity, the saturation of receptors, a non-linear dose–response relationship, pharmacokinetic difference, and pharmacodynamic difference [38]. Further studies are needed to determine an accurate dosage of PV extract as a therapeutic agent for BPH.

The most used medications are 5-ARIs, α1-blockers, and cocktails of the two combined (tamsulosin and dutasteride), and the most common mechanism of these drugs is inhibiting the conversion of testosterone to DHT by inhibiting the 5αR enzyme [16–18]. According to the previous literature, for treating BPH, the most used herbal plants are *Serenoa repens, Prunus africana, Urtica dioica, Cucurbita pepo,* and *Secale cereale* [56,57]. Based on earlier studies, these plants have similar mechanisms of action, such as inhibiting the conversion of testosterone to DHT, and anti-inflammatory effects [56,57]. According to our study, PV extract shows potential in treating BPH. While it is not necessarily "more effective" than all other plant materials, it possesses several properties that make it a promising option, such as regulating androgen levels, antiproliferative effects, apoptosis, and anti-growth factor effects. It can be a potential candidate in treating BPH, as a multi-targeted natural product.

4. Materials and Methods

4.1. Preparation of PV Extract

PV was purchased from Jecheon Herbal Market (Jecheon, Chungbuk, Republic of Korea), and voucher specimens (No. 2022-HF001, confirmed) were deposited at the college of pharmacy, Han Yang University (Seoul, Republic of Korea). PV was extracted as follows: dried PV spikes were macerated in 70% ethanol at 50 °C for 8 h, the remnant was extracted a second time with 50% ethanol at 50 °C for 15 h, the two infusions were mixed and concentrated under reduced pressure, and the concentrate was lyophilized. The PV extract was produced in Huons Foodience under principles of Good Manufacturing Practice (GMP) and stored at −20 °C for further analysis.

4.2. HPLC Analysis

The extract (1 g) was dissolved in a 100-mL volumetric flask using methanol, filtered through a 0.45 μm PDVF filter, and injected into an Agilent 1260 series HPLC system equipped with a DAD (diode array detector). Chromatographic separation was performed on an Acclaim C30 column (250 × 4.6 mm, 5 μm) with the column temperature maintained at 25 °C. The detection wavelength was set at 210 nm, and the injection volume was 10 μL. An isocratic mobile phase of methanol/0.2% ammonium acetate was used, with a flow rate of 0.4 mL/min. The standards of OA (O5504) and UA (U6753), (purity 99% or higher) were purchased from Sigma Aldrich (Saint Louis, MO, USA). The OA and UA in the extract were identified based on their retention times and spectrums, compared with those of their respective standards.

4.3. Animals

Sprague Dawley male rats (n = 25, 7 weeks old) were obtained from Orient Bio (Seongnam, Republic of Korea), and the mice were divided into numbers of 5 for each group and maintained under standard laboratory conditions (22 ± 2 °C; relative humidity, 50 ± 5%; 12 h light/dark cycle); standard rodent dietary formulations were fed to them, and they had ad libitum access to sterilized tap water. The methodologies for the experimental animal study received endorsement from the Animal Experimentation Ethics Committee at Chungnam National University in Daejeon, Republic of Korea.

4.4. Initiation of BPH in Rats and Treatment Design

Rats were randomly divided into four groups and administrated the following dosage regimens: (1) the NC group received a subcutaneous (SC) injection of corn oil (as a vehicle control) and oral gavage of PBS (as a vehicle control); (2) the BPH group received an SC injection of 3 mg/kg TP (Tokyo Chemicals Ind. Co., Chuo ku, Tokyo, Japan) and oral gavage of PBS; (3) the BPH plus finasteride (BPH + FIN) group (positive control), received an SC injection of TP and oral gavage of finasteride (10 mg/kg; Sigma); and (4) the BPH + PV group received an SC injection of TP and oral gavage of PV (60 mg/kg or 80 mg/kg). All treatments were given daily for 4 weeks; the treatment volumes were 5 mL/kg for oral gavage (PBS, finasteride, and PV) and 3 mL/kg for SC injections. The lyophilized PV extract was dissolved in PBS. A single batch of PV was prepared for the rats' oral gavage, which was adequate for a 4-week duration. The body mass of the experimental rats was assessed on a weekly basis throughout the duration of the study, in addition to being recorded on the day designated for necropsy. Following the final administration of the injection, the rats were humanely euthanized, and blood samples were procured from the vena cava. Serum was subsequently extracted from the whole blood and preserved at a temperature of −70 °C. The prostate tissues were meticulously excised and weighed.

4.5. Analysis Serum of DHT and Testosterone Levels

Commercial assay kits were used to determine the serum levels of testosterone (Cayman Chemicals, Ann Arbor, MI, USA) and serum DHT (ALPCO Diagnostics, Salem, NH, USA). All procedures were performed according to the manual. In summary, the serum specimens underwent incubation with enzyme conjugates, were washed, and exposed to substrates, and the testosterone and DHT concentrations were determined by assessing absorbance at 412 and 450 nm, respectively.

4.6. Histopathology

Prostatic tissues were preserved in a 10% buffered formalin solution, subsequently embedded in paraffin wax, sectioned to a thickness of 4 μm, and subjected to staining with hematoxylin and eosin (H&E). The measurement of epithelial thickness was conducted in the ventral lobe of each prostate in accordance with previously established methodologies [13]. To summarize, the epithelial structures in five randomly selected microscopic fields (×400) from each rat (n = 5 per group) were quantified utilizing Image J software (version 46a; NIH, Bethesda, MD, USA).

4.7. Immunohistochemical (IHC) Staining of Proliferative Cell Nuclear Antigen (PCNA)

Briefly, sections were de-paraffinized by xylene and rehydrated in an ethanol series. Following the process of heat-induced antigen retrieval, the specimens underwent blocking with normal goat serum (Vectastain, Cambridge, UK) and were subsequently incubated overnight in the presence of a primary antibody targeting proliferative cell nuclear antigen (PCNA, dilution 1:10,000; Abcam, Cambridge, UK), alongside a secondary antibody (Vectastain). The detection of avidin–biotin complexes was accomplished utilizing diaminobenzidine (DAB; Vector Laboratories, Newark, CA, USA) reagent. Five randomly selected regions (×400) were observed for each rat (n = 5 per group), and the numbers of PCNA-positive cells per 100 cells were counted.

4.8. TUNEL Assay

The TUNEL assay was performed using a commercial kit (Merck Millipore Corporation, Burlington, MA, USA) according to the manufacturer's manual. Briefly, sections were de-paraffinized by xylene, rehydrated with an ethanol series, pretreated with Proteinase K enzyme (Merck Millipore Corporation, MA, USA), and subjected to the inactivation of endogenous peroxides using 3.0% hydrogen peroxide (SAMCHUN Chemical Co., Ltd., Bongeunsa ro 37 gil, Seoul, Republic of Korea). Biotinylated dUTP was incorporated onto the 3′ ends of fragmented DNA in a reaction mixture containing TdT enzyme (Merck Millipore Corporation), DAB reagent was used to observe the immune complexes, and the sections were further stained with hematoxylin. TUNEL-positive cells were counted in five randomly selected fields per slide (×400), and the results were reported as the number of TUNEL-positive cells per 100 cells.

4.9. Western Blot Analysis

Prostate tissues underwent homogenization utilizing RIPA lysis buffer (Cell Signaling, Danvers, MA, USA) to facilitate the extraction of proteins. An equal quantity of total protein (15 μg) was subjected to resolution via SDS-PAGE, following which the resolved proteins were transferred onto membranes, which were subsequently incubated overnight with the specified primary antibodies: anti-cyclin D1, anti-cleaved caspase 3, anti-JNK, anti-P-JNK, and anti-β-actin (Cell Signaling). After that, the membranes were exposed to secondary antibodies at room temperature for a duration of 2 h, with the resultant signals being detected through a chemiluminescence detection kit and quantified employing a CSAnalyzer4 (Atto, Tokyo, Japan).

4.10. Quantitative Real-Time PCR (RT-qPCR)

Total RNA was isolated from prostate tissues utilizing TRIzol reagent (Thermo Scientific, Waltham, MA, USA). Equivalent quantities of total RNA (1.4 μg) derived from the prostate tissues of each individual rat were exposed to reverse transcription (RT), employing a commercial RT kit (Toyobo, Osaka, Japan). A quantitative real-time PCR was executed utilizing SYBR Green Master Mix (Thermo Scientific, MA, USA) alongside the designated PCR primers. TGF-β, f:5′-AGGGCTCAACACATGGAC-3′ and r: 5′-GGGCCCCACACAGGAGTT-3′; IGF, f:5′-GTCTGTGGCTCAGGCTCTTC-3′ and r: 5′-CCCATTTGGGAACTTCGCCT-3′; FGF, f: 5′-GAGGAAAGGGAAAGGGTCAAAA-3′ and r: 5′-CACAGTGAACGCTCCAGGATT-3′; GAPDH f:5′-CAACTCCCTCAAGATTGTCAGC AA-3′ and r: 5′-GGCATGGACTGTGGTCATGA-3′. The fold change in the expression levels of each target gene in relation to that of the endogenous control (GAPDH) was computed employing the $2^{-\Delta\Delta Ct}$ method.

4.11. Statistical Analysis

A series of multiple comparisons were conducted utilizing a one-way analysis of variance (ANOVA), subsequently accompanied by Dunnett's post hoc test. The threshold for statistical significance was established at $p < 0.05$. The statistical analyses were executed employing GraphPad Prism 9 (GraphPad Software Inc., Boston, MA, USA). The data are represented as the average ± standard deviation (SD).

5. Conclusions

The current study demonstrated that the therapeutic treatment of PV extract in rats hindered the development of testosterone-induced BPH, as evidenced by decreases in the weight and hyperplasia of the prostate. This impact can be partly attributed to PV extract-induced decreases in serum levels of DHT and testosterone, as well as its anti-proliferative, pro-apoptotic, and anti-growth properties. These results indicate that PV extract may be utilized as a novel agent for BPH treatment. Further research, such as studies using larger sample sizes, less variable sample knockout models, and/or functional analyses, will be needed to assess the clinical value of PV.

Author Contributions: Conceptualization: H.-J.K.; methodology: P.K., E.-B.B. and E.-J.H.; formal analysis: P.K., E.-B.B., E.-J.H., J.-Y.S., Y.-G.K., M.-R.J. and H.-S.J.; investigation: P.K., E.-B.B. and E.-J.H.; writing—original draft preparation: P.K.; writing—review and editing: P.K., E.-B.B. and H.-J.K.; supervision: H.-J.K. All authors have read and agreed to the published version of the manuscript.

Funding: This work was supported by the Korea Institute of Planning and Evaluation for Technology in Food, Agriculture, and Forestry (IPET) through the Technology Commercialization Support Program, funded by the Ministry of Agriculture, Food, and Rural Affairs (MAFRA) (1220453).

Institutional Review Board Statement: The experimental protocol was conducted in accordance with the Guide for the Care and Use of Laboratory Animals (NIH publication, 1996), and the animal study protocol was approved by the Animal Experimental Ethics Committee of 27 April 2023, Chungnam National University, with the approval number 20230A-CNU-070.

Informed Consent Statement: Not applicable.

Data Availability Statement: The data that support the findings of this study are available from the corresponding author upon reasonable request.

Conflicts of Interest: Author Youn Gil Kwak, Mi Ran Jang, and Hyo Seong Ji were employed by the company Huons Foodience Co., Ltd. The remaining authors declare that the research was conducted in the absence of any commercial or financial relationships that could be construed as a potential conflict of interest.

Abbreviations

5-αR, 5α-reductase; 5-ARIs, 5α-reductase inhibitors; α1-blockers, alpha1-adrenergic antagonists; AR, androgen receptor; BPH, benign prostatic hyperplasia; DHT, dihydrotestosterone; H&E, hematoxylin and eosin; FGF, fibroblast growth factor; GMP, Good Manufacturing Practice; IGFs, insulin-like growth factors; JNK, c-Jun N-terminal kinase; LUTS, lower urinary tract symptoms; MAPK, mitogen-activated protein kinase; OA, oleanolic acid, PCNA, proliferating cell nuclear antigen; PDE5Is, phosphodiesterase 5 inhibitors; PV, *Prunella vulgaris* L.; PSA, prostate-specific antigen; SC, subcutaneous; TUNEL, terminal deoxynucleotidyl transferase dUTP nick-end labeling; TP, testosterone propionate; TGF- β, transforming growth factor beta; UA, ursolic acid.

References

1. Chughtai, B.; Forde, J.C.; Thomas, D.D.M.; Laor, L.; Hossack, T.; Woo, H.H.; Te, A.E.; Kaplan, S.A. Benign prostatic hyperplasia. *Nat. Rev. Dis. Primers* **2016**, *2*, 16031. [CrossRef] [PubMed]
2. Berry, S.J.; Coffey, D.S.; Walsh, P.C.; Ewing, L.L. The development of human benign prostatic hyperplasia with age. *J. Urol.* **1984**, *132*, 474–479. [CrossRef] [PubMed]
3. Barry, M.J.; Fowler, F.J.; O'leary, M.P.; Bruskewitz, R.C.; Holtgrewe, H.L.; Mebust, W.K.; Cockett, A.T. The American Urological Association symptom index for benign prostatic hyperplasia. *J. Urol.* **1992**, *148*, 1549–1557. [CrossRef] [PubMed]
4. Bushman, W. Etiology, epidemiology, and natural history of benign prostatic hyperplasia. *Urol. Clin. N. Am.* **2009**, *36*, 403–415. [CrossRef] [PubMed]
5. Bartsch, G.; Rittmaster, R.; Klocker, H. Dihydrotestosterone and the concept of 5α-reductase inhibition in human benign prostatic hyperplasia. *World J. Urol.* **2002**, *19*, 413–425. [CrossRef]
6. Chatterjee, B. The role of the androgen receptor in the development of prostatic hyperplasia and prostate cancer. *Mol. Cell. Biochem.* **2003**, *253*, 89–101. [CrossRef]

7. Lloyd, G.L.; Marks, J M.; Ricke, W.A. Benign Prostatic Hyperplasia and Lower Urinary Tract Symptoms: What Is the Role and Significance of Inflammation? *Curr. Urol. Rep.* **2019**, *20*, 54. [CrossRef]
8. McConnell, J.D. The pathophysiology of benign prostatic hyperplasia. *J. Androl.* **1991**, *12*, 356–363. [CrossRef]
9. Isaacs, J.T.; Coffey, D.S. Etiology and disease process of benign prostatic hyperplasia. *Prostate* **1989**, *15*, 33–50. [CrossRef]
10. Lawson, R.K. Role of growth factors in benign prostatic hyperplasia. *Eur. Urol.* **1997**, *32* (Suppl. S1), 22–27.
11. Scott Lucia, M.; Lambert, J.R. Growth factors in benign prostatic hyperplasia: Basic science implications. *Curr. Urol. Rep.* **2008**, *9*, 272–278. [CrossRef] [PubMed]
12. McLaren, I.D.; Jerde, T.J.; Bushman, W. Role of interleukins, IGF and stem cells in BPH. *Differentiation* **2011**, *82*, 237–243. [CrossRef] [PubMed]
13. Shrivastava, A.; Gupta, V.B. Various treatment options for benign prostatic hyperplasia: A current update. *J. Mid-Life Health* **2012**, *3*, 10–19. [CrossRef] [PubMed]
14. Steers, W.D. 5α-reductase activity in the prostate. *Urology* **2001**, *58*, 17–24. [CrossRef] [PubMed]
15. Blankstein, U.; BAsseldonk, V.; Elterman, D.S. BPH update: Medical versus interventional management. *Can. J. Urol.* **2016**, *23* (Suppl. S1), 10–15. [PubMed]
16. Quaresma, B.M.C.S.; Pimenta, A.R.; da Silva, A.C.S.; Pupo, A.S.; Romeiro, L.A.S.; Silva, C.L.M.; Noël, F. Revisiting the Pharmacodynamic Uroselectivity of α (1)-Adrenergic Receptor Antagonists. *J. Pharmacol. Exp. Ther.* **2019**, *371*, 106–112. [CrossRef]
17. Kulig, K.; Malawska, B. Trends in the development of new drugs for treatment of benign prostatic hyperplasia. *Curr. Med. Chem.* **2006**, *13*, 3395–3416. [CrossRef]
18. Facio, F.; Kashiwabuschi, R.; Nishi, Y.; Leao, R.; Mcdonnell, P.; Burnett, A. Benign prostatic hyperplasia. Clinical treatment can complicate cataract surgery. *Int. Braz. J. Urol.* **2010**, *36*, 563–570. [CrossRef]
19. Wong, P.; Lawrentschuk, N.; Bolton, D.M. Phosphodiesterase 5 inhibitors in the management of benign prostatic hyperplasia and erectile dysfunction: The best of both worlds. *Curr. Opin. Urol.* **2009**, *19*, 7–12. [CrossRef]
20. Laufer, M.; Shoenfeld, S. Phytotherapy and Natural Agents in Symptomatic Benign Prostatic Hyperplasia (BPH). *Harefuah* **2024**, *163*, 50–53.
21. Pan, J.; Wang, H.; Chen, Y. *Prunella vulgaris* L.—A review of its ethnopharmacology, phytochemistry, quality control and pharmacological effects. *Front. Pharmacol.* **2022**, *13*, 903171. [CrossRef] [PubMed]
22. Sukjamnong, S.; Chen, H.; Saad, S.; Santiyanont, R. Fimbristylis ovata and Artemisia vulgaris extracts inhibited AGE-mediated RAGE expression, ROS generation, and inflammation in THP-1 cells. *Toxicol. Res.* **2022**, *38*, 331–343. [CrossRef] [PubMed]
23. Wang, S.-J.; Wang, X.-H.; Dai, Y.-Y.; Ma, M.-H.; Rahman, K.; Nian, H.; Zhang, H. Prunella vulgaris: A comprehensive review of chemical constituents, pharmacological effects and clinical applications. *Curr. Pharm. Des.* **2019**, *25*, 359–369. [CrossRef] [PubMed]
24. Rasool, R.; Ganai, B.A. *Prunella vulgaris* L.: A literature review on its therapeutic potentials. *Pharmacologia* **2013**, *4*, 441–448. [CrossRef]
25. Mîrza, C.M.; Mîrza, T.-V.; Odagiu, A.C.M.; Uifălean, A.; But, A.E.; Pârvu, A.E.; Bulboacă, A.-E. Phytochemical Analysis and Antioxidant Effects of Prunella vulgaris in Experimental Acute Inflammation. *Int. J. Mol. Sci.* **2024**, *25*, 4843. [CrossRef]
26. Similie, D.; Minda, D.; Bora, L.; Kroškins, V.; Lugiņina, J.; Turks, M.; Dehelean, C.A.; Danciu, C. An Update on Pentacyclic Triterpenoids Ursolic and Oleanolic Acids and Related Derivatives as Anticancer Candidates. *Antioxidants* **2024**, *13*, 952. [CrossRef]
27. Zhang, Q.; Chen, X.; Palen, K.; Johnson, B.; Bui, D.; Xiong, D.; Pan, J.; Hu, M.; Wang, Y.; You, M. Cancer chemoprevention with PV-1, a novel Prunella vulgaris-containing herbal mixture that remodels the tumor immune microenvironment in mice. *Front. Immunol.* **2023**, *14*, 1196434. [CrossRef]
28. Ning, N.; Nan, Y.; Chen, G.; Huang, S.; Lu, D.; Yang, Y.; Meng, F.; Yuan, L. Anti-Tumor Effects and Toxicity Reduction Mechanisms of Prunella vulgaris: A Comprehensive Review. *Molecules* **2024**, *29*, 1843. [CrossRef]
29. Asiedu, B.; Anang, Y.; Nyarko, A.; Doku, D.A.; Amoah, B.Y.; Santa, S.; Ngala, R.A.; Asare, G.A. The role of sex steroid hormones in benign prostatic hyperplasia. *Aging Male* **2017**, *20*, 17–22. [CrossRef]
30. Lee, G.H.; Lee, H.-Y.; Zhao, L.; Rashid, M.M.U.; Kim, M.K.; Jeong, Y.B.; Chae, H.-J.; Shin, Y.S. The Role of Reactive Oxygen Species, Inflammation, and Endoplasmic Reticulum Stress Response in the Finasteride Protective Effect against Benign Prostate Hyperplasia. *World J. Mens. Health* **2024**, *42*, 600–609. [CrossRef]
31. Traish, A.M. Health Risks Associated with Long-Term Finasteride and Dutasteride Use: It's Time to Sound the Alarm. *World J. Mens. Health* **2020**, *38*, 323–337. [CrossRef] [PubMed]
32. An, J.; Song, Y.; Kim, S.; Kong, H.; Kim, K. Alteration of Gut Microbes in Benign Prostatic Hyperplasia Model and Finasteride Treatment Model. *Int. J. Mol. Sci.* **2023**, *24*, 5904. [CrossRef] [PubMed]
33. Busetto, G.M.; Del Giudice, F.; D'Agostino, D.; Romagnoli, D.; Minervini, A.; Rocco, B.; Antonelli, A.; Celia, A.; Schiavina, R.; Cindolo, L.; et al. Efficacy and safety of Finasteride (5 alpha-reductase inhibitor) monotherapy in patients with benign prostatic hyperplasia: A critical review of the literature. *Arch. Ital. Urol. Androl.* **2020**, *91*, 205–210. [CrossRef] [PubMed]
34. Hegazi, M.; Taverna, G.; Grizzi, F. Is Artificial Intelligence the Key to Revolutionizing Benign Prostatic Hyperplasia Diagnosis and Management. *Arch. Esp. Urol.* **2023**, *76*, 643–656. [CrossRef] [PubMed]
35. D'Amico, R.; Genovese, T.; Cordaro, M.; Siracusa, R.; Gugliandolo, E.; Peritore, A.F.; Interdonato, L.; Crupi, R.; Cuzzocrea, S.; Di Paola, R.; et al. Palmitoylethanolamide/Baicalein Regulates the Androgen Receptor Signaling and NF-κB/Nrf2 Pathways in Benign Prostatic Hyperplasia. *Antioxidants* **2021**, *10*, 1014. [CrossRef]

36. He, Y.; Franco, O.E.; Jiang, M.; Williams, K.; Love, H.D.; Coleman, I.M.; Nelson, P.S.; Hayward, S.W. Tissue-specific consequences of cyclin D1 overexpression in prostate cancer progression. *Cancer Res.* **2007**, *67*, 8188–8197. [CrossRef]
37. Chen, L.M.; Hatfield, M.L.; Fu, Y.; Chai, K.X. Prostasin regulates iNOS and cyclin D1 expression by modulating protease-activated receptor-2 signaling in prostate epithelial cells. *Prostate* **2009**, *69*, 1790–1801. [CrossRef]
38. Zhang, M.; Hwang, E.; Lin, P.; Gao, W.; Ngo, H.T.; Yi, T.H. Prunella vulgaris L. Exerts a Protective Effect Against Extrinsic Aging Through NF-κB, MAPKs, AP-1, and TGF-β/Smad Signaling Pathways in UVB-Aged Normal Human Dermal Fibroblasts. *Rejuvenation Res.* **2018**, *21*, 313–322. [CrossRef]
39. Caggia, S.; Libra, M.; Malaponte, G.; Cardile, V. Modulation of YY1 and p53 expression by transforming growth factor-β3 in prostate cell lines. *Cytokine* **2011**, *56*, 403–410. [CrossRef]
40. Gong, G.Y.; Xi, S.-Y.; Li, C.-C.; Tang, W.-L.; Fu, X.-M.; Huang, Y.-P. Bushen Tongluo formula ameliorated testosterone propionate-induced benign prostatic hyperplasia in rats. *Phytomedicine* **2023**, *120*, 155048. [CrossRef]
41. Sinowatz, F.; Schams, D.; Einspanier, R.; Arnold, G.; Pfeffer, M.; Temmim-Baker, L.; Amselgruber, W.; Plendl, J. Cellular localization of fibroblast growth factor 2 (FGF-2) in benign prostatic hyperplasia. *Histol. Histopathol.* **2000**, *15*, 475–481. [PubMed]
42. Correa, L.L.; Neto, L.V.; Lima, G.A.B.; Gabrich, R.; de Miranda, L.C.D.; Gadelha, M.R. Insulin-like growth factor (IGF)-I, IGF binding protein-3, and prostate cancer: Correlation with Gleason score. *Int. Braz. J. Urol.* **2015**, *41*, 110–115. [CrossRef] [PubMed]
43. Khosravi, J.; Diamandi, A.; Mistry, J.; Scorilas, A. Insulin-like growth factor I (IGF-I) and IGF-binding protein-3 in benign prostatic hyperplasia and prostate cancer. *J. Clin. Endocrinol. Metab.* **2001**, *86*, 694–699. [CrossRef] [PubMed]
44. Gnanapragasam, V.J.; Mccahy, P.; Neal, D.; Robson, C. Insulin-like growth factor II and androgen receptor expression in the prostate. *BJU Int.* **2000**, *86*, 731–735. [CrossRef]
45. Ho, P.J.; Baxter, R.C. Insulin-like growth factor-binding protein-2 in patients with prostate carcinoma and benign prostatic hyperplasia. *Clin. Endocrinol.* **1997**, *46*, 145–154. [CrossRef]
46. Story, M.T.; Hopp, K.A.; Molter, M. Expression of transforming growth factor beta 1 (TGF beta 1), -beta 2, and- beta 3 by cultured human prostate cells. *J. Cell Physiol.* **1996**, *169*, 97–107. [CrossRef]
47. Wu, X.-Z.; Zhang, S.-X.; Zhu, C.; Chen, D. Effects of sulfated polysaccharide extracted from Prunella vulgaris on endothelial cells. *J. Med. Plants Res.* **2011**, *5*, 4218–4223.
48. Fan, J.; Ren, D.; Wang, J.; Liu, X.; Zhang, H.; Wu, M.; Yang, G. Bruceine D induces lung cancer cell apoptosis and autophagy via the ROS/MAPK signaling pathway in vitro and in vivo. *Cell Death Dis.* **2020**, *11*, 126. [CrossRef]
49. Lee, E.H.; Kim, H.T.; Chun, S.Y.; Chung, J.-W.; Choi, S.H.; Lee, J.N.; Kim, B.S.; Yoo, E.S.; Kwon, T.G.; Kim, T.-H.; et al. Role of the JNK Pathway in Bladder Cancer. *OncoTargets Ther.* **2022**, *15*, 963–971. [CrossRef]
50. Yan, H.; He, L.; Lv, D.; Yang, J.; Yuan, Z. The Role of the Dysregulated JNK Signaling Pathway in the Pathogenesis of Human Diseases and Its Potential Therapeutic Strategies: A Comprehensive Review. *Biomolecules* **2024**, *14*, 243. [CrossRef]
51. Wijerathne, C.U.; Park, H.-S.; Jeong, H.-Y.; Song, J.-W.; Moon, O.-S.; Seo, Y.-W.; Won, Y.-S.; Son, H.-Y.; Lim, J.-H.; Yeon, S.-H.; et al. Quisqualis indica improves benign prostatic hyperplasia by regulating prostate cell proliferation and apoptosis. *Biol. Pharm. Bull.* **2017**, *40*, 2125–2133. [CrossRef] [PubMed]
52. Zhao, R.; Wang, X.; Jiang, C.; Shi, F.; Zhu, Y.; Yang, B.; Zhuo, J.; Jing, Y.; Luo, G.; Xia, S.; et al. Finasteride accelerates prostate wound healing after thulium laser resection through DHT and AR signalling. *Cell Prolif.* **2018**, *51*, e12415. [CrossRef] [PubMed]
53. Rodríguez-Berriguete, G.; Fraile, B.; Martínez-Onsurbe, P.; Olmedilla, G.; Paniagua, R.; Royuela, M. MAP kinases and prostate cancer. *J. Signal Transduct.* **2012**, *2012*, 169170. [CrossRef] [PubMed]
54. Martínez-Martínez, D.; Toledo Lobo, M.-V.; Baquero, P.; Ropero, S.; Angulo, J.C.; Chiloeches, A.; Lasa, M. Downregulation of Snail by DUSP1 impairs cell migration and invasion through the inactivation of JNK and ERK and is useful as a predictive factor in the prognosis of prostate cancer. *Cancers* **2021**, *13*, 1158. [CrossRef] [PubMed]
55. Wu, H.; Gao, M.; Ha, T.; Kelley, J.; Young, A.; Breuel, K. Prunella vulgaris aqueous extract attenuates IL-1β-induced apoptosis and NF-κB activation in INS-1 cells. *Exp. Ther. Med.* **2012**, *3*, 919–924. [CrossRef]
56. Dvorkin, L.; Song, K.Y. Herbs for benign prostatic hyperplasia. *Ann. Pharmacother.* **2002**, *36*, 1443–1452. [CrossRef]
57. Ney, J.P.; Joseph, K.R. Neurologic uses of botulinum neurotoxin type A. *Neuropsychiatr. Dis. Treat.* **2007**, *3*, 785–798. [CrossRef]

pharmaceuticals

MDPI

Article

Vernonanthura tweediana (Baker) H. Rob. (Asteraceae), an Ordinary Bush or an Anti-Inflammatory and Immunomodulator Aromatic Species?

Isabel D. Machado [1], Pâmela P. Borges [1], Larissa J. A. Giacomozzi [2], Larissa Benvenutti [3], José R. Santin [3], Sarah C. dos Santos [4], Martinho Rau [4], Iêda M. Begnini [4], Ricardo A. Rebelo [4,*], Henrique D. M. Coutinho [5], Clara M. G. Lima [6] and Talha B. Emran [7,8,9]

1 Postgraduate Program in Biodiversity, Regional University of Blumenau, Rua Antônio da Veiga, 140, Itoupava Seca, Blumenau 89030-903, Brazil; isabelm@furb.br (I.D.M.); ppborges@furb.br (P.P.B.)
2 Laboratory of Synthesis and Technology, T-313, Regional University of Blumenau, Blumenau 89030-903, Brazil; ljagiacomozzi@furb.br
3 Postgraduate Program in Pharmaceutical Sciences, University of Vale do Itajaí-UNIVALI, Itajaí 88302-901, Brazil; larabenv@gmail.com (L.B.); jrs.santin@univali.br (J.R.S.)
4 Postgraduate Program in Chemistry, Regional University of Blumenau, Blumenau 89030-903, Brazil; sarahcastro.chemistry@gmail.com (S.C.d.S.); mrau@furb.br (M.R.); ieda@furb.br (I.M.B.)
5 Department of Biological Chemistry, Cariri Regional University, Crato 63105-000, Brazil; hdmcoutinho@gmail.com
6 Department of Food Science, Federal University of Lavras, Lavras 37200-900, Brazil; claramarianalima@gmail.com
7 Department of Pathology and Laboratory Medicine, Warren Alpert Medical School, Brown University, Providence, RI 02912, USA; talha_bin_emran@brown.edu
8 Legorreta Cancer Center, Brown University, Providence, RI 02912, USA
9 Department of Pharmacy, Faculty of Allied Health Sciences, Daffodil International University, Dhaka 1207, Bangladesh
* Correspondence: ricardorebelo@furb.br

Citation: Machado, I.D.; Borges, P.P.; Giacomozzi, L.J.A.; Benvenutti, L.; Santin, J.R.; dos Santos, S.C.; Rau, M.; Begnini, I.M.; Rebelo, R.A.; Coutinho, H.D.M.; et al. *Vernonanthura tweediana* (Baker) H. Rob. (Asteraceae), an Ordinary Bush or an Anti-Inflammatory and Immunomodulator Aromatic Species? *Pharmaceuticals* **2024**, *17*, 1492. https://doi.org/10.3390/ph17111492

Academic Editors: Elena Y. Enioutina, Catherine Sherwin and Kathleen M. Job

Received: 29 September 2024
Revised: 23 October 2024
Accepted: 26 October 2024
Published: 7 November 2024

Abstract: Background: Oral traditional knowledge disseminates the use of young leaves of *Vernonanthura tweediana* (Asteraceae) as poultice in feverish cases among family farmers in Santa Catarina, Brazil, but there is a lack of phytochemistry and pharmacological studies on this species, especially those related to volatile organic compounds. **Methods:** In the present study, the dry leaves of *V. tweediana* were subjected to hydrodistillation for the extraction of essential oil. Sample characterization was conducted using GC-FID and GC-MS. To evaluate anti-inflammatory and immunomodulatory activities, the air pouch method was used, and with the exudate obtained, total and differential leukocyte counts were performed, as well as the quantification of total proteins, interleukin (IL) 1β, IL-6, and tumor necrosis factor (TNF). **Results:** The essential oil yield extraction was 0.13%, and sesquiterpenes were the main constituents: α-copaene (5.1%), β-caryophyllene (27.77%), α-caryophyllene (15.1%), germacrene D (14.0%), and bicyclogermacrene (13.3%). A sample was subjected to biological tests, with a reduction in leukocyte migration to the inflammatory focus. The immunomodulatory activity was also pronounced, as the oil modulated all cytokine secretions measured when compared to the control. The high concentration of caryophyllenes might explain these findings. **Conclusions:** Future studies will consider the fractionation of the essential oil to establish the degree of synergism between the constituents.

Keywords: hydrodistillation; essential oil; chromatographic characterization; caryophyllenes; leukocytes and cytokines

1. Introduction

The Asteraceae family encompasses many species, with several examples within the genus *Vernonanthura* with proven therapeutic activity. Among them, the following members and properties can be highlighted: *V. colorata*, antibacterial and anti-inflammatory [1], *V. cinerea*, analgesic, antipyretic, anti-inflammatory, and cytotoxic [2], *V. phosphorica*, antimicrobial, leishmanicidal, antinociceptive, and anti-inflammatory [3], and *V. montevidensis*, moderate antimycobacterial [4].

V. tweediana, popularly known as "chamarritão" or "figatil", is used by different populations to treat stomach and liver pain [5]. Also known as "assa-peixe", "chamarrita", and "mata-pasto", it is popularly used by different communities for treating respiratory problems [6]. There are reports on the biological activities of *V. tweediana* extracts, such as antibacterial [7], antifungal [8], antioxidant [9], immunomodulatory in mice [10], antinociceptive, and anti-edematogenic [11]; in addition, it presents weak toxicity against *Artemisa salina* and allelopathic activity [12]. Among family farmers in the interior community of the Itajaí Valley of Santa Catarina, southern Brazil, young fresh leaves were used as poultice in feverish cases (RAR, personal communication, 19 October 2019).

The treatment of inflammatory conditions is based on steroidal and non-steroidal anti-inflammatory drugs; however, prolonged use of these medications can cause harmful effects, such as gastrointestinal, cardiovascular, and hepatic disorders. Prospecting new bioactive natural products and extracts, especially those capable of acting in multiple biological pathways, is very attractive, and essential oils commonly composed of several chemical structures may well fit in the search for multitargeted therapy [13]. The anti-inflammatory and immunomodulatory effects of essential oils and their components are known for their potential to reduce oxidative stress through the scavenging of reactive oxygen species (ROS), reducing immune cell activation, and modulating pro-inflammatory responses. Furthermore, essential oils influence the expression of inflammatory mediators such as inducible nitric oxide synthase (iNOS) and cyclooxygenase-2 (COX-2), which play a role in producing gaseous and eicosanoid pro-inflammatory molecules, respectively. Additionally, research evidence indicates that essential oils can inhibit the activation of NF-κB and MAPKs, resulting in a reduction in pro-inflammatory cytokines and chemokines. These targets are essential for regulating the inflammatory process as they operate across various pathways involved in cellular and molecular signaling [14,15].

Given the lack of studies related to the volatile constituents of this species, this work investigates the chemical composition of the essential oil from *V. tweediana* leaves and its anti-inflammatory and immunomodulatory activity, aiming to support its use in folk medicine. In addition, it will provide the scientific basis for the potential use of its essential oil in pharmaceutical formulations, resulting in the valorization of Atlantic Forest biodiversity and stimulating research on the development of phytotherapics.

Biological assays demonstrated notable anti-inflammatory and immunomodulatory activities, including reduced leukocyte migration and modulated cytokine secretion. These effects are likely linked to the high caryophyllene content.

2. Results

The investigation conducted is presented in two main headings, extraction of the essential oil of *V. tweediana* and its chemical characterization and the biological assays associated with the air pouch model.

2.1. Extraction and Chemical Characterization of Essential Oil from V. tweediana

To extract the essential oil (EO), the hydrodistillation technique was used, which consists of heating the plant material in direct contact with distilled water. The hydrodistillation product was isolated using liquid–liquid extraction with bidistilled dichloromethane as an extracting solvent. The removal of the solvent and traces of water gave pure essential oil in 0.13% yield.

The sample was analyzed via gas chromatography using a flame ionization detector (GC-FID) and a mass detector (GC-MS). These techniques in association with the arithmetic retention index (AI) are very efficient for the characterization of organic volatile compounds. The corresponding GC-FID and GC-MS chromatograms are given as Supplementary Material (SM)

(Figures S1 and S2). Although mass spectrometry can detect very low analyte concentrations in a complex mixture such as essential oils, its use for quantification is compromised because ionization efficiencies are variable among other factors. GC-FID gives a better correlation between a peak area of a given constituent and its concentration; furthermore, outstanding reproducibility can be achieved. This can be confirmed by the standard deviation observed in Table 1.

Table 1. Chemical composition of the essential oils from the dry leaves of *V. tweediana* (Baker) H. Rob. (Asteraceae).

Entry	Constituents	AI_{exp}	AI_{lit}	[%] SD
1	α-pinene	935	932	0.27 ± 0.01
2	benzaldehyde	974	952	0.15 ± 0.01
3	β-pinene	980	974	0.58 ± 0.01
4	β-myrcene	991	988	0.27 ± 0.00
5	α-phellandrene	1009	1002	0.30 ± 0.01
6	cymene [1]	1026	1020 [2]/1022 [3]	0.39 ± 0.01
7	limonene	1030	1024	0.37 ± 0.01
8	*Z*−β−ocimene	1035	1032	0.67 ± 0.01
9	*E*- β-ocimene	1046	1044	0.22 ± 0.01
10	γ-terpinene	1059	1054	0.09 ± 0.00
11	terpinen-4-ol	1188	1174	0.16 ± 0.01
12	β-cyclocitral	1229	1217	0.09 ± 0.00
13	safrole	1298	1285	0.08 ± 0.00
14	δ-elemene	1334	1335	0.64 ± 0.00
15	α-copaene	1373	1374	5.07 ± 0.01
16	β-bourbonene	1380	1387	0.37 ± 0.01
17	β-elemene	1388	1389	0.59 ± 0.00
18	β-caryophyllene	1419	1417	27.73 ± 0.02
19	α-caryophyllene	1454	1452	15.12 ± 0.03
20	*allo*-aromadendrene	1457	1458	1.57 ± 0.01
21	germacrene D	1479	1480	13.98 ± 0.01
22	*E*-β-ionone	1487	1487	0.26 ± 0.02
23	bicyclogermacrene	1495	1500	13.32 ± 0.00
24	α-muurolene	1497	1500	2.56 ± 0.00
25	*E,E*−α−farnesene	1505	1505	0.28 ± 0.01
26	β-bisabolene	1507	1505	0.18 ± 0.00
27	δ-cadinene	1519	1522	1.99 ± 0.03
28	*E*-nerolidol	1565	1561	0.34 ± 0.01
29	spathulenol	1580	1577	2.94 ± 0.00
30	caryophyllene oxide	1583	1582	3.24 ± 0.00
31	humulene-1,2-epoxide	1611	1608	1.07 ± 0.04
32	τ-muurolol	1647	1640	0.48 ± 0.02
33	α-muurolol	1651	1644	0.48 ± 0.00
34	α-cadinol	1658	1652	0.78 ± 0.01
35	6*R*,7*R*-bisabolone	1748	1740	0.21 ± 0.01
36	kaurene [4]	-	2042	0.20 ± 0.01
	Total			94.07
	HM			3.16
	OM			0.25
	HS			83.40
	OS			9.80
	HD			0.20
	Others			0.23

[1] It was not possible to discriminate between the two isomers: [2] *para* and [3] *ortho*; AI_{exp}: experimental arithmetic retention indices; AI_{lit}: arithmetic retention indices from the literature [16]; [4] Based on MS analysis; HM: hydrocarbon monoterpenes; OM: oxygenated monoterpenes; HS: hydrocarbon sesquiterpenes; OS: oxygenated sesquiterpenes; HD: hydrocarbon diterpene.

Figure 1 shows a selected expanded chromatogram (18–36 min) and peaks are assigned with the entries 14–35. The peaks 15, 18, 19, 21, and 23 correspond to the major constituents. Expanded GC-MS chromatograms covering entries 1–36 are given as SM (Figure S3A–C).

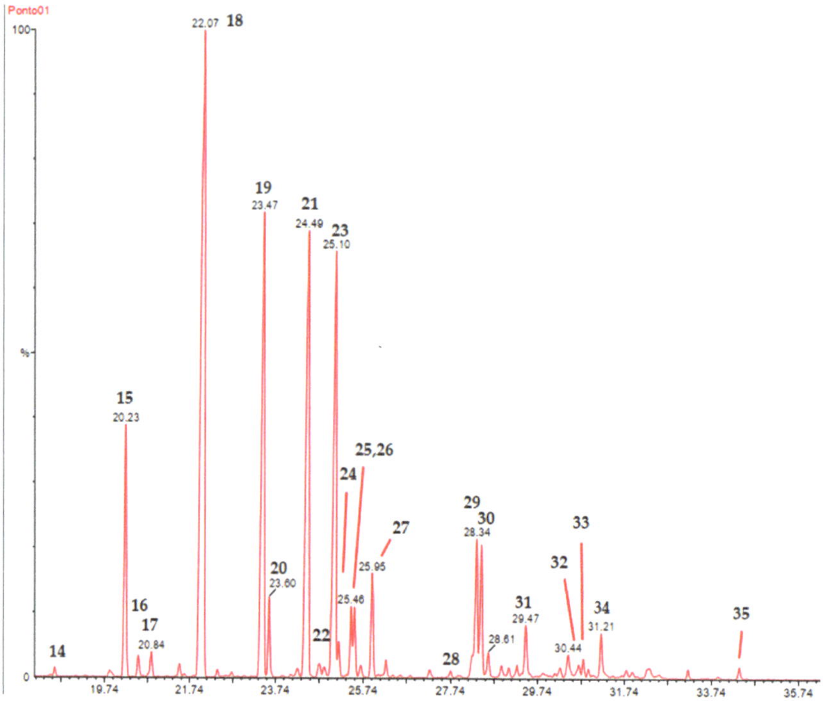

Figure 1. Expanded GC-MS chromatogram of the essential oil from the dry leaves of *V. tweediana*. In the selected region, 18–36 min are the major constituents of the essential oil. Peaks are assigned with entries 14–34.

Based on the chromatogram profile, expressed in the retention times observed in association with the selected analytical conditions [16], it is possible to assert that the essential oil is poor in hydrocarbon and oxygenated monoterpenes since most of them eluted below 18 min. Above 18 min are the hydrocarbon and oxygenated sesquiterpenes, along with the majority of the arylpropanoids. This was confirmed through GC-MS analysis and AIs.

For the identification of each constituent, mass spectra and arithmetic retention indices (AIs) were considered. Table 1 shows the identified constituents with their corresponding AI and concentration. The MS spectra of the constituents and the MS spectra of the identified compound from the NIST library are given as SM (MS Data).

Hydrocarbon sesquiterpene was the main class of secondary metabolites among the 36 compounds characterized, with safrole as the only representative of arylpropanoids but in very low concentration. The caryophyllenes (α and β) comprise approximately 43% of the sample and were the two major constituents, followed by germacrene D (14%) and bicyclogermacrene (13%). Spathulenol and caryophyllene oxide were the main bioactive oxygenated sesquiterpenes found in the sample, however in much lower concentrations, about 3% each.

Infrared Analysis of the Essential Oil

Pure samples provided a spectrum typical of hydrocarbons with a certain degree of unsaturation (Figure 2). Absorptions at 2925 cm^{-1} and 2856 cm^{-1} refer to the Csp^3-

H stretching vibrations, and those at 1448 cm^{-1}, 1382 cm^{-1} and 1357 cm^{-1} are Csp^3-H bend vibrations. The very weak bands at 1633 cm^{-1} and just above 3000 cm^{-1} might be associated with Csp^2-H vibrations, which are comparably less intense due to the low degree of unsaturation in the sample. The presence of C=C bonds is further evidenced by the intense absorption at 738 and 705 cm^{-1}, referring to the =C-H out-of-plane bending.

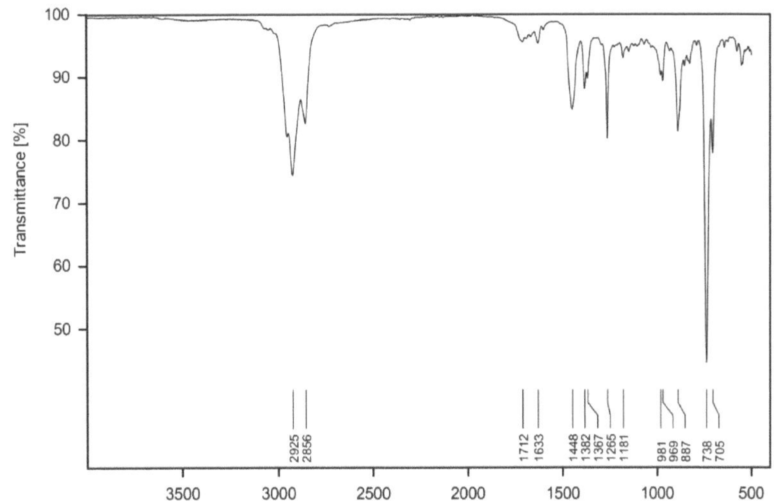

Figure 2. Infrared spectrum of the pure essential oil of *V. tweediana*.

2.2. Biological Assays of Essential Oil from *V. tweediana*

We evaluated the effects of *V. tweediana* essential oil on neutrophil migration in the air pouch model using carrageenan as a phlogistic agent. To assess the in vivo impact, we analyzed histological sections of air pouch tissue from vehicle-treated animals challenged with carrageenan (Figure 3A–C). These sections revealed typical morphological changes associated with inflammation, such as thickening of the air pouch membrane, intense edema, fibrin-hemorrhagic exudate, leukocyte accumulation, and tissue injury. Most of the inflammatory cells observed were neutrophils, identifiable by their lobulated nuclei. These cells were present in high numbers in the injured tissue and distributed throughout the adjacent muscular fibers.

Compared to mice injected with the vehicle, those treated with indomethacin displayed a reduction in the thickness of air pouch membranes challenged with carrageenan (Figure 3L–N). Furthermore, edema was restricted to specific regions, and there was a noticeable decrease in the number of neutrophils infiltrating the area. In addition to fibroblasts and neutrophils, few normal and foamy macrophages were present in the pouch membrane.

Animals treated with *V. tweediana*, particularly those treated with a dosage of 300 mg kg^{-1}, displayed a noticeable reduction in the thickness of air pouches challenged with carrageenan (Figure 3I–K). The pouch wall was formed by loose connective tissue and newly formed blood vessels, and no edema was observed. Additionally, the number of neutrophils and macrophages were significantly decreased compared to the negative control group, and a lining of fibroblast-like cells with no directional orientation was observed. These histological observations suggest that *V. tweediana* essential oil effectively suppresses the acute inflammatory response in the pouch wall.

Figure 4A shows that the *V. tweediana* extract, administered at a dose of 300 mg kg^{-1}, was able to reduce cell counts in the exudate similarly to indomethacin when compared to the control group. Furthermore, differential cell analysis indicated that both *V. tweediana* and indomethacin primarily affected neutrophils (Figure 4B).

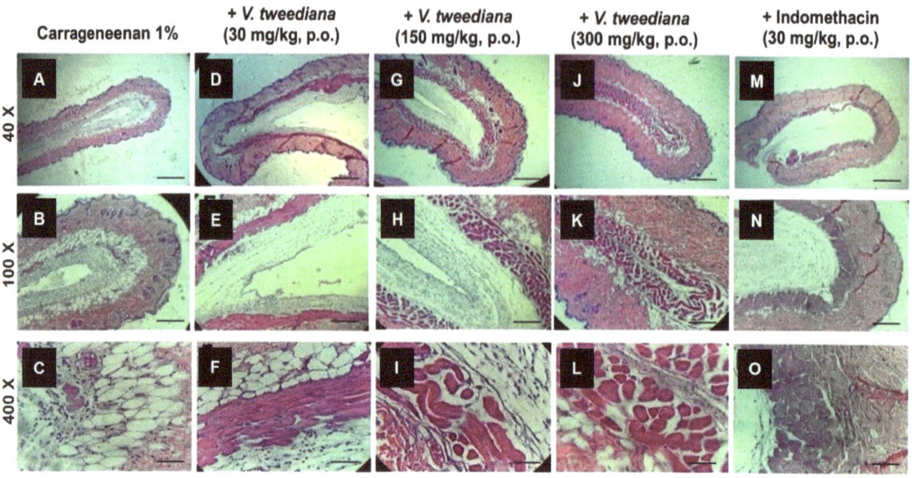

Figure 3. Air pouches were induced in the dorsal subcutaneous tissue of Swiss mice. Illustrative figures of air pouches tissues obtained from animals treated orally with (**A–C**) vehicle, (**D–F**) *V. tweediana* 30 mg/kg, (**G–I**) *V. tweediana* 150 mg/kg, (**J–L**) *V. tweediana* 300 mg/kg, (**M–O**) Indomethacin 30 mg/kg one hour before the injection of 2 mL of carrageenan (1%). Representative H.E. histological sections of skin biopsies obtained from mice with air pouches (40, 100, and 400×). Scale bar = 100 μm.

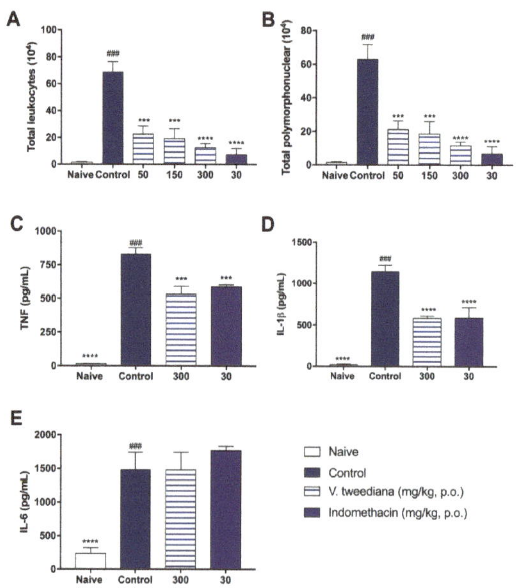

Figure 4. An air pouch was induced in the dorsal subcutaneous tissue of Swiss mice. The animals were treated orally one hour before the injection of 2 mL of carrageenan (1%). The lavage of the inflammatory infiltrate was collected 4 h after the injection of carrageenan into the air pouch. The determination of the (**A**) total number of exudate cells was performed in a Neubauer chamber and the (**B**) differential value was determined. The levels of (**C**) TNF, (**D**) IL-1β, and (**E**) IL-6 were determined using the ELISA method. Values are expressed as the mean ± S. E. M. of tests performed with the inflammatory exudate obtained from 6 animals per group. *** $p < 0.001$ and **** $p < 0.0001$ vs. the control group significantly different from the naïve group ### $p < 0.0001$ (one-way ANOVA followed by Tukey's post hoc test).

In addition to reducing cell counts in the exudate, *V. tweediana* extract at a dose of 300 mg kg^{-1} also decreased the levels of TNF and IL-1β compared to carrageenan-injected mice, as shown in Figure 4C,D. Indomethacin-treated animals exhibited similar results. However, neither the essential oil nor indomethacin influenced IL-6 production, as demonstrated in Figure 4E.

3. Discussion

3.1. Essential Oil Extraction and Chemical Characterization

The dry leaves of *V. tweediana* when submitted to hydrodistillation provided essential oil in yield similar to other species of this genus. For instance, yields of 0.10 and 0.15% were observed for *V. brasiliana* [17] and *V. phosphorica* [18], respectively. On the other hand, *V. montevidensis* gave yields ranging from 0.19–0.21% for fresh leaves [4]. Nevertheless, these yields are considerably lower when compared to representatives of aromatic plants such as the genus *Piper* (Piperaceae), which can reach values of 0.96%, as observed for *P. mikanianum* [19].

The general methodology used to characterize the essential oil, which consisted of gas-phase chromatography with FID and MS detectors, was suitable and provided a level of characterization of 97.04%.

Terpenes were the main class of secondary metabolites present in the analyzed sample, with the predominance of hydrocarbon sesquiterpenes. Identical results were observed in the literature [17,18], except that the hydrocarbon monoterpenes β-pinene and myrcene were the major compounds in *V. montevidensis* [18] and in one work related to *V. phosphorica* [20], respectively. However, the major caryophyllenes (α and β), bicyclogermacrene, germacrene D, and spathulenol are common to this genus.

In contrast, the IR spectrum (Figure 2) does not allow for the identification of single compounds but instead provides a fingerprint of the mixture, which is useful as a preliminary analysis. Furthermore, it is a very accessible instrument, and the IR-ATR technique does not require any additional work during sample preparation.

3.2. Biological Assays

To investigate the anti-inflammatory effects of *V. tweediana*, an in vivo experiment using the air pouch model induced by carrageenan was performed. Carrageenan is known to activate transcription factors such as STAT3 and NF-κB [21], leading to the production and secretion of various inflammatory mediators. The differential analysis of the air pouch-migrated cells, based on the total leukocyte count, showed that the reduction in leukocytes was mainly due to the decrease in polymorphonuclear cells, particularly neutrophil migration. Moreover, histological analyses of the pouch tissue revealed a significant reduction in leukocyte migration and connective tissue edema when compared to the carrageenan group.

During the inflammatory process, the production and release of inflammatory cytokines and chemokines, including TNF, IL-1β, and IL-6, are significantly increased [22]. The findings obtained in this study indicate that treatment with *V. tweediana* extract led to a significant decrease in TNF and IL-1β levels, but no effect on IL-6 was observed. TNF and IL-1β are pro-inflammatory cytokines that play a pivotal role in the initiation and progression of inflammation. They can induce the production and secretion of other cytokines and chemokines, the expression of adhesion molecules, and angiogenesis and mediate systemic inflammatory effects, such as fever, hypotension, and the promotion of neutrophilia. The reduction of TNF and IL-1β levels directly implies a decrease in the progression of the inflammatory process. This reduction results in decreased cell migration and production/secretion of inflammatory cytokines, which in turn contributes to the restoration of homeostasis [23]. IL-6 is a cytokine that is not only released by neutrophils but also by other cell types such as keratinocytes, fibroblasts, and endothelial cells. This broad release by multiple cell types justifies its increased levels in the in vivo model [24].

IL-6 is generally considered a pro-inflammatory cytokine; however, there is some evidence indicating that under certain conditions, it possesses anti-inflammatory properties [25].

The effect observed could be correlated with the presence of β-caryophyllene, which is a bicyclic sesquiterpene that has garnered Food and Drug Administration approval for its promising therapeutic potential. β-caryophyllene binds to cannabinoid receptor type 2 (CB2), primarily expressed in immune and immune-derived cells, which modulate inflammatory responses. Studies on arthritic rats showed that β-caryophyllene possesses analgesic, anti-inflammatory, and antioxidant properties. Recent research suggests that β-caryophyllene's interaction with peroxisome proliferator-activated receptor gamma (PPARγ) may provide some explanation [26].

Furthermore, the essential oil studied herein presents other compounds that may be responsible for its anti-inflammatory activity, such as α-caryophyllene [27], spathulenol [28], and germacrene [29].

Finally, the use of *V. tweediana* as a phytoterapic is consistent with the present findings and might be related to an agonist synergism involving volatiles and non-volatile metabolites [10].

4. Materials and Methods

4.1. Plant Material

The collection of leaves was carried out on 12 October 2019 on the banks of Rua Presidente Costa e Silva, n° 22, Testo Rega, Pomerode, SC (26°42′42.5″ South Latitude and 49°09′51.1″ West Longitude). The intact leaves were placed to dry on a bench at room temperature and in the shade, remaining there until constant mass. Exsiccates of *V. tweediana* were deposited in the Dr. Roberto Miguel Klein herbarium under the code FURB63250 under the supervision of the curator prof. Dr. André Luís de Gasper.

4.2. Essential Oil Extraction

After drying, the leaves were cut into pieces and subjected to hydrodistillation in a modified Clevenger apparatus for 4 h. A proportion of 50 g of plant material to 1 L of deionized water was used. To isolate the EO, the liquid-liquid extraction technique was used with bidistilled dichloromethane as the extracting solvent. The essential oil and hydrolate were transferred to a separation funnel and subjected to 3 (three) successive extractions. The organic fractions were combined in an Erlenmeyer flask, with portions of desiccant agent (magnesium sulfate) added to the flask. The mixture was then filtered into a round-bottom flask and concentrated in a rotary evaporator. The vial containing the EO was kept in a desiccator under vacuum and subsequently weighed to ensure the complete removal of the solvent. The percentage extraction yield was the quotient of the mass of the isolated oil by the mass of the plant material used in the extraction times 100 (one hundred). The oil was stored in a vial and kept refrigerated until analysis.

4.3. Chemical Characterization of the Essential Oil

For the quantification of the EO constituents, a semi-quantitative method was used based on their peak areas without correcting response factors. The concentrations are the mean values of the two analyses. This was carried out using a GC-FID, using an instrument from the Perkin-Elmer brand, model Clarus 600. For the identification of its constituents, we used a Perkin-Elmer gas chromatograph, model Clarus 680 coupled to a Perkin-Elmer model 600T mass detector.

The sample was diluted in an appropriate vial with double-distilled dichloromethane at a concentration of approximately 1% (m/m). The total analysis time was 62 min for both detectors. The injection volume of the samples was 1 microliter in split mode 1:20, with helium as the carrier gas in a flow of 1 mL min^{-1} and DB5 type column measuring 30 m (length), 0.25 mm (internal diameter) and 0.25 μm (thickness of stationary phase). The instruments operated in temperature gradient mode according to Adams [16]: initial column temperature of 60 °C, with a heating rate of 3 °C min^{-1} reaching 240 °C, remaining at that temperature for 2 min. In the GC-FID analysis, the injector temperature was 220 °C and 280 °C for the detector. In the GC-MS analysis, the temperature of the ion source and the transfer line were 250 °C and 240 °C, respectively, and the instrument operated in electron impact mode, with a collision energy of 70 eV, under the same analytical conditions described for GC-FID.

The arithmetic retention index (AI) of each constituent present in the sample was experimentally determined in GC-FID using a homologous series of linear alkanes and applying the Van den Dool and Kratz Equation (1) [16]:

$$AI = 100Z + 100\,(RT_X - RT_Z/RT_{(Z+1)} - RT_Z) \quad (1)$$

where Z: alkane with Z carbons; (Z + 1): alkane with Z + 1 carbons; RT_Z: retention time of the alkane with Z carbons; TR_{Z+1}: retention time of the alkane with Z + 1 carbons; and TR_X: retention time of the constituent x.

Identification of the constituents was carried out using an automatic interpretive program of the NIST spectra library (2008) by visual comparison of the spectra obtained and those available in the literature and by comparing the experimental AI for each of the constituents and those from the literature [16].

Finally, to establish the spectroscopic profile of the essential oil and the identification of its main functional groups, infrared spectroscopy with attenuated total reflectance (IR-ATR) was conducted using Bruker equipment, model Vertex 70.

4.4. Animals

Experiments were performed in male Swiss mice, 6–8 weeks old, (n = 6). All animals were obtained from the Central Animal Facility of the Universidade Regional de Blumenau (FURB) and kept in a climate-controlled room at 22 ± 2°C, under a light/dark (12:12 h) cycle, with water and food ad libitum.

4.5. Leukocyte Migration: Air Pouch Model

Air pouches were produced on the back of the mice. Briefly, the animals were orally treated by gavage with *V. tweediana* essential oil at doses of 50, 150, or 300 mg kg^{-1}, indomethacin (30 mg kg^{-1}, positive control), or vehicle (PBS; 10 mL kg^{-1}). After 1 h, carrageenan (1%; 3 mL/cavity) was injected directly into the air pouch chamber. Four hours later, a small incision was made in the air pouch, the cavity was washed with 3 mL of PBS, and the inflammatory infiltrate was collected for analysis. Total and differential cell counts were performed, and the rest of the exudate was kept for further analysis of cytokines.

4.6. Histological Analysis

The air pouch lining tissue was collected for histological analysis and preserved in formaldehyde solution until the blades were made. The preparation consisted of inserting the tissue fragment into a cassette. The sample was submitted to a 1 h dehydration process in increasing concentrations of ethanol (70%, 96%, and absolute ethanol). Subsequently, each sample was placed in xylol and then in a paraffin bath. After this process, the cassette with the sample was placed in a microtome where serial sections of 3 or 4 µm were made. The sections were placed on slides and stained with hematoxylin and eosin. The samples were then analyzed via optical microscopy (4, 10 and 40×).

4.7. Cytokines Quantification

The levels of tumor necrosis factor (TNF), interleukin (IL)-6, and IL-1β were analyzed in the exudate samples from the air pouch model. The assays were performed according to the manufacturer's instructions (DuoSet R&D Systems—Minneapolis, MN, USA), and the results are expressed in pg mL^{-1}.

4.8. Statistical Analysis

The obtained results are expressed as the mean ± standard error of the mean (SEM) and were statistically analyzed using analysis of variance with multiple comparisons (ANOVA), and, when necessary, the Tukey–Kramer or Dunnett's post hoc test was used. The data were analyzed using the GraphPadPrism® program, assuming $p < 0.05$ as statistically significant.

5. Conclusions

The essential oil from the leaves of *V. tweediana* was characterized by means of GC-FID, GC-MS, and IR-ATR techniques, and hydrocarbon sesquiterpenes make up the largest group present. Biological assays demonstrated notable anti-inflammatory and immunomodulatory activities, including reduced leukocyte migration and modulated cytokine secretion (IL-1β, IL-6, and TNF). These effects are likely linked to the high caryophyllene content. The research suggests the necessity of further studies to assess the synergism between the oil's constituents and to determine the influence of seasonality and circadian rhythm on its chemical composition and production.

The current work is another example of the importance of plant biodiversity, its study, and preservation.

Supplementary Materials: The following supporting information can be downloaded at: https://www.mdpi.com/article/10.3390/ph17111492/s1. Figure S1: GC-FID chromatogram of the essential oil of dry leaves from *Vernonanthura tweediana*, Pomerode, SC-Brazil; Figure S2: GC-MS chromatogram of the essential oil of dry leaves from *Vernonanthura tweediana*, Pomerode, SC-Brazil; Figure S3: A. Expanded GC-MS chromatogram of the essential oil from dried leaves from *Vernonanthura tweediana* (4.65–18.80 min). Identified peaks are assigned with the entries 1–14; B. Expanded GC-MS chromatogram of the essential oil of dry leaves from *Vernonanthura tweediana* (19.59–25.95 min). Identified peaks are assigned with the entries 15–27; C. Expanded GC-MS chromatogram of the essential oil of dry leaves from *Vernonanthura tweediana* (27.20–47.88 min). Identified peaks are assigned with the entries 28–36.

Author Contributions: Conceptualization, R.A.R. and I.D.M.; methodology, R.A.R., I.D.M. and M.R.; validation, R.A.R., I.D.M., I.M.B., M.R., J.R.S., H.D.M.C., C.M.G.L. and T.B.E.; formal analysis, R.A.R., I.D.M., I.M.B. and M.R.; investigation, P.P.B., L.J.A.G., S.C.d.S., L.B., M.R., I.D.M. and R.A.R.; resources, R.A.R., I.D.M., J.R.S. and T.B.E.; writing—original draft preparation, R.A.R., I.D.M. and I.M.B.; writing—review and editing, R.A.R., I.D.M., H.D.M.C., C.M.G.L. and T.B.E.; visualization, R.A.R. and I.D.M.; supervision, R.A.R., I.D.M., M.R. and J.R.S.; project administration, R.A.R. and I.D.M.; funding acquisition, R.A.R. All authors have read and agreed to the published version of the manuscript.

Funding: This research was funded by CNPq-Conselho Nacional de Desenvolvimento Científico e Tecnológico, Brazil, proc. number 444061/2018-5, FAPESC-Fundação de Amparo à Pesquisa e Inovação do Estado de Santa Catarina, proc. number TO-N2019TR0847, and CAPES-Fundação Coordenação de Aperfeiçoamento de Pessoal de Nível Superior, proc. number 88881-848146/2023-01.

Institutional Review Board Statement: All experiments were approved by the local ethics committee (CEUA—Ethics Committee on the Use of Animals/FURB: 002/22).

Informed Consent Statement: Not applicable.

Data Availability Statement: The original contributions presented in this study are included in the article/Supplementary Material. Further inquiries can be directed to the corresponding author(s).

Acknowledgments: We acknowledge the technical support and instrumentation facilities provided by CLAIMS—Instrumental Analysis Laboratory Center, Department of Chemistry-FURB. S.Cd.S. was supported by CAPES (grant Social Demand, proc. number 88882-442473/2019-01). We also acknowledge the scientific and technical support provided by INCT-Catalysis.

Conflicts of Interest: The authors declare no conflicts of interest.

References

1. Rabe, T.; Mullholland, D.; Staden, J. Isolation and identification of antibacterial compounds from *Vernonia colorata* leaves. *J. Ethnopharmacol.* **2002**, *80*, 91–94. [CrossRef] [PubMed]
2. Iwalewa, E.O.; Iwalewa, O.J.; Adeboye, J.O. Analgesic, antipyretic, antiinflammatory effects of methanol, chloroform and ether extracts of *Vernonia cinerea* Less. Leaf. *J. Ethnopharmacol.* **2003**, *86*, 229–234. [CrossRef] [PubMed]
3. Souza, P.V.R.; Mazzei, J.L.; Siani, A.C.; Behrens, M.D. *Vernonia polyanthes* (Spreng.) Less.: Uma visão geral da sua utilização como planta medicinal, composição química e atividades farmacológicas. *Rev. Fitos.* **2017**, *11*, 105–115. [CrossRef]
4. Rebelo, R.A.; Tizziani, T.; Begnini, I.M.; Crestani, I.; Dognini, J.; Gasper, A.L.; Cordova, C.M.M.; Santos, L.; Hochheim, S.; Baldovini, N. Essential oils from leaves of *Vernonanthura montevidensis* (Spreng.) H. Rob.: Chemical profile and antimollicute potential. *Nat. Prod. Res.* **2022**, *36*, 2393–2398. [CrossRef]
5. Tribess, B.; Pintarello, G.B.; Bini, L.A.; Camargo, A.; Funez, L.A.; Gasper, A.L.; Zeni, A.L.B. Ethnobotanical study of plants used for therapeutic purposes in the Atlantic Forest region, Southern Brazil. *J. Ethnopharmacol.* **2015**, *164*, 136–146. [CrossRef] [PubMed]
6. Silva, L.A.L.; Faqueti, L.G.; Reginatto, F.H.; Santos, A.D.C.; Barison, A.; Biavatti, M.W. Phytochemical analysis of *Vernonanthura tweedieana* and a validated UPLC-PDA method for the quantification of eriodictyol. *Rev. Bras. Farmacogn.* **2015**, *25*, 375–381. [CrossRef]
7. Diaz, G.; Nogueira, M.A.; Olguin, C.F.A.; Somensi, A.; Vidotti, G.J. Estudo fitoquímico e biológico de *Vernonia tweediana* Bakes (Asteraceae). *Lat. Am. J. Pharm.* **2008**, *27*, 56–61.
8. Portillo, A.; Vila, R.; Freixa, B.; Ferro, E.; Parella, T.; Casanova, J.; Cañigueral, S. Antifungal sesquiterpene from the root of *Vernonanthura tweedieana*. *J. Ethnophamacol.* **2005**, *97*, 49–52. [CrossRef]
9. Zanon, R.B.; Pereira, D.F.; Boschetti, T.K.; Santos, M.; Athayde, M.L. Phytoconstituents isolated from dichloromethane fraction of *Vernonia tweediana* Baker leaves. *Rev. Bras. Farmacogn.* **2008**, *18*, 226–229.
10. Petri, R.D.; Pletsch, M.U.; Zeifert, M.; Schweigert, I.D. Efeito de extratos hidroetanólicos de *Vernonia tweedieana* e *Vernonia cognata* sobre imunidade de camundongos. *Rev. Bras. Farmacogn.* **2008**, *89*, 139–141.
11. Trevisan, G.; Rossato, M.F.; Walker, C.I.B.; Klafke, J.Z.; Rosa, F.; Oliveira, S.M.; Tonello, R.; Guerra, G.P.; Boligon, A.A.; Zanon, R.B.; et al. Identification of the plant steroid α-spinasterol as a novel transient receptor potential vanilloid 1 antagonist with antinociceptive properties. *J. Pharmacol. Exp. Ther.* **2012**, *343*, 258–269. [CrossRef] [PubMed]
12. Olguin, C.F.A.; Hamerski, L.; Percio, M.F.; Somensi, A. Avaliação do potencial biológico alelopático dos extratos fracionados da raiz de *Vernonia tweediana* baker. *Rev. Varia Sci.* **2005**, *5*, 137–143. Available online: https://e-revista.unioeste.br/index.php/variascientia/article/view/252 (accessed on 28 October 2024).
13. Bunse, M.; Daniels, R.; Gründemann, C.; Heilmann, J.; Kammerer, D.R.; Keusgen, M.; Lindequist, U.; Melzig, M.F.; Morlock, G.E.; Schulz, H.; et al. Essential Oils as Multicomponent Mixtures and Their Potential for Human Health and Well-Being. *Front. Pharmacol.* **2022**, *13*, 956541. [CrossRef]
14. Fullerton, J.N.; Gilroy, D.W. Resolution of inflammation: A new therapeutic frontier. *Nat. Rev. Drug Discov.* **2016**, *15*, 551–567. [CrossRef]
15. Miguel, M.G. Antioxidant and anti-inflammatory activities of essential oils: A short review. *Molecules* **2010**, *15*, 9252–9287. [CrossRef] [PubMed]
16. Adams, R.P. *Identification of Essential Oils Components by Gas Chromatography, Mass Spectroscopy*, 4th ed.; Allured Publishing: Carol Stream, IL, USA, 2017; 809p.
17. Maia, A.I.V.; Torres, M.C.M.; Pessoa, O.D.L.; de Menezes, J.E.S.A.; Costa, S.M.O.; Nogueira, V.L.R.; Melo, V.M.M.; de Souza, E.B.; Cavalcante, M.G.B.; Albuquerque, M.R.J.R. Óleos essenciais das folhas de *Vernonia remotiflora* e *Vernonia brasiliana*: Composicão química e atividade biológica. *Quím. Nova* **2010**, *33*, 584–586. [CrossRef]
18. Barbosa, L.N.; Probst, I.S.; Andrade, B.F.M.T.; Alves, F.C.B.; Albano, M.; da Cunha, M.L.R.S.; Doyama, J.T.; Rall, V.L.M.; Junior, A.F. In vitro antibacterial and chemical properties of essential oils including native plants from Brazil against pathogenic and resistant bacteria. *J. Oleo Sci.* **2015**, *64*, 289–298. [CrossRef]
19. Carneiro, J.N.P.; Cruza, R.P.; Campina, F.F.; Costa, M.S.; Santos, A.T.L.; Sales, D.L.; Bezerra, C.F.; Silva, L.E.; Araujo, J.P.; Amaral, W.; et al. GC/MS analysis and antimicrobial activity of the *Piper mikanianum* (Kunth) Steud. essential oil. *Food Chem. Toxicol.* **2020**, *135*, 110987. [CrossRef]
20. Moreira, R.R.D.; Martins, G.Z.; Varandas, R.; Cogo, J.; Perego, C.H.; Roncoli, G.; Sousa, M.C.; Nakamura, C.V.; Salgueiro, L.; Cavaleiro, C. Composition and leishmanicidal activity of the essential oil of *Vernonia polyanthes* Less (Asteraceae). *Nat. Prod. Res.* **2017**, *31*, 2905–2908. [CrossRef]
21. Fathi, M.A.A.; El-Hafeez, A.A.A.; Abdelhamid, D.; Abbas, S.H.; Montano, M.M.; Mohamed Abdel-Aziz, M. 1,3,4-oxadiazole/chalcone hybrids: Design, synthesis, and inhibition of leukemia cell growth and EGFR, Src, IL-6 and STAT3 activities. *Bioorg. Chem.* **2019**, *84*, 150–163. [CrossRef]
22. Rosales, C. Neutrophil: A cell with many roles in inflammation or several cell types? *Front. Physiol.* **2018**, *9*, 113. [CrossRef] [PubMed]
23. Rea, I.M.; Gibson, D.S.; McGilligan, V.; McNerlan, S.E.; Alexander, H.D.; Ross, O.A. Age and Age-Related Diseases: Role of Inflammation Triggers and Cytokines. *Front. Immunol.* **2018**, *9*, 586. [CrossRef] [PubMed]
24. Sproston, N.R.; Ashworth, J.J. Role of C-reactive protein at sites of inflammation and infection. *Front. Immunol.* **2018**, *9*, 754. [CrossRef] [PubMed]

25. Xing, Z.; Gauldie, J.; Cox, G.; Baumann, H.; Jordana, M.; Lei, X.F.; Achong, M.K. IL-6 is an anti-inflammatory cytokine required for controlling local or systemic acute inflammatory responses. *J. Clin. Investig.* **1998**, *101*, 311–312. [CrossRef]
26. Irrera, N.; D'Ascola, A.; Pallio, G.; Bitto, A.; Mazzon, E.; Mannino, F.; Squadrito, V.; Arcoraci, V.; Minutoli, L.; Campo, G.M.; et al. β-Caryophyllene Mitigates Collagen Antibody Induced Arthritis (CAIA) in Mice Through a Cross-Talk Between CB2 and PPAR-γ Receptors. *Biomolecules* **2019**, *9*, 326. [CrossRef] [PubMed]
27. Viveiros, M.M.H.; Silva, M.G.; da Costa, J.G.M.; de Oliveira, A.G.; Rubio, C.; Padovani, C.R.; Rainho, C.A.; Schellini, S.A. Anti-inflammatory effects of α-humulene and β-caryophyllene on pterygium fibroblasts. *Int. J. Ophthalmol.* **2022**, *15*, 1903–1907. [CrossRef]
28. do Nascimento, K.F.; Moreira, F.M.F.; Santos, J.A.; Kassuya, C.A.L.; Croda, J.H.R.; Cardoso, C.A.L.; Vieira, M.D.C.; Góis Ruiz, A.L.T.G.; Foglio, M.A.; de Carvalho, J.E.; et al. Antioxidant, anti-inflammatory, antiproliferative and antimycobacterial activities of the essential oil of *Psidium guineense* Sw. and spathulenol. *J. Ethnopharmacol.* **2018**, *10*, 351–358. [CrossRef]
29. Tosun, A.; Chun, J.; Jerković, I.; Marijanović, Z.; Fenu, M.A.; Aslan, S.S.; Tuberoso, C.I.G.; Kim, Y.S. Chemical Profiles and Anti-inflammatory Activity of the Essential Oils from *Seseli gummiferum* and *Seseli corymbosum* subsp. *corymbosum*. *Nat. Prod. Commun.* **2016**, *11*, 1523–1526. [CrossRef] [PubMed]

pharmaceuticals

Article

Antidepressant-like Effects of *Cannabis sativa* L. Extract in an Lipopolysaccharide Model: Modulation of Mast Cell Activation in Deep Cervical Lymph Nodes and Dura Mater

Joonyoung Shin [1,†], Dong-Uk Kim [2,†], Gi-Sang Bae [2], Ji-Ye Han [3], Do-Won Lim [3], Young-Mi Lee [3], Eunjae Kim [4], Eunjeong Kwon [4], Dongwoon Han [1,5] and Sungchul Kim [1,*]

1 Institute for Global Rare Disease Network, Professional Graduate School of Korean Medicine, Wonkwang University, Iksan 54538, Republic of Korea; spm1219@naver.com (J.S.); dwhan@hanyang.ac.kr (D.H.)
2 Department of Pharmacology, School of Korean Medicine, Wonkwang University, Iksan 54538, Republic of Korea; ckck202@naver.com (D.-U.K.); baegs888@wku.ac.kr (G.-S.B.)
3 Department of Oriental Pharmacy, Wonkwang-Oriental Medicines Research Institute, College of Pharmacy, Wonkwang University, Iksan 54538, Republic of Korea; hsue0112@gmail.com (J.-Y.H.); limsc05@wku.ac.kr (D.-W.L.); ymlee@wku.ac.kr (Y.-M.L.)
4 College of Pharmacy, Kyung Hee University, Seoul 02447, Republic of Korea; dmswo3537@naver.com (E.K.); dmswjd4876@naver.com (E.K.)
5 Department of Global Health and Development, Hanyang University, Seoul 04763, Republic of Korea
* Correspondence: kscndl@naver.com; Tel.: +82-63-850-7562
† These authors contributed equally to this work.

Abstract: Background: Lipopolysaccharide (LPS)-induced neuroinflammation is a well-established model for studying depression-like behavior, driven by pro-inflammatory cytokines such as TNF-α and IL-1β. Mast cells (MCs) contribute to neuroinflammation by releasing mediators that exacerbate depressive-like symptoms. This study evaluates the antidepressant-like and anti-inflammatory effects of *Cannabis sativa* L. inflorescence extract (CSL) in an LPS-induced neuroinflammation model. Methods: Male C57BL/6 mice were intraperitoneally injected with CSL at doses of 10, 20, and 30 mg/kg, 30 min prior to LPS (0.83 mg/kg) administration. Depressive behaviors were assessed using the sucrose preference test (SPT), tail suspension test (TST), and forced swimming test (FST). The neutrophil-to-lymphocyte ratio (NLR) was measured to assess systemic inflammation. Cytokine levels in the prefrontal cortex (PFC) were measured, and mast cell degranulation in the lymph nodes and dura mater was analyzed histologically (approval number: WKU24-64). Results: CSL significantly improved depressive-like behaviors and decreased the NLR, indicating reduced systemic inflammation. CSL also significantly reduced TNF-α and IL-1β levels in the PFC. Furthermore, CSL inhibited MC degranulation in the deep cervical lymph nodes and dura mater, with the strongest effects observed at 30 mg/kg. Conclusions: CSL demonstrated antidepressant-like and anti-inflammatory effects in an LPS-induced neuroinflammation model, likely through the modulation of cytokine expression and mast cell activity. These results suggest the potential of CSL as a therapeutic option for treating inflammation-related depression.

Keywords: *Cannabis sativa* L. inflorescence extract; lipopolysaccharide; mast cells; cytokine; deep cervical lymph nodes; dura mater

Citation: Shin, J.; Kim, D.-U.; Bae, G.-S.; Han, J.-Y.; Lim, D.-W.; Lee, Y.-M.; Kim, E.; Kwon, E.; Han, D.; Kim, S. Antidepressant-like Effects of *Cannabis sativa* L. Extract in an Lipopolysaccharide Model: Modulation of Mast Cell Activation in Deep Cervical Lymph Nodes and Dura Mater. *Pharmaceuticals* **2024**, *17*, 1409. https://doi.org/10.3390/ph17101409

Academic Editors: Catherine Sherwin, Elena Y. Enioutina and Kathleen M. Job

Received: 24 September 2024
Revised: 16 October 2024
Accepted: 18 October 2024
Published: 21 October 2024

1. Introduction

Major Depressive Disorder (MDD) is a widespread and severe mental health condition, characterized by persistent symptoms. These include profound sadness, loss of interest in previously pleasurable activities (anhedonia), motor agitation or slowing, feelings of guilt or worthlessness, difficulty focusing, and recurring thoughts of death or suicide [1]. Recent studies are exploring the connection between elevated levels of pro-inflammatory cytokines, including tumor necrosis factor-alpha (TNF-α), Interleukin 1 beta (IL-1β), and

IL-6, and the development of MDD [2,3]. Mast cells (MCs), key components of the innate immune system, have been implicated in these neuroinflammatory processes by releasing cytokines, chemokines, and other pro-inflammatory mediators [4]. These immune activities are thought to contribute to psychiatric disorders like MDD by interacting with the brain's immune system, potentially triggering neuroinflammatory responses that lead to depressive symptoms [5–7]. A well-known trigger of immune responses is lipopolysaccharide (LPS), a component of bacterial cell walls. Studies have shown that administering LPS can lead to sickness behaviors in animal models, such as depression-like behavior, anhedonia, and increased anxiety [8,9]. Similarly, LPS has also been associated with depressive symptoms in humans [10,11]. Notably, mice administered LPS (5 mg/kg, i.p.) exhibited dysfunction in deep cervical lymph nodes (dcLNs) and alterations in meningeal lymphatic drainage and morphology, leading to heightened neuroinflammation and cognitive impairment [12]. These findings suggest a critical role for immune system dysfunction in the development and exacerbation of depressive symptoms in MDD.

Cannabis sativa L. is a dioecious annual plant known for its diverse pharmacological properties. Cultivated primarily in Central Asia, particularly in regions like India and China, since ancient times [13], *Cannabis sativa* L. contains bioactive compounds, including cannabinoids such as cannabidiol (CBD) and delta-9-tetrahydrocannabinol (Δ9-THC) [14]. These cannabinoids are especially significant because of their therapeutic potential. Δ9-THC, a psychoactive compound, and CBD, a non-psychoactive compound, both interact with endocannabinoid receptors [15], offering therapeutic effects for various conditions, including epilepsy, inflammation, and MDD [16–18]. Additionally, cannabidiolic acid methyl ester, a derivative of cannabidiolic acid (CBDA), has demonstrated the ability to reduce stress-induced anxiety-like behaviors in depressed rat models [19]. In addition to cannabinoids, *Cannabis sativa* L. is rich in terpenes, which play a significant role in its wide-ranging pharmacological effects, including anti-inflammatory and pain-relieving properties [20]. Terpenes are among the most varied plant compounds, with key constituents such as α-pinene, β-pinene, myrcene, limonene, β-caryophyllene, and α-humulene. These terpenes offer a wide range of health benefits, including anti-inflammatory, anticancer, and antibacterial effects [21,22]. Interestingly, myrcene has been shown to reduce the expression of pro-inflammatory cytokines such as IL-1β, IL-6, IL-8, and TNF-α [23]. In addition, α-pinene reduces Parkinson's disease symptoms [24], and alleviates postpartum depression through its antioxidant properties [25]. These findings highlight the diverse bioactive compounds in *Cannabis sativa* L. and their potential role in managing inflammation.

This study aimed to evaluate the effects of *Cannabis sativa* L. inflorescence extract (CSL) on LPS-induced depressive-like behaviors in mice. Additionally, the study assessed the ability of CSL to modulate MC activation in the dcLNs and dura mater, regions known to be involved in neuroinflammation, as well as its impact on the neutrophil-to-lymphocyte ratio (NLR) as an inflammatory marker. Furthermore, we examined the inhibitory effect of CSL on pro-inflammatory cytokines (TNF-α, and IL-1β) in the prefrontal cortex (PFC). These findings suggest that CSL may offer valuable insights into the interactions between mast cell activation and inflammation in neuroinflammatory conditions.

2. Results

2.1. Cannabinoids and Terpenes Contents in CSL

A typical total ion chromatogram (TIC) for the conversion products of CSL under acidic reaction conditions, as analyzed in gas chromatography–mass spectrometry (GC-MS) scan mode, is shown in Figure 1a. CBDA (peak 6, 1209.39 μg/mg), and CBCA (peak 8, 18.99 μg/mg) were detected as major cannabinoid components of CSL (Figure 1a). Terpenes were detected in CSL using headspace–gas chromatography/mass spectrometry (HS-GC/MS). Myrcene (peak 3, 2284.17 μg/mg) and α-Pinene (peak 1, 1115.25 μg/mg) were detected as major terpenes of CSL (Figure 1b).

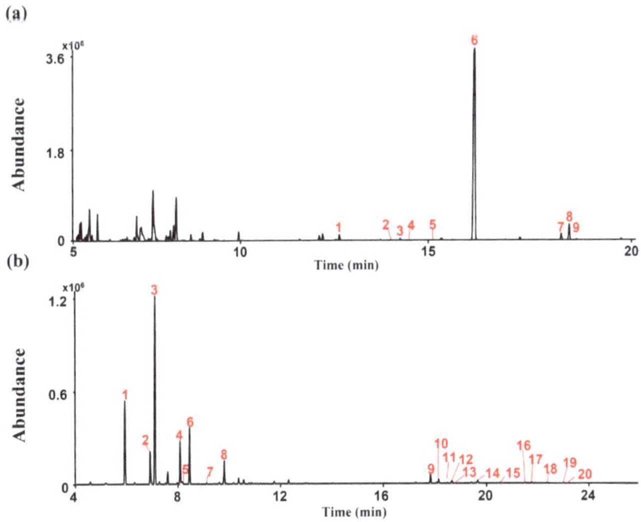

Figure 1. Total ion chromatograms (TICs) of CSL. (**a**) Peak identities by GC-MS are as follows: 1. CBD; 2. CBC; 3. Δ8-THC; 4. Δ9-THC; 5. CBG; 6. CBDA; 7. THCA; 8. CBCA; 9. CBGA. (**b**) Peak identities by headspace GC-MS are as follows: 1. α-Pinene; 2. β-Pinene; 3. Myrcene; 4. D-Limonene; 5. Eucalyptol; 6. β-Ocimene; 7. γ-Terpinene; 8. Sabienen hydrate; 9. β-Caryophyllene; 10. trans-α-Bergamotene; 11. E-β-Farnesene; 12. α-Humulene; 13. Alloaromadrene; 14. β-Bisabolene; 15. cis-α-Bisabolene; 16.Carophyllene oxid; 17 Guaiol; 18. γ-Eudesmol; 19. α-Eudesmol; 20.Bulnesol.

2.2. Antidepressant-like Effect of CSL in the LPS Model

In the sucrose preference test (SPT), the LPS group presented a decreased sucrose preference (45.35 ± 4.30%) compared to the control (CON) group (77.71 ± 6.86%, $p < 0.001$, Figure 2a). CSL administration significantly increased sucrose preference in a dose-dependent manner compared to the LPS group. The sucrose preference for the 10 mg/kg CSL + LPS group was 58.85 ± 4.58% ($p < 0.05$), for the 20 mg/kg CSL + LPS group was 63.96 ± 10.65% ($p < 0.001$), and for the 30 mg/kg CSL + LPS group was 67.86 ± 5.55% ($p < 0.001$). No significant differences were observed between the CSL + LPS groups.

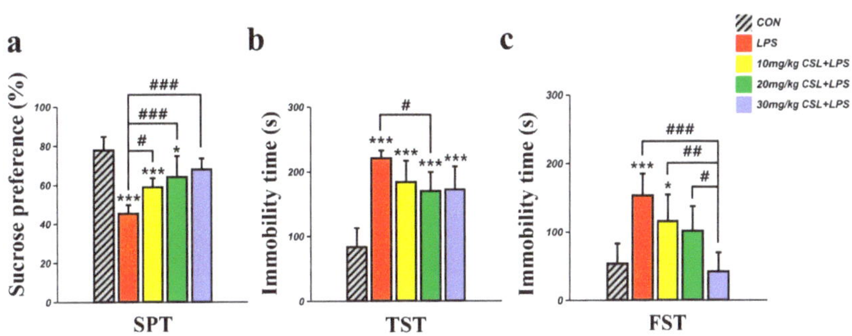

Figure 2. Behavioral effect of CSL administration in the LPS model. (**a**) Sucrose preference test, (**b**) immobility time in the tail suspension test (TST), and (**c**) immobility time in the forced swimming test (FST). Results are expressed as mean ± standard deviation (S.D.). One-way ANOVA followed by Tukey's post hoc test. *, compared with the CON group; #, compared between the groups. */#, $p < 0.05$; ##, $p < 0.01$; ***/###, $p < 0.001$. (n = 6 per group).

In the tail suspension test (TST), the LPS group presented an increased immobility time (220.38 ± 11.84 s) compared to the CON group (82.81 ± 29.56 s, $p < 0.001$, Figure 2b). CSL administration reduced immobility time across all groups compared to the LPS group, but a significant reduction was observed only in the 20 mg/kg CSL + LPS group. The immobility time for the 10 mg/kg CSL + LPS group was 183.36 ± 32.75 s, for the 20 mg/kg CSL + LPS group was 169.81 ± 29.20 s ($p < 0.05$), and for the 30 mg/kg CSL + LPS group was 171.93 ± 35.53 s. No significant differences were observed between the CSL + LPS groups.

In the forced swimming test (FST), the LPS group presented an increased immobility time (152.93 ± 31.68 s) compared to the CON group (52.76 ± 29.53 s, $p < 0.001$, Figure 2c). CSL administration reduced immobility time in a dose-dependent manner compared to the LPS group, but a significant reduction was observed only in the 30 mg/kg CSL + LPS group. The immobility time for the 10 mg/kg CSL group was 115.28 ± 38.77 s, for the 20 mg/kg CSL + LPS group was 101.13 ± 35.91 s, and for the 30 mg/kg CSL + LPS group was 41.56 ± 27.46 s ($p < 0.001$). Notably, the 30 mg/kg CSL + LPS group showed a significantly lower immobility time compared to the other CSL + LPS groups: 10 mg/kg CSL + LPS group ($p < 0.01$) and 20 mg/kg CSL + LPS group ($p < 0.05$).

2.3. Hematological Inflammatory Markers: NLR, Monocytes, Eosinophils, and Basophils

The LPS group (2.64 ± 1.25) presented increased neutrophil to lymphocyte ratio (NLR) values compared to the CON group (0.23 ± 0.04, Figure 3a). CSL administration reduced NLR values in a dose-dependent manner compared to the LPS group, with a significant reduction observed in all CSL + LPS groups except the 10 mg/kg CSL + LPS group. The NLR values were 1.81 ± 0.98 for the 10 mg/kg CSL + LPS group, 0.66 ± 0.15 for the 20 mg/kg CSL + LPS group ($p < 0.001$), and 0.52 ± 0.20 for the 30 mg/kg CSL + LPS group ($p < 0.001$). Notably, the 30 mg/kg CSL + LPS group showed significantly lower NLR values compared to the 10 mg/kg CSL + LPS groups ($p < 0.05$, Figure 3a). The LPS group presented increased monocyte (MONO) values (6.00 ± 3.07) compared to the CON group (1.03 ± 0.39, $p < 0.001$, Figure 3b). CSL administration reduced MONO values in a dose-dependent manner compared to the LPS group, but there were no significant differences (Figure 3b). The MONO values were 5.00 ± 2.05 for the 10 mg/kg CSL + LPS group, 4.48 ± 0.95 for the 20 mg/kg CSL + LPS group, and 4.10 ± 1.69 for the 30 mg/kg CSL + LPS group. For eosinophils (EOS) and basophils (BASO), no significant differences in values were observed between each group.

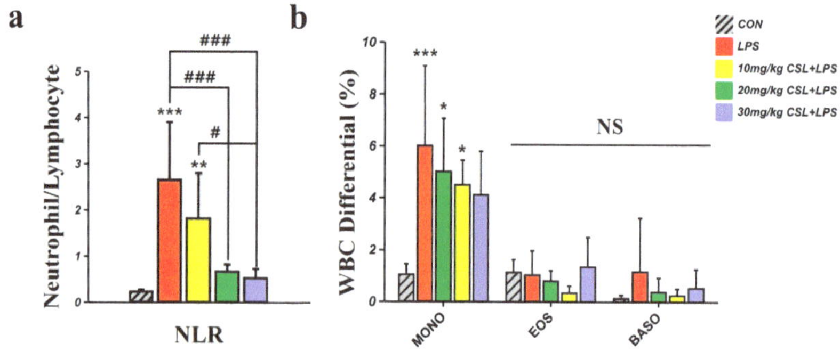

Figure 3. Hematological inflammatory markers following CSL administration in the LPS model. (**a**) Neutrophil to lymphocyte ratio (NLR), (**b**) monocytes (MONO), eosinophils (EOS), and basophils (BASO). Results are expressed as mean ± standard deviation (S.D.). One-way ANOVA followed by Tukey's post hoc test. *, compared with the CON group; #, compared between the groups; NS, not significant. */#, $p < 0.05$; **, $p < 0.01$; ***/###, $p < 0.001$. ($n = 6$ per group).

2.4. Activation of Mast Cells (MCs) in Lymph Nodes (LNs)

The LPS administration showed no significant differences in the area of lymph nodes (LNs) and the number of MCs in both the dcLNs and submandibular lymph nodes (smLNs) compared to the CON group (Figure 4b,c). CSL administration also did not result in significant differences in LN size or MC counts in either LN type. On the other hand, CSL significantly decreased the degranulation rate of MCs in both node types compared to the LPS group.

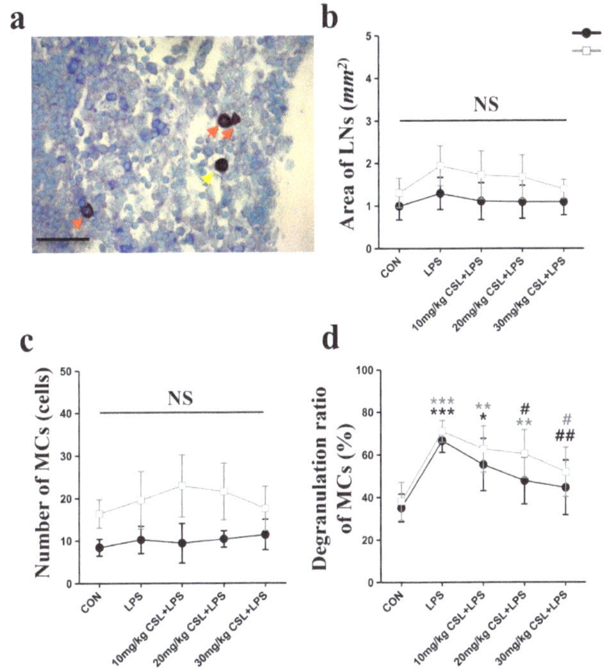

Figure 4. Effects of CSL on mast cell (MC) activation in deep cervical lymph nodes (dcLNs) and submandibular lymph nodes (smLNs) in the LPS model. (**a**) Representative LN image showing mast cell degranulation (red arrows: degranulated MCs, yellow arrow: non-degranulated MCs, scale bar: 100 μm), (**b**) area of LNs, (**c**) number of MCs, (**d**) degranulation ratio of MCs. Results are expressed as mean ± standard deviation (S.D.). One-way ANOVA followed by Tukey's post hoc test. *, compared with the CON group; #, compared with the LPS group; NS, not significant. */#, $p < 0.05$; **/##, $p < 0.01$; ***, $p < 0.001$. ($n = 6$ per group).

In the smLNs, the LPS group exhibited an increased degranulation rate (70.82 ± 5.09%) compared to the CON group (38.01 ± 8.93%, $p < 0.001$, Figure 4d). CSL administration reduced the degranulation rate in a dose-dependent manner, but a significant reduction was observed only in the 30 mg/kg CSL + LPS group. The degranulation rates were 62.51 ± 10.77% for the 10 mg/kg CSL group, 62.71 ± 10.16% for the 20 mg/kg CSL + LPS group, and 51.65 ± 11.53% for the 30 mg/kg CSL + LPS group ($p < 0.05$).

In the dcLNs, the LPS group showed a higher degranulation rate (66.40 ± 5.43%) compared to the CON group (34.93 ± 6.53%, $p < 0.001$, Figure 4d). CSL reduced the degranulation rate in a dose-dependent manner, with significant reductions observed in all groups except the 10 mg/kg CSL + LPS group. The degranulation rates were 55.16 ± 12.24% for the 10 mg/kg CSL group, 47.60 ± 10.96% for the 20 mg/kg CSL + LPS group ($p < 0.05$), and 44.33 ± 12.81% for the 30 mg/kg CSL + LPS group ($p < 0.01$). Although smLNs generally showed higher values than dcLNs for LN area, MC count, and degranulation rate, these differences were not statistically significant.

2.5. Activation of Mast Cells (MCs) in Dura Mater

The LPS administration did not result in significant differences in the number of MCs in both the parietal and superior sagittal sinus (SSS) regions of the dura mater. CSL administration also did not result in significant differences in MC counts in either dura mater region. However, consistent with the LN results, CSL significantly decreased the degranulation rate of MCs in both regions compared to the LPS group.

In the parietal region, the LPS group exhibited a higher degranulation rate (44.30 ± 12.33%) compared to the CON group (26.86 ± 7.26%, $p < 0.01$, Figure 5e). CSL administration reduced the degranulation rate in a dose-dependent manner, with a significant reduction observed only in the 30 mg/kg CSL + LPS group. The degranulation rates were 37.01 ± 6.28% for the 10 mg/kg CSL group, 32.55 ± 3.61% for the 20 mg/kg CSL + LPS group, and 30.14 ± 5.03% for the 30 mg/kg CSL + LPS group ($p < 0.05$).

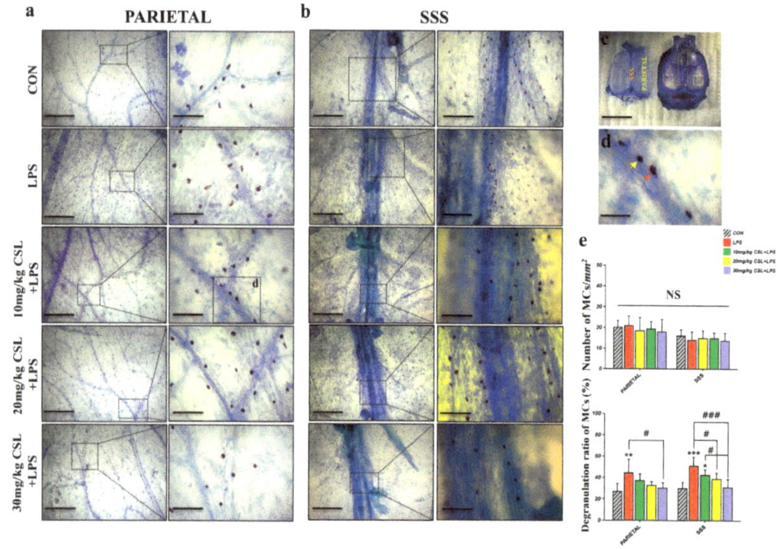

Figure 5. Effects of CSL on mast cell (MC) activation in the dura mater of the LPS model. (**a**) Representative images of MCs in the parietal region and (**b**) in the superior sagittal sinus (SSS) region. The right side of each image is a magnified view of the area highlighted by the dashed box. Scale bar: (**a**) left: 1 mm, right: 200 µm; (**b**) left: 1 mm, right (CON and LPS groups): 400 µm, (CSL groups): 200 µm. (**c**) Dura mater separated from the skull, with the parietal region marked by a yellow dashed box and the SSS region by an orange dashed box. Scale bar: 10 mm. (**d**) Representative image of MCs in the dura mater (red arrow: degranulated MCs, yellow arrow: non-degranulated MCs, scale bar: 100 µm). (**e**) Number of MCs/mm^2, and degranulation ratio of MCs. Results are expressed as mean ± standard deviation (S.D.). One-way ANOVA followed by Tukey's post hoc test. *, compared with the CON group; #, compared between the groups; NS, not significant. */#, $p < 0.05$; **, $p < 0.01$; ***/###, $p < 0.001$. (n = 6 per group).

In the SSS region, the LPS group showed an increased degranulation rate (50.79 ± 8.36%) compared to the CON group (29.69 ± 6.03%, $p < 0.001$, Figure 5e). CSL administration reduced the degranulation rate in a dose-dependent manner, with significant reductions observed in all CSL + LPS groups, except the 10 mg/kg CSL + LPS group. The degranulation rates were 42.45 ± 4.92% for the 10 mg/kg CSL group, 36.90 ± 6.86% for the 20 mg/kg CSL + LPS group ($p < 0.05$), and 30.66 ± 7.76% for the 30 mg/kg CSL + LPS group ($p < 0.001$). Notably, the 30 mg/kg CSL + LPS group exhibited a significantly lower degranulation rate compared to the 10 mg/kg CSL + LPS group ($p < 0.05$, Figure 5e).

2.6. Inhibitory Effect of CSL on the Expression of TNF-α, and IL-1β in the PFC

The LPS group presented an increased TNF-α mRNA level, compared to the CON group ($p < 0.001$, Figure 6a). CSL administration reduced TNF-α mRNA levels in a dose-dependent manner compared to the LPS group, with a significant reduction observed in the 20 mg/kg CSL + LPS group ($p < 0.01$) and the 30 mg/kg CSL + LPS group ($p < 0.01$). The LPS group presented increased IL-1β mRNA level, compared to the CON group ($p < 0.001$, Figure 6b). CSL administration reduced IL-1β mRNA levels in a dose-dependent manner compared to the LPS group, while a significant reduction was observed only in the 30 mg/kg CSL + LPS group ($p < 0.05$).

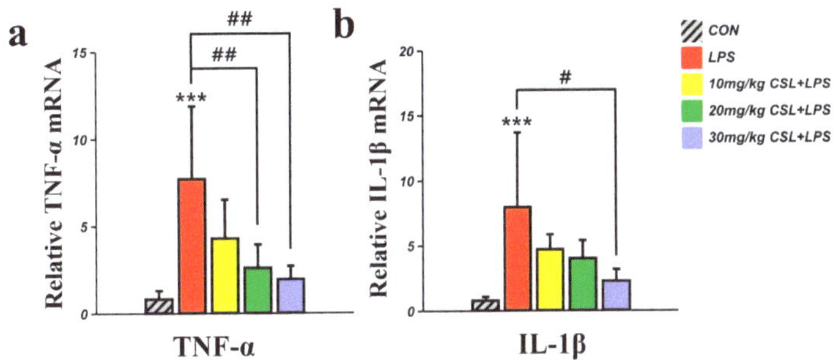

Figure 6. Inhibitory effects of CSL on the expression of pro-inflammatory cytokines in the prefrontal cortex (PFC) of the LPS model. (**a**) TNF-α mRNA level and (**b**) IL-1β mRNA level in the PFC. CSL administration significantly reduced the expression of TNF-α and IL-1β in a dose-dependent manner compared to the LPS group. Results are expressed as mean ± standard deviation (S.D.). One-way ANOVA followed by Tukey's post hoc test. *, compared with the CON group; #, compared between the groups. #, $p < 0.05$; ##, $p < 0.01$; ***, $p < 0.001$. ($n = 6$ per group).

3. Discussion

This study investigated the antidepressant-like effects of CSL in an LPS-induced depression model. The results from the SPT, TST, and FST indicated that CSL significantly reduced depressive-like behaviors. Furthermore, CSL notably modulated mast cell (MC) activation in the smLNs, dcLNs, and dura mater. Hematological analysis demonstrated that CSL effectively lowered the neutrophil-to-lymphocyte ratio (NLR), and analysis of the PFC revealed a significantly inhibited expression of pro-inflammatory cytokines like TNF-α and IL-1β.

Behavioral tests such as the SPT, TST, and FST are well-recognized tools for evaluating depression-like behaviors in preclinical models of depression. Anhedonia, characterized by a diminished capacity to experience pleasure, is a core symptom of depression and can be effectively modeled using the SPT, where a reduction in sucrose preference is indicative of anhedonia [26]. Conversely, the TST and FST are designed to assess behavioral despair, with increased immobility interpreted as a lack of escape-driven behavior, a feature commonly associated with depression [27,28]. LPS-induced depression models are widely used to replicate inflammation-related depressive conditions, as LPS administration elicits sickness behaviors, including decreased sucrose preference and increased immobility, by activating peripheral and central inflammatory responses. [29]. In our study, LPS administration led to decreased sucrose preference in the SPT and heightened immobility in both the TST and FST, aligning with its established depressive-like effects [18,30]. Treatment with CSL reversed these effects in a dose-dependent manner, restoring sucrose preference and reducing immobility, which suggests an antidepressant-like action. These results are consistent with previous research showing the efficacy of cannabinoids in mitigating inflammation-induced behavioral changes, likely through the modulation of neuroimmune pathways [14,18,31]. However, it is important to note that while a clear dose-dependent effect of CSL was observed in the FST and SPT, the TST did not demonstrate the same level of dose-dependency at the 30 mg/kg dose. This discrepancy may be attributed to the TST's lower sensitivity to cannabinoid effects compared to the FST and SPT, which may engage distinct neurobiological pathways [17]. Additionally, pharmacokinetic factors, such as the distribution and metabolism of cannabinoids, could influence receptor activation differently across these tests [32]. Further investigations are warranted to explore these differences, with future studies incorporating additional dosing regimens and behavioral assays to more comprehensively assess the therapeutic potential of CSL.

The NLR is gaining recognition as a reliable indicator of systemic inflammation and is widely used in clinical and preclinical models to assess immune responses during stress conditions [33]. An elevated NLR reflects a disruption in immune regulation, primarily resulting from increased neutrophil activity and decreased lymphocyte levels, both indicative of heightened inflammatory responses [34]. Neutrophils function as the primary line of defense in the host immune response against pathogens, utilizing mechanisms such as chemotaxis, phagocytosis, and the release of reactive oxygen species (ROS), granular proteins, and cytokines [35]. As essential regulators of innate immunity, neutrophils recruit, activate, and modulate the functions of other immune cells through the secretion of pro-inflammatory and immunomodulatory cytokines and chemokines. This activity promotes the recruitment and activation of immune cells such as dendritic cells, natural killer (NK) cells, and CD4 and CD8 T cells [36]. In animal models, the administration of LPS is known to cause systemic inflammation, as evidenced by elevated NLR, indicating a peripheral inflammatory burden [37]. LPS activates various immune cells, including MCs and neutrophils [38,39]. Specifically, LPS binds to receptors on leukocytes, inducing the release of pro-inflammatory cytokines such as TNF-α, IL-6, and IL-1β [40]. NLR has been shown to change in MDD and has been associated with various factors, including chronic stress and impulsivity, both of which have been previously linked to suicidal behavior [41]. In our study, LPS administration significantly elevated NLR, indicating increased systemic inflammation. However, CSL treatment dose-dependently reduced NLR, suggesting a potential immunomodulatory effect. This reduction in NLR implies that CSL may help mitigate systemic inflammation, which plays a crucial role in inflammation-driven psychiatric disorders such as depression. Given that the endocannabinoid system regulates immune cell activity through cannabinoid receptors, it is plausible that CSL has an effect by inhibiting neutrophil activation and reducing cytokine production. While further research is needed, these findings suggest that CSL could be a promising therapeutic approach for managing inflammation-induced depressive disorders [42].

MCs are prevalent in nearly all vascularized tissues. Their close anatomical relationship with lymphatic vessels, combined with their capacity to synthesize, store, and release a wide range of inflammatory and vasoactive mediators, highlights their crucial role in regulating lymphatic vascular functions [43]. Recent studies suggest that MCs function as immune sentinels by presenting antigens through the expression of major histocompatibility complex II (MHC II) molecules. Additionally, they regulate the activity of various immune cells, including macrophages, dendritic cells (DCs), eosinophils, fibroblasts, and both T and B lymphocytes [44–47]. MC-derived histamine is essential for the LPS-induced phosphorylation of NF-κB [48]. LPS stimulates TLR4, initiating the histamine- and NF-κB-dependent production and secretion of various cytokines by MCs and surrounding tissue [48]. Upon encountering Gram-negative bacteria, MCs release inflammatory mediators, including TNFα, IL-6, and IL-1β. This response facilitates the chemotactic migration of NK cells, eosinophils, and neutrophils, while also enhancing the expression of adhesion molecules and chemokine ligands in lymphatic and blood vessels [49]. Additionally, MC-derived mediators affect lymphatic pumping by modulating the contractility of lymphatic muscle cells, which can either enhance or delay the transport of pathogens and immune cells to draining LNs [48,50]. In our study, the administration of CSL significantly inhibited excessive MC degranulation in both the smLNs and dcLNs, which are draining LNs connected to the meningeal lymphatic system [51,52]. Particularly, dcLNs are more directly connected to the meningeal lymphatic vessels and function as drainage LNs for macromolecules, cellular waste, toxic substances, and immune cells [52]. Aging is acknowledged as a significant risk factor for neurodegenerative disorders, including Alzheimer's disease [53]. In aged mice, lymphatic drainage becomes compromised, resulting in a reduction diameter and coverage of meningeal lymphatic vessels, as well as diminished transport of CSF macromolecules to dcLNs [54]. Additionally, MC numbers in cervical lymph nodes are lower in young rats (2 months old) compared to other lymph nodes, but a more pronounced increase in MC density is observed in older rats (12 months old) [55]. Aging also leads to the basal activation of peri-lymphatic MCs, hindering the recruitment and activation of immune cells and potentially exacerbating inflammatory responses in these areas [56,57]. While this study was conducted on young healthy animals, the findings provide a baseline understanding of how CSL affects MC degranulation and neuroinflammation. The potential anti-inflammatory and neuroprotective effects observed in this context suggest that CSL may also have therapeutic relevance for age-related increases in MC activation and inflammation. Future studies should investigate whether these effects are preserved or enhanced in aging models, where chronic inflammation and impaired lymphatic function are more pronounced. MCs express both CB1 and CB2 cannabinoid receptors, and they exhibit diverse responses to cannabinoid exposure [58–60]. MCs also produce endocannabinoids, including an andamide, palmitoylethanolamide (PEA), suggesting the presence of a potential autocrine regulatory mechanism. Notably, CB1 possesses a unique ability to suppress FcεRI-induced secretory responses in MCs [61]. The inhibition of degranulation in dcLNs is consistent with our previous study on another species of *Cannabis sativa* L. [62], suggesting that CSL regulates MC activity in drainage LNs. Further research is needed to determine whether this regulation is associated with CSF drainage functions in the meningeal lymphatic system.

The vascularized meninges of the central nervous system (CNS) are essential for the protection, development, and maintenance of neural parenchyma [63]. The meninges are normal residents of innate immune cells, including macrophages, MCs, and innate lymphoid cells (ILCs). Additionally, circulating immune cells like neutrophils and T cells pass through the meninges as part of routine immunosurveillance [64–66]. Within the dura mater, the meningeal layer closest to the skull, MC distribution varies notably, with the highest density found in the interparietal region and the most pronounced activation occurring in the transverse region [67]. In humans, MCs in the convexity of the intracranial dura mater are situated near arterial and venous vessels, with a greater concentration observed around venous vessels within the periosteal layers and near the SSS [68]. In our study, MCs were more densely distributed in the parietal region compared to the SSS region, which is consistent with previous research [68]. No significant changes in MC number were observed following LPS or CSL administration. However, a notable increase in the degranulation ratio was observed in both regions, with the SSS region exhibiting a higher degranulation ratio after LPS administration. CSL treatment showed a dose-dependent suppression of degranulation in the SSS region. This suggests that the regulation of MC activation in the SSS region is functionally important, as this area is not only a venous site, but is also a critical region for the meningeal lymphatics. Since the discovery of meningeal lymphatics in 2015, an increasing body of evidence has highlighted the essential role of the meningeal lymphatics in regulating immune responses and inflammation within the central nervous system [52,54,69–72]. Moreover, recent studies suggest that the drainage of meningeal lymphatics, driven by VEGF-C, plays a crucial role in regulating depression-like behavior and enhancing the immune response against brain tumors [73–75]. MCs in the meninges may play a critical regulatory role in controlling brain inflammation and the progression of injury following a stroke [76]. Also, aging triggers the basal activation of perilymphatic MCs, which subsequently limits the recruitment and activation of various immune cell types within perilymphatic tissues [77]. CSL effectively suppressed the degranulation of MCs in the dura mater, particularly in the SSS region, suggesting that it plays a critical role in modulating mast cell activation in this area. These findings imply a complex interaction between mast cell activity and meningeal lymphatic drainage, which may serve as a crucial mechanism for regulating immune responses and inflammation in the central nervous system. Future studies should focus on elucidating the mechanisms by which CSL regulates meningeal lymphatic pathways through mast cell modulation, with particular emphasis on the VEGF-C-mediated pathway and its potential connections to neuroinflammatory or neurodegenerative diseases. Furthermore, it will be important to investigate how the basal activation of dural MCs during aging progresses and how CSL affects this activation. These studies could provide vital insights into developing preventive or therapeutic strategies for age-related neurological disorders and inflammatory diseases.

Pro-inflammatory cytokines such as TNF-α and IL-1β are pivotal in the neuroinflammatory response observed in LPS models, playing critical roles in the pathogenesis of neurodegenerative and psychiatric disorders, including depression and cognitive impairments. Our study demonstrates a significant increase in TNF-α and IL-1β expression in the PFC following LPS administration, consistent with previous reports in LPS models [18,29,30]. The administration of CSL markedly reduced these pro-inflammatory cytokines in a dose-dependent manner, particularly at the 30 mg/kg dose. This aligns with studies showing that cannabinoids like CBD and Δ9-THC, along with terpenes such as β-caryophyllene, exert potent anti-inflammatory and antidepressant effects in LPS-induced models by inhibiting pro-inflammatory cytokines through modulation of the NF-κB pathway and interactions with CB1 and CB2 receptors [78,79]. Further studies should focus on the precise mechanisms by which CSL exerts its anti-inflammatory and antidepressant effects. Investigating how CSL modulates the endocannabinoid system, including enzymes like FAAH and receptors such as GPR55, would provide key insights [80]. Additionally, exploring the roles of PPAR-γ, TRPV1, and the inhibition of NF-κB signaling in reducing cytokine expression and oxidative stress is needed [78–80].

Studies on the therapeutic potential of cannabis have predominantly focused on isolated cannabinoids, such as CBD and Δ9-THC, to explore their pharmacological properties. However, an increasing amount of evidence shows that treatments using the whole cannabis plant tend to produce more effective therapeutic outcomes compared to those relying solely on purified cannabinoids [81–85]. This superior efficacy is attributed to the "entourage effect," a synergistic interaction between multiple bioactive compounds, including cannabinoids, terpenes, and flavonoids. In our study, we identified a variety of bioactive components in CSL, such as CBDA, CBCA, myrcene, and α-Pinene, which are likely to work together to produce the antidepressant-like effects observed. We propose that this synergistic interaction amplifies the therapeutic benefits, supporting the idea that whole plant formulations may offer superior efficacy for managing depression-like symptoms.

The limitations of our study include several important factors. First, we relied on the LPS-induced neuroinflammation model to assess the anti-inflammatory and antidepressant effects of CSL, which may not fully capture the complexity of depressive disorders in humans. Second, while CSL demonstrated significant effects on cytokine levels and behavior, the exact molecular pathways, particularly the interactions between cannabinoids and signaling mechanisms such as NF-κB and PPAR-γ, remain unclear. Furthermore, we did not assess the long-term effects or potential side effects of CSL, nor its efficacy in chronic depression models. Future studies should incorporate additional depression models and explore these mechanisms in greater depth to improve the translational relevance of our findings.

4. Materials and Methods

4.1. Animals

Male C57BL/6 mice (8 weeks old, 25–27 g) were obtained from Samtaco BIO (Gyeonggi-do, Republic of Korea) and housed in groups of 3–4 under a 12 h light–dark cycle with free access to food and water. All animal experiments were conducted in accordance with guidelines approved by the Wonkwang University Animal Experiment Ethics Committee (WKU24-64).

4.2. Experimental Design

A graphical representation of the experimental procedure is shown in Figure 7. Mice were randomly assigned to five groups (n = 6 per group): (i) CON group (vehicle), (ii) LPS group (LPS only), (iii) 10 mg/kg CSL + LPS group (administered 10 mg/kg of CSL 30 min prior to 0.83 mg/kg LPS), (iv) 20 mg/kg CSL + LPS group (administered 20 mg/kg of CSL 30 min prior to 0.83 mg/kg LPS), and (v) 30 mg/kg CSL + LPS group (administered 30 mg/kg of CSL 30 min prior to 0.83 mg/kg LPS). Both CSL and LPS were administered i.p. at a dose of 10 μL/g of body weight. Mice that did not receive CSL or LPS were injected with the corresponding vehicle. Anesthesia was administered via intramuscular injection of an anesthetic cocktail containing Zoletil (20 mg/kg, Virbac, Carros, France) and xylazine (5 mg/kg, Bayer, Leverkusen, Germany). One week before the experiment, the mice were individually housed and habituated to a free choice of 1% sucrose solution and water. CSL was administered 30 min before the LPS injection. The TST and the FST were performed 24 h after LPS administration. SPT was assessed during that 24 h period. After the behavioral tests, blood, LNs, dura mater, and PFC samples were collected for the different analyses.

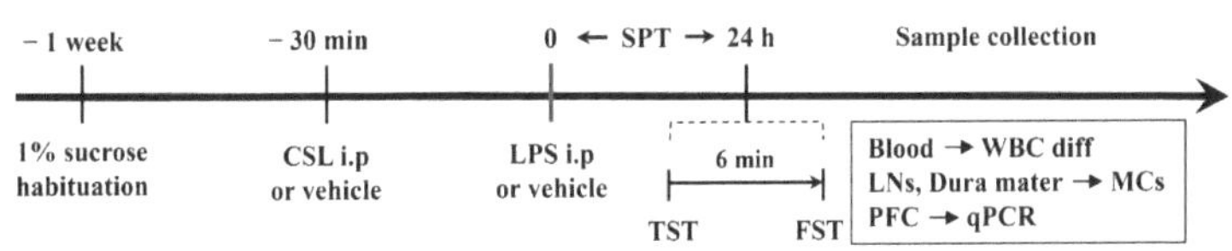

Figure 7. Experimental procedure of drug administration and behavioral tests performed in this study, and sample collection for the different analyses. CSL: *Cannabis sativa* L. inflorescence extract, LPS: lipopolysaccharide, SPT: sucrose preference test, TST: tail suspension test, FST: forced swimming test, WBC diff: white blood cell differential, LNs: lymph nodes, MCs: mast cells, PFC: prefrontal cortex, qPCR: quantitative PCR.

4.3. Drugs

Cannabis sativa L. inflorescence samples of the species 'V1' [86] were obtained from Nongboomind Company (Seoul, Republic of Korea) under the permission of the Ministry of Food and Drug Safety. *Cannabis sativa* L. was extracted with 70% ethanol. First, 300 mL of 70% ethanol was added to a flask containing 20.4 g of *Cannabis sativa* L. The *Cannabis sativa* L. soaked in 70% ethanol was ultrasonicated (frequency 40 kHz bath) at 40 °C for 30 min using an ultrasonicator (POWERSONIC 410, Hwashin Technology, Seoul, Republic of Korea). The extraction process was repeated three times. The extracted solution was then filtered through a 5 μM pore-size qualitative filter paper (ADVANTEC, Tokyo, Japan). The extract was concentrated under reduced pressure at 40 °C using a rotary vacuum evaporator (EYELA N-1110, Tokyo, Japan). Subsequently, the extract was freeze-dried at −80 °C and stored at −20 °C until use. A final 3.13 g dried powder was obtained from 20.4 g of *Cannabis sativa* L., and the final yield was 15.62%. For administration, the CSL was dissolved in a solution of 2% Tween 80 (Duksan, Seoul, Republic of Korea), 5% Propylene Glycol (Duksan, Seoul, Republic of Korea), and saline, and administered at doses of 10, 20, and 30 mg/kg [62]. LPS (Lipopolysaccharides from Escherichia coli O55:B5, Sigma-Aldrich, Darmstadt, Germany) was dissolved in saline and used at a dose of 0.83 mg/kg [29]. Identification and quantification of cannabinoids in CSL was analyzed using GC-MS, as previously reported [87]. The analyzed cannabinoids were a reference standard mixture of eight neutral cannabinoids (purity ≥ 99.0%) [cannabidivarin (CBDV), tetrahydrocannabivarin (THCV), cannabidiol (CBD), cannabinol (CBN), delta-9-tetrahydrocannabinol (Δ9-THC), delta-8-tetrahydrocannabinol (Δ8-THC), cannabichromene (CBC), cannabigerol (CBG)] and a standard mixture of 6 acidic cannabinoids (purity ≥ 98.5%) [cannabichromenic acid (CBCA), cannabidivarinic acid (CBDVA), cannabidiolic acid (CBDA), cannabigerolic acid (CBGA), tetrahydrocannabivarinic acid

(THCVA), and tetrahydrocannabinolic acid-A (THCA-A)], and isotopically labeled internal standards such as Δ9-THC-d3, CBD-d3, CBDA-d3, and THCA-d3 (purity $\geq$ 99.9%). And HS-GC/MS was employed to identify the major terpenes in the CSL [86]. Quantitative analysis was performed on α- and β-pinene, myrcene, limonene, β-caryophyllene, α-humulene, etc., which are known as the major terpenes in *Cannabis sativa* L., in order to investigate terpenes.

4.4. Sucrose Preference Test (SPT)

This test was used to assess anhedonia. Prior to the experiment, animals were housed individually and given unrestricted access to both water and a 1% sucrose solution for one week to acclimate them to the availability of both liquids, as described in previous studies [26]. The positions of the two bottles were alternated daily to prevent any positional preference. Sucrose preference was measured 24 h after LPS injection by calculating the percentage of sucrose solution consumed relative to the total liquid intake during that time period [88].

4.5. Tail Suspension Test (TST)

Mice were suspended by the tail and video recorded for 6 min using a webcam (APC930U, ABKO, Seoul, Republic of Korea). Immobility time was defined as the period when the mice hung passively and remained completely motionless, indicating behavioral despair, following standard protocols [27].

4.6. Forced Swimming Test (FST)

The Forced Swim Test (FST) was performed according to established protocols [28]. The apparatus consisted of a transparent cylindrical glass container (15 cm in diameter, 20 cm deep) filled with water maintained at 23–25 °C, with a webcam (APC930U, ABKO, Seoul, Republic of Korea) positioned in front of the container for recording. The immobility time of the mice was recorded over a 6 min period, with the data analyzed during the last 4 min, excluding the initial 2 min for acclimatization. Immobility time was defined as the period when the mouse was floating with minimal movement, except those required to keep its nose above water, indicating behavioral despair.

4.7. Hematological Inflammatory Markers Analysis

In total, 150 μL of blood sample was collected from the heart following an abdominal incision and the careful removal of the ribs and diaphragm to ensure optimal access. This procedure was performed prior to perfusion for PFC sampling. The collected blood was immediately transferred into EDTA tubes (Greiner Bio-One, Chonburi, Thailand), kept refrigerated, and sent to the Korea Non-Clinical Technology Solution Center (KNTSC) for hematological analysis. The analysis focused on white blood cell differential counts, including neutrophils, lymphocytes, monocytes, eosinophils, and basophils. The NLR was calculated by dividing the neutrophil count by the lymphocyte count.

4.8. Staining of Mast Cells (MCs) in LNs

All procedures were performed under a stereomicroscope (SZX16, Olympus, Tokyo, Japan) for precise observation. Once deep anesthesia was confirmed, the mice's legs were secured using tape to maintain positioning. The neck region was shaved with a razor blade to create a clear surgical area. A midline skin incision was made along the neck, allowing for access to the smLNs and dcLNs. The smLNs were the first to be identified and excised, as they are located superficially above the submandibular gland. Following this, the incision was deepened to access and collect the dcLNs, located deeper beneath the sternocleidomastoid muscle. Both the dcLNs and smLNs were fixed overnight in 10% neutral buffered formalin (NBF) for tissue preservation. The samples were subsequently dehydrated in a graded series of alcohols, cleared in xylene, and embedded in paraffin. Paraffin blocks were sectioned at 4 μm using a microtome and mounted onto slides for staining. MCs were stained using 0.5% toluidine blue in 0.5 N hydrochloric acid, as described in previous studies [89]. The LN area and MC count were evaluated using a phase contrast microscope (BX51, Olympus, Tokyo, Japan). The degranulation rate was calculated as the ratio of degranulated MCs to the total number of MCs in each LN.

4.9. Staining of Mast Cells (MCs) in Dura Mater

Following perfusion, the neck was severed, and the scalp was carefully incised to expose the skull. The skull, with the dura mater intact, was excised and fixed in 10% NBF for 24 h. To stain mast cells, the skulls were immersed in 0.5% acidic toluidine blue for 30 s and subsequently rinsed with phosphate-buffered saline (PBS, Gibco, Grand Island, USA) [67,90]. The dura mater was carefully separated from the skull, mounted onto glass slides, and coverslipped using mounting medium. For mast cell analysis, the dura mater was divided into two regions: the parietal and the SSS. In total, 8 non-overlapping 1 mm^2 boxes were selected per region, and the average number of MCs was calculated. Quantification was performed using a phase contrast microscope (BX51, Olympus, Tokyo, Japan), and the degranulation rate was determined by calculating the ratio of degranulated MCs to the total number of MCs within each counting region.

4.10. Quantitative PCR (qPCR)

To prepare brain tissues for molecular analysis, the animals were perfused with cold PBS through the heart under deep anesthesia to remove circulating blood, ensuring clean tissue samples. After perfusion, the skull was carefully opened and the entire brain was removed. The prefrontal cortex (PFC) was then precisely dissected from the extracted brain. The isolated PFC tissues were immediately flash-frozen in liquid nitrogen and stored at −80 °C until RNA extraction. Total RNA was extracted from the PFC using the Easy-BlueTM RNA extraction kit (iNtRON Biotechnology, Sungnam, Republic of Korea). Reverse transcription of RNA to cDNA was performed using the ReverTra Ace qPCR RT Kit (Toyobo, Osaka, Japan). The ABI StepOne Plus detection system was used to perform TaqMan quantitative RT-PCR according to the manufacturer's protocol. The housekeeping gene, β-actin, was used for normalizing the mRNA levels of the target genes. The PCR cycling conditions were as follows: 95 °C for 3 min, 60 cycles of 95 °C for 10 s, 60 °C for 10 s, and 72 °C for 20 s. The sequences of primers used for qPCR are shown in Table 1.

Table 1. Sequences of primers used for qPCR.

Gene	Primer
TNF-α (F)	5′-TAC CTT GTC TAC TCC CAG GTT CTC-3′
TNF-α (R)	5′-GTG TGG GTG AGG AGC ACG TA-3′
IL-1β (F)	5′-ACC TGC TGG TGT GTG ACG TT-3′
IL-1β (R)	5′-TCG TTG CTT GGT TCT CCT TG-3′
β-actin (F)	5′-ATC ACT ATT GGC AAC GAG CG-3′
β-actin (R)	5′-TCA GCA ATG CCT GGG TAC AT-3′

4.11. Statistical Analysis

All data are expressed as mean ± standard deviation (SD). Statistical analyses were performed using one-way analysis of variance (ANOVA) followed by Tukey's post hoc test in SPSS for Windows (version 26.0; IBM Corp., Armonk, NY, USA). A p-value of <0.05 was considered statistically significant.

5. Conclusions

We demonstrated that CSL exhibits significant antidepressant-like and anti-inflammatory effects in an LPS-induced neuroinflammatory model. CSL administration effectively reduced depressive-like behaviors, as observed in the SPT, TST, and FST, and modulated the degranulation of MCs in LNs and the dura mater. Furthermore, CSL decreased the expression of pro-inflammatory cytokines TNF-α and IL-1β in the PFC in a dose-dependent manner. These findings suggest that CSL acts both through immune modulation and neuroinflammation suppression, possibly via the endocannabinoid system and pathways such as NF-κB, PPAR-γ, and VEGF-C. The synergistic interaction between cannabinoids and terpenes in CSL likely contributes to its therapeutic potential, supporting the notion of the "entourage effect". While these results are promising, further studies are required to clarify the exact mechanisms involved and to assess the long-term safety and efficacy of CSL in chronic depression models.

Author Contributions: Conceptualization, J.S. and D.-U.K.; Formal analysis, E.K. (Eunjae Kim); Investigation, J.S., D.-U.K., J.-Y.H., D.-W.L. and E.K. (Eunjeong Kwon); Resources, D.H. and S.K.; Supervision, and S.K.; Writing—original draft, J.S., D.-U.K. and J.-Y.H.; Writing—review and editing, G.-S.B., Y.-M.L., D.H. and S.K. All authors have read and agreed to the published version of the manuscript.

Funding: This study was supported by a grant from the Rural Development Administration [PJ017015 (RS2022RD010270)].

Institutional Review Board Statement: This research was approved by the Wonkwang University Animal Experiment Ethics Committee (WKU24-64).

Informed Consent Statement: Not applicable.

Data Availability Statement: Data are contained within the article.

Conflicts of Interest: The authors declare no conflicts of interest.

References

1. American Psychiatric Association. *Task DSM-5Force, Diagnostic and Statistical Manual of Mental Disorders: DSM-5™*, 5th ed.; American Psychiatric Publishing, Inc.: Arlington, VA, USA, 2013.
2. Dregan, A.; Matcham, F.; Harber-Aschan, L.; Rayner, L.; Brailean, A.; Davis, K.; Hatch, S.; Pariante, C.; Armstrong, D.; Stewart, R.; et al. Common mental disorders within chronic inflammatory disorders: A primary care database prospective investigation. *Ann. Rheum. Dis.* **2019**, *78*, 688–695. [CrossRef] [PubMed]
3. Dowlati, Y.; Herrmann, N.; Swardfager, W.; Liu, H.; Sham, L.; Reim, E.K.; Lanctôt, K.L. A Meta-Analysis of Cytokines in Major Depression. *Biol. Psychiatry* **2009**, *67*, 446–457. [CrossRef] [PubMed]
4. Mukai, K.; Tsai, M.; Saito, H.; Galli, S.J. Mast cells as sources of cytokines, chemokines, and growth factors. *Immunol. Rev.* **2018**, *282*, 121–150. [CrossRef] [PubMed]
5. Xiao, B.-G.; Link, H. IFN-γ production of adult rat astrocytes triggered by TNF-α. *Neuroreport* **1998**, *9*, 1487–1490. [CrossRef]
6. Maier, S.F. Bi-directional immune–brain communication: Implications for understanding stress, pain, and cognition. *Brain Behav. Immun.* **2003**, *17*, 69–85. [CrossRef]
7. Connor, T.J.; Starr, N.; O'Sullivan, J.B.; Harkin, A. Induction of indolamine 2, 3-dioxygenase and kynurenine 3-monooxygenase in rat brain following a systemic inflammatory challenge: A role for IFN-γ? *Neurosci. Lett.* **2008**, *441*, 29–34. [CrossRef]
8. Leonard, B.; Maes, M. Mechanistic explanations how cell-mediated immune activation, inflammation and oxidative and nitrosative stress pathways and their sequels and concomitants play a role in the pathophysiology of unipolar depression. *Neurosci. Biobehav. Rev.* **2011**, *36*, 764–785. [CrossRef]
9. Maes, M.; Berk, M.; Goehler, L.; Song, C.; Anderson, G.; Gałecki, P.; Leonard, B. Depression and sickness behavior are Janus-faced responses to shared inflammatory pathways. *BMC Med.* **2012**, *10*, 66. [CrossRef]
10. Engler, H.; Brendt, P.; Wischermann, J.; Wegner, A.; Röhling, R.; Schoemberg, T.; Meyer, U.; Gold, R.; Peters, J.; Benson, S.; et al. Selective increase of cerebrospinal fluid IL-6 during experimental systemic inflammation in humans: Association with depressive symptoms. *Mol. Psychiatry* **2017**, *22*, 1448–1454. [CrossRef]
11. Engler, H.; Benson, S.; Wegner, A.; Spreitzer, I.; Schedlowski, M.; Elsenbruch, S. Men and women differ in inflammatory and neuroendocrine responses to endotoxin but not in the severity of sickness symptoms. *Brain Behav. Immun.* **2016**, *52*, 18–26. [CrossRef]
12. Dong, H.; Dai, X.; Zhou, Y.; Shi, C.; Bhuiyan, P.; Sun, Z.; Li, N.; Jin, W. Enhanced meningeal lymphatic drainage ameliorates lipopolysaccharide-induced brain injury in aged mice. *J. Neuroinflamm.* **2024**, *21*, 36. [CrossRef] [PubMed]
13. Ren, M.; Tang, Z.; Wu, X.; Spengler, R.; Jiang, H.; Yang, Y.; Boivin, N. The origins of cannabis smoking: Chemical residue evidence from the first millennium BCE in the Pamirs. *Sci. Adv.* **2019**, *5*, eaaw1391. [CrossRef] [PubMed]
14. Ashton, J.C. Cannabinoids for the treatment of inflammation. *Curr. Opin. Investig. Drugs* **2007**, *8*, 373–384. [PubMed]
15. Mechoulam, R.; Parker, L.A. The endocannabinoid system and the brain. *Annu. Rev. Psychol.* **2013**, *64*, 21–47. [CrossRef]
16. Russo, E.B. Taming THC: Potential cannabis synergy and phytocannabinoid-terpenoid entourage effects. *Br. J. Pharmacol.* **2011**, *163*, 1344–1364. [CrossRef]

17. El-Alfy, A.T.; Ivey, K.; Robinson, K.; Ahmed, S.; Radwan, M.; Slade, D.; Khan, I.; ElSohly, M.; Ross, S. Antidepressant-like effect of Δ9-tetrahydrocannabinol and other cannabinoids isolated from *Cannabis sativa* L. *Pharmacol. Biochem. Behav.* **2010**, *95*, 434–442. [CrossRef]
18. Florensa-Zanuy, E.; Garro-Martínez, E.; Adell, A.; Castro, E.; Díaz, Á.; Pazos, Á.; Mac-Dowell, K.S.; Martín-Hernández, D.; Pilar-Cuéllar, F. Cannabidiol antidepressant-like effect in the lipopolysaccharide model in mice: Modulation of inflammatory pathways. *Biochem. Pharmacol.* **2021**, *185*, 114433. [CrossRef]
19. Hen-Shoval, D.; Amar, S.; Shbiro, L.; Smoum, R.; Haj, C.G.; Mechoulam, R.; Zalsman, G.; Weller, A.; Shoval, G. Acute oral cannabidiolic acid methyl ester reduces depression-like behavior in two genetic animal models of depression. *Behav. Brain Res.* **2018**, *351*, 1–3. [CrossRef]
20. Liktor-Busa, E.; Keresztes, A.; LaVigne, J.; Streicher, J.M.; Largent-Milnes, T.M. Analgesic Potential of Terpenes Derived from *Cannabis sativa*. *Pharmacol. Rev.* **2021**, *73*, 1269–1297. [CrossRef]
21. Surendran, S.; Qassadi, F.; Surendran, G.; Lilley, D.; Heinrich, M. Myrcene—What Are the Potential Health Benefits of This Flavouring and Aroma Agent? *Front. Nutr.* **2021**, *8*, 699666. [CrossRef]
22. Rufino, A.T.; Ribeiro, M.; Sousa, C.; Judas, F.; Salgueiro, L.; Cavaleiro, C.; Mendes, A.F. Evaluation of the anti-inflammatory, anti-catabolic and pro-anabolic effects of E-caryophyllene, myrcene and limonene in a cell model of osteoarthritis. *Eur. J. Pharmacol.* **2015**, *750*, 141–150. [CrossRef] [PubMed]
23. Islam, A.U.S.; Hellman, B.; Nyberg, F.; Amir, N.; Jayaraj, R.L.; Petroianu, G.; Adem, A. Myrcene Attenuates Renal Inflammation and Oxidative Stress in the Adrenalectomized Rat Model. *Molecules* **2020**, *25*, 4492. [CrossRef] [PubMed]
24. Goudarzi, S.; Rafieirad, M. Evaluating the effect of α-pinene on motor activity, avoidance memory and lipid peroxidation in animal model of Parkinson disease in adult male rats. *Res. J. Pharmacogn.* **2017**, *4*, 53–63.
25. Elahinia, A.; Hassanpour, S.; Asghari, A.; Khaksar, E. Effects of α-pinene Administration During Pregnancy on Depressive-like Behavior Following Delivery in Mice. *Iran. J. Vet. Med.* **2023**, *17*, 253–262. [CrossRef]
26. Liu, M.-Y.; Yin, C.-Y.; Zhu, L.-J.; Zhu, X.-H.; Xu, C.; Luo, C.-X.; Chen, H.; Zhu, D.-Y.; Zhou, Q.-G. Sucrose preference test for measurement of stress-induced anhedonia in mice. *Nat. Protoc.* **2018**, *13*, 1686–1698. [CrossRef]
27. Ferrés-Coy, A.; Galofré, M.; Pilar-Cuéllar, F.; Vidal, R.; Paz, V.; Ruiz-Bronchal, E.; Campa, L.; Pazos, Á.; Caso, J.R.; Leza, J.C.; et al. Therapeutic antidepressant potential of a conjugated siRNA silencing the serotonin transporter after intranasal administration. *Mol. Psychiatry* **2015**, *21*, 328–338. [CrossRef]
28. Yao, H.; Shen, H.; Yu, H.; Wang, C.; Ding, R.; Lan, X.; Tash, D.; Wu, X.; Wang, X.; Zhang, G. Chronic ethanol exposure induced depressive-like behavior in male C57BL/6 N mice by downregulating GluA1. *Physiol. Behav.* **2021**, *234*, 113387. [CrossRef]
29. Yin, R.; Zhang, K.; Li, Y.; Tang, Z.; Zheng, R.; Ma, Y.; Chen, Z.; Lei, N.; Xiong, L.; Guo, P.; et al. Lipopolysaccharide-induced depression-like model in mice: Meta-analysis and systematic evaluation. *Front. Immunol.* **2023**, *14*, 1181973. [CrossRef]
30. Cheng, L.; Huang, C.; Chen, Z. Tauroursodeoxycholic Acid Ameliorates Lipopolysaccharide-Induced Depression Like Behavior in Mice via the Inhibition of Neuroinflammation and Oxido-Nitrosative Stress. *Pharmacology* **2018**, *103*, 93–100. [CrossRef]
31. Gáll, Z.; Farkas, S.; Albert, Á.; Ferencz, E.; Vancea, S.; Urkon, M.; Kolcsár, M. Effects of Chronic Cannabidiol Treatment in the Rat Chronic Unpredictable Mild Stress Model of Depression. *Biomolecules* **2020**, *10*, 801. [CrossRef]
32. Vieira, G.; Cavalli, J.; Gonçalves, E.C.D.; Braga, S.F.P.; Ferreira, R.S.; Santos, A.R.S.; Cola, M.; Raposo, N.R.B.; Capasso, R.; Dutra, R.C. Antidepressant-Like Effect of Terpineol in an Inflammatory Model of Depression: Involvement of the Cannabinoid System and D2 Dopamine Receptor. *Biomolecules* **2020**, *10*, 792. [CrossRef] [PubMed]
33. Paul, A.M.; Mhatre, S.D.; Cekanaviciute, E.; Schreurs, A.-S.; Tahimic, C.G.T.; Globus, R.K.; Anand, S.; Crucian, B.E.; Bhattacharya, S. Neutrophil-to-Lymphocyte Ratio: A Biomarker to Monitor the Immune Status of Astronauts. *Front. Immunol.* **2020**, *11*, 564950. [CrossRef] [PubMed]
34. Cho, I.R.; Park, J.C.; Park, C.H.; Jo, J.H.; Lee, H.J.; Kim, S.; Shim, C.N.; Lee, H.; Shin, S.K.; Kil Lee, S.; et al. Pre-treatment neutrophil to lymphocyte ratio as a prognostic marker to predict chemotherapeutic response and survival outcomes in metastatic advanced gastric cancer. *Gastric Cancer* **2014**, *17*, 703–710. [CrossRef] [PubMed]
35. Mortaz, E.; Alipoor, S.D.; Adcock, I.M.; Mumby, S.; Koenderman, L. Update on Neutrophil Function in Severe Inflammation. *Front. Immunol.* **2018**, *9*, 2171. [CrossRef]
36. Li, Y.; Wang, W.; Yang, F.; Xu, Y.; Feng, C.; Zhao, Y. The regulatory roles of neutrophils in adaptive immunity. *Cell Commun. Signal.* **2019**, *17*, 147. [CrossRef]
37. Rose, R.; Banerjee, A.; Ramaiah, S.K. Characterization of a lipopolysaccharide mediated neutrophilic hepatitis model in Sprague Dawley rats. *J. Appl. Toxicol.* **2007**, *27*, 602–611. [CrossRef]
38. Shakoory, B.; Fitzgerald, S.M.; Lee, S.A.; Chi, D.S.; Krishnaswamy, G. The Role of Human Mast Cell-Derived Cytokines in Eosinophil Biology. *J. Interf. Cytokine Res.* **2004**, *24*, 271–281. [CrossRef]
39. Hailman, E.; Vasselon, T.; Kelley, M.; A Busse, L.; Hu, M.C.; Lichenstein, H.S.; A Detmers, P.; Wright, S.D. Stimulation of macrophages and neutrophils by complexes of lipopolysaccharide and soluble CD14. *J. Immunol.* **1996**, *156*, 4384–4390. [CrossRef]
40. Zhou, J.; Schmidt, M.; Johnston, B.; Wilfart, F.; Whynot, S.; Hung, O.; Murphy, M.; Černý, V.; Pavlovic, D.; Lehmann, C. Experimental Endotoxemia Induces Leukocyte Adherence and Plasma Extravasation within the Rat Pial Microcirculation. *Physiol. Res.* **2011**, *60*, 853. [CrossRef]

41. Ekinci, O.; Ekinci, A. The connections among suicidal behavior, lipid profile and low-grade inflammation in patients with major depressive disorder: A specific relationship with the neutrophil-to-lymphocyte ratio. *Nord. J. Psychiatry* **2017**, *71*, 574–580. [CrossRef]
42. Paland, N.; Pechkovsky, A.; Aswad, M.; Hamza, H.; Popov, T.; Shahar, E.; Louria-Hayon, I. The Immunopathology of COVID-19 and the Cannabis Paradigm. *Front. Immunol.* **2021**, *12*, 631233. [CrossRef] [PubMed]
43. Pal, S.; Nath, S.; Meininger, C.J.; Gashev, A.A. Emerging Roles of Mast Cells in the Regulation of Lymphatic Immuno-Physiology. *Front. Immunol.* **2020**, *11*, 1234. [CrossRef] [PubMed]
44. Abraham, S.N.; John, A.L.S. Mast cell-orchestrated immunity to pathogens. *Nat. Rev. Immunol.* **2010**, *10*, 440–452. [CrossRef] [PubMed]
45. Dudeck, J.; Medyukhina, A.; Fröbel, J.; Svensson, C.-M.; Kotrba, J.; Gerlach, M.; Gradtke, A.-C.; Schröder, B.; Speier, S.; Figge, M.T.; et al. Mast cells acquire MHCII from dendritic cells during skin inflammation. *J. Exp. Med.* **2017**, *214*, 3791–3811. [CrossRef] [PubMed]
46. St John, A.L.; Abraham, S.N. Innate immunity and its regulation by mast cells. *J. Immunol.* **2013**, *190*, 4458–4463. [CrossRef]
47. Urb, M.; Sheppard, D.C. The Role of Mast Cells in the Defence against Pathogens. *PLoS Pathog.* **2012**, *8*, e1002619. [CrossRef]
48. Nizamutdinova, I.T.; Dusio, G.F.; Gasheva, O.Y.; Skoog, H.; Tobin, R.; Peddaboina, C.; Meininger, C.J.; Zawieja, D.C.; Newell-Rogers, M.K.; Gashev, A.A. Mast cells and histamine are triggering the NF-κB-mediated reactions of adult and aged perilymphatic mesenteric tissues to acute inflammation. *Aging* **2016**, *8*, 3065. [CrossRef]
49. Kunder, C.A.; John, A.L.S.; Abraham, S.N. Mast cell modulation of the vascular and lymphatic endothelium. *Blood* **2011**, *118*, 5383–5393. [CrossRef]
50. Plaku, K.J.; Von Der Weid, P. Mast Cell Degranulation Alters Lymphatic Contractile Activity Through Action of Histamine. *Microcirculation* **2006**, *13*, 219–227. [CrossRef]
51. Mathieu, E.; Gupta, N.; Macdonald, R.L.; Ai, J.; Yücel, Y.H. In Vivo Imaging of Lymphatic Drainage of Cerebrospinal Fluid in Mouse. *Fluids Barriers CNS* **2013**, *10*, 35. [CrossRef]
52. Louveau, A.; Smirnov, I.; Keyes, T.J.; Eccles, J.D.; Rouhani, S.J.; Peske, J.D.; Derecki, N.C.; Castle, D.; Mandell, J.W.; Lee, K.S.; et al. Structural and functional features of central nervous system lymphatic vessels. *Nature* **2015**, *523*, 337–341. [CrossRef] [PubMed]
53. das Neves, S.P.; Delivanoglou, N.; Da Mesquita, S. CNS-draining meningeal lymphatic vasculature: Roles, conundrums and future challenges. *Front. Pharmacol.* **2021**, *12*, 655052. [CrossRef] [PubMed]
54. Da Mesquita, S.; Louveau, A.; Vaccari, A.; Smirnov, I.; Cornelison, R.C.; Kingsmore, K.M.; Contarino, C.; Onengut-Gumuscu, S.; Farber, E.; Raper, D.; et al. Functional aspects of meningeal lymphatics in ageing and Alzheimer's disease. *Nature* **2018**, *560*, 185–191. [CrossRef] [PubMed]
55. Sainte-Marie, G.; Peng, F.S. Mast cells and fibrosis in compartments of lymph nodes of normal, gnotobiotic, and athymic rats. *Cell Tissue Res.* **1990**, *261*, 1–15. [CrossRef] [PubMed]
56. Chatterjee, V.; Gashev, A.A. Aging-associated shifts in functional status of mast cells located by adult and aged mesenteric lymphatic vessels. *Am. J. Physiol. Circ. Physiol.* **2012**, *303*, H693–H702. [CrossRef]
57. Chatterjee, V.; Gashev, A.A. Mast Cell-Directed Recruitment of MHC Class II Positive Cells and Eosinophils Towards Mesenteric Lymphatic Vessels in Adulthood and Elderly. *Lymphat. Res. Biol.* **2014**, *12*, 37–47. [CrossRef]
58. Facci, L.; Toso, R.D.; Romanello, S.; Buriani, A.; Skaper, S.D.; Leon, A. Mast cells express a peripheral cannabinoid receptor with differential sensitivity to anandamide and palmitoylethanolamide. *Proc. Natl. Acad. Sci. USA* **1995**, *92*, 3376–3380. [CrossRef]
59. Granberg, M.; Fowler, C.J.; Jacobsson, S.O. Effects of the cannabimimetic fatty acid derivatives 2-arachidonoylglycerol, anandamide, palmitoylethanolamide and methanandamide upon IgE-dependent antigen-induced β-hexosaminidase, serotonin and TNFα release from rat RBL-2H3 basophilic leukaemia cells. *Naunyn-Schmiedebergs Arch. Pharmacol.* **2001**, *364*, 66–73.
60. Bisogno, T.; Maurelli, S.; Melck, D.; De Petrocellis, L.; Di Marzo, V. Biosynthesis, Uptake, and Degradation of Anandamide and Palmitoylethanolamide in Leukocytes. *J. Biol. Chem.* **1997**, *272*, 3315–3323. [CrossRef]
61. Samson, M.-T.; Small-Howard, A.; Shimoda, L.M.N.; Koblan-Huberson, M.; Stokes, A.J.; Turner, H. Differential Roles of CB1 and CB2 Cannabinoid Receptors in Mast Cells. *J. Immunol.* **2003**, *170*, 4953–4962. [CrossRef]
62. Shin, J.; Choi, S.; Park, A.Y.; Ju, S.; Kweon, B.; Kim, D.-U.; Bae, G.-S.; Han, D.; Kwon, E.; Hong, J.; et al. In Vitro and In Vivo Anti-Inflammatory and Antidepressant-like Effects of *Cannabis sativa* L. Extracts. *Plants* **2024**, *13*, 1619. [CrossRef] [PubMed]
63. Rozniecki, J.J.; Dimitriadou, V.; Lambracht-Hall, M.; Pang, X.; Theoharides, T.C. Morphological and functional demonstration of rat dura mater mast cell–neuron interactions in vitro and in vivo. *Brain Res.* **1999**, *849*, 1–15. [CrossRef] [PubMed]
64. Decimo, I.; Fumagalli, G.; Berton, V.; Krampera, M.; Bifari, F. Meninges: From protective membrane to stem cell niche. *Am. J. Stem Cells* **2012**, *1*, 92–105. [PubMed]
65. Kivisäkk, P.; Imitola, J.; Rasmussen, S.; Elyaman, W.; Zhu, B.; Ransohoff, R.M.; Khoury, S.J. Localizing central nervous system immune surveillance: Meningeal antigen-presenting cells activate T cells during experimental autoimmune encephalomyelitis. *Ann. Neurol.* **2009**, *65*, 457–469. [CrossRef]
66. Walker-Caulfield, M.E.; Hatfield, J.K.; Brown, M.A. Dynamic changes in meningeal inflammation correspond to clinical exacerbations in a murine model of relapsing–remitting multiple sclerosis. *J. Neuroimmunol.* **2014**, *278*, 112–122. [CrossRef]
67. Duque-Wilckens, N.; Teis, R.; Sarno, E.; Stoelting, F.; Khalid, S.; Dairi, Z.; Douma, A.; Maradiaga, N.; Hench, S.; Dharshika, C.D.; et al. Early life adversity drives sex-specific anhedonia and meningeal immune gene expression through mast cell activation. *Brain Behav. Immun.* **2022**, *103*, 73–84. [CrossRef]

68. Rosas, E.P.; Paz, S.T.; Costa, R.F.; da Silva, R.L.; da Silva, A.P.F.; da Silva, S.R.S.; de Medeiros, P.L.; de Freitas, M.F.L.; Valença, M.M. Histomorphometry of mast cells in the convexity of human intracranial dura mater. *Am. J. Anat.* **2021**, *240*, 724–734. [CrossRef]
69. Harrison, I.F.; Ismail, O.; Machhada, A.; Colgan, N.; Ohene, Y.; Nahavandi, P.; Ahmed, Z.; Fisher, A.; Meftah, S.; Murray, T.K.; et al. Impaired glymphatic function and clearance of tau in an Alzheimer's disease model. *Brain* **2020**, *143*, 2576–2593. [CrossRef]
70. Da Mesquita, S.; Papadopoulos, Z.; Dykstra, T.; Brase, L.; Farias, F.G.; Wall, M.; Jiang, H.; Kodira, C.D.; de Lima, K.A.; Herz, J.; et al. Meningeal lymphatics affect microglia responses and anti-Aβ immunotherapy. *Nature* **2021**, *593*, 255–260. [CrossRef]
71. Bolte, A.C.; Dutta, A.B.; Hurt, M.E.; Smirnov, I.; Kovacs, M.A.; McKee, C.A.; Ennerfelt, H.E.; Shapiro, D.; Nguyen, B.H.; Frost, E.L.; et al. Meningeal lymphatic dysfunction exacerbates traumatic brain injury pathogenesis. *Nat. Commun.* **2020**, *11*, 4524. [CrossRef]
72. Louveau, A.; Herz, J.; Alme, M.N.; Salvador, A.F.; Dong, M.Q.; Viar, K.E.; Herod, S.G.; Knopp, J.; Setliff, J.C.; Lupi, A.L.; et al. CNS lymphatic drainage and neuroinflammation are regulated by meningeal lymphatic vasculature. *Nat. Neurosci.* **2018**, *21*, 1380–1391. [CrossRef] [PubMed]
73. Song, E.; Mao, T.; Dong, H.; Boisserand, L.S.B.; Antila, S.; Bosenberg, M.; Alitalo, K.; Thomas, J.-L.; Iwasaki, A. VEGF-C-driven lymphatic drainage enables immunosurveillance of brain tumours. *Nature* **2020**, *577*, 689–694. [CrossRef]
74. Hu, X.; Deng, Q.; Ma, L.; Li, Q.; Chen, Y.; Liao, Y.; Zhou, F.; Zhang, C.; Shao, L.; Feng, J.; et al. Meningeal lymphatic vessels regulate brain tumor drainage and immunity. *Cell Res.* **2020**, *30*, 229–243. [CrossRef] [PubMed]
75. Dai, W.; Yang, M.; Xia, P.; Xiao, C.; Huang, S.; Zhang, Z.; Cheng, X.; Li, W.; Jin, J.; Zhang, J.; et al. A functional role of meningeal lymphatics in sex difference of stress susceptibility in mice. *Nat. Commun.* **2022**, *13*, 4825. [CrossRef] [PubMed]
76. Arac, A.; Grimbaldeston, M.A.; Nepomuceno, A.R.; Olayiwola, O.; Pereira, M.P.; Nishiyama, Y.; Tsykin, A.; Goodall, G.J.; Schlecht, U.; Vogel, H.; et al. Evidence that Meningeal Mast Cells Can Worsen Stroke Pathology in Mice. *Am. J. Pathol.* **2014**, *184*, 2493–2504. [CrossRef]
77. Pal, S.; Meininger, C.J.; Gashev, A.A. Aged Lymphatic Vessels and Mast Cells in Perilymphatic Tissues. *Int. J. Mol. Sci.* **2017**, *18*, 965. [CrossRef]
78. Al-Khazaleh, A.K.; Zhou, X.; Bhuyan, D.J.; Münch, G.W.; Al-Dalabeeh, E.A.; Jaye, K.; Chang, D. The Neurotherapeutic Arsenal in *Cannabis sativa*: Insights into Anti-Neuroinflammatory and Neuroprotective Activity and Potential Entourage Effects. *Molecules* **2024**, *29*, 410. [CrossRef]
79. Suryavanshi, S.V.; Kovalchuk, I.; Kovalchuk, O. Cannabinoids as Key Regulators of Inflammasome Signaling: A Current Perspective. *Front. Immunol.* **2021**, *11*, 613613. [CrossRef]
80. Askari, V.R.; Shafiee-Nick, R. Promising neuroprotective effects of β-caryophyllene against LPS-induced oligodendrocyte toxicity: A mechanistic study. *Biochem. Pharmacol.* **2018**, *159*, 154–171. [CrossRef]
81. Ferber, S.G.; Namdar, D.; Hen-Shoval, D.; Eger, G.; Koltai, H.; Shoval, G.; Shbiro, L.; Weller, A. The "Entourage Effect": Terpenes Coupled with Cannabinoids for the Treatment of Mood Disorders and Anxiety Disorders. *Curr. Neuropharmacol.* **2020**, *18*, 87–96. [CrossRef]
82. Mechoulam, R.; Ben-Shabat, S. From gan-zi-gun-nu to anandamide and 2-arachidonoylglycerol: The ongoing story of cannabis. *Nat. Prod. Rep.* **1999**, *16*, 131–143. [CrossRef] [PubMed]
83. Lewis, M.A.; Russo, E.B.; Smith, K.M. Pharmacological Foundations of Cannabis Chemovars. *Planta Med.* **2018**, *84*, 225–233. [CrossRef] [PubMed]
84. McPartland, J.M.; Russo, E.B. Cannabis and cannabis extracts: Greater than the sum of their parts? *J. Cannabis Ther.* **2001**, *1*, 103–132. [CrossRef]
85. Namdar, D.; Anis, O.; Poulin, P.; Koltai, H. Chronological Review and Rational and Future Prospects of Cannabis-Based Drug Development. *Molecules* **2020**, *25*, 4821. [CrossRef]
86. Lee, S.; Kim, E.J.; Kwon, E.; Oh, S.J.; Cho, M.; Kim, C.M.; Lee, W.; Hong, J. Identification of Terpene Compositions in the Leaves and Inflorescences of Hybrid *Cannabis* Species Using Headspace-Gas Chromatography/Mass Spectrometry. *Molecules* **2023**, *28*, 8082. [CrossRef]
87. Jeong, M.; Lee, S.; Seo, C.; Kwon, E.; Rho, S.; Cho, M.; Kim, M.Y.; Lee, W.; Lee, Y.S.; Hong, J. Chemical transformation of cannabidiol into psychotropic cannabinoids under acidic reaction conditions: Identification of transformed products by GC-MS. *J. Food Drug Anal.* **2023**, *31*, 165–176. [CrossRef]
88. Markov, D.D. Sucrose Preference Test as a Measure of Anhedonic Behavior in a Chronic Unpredictable Mild Stress Model of Depression: Outstanding Issues. *Brain Sci.* **2022**, *12*, 1287. [CrossRef]
89. Wang, H.W.; Tedla, N.; Lloyd, A.R.; Wakefield, D.; McNeil, P.H. Mast cell activation and migration to lymph nodes during induction of an immune response in mice. *J. Clin. Investig.* **1998**, *102*, 1617–1626. [CrossRef]
90. Christy, A.L.; Walker, M.E.; Hessner, M.J.; Brown, M.A. Mast cell activation and neutrophil recruitment promotes early and robust inflammation in the meninges in EAE. *J. Autoimmun.* **2013**, *42*, 50–61. [CrossRef]

pharmaceuticals

MDPI

Article

High-CBD Extract (CBD-X) in Asthma Management: Reducing Th2-Driven Cytokine Secretion and Neutrophil/Eosinophil Activity

Miran Aswad [1,2], Antonina Pechkovsky [1,2], Narmeen Ghanayiem [1,2], Haya Hamza [1,2], Yaniv Dotan [2,3] and Igal Louria-Hayon [1,2,*]

1 Medical Cannabis Research and Innovation Center, Rambam Health Care Campus, Haifa 3109601, Israel
2 Clinical Research Institute at Rambam (CRIR), Rambam Health Care Campus, Haifa 3109601, Israel
3 Institute of Pulmonology, Rambam Health Care Campus, Haifa 3109601, Israel
* Correspondence: i_louriahayon@rambam.health.gov.il; Tel.: +972-4-7771114

Abstract: Background/Objectives: Asthma is a chronic inflammatory disorder of the airways affecting over 10% of the global population. It is characterized by airway inflammation, mucus hypersecretion, and bronchial hyperresponsiveness, driven predominantly by type 2 helper T cells (Th2) and type 2 innate lymphoid cells (ILC2s) in a subset of patients. However, a significant portion of asthmatic individuals present with "type 2-low" asthma that is often refractory to standard inhaled corticosteroid (ICS) therapy. Therefore, developing innovative therapeutic strategies has become essential. Recent studies have highlighted cannabidiol (CBD) as a promising anti-inflammatory agent capable of modulating immune responses. This study investigates the therapeutic potential of a high-CBD extract (CBD-X) in asthma. Methods: We evaluated the effects of CBD-X on cells involved in asthma pathogenesis using primary human Th2 cells, neutrophils, and asthma mouse model. Results: Our findings indicate that CBD-X extract inhibits Th2 differentiation and reduces the secretion of IL-5 and IL-13, which are crucial cytokines in asthma. Additionally, CBD-X significantly reduces pro-inflammatory cytokines IL-8 and IL-6 in neutrophils and impairs their migration, a critical step in airway inflammation. In a murine asthma model, CBD-X administration led to marked downregulation of IgE and pro-asthmatic cytokines, along with reduced leukocyte, eosinophil, and neutrophil infiltration in lung tissues. Conclusions: These results suggest that CBD-X extract could offer a novel and complementary approach to managing both type 2-high and type 2-low asthma by targeting key inflammatory pathways and modulating immune cell behavior.

Keywords: CBD extracts; asthma; type 2 helper T cells (Th2); neutrophil; eosinophil; OVA-induced asthmatic mouse model; cytokines; migration; IgE

Citation: Aswad, M.; Pechkovsky, A.; Ghanayiem, N.; Hamza, H.; Dotan, Y.; Louria-Hayon, I. High-CBD Extract (CBD-X) in Asthma Management: Reducing Th2-Driven Cytokine Secretion and Neutrophil/Eosinophil Activity. *Pharmaceuticals* **2024**, *17*, 1382. https://doi.org/10.3390/ph17101382

Academic Editors: Elena Y. Enioutina, Kathleen M. Job and Catherine Sherwin

Received: 10 September 2024
Revised: 9 October 2024
Accepted: 12 October 2024
Published: 17 October 2024

1. Introduction

Asthma is a chronic inflammatory condition of the airways, characterized by coughing, wheezing, shortness of breath, and chest tightness. More than 10% of the global population is affected by this disease [1]. The pathophysiology of asthma involves airway inflammation that leads to increased mucus production [2], remodeling of the airway wall [3], and bronchial hyper-responsiveness (BHR) [4], which is the tendency of airway smooth muscle cells to react to non-specific stimuli such as allergens and cold air [5]. In many asthmatic individuals, chronic airway inflammation is primarily driven by type 2 helper T cells (Th2) or innate lymphoid cells type 2 (ILC2s) producing cytokines such as IL-4, IL-5, and IL-13 [6,7]. These type 2 cytokines are central to the disease's hallmark features, including eosinophilia [8], IgE production [9], and increased susceptibility to exacerbations [10]. However, only approximately 50% of asthmatic patients exhibit this "type 2-high" signature. The remaining patients often present with "type 2-low" asthma, which is frequently associated with obesity, neutrophilic inflammation, and poor response to corticosteroids, the conventional treatment for asthma [11].

Inhaled corticosteroids (ICS) remain the cornerstone of therapy for persistent asthma, supplemented by inhaled short acting bronchodilators for acute relief and long acting bronchodilators for prolonged effect [12]. Despite these treatments, many patients continue to experience inadequate asthma control due to factors such as refractory disease, ineffective treatment regimens, non-adherence, and comorbid conditions [13], highlighting the urgent need to identify new and more effective treatments for asthma.

Recent interest has emerged in the potential therapeutic role of cannabis, particularly cannabidiol (CBD), in managing inflammation. Studies indicate that CBD can reduce pro-inflammatory cytokine levels and cytokine storm [14], inhibit T cell proliferation, induce T cell apoptosis [15], effect macrophages function [16,17], and decrease immune cell migration and adhesion [18]. Moreover, CBD has demonstrated anti-oxidative [19] and anti-inflammatory properties in various autoimmune conditions, including rheumatoid arthritis, allergic contact dermatitis, and multiple sclerosis [20–23].

CBD interacts with CB1 and CB2 receptors as antagonist [24], which are highly expressed in the central nervous system and immune system, but also found in other tissues [25]. Additionally, CBD modulates redox balance and inflammation through transient receptor potential (TRP) channels, PPARγ receptors, GPR receptors, 5-HT1A receptors, and adenosine A2A receptors [20,26].

CBD administration has demonstrated significant potential in treating asthma. In experimental models of allergic asthma, CBD has been shown to reduce airway inflammation and fibrosis [27,28]. Additionally, CBD has been observed to lower cytokine levels in asthma models, suggesting its ability to modulate the immune response effectively [29].

Our recent findings further support this potential. High-CBD extract (CBD-X) has been found to effectively downregulate cytokine storm both systemically and locally in inflamed lungs [30].

2. Results

2.1. CBD-X Extract Impairs Differentiation of Human CD4 T Cells into Th2 Cells and Downregulates IL-5 and IL-13 Secretion

Based on our previous research on the effects of CBD-X extracts from the High CBD-cannabis strain, on cytokine storms and lung disease [30], we were prompted to investigate its impact on chronic lung diseases such as asthma. Th2 cells play a critical role in asthma development [31], secreting the pro-inflammatory type 2 cytokines IL-5 and IL-13 [6,7]. Moreover, Th2 cells differentiate from CD4 T cells in response to cytokines such as IL-4 [32].

We first analyzed the effect of CBD-X extract on the differentiation of CD4 T cells into Th2 cells ex vivo. Isolated CD4 T cells were treated with the high-CBD extract CBD-X. The cells were then differentiated into Th2 cells over six days. Cells were subjected to flow cytometry analysis using CD4, CCR4, and CCR6 markers. The percentage of CCR4+CCR6- in the CD4 population, termed Th2 cells, was determined.

Differentiated Th2 cells showed a fourfold increase in the percentage of CCR4+CCR6- cells compared to inactivated cells. However, CBD-X significantly reduced the capacity of CD4 T cells to differentiate into Th2 cells back to baseline levels (Figure 1a). The flow cytometry analysis demonstrated a marked decrease in the proportion of Th2 cells among CBD-X-treated CD4 T cells compared to the differentiated control group. Representative results of Th2 cell flow cytometry analysis are shown in three groups: inactivated, differentiated, and CBD-X differentiated cells (Figure 1b).

Given that Th2 cells secrete IL-5 and IL-13 during asthma exacerbation, we further examined the effect of CBD-X extract on the secretion of these cytokines. Differentiated Th2 cells significantly increased the secretion of IL-5 and IL-13 by threefold, compared to the control. However, CBD-X-treated Th2 cells exhibited a substantial reduction in the levels of these cytokines (Figure 1c,d).

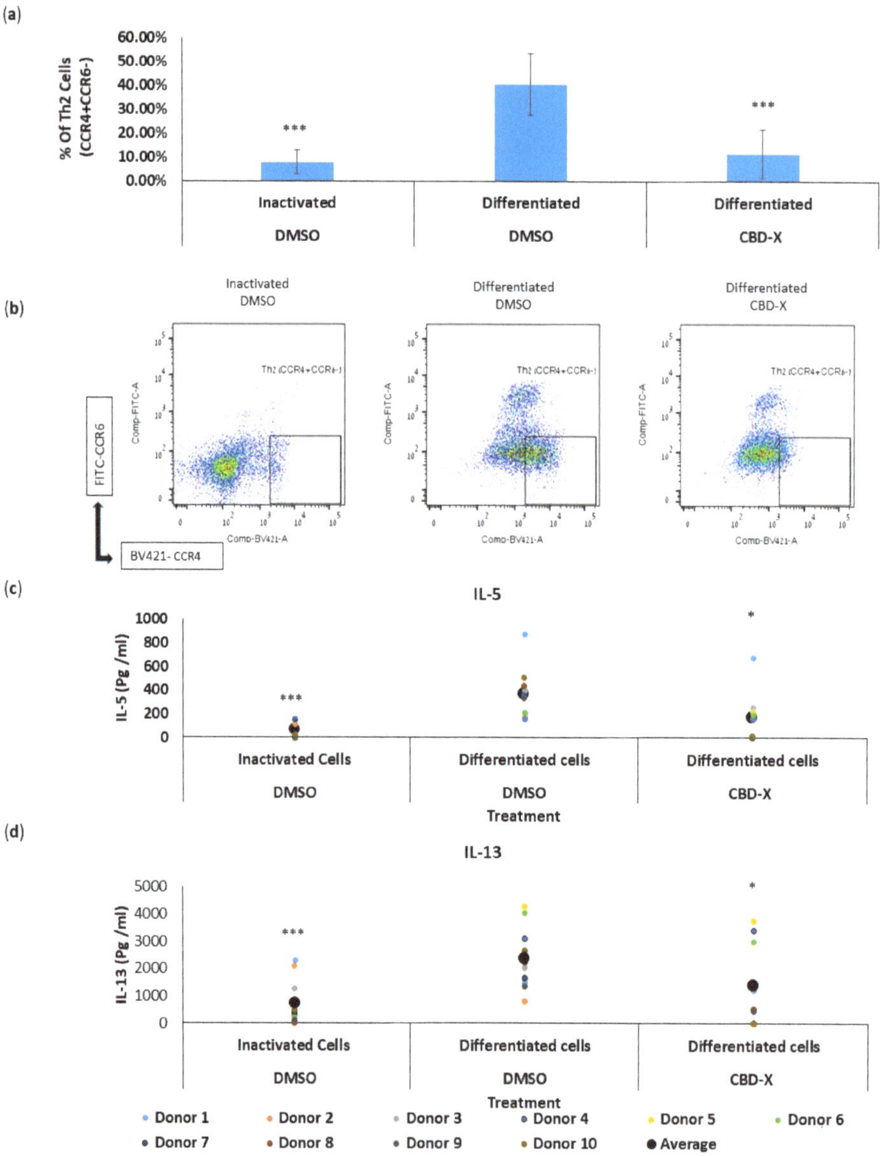

Figure 1. CBD-X extract attenuates the differentiation and cytokine release of human T helper 2 (Th2) cells. CBD-X extract was added to isolated differentiated CD4 T cells. Then, Th2 cells were subjected to flow cytometry analysis. CBD-X-treated cells and their control cells were stained with human APC-CD4, BV421- CCR4 and FITC-CCR6. The means and standard deviations of the percentage of Th2 (CCR4+CCR6-) from CD4 population were calculated. (**a**) The means were calculated from three different experiments of ten healthy donors. Data were analyzed in comparison to differentiated DMSO treatment representative results for CBD-X-treated cells and their control cells are shown (**b**). Moreover, supernatants were collected and levels of pro-inflammatory cytokines IL5 (**c**) and IL-13 (**d**) were detected via ELISA. The means were calculated from healthy donors (black big dot); each dot represents one case. Data were normalized to differentiated cell groups and analyzed via one-way ANOVA (Fisher's LSD test with values $p < 0.05$ considered statistically significant, (* $p < 0.05$, *** $p < 0.001$).

To exclude the possibility that this observation was due to a cytotoxic effect of the added extract, cell viability was measured via Alamar Blue assay. Cell viability was not reduced with the addition of the cannabinoid samples, allowing us to conclude that the reduction in differentiation and cytokine secretion was due to a regulatory effect of CBD-X (Figure S1).

These results indicate that CBD-X extract not only impairs the differentiation process but also diminishes the functional capacity of Th2 cells, potentially impacting Th2-mediated immune responses in chronic lung diseases like asthma.

2.2. CBD-X Extract Attenuates the Secretion of Pro-Inflammatory Cytokines from PBMC Derived Neutrophils

Some asthma patients exhibit elevated neutrophil counts in their airway secretions [33], which often show resistance to steroid treatments [34]. Neutrophilia in asthma is linked to factors such as IL-8, IL-17, and granulocyte-colony stimulating factor (G-CSF). The production of IL-8 is increased in some asthma patients [35,36], and clinical data reveal that IL-8 can serve as a marker for type 2-low asthma [37]. IL-8 is a crucial chemokine responsible for recruiting and activating neutrophils. Additionally, it is secreted by activated neutrophils, further amplifying the inflammatory response. To further investigate the role of CBD-X extract in this context, we examined its effect on neutrophils. Isolated human-derived neutrophils were pre-treated with 2 mg/mL CBD-X extract or vehicle as a control and then activated with 100 ng/mL lipopolysaccharide (LPS) overnight to induce cytokine secretion. The levels of IL-8 and IL-6 were analyzed. Our results demonstrate that LPS significantly increased the release of the pro-inflammatory cytokines IL-8 and IL-6 by about fourfold compared to the control (Figure 2a,b). However, CBD-X-treated neutrophils exhibited a significantly reduced capacity to secrete both cytokines. It is worth noting that the viability of neutrophils was not affected by the CBD-X extract at the concentration used, as determined via the Alamar Blue assay (Figure S2).

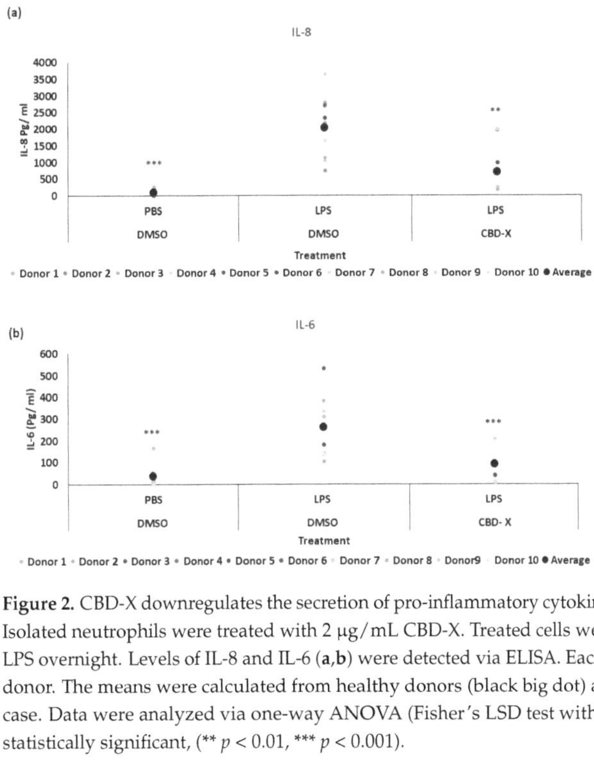

Figure 2. CBD-X downregulates the secretion of pro-inflammatory cytokines from human neutrophils. Isolated neutrophils were treated with 2 μg/mL CBD-X. Treated cells were activated via 100 ng/mL LPS overnight. Levels of IL-8 and IL-6 (**a**,**b**) were detected via ELISA. Each colored dot represents one donor. The means were calculated from healthy donors (black big dot) and each dot represents one case. Data were analyzed via one-way ANOVA (Fisher's LSD test with values $p < 0.05$ considered statistically significant, (** $p < 0.01$, *** $p < 0.001$).

2.3. CBD-X Extract Inhibits IL-8 Induced Migration of Neutrophils

Neutrophils are recruited to the airways of asthma patients in response to various chemokines, with IL-8 being particularly crucial for their recruitment [38,39]. IL-8 plays a significant role in asthma pathology by promoting increased neutrophilic infiltration into the lungs and exacerbating lung damage [40]. To determine whether CBD-X extract affects the migration capacity of neutrophils towards IL-8, PBMC-derived neutrophils were treated with 1 or 2 μg/mL CBD-X extract. Their ability to migrate towards IL-8 across a Boyden chamber was tested. Cells that migrated through the pores into the lower chamber were collected and subjected to flow cytometry analysis. IL-8 induced neutrophil migration significantly compared to the control. However, CBD-X extract inhibited the migration of neutrophils towards IL-8 in a dose-dependent manner (Figure 3). Neutrophil migration was inhibited by 2.5-fold and 3.5-fold with 1 and 2 μg/mL CBD-X extract, respectively (Figure 3a,b), effectively attenuating the IL-8 induced migration capacity.

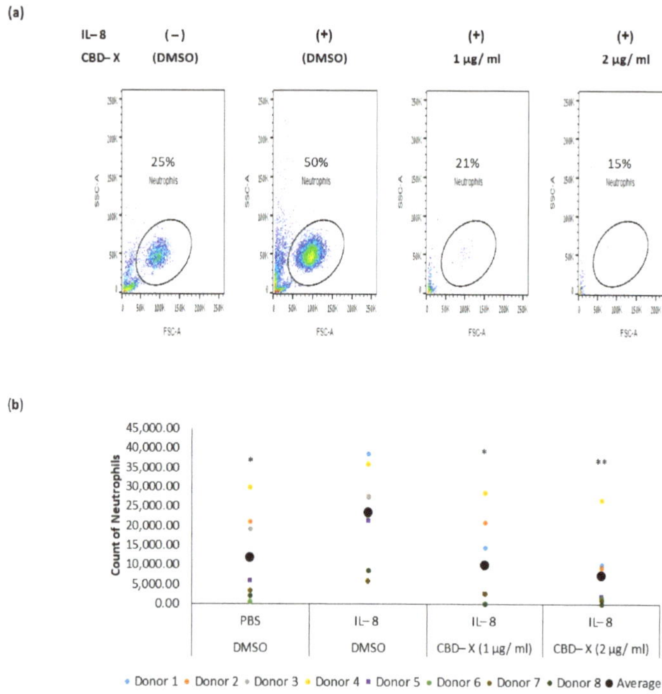

Figure 3. CBD-X extract inhibits the migration of neutrophils induced by IL-8. CBD-X-treated neutrophils were seeded onto the 3 μm pore polyester membrane in the upper chamber of a 24-well Boyden chamber. Human IL-8 in a concentration of 1 ng/mL was placed in the lower chamber. After three hours, cells that had migrated through the pores into the lower chamber were collected and subjected to flow cytometry analysis. (**a**) Representative results for migrated neutrophils toward IL-8 after treatment with (1 and 2 μg/mL) CBD-X. The colors in the dot plots represent the quantity of the cells. The lightest color (i.e., blue) would represent the low number of cells. In contrast, green, yellow and red would represent increasing values, with red indicating the highest values. (**b**) The number of migrated neutrophils. The means were calculated from healthy donors (black big dot) and each dot represents one case. Data were analyzed in comparison to the "IL-8, DMSO" group and analyzed via One-way ANOVA (Fisher's LSD test with values $p < 0.05$ considered statistically significant, (* $p < 0.05$, ** $p < 0.01$).

These results, combined with the observed downregulation of IL-8 and IL-6 secretion by CBD-X-treated neutrophils, suggest that CBD-X may modulate the inflammatory response by impairing both neutrophil recruitment and activity. This could potentially offer a therapeutic strategy for managing conditions characterized by excessive neutrophilic inflammation, such as type 2-low asthma.

2.4. CBD-X Extract Modulates IgE Levels and Cytokine Secretion in a Murine Model of Asthma

We investigated the therapeutic potential of CBD-X extract in an in vivo mouse model of asthma. BALB/c mice were sensitized with ovalbumin (OVA, grade V) to induce an allergic response. To assess the effects of CBD-X extract, lung fluids and blood were collected and analyzed (Figure 4).

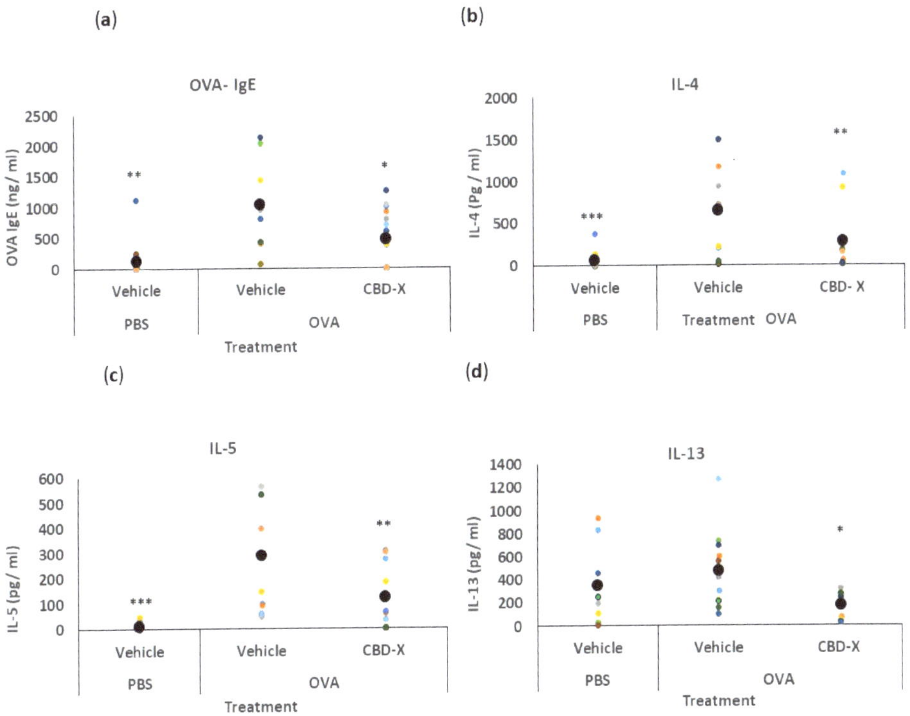

Figure 4. CBD-X extract attenuates serum OVA- IgE and BALF cytokine levels in an asthma mouse model. BALB/c mice were induced with OVA and were treated with 150 mg/kg CBD-X extract. Mice were euthanized, blood and lung fluids were collected. Levels of serum OVA- IgE (**a**) were detected via ELISA. Alternatively, levels of the pro-inflammatory IL-4 (**b**), IL-5 (**c**), and IL-13 (**d**) were also detected in the lung fluids via ELISA. Each colored dot represents one mouse. Standard deviations were calculated as the means of three biologically independent experiments (black big dot); $n = 10$. Data were analyzed via one-way ANOVA (Fisher's LSD test with values $p < 0.05$ considered statistically significant, (* $p < 0.05$, ** $p < 0.01$, *** $p < 0.001$).

We first quantified serum IgE levels, given its role as a marker of allergic asthma [41]. The secretion of OVA-IgE levels in the serum was detected via ELISA. The increased levels of OVA-IgE in the serum of OVA-treated mice were reduced by more than twofold with the CBD-X extract (Figure 4a).

Next, we analyzed cytokine levels in the bronchoalveolar lavage fluid (BALF) from the lungs. Remarkably, the CBD-X extract led to a substantial reduction in the pro-asthmatic cytokines IL-4, IL-5, and IL-13 compared to the OVA-treated mice (Figure 4b–d).

These results indicate that CBD-X extract effectively attenuates both systemic and localized inflammatory responses associated with allergic asthma.

2.5. CBD-X Extract Inhibits Migration of Leukocytes to OVA-Induced Asthmatic Lungs

The asthmatic airway is characterized by chronic inflammation of the airway wall due to a complex infiltration and interplay of immune cells [11]. Therefore, we examined whether CBD-X extract affected leukocyte migration into the lungs in an OVA-treated mouse asthma model. Lung fluids were collected and immune cells were marked with anti-mouse APC-CD45, anti-mouse FITC-F4/80, anti-mouse BV786-LY6G, and PE-Siglec F for flow cytometry analysis.

Examination of lung immune cell populations revealed that control mice with asthma (OVA-treated mice) exhibited elevated numbers of leukocytes, and eosinophils, while neutrophil and macrophage numbers remained unchanged (Figure 5). In contrast, CBD-X-treated mice showed a significant reduction in leukocyte and eosinophil counts by 51% and 58%, respectively (Figure 5a), suggesting a targeted attenuation of the inflammatory response. Macrophage and neutrophil numbers were unaffected, indicating that CBD-X extract modulates specific immune cell populations rather than broadly suppressing immune activity.

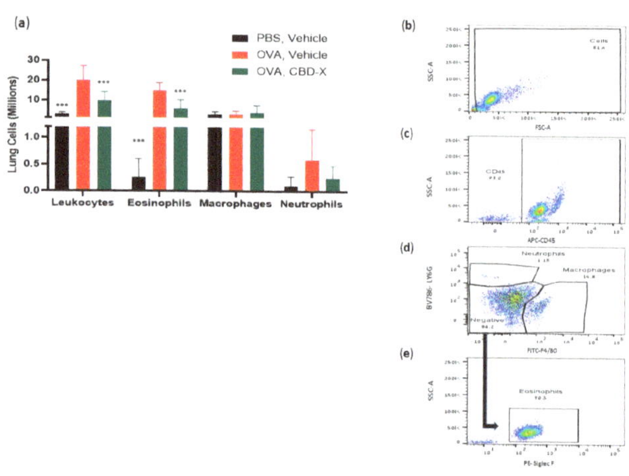

Figure 5. CBD-X extract inhibits migration of leukocytes to OVA-induced asthma lungs. Mice were induced with OVA-induced asthma and were treated with 150 mg/kg of CBD-X extract. Then, mice were sacrificed and lung fluids were collected. (**a**) Cells in the lung fluids were stained with anti-mouse APC-CD45, anti-mouse FITC- F480, anti-mouse BV786-LY6G, and PE- Siglec F for flow cytometry analysis. Numbers of leukocytes, eosinophils, macrophages, and neutrophils were calculated in the three different treatments; PBS- vehicle (Black bars), OVA- vehicle (Red bars) and OVA- CBD-X (green bars) (**a**). The gating strategy is (**b**) FSC vs. SSC, (**c**) APC-CD45 vs. SSC, and (**d**) BV786-LY6G vs. FITC-F4/80. (**e**) PE- Siglec F vs. SSC out of the negative population gate in (**d**). The colors in the dot plots represent the quantity of the cells. The lightest color (i.e., blue) would represent the low number of cells. In contrast, green, yellow and red would represent increasing values, with red indicating the highest values. Averages and standard deviations were calculated as the means of two biologically independent experiments, each experiment included five mice per group. Data were analyzed via mixed-effects model (Fisher's LSD test with values $p < 0.05$ considered statistically significant, (*** $p < 0.001$).

The gating strategy of representative results is shown (Figure 5b–e). Collectively, these findings demonstrate that CBD-X treatment effectively alleviates asthma symptoms in the mouse model. The reduction in IgE levels and pro-inflammatory cytokines, along with the decreased recruitment of inflammatory cells, underscores the potential of CBD-X extract as a therapeutic agent for asthma, targeting both systemic and localized inflammatory processes.

3. Discussion

Asthma is a chronic inflammatory disease of the airways characterized by wheezing, shortness of breath, chest tightness, and coughing. Current treatments, such as inhaled corticosteroids (ICS), long-acting beta-agonists (LABAs), leukotriene modifiers, and biologics, aim to control symptoms and prevent exacerbations [42]. While these treatments are effective, they can have side effects ranging from oral thrush, increased risk of pneumonia, and in high doses, to systemic effects of steroids due to absorption from the lungs to the blood circuit, [43], highlighting the need for novel therapies with fewer adverse effects.

Here, we showed that the CBD-X extract of the high CBD cannabis strain, presents significant therapeutic potential in managing chronic lung diseases, particularly asthma. Our previous findings indicated that CBD-X extract had beneficial effects on cytokine storms and acute lung disease [30], which prompted us to explore its efficacy in a chronic lung disease model.

We first examined the effect of the CBD-X extract on primary human Th2 cells, as their cytokines play a central role in asthma and drive key features of the disease, including eosinophilia, mucus hypersecretion, bronchial hyper-responsiveness (BHR), IgE production, and increased susceptibility to exacerbations [11]. We observed that CBD-X extract markedly reduced the differentiation capacity of CD4 T cells into Th2 cells. This was demonstrated by a significant decrease in the proportion of Th2 cells among CBD-X-treated CD4 T cells compared to the differentiated control group. These findings suggest that CBD-X extract impaired the CD4 to Th2 differentiation process, potentially mitigating the Th2-mediated immune responses that exacerbate asthma symptoms. Th2 cells are crucial in the pathogenesis of asthma due to their secretion of IL-5 and IL-13, which promote eosinophilic inflammation and BHR.

Further analysis revealed that CBD-X-treated Th2 cells exhibited a substantial reduction in IL-5 and IL-13 secretion, underscoring the functional impairment of Th2 cells induced by CBD-X extract. Our results indicate that CBD-X not only affects the differentiation of Th2 cells but also diminishes their functional activity, thereby potentially reducing the inflammatory milieu characteristic of type 2-high asthma.

Asthma pathology is often complicated by the presence of elevated eosinophil and/or neutrophil counts in the airways, particularly in patients resistant to steroid treatments for the latter [33]. 'Type 2-low' asthma is more associated with obesity, presence of neutrophils, and unresponsiveness to corticosteroids [11]. Our study shows that CBD-X significantly reduces the secretion of type 2-low cytokines such as IL-8 and IL-6 from human-derived neutrophils. IL-8 is pivotal in recruiting neutrophils to the airways, thereby amplifying inflammation and lung damage [36]. CBD-X-treated neutrophils demonstrated a dose-dependent inhibition of migration towards IL-8, as shown via the Boyden chamber assay. These findings suggest that CBD-X modulates the inflammatory response by impairing neutrophil recruitment and activity, offering a novel approach to managing neutrophil-dominated inflammation in asthma. In our in vivo studies using an asthma mouse model, CBD-X treatment resulted in a notable reduction in IgE levels in the blood, a key indicator of allergic responses. Additionally, cytokine analysis of bronchoalveolar lavage fluid (BALF) from the lungs of CBD-X-treated mice revealed significant reductions in IL-4, IL-5, and IL-13 levels compared to asthmatic controls. Examination of immune cell populations in the lungs showed that control sick mice exhibited elevated numbers of leukocytes and eosinophils, but not macrophages and neutrophils. In contrast, CBD-X-treated mice demonstrated a reduction in leukocytes and eosinophils, while macrophage and neutrophil numbers remained unchanged. This selective modulation of immune cell populations by CBD-X extract highlights its potential to alleviate asthma symptoms by targeting key inflammatory pathways. Interestingly, these results align with previously reported effects of CB2 antagonists on eosinophil counts [44] and cytokine secretion [45]. This alignment may partially explain the effects of CBD-X, as CBD is known to act as a CB2 antagonist [24]. In most individuals, asthma is easily controlled with inhaled corticosteroids (ICS) and bronchodilators, usually combined in a single inhaler. However, many asthmatics do not respond adequately to these therapies and have persistent symptoms and/or exacerbations that require systemic steroids and/or hospitalization [46].

The acknowledgment that asthma is a heterogeneous disease has prompted pharmaceutical companies to develop new drugs to specifically target eosinophils, IL-5, IL4 receptor, and IgE involved in different types of asthma [11].

This evidence underscores the growing interest in CBD as a complementary treatment for asthma, highlighting its capability to address both inflammation and immune response in respiratory conditions.

In this study, we explored the therapeutic potential of CBD-X extract by examining its effects on cells involved in the asthmatic process. We utilized two ex vivo cell models—primary human Th2 cells and neutrophils—to evaluate the anti-inflammatory properties of CBD-X. Our findings revealed that CBD-X extract inhibits the differentiation of CD4+ cells into Th2 cells, leading to a reduction in the secretion of pro-asthmatic cytokines IL-5 and IL-13. Additionally, CBD-X extract decreases the levels of pro-inflammatory cytokines IL-8 and IL-6 in primary human neutrophils and impairs their migration towards IL-8. This reduction impairs the communication between immune cells, which is crucial in the development and exacerbation of asthma. Moreover, in a murine model of asthma, CBD-X administration significantly downregulated key asthma markers such as IgE and pro-asthmatic cytokines IL-4, IL-5, and IL-13 in both blood and lung tissues, and inhibited the migration of leukocytes, eosinophils, and neutrophils to lung tissues.

These results pave the way for further clinical studies to validate the efficacy and safety of CBD-X extract as a potential treatment for asthma and other chronic inflammatory lung diseases.

4. Materials and Methods

4.1. Reagents

ELISA kits for human IL-5, IL-13, IL-8, and IL-6 or mouse IL-4, IL-5, and IL-13 were obtained from R&D System (Minneapolis, MN, USA). The Mouse Anti-OVA IgE Antibody Assay Kit was obtained from Chondrex, Inc (Woodinville, WA, USA). Human TruStain FcX™ (Fc Receptor Blocking Solution), anti-human CD3 (mouse, IgG2a, κ, clone OKT3), anti-human CD28 (mouse, IgG1, κ, clone CD28.2), human IL-2 and anti-human IFN-γ (Mouse IgG1, κ, clone B27), APC anti-human CD4, (mouse, IgG2b, κ, clone A17070D), Brilliant Violet 421 anti-human CD194 (CCR4, Mouse IgG1, κ, clone L291H4) and FITC anti-human CD196 (CCR6, Mouse IgG2b, κ, clone G034E3), TruStain FcX™ (rat anti-mouse CD16/32, IgG2a, Λ, a) and APC anti-mouse CD45 (rat, IgG2b, κ, clone 30/F11), FITC anti-mouse F4/80 recombinant (Mouse IgG1, κ, clone QA17A29), Brilliant Violet 785 anti-mouse Ly-6G (Rat IgG2a, κ, clone 1A8), and PE anti-human Siglec-8 (Mouse IgG1, κ, clone 7C9) were purchased from BioLegend (San Diego, CA, USA). The media RPMI 1640 Medium with L-Glutamine were obtained from Sartorius, Beit Haemek, Israel and the medium X-VIVO 15 with gentamicin and phenol red was obtained from Lonza (Basel, Switzerland). The Human Neutrophil Isolation Kit and the Human CD4+ T -Cell Isolation Kit were obtained from STEMCELL Technologies, Vancouver, BC, Canada. Millicell Hanging Cell Culture Inserts, PET 3 μm, and the 24-well were purchased from Merck (Rahway, NJ, USA). Lipopolysaccharide (LPS) was obtained from Santa Cruz (CA, USA). Human IL4 and IL8 were obtained from PeproTech (London, UK). Fetal bovine serum (FBS), glutamine and penicillin, and 100 U/mL streptomycin were purchased from Biological Industries, Beit Haemek (Israel). Albumin from chicken egg white and lyophilized powder (Ovalbumin) were purchased from Merck (Rahway, NJ, USA). Imject™ Alum Adjuvant was purchased from Thermo Fisher Scientific (Waltham, MA, USA).

4.2. Cannabis Extracts

Cannabis extracts were kindly provided by Raphael Pharmaceutical, Inc (Las Vegas, NV, USA). The strains were cultivated and grown by WOLC-Way Of Life Cannabis (Israel). A concentration of 1 μg/mL CBD-X contained 35% CBD, 0.3% THC, 0% CBN, and 0.3% CBG.

4.3. Human Peripheral Blood Samples

Human peripheral blood samples were provided by the Israeli National Biobank for Research (MIDGAM) at Rambam Health Care Campus. The experiments were authorized by the Helsinki Committee at Rambam Health Care Campus (Authorization No. 0442-20 RMB).

4.4. Mice

BALB/c mice at the age of 8 to 10 weeks were purchased from Envigo, Israel. All mice were housed at a barrier-free and specific pathogen-free animal facility at the Pre-Clinical Research Authority, Technion-Israel Institute of Technology in Haifa, Israel. All experiments were performed according to the regulations of the Inspection Committee on the Constitution of the Animal Experimentation of the Technion-Israel Institute of Technology in Haifa, Israel from which authorization for performing animal studies was approved (Authorization No. IL-1330221). Experiments conformed to the regulations in the Prevention of Cruelty to Animals Law (Experiments on Animals) 5754-1994 and the Prevention of Cruelty to Animals Rules (Experiments on Animals) 5761-2001 (correct as of 1 December 2005).

4.5. Isolation of Immune Cells from Blood

Peripheral blood samples of healthy volunteers were collected in EDTA-containing tubes.

4.5.1. CD4 Cell Isolation

CD4+ T cells were isolated via an EasySep Direct Human CD4+ T-cell Isolation Kit according to the manufacturer's instructions (STEMCELL Technologies). In brief, isolation cocktail (50 μL/mL) and RapidSpheres (50 μL/mL) were added to the blood samples for 5 min. Samples were topped up with the recommended medium. The sample tubes were inserted into the magnet for a further 5 min. The samples were transferred to a new tube. RapidSpheres (50 μL/mL) were once more added to the samples. These were inserted into the magnet for another 5 min. The final step was repeated to produce a clear fraction.

4.5.2. Neutrophil Cell Isolation

Neutrophils were isolated from blood samples via negative magnetic selection with the EasySep Direct Human Neutrophil Isolation Kit (STEMCELL Technologies) according to the manufacturer's instructions. Briefly, Isolation Cocktail (50 μL/mL) and RapidSpheres (50 μL/mL) were added to a whole blood sample tube for 5 min. The sample tube was topped up with recommended medium and inserted into the magnet for 10 min. Then, the sample was transferred to a new tube and RapidSpheres (50 μL/mL) were added for an additional 5 min of incubation. The sample with the RapidSpheres was inserted into the magnet for 5 min and sample was transferred to a third tube. The last step was repeated to obtain a final clear fraction.

4.6. Cell Culture and Treatment of the Cells with Cannabis Extracts

4.6.1. Th2 Cells

Firstly, 0.2×10^6 Isolated CD4+ T cells were treated with 2 μg/mL cannabis extract or DMSO as a control for two hours. CD4+ T cells were cultured in RPMI 1640 or neutrophils in X-VIVO 15. After incubation, CBD-X-treated cells and control cells were centrifuged and activated or left untreated. CD4+ T cells were differentiated by seeding them on a plate coated with 2.5 μg/mL anti-human CD3 to which were added 2.5 μg/mL anti-CD28, 125 units/mL hIL-2, 20 ng/mL hIL-4, and 1 μg/mL anti-human IFN-γ in complete RPMI 1640 medium for six days. Cells were refreshed with complete RPMI 1640 medium which included hIL-2, hIL-4, and anti-human IFN-γ every three days. Then, cells were centrifuged, supernatants were collected, and levels of IL-5 and Il 13 were detected via enzyme-linked immunosorbent assay (ELISA) according to the manufacturer's instructions (R&D System).

4.6.2. Neutrophil Cells

Firstly, 0.2×10^6 Isolated neutrophils were treated with 2 μg/mL cannabis extract or DMSO as a control for two hours. Then, neutrophils were activated with 100 ng/mL LPS in X-VIVO 15 medium overnight. Cells were centrifuged, supernatants were collected, and levels of IL-8 and IL-6 were detected via ELISA [30].

4.7. Cell Viability Measurement

CBD-X-treated Th2 or neutrophils were washed, and medium was added to the cells with 10% Alamar Blue solution. As a negative control, Alamar Blue was added to the medium without cells. The cells were further incubated for another four hours at 37 °C. The absorbance of the test and control wells was read at 570 nm and 600 nm with a standard spectrophotometer [30].

4.8. Cell Migration

For the cell migration experiments, 3 μm 24-well Boyden chambers were used. A total of 0.25–0.5×10^6 cells/mL of neutrophils were seeded in the upper chamber of the 24-well Boyden chamber in medium. In the lower chamber, 100 ng/mL of hIL-8 were placed. Increased concentrations of cannabis extract (1 and 2 μg/mL) or DMSO as a vehicle functioning as a negative control were added to the cells. Three hours later, cells that were migrated through the pores into the lower chamber were collected and counted via flow cytometry [30].

4.9. Asthma Mouse Model

BALB/c mice were intraperitoneally (i.p) injected with 100 μg albumin, chicken egg grade V (OVA), 3 mg/mL Inject Alum (aluminum hydroxide (40 mg/mL), and magnesium hydroxide (40 mg/mL) on days 1, 7, and 14 [47,48]. Then, mice were challenged intranasally (i.n) with 150 μg OVA or PBS on days 21, 23, and 26. Mice were treated intraperitoneally with 300 mg/kg CBD-X extract or vehicle (5% kolliphor, 5% ethanol, 90% of 0.9% NaCl in sterile water for injections) as a control on days 20, 21, 23, and 26 (Figure 6). After 3 h of the last challenge, the mice were euthanized. Then, lung fluids were collected using PBS through lavage and blood was drained from the heart. Samples were centrifuged and supernatants were collected and stored at −20 °C. Levels of OVA-IgE were detected in the serum and cytokines of IL-4, IL-5, and IL-13 levels were detected in the lung fluids via ELISA. Moreover, cells in the lung fluids were stained with TruStain FcX™ (anti-mouse CD16/32) and anti-mouse APC-CD45, anti-mouse FITC- F4/80, anti-mouse BV786-LY6G, and PE- Siglec F for flow cytometry analysis.

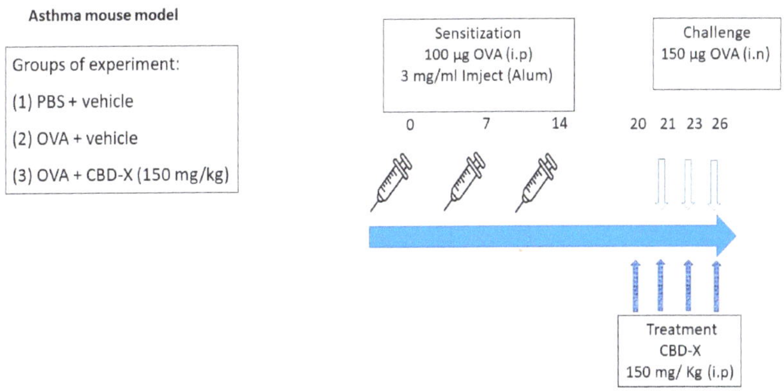

Figure 6. CBD-X treatment in a mouse model of OVA-induced asthma. For sensitization, BALB/c mice received an i.p injection of OVA (100 µg) with 3 mg/mL Inject (Alum) (aluminum hydroxide (40 mg/mL) and magnesium hydroxide (40 mg/mL) on days 1, 7, and 14. PBS was injected as a control. The mice were challenged with an (intranasal) i.n injection of OVA (150 µg) or PBS on days 21, 23, and 26. Mice were injected intraperitoneally with 150 mg/kg CBD-X extract or vehicle as a control on days 20, 21, 23, and 26. After 3 h of the last challenge, mice were euthanized and lung fluids were collected using PBS through lavage.

5. Statistical Analysis

For statistical analysis, the ex vivo experiments data were analyzed in comparison to activated treatment as a baseline. In the case of TH2 cells, significance was determined in comparison to the "Differentiated, DMSO" group. TH2 differentiation was performed for anti-CD3, anti-CD28, hIL-2, hIL-4, and anti-IFN-γ. While in neutrophils, the significance was determined in comparison to the "LPS, DMSO" group.

In the in vivo experiments, data were analyzed in comparison to OVA-induced mice as a baseline named "OVA, Vehicle" group. Means were calculated for at least three biologically independent experiments. When each experiment included three to five mice in each group. Data were analyzed via one-way ANOVA (Fisher's LSD test with values $p < 0.05$ considered statistically significant, (* $p < 0.05$, ** $p < 0.01$, *** $p < 0.001$).

6. Conclusions

This study reveals novel roles of high CBD (CBD-X) extract in regulating human Th2 cell differentiation and its subsequent suppression of IL-5 and IL-13 production. In addition to inhibiting cytokine secretion, CBD-X also reduces neutrophil migration to inflamed tissues, indicating its promising therapeutic potential. The ability of CBD-X to reduce key inflammatory markers of asthma—such as IgE, IL-4, IL-5, and IL-13—in a murine asthma model further supports its anti-inflammatory effects. Additionally, CBD-X modulates immune cell recruitment to the lungs, suggesting its potential in developing new cannabis-based therapies for inflammatory disorders.

These findings indicate that CBD-X extract may provide a novel, complementary approach to managing both type 2-high and type 2-low asthma by targeting key inflammatory pathways and modulating immune responses. Further research is required to explore the molecular mechanisms underlying CBD-X's effects. Specifically, experiments will involve treating Th2 cells and neutrophils with CBD-X to evaluate downstream inflammatory pathways. Given its therapeutic potential, CBD-X will be tested in clinical trials to assess its efficacy and safety for asthma patients.

Supplementary Materials: The following supporting information can be downloaded at: https://www.mdpi.com/article/10.3390/ph17101382/s1, Figure S1: CBD-X have no cytotoxic effect on the viability of Th2 cells; Figure S2: Cannabinoids have no cytotoxic effect on the viability of human neutrophils.

Author Contributions: Conceptualization, M.A. and I.L.-H.; methodology, M.A.; software, M.A.; validation, M.A., A.P. and N.G.; formal analysis, H.H. and M.A.; investigation, M.A., H.H. and I.L.-H.; resources, I.L.-H.; data curation, M.A.; writing—original draft preparation, M.A. and I.L.-H.; writing—review and editing, M.A., A.P., Y.D. and I.L.-H.; visualization, M.A.; supervision, I.L.-H.; project administration, I.L.-H.; funding acquisition, I.L.-H. All authors have read and agreed to the published version of the manuscript.

Funding: This research was funded by Raphael Pharmaceutical Inc. grant for cannabis and inflammation. In addition to RAMBAM- MED-TECH, Nitzots grant for cannabis and immunology.

Institutional Review Board Statement: The study was conducted in accordance with the Declaration of Helsinki, and approved by the Institutional Review Board (or Ethics Committee) of (MIDGAM) at Rambam Health Care Campus in Haifa, Israel (protocol code No. 0442-20 RMB and date of approval 21 March 22). The animal study protocol was approved by the Institutional Review Board (or Ethics Committee) of the Animal Experimentation of the Technion-Israel Institute of Technology in Haifa, Israel (protocol code No. IL-1330221 and date of approval 10 October 21).

Informed Consent Statement: Informed consent was obtained from all subjects involved in the study. Written informed consent has been obtained from the patient(s) to publish this paper.

Data Availability Statement: The data presented in this study are available on request from the corresponding author.

Acknowledgments: We want to thank Raphael Pharmaceutical Inc. for supporting this study and for providing the CBD-X cannabis extracts.

Conflicts of Interest: This study received funding from Raphael Pharmaceutical Inc. The funders were not involved in any aspect of the study. The authors declare no conflicts of interest.

References

1. Song, P.; Adeloye, D.; Salim, H.; Dos Santos, J.P.; Campbell, H.; Sheikh, A.; Rudan, I. Global, Regional, and National Prevalence of Asthma in 2019: A Systematic Analysis and Modelling Study. *J. Glob. Health* **2022**, *12*, 04052. [CrossRef] [PubMed]
2. Evans, C.M.; Kim, K.; Tuvim, M.J.; Dickey, B.F. Mucus Hypersecretion in Asthma: Causes and Effects. *Curr. Opin. Pulm. Med.* **2009**, *15*, 4–11. [CrossRef]
3. Fehrenbach, H.; Wagner, C.; Wegmann, M. Airway Remodeling in Asthma: What Really Matters. *Cell Tissue Res.* **2017**, *367*, 551–569. [CrossRef] [PubMed]
4. Chapman, D.G.; Irvin, C.G. Mechanisms of Airway Hyper-responsiveness in Asthma: The Past, Present and yet to Come. *Clin. Exp. Allergy* **2015**, *45*, 706–719. [CrossRef]
5. Wu, W.; Bang, S.; Bleecker, E.R.; Castro, M.; Denlinger, L.; Erzurum, S.C.; Fahy, J.V.; Fitzpatrick, A.M.; Gaston, B.M.; Hastie, A.T.; et al. Multiview Cluster Analysis Identifies Variable Corticosteroid Response Phenotypes in Severe Asthma. *Am. J. Respir. Crit. Care Med.* **2019**, *199*, 1358–1367. [CrossRef] [PubMed]
6. Nakayama, T.; Hirahara, K.; Onodera, A.; Endo, Y.; Hosokawa, H.; Shinoda, K.; Tumes, D.J.; Okamoto, Y. Th2 Cells in Health and Disease. *Annu. Rev. Immunol.* **2017**, *35*, 53–84. [CrossRef]
7. Lambrecht, B.N.; Hammad, H.; Fahy, J.V. The Cytokines of Asthma. *Immunity* **2019**, *50*, 975–991. [CrossRef]
8. Hussain, M.; Liu, G. Eosinophilic Asthma: Pathophysiology and Therapeutic Horizons. *Cells* **2024**, *13*, 384. [CrossRef]
9. Platts-Mills, T.A.E. The Role of Immunoglobulin E in Allergy and Asthma. *Am. J. Respir. Crit. Care Med.* **2001**, *164*, S1–S5. [CrossRef]
10. Castillo, J.R.; Peters, S.P.; Busse, W.W. Asthma Exacerbations: Pathogenesis, Prevention, and Treatment. *J. Allergy Clin. Immunol. Pract.* **2017**, *5*, 918–927. [CrossRef]
11. Hammad, H.; Lambrecht, B.N. The Basic Immunology of Asthma. *Cell* **2021**, *184*, 1469–1485. [CrossRef] [PubMed]
12. Kearns, N.; Maijers, I.; Harper, J.; Beasley, R.; Weatherall, M. Inhaled Corticosteroids in Acute Asthma: A Systemic Review and Meta-Analysis. *J. Allergy Clin. Immunol. Pract.* **2020**, *8*, 605–617. [CrossRef] [PubMed]
13. Bleecker, E.R.; Al-Ahmad, M.; Bjermer, L.; Caminati, M.; Canonica, G.W.; Kaplan, A.; Papadopoulos, N.G.; Roche, N.; Ryan, D.; Tohda, Y.; et al. Systemic Corticosteroids in Asthma: A Call to Action from World Allergy Organization and Respiratory Effectiveness Group. *World Allergy Organ. J.* **2022**, *15*, 100726. [CrossRef] [PubMed]
14. Paland, N.; Pechkovsky, A.; Aswad, M.; Hamza, H.; Popov, T.; Shahar, E.; Louria-Hayon, I. The Immunopathology of COVID-19 and the Cannabis Paradigm. *Front. Immunol.* **2021**, *12*, 631233. [CrossRef]

15. Rieder, S.A.; Chauhan, A.; Singh, U.; Nagarkatti, M.; Nagarkatti, P. Cannabinoid-Induced Apoptosis in Immune Cells as a Pathway to Immunosuppression. *Immunobiology* **2010**, *215*, 598–605. [CrossRef] [PubMed]
16. Yekhtin, Z.; Khuja, I.; Meiri, D.; Or, R.; Almogi-Hazan, O. Differential Effects of D9 Tetrahydrocannabinol (THC)- and Cannabidiol (CBD)-Based Cannabinoid Treatments on Macrophage Immune Function In Vitro and on Gastrointestinal Inflammation in a Murine Model. *Biomedicines* **2022**, *10*, 1793. [CrossRef]
17. Zaiachuk, M.; Suryavanshi, S.V.; Pryimak, N.; Kovalchuk, I.; Kovalchuk, O. The Anti-Inflammatory Effects of Cannabis Sativa Extracts on LPS-Induced Cytokines Release in Human Macrophages. *Molecules* **2023**, *28*, 4991. [CrossRef]
18. Pagano, S.; Coniglio, M.; Valenti, C.; Federici, M.I.; Lombardo, G.; Cianetti, S.; Marinucci, L. Biological Effects of Cannabidiol on Normal Human Healthy Cell Populations: Systematic Review of the Literature. *Biomed. Pharmacother.* **2020**, *132*, 110728. [CrossRef]
19. Krzyżewska, A.; Baranowska-Kuczko, M.; Jastrząb, A.; Kasacka, I.; Kozłowska, H. Cannabidiol Improves Antioxidant Capacity and Reduces Inflammation in the Lungs of Rats with Monocrotaline-Induced Pulmonary Hypertension. *Molecules* **2022**, *27*, 3327. [CrossRef]
20. Atalay, S.; Jarocka-Karpowicz, I.; Skrzydlewska, E. Antioxidative and Anti-Inflammatory Properties of Cannabidiol. *Antioxidants* **2019**, *9*, 21. [CrossRef]
21. Lowin, T.; Tingting, R.; Zurmahr, J.; Classen, T.; Schneider, M.; Pongratz, G. Cannabidiol (CBD): A Killer for Inflammatory Rheumatoid Arthritis Synovial Fibroblasts. *Cell Death Dis.* **2020**, *11*, 714. [CrossRef] [PubMed]
22. Paland, N.; Hamza, H.; Pechkovsky, A.; Aswad, M.; Shagidov, D.; Louria-Hayon, I. Cannabis and Rheumatoid Arthritis: A Scoping Review Evaluating the Benefits, Risks, and Future Research Directions. *Rambam Maimonides Med. J.* **2023**, *14*, e0022. [CrossRef]
23. Mecha, M.; Feliú, A.; Iñigo, P.M.; Mestre, L.; Carrillo-Salinas, F.J.; Guaza, C. Cannabidiol Provides Long-Lasting Protection against the Deleterious Effects of Inflammation in a Viral Model of Multiple Sclerosis: A Role for A2A Receptors. *Neurobiol. Dis.* **2013**, *59*, 141–150. [CrossRef]
24. Thomas, A.; Baillie, G.L.; Phillips, A.M.; Razdan, R.K.; Ross, R.A.; Pertwee, R.G. Cannabidiol Displays Unexpectedly High Potency as an Antagonist of CB_1 and CB_2 Receptor Agonists *In Vitro*. *Br. J. Pharmacol.* **2007**, *150*, 613–623. [CrossRef] [PubMed]
25. An, D.; Peigneur, S.; Hendrickx, L.A.; Tytgat, J. Targeting Cannabinoid Receptors: Current Status and Prospects of Natural Products. *Int. J. Mol. Sci.* **2020**, *21*, 5064. [CrossRef] [PubMed]
26. Ribeiro, A.; Ferraz-de-Paula, V.; Pinheiro, M.L.; Vitoretti, L.B.; Mariano-Souza, D.P.; Quinteiro-Filho, W.M.; Akamine, A.T.; Almeida, V.I.; Quevedo, J.; Dal-Pizzol, F.; et al. Cannabidiol, a Non-Psychotropic Plant-Derived Cannabinoid, Decreases Inflammation in a Murine Model of Acute Lung Injury: Role for the Adenosine A2A Receptor. *Eur. J. Pharmacol.* **2012**, *678*, 78–85. [CrossRef]
27. Vuolo, F.; Abreu, S.C.; Michels, M.; Xisto, D.G.; Blanco, N.G.; Hallak, J.E.; Zuardi, A.W.; Crippa, J.A.; Reis, C.; Bahl, M.; et al. Cannabidiol Reduces Airway Inflammation and Fibrosis in Experimental Allergic Asthma. *Eur. J. Pharmacol.* **2019**, *843*, 251–259. [CrossRef]
28. Menezes, P.M.N.; Araújo, T.C.D.L.; Pereira, E.C.V.; Neto, J.A.; Silva, D.S.; Brito, M.C.; Lima, K.S.B.; Monte, A.P.O.D.; Matos, M.H.T.D.; Lima, R.S.D.; et al. Investigation of Antinociceptive, Antipyretic, Antiasthmatic, and Spasmolytic Activities of Brazilian *Cannabis Sativa* L. Roots in Rodents. *J. Ethnopharmacol.* **2021**, *278*, 114259. [CrossRef]
29. Vuolo, F.; Petronilho, F.; Sonai, B.; Ritter, C.; Hallak, J.E.C.; Zuardi, A.W.; Crippa, J.A.; Dal-Pizzol, F. Evaluation of Serum Cytokines Levels and the Role of Cannabidiol Treatment in Animal Model of Asthma. *Mediat. Inflamm.* **2015**, *2015*, 538670. [CrossRef]
30. Aswad, M.; Hamza, H.; Pechkovsky, A.; Zikrach, A.; Popov, T.; Zohar, Y.; Shahar, E.; Louria-Hayon, I. High-CBD Extract (CBD-X) Downregulates Cytokine Storm Systemically and Locally in Inflamed Lungs. *Front. Immunol.* **2022**, *13*, 875546. [CrossRef]
31. Harker, J.A.; Lloyd, C.M. T Helper 2 Cells in Asthma. *J. Exp. Med.* **2023**, *220*, e20221094. [CrossRef] [PubMed]
32. Stark, J.M.; Tibbitt, C.A.; Coquet, J.M. The Metabolic Requirements of Th2 Cell Differentiation. *Front. Immunol.* **2019**, *10*, 2318. [CrossRef] [PubMed]
33. Moore, W.C.; Hastie, A.T.; Li, X.; Li, H.; Busse, W.W.; Jarjour, N.N.; Wenzel, S.E.; Peters, S.P.; Meyers, D.A.; Bleecker, E.R. Sputum Neutrophil Counts Are Associated with More Severe Asthma Phenotypes Using Cluster Analysis. *J. Allergy Clin. Immunol.* **2014**, *133*, 1557–1563.e5. [CrossRef] [PubMed]
34. Nabe, T. Steroid-Resistant Asthma and Neutrophils. *Biol. Pharm. Bull.* **2020**, *43*, 31–35. [CrossRef]
35. Mohamed, S.F.; Abd-Elwahab, F.M.; Shokry, D.M.; Samy, W.M. Relation between Interleukin 8 and Bronchial Asthma in Children: Review Article. *Egypt. J. Hosp. Med.* **2021**, *85*, 3621–3623. [CrossRef]
36. Gibson, P.G.; Simpson, J.L.; Saltos, N. Heterogeneity of Airway Inflammation in Persistent Asthma. *Chest* **2001**, *119*, 1329–1336. [CrossRef]
37. Garth, J.; Barnes, J.W.; Krick, S. Targeting Cytokines as Evolving Treatment Strategies in Chronic Inflammatory Airway Diseases. *Int. J. Mol. Sci.* **2018**, *19*, 3402. [CrossRef]
38. Jatakanon, A.; Uasuf, C.; Maziak, W.; Lim, S.; Chung, K.F.; Barnes, P.J. Neutrophilic Inflammation in Severe Persistent Asthma. *Am. J. Respir. Crit. Care Med.* **1999**, *160*, 1532–1539. [CrossRef]
39. Hosoki, K.; Itazawa, T.; Boldogh, I.; Sur, S. Neutrophil Recruitment by Allergens Contribute to Allergic Sensitization and Allergic Inflammation. *Curr. Opin. Allergy Clin. Immunol.* **2016**, *16*, 45–50. [CrossRef]

40. Simpson, J.L.; Phipps, S.; Gibson, P.G. Inflammatory Mechanisms and Treatment of Obstructive Airway Diseases with Neutrophilic Bronchitis. *Pharmacol. Ther.* **2009**, *124*, 86–95. [CrossRef]
41. Gevaert, P.; Wong, K.; Millette, L.A.; Carr, T.F. The Role of IgE in Upper and Lower Airway Disease: More Than Just Allergy! *Clin. Rev. Allerg. Immunol.* **2022**, *62*, 200–215. [CrossRef] [PubMed]
42. Miller, R.L.; Grayson, M.H.; Strothman, K. Advances in Asthma: New Understandings of Asthma's Natural History, Risk Factors, Underlying Mechanisms, and Clinical Management. *J. Allergy Clin. Immunol.* **2021**, *148*, 1430–1441. [CrossRef] [PubMed]
43. Papi, A.; Brightling, C.; Pedersen, S.E.; Reddel, H.K. Asthma. *Lancet* **2018**, *391*, 783–800. [CrossRef] [PubMed]
44. Frei, R.B.; Luschnig, P.; Parzmair, G.P.; Peinhaupt, M.; Schranz, S.; Fauland, A.; Wheelock, C.E.; Heinemann, A.; Sturm, E.M. Cannabinoid Receptor 2 Augments Eosinophil Responsiveness and Aggravates Allergen-induced Pulmonary Inflammation in Mice. *Allergy* **2016**, *71*, 944–956. [CrossRef] [PubMed]
45. Kwon, E.-K.; Choi, Y.; Sim, S.; Ye, Y.-M.; Shin, Y.S.; Park, H.-S.; Ban, G.-Y. Cannabinoid Receptor 2 as a Regulator of Inflammation Induced Oleoylethanolamide in Eosinophilic Asthma. *J. Allergy Clin. Immunol.* **2024**, *153*, 998–1009. [CrossRef]
46. Moore, W.C.; Peters, S.P. Severe Asthma: An Overview. *J. Allergy Clin. Immunol.* **2006**, *117*, 487–494. [CrossRef]
47. Kim, D.I.; Song, M.-K.; Lee, K. Comparison of Asthma Phenotypes in OVA-Induced Mice Challenged via Inhaled and Intranasal Routes. *BMC Pulm. Med.* **2019**, *19*, 241. [CrossRef]
48. Kim, B.-G.; Park, M.-K.; Lee, P.-H.; Lee, S.-H.; Hong, J.; Aung, M.M.M.; Moe, K.T.; Han, N.Y.; Jang, A.-S. Effects of Nanoparticles on Neuroinflammation in a Mouse Model of Asthma. *Respir. Physiol. Neurobiol.* **2020**, *271*, 103292. [CrossRef]

pharmaceuticals

Article

Unraveling the Impact of Six Pentacyclic Triterpenes Regulating Metabolic Pathways on Lung Carcinoma Cells

Anamaris Torres-Sanchez [1,2], Grace Torres [3], Sthephanie Estrada [4], Daraishka Perez [3], Carlos Garcia [5], Melissa Milian [3], Eddian Velazquez [3], Valerie Molina [3] and Yamixa Delgado [3,*]

1 Biology Department, University of Puerto Rico-Rio Piedras, San Juan, PR 00931, USA; anamaris.torres@upr.edu
2 Biochemistry Department, University of Puerto Rico-Medical Sciences Campus, San Juan, PR 00936, USA
3 Biochemistry & Pharmacology Department, San Juan Bautista School of Medicine, Caguas, PR 00726, USA; daraishkapc@sanjuanbautista.edu (D.P.); eddianva@sanjuanbautista.edu (E.V.); valeriemp@sanjuanbautista.edu (V.M.)
4 Biology Department, University of Puerto Rico-Cayey, Cayey, PR 00736, USA; sthephanie.estrada@upr.edu
5 Medical Program, Ponce Health Science University, Ponce, PR 00716, USA
* Correspondence: ydelgado@sanjuanbautista.edu

Abstract: Recently, there has been great interest in plant-derived compounds known as phytochemicals. The pentacyclic oleanane-, ursane-, and lupane-type triterpenes are phytochemicals that exert significant activity against diseases like cancer. Lung cancer is the leading cause of cancer-related death worldwide. Although chemotherapy is the treatment of choice for lung cancer, its effectiveness is hampered by the dose-limiting toxic effects and chemoresistance. Herein, we investigated six pentacyclic triterpenes, oleanolic acid, ursolic acid, asiatic acid, betulinic acid, betulin, and lupeol, on NSCLC A549 cells. These triterpenes have several structural variations that can influence the activation/inactivation of key cellular pathways. From our results, we determined that most of these triterpenes induced apoptosis, S-phase and G2/M-phase cycle arrest, the downregulation of ribonucleotide reductase (RR), reactive oxygen species, and caspase 3 activation. For chemoresistance markers, we found that most triterpenes downregulated the expression of MAPK/PI3K, STAT3, and PDL1. In contrast, UrA and AsA also induced DNA damage and autophagy. Then, we theoretically determined other possible molecular targets of these triterpenes using the online database ChEMBL. The results showed that even slight structural changes in these triterpenes can influence the cellular response. This study opens up promising perspectives for further research on the pharmaceutical role of phytochemical triterpenoids.

Keywords: pentacyclic triterpenes; non-small cell lung carcinoma; phytochemicals; chemoresistance

Citation: Torres-Sanchez, A.; Torres, G.; Estrada, S.; Perez, D.; Garcia, C.; Milian, M.; Velazquez, E.; Molina, V.; Delgado, Y. Unraveling the Impact of Six Pentacyclic Triterpenes Regulating Metabolic Pathways on Lung Carcinoma Cells. *Pharmaceuticals* **2024**, *17*, 694. https://doi.org/10.3390/ph17060694

Academic Editors: Daniela De Vita, Catherine Sherwin, Elena Y. Enioutina and Kathleen M. Job

Received: 18 March 2024
Revised: 11 May 2024
Accepted: 21 May 2024
Published: 28 May 2024

1. Introduction

Cancer is a leading cause of death around the world, where lung cancer is the most common cause of cancer-related deaths. Approximately 85% of all lung cancers are non-small cell lung carcinoma (NSCLC) [1]. Unfortunately, existing therapies do not cure most NSCLC patients. Even chemotherapy (e.g., platinum-based drugs such as cisplatin (CisPt)), the preferred and most effective treatment for lung cancer, only shows a complete response in 30% of individuals with NSCLC [2]. Additionally, chemoresistance, which results in more aggressive cancer cells, limits the efficacy of chemotherapy. Approximately 10–15% of patients receiving CisPt will relapse and invariably develop chemoresistance, with an expected survival time of no longer than a year [3]. In the last decade, the approvals for novel targeted and immunogenic anticancer agents have increased exponentially. From 2020 to 2023, sixteen of these new drugs were approved for the treatment of lung cancer, e.g., nivolumab (Opdivo®) and ipilimumab (Yervoy®) combined with a platinum-based drug is the first-line therapy for PDL1+ NSCLC [4]. For these reasons, new and adjuvant therapies are still needed. Phytochemicals such as triterpenes have demonstrated great potential against different cancers [5] and could work to overcome drug resistance mechanisms [6].

Triterpenes are secondary metabolites abundantly found in numerous plant species and composed of six isoprene units, resulting in a total of 30 carbon atoms in their molecular structure (see Figure 1A). Among the various triterpenes, pentacyclic triterpenoids exhibit approximately 200 different skeletons, showcasing remarkable structural diversity and potent biomedical activity [7]. Pentacyclic triterpenes that possess either five six-carbon (C_6) rings (C 6-6-6-6-6) or four six-carbon (C_6) rings and one five-carbon (C_5) ring (C 6-6-6-6-5) are considered the most bioactive triterpenoids [8].

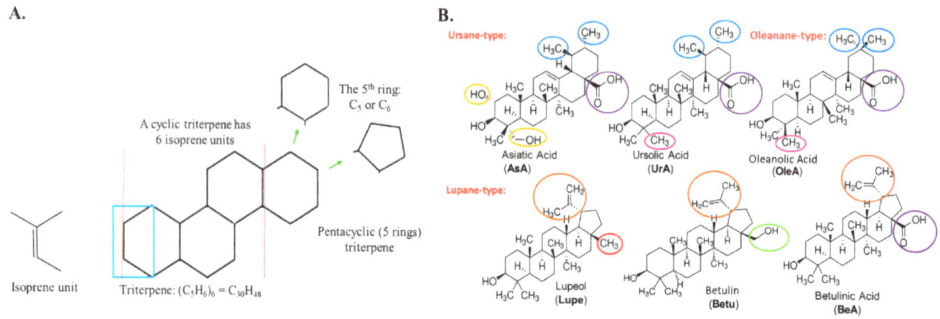

Figure 1. Structural representation of triterpenes. (**A**) Basic structure of a pentacyclic triterpene; (**B**) six pentacyclic triterpenes with their key substituents highlighted in color.

The ursane, lupane, and oleanane types are widely distributed within higher plants, including edible species. Within the ursane and oleanane types, asiatic acid (AsA), ursolic acid (UrA), and oleanolic acid (OleA) present a C 6-6-6-6-6 structural arrangement. These compounds exhibit very similar structures, with only slight variations in the substituent groups of the fifth C_6 ring. For instance, AsA possesses an additional hydroxyl group at position 2 and a hydroxymethyl substituent at position 4. On the other hand, OleA differs from UrA in that a methyl substituent has been moved from position 19 to position 20. Interestingly, the lupane-type pentacyclic triterpenes, namely lupeol (Lupe), betulin (Betu), and betulinic acid (BeA), exhibit a C 6-6-6-6-5 structural arrangement. The primary distinction among these three compounds lies in the substituent group at position 17. Specifically, Lupe possesses a methyl group, Betu contains a hydroxymethyl group, and BeA features a carboxylic acid group at this position. These subtle but specific variations among these six pentacyclic triterpenoids may play a crucial role in their activity across metabolic pathways, especially in cancer [9]. Figure 1B provides a visual representation highlighting the differences between these pentacyclic triterpenes.

Herein, we investigated a library of six structurally similar pentacyclic triterpenes, AsA, UrA, OleA, Lupe, Betu, and BeA, against NSCLC. To study their cellular mechanistic effects, we determined the impact on the cell cycle, DNA, production of reactive oxygen (ROS), and activation of apoptosis and autophagy. In addition, we determined the protein expression of the mitogen-activated protein kinase/phosphatidylinositol 3-kinase (MAPK/PI3K) and the gene expression of ribonucleotide reductase (RR), programmed death-ligand 1 (PDL1), and signal transducer and activator of transcription 3 (STAT3), key markers of chemoresistance in NSCLC. This study opens up promising perspectives for further research on the role of triterpenoids as therapeutics, which ultimately will contribute to their more rational application in lung cancer therapy.

2. Results

2.1. Cytotoxicity and Therapeutic Index (TI)

The MTS/PMS colorimetric assay was used to determine the viability of cells exposed to the triterpenes, generating a dose–response curve for NSCLC A549 cells and normal lung fibroblast MRC5 cells. Each triterpene was incubated at several μM concentrations for 24 h to determine the IC_{50}. As expected, the cell viability decreased at increasing drug concentrations (Figure 2). The IC_{50} values were calculated using the data from Figure 2 and are summarized in Table 1. UrA was the most cytotoxic triterpene in MRC5 cells, and BeA was the most cytotoxic in the A549 cell line. In contrast, Lupe was the least cytotoxic in both cell lines.

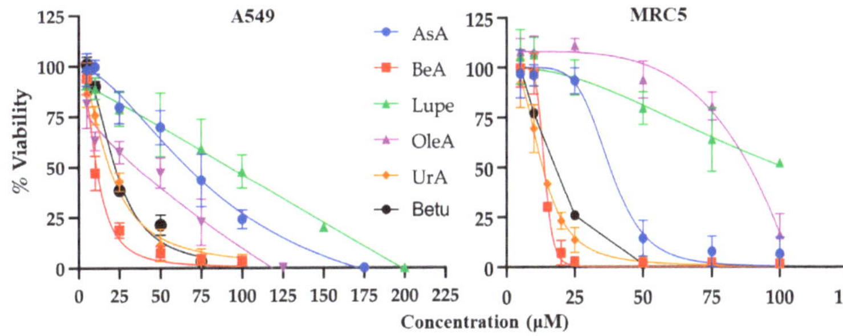

Figure 2. Cell death assays. MTS/PMS viability. Triterpenes were incubated for 24 h in A549 and MRC5 cells. Data show the average of eight measurements for each treatment (mean ± SD) in at least three independent experiments. All triterpenes were cytotoxic to A549 and MRC5 cells at a micromolar range. Both graphs show normalized data.

Table 1. IC_{50} and TI in A549 and MRC5 cells for each pentacyclic triterpene under study.

Triterpene	A549 IC_{50} (μM)	MRC5 IC_{50} (μM)	TI #
AsA	59 ± 6 *	38 ± 2	0.64
OleA	43 ± 5 *	86 ± 2	2.00
UrA	23 ± 1 *	13 ± 1	0.57
BeA	15 ± 0.7 *	19 ± 0.4	1.27
Lupe	80 ± 6 *	101 ± 8	1.26
Betu	22 ± 1	16 ± 0.5	0.73

* These results have already been obtained by the authors [10]. # TI = MRC5 IC_{50}/A549 IC_{50}, where >1 means higher selectivity.

The therapeutic index (TI) is a measurement of selectivity, comparing the IC_{50} of a drug against non-cancerous vs. cancerous cells. The OleA showed the highest TI (=2), while UrA showed the lowest TI (=0.57). Interestingly, Lupe and BeA had the same TI but BeA had the lowest IC_{50} for both cell lines.

2.2. Cell Cycle Arrest, DNA Damage, and Ribonucleotide Reductase (RR) Expression

To characterize the effects of these triterpenes on nuclear processes, we evaluated the cell cycle populations and DNA damage machinery. Figure 3A demonstrates that all pentacyclic triterpenes produced cell cycle arrest in A549 cells at the S phase and G2/M phase in comparison to the negative control (untreated cells) and greater cycle arrest in G2/M in comparison to CisPt. In contrast, only UrA and AsA caused the activation of the DNA damage machinery compared to the negative control (untreated cells), as shown in Figure 3B. UrA was demonstrated to induce a similar DNA damage extent to CisPt chemotherapy. After we found these nuclear effects, we decided to test whether the expression of RR was also affected. Figure 3C shows the significant downregulation of the RRM1 gene compared to untreated cells, being more potent than CisPt. Only OleA did not downregulate RR.

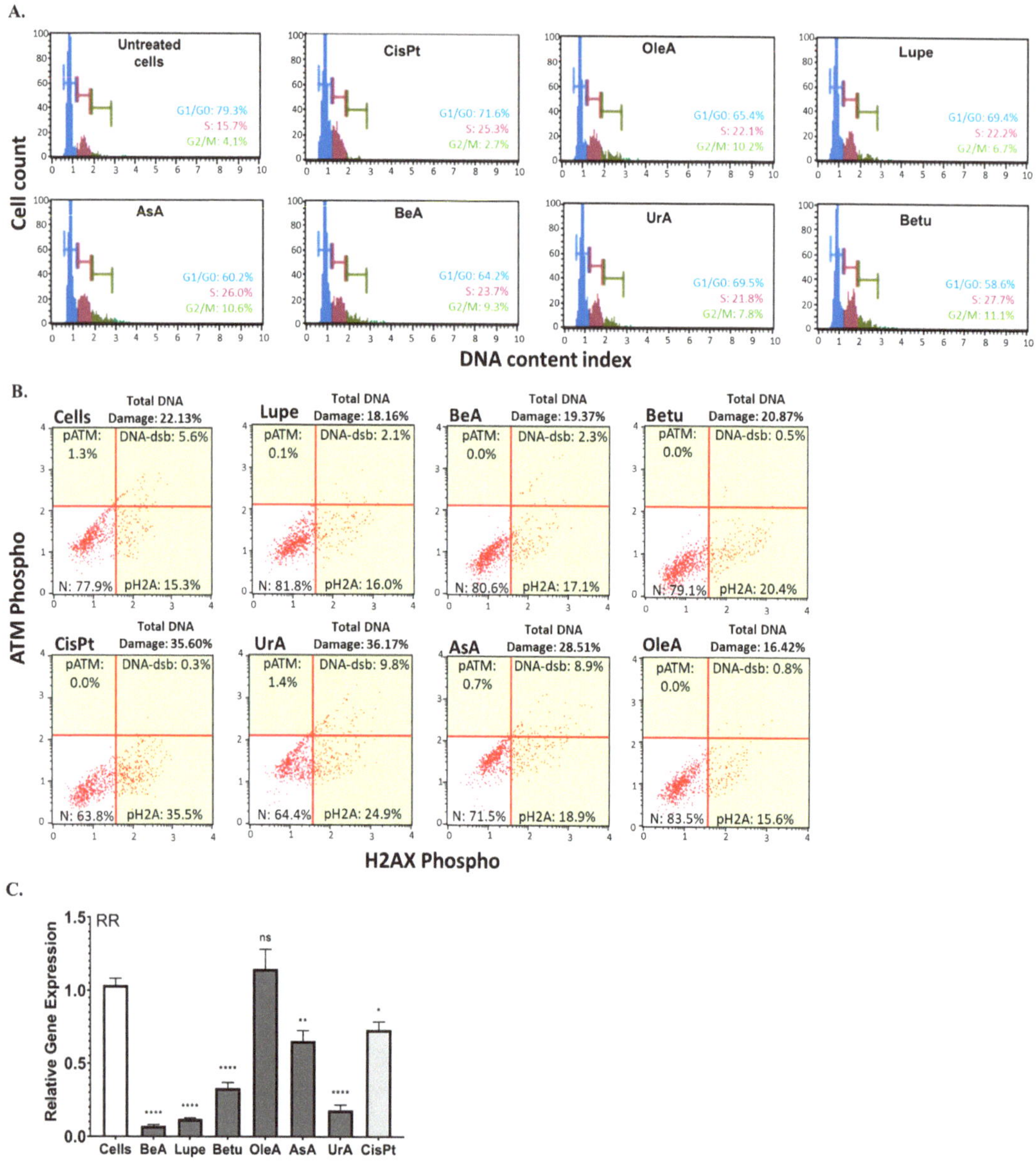

Figure 3. DNA-related pathways. (**A**). Cell cycle arrest assay. All pentacyclic triterpenes induced cell cycle arrest at the S phase and G2/M. (**B**). DNA damage assay. Only UrA and AsA induced the activation of the DNA damage machinery. (**C**). Gene expression of RR. Each assay was run in at least two independent experiments and samples were analyzed in triplicate. The statistical significance for p values was defined as **** < 0.0001, ** from 0.001 to 0.01, * from 0.01 to 0.05, and non-significant (ns) ≥ 0.05.

2.3. Apoptosis: Externalization of PS and Caspase 3 Activity

Given the importance of the activation apoptotic processes to eradicate cancer cells, we chose to determine the markers of early apoptosis and intrinsic apoptosis pathways after 24 h in NSCLC cells. We used confocal microscopy to identify the activation of the apoptotic machinery by the externalization of PS on the cell membrane using Annexin V dye and

NucBlue DAPI as the nuclear markers. In Figure 4A, we demonstrate that all triterpenes showed early apoptosis activity (green marker), similarly to CisPt. The complete set of images for each individual channel can be found in the Supporting Information (Figure S1). Qualitatively, we observed that UrA and Betu showed the strongest activation and Lupe and BeA the lowest.

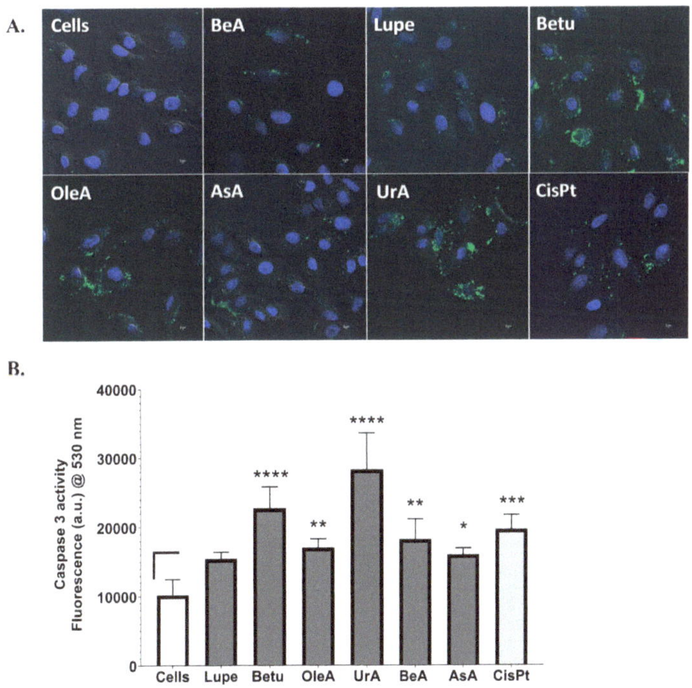

Figure 4. Apoptotic-related pathways. (**A**). Externalization of phosphatidylserine. Triterpenes were incubated for 24 h in A549 and then with Annexin V (green) and NucBlue DAPI (blue); scale bars are shown (2 μm). The brightfield, green, and blue fluorescence channels are overlaid in these images. All triterpenes showed the activation of early apoptosis to A549. Each sample was analyzed in duplicate in two independent experiments. The images shown were selected arbitrarily. All images were taken at 20× magnification. (**B**). Caspase 3 activity assay. All triterpenes activated caspase 3, except Lupe. UrA and Betu showed the highest activation. Data shown as mean ± SD in three independent experiments and samples were analyzed in triplicate. The statistical significance for p values was defined as **** < 0.0001, *** from 0.001 to 0.0001, ** from 0.001 to 0.01, * from 0.01 to 0.05, and non-significant (ns) ≥ 0.05.

Figure 4B shows that all triterpenes activated the caspase 3 enzymatic machinery during a 24 h treatment period, except for Lupe, compared to the negative control (untreated cells). However, UrA and Betu produced higher caspase 3 activation than CisPt, where UrA was the highest.

2.4. Total ROS and Mitochondrial ROS Production and Autophagy

Oxidative stress, as ROS, plays an interesting role by regulating cell death mechanisms such as autophagy [8]. Thus, we determined the effect of these triterpenes on this process. Figure 5A shows that all triterpenes increased the superoxide ROS generated from mitochondria compared with the negative control, and some of their levels were higher than that of CisPt. BeA caused the largest level of mROS, whereas the lowest was produced by AsA. Then, we measured the total amount of ROS to confirm our results for mROS.

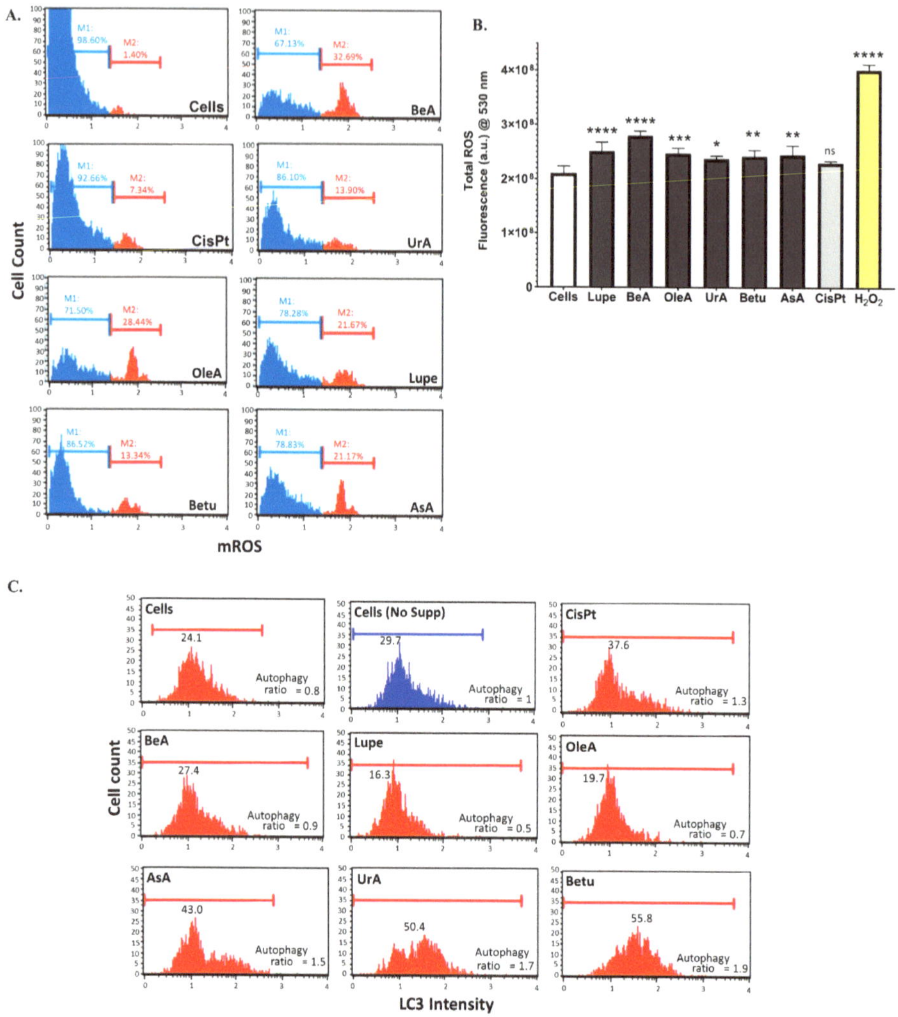

Figure 5. Oxidative stress-related processes. (**A**). Mitochondrial ROS production assay. Dihydroethidium (DHE) dye reacts with the superoxide species mostly produced by mitochondrial damage. All six triterpenes induced the production of mROS. Each assay was run in at least two independent experiments and samples were analyzed in triplicate in the instrument. (**B**). Total ROS production assay. DCF dye reacts with the peroxide (H_2O_2) species as the final product during oxidation in cells. All six triterpenes induced the production of ROS. Data shown as mean ± SD in three independent experiments and samples were analyzed in triplicate. (**C**). Autophagy induction assay. For this experiment, we included a positive control (No supp) by removing the serum from the culturing medium (starvation) of the untreated cells. Betu, AsA, and UrA activated the autophagic response. Each assay was run at least in two independent experiments and samples were analyzed in triplicate in the instrument. The statistical significance for p values was defined as **** < 0.0001, *** from 0.001 to 0.0001, ** from 0.001 to 0.01, * from 0.01 to 0.05, and non-significant (ns) ≥ 0.05.

Figure 5B showed a very similar tendency in the mROS results. All triterpenes induced an increase in the total ROS from peroxide species. In the case of CisPt, the increase in the total ROS was not statistically significant. For this assay, we used cells incubated with 3 μM of H_2O_2 as a positive control.

Figure 5C shows that Betu, AsA, and UrA induced an autophagic response similar to that of CisPt, compared to the controls (negative control untreated cells, ratio = 0.8, and positive control untreated starving cells, ratio = 1). BeA had a similar ratio to the untreated cells, while Lupe and OleA were shown to inhibit the LC3-II activity.

2.5. MAPK/PI3K Protein Expression and PDL1 and STAT3 Gene Expression

The MAPK, PI3K, PDL1, and STAT3 pathways are commonly studied in cancer due to their involvement in several cellular processes, especially chemoresistance [9]. These were assessed in this study in A549 cells after 24 h incubation with the triterpenes. Figure 6A shows that UrA was the only one that induced the simultaneous expression of MAPK and PI3K, similarly to CisPt, while Betu could slightly inhibit the total expression of MAPK/PI3K, compared to untreated cells. In contrast, BeA, AsA, Lupe, and OleA did not affect the expression of MAPK/PI3K.

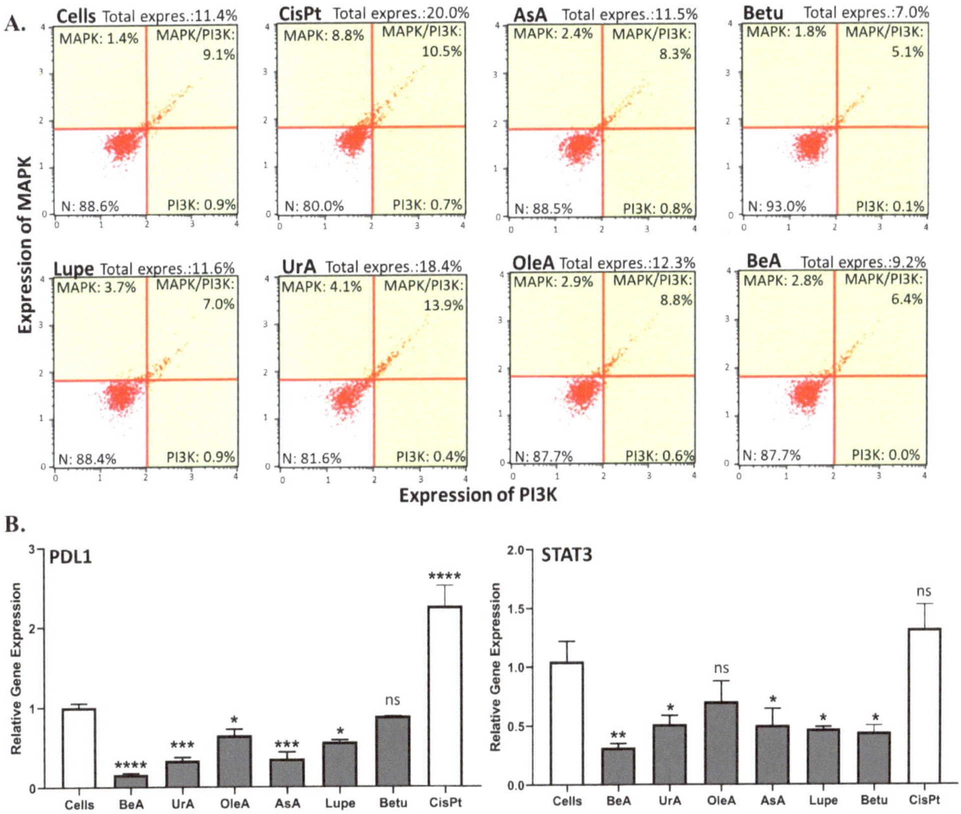

Figure 6. Protein and gene expression assays. (**A**). MAPK/PI3K protein expression. Only UrA increased and Betu diminished MAPK/PI3K expression. Each assay was run at least in two independent experiments and samples were analyzed in triplicate in the instrument. (**B**). PDL1 and STAT3 gene expression using real-time qPCR. Only OleA and Betu did not inhibit the STAT3 and PDL1 genes, respectively. The data were analyzed in triplicate and are expressed as the mean ± SD of three independent experiments. The statistical significance for p values was defined as **** < 0.0001, *** from 0.001 to 0.0001, ** from 0.001 to 0.01, * from 0.01 to 0.05, and non-significant (ns) ≥ 0.05.

In the RT-qPCR gene expression assays (Figure 6B), most triterpenes significantly inhibited PDL1 and STAT3. OleA and Betu, on the other hand, did not inhibit the STAT3 and PDL1 genes, respectively. The lupane-type BeA is superior in suppressing both genes.

2.6. Theoretical Predictions of Molecular Targets

Theoretical analysis not only enriches our understanding of the pharmacokinetic properties of drugs, but also provides insights into possible protein targets, thereby increasing the robustness of the experimental results. Based on the results of our experiments, we decided to incorporate a theoretical prediction analysis of possible molecular targets using the comprehensive ChEMBL database.

From the results of this theoretical analysis of 339 biological targets, the program predicted more than 20 targets for each triterpene, with different confidence levels. We selected only those targets that met the three confidence levels (70, 80, 90%) and had the strongest activity thresholds (5–6 numerical values). The whole set of targets (~10) that fulfilled the strict criteria are shown in the Supporting Information, Table S1. From this whole set, we summarize the targets related to cancer metabolism, chemoresistance, and metastatic processes in Table 2. We use different colors to match the same targets across the different triterpenes. ChEMBL only predicts the interactions of the two molecules in the comparison and not the activation or inhibition of these targets per se.

Table 2. Cancer-related targets that are theoretically predicted to interact with the six pentacyclic triterpenes.

BeA Target ID: CHEMBL269277	Confidence 70, 80, 90%	Activity Threshold	OleA Target ID: CHEMBL168	Confidence 70, 80, 90%	Activity Threshold
Interleukin-2	active	6	Interleukin-2	active	6
TNF-alpha	active	6	TNF-alpha	active	6
Dihydrofolate reductase	active	6	Dihydrofolate reductase	active	6
Adenosine deaminase	active	6	WD repeat-containing protein 5	active	6
WD repeat-containing protein 5	active	6			
LSD1/CoREST complex	active	6			
Lupe Target ID: CHEMBL289191	**Confidence 70, 80, 90%**	**Activity Threshold**	**UrA Target ID: CHEMBL169**	**Confidence 70, 80, 90%**	**Activity Threshold**
Interleukin-2	active	6	Interleukin-2	active	6
Dihydrofolate reductase	active	6	TNF-alpha	active	6
Adenosine deaminase	active	6	Dihydrofolate reductase	active	6
WD repeat-containing protein 5	active	6	WD repeat-containing protein 5	active	6
LSD1/CoREST complex	active	6			
Carbonic anhydrase IX	active	6			
Betu Target ID: CHEMBL23236	**Confidence 70, 80, 90%**	**Activity Threshold**	**AsA Target ID: CHEMBL404313**	**Confidence 70, 80, 90%**	**Activity Threshold**
Interleukin-2	active	6	Interleukin-2	active	6
Dihydrofolate reductase	active	6	TNF-alpha	active	6
Adenosine deaminase	active	6	LSD1/CoREST complex	active	6
WD repeat-containing protein 5	active	6	Mucosa-associated lymphoid tissue lymphoma translocation protein 1	active	6
LSD1/CoREST complex	active	6	Gamma-secretase	active	5

Matching colors are used to show similarities between the six triterpenes. Molecules in black show unique targets among the six triterpenes.

2.7. Results Summary

Table 3 summarizes the findings from all of the experimental mechanistic pathways studied in this project. The lupane-type BeA is the pentacyclic triterpene that affects most of the key pathways with a lower concentration (lowest IC_{50}) and is the most potent in the production of total and mROS and the downregulation of STAT3 and PDL1 in the NSCLC A549 cells. These results indicate that the structure of the triterpene affects its interaction with different pathways.

Table 3. Summary of the six pentacyclic triterpenes' results against NSCLC A549 cells.

Mechanism	UrA	AsA	OleA	Lupe	BeA	Betu	Highest	Lowest
Cytotoxicity	✔	✔	✔	✔	✔	✔	BeA	Lupe
TI > 1	-	-	✔	✔	✔	-	OleA	UrA
Early apoptosis	✔	✔	✔	✔	✔	✔	UrA	Lupe
Caspase 3 activation	✔	✔	✔	-	✔	✔	UrA	Lupe
Cell cycle arrest	✔	✔	✔	✔	✔	✔	Betu	UrA
DNA damage	✔	✔	-	-	-	-	UrA	OleA
RRM1 downregulation	✔	✔	-	✔	✔	✔	BeA	OleA
Total ROS production	✔	✔	✔	✔	✔	✔	BeA	UrA
mROS production	✔	✔	✔	✔	✔	✔	BeA	Betu
Autophagy inhibition	-	-	✔	✔	✔	-	Lupe	Betu
MAPK/PI3K inhibition	-	-	-	-	-	✔	Betu	UrA
PDL1 downregulation	✔	✔	✔	✔	✔	-	BeA	Betu
STAT3 downregulation	✔	✔	-	✔	✔	✔	BeA	OleA

"✔" means induction and "-" means non-induction of any of the tested processes.

3. Discussion

Triterpenes are known for their wide range of benefits, including their anti-inflammatory, antimicrobial, antiviral, analgesic, anti-tumorigenic, and immunomodulatory characteristics [5–8,11]. For this project, we aimed to study a library of six pentacyclic triterpenes with similar structures to determine which one was the most potent against lung carcinoma, one of the deadliest cancers. While previous research has demonstrated the potency of these triterpenes, our study aimed to determine which one had the most effective structural arrangement for potency, selectivity, and the targeting of key pathways against chemoresistance, the major problem contributing to chemotherapy failure. We selected pentacyclic triterpenes because, in our previous study, we found that the fifth ring of the structure is essential for the cytotoxic activity in NSCLC A549 cells. For instance, even at the highest concentration of 100 μM, β-sitosterol and cholesterol (tetracyclic triterpenes) did not kill A549 cells [10]. Thus, this study explored the underlying mechanistic principles (Figure 7) with a particular emphasis on key pathways to induce cell death (i.e., cell cycle arrest, expression of RR, DNA damage, activation of caspase 3, and oxidative stress) but also in chemoresistance-related processes (i.e., inhibition of autophagy; MAPK, PI3K, STAT3, and PDL1 expression).

Our experimental results revealed distinct patterns in the response of NSCLC cells to the six pentacyclic triterpenes under scrutiny. The viability assays demonstrated that Lupe had the highest IC_{50}, OleA had the best TI, and BeA had the lowest IC_{50} with a TI >1. Normal lung cells such as MRC5 have been considered as cancer-associated fibroblasts (CAF), even when they are non-cancerous cells [12]. This means that an effective therapy must kill both cell lines (NSCLC and CAF) but behave aggressively towards cancerous cells. In this context, BeA showed the lowest IC_{50} to kill both cell lines (NSCLC and CAF) but behaved more aggressively towards the NSCLC A549 cells among the six triterpenes. These results suggest that a methyl substituent in lupane-type triterpenes, instead of carboxylic acid or hydroxyl, can drastically diminish their cytotoxicity. On the other hand, changes in the methyl substituents in OleA (vs. UrA) diminished their cytotoxicity in cells but increased their selectivity. Previous studies have found similar IC_{50} values in the μM range in a 24 h treatment period for the six selected pentacyclic triterpenes exposed to different cancer cell types [13–18]. This highlights the versatility of using triterpenes against cancer in different organs and tissues.

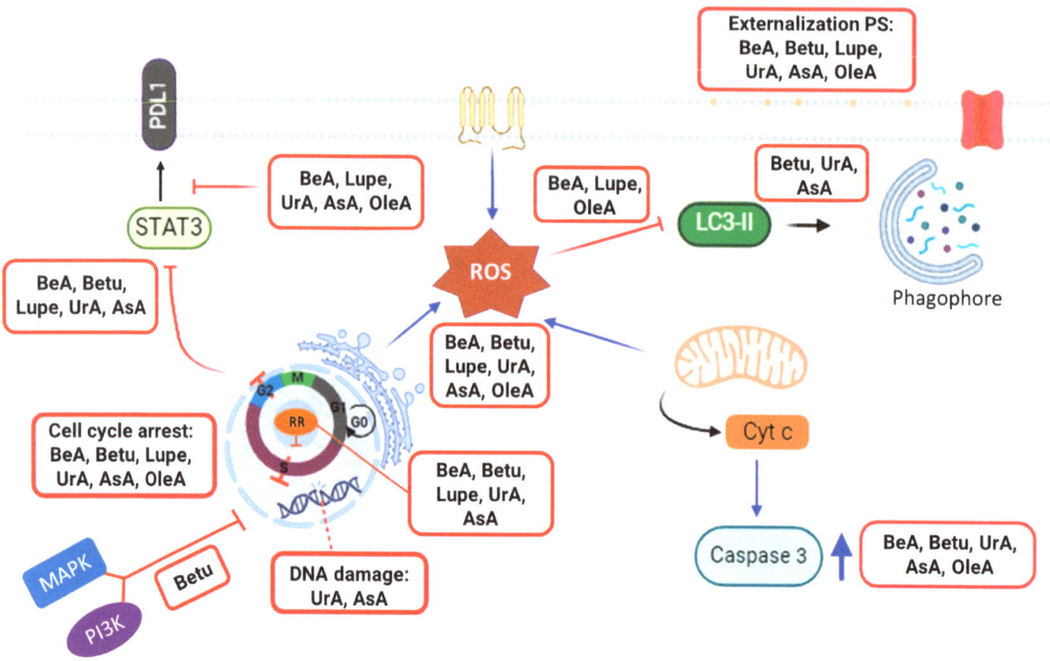

Figure 7. Summary of the experimental pathways' relationships as activated or inhibited by the six pentacyclic triterpenes against NSCLC.

Nuclear processes such as the cell cycle are important pathways that promote cancer progression. Cell cycle arrest in response to DNA damage is a critical mechanism that helps to prevent the propagation of cancer cells and to induce apoptosis [19]. In this study, all triterpenes produced cell cycle arrest in the S phase and G2/M phase. There are several studies that have shown similar results, where these triterpenes exhibited S-phase and G2/M-phase arrest in myeloma, gastric, breast, and lung cancer cells [20–23]. These results suggest that, regardless of their structural variations, these six pentacyclic triterpenes may trigger cell cycle arrest in these two critical divisions in NSCLC, implying that they all may be able to prevent the proliferation of these cancer cells. In addition, only the ursane-type UrA and AsA caused DNA damage, implying their other potential targets to kill cancer cells compared to the other four triterpenes. These results revealed that, unlike lupane-type triterpenes, ursane-type triterpenes might employ DNA damage machinery to induce apoptosis. These results support previous studies that highlight UrA's ability to increase DNA damage and chemosensitize A549 cells [24]. In contrast, there are several studies that have demonstrated that lupane-type triterpenes are able to cause DNA damage [25,26]. RR is an enzyme complex composed of two subunits: a catalytic alpha subunit (RRM1) and a radical-generating beta subunit (RRM2). These subunits are responsible for catalyzing the rate-limiting step for DNA synthesis and are known to be elevated in a variety of cancers because of their influence on invasion, including NSCLC [27]. This study found that the lupane- and ursane-type triterpenes downregulated the RRM1 subunit gene. No previous studies have demonstrated that these pentacyclic triterpenes affect RR. However, the literature indicates that another pentacyclic (C6-6-6-6-6) triterpene, celastrol, downregulates RRM2 [28].

Another important pathway is the activation of apoptosis through the mitochondrial response and the externalization of PS on the cell membrane. The disruption of the mitochondrial membrane potential can lead to the release of cytochrome c, which activates caspase 3, initiating intrinsic apoptosis and, then, cell death [29]. Another explanation for this mechanism is that the proapoptotic protein Bid can directly activate caspase 8 or translocate to the mitochondrion, leading to the release of cytochrome c to activate caspases 3/7, regardless of the mitochondrial potential [30]. Most studies in the literature show that pentacyclic triterpenes induce both intrinsic and extrinsic apoptosis by caspase 3 and caspase 8, respectively [31]. In the current study, all triterpenes except Lupe activated caspase 3. In addition, all triterpenes activated the early apoptotic cellular process on the A549 cells, where Lupe and BeA induced the lowest level of activation. Interestingly, BeA demonstrated the low activation of early apoptosis and caspase 3 and no DNA damage, while UrA showed the activation of the DNA damage machinery, as well as the strongest activation of caspase 3 and the externalization of PS. Structurally, BeA and UrA were demonstrated to more aggressively attack different pathways in NSCLC.

Oxidative stress, such as ROS levels, can modulate autophagy. Mild amounts of ROS promote the autophagic response, while high concentrations inhibit autophagy and promote cell death [32]. To determine the mROS, we used the DHE dye, which reacts mainly with superoxide species [33]. Although all triterpenes produced mROS, compared to the untreated cells, the amounts of mROS from BeA, OleA, and Lupe were, on average, 26.2%, while Betu, AsA, and UrA showed an average of 10.1%. Thus, BeA, OleA, and Lupe did not activate autophagy because of the high concentration of ROS. On the other hand, Betu, AsA, and UrA activated the autophagic response via the lower levels of ROS. Although mitochondria are the main suppliers of ROS, other organelles, such as the endoplasmic reticulum, also play important roles in ROS production [34]. Thus, we decided to test the total amount of ROS using the DCF dye, which labels mostly the peroxide species as the end products of free radicals during oxidation reactions. Again, BeA showed the highest increase in total ROS, in agreement with the increase in mROS. Numerous studies agree with our results showing that triterpenes can induce cell death via the production of ROS, as summarized in the review in [31]. It is important to understand that autophagy can suppress tumor development in the early stages, but, once the tumor is established, it promotes chemotherapy resistance [35]. Based on the structural aspects of these triterpenes, our results suggest that the skeletal carbon ring structure of the pentacyclic triterpenes is essential in triggering the formation of mROS. Moreover, the results revealed that most of the differences in the six pentacyclic triterpenes' structures and their substituents changed the ROS production levels, but this was not sufficient to inhibit this process. A possible explanation is that these triterpenes inactivate iron complex I and iron complex III in the electron transport chain. Thus, under increased ROS levels, iron is released from these complexes and apoptosis is switched to a process called ferroptosis, which depends on the presence of free iron and high oxidant conditions [36]. In this way, BeA can activate apoptosis but mostly ferroptosis by high ROS and no autophagy. In contrast, UrA can activate mostly apoptosis and autophagy by DNA damage and moderate levels of ROS.

MAPK/PI3K has been linked to the upregulation of PDL1, which leads to immune suppression and chemoresistance [9,37]. Meanwhile, the STAT3-mediated upregulation of PDL1 expression in cancer cells has been observed [37]. In our experiments, only UrA slightly increased the expression of MAPK/PI3K when compared to the negative (untreated cells) and positive (CisPt) controls. These results suggest that lupane-type triterpenes with a 6-6-6-6-5 structural arrangement (where Betu < BeA < Lupe) are superior in limiting cell progression and survival by MAPK/PI3K. Regarding the chemoresistance markers STAT3 and PDL1, our results revealed that most of the pentacyclic triterpenes suppressed these two genes, where the chemotherapy CisPt clearly upregulated PDL1. However, BeA was the greater inhibitor of PDL1 and STAT3 gene expression, while it did not increase MAPK/PI3K expression. This outcome is also in agreement with our hypothesis of the activation of ferroptosis, which may sensitize chemoresistant cancer cells [36]. In the literature, we found similar results for MAPK, PI3K, PDL1, and STAT3 after BeA treatment [38,39]. UrA was also shown to downregulate STAT3 and PDL1 [40].

Computational approaches provide detailed information to predict the pharmacokinetic properties, biological activity, and molecular mechanisms of small molecules, including their interactions with specific protein targets with associated signaling pathways [41]. For example, from a database of 339 proteins, ChEMBL predicted interactions with approximately 25 targets with an activity threshold of 5–7.5. In evaluating the data, we selected targets with stronger predictive properties: lower activity threshold values and confidence intervals of 70, 80, and 90%. These protein targets were of the following types: (a) membrane-associated proteins, receptors, and ion channels; (b) nuclear proteins; (c) cytoplasmic enzymes; and (d) cytokines and signaling molecules (shown in Table S1). Thus, Table 2 shows only the cancer-related targets (~five for each triterpene). Most of these triterpenes have very similar targets. Interleukin-2 is a common target of all six triterpenes. Dihydrofolate reductase and WD repeat-containing protein 5 are targeted by all except AsA. TNF-alpha is targeted by all except Lupe and Betu. The LSD1/CoREST complex is targeted by all except OleA and UrA. Adenosine deaminase is only targeted by lupane-type triterpenes. On the other hand, mucosa-associated lymphoid tissue lymphoma translocation protein 1 (MALT1) and gamma-secretase are only targeted by AsA, and carbonic anhydrase IX is only targeted by Lupe. Knowing that ChEMBL calculates the probability of each triterpene interacting with the protein targets in the database (not their specific activation or inhibition), we can make several important connections based on the molecules predicted to be targeted. The most important findings from these predictions are that these pentacyclic triterpenes have the ability to trigger an inflammatory response (IL-2 and TNF-alpha) by the activation of adenosine deaminase. This process may induce immunostimulation to attack tumor cells [42]. In addition, only AsA could target MALT1, which acts as a scaffolding protein to drive immune activation [43]. This prediction confirmed our experimental results on the downregulation of PDL1 and STAT3. Furthermore, these triterpenes can interact with proteins such as the LSD1/CoREST complex, WD repeat-containing protein 5, and dihydrofolate reductase, which regulate the cell cycle, DNA synthesis, and genomic instability [19]. This prediction could explain our experimental results regarding cell cycle arrest in the S phase and G2/M. Similarly, targeting carbonic anhydrase IX could disrupt the stability of the hypoxic tumor environment. Targeting carbonic anhydrase IX is a potential therapeutic strategy to starve tumors and limit their spread [44]. In particular, AsA is predicted to interact with gamma-secretase, which is a novel therapeutic strategy in cancer that involves blocking Notch cleavage [45].

In summary, BeA emerges as the triterpene exerting the most widespread influence on several key pathways related to ROS-mediated cell death, with the lowest IC_{50} and a TI > 1, and inhibits the chemoresistance-related genes STAT3 and PDL1. Theoretically, BeA can also modulate the immune response by interacting with IL-2, TNF-alpha, and adenosine deaminase. Based on the structure, the C 6-6-6-6-5 arrangement substituted with a carboxylic acid and a HC=C-CH_2 group is the most potent against NSCLC. These findings collectively indicate that triterpenes impact different pathways depending on the substituents of their rings. While BeA has the lower IC_{50} of 11 μM, it is important to note that its TI is narrow but above 1. However, OleA showed the best TI (= 2), making it a promising candidate for derivatization. A low IC_{50} reflects the potency of a drug in inhibiting cancer cell growth, while a high TI is crucial in ensuring the safety and tolerability of the drug. Both parameters are important considerations in cancer therapeutics, with the ideal drug having both a low IC_{50} and a high TI. However, MEK inhibitors, clinically approved chemotherapeutics, have a TI ~ 1 [46]. Based on these findings, future research can utilize the most effective patterns of parent molecules BeA and OleA for derivatization. Specifically, the alternate methyl groups of the fifth C_6 ring of OleA could be the key to higher selectivity. A possibility to consider is a BeA derivative that includes the original substituent of the HC=C-CH_2 group in the fifth C_5 ring to maintain the potency, as well as the alternate methyl groups of OleA to increase the selectivity. To validate our arguments about OleA, two synthetic derivatives of OleA, CDDO-Me and CDDO-Im, were studied in phase I clinical trials [47,48]. Furthermore, OleA in combination with curcumin was examined in a phase I clinical trial [49]. On the other hand, selectivity of BeA could be increased by its encapsulation into a targeted drug delivery system (DDS). Thus, we previously loaded BeA in a protein-based DDS, demonstrating that BeA was synergized with doxorubicin chemotherapy in A549 cells [50].

4. Materials and Methods

4.1. Chemicals and Reagents

Aqueous solutions were prepared with sterile (autoclave conditions: 121 °C and 18 PSI), high-quality nanopure water (18.2 MΩ cm resistivity, Thermo Scientific™ Barnstead™ Easypure™ II system (Thermo Fisher Scientific, Waltham, MA, USA)).

Asiatic acid, ursolic acid, oleanolic acid, betulin, lupeol, betulinic acid, 2′,7′-dichlorodihydrofluorescein diacetate (DCF) and cis-diamminedichloroplatinum (II) (cisplatin, CisPt) were purchased from Sigma-Aldrich (St. Louis, MO, USA). The cell lines A549 (human lung adenocarcinoma; ATCC CCL-185) and MRC5 (human fibroblast-like cells; ATCC CCL-171) were obtained from the American Type Culture Collection (Manassas, VA, USA). The CellTiter 96 Aqueous Non-Radioactive Cell Proliferation Assay (3-(4,5-dimethylthiazol-2-yl)-5-(3-carboxymethoxyphenyl)-2-(4-sulfophenyl)-2H-tetrazolium (MTS) reagent) was obtained from the Promega Corporation (Madison, WI, USA). The cell cycle, MAPK/PI3K expression, DNA damage, and mitochondrial oxidative stress assays were obtained from the Luminex Corporation (Austin, TX, USA). Reagents for Taqman gene expression assays were purchased from Applied Biosystems (Waltham, MA, USA). All other chemicals were purchased from various suppliers, of analytical grade, and used without further purification.

4.2. Cell Culture Conditions

The human NSCLC A549 and normal lung MRC5 cell lines were maintained following the ATCC protocols. These cells were cultured in Dulbecco's Modified Eagle's Medium (DMEM-high glucose) containing 1% L-glutamine, 10% fetal bovine serum (FBS), and 1% penicillin/streptomycin. Cells were kept in a humidified incubator under 5% CO_2 and 95% air at 37 °C. We conducted all of the experiments before the cells reached 25 passages. For all experiments, the triterpenes were initially dissolved in pure dimethylformamide (DMF) and subsequently diluted in phosphate-buffered saline (PBS), ensuring a final DMF concentration in the cells of less than 1%. CisPt (25 μM) was included as a control to compare the effects of the triterpenes with the most used chemotherapy in NSCLC.

4.3. Cell Viability

The 50% inhibitory concentration (IC_{50}) of some of these triterpenes in A549 NSCLC cells were previously determined by us [10]. A similar procedure was performed to determine the IC_{50} of the triterpenes in a normal lung fibroblast cell line (MRC5). In brief, the A549 and MRC5 cells were seeded into 96-well plates at a density of 1×10^5 cells/mL in supplemented DMEM medium. The cells were treated with specific concentrations (A549: 5, 10, 25, 50, 75, 100, 125,150, 175, 200 μM; MRC5: 5, 10, 25, 50, 75, 100 μM) of the triterpenes and incubated for 24 h. Then, 10 uL of the MTS reagent from the CellTiter 96® Aqueous Non-Radioactive Cell Proliferation Assay (Promega G5421) was added to each well. Then, we incubated the plates at 37 °C and in a 5% CO_2 atmosphere for 1 h. After incubation, the absorbance was measured at 492 nm (n = 8) in a microplate reader spectrophotometer (Thermoscientific Multiskan FC). The cell viability was calculated as follows:

$$\% \text{ Viability} = (\text{sample absorbance} - \text{sample media absorbance})/(\text{untreated cells' absorbance} - \text{untreated cells' media absorbance}) \times 100$$

The cell viability data were presented by plotting the values with an average of eight measurements for each treatment (mean ± SD) in at least three independent experiments.

The IC_{50} values were calculated with the GraphPad Prism 9 software (Prism 9; GraphPad by Dotmatics, San Diego, CA, USA) using the dose–response curve. The data were normalized by the non-linear fit of the log (drug inhibition) vs. normalized response variable slope to obtain the best fit IC_{50} and R-squared values.

4.4. Apoptosis Externalization of Phospatidylserine (PS) Annexin V Assay

Early apoptotic activity was evaluated by the externalization of PS using the Alexa Fluor® 488 Annexin V Apoptosis Reagent (Molecular Probes™) and NucBlue ReadyProbes Reagent™ (Thermo Fisher Scientific). For this assay, A549 cells were seeded in 8-well cover slip plates with a density of 1×10^5 cells/mL for 24 h in supplemented DMEM. Then, the A549 cells were incubated with the triterpenes (IC_{25}) and controls for 24 h. Afterward, the cells were washed with 1× PBS and incubated with NucBlue (DAPI analog) and Annexin V for 15 min in the dark. The cells were fixed with 3.7% formaldehyde solution for 15 min, washed three times with 1× PBS, and covered with glycerol before visualization. The plates were observed by confocal microscopy using a Nikon Eclipse Ti microscope (Nikon Instruments Inc., El Segundo, CA, USA), utilizing a 20× oil objective with filter sets compatible with DAPI (Ex/Em = 405/460 nm) and Annexin V Alexa Fluor (Ex/Em = 488/525 nm). The fluorescence intensity was analyzed using the NIS-Elements Viewer program (version 5.21 64-bit) (Nikon Instruments Inc.). Each sample was analyzed in duplicate in two independent experiments. The fluorescence intensity was adjusted using untreated cells for each fluorescence channel (green and blue). Subsequently, this calibrated intensity was applied for the analysis of all treated cells.

4.5. Caspase 3 Activity Assay

The intrinsic apoptosis activity was evaluated by the quantification of caspase 3 enzymatic activity using the Apo-ONE® Homogeneous Caspase-3/7 Assay (Promega G7792). A549 cells were seeded in a concentration of 1×10^5 cells/mL into black 96-well plates with a clear bottom. After 24 h, the cells were incubated with the triterpenes (IC_{50}) and controls for 24 h. After the completion of the incubation, 50 µL of Apo-ONE® Caspase-3/7 Reagent (1:100 rhodamine 110 bis-(N-CBZ-l-aspartyl-l-glutamyl-l-valyl-aspartic acid amide) (Z-DEVD-R110) substrate diluted in lysis buffer) was added to each well. The plate was gently mixed using a plate shaker at 150 rpm for 2 h at room temperature. Then, the fluorescence of each well was measured (Ex/Em = 485/530 nm) in the Tecan® M200 plate reader.

The caspase 3 activity experiments were performed in triplicate. All data were expressed by plotting the values with an average of three measurements for each treatment condition as the mean ± SD and analyzed with the software GraphPad Prism 9 (San Diego, CA, USA). Statistical analysis was performed using one-way analysis of variance (ANOVA) to compare the mean value of each type of treated cells versus the control (untreated cells). The statistical significance defined by the software for p values was **** < 0.0001, *** from 0.001 to 0.0001, ** from 0.001 to 0.01, * from 0.01 to 0.05, and non-significant (ns) $\geq$ 0.05.

4.6. Flow Cytometry Analysis

We used flow cytometry to analyze several cellular mechanistic pathways in A549 cells after incubation with the triterpenes. In general, the cells were seeded in a 6-well plate at a density of 1×10^6 cells/mL and incubated for 24 h in supplemented DMEM. After 24 h, the A549 cells were treated with the triterpenes, following each manufacturer's protocol. All of the following experiments were performed in a Muse® Cell Analyzer (EMD Millipore Corporation, Temecula, CA). The instrument was calibrated before each assay using the Muse® System Check Kit (Luminex MCH100101, Luminex Corporation). Each assay was run at least in two independent experiments. For each experiment, all samples were analyzed in triplicate in the instrument and the capillary line was washed after each sample run to avoid artifacts. In addition, to address the issue of cell doublets, we used the Muse® Cell Dispersal Reagent (Luminex Corporation) in all experiments.

The concentration of the triterpenes in each assay was selected depending on the cellular concentration necessary to generate the gain signal in the instrument. This means that we attempted to select concentrations avoiding excessive cytotoxicity to accurately determine the respective signal from each assay.

4.6.1. Cell Cycle Arrest

A549 cells were incubated with the triterpenes (IC_{25}) for 24 h. Then, the cells were scraped, centrifuged, and fixed using cold 70% ethanol. Afterward, the fixed cell pellet was incubated with the propidium iodide (PI)-based cell cycle reagent (Luminex MCH100106 kit, Luminex Corporation) for 30 min for immediate measurement.

4.6.2. DNA Damage Induction

A549 cells were incubated with the triterpenes (IC_{50}) for 24 h. Then, the A549 cells were scraped and centrifuged. The pellet was suspended in the assay buffer from the Luminex MCH200107 kit (Luminex Corporation). Later, the cell pellet was fixed and permeabilized. Afterward, the antibodies anti-pH2AX (histone) and anti-pATM (ataxia-telangiectasia mutated) were added and incubated for 30 min. Next, the cell pellet was washed and suspended in fresh assay buffer for measurement.

4.6.3. Mitochondrial Oxidative Stress

The production of reactive oxygen species (ROS) by mitochondria was determined using the Oxidative Stress Kit (Luminex MCH100111, Luminex Corporation). After the A549 cells were treated with the triterpenes (IC_{25}) for 24 h, the cells were scraped and centrifuged. For ROS, the cell pellet was incubated with dihydroethidium (DHE) dye for 1 h at 37 °C.

4.6.4. Autophagy Activation

The Muse® Autophagy LC3 Antibody-Based Kit (Luminex MCH200109, Luminex Corporation) was used to determine autophagy activation by monitoring lipidated LC3-II. After the A549 cells were treated with the triterpenes (IC_{25}) for 24 h, autophagy reagent A was added for 4 h to prevent the lysosomal degradation of LC3-II. Then, the cells were detached and centrifuged. The pellet was suspended and incubated for 30 min in the autophagy reagent B containing anti-LC3-II mouse monoclonal antibody. Finally, the cell pellet was washed and suspended in fresh assay buffer for measurement. The autophagy response was calculated using the following formula:

Autophagy ratio = mean autophagy value of treated or untreated cells/mean autophagy value of starving cells.

The starving cells were labeled 'No supp' as non-supplemented cells. These served as the positive signal for autophagy and were designated a ratio of 1 since they were compared to themselves. A ratio $\geq$1 indicates the activation of the autophagic response.

4.6.5. MAPK/PI3K Expression

The Muse® P13K/MAPK Dual Pathway Activation Kit (Luminex MCH200108, Luminex Corporation) was used to determine MAPK/PI3K expression. After the incubation treatment with the triterpenes (IC_{25}) for 24 h, the A549 cells were scraped, centrifuged, and washed once with 1× PBS. Next, the fixation buffer was incubated for 10 min and then the permeabilization buffer for another 10 min. Both incubations were performed on ice. Later, the antibody cocktail containing anti-phospho-Akt and anti-phospho-ERK1/2 was incubated for 30 min. Afterward, the cell pellet was washed and suspended in fresh assay buffer for measurement.

4.7. Total Oxidative Stress

The production of total ROS was determined using the 2′,7′-dichlorodihydrofluorescein diacetate (DCF) fluorescent dye. A549 cells were seeded in a concentration of 1×10^5 cells/mL into black 96-well plates with a clear bottom. After 24 h, the cells were incubated with the triterpenes (IC_{25}) and controls for 24 h. Then, 50 μL of DCF (10 μM) was added to each well and they were incubated for 1 h at room temperature. Then, the fluorescence of each well was measured (Ex/Em = 485/530 nm) in the Tecan® M200 plate reader.

This experiment was performed in triplicate. All data were expressed by plotting the values as an average of three measurements for each treatment condition as the mean ± SD and analyzed with the software GraphPad Prism 9. Statistical analysis was performed using one-way analysis of variance (ANOVA) to compare the mean value of each treated type of cells versus the control (untreated cells). The statistical significance defined by the software for p values was **** < 0.0001, *** from 0.001 to 0.0001, ** from 0.001 to 0.01, * from 0.01 to 0.05, and non-significant (ns) ≥ 0.05.

4.8. RNA Extraction and Real-Time (RT) Quantitative PCR

A549 cells were seeded into 6-well plates at a density of 1×10^6 cells/mL in supplemented DMEM. The cells were incubated with the triterpenes (IC_{25}) for 24 h. Total RNA was extracted from the cells using the TRIzol reagent (Invitrogen Corporation, Carlsbad, CA, USA) according to the manufacturer's instructions. The purity and concentration of RNA were assessed using a NanoDrop spectrophotometer (Thermo Fisher Scientific). cDNA was synthesized using the High-Capacity cDNA Reverse Transcription Kit (Applied Biosystems) according to the manufacturer's instructions.

RT-qPCR was performed on a StepOnePlus® Real-Time PCR System (Thermo Fisher Scientific) using TaqMan Gene Expression Assays (Applied Biosystems) for PDL1 (CD274; Assay ID: Hs01125297_m1), ribonucleotide reductase (RR) M1 (Assay ID: Hs01040697_m1), and STAT3 (Assay ID: Hs01047586_g1). Each reaction consisted of 10 ng of cDNA, TaqMan Gene Expression Master Mix (Applied Biosystems), and TaqMan probes. The PCR cycling conditions were as follows: 95 °C for 10 min, followed by 40 cycles of 95 °C for 15 s and 60 °C for 60 s. The relative gene expression levels were calculated using the ΔΔCt method. GAPDH (Assay ID: Hs02758991_g1) was used as the endogenous control for normalization.

All RT-qPCR experiments were performed at least in triplicate. All data were expressed by plotting values with an average of four measurements for each treatment condition as the mean ± SD and analyzed with the software GraphPad Prism 9. Statistical analysis was performed using one-way analysis of variance (ANOVA) to compare the mean value of each treated type of cells versus the control (untreated cells). The statistical significance defined by the software for p values was **** < 0.0001, *** from 0.001 to 0.0001, ** from 0.001 to 0.01, * from 0.01 to 0.05, and non-significant (ns) ≥ 0.05.

4.9. Theoretical Target Predictive Analysis

Computational analysis is an approach that helps to identify novel targets from extensive databases. We selected the curated database of bioactive molecules ChEMBL (from EMBL's European Bioinformatics Institute) for our analysis. ChemBL was accessed through the online platform (https://www.ebi.ac.uk/chembl/) (accessed on 1 May 2024), where we searched the chemical structures and ChemIDs of the six pentacyclic triterpenes of interest. By applying filters such as human species specificity, active/inactive, confidence levels, and activity thresholds (logarithmic potency values), we retrieved the predictive information on the targets, including the protein names and triterpene compound IDs. The target prediction returned a result of 'active' or 'inactive' depending on whether the compound was predicted to interact or not with the target, 'empty' if the model was unable to make a prediction, or 'both' if it could not make a conclusion.

5. Conclusions

This investigation significantly advances our understanding of the promising therapeutic implications of pentacyclic triterpenoids in cancer treatment. By dissecting the structural differences associated with the regulation of cellular processes, we lay the groundwork for the strategic development of triterpene derivatives with superior efficacy. For instance, the basic structure of BeA provides a promising scaffold for the synthesis of novel lung cancer therapies, where substituent manipulations can be explored to enhance its activity. Similarly, OleA emerges as a focal point in unraveling the structural specificities that govern its selective effects on cancer cells. Our findings suggest opportunities for future research to delve deeper into the regulatory mechanisms influencing chemoresistance in these triterpenes. Towards clinical translation, it is imperative to develop derivatives that integrate the structural patterns of OleA and BeA to position them as robust future candidates.

Supplementary Materials: The following supporting information can be downloaded at: https://www.mdpi.com/article/10.3390/ph17060694/s1, Figure S1: Confocal microscopy images of the A549 cells (2 μm) treated with the six triterpenes. Table S1. Whole set of molecular targets which are predicted to interact with the six pentacyclic triterpenes generated using ChEMBL.

Author Contributions: Conceptualization, Y.D.; formal analysis, A.T.-S., C.G., D.P., G.T., S.E., E.V., M.M. and Y.D.; funding acquisition, Y.D.; investigation, Y.D.; methodology, A.T.-S., D.P., G.T., S.E., M.M., E.V., V.M. and Y.D.; project administration, Y.D.; resources, Y.D.; supervision, Y.D.; validation, Y.D.; visualization, Y.D.; writing—original draft, C.G. and Y.D.; writing—review and editing, A.T.-S. and Y.D. All authors have read and agreed to the published version of the manuscript.

Funding: This project was supported by the Sloan Scholars Mentoring Network Seed Grant, Cancer Prevention and Control (CAPAC) Research Training Program (grant number: R25CA240120) from the National Cancer Institute (NCI), the National Institute of General Medical Sciences (NIGMS) of the National Institutes of Health (NIH) (award number P20GM103475), the Neuroimaging and Electrophysiology Facility (NIEF) supported by the NIGMS of the NIH (award number: P20GM103642), and Fundación Intellectus. The content is solely the responsibility of the authors and does not necessarily represent the official views of the sponsoring agencies.

Institutional Review Board Statement: Not applicable.

Informed Consent Statement: Not applicable.

Data Availability Statement: Data are available upon reasonable request.

Acknowledgments: The authors would like to thank Estela Estapé for her outstanding dedication and service as a senior advisor in the writing process of this paper. We acknowledge the dedicated contribution of the confocal microscopy specialist Bismark Madera, MS, MT at the Neuroimaging and Electrophysiology Facility (NIEF) to this publication. We also thank the San Juan Bautista School of Medicine for supporting this publication.

Conflicts of Interest: The authors declare no conflicts of interest. The funders had no role in the design of the study; in the collection, analyses, or interpretation of data; in the writing of the manuscript; or in the decision to publish the results.

References

1. Sung, H.; Ferlay, J.; Siegel, R.L.; Laversanne, M.; Soerjomataram, I.; Jemal, A.; Bray, F. Global cancer statistics 2020: GLOBOCAN estimates of incidence and mortality worldwide for 36 cancers in 185 countries. *CA Cancer J. Clin.* **2021**, *71*, 209–249. [CrossRef] [PubMed]
2. Baxevanos, P.; Mountzios, G. Novel chemotherapy regimens for advanced lung cancer: Have we reached a plateau? *J. Transl. Med.* **2018**, *6*, 139. [CrossRef] [PubMed]
3. Ranasinghe, R.; Mathai, M.L.; Zulli, A. Cisplatin for cancer therapy and overcoming chemoresistance. *Heliyon* **2022**, *8*, e10608. [CrossRef] [PubMed]
4. Lung Cancer Research Foundation. October 2023. Available online: https://www.lungcancerresearchfoundation.org/research/why-research/treatment-advances/ (accessed on 4 April 2024).
5. Dong, L.; He, J.; Luo, L.; Wang, K. Targeting the Interplay of Autophagy and ROS for Cancer Therapy: An Updated Overview on Phytochemicals. *Pharmaceuticals* **2023**, *16*, 92. [CrossRef]
6. Yan, X.-J.; Gong, L.-H.; Zheng, F.-Y.; Cheng, K.-J.; Chen, Z.-S.; Shi, Z. Triterpenoids as reversal agents for anticancer drug resistance treatment. *Drug Discov. Today* **2014**, *19*, 482–488. [CrossRef] [PubMed]
7. Xu, R.; Fazio, G.C.; Matsuda, S.P.T. On the origins of triterpenoid skeletal diversity. *Phytochemistry* **2004**, *65*, 261–291. [CrossRef] [PubMed]
8. Ren, Y.; Kinghorn, A.D. Natural product triterpenoids and their semi-synthetic derivatives with potential anticancer activity. *Planta Med.* **2019**, *85*, 802–814. [CrossRef]

9. Vo, N.N.Q.; Nomura, Y.; Muranaka, T.; Fukushima, E.O. Structure-activity relationships of pentacyclic triterpenoids as inhibitors of cyclooxygenase and lipoxygenase enzymes. *J. Nat. Prod.* **2019**, *82*, 3311–3320. [CrossRef]
10. Delgado, Y.; Torres, A.; Milian, M. Data on cytotoxic pattern of cholesterol analogs for lung adenocarcinoma cells. *Data Brief.* **2019**, *25*, 104179. [CrossRef]
11. Rufino-Palomares, E.E.; Pérez-Jiménez, A.; García-Salguero, L.; Mokhtari, K.; Reyes-Zurita, F.J.; Peragón-Sánchez, J.; Lupiáñez, J.A. Nutraceutical role of polyphenols and triterpenes present in the extracts of fruits and leaves of *Olea europaea* as antioxidants, anti-infectives and anti-cancer agents on healthy growth. *Molecules* **2022**, *27*, 2341. [CrossRef]
12. Ding, S.M.; Lu, A.L.; Zhang, W.; Zhou, L.; Xie, H.Y.; Zheng, S.S.; Li, Q.Y. The role of cancer-associated fibroblast MRC-5 in pancreatic cancer. *J. Cancer* **2018**, *9*, 614–628. [CrossRef] [PubMed]
13. Guo, W.; Xu, B.; Wang, X.; Zheng, B.; Du, J.; Liu, S. The analysis of the anti-tumor mechanism of ursolic acid using connectively map approach in breast cancer cells line MCF-7. *Cancer Manag. Res.* **2020**, *12*, 3469–3476. [CrossRef] [PubMed]
14. Wróblewska-Łuczka, P.; Cabaj, J.; Bąk, W.; Bargieł, J.; Grabarska, A.; Góralczyk, A.; Łuszczki, J.J. Additive interactions between betulinic acid and two taxanes in in vitro tests against four human malignant melanoma cell lines. *Int. J. Mol. Sci.* **2022**, *23*, 9641. [CrossRef] [PubMed]
15. Pantia, S.; Kangsamaksin, T.; Janvilisri, T.; Komyod, W. Asiatic acid inhibits nasopharyngeal carcinoma cell viability and migration via suppressing STAT3 and Claudin-1. *Pharmaceuticals* **2023**, *16*, 902. [CrossRef] [PubMed]
16. Gao, C.; Li, X.; Yu, S.; Liang, L. Inhibition of cancer cell growth by oleanolic acid in multidrug resistant liver carcinoma is mediated via suppression of cancer cell migration and invasion, mitochondrial apoptosis, G2/M cell cycle arrest and deactivation of JNK/p38 signalling pathway. *J. BUON* **2019**, *24*, 1964–1969. [PubMed]
17. Król, S.K.; Kiełbus, M.; Rivero-Müller, A.; Stepulak, A. Comprehensive review on betulin as a potent anticancer agent. *Biomed. Res. Int.* **2015**, *2015*, 584189. [CrossRef] [PubMed]
18. Pitchai, D.; Roy, A.; Ignatius, C. In vitro evaluation of anti-cancer potentials of lupeol isolated from *Elephantopus scaber* L. on MCF-7 cell line. *J. Adv. Pharm. Technol. Res.* **2014**, *5*, 179–184. [CrossRef]
19. Ford, J.M.; Kastan, M.B. 11—DNA Damage Response Pathways and Cancer. In *Abeloff's Clinical Oncology*, 5th ed.; Niederhuber, J.E., Armitage, J.O., Doroshow, J.H., Kastan, M.B., Tepper, J.E., Eds.; Churchill Livingstone: Philadelphia, PA, USA, 2014; pp. 142–153.e143.
20. Zhan, X.K.; Li, J.L.; Zhang, S.; Xing, P.Y.; Xia, M.F. Betulinic acid exerts potent antitumor effects on paclitaxel-resistant human lung carcinoma cells (H460) via G2/M phase cell cycle arrest and induction of mitochondrial apoptosis. *Oncol. Lett.* **2018**, *16*, 3628–3634. [CrossRef] [PubMed]
21. Shen, M.; Hu, Y.; Yang, Y.; Wang, L.; Yang, X.; Wang, B.; Huang, M. Betulinic acid induces ROS-dependent apoptosis and S-phase arrest by inhibiting the NF-kappaB pathway in human multiple myeloma. *Oxid. Med. Cell Longev.* **2019**, *2019*, 5083158. [CrossRef]
22. Weng, H.; Tan, Z.J.; Hu, Y.P.; Shu, Y.J.; Bao, R.F.; Jiang, L.; Wu, X.S.; Li, M.L.; Ding, Q.; Wang, X.A.; et al. Ursolic acid induces cell cycle arrest and apoptosis of gallbladder carcinoma cells. *Cancer Cell Int.* **2014**, *14*, 96. [CrossRef]
23. Zhang, Y.; Ma, X.; Li, H.; Zhuang, J.; Feng, F.; Liu, L.; Liu, C.; Sun, C. Identifying the effect of ursolic acid against triple-negative breast cancer: Coupling network pharmacology with experiments verification. *Front. Pharmacol.* **2021**, *12*, 685773. [CrossRef] [PubMed]
24. Kim, S.H.; Ryu, H.G.; Lee, J.; Shin, J.; Harikishore, A.; Jung, H.Y.; Kim, Y.S.; Lyu, H.N.; Oh, E.; Baek, N.I.; et al. Ursolic acid exerts anti-cancer activity by suppressing vaccinia-related kinase 1-mediated damage repair in lung cancer cells. *Sci. Rep.* **2015**, *5*, 14570. [CrossRef] [PubMed]
25. Park, C.; Jeong, J.W.; Han, M.H.; Lee, H.; Kim, G.Y.; Jin, S.; Park, J.H.; Kwon, H.J.; Kim, B.W.; Choi, Y.H. The anti-cancer effect of betulinic acid in u937 human leukemia cells is mediated through ROS-dependent cell cycle arrest and apoptosis. *Anim. Cells Syst.* **2021**, *25*, 119–127. [CrossRef]
26. Goswami, P.; Paul, S.; Banerjee, R.; Kundu, R.; Mukherjee, A. Betulinic acid induces DNA damage and apoptosis in SiHa cells. *Mutat. Res. Genet. Toxicol. Environ. Mutagen.* **2018**, *828*, 1–9. [CrossRef]
27. Huff, S.E.; Winter, J.M.; Dealwis, C.G. Inhibitors of the cancer target ribonucleotide reductase, past and present. *Biomolecules* **2022**, *12*, 815. [CrossRef]
28. Youns, M.; Askoura, M.; Abbas, H.A.; Attia, G.H.; Khayyat, A.N.; Goda, R.M.; Almalki, A.J.; Khafagy, E.S.; Hegazy, W.A.H. Celastrol modulates multiple signaling pathways to inhibit proliferation of pancreatic cancer via DDIT3 and ATF3 up-regulation and RRM2 and MCM4 downregulation. *OncoTargets Ther.* **2021**, *14*, 3849–3860. [CrossRef]
29. Wang, C.; Youle, R.J. The role of mitochondria in apoptosis. *Annu. Rev. Genet.* **2009**, *43*, 95–118. [CrossRef] [PubMed]
30. Bhadra, K. A mini review on molecules inducing caspase-independent cell death: A new route to cancer therapy. *Molecules* **2022**, *27*, 6401. [CrossRef]
31. Ling, T.; Boyd, L.; Rivas, F. Triterpenoids as reactive oxygen species modulators of cell fate. *Chem. Res. Toxicol.* **2022**, *35*, 569–584. [CrossRef]
32. Redza-Dutordoir, M.; Averill-Bates, D.A. Interactions between reactive oxygen species and autophagy: Special issue: Death mechanisms in cellular homeostasis. *Biochim. Biophys. Acta Mol. Cell Res.* **2021**, *1868*, 119041. [CrossRef]
33. Wang, Q.; Zou, M.H. Measurement of reactive oxygen species (ROS) and mitochondrial ROS in AMPK knockout mice blood Vessels. *Methods Mol. Biol.* **2018**, *1732*, 507–517. [CrossRef]

34. Napolitano, G.; Fasciolo, G.; Venditti, P. Mitochondrial management of reactive oxygen species. *Antioxidants* **2021**, *10*, 1824. [CrossRef]
35. Yun, C.W.; Lee, S.H. The roles of autophagy in cancer. *Int. J. Mol. Sci.* **2018**, *19*, 3466. [CrossRef]
36. Perillo, B.; Di Donato, M.; Pezone, A.; Di Zazzo, E.; Giovannelli, P.; Galasso, G.; Castoria, G.; Migliaccio, A. ROS in cancer therapy: The bright side of the moon. *Exp. Mol. Med.* **2020**, *52*, 192–203. [CrossRef] [PubMed]
37. Liu, Z.; Yu, X.; Xu, L.; Li, Y.; Zeng, C. Current insight into the regulation of PD-L1 in cancer. *Exp. Hematol. Oncol.* **2022**, *11*, 44. [CrossRef] [PubMed]
38. Kutkowska, J.; Strzadala, L.; Rapak, A. Sorafenib in combination with betulinic acid synergistically induces cell cycle arrest and inhibits clonogenic activity in pancreatic ductal adenocarcinoma cells. *Int. J. Mol. Sci.* **2018**, *19*, 3234. [CrossRef]
39. Pandey, M.K.; Sung, B.; Aggarwal, B.B. Betulinic acid suppresses STAT3 activation pathway through induction of protein tyrosine phosphatase SHP-1 in human multiple myeloma cells. *Int. J. Cancer* **2010**, *127*, 282–292. [CrossRef]
40. Kang, D.Y.; Sp, N.; Lee, J.M.; Jang, K.J. Antitumor effects of ursolic acid through mediating the inhibition of STAT3/PD-L1 signaling in non-small cell lung cancer cells. *Biomedicines* **2021**, *9*, 297. [CrossRef] [PubMed]
41. Myung, Y.; de Sá, A.G.C.; Ascher, D.B. Deep-PK: Deep learning for small molecule pharmacokinetic and toxicity prediction. *Nucleic Acids Res.* **2024**, gkae254. [CrossRef]
42. Azambuja, J.H.; Ludwig, N.; Braganhol, E.; Whiteside, T.L. Inhibition of the adenosinergic pathway in cancer rejuvenates innate and adaptive immunity. *Int. J. Mol. Sci.* **2019**, *20*, 5698. [CrossRef]
43. O'Neill, T.J.; Tofaute, M.J.; Krappmann, D. Function and targeting of MALT1 paracaspase in cancer. *Cancer Treatment Rev.* **2023**, *117*, 102568. [CrossRef] [PubMed]
44. McDonald, P.C.; Chafe, S.C.; Supuran, C.T.; Dedhar, S. Cancer therapeutic targeting of hypoxia induced carbonic anhydrase IX: From bench to bedside. *Cancers* **2022**, *14*, 3297. [CrossRef] [PubMed]
45. Song, C.; Zhang, J.; Xu, C.; Gao, M.; Li, N.; Geng, Q. The critical role of γ-secretase and its inhibitors in cancer and cancer therapeutics. *Int. J. Biol. Sci.* **2023**, *19*, 5089–5103. [CrossRef] [PubMed]
46. Welsh, S.J.; Corrie, P.G. Management of BRAF and MEK inhibitor toxicities in patients with metastatic melanoma. *Ther. Adv. Med. Oncol.* **2015**, *7*, 122–136. [CrossRef] [PubMed]
47. Zuo, Z.; Liu, J.; Sun, Z.; Silverstein, R.; Zou, M.; Finkel, T.; Bugge, T.H.; Leppla, S.H.; Liu, S. A potent tumor-selective ERK pathway inactivator with high therapeutic index. *PNAS Nexus* **2022**, *1*, 104. [CrossRef] [PubMed]
48. Hong, D.S.; Kurzrock, R.; Supko, J.G.; He, X.; Naing, A.; Wheler, J.; Lawrence, D.; Eder, J.P.; Meyer, C.J.; Ferguson, D.A.; et al. A phase I first-in-human trial of bardoxolone methyl in patients with advanced solid tumors and lymphomas. *Clin. Cancer Res.* **2012**, *18*, 3396–3406. [CrossRef]
49. Clinical Trials Study Records. 16 September 2021. Available online: https://clinicaltrials.gov/study/NCT04403568?term=NCT04403568&rank=1 (accessed on 29 April 2024).
50. Torres-Martinez, Z.; Pérez, D.; Torres, G.; Estrada, S.; Correa, C.; Mederos, N.; Velazquez, K.; Castillo, B.; Griebenow, K.; Delgado, Y. A synergistic pH-responsive serum albumin-based drug delivery system loaded with doxorubicin and pentacyclic triterpene betulinic acid for potential treatment of NSCLC. *BioTech* **2023**, *12*, 13. [CrossRef]

pharmaceuticals

Article

Effects of Chicory (*Cichorium intybus* L.) Extract on Male Rat Reproductive System, Pregnancy and Offspring Development

Alexandra N. Babenko [1], Lubov V. Krepkova [1], Marina V. Borovkova [1], Olga S. Kuzina [1], Vladimir A. Mkhitarov [2], Kathleen M. Job [3] and Elena Y. Enioutina [3,*]

1 All-Russian Institute of Medicinal and Aromatic Plants (VILAR), Moscow 113628, Russia; alexandra.mogileva@gmail.com (A.N.B.); krepkowa2011@yandex.ru (L.V.K.); borovkova_65@mail.ru (M.V.B.); oskt@list.ru (O.S.K.)
2 FSBI "Research Institute of Human Morphology", Moscow 117418, Russia; mkhitarov@mail.ru
3 Division of Clinical Pharmacology, Department of Pediatrics, School of Medicine, University of Utah, Salt Lake City, UT 84108, USA; kate.job@hsc.utah.edu
* Correspondence: elena.enioutina@hsc.utah.edu

Abstract: Background: We recently reported that extract prepared from the aerial part of *Cichorium intybus* L. (CE) possesses hepatoprotective, hypolipidemic, and hypoglycemic properties. This paper focuses on the effects of CE on the male rat reproductive system and the effects of this treatment on pregnancy and offspring development. Methods: The experimental male rats received 100 mg/kg bw/day, 500 mg/kg bw/day, and 1000 mg/kg bw/day of CE orally for 60 consecutive days. Rats that received tap water were used as controls. After treatment, we evaluated the effects of CE on the male reproductive system, fertility, and offspring development. Results: For CE-treated male rats, there was a significant increase in the (1) diameter of seminiferous tubules, (2) spermatogenic index, (3) number of total and motile spermatozoa, and (4) testosterone levels. Additionally, there was a decrease in the pre- and post-implantation death of the embryos in the CE-treated group. All pups born from CE-treated males demonstrated normal development. Conclusions: CE treatment significantly improved male reproductive functions. No adverse effects on pregnancy and offspring development were observed when males were treated with CE. Further clinical evaluation of CE should lead to the development of a safe and effective phytodrug for treating male infertility.

Keywords: chicory extract; male reproductive system; spermatogenesis; fertility; offspring development

Citation: Babenko, A.N.; Krepkova, L.V.; Borovkova, M.V.; Kuzina, O.S.; Mkhitarov, V.A.; Job, K.M.; Enioutina, E.Y. Effects of Chicory (*Cichorium intybus* L.) Extract on Male Rat Reproductive System, Pregnancy and Offspring Development. *Pharmaceuticals* **2024**, *17*, 700. https://doi.org/10.3390/ph17060700

Academic Editor: Michael Danilenko

Received: 28 March 2024
Revised: 21 May 2024
Accepted: 22 May 2024
Published: 28 May 2024

1. Introduction

Over the past several decades, the total fertility rates in Europe, North America, and Australia dropped below the rate necessary to maintain the population rate [1–3]. Reasons for decreasing fertility rates is the growing number of both male and female infertility cases. About one-third of infertility cases were associated with changes in the male reproductive system, and an additional 30% were related to problems in male and female reproductive systems [3]. The increase in infertility is likely due to lifestyle changes (e.g., reduced sleep time, dietary changes, use of alcohol, tobacco, and narcotics), poor health conditions (e.g., obesity), or environmental pollution (e.g., industrial chemical exposure, heavy household chemical use) [2,4]. These reasons for infertility are unlikely to change in the near future. Therefore, medical interventions are being pursued to return the fertility rates to maintenance levels.

Several pharmacological and microsurgical methods are available for the treatment of male infertility [5]. Treatments include microsurgical testicular sperm extraction, hormonal therapy (e.g., the use of gonadotropins and selective estrogen receptor modulators), and the use of aromatase inhibitors [5].

Many patients, however, prefer to use traditional methods of treatment, including the use of acupuncture and phytodrugs. Multiple studies have presented the positive effects of various medicinal plants or extracts prepared from them on the male reproductive system. Medicinal plants such as Tribulus (*Tribulus terrestris*), bananas (e.g., *Musa acuminata*), nigella (*Nigella sativa*), burdock (*Arctium lappa*), and fenugreek *Trigonella foenum-graecum* may stimulate spermatogenesis [6,7]. There are also reports that the use of *Panax ginseng* C.A.Mey, *Dáucus caróta*, *Passiflora incarnata*, *Rhaponticum carthamoides* (Willd.), *Allium cepa* L., *Állium satívum*, *Camellia sinensis*, *Amaranthus spinosus*, *Lepidium meyenii*, *Morinda officinalis*, *Schisandrae chinensidis* plant, root or seed extracts may improve semen parameters, hormonal levels, and sexual dysfunctions in both humans and experimental animals [7–12].

Recently, we conducted a preclinical evaluation of a highly purified extract prepared from the aerial part of wild chicory (*Cichorium intybus* L., CE). The extract demonstrated hepatoprotective, hypolipidemic, and hypoglycemic effects [13].

Our present studies have evaluated the impact of CE treatment on male rats' reproductive functions and fertility. We determined that treatment with CE improved the male rat reproductive system functions, evidenced by an increase in the diameter of seminiferous tubules, spermatogenic index, number of total and motile spermatozoa, and testosterone levels. Another research group has reported that the treatment of male rats with a different extract prepared from chicory leaves increased the weight of testes and epididymis, stimulated the production of morphologically normal sperm, and increased serum testosterone levels [14]. The authors attributed the gonadotropic effects to the antioxidant properties of the bioactive components present in the extract. While the extracts were prepared using different extraction methods and the extracts' compositions can differ significantly, the findings show that extracts prepared from the aerial part of chicory may stimulate spermatogenesis in male rats.

To the best of our knowledge, there were no reported studies investigating the effects of the phytodrug impacting male reproductive function on pregnancy or postnatal offspring development. This study additionally examines the impact of CE treatment of male rats on pregnancy and offspring development. The study results show that male rat treatment with CE did not affect pregnancy and offspring development.

2. Results

As part of the CE preclinical pharmacological and safety studies, we have investigated its effects on the reproductive function of male rats, fertility, and effects on offspring development.

2.1. The Effect of CE on the Reproductive Function of Male Rats

One of the most critical indicators that characterize the testes' morphological state is its relative mass. It is defined as the ratio of organ mass to body mass, expressed as a percentage. The administration of CE for 60 consecutive days to male rats in doses of 100, 500, and 1000 mg/kg bw/day had no significant effect on relative testicular weight (Table 1).

Table 1. The effect of CE on the weight of testes of male rats.

Parameters	Experimental Groups [a]			
	Control (H_2O)	CE 100 mg/kg bw/day	CE 500 mg/kg bw/day	CE 1000 mg/kg bw/day
Number of animals evaluated	10	10	10	10
Weight of testes (g) [b]	3.21 ± 0.20	3.20 ± 0.21 [ns]	3.20 ± 0.07 [ns]	3.20 ± 0.14 [ns]
Relative weight (%) [b]	0.96 ± 0.04	0.96 ± 0.04 [ns]	0.94 ± 0.09 [ns]	0.98 ± 0.08 [ns]

[a]—Male rats were treated with either H_2O (control) or CE (100, 500, or 1000 mg/kg bw/day) for 60 days before mating; [b]—mean ± SE. [ns]—the differences between the CE-treated and control groups were not statistically significant.

There is evidence of active spermatogenesis at different stages of development in control and experimental groups. The morphological structure of the testes of male rats receiving CE at 100, 500, or 1000 mg/kg bw/day for 60 consecutive days appeared normal and was not different from the control group (Figure 1). The testes have a dense connective tissue membrane, from which connective tissue septa extend to the center. The septa contain numerous elastic fibers dividing the organ into lobules. The inner side of the seminiferous tubules is covered with spermatogenic epithelium, which contains morphologically normal spermatogenic cells.

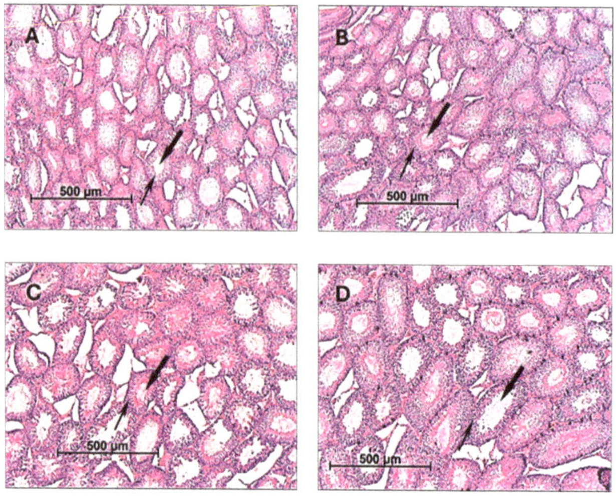

Figure 1. The morphological structure of testes of male rats. Male rats were orally treated for 60 days with (**A**)—H_2O (control); (**B**)—CE 100 mg/kg bw/day; (**C**)—500 mg/kg bw/day; and (**D**)—1000 mg/kg bw/day. Thin arrow—seminiferous spermatogenic epithelium of the testes; bold arrow—lumens of the seminiferous tubule. Staining hematoxylin/eosin; magnification ×50.

The productive function of the testes was investigated based on three parameters: the diameter and cross-sectional area of the convoluted seminiferous tubules and the spermatogenesis index. The highest dose CE (1000 mg/kg bw/day) treatment significantly increased the diameter of the seminiferous tubules in the rats (Figure 2) when compared to the control group (p = 0.0339).

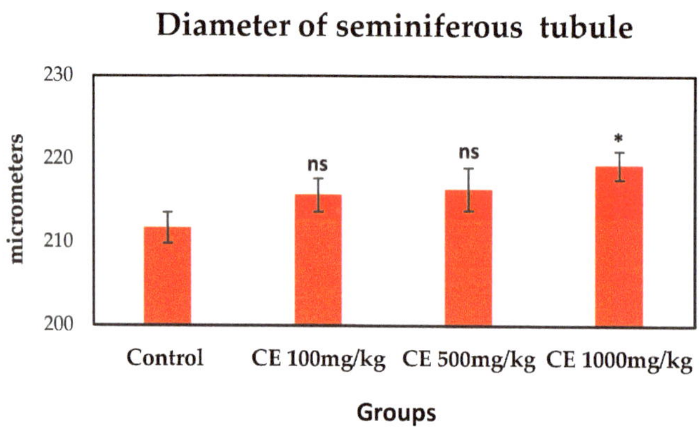

Figure 2. Effect of CE treatment on the diameter of seminiferous tubules. Control rats were orally treated with H_2O for 60 days; experimental rats received 100, 500, and 1000 mg/kg bw/day of CE by gavage for 60 days. *—differences are statistically different compared to control (p = 0.0339). ^{ns}—the differences between the CE-treated and control groups were not statistically significant.

CE treatment increased the total area of the spermatogenic epithelium compared to control; however, statistically significant differences were observed only in doses of 500 ($p = 0.0019$) and 1000 mg/kg bw/day ($p = 0.0001$) (Figure 3). Representative morphological structures of spermatogenic epithelia are presented in Figure 3.

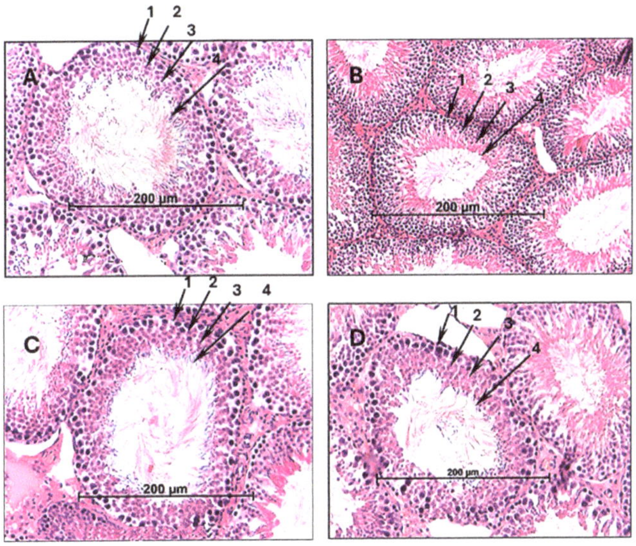

Area of the spermatogenic epithelium (μm²)

Control	CE 100mg/kg	CE 500 mg/kg	CE 1000 mg/kg
35652.7±680.8	37381.6±694.7	38982.8±707.4*	39891.3±920.1†

* p=0.0019; † p=0.0001

Figure 3. The effects of CE treatment on spermatogenic epithelia. Male rats were orally treated for 60 days with (**A**)—H_2O (control); (**B**)—CE 100 mg/kg bw/day; (**C**)—500 mg/kg bw/day; and (**D**)—1000 mg/kg bw/day 1—spermatogonia; 2—spermatocytes; 3—spermatids; 4—spermatozoa. Staining hematoxylin/eosin; magnification ×200.

The spermatogenesis index is an essential marker of the testes' reproductive function and demonstrates the spermatogenic epithelium's functional activity. The oral administration of CE in doses 500 and 1000 mg/kg bw/day stimulated spermatogenesis in male rat testes; the differences were statistically significant ($p = 0.001$–0.002, Table 2).

Table 2. The CE effect on the spermatogenesis index.

Parameters	Experimental Groups [a]			
	Control (H_2O)	CE 100 mg/kg bw/day	CE 500 mg/kg bw/day	CE 1000 mg/kg bw/day
Number of animals evaluated	10	10	10	10
Spermatogenesis index [b]	3.47 ± 0.02	3.49 ± 0.02 [ns]	3.71 ± 0.02 *	3.76 ± 0.02 **

[a]—Male rats were orally treated with either H_2O (control) or CE (100, 500, or 1000 mg/kg bw/day) for 60 days; [b]—mean ± SE. * $p = 0.001$, ** $p = 0.002$; [ns]—the differences between the CE-treated and control groups were not statistically significant.

2.2. The Effect of CE on Morpho-Functional Parameters of Epididymal Spermatozoa of Male Rats

The condition of spermatozoa was assessed by counting the total and motile number of spermatozoa, the duration of movement, and the number of pathological forms. The oral administration of CE (100, 500, and 1000 mg/kg bw/day) for 60 consecutive days to male rats had a significant positive effect on the main morpho-functional parameters of spermatozoa (Table 3). The CE treatment increased the total number of spermatozoa. Differences between the CE-treated and control groups were statistically significant ($p < 0.05$). The number of motile spermatozoa in the homogenate of the epididymis from CE-treated groups has been increased compared to those in the control group. The duration of movement and the number of pathological forms of spermatozoa in CE-treated groups were not different from those in the control group. These results indicate that CE at the tested doses had a stimulating effect on spermatogenesis.

Table 3. The CE effect on the spermatogenesis of male rats.

Parameters	**Groups** [a]			
	Control (H_2O)	**CE 100 mg/kg bw/day**	**CE 500 mg/kg bw/day**	**CE 1000 mg/kg bw/day**
The number of animals evaluated	10	10	10	10
Total number of spermatozoa ($\times 10^6$) [b]	23.5 ± 2.4	36.3 ± 3.3 *	37.4 ± 3.6 *	40.0 ± 4.6 *
Motile spermatozoa ($\times 10^6$) [b]	17.2 ± 1.7	23.7 ± 2.4 *	23.8 ± 2.2 *	32.9 ± 2.6 *
Duration of spermatozoon movement (min.) [b]	360.0 ± 23.5	362.2 ± 26.0 [ns]	345.3 ± 25.6 [ns]	352.7 ± 23.5 [ns]
Pathologic forms of spermatozoa (%)	1.5 ± 0.2	1.7 ± 0.2 [ns]	1.6 ± 0.1 [ns]	1.7 ± 0.2 [ns]

[a]—male rats were orally treated with either H_2O (control) or CE (100, 500, or 1000 mg/kg bw/day) for 60 days before mating; [b]—mean ± SE. * $p < 0.05$, [ns]—the differences between the CE-treated and control groups were not statistically significant.

2.3. Characteristics of the Functional State of Leydig Cells

Testosterone is one of the most essential androgenic hormones that regulate fertility, development, and maintenance of the male reproductive system and sexual function [15]. Testosterone is secreted by endocrinocytes, also called Leydig cells, located in the interstitial connective tissue of the testes. One of the indicators of the functional activity of Leydig cells is the surface area of their nuclei. The treatment of male rats with CE did not increase the surface areas of nuclei compared with the control group (Figure 4).

Serum testosterone concentrations were significantly higher in the animals receiving CE at all tested doses than in control animals (Figure 5). These results may suggest an increase in the level of sexual activity and fertility of males treated with CE.

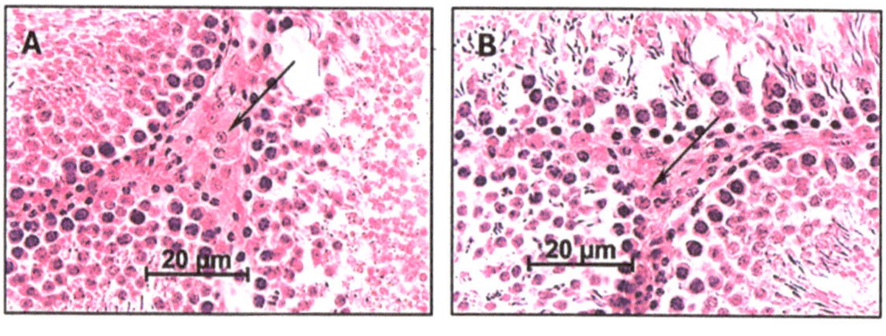

Figure 4. *Cont.*

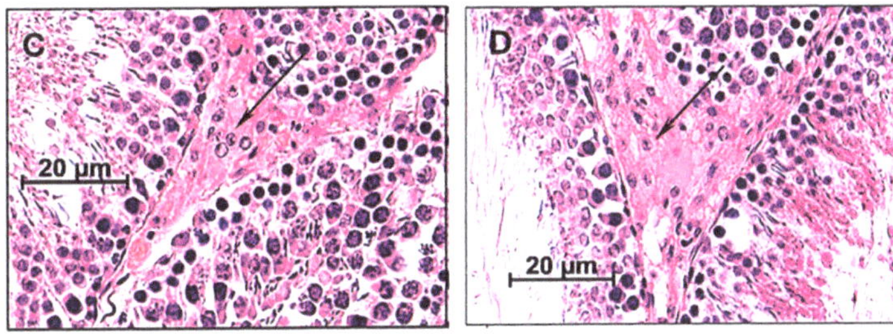

Leydig cells' surface areas of nuclei (µm²)

Control	CE, 100 mg/mg	CE, 500 mg/kg	CE, 1000 mg/kg
24. 80 ± 0.36	24.40 ± 0.36	24.53 ± 0.35	24.45 ± 0.29

Figure 4. The effects of CE treatment on Leydig cells. Male rats were orally treated for 60 days with (**A**)—H_2O (control); (**B**)—CE 100 mg/kg bw/day; (**C**)—500 mg/kg bw/day; and (**D**)—1000 mg/kg bw/day. Arrows—Leydig cells. Staining hematoxylin/eosin; magnification × 640.

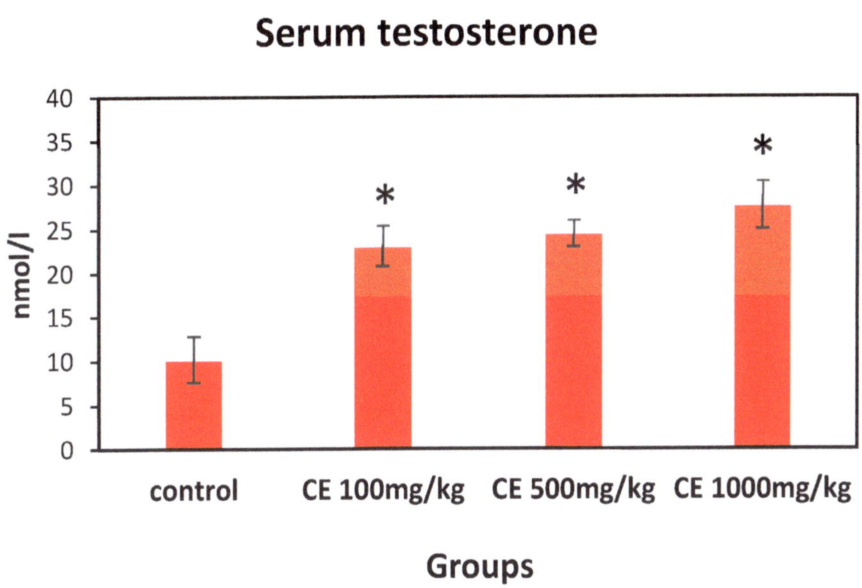

Figure 5. The effect of CE treatment on serum testosterone levels. Control rats were orally treated with H_2O for 60 days; experimental rats received 100, 500, and 1000 mg/kg bw/day of CE by gavage for 60 days. The serum total testosterone concentrations were measured on day 60 of treatment. *—$p < 0.05$.

2.4. *Effects of CE on Male Rat Fertility*

The fertility indicator is an integral criterion of the effectiveness of spermatogenesis and its sensitivity to harmful factors. The fertility of experimental animals was determined by mating intact female rats with control or CE-treated mature male rats. Subsequently, the fertility and pregnancy index was calculated.

The oral CE administration (100, 500, and 1000 mg/kg bw/day) to male rats for 60 days before mating with intact females did not affect the body weight dynamics of pregnant female rats after their impregnation. The fertility index was consistent between groups of female rats mated with CE-treated males and female rats mated with control males (Table 4). All females mated with CE-treated or control male rats became pregnant (Table 4).

Table 4. Effects of CE on male rat fertility.

Parameters	Experimental Groups [a]			
	♂ × ♀	♂ × ♀	♂ × ♀	♂ × ♀
	H_2O × Intact	**CE, 100 mg/kg × Intact**	**CE, 500 mg/kg × Intact**	**CE, 1000 mg/kg × Intact**
Number of mated females	15	15	15	15
Number of fertile females	14	14	14	14
Number of pregnant females	14	14	14	14
Fertility index (%)	93.3	93.3	93.3	93.3
Pregnancy index (%)	100	100	100	100

[a]—male rats were orally treated with either H_2O (control) or CE (100, 500, or 1000 mg/kg bw/day) for 60 days before mating.

The effects of CE treatment of male rats before mating on pre- and post-implantation embryonic death were investigated on day 20 of pregnancy (Table 5). CE treatment did not significantly change embryonic pre- and post-implantation death compared to the control group. However, pregnant females who were mated with males treated with 500 mg/mL and 1000 mg/mL tended to have less embryonic pre- and post-implantation death. Fetal weight on day 20 of pregnancy was similar in all treatment groups compared to the control group (Table 5).

Table 5. Effect of CE treatment of male rates on embryonic pre- and post-implantation death of day 20 of pregnancy.

Parameters		Experimental Groups [a]			
		♂ × ♀	♂ × ♀	♂ × ♀	♂ × ♀
		H_2O × Intact	**CE, 100 mg/kg × Intact**	**CE, 500 mg/kg × Intact**	**CE, 1000 mg/kg × Intact**
Number of pregnant female rats investigated		7	7	7	7
Embryonic Death (%) [b]	Pre-implantation	7.7 ± 0.8	7.6 ± 0.7 [ns]	7.2 ± 0.3 [ns]	6.4 ± 0.6 [ns]
	Post-implantation	4.7 ± 0.5	4.5 ± 0.3 [ns]	4.2 ± 0.3 [ns]	3.8 ± 0.4 [ns]
Embryonic weight on day 20 (g) [b]		2.4 ± 0.1	2.3 ± 0.1 [ns]	2.4 ± 0.03 [ns]	2.3 ± 0.1 [ns]

[a]—male rats were orally treated with either H_2O (control) or CE (100, 500, or 1000 mg/kg bw/day) for 60 days before mating; [b]—mean ± SE. [ns]—the differences between the CE-treated and control groups were not statistically significant.

2.5. The Effect of CE Male Rat Treatment on Offspring Development

The parameters for postnatal offspring development (the number of newborns in litters, the number of surviving pups, and their body weights in all experimental groups) in CE-male-treated groups were not statistically different compared to the control group (Table 6). However, the number of newborn pups was slightly higher in the groups born from male rats treated with 500 mg/kg bw/day and 1000 mg/kg bw/day. The number of surviving pups in the groups born from male rats treated with 500 mg/kg bw/day and 1000 mg/kg bw/day was higher compared to the control group, and all pups survived in the group born from male rats treated with 1000 mg/kg bw/day.

Table 6. The effect of CE treatment of male rats on the postnatal offspring development.

Parameters			Experimental Groups [a]			
			♂ × ♀	♂ × ♀	♂ × ♀	♂ × ♀
			H_2O × Intact	CE, 100 mg/kg × Intact	CE, 500 mg/kg × Intact	CE, 1000 mg/kg × Intact
Number of litters evaluated			7	7	7	7
Number of newborn pups in the litter [b]			8.4 ± 0.4	8.1 ± 0.7 [ns]	8.5± 0.3 [ns]	9.3 ± 0.8 [ns]
Number of surviving pups per female rat post-delivery	Day 7	Number [b]	8.1 ± 0.6	8.1 ± 0.7 [ns]	8.5± 0.3 [ns]	9.3 ± 0.8 [ns]
		%	96.4	100	100	100
	Day 14	Number [b]	8.1 ± 0.6	7.9 ± 0.6 [ns]	8.5± 0.3 [ns]	9.3 ± 0.8 [ns]
		%	96.4	97.5	100	100
	Day 21	Number [b]	7.9 ± 0.6	7.7 ± 0.6 [ns]	8.3 ± 0.4 [ns]	9.3 ± 0.8 [ns]
		%	94.0	95.1	98.0	100
Pups weight (g) [b]	Day 1		6.2 ± 0.2	6.3 ± 0.3 [ns]	6.1± 0.4 [ns]	6.0 ± 0.2 [ns]
	Day 4		9.1 ± 0.5	9.0 ± 0.5 [ns]	8.9 ± 0.7 [ns]	8.9 ± 0.3 [ns]
	Day 7		12.3 ± 0.8	12.7 ± 1.1 [ns]	11.9 ± 0.5 [ns]	11.8 ± 0.6 [ns]
	Day 14		22.6 ± 0.9	22.9 ± 0.9 [ns]	20.9 ±1.5 [ns]	20.9 ± 1.3 [ns]
	Day 21		32.4 ± 2.2	33.2± 2.0 [ns]	32.2 ± 3.4 [ns]	31.2 ± 3.0 [ns]

[a]—male rats were orally treated with either H_2O (control) or CE (100, 500, or 1000 mg/kg bw/day) for 60 days before mating; [b]—mean ± SE. [ns]—the differences between the CE-treated and control groups were not statistically significant.

The physical development (e.g., pinna detachment, fur appearance, and eye-opening) in pups of all experimental groups was similar to the pups in the control group and corresponded to the physiological norm. There were no statistically significant differences in the negative geotaxis skills of experimental rat pups compared to the control animals (Table 7). The negative geotaxis test examines the maturity of motor skills and cerebellar integration in pups [16,17]. While there were no statistically significant differences in the open-field test between pups born from rat males treated with CE and control pups, the pups born from males treated with CE were more active, as evidenced by increased numbers of square crossing, head dipping and their emotional status (i.e., frequency of defecation) (Table 7).

Table 7. Postnatal offspring development.

Parameters			Groups [a]			
			Control (H_2O)	CE 100 mg/kg	CE 500 mg/kg	CE 1000 mg/kg
Number of pups evaluated			51	52	50	54
Time of cliff avoidance (sec.) [b]			5.0 ± 0.6	4.7 ± 0.4 [ns]	6.2 ± 0.5 [ns]	5.3 ± 0.5 [ns]
Flip/roll over onto all four paws	Pups with positive reaction	No.	51	52	50	54
		%	100	100	100	100
Negative geotaxis (sec) [b]			11.3 ± 1.2	10.9 ± 1.1 [ns]	11.5 ±1.3 [ns]	10.9 ± 1.0 [ns]
Open-field test	Total squares crossed [b]		32.9 ± 3.2	37.6 ± 3.9 [ns]	37.8 ± 4.0 [ns]	38.0 ± 3.7 [ns]
	Head dipping [b]		3.17 ± 0.35	3.20 ± 0.33 [ns]	3.50 ± 0.35 [ns]	3.60 ± 0.35 [ns]
	Grooming frequency [b]		1.20 ± 0.13	1.20 ± 0.12 [ns]	1.10 ± 0.11 [ns]	1.10 ± 0.13 [ns]
	Defecation [b]		2.90 ± 0.22	3.10 ± 0.30 [ns]	3.40 ± 0.34 [ns]	3.60 ± 0.41 [ns]
	Rearing frequency [b]		0.10 ± 0.10	0.20 ± 0.13 [ns]	0.20 ± 0.13 [ns]	0.20 ± 0.13 [ns]

[a]—male rats were orally treated with either H_2O (control) or CE (100, 500, or 1000 mg/kg bw/day) for 60 days before mating; [b]—mean ± SE. [ns]—the differences between the CE-treated and control groups were not statistically significant.

3. Discussion

Multiple studies have reported the enhancement of spermatogenesis by phytodrugs or extracts from medicinal plants, including extracts from various species of chicory [6–8,12,14,18–20]. One difficulty in comparing the pharmacological effects of phytodrugs or extracts obtained from the same medicinal herb is that the studies may use extracts from different plant parts (e.g., whole plant, aerial part of the plant, or roots). The composition of the biologically active constituents in various plant parts varies significantly. For example, the HPLC fingerprinting analysis of different parts of chicory (e.g., flowers, stems, leaves, and roots) established that the highest amount of bioactive constituents is present in flowers, followed by stems, leaves, roots, and seeds [21]. The leaves and stems had the highest amounts of cichoric acid, flowers had the highest levels of esculin, and roots were rich in chlorogenic acid. Additionally, the extract composition may differ significantly depending on the extraction methods (e.g., water, ethanol, or a mixture of water and ethanol).

One of the first publications by Roy-Choudhury A. and Venkatakrishna-Bhatt H. on the effects of chicory extracts on reproductive functions of male animals showed that *Cichorium intybus* L. "aqueous root suspension" suppressed spermatogenesis in mice [22]. Our data demonstrate that the CE treatment improved the reproductive function of male rats. CE was prepared from the *Cichorium intybus* L. aerial part, which included stems, leaves, and flowers. The therapy with CE increased spermatogenesis and testosterone levels in healthy male rats. Another publication also showed chicory extract's stimulatory effects on the male rats' reproductive system [14]. The extract was prepared from the dried *Cichorium intybus* L. leaves by extraction of bioactive compounds with ethanol. The extract was orally administered to healthy adult male rats at doses 50, 100, and 200 mg/kg daily for 70 consecutive days. Unlike in our study, the chicory ethanolic extract administration significantly increased the testicular and epididymal weights. The authors reported a statistically significant increase in "sperm density" and a reduction in morphologically abnormal forms of spermatozoa. Spermatozoa motility in extract-treated rats were similar to the control group. Our study found an increase in the total number of spermatozoa and motile forms. Both studies showed an increase in testosterone levels. Different bioactive molecules in the extracts could explain the observed difference in the effects of chicory extract obtained by ethanol extraction and CE on the male reproductive system. Unfortunately, we could not find more details on the extraction method and extract's chemical composition. The mechanism of action of the chicory ethanolic extract was potentially associated with the extract's antioxidant properties [14].

Koloko B. et al. investigated the effect of *Rauvolfia vomitoria* ethanolic extract on reproductive activity and sexual performance of healthy male rats [20]. Rats were treated with the extract at doses of 50, 100, and 200 mg/kg bw/day for 22 days. The *Rauvolfia* extract increased the spermatozoa count and their motility. *Rauvolfia* extract-treated male rats demonstrated an increase in sexual activity. The mount latency, intromission latency, and post-ejaculatory intervals were significantly reduced, while ejaculation latency, mount frequency, intromission frequency, and ejaculation frequency were significantly increased compared to control animals.

Exposure to metal particles (e.g., lead, cadmium, aluminum, arsenic, and chromium) through air pollution may lead to male infertility [23]. Lead is a well-known environmental pollutant. Lead significantly decreased the spermatozoa concentrations and the number of motile spermatozoa in male rats [18]. Co-administration of chicory extract with lead restored the number of motile spermatozoa to control group levels and reduced the number of abnormal forms. Humans are frequently exposed to aluminum particles through air pollution, antiperspirants, cooking containers, canned food, and cosmetics. Aluminum exposure may result in damaging effects on the male reproductive system [24]. The exposure of male rats to aluminum chloride at a dose of 50 mg/kg bw/day for 70 days resulted in decreased spermatozoa count and motility and an increase in dead cells and morphologically abnormal forms of spermatozoa. Treatment with esculetin, a coumarin derivative, ameliorated adverse aluminum chloride effects on the male rat reproductive system.

Tobacco smoke is another air pollutant that produces fine particles. Hashemi M. et al. evaluated the effect of 70% ethanol/water chicory extract on the reproductive function of male rats exposed to cigarette smoke [25]. The treatment with the chicory extract reduced damage from cigarette smoke to male rat reproductive functions. The chicory treatment of rats exposed to smoke increased the number of Sertoli cells, spermatogonia, and spermatocytes and reduced the number of apoptotic cells otherwise damaged by exposure to smoke.

Certain drugs may have adverse effects on the male reproductive system. It has been reported that aldosterone inhibits stem Leydig cell proliferation, while dexamethasone inhibits their differentiation [26]. Animal studies determined that prenatal exposure to dexamethasone leads to spermatozoa quality in male offspring [27]. It has been proposed that these changes are associated with epigenetic programming of the Sertoli cells. *Portulaca oleracea* and *Cichorium intybus* extracts synergistically enhanced male rat fertility in the dexamethasone-induced testicular and autophagy dysfunction model. The treatment with these extracts of dexamethasone-exposed male rats increased sperm motility and showed a protective effect on seminiferous tubules. The potential mechanism of action of the *Portulaca oleracea* and *Cichorium intybus* is proposed through attenuating oxidative stress and autophagy. *Ocimum tenuiflorum*, a medicinal plant with antioxidant properties, protected spermatozoa and germ cells from filgrastim damaging effects [28].

Excessive oxidative stress is one of the mechanisms responsible for male infertility [29–31]. It damages spermatozoan activities and male fertility. Reactive oxygen species (ROS) are produced during the maturation and capacitation of spermatozoa, as well as by the prostate and seminal vesicles. Excessive ROS production may reduce sperm motility and viability and damage DNA and other cellular components. Chronic inflammation also plays a significant role in male infertility. Mehran Dorostghoal and colleagues investigated the mechanisms of the gonadotropic effect of the chicory leaf extract. They determined that the extract reduced malondialdehyde levels and increased superoxide dismutase and glutathione peroxidase activity in the testicles of treated rats [14]. The authors suggested that the improvements in male reproductive health may be associated with the extract's antioxidant and androgenic properties. Other investigators agree that the antioxidant and anti-inflammatory properties of medicinal plants such as cinnamon (*Cinnamomum verum*), grape (*Vitis vinifera*), onion (*Allium cepa*), garlic (*Allium sativum*), apricot (*Prunus armeniaca*), dogwood (*Cornus florida*) are responsible for the improve sperm quality and the number of motile sperm in patients with asthenozoospermia [6]. The modulations of extracellular-regulated kinase (ERK), protein kinase B (PKB), and NF-kB signaling pathways by the phytodrugs are mechanisms regulating male fertility [8]. Another potential mechanism responsible for the anti-infertility properties of the phytodrugs is smooth muscle-relaxing properties, which could help reduce male infertility [31].

Most of the above-presented studies focused on the effects of herbal extracts on the male reproductive system. Occasionally, medicinal herbs and phytodrugs may represent a potential risk to the childbearing mother, the fetuses, and offspring born from mother or father exposed to herbal remedies. Our study also demonstrated that male exposure to CE did not affect pregnancy development; CE male treatment reduced pre- and post-implantation embryonic death. The systematic review investigating the effect of an oral antioxidant, *Satureja khuzestanica,* on male infertility and pregnancy rate concluded that the plant increases spermatozoa quality and pregnancy rate [32]. The bioflavonoid composition from the roots of *Scutellaria baicalensis* and the heartwoods of *Acacia catechu* administered to either male rats for 4 weeks or female rats for 2 weeks before mating at the highest dose of 1000 mg/kg had no significant effects on male fertility indexes, but it appears that increased implantation rate and reduced embryo mortality [33].

Our current study also reported that CE treatment of male rats had no significant effect on offspring development. However, there is a limitation to this study. The International Standard OECD Test No. 416:2001 Two-Generation Reproduction Toxicity Study requires evaluation of reproductive toxicity on two generations of laboratory animals to provide information regarding the effects of the test substance on the development of F1 and F2 offspring. We assessed the CE effects on the growth and development of one F1 generation.

Animal studies demonstrate that herbal extracts have great potential to improve male reproductive health. Unfortunately, very few high-quality clinical trials were conducted to determine whether these herbal extracts can help to overcome male infertility in human patients. A meta-analysis of the effect of ginseng on erectile dysfunction analyzed data from randomized and semi-randomized trials [34]. The investigators concluded that the ginseng treatment had minimal adverse reactions; however, it had a "trivial effect" on erectile function, as evidenced by the measurements of the index of erectile function. Salgado R. et al. reported that *Tribulus terrestris* given to men with abnormal spermatogenesis increased dihydrotestosterone levels, enhanced sperm concentration, and motility [35]. Protodioscin, a bioactive *Tribulus* constituent, stimulated germ cell proliferation and growth of seminiferous tubules. Another review, however, concluded that *Tribulus terrestris* and *Lepidium meyenii* Walp treatment did not stimulate testosterone production in men [7].

Hsieh C. et al. investigated the impact of herbal formula as an adjunct therapy in males with impotence [36]. The herb formula was comprised of seven ingredients: *Astragalus membranaceus*, *Lepidium meyenii* Walp., *Ophiocordyceps sinensis*, *Panax quiquefolium* (American ginseng) 1, *Piper nigrum*, *Rhodiola rosea* and *Serpentes cnidium monnieri*. Males who had impotence and were refractory to conventional drug treatment underwent penile venous stripping surgery, an effective technique for the treatment of impotence. Those patients who were unsatisfied with the procedure results were randomly assigned to either an herbal formula or placebo treatment group. The combinational treatment of these patients improved the index of erectile function compared to the procedure alone.

A large body of preclinical evidence demonstrates the effectiveness of phytodrugs in improving animal reproductive functions. In our opinion, phytodrugs can be used as effective treatments for minor or moderate male reproductive functions in men. Additionally, the phytodrugs can be used as an adjunct therapy in severe cases of reproductive system dysfunctions.

Metabolic syndrome is a common disorder in men. The syndrome is presented with hypertension, dyslipidemia, and altered glucose metabolism. Smoking, excessive alcohol use, and limited physical activity are shared risk factors for the development of metabolic syndrome and male infertility [37]. The advantage of CE use is that CE targets multiple organs and systems. It possesses hepatoprotective, hypolipidemic, hypoglycemic, and male reproductive system-enhancing properties [13,38]. Treatment with CE can benefit patients with metabolic syndrome and developing infertility.

CE and other phytodrugs enhancing male fertility may be of interest to andrologists and patients as a mono or adjuvant therapy. More high-quality clinical trials are needed to introduce these phytodrugs to clinical practice.

4. Materials and Methods

4.1. Phytodrug

During the flowering period, the aerial part of wild chicory (*Cichorium intybus* L.) was collected and used to prepare the dry extract (CE) used in this study. CE was developed at the Institute of Medicinal and Aromatic Plants, VILAR. The plant material was harvested from 2020 to 2021 in the Ryazan region. CE was obtained by extracting bioactive constituencies with 70% v/v ethyl alcohol at 50 ± 5 °C. CE was standardized by the phenolic constituents calculated as chicoric acid. The extract used in the current study contained 9.20 + 0.46% w/w of phenolic constituents. Additional details on the extract preparation and chemical analysis can be found in the recently published article by Krepkova et al. [13].

4.2. Experimental Animals

CE effects on the male reproductive system, male fertility, and offspring development were investigated in Wistar rats obtained from the animal nursery "Andreevka", Moscow, Russia. Three-to-four-month-old females (180–200 g) and males (200–250 g) were used in the study. Animals were housed in plastic cages with 4–5 rats per cage. Animals were kept under controlled environmental conditions of light (12 h light cycle), temperature (20–22 °C), and humidity (40–60%) with free access to Laboratorkorm standard chow for laboratory rats and tap water. After two weeks of acclimation, rats were used in the study. Following short procedures, rats were lightly anesthetized with isoflurane using a drop jar method to minimize unnecessary stress. At the end of each experiment, adult animals and offspring were euthanized by CO_2 inhalation. Feti were considered to be euthanized after the confirmed death of the mother.

All studies were conducted according to the "Guidelines for conducting preclinical studies of drugs" implemented by the Ministry of Public Health of the Russian Federation [39]. The study protocols No 42 from 2 May 2021, No 43 from 3 March 2021, and No 59 from 11 August 2021 had been approved by the VILAR Ethical Committee on Animal Experimentation and carried out per the "European Convention for the Protection of Vertebrate Animals Used for Experimental and Other Scientific Purposes (ETS 123). Strasbourg, 1986" [40]. The numbers of experimental animals were chosen in accordance with the National Standard of the Russian Federation (GOST 56698-2015), identical to the International Guidelines OECD Test No. 416:2001 Two-Generation Reproduction Toxicity Study, IDT.

4.3. CE Treatment

Male rats were randomly assigned into four groups to evaluate the effects of CE on the male reproductive system, fertility, and offspring development. Rats were lightly anesthetized before CE or water administration by gavage. Control animals (18 per group) received tap water by gavage for 60 consecutive days. The experimental rats (18 per group) received 100 mg/kg bw/day, 500 mg/kg bw/day, and 1000 mg/kg bw/day of the 10% aqueous solution of CE orally for 60 consecutive days. The 10% aqueous CE solution was prepared daily. The experimental doses were chosen based on the pharmacological activity of the drug (hepatoprotective activity) and the evaluation of the safety profile of phytodrug in chronic experiments. It has been determined that the hepatoprotective therapeutic daily dose in rats was 100 mg/kg bw/day [13,41]. The doses exceeding the therapeutic dose 5- and 10-fold (500 and 1000 mg/kg bw/day, respectively) were well tolerated by rats in chronic experiments. Therefore, we have chosen these doses to evaluate the effects of CE on reproductive functions. The amount of the drug was calculated for each animal based on the body weight determined at the last weighing.

4.4. Analysis of CE Effects on the Male Reproductive System

Evaluation of the gonadotropic effects of CE was conducted the next day after treatment completion (day 61). Sperm was obtained from 10 male rats in each group by vortexing a longitudinally cut-open epididymis in 10 mL of 0.9% sodium chloride for two minutes. At least 200 spermatozoa per animal were counted to enumerate total and motile spermatozoon numbers. Sperm motility was presented as a percentage of motile sperm in a sample. The sperm motility time was determined by placing a drop of sperm suspension onto a slide in a humid chamber at ~37 °C. Sperm motility was monitored every 5–7 min until complete cessation of all sperm movement.

Another drop of sperm suspension was placed onto the histological slide, fixed with ethanol for 10 min, air-dried, and stained with Giemsa staining to assess the presence of pathologic forms of spermatozoa. The fixed slides were reviewed under a microscope (magnification ×200–400). A minimum of five to seven view fields was counted.

The testes' absolute and relative weights were initially determined following morphometric analysis of the testes. Then, ten-millimeter testicular pieces were fixed in 10% neutral formalin, embedded in paraffin, and sectioned to assess the testicular morphology. Sections of 10 μm were stained with hematoxylin and eosin. The sections were microfilmed on an Axioplan 2 Imaging Zeiss microscope equipped with an AxioCam HRc video camera at various magnifications with a 2776 × 2080 pixels/inch resolution. All measurements described below were conducted using the Image-Pro Plus 6.0 program (Media Cybernetics, Rockville, MD, USA), the "Measurement" function.

The tubules' diameter was assessed at a magnification of ×50. Only the diameters of tubules cut tangentially were measured: 20 tubules per animal and 100 per group.

Twenty tangential sections of the seminiferous tubules were evaluated at a magnification of x200 to calculate the area of the spermatogenic epithelium. The area of the seminiferous tubule and lumen in μm^2 was measured. The area of the spermatogenic epithelium was calculated as the area of the seminiferous tubule minus the luminal area.

The microfilms of twenty endocrinocytes (Leydig cells) per group were evaluated at a magnification of ×640 to measure the surface nuclear areas of Leydig cells. The surface nuclear areas were measured by manual nucleus contouring.

The spermatogenesis index was used to quantitatively assess the spermatogenic competence of the testes. The number of spermatogenic epithelium layers was counted in 100 convoluted seminiferous tubules per group. The index of spermatogenesis was calculated using the formula $I = \sum n/N$, where n is the number of layers of spermatogenic epithelium (spermatogonia, spermatocytes, spermatids, and spermatozoa) in one tubule, N is the number of tubules examined.

The total testosterone concentrations in male rats' serum were measured using an enzyme immunoassay using ImmunoChem-2100 (High Technology, Inc., North Attleborough, MA, USA) and a set of reagents (ZAO NVO Immunotech, Moscow, Russia).

4.5. Analysis of CE Effects on Male Fertility

In total, 15 intact females were mated with 7–8 males CE treated or control males. The effects of CE treatment on male fertility were evaluated by measuring fertility and pregnancy indexes. The fertility index was calculated as follows: the number of pregnant rats divided by the number of fertilized rats multiplied by 100. The pregnancy index was calculated as a ratio between the number of delivered dams and the number of pregnant dams multiplied by 100.

4.6. Investigation of PADE Effects on Fetal and Offspring Development

Pregnant rats were divided into two cohorts. Female rats from Cohort 1 were used to investigate CE effects on fetal growth, and female rats from Cohort 2 were used to analyze the impact of CE male treatment on offspring development. Pregnant rats of Cohort 1 (7 dams in each group) were sacrificed on day 20 of pregnancy by carbon dioxide asphyxiation. The number of corpora lutea, the status of each implant site (live/dead embryo, early/late resorption), and embryo body weight were determined. Cohort 2 (7 dams in each group) delivered their offspring by natural route. Weight gain and survival of the born offspring were assessed and recorded on day 21 after birth. Pups (47–51 in each group) were evaluated for reflex maturity: flip/roll over onto all four paws (day 7 after birth), time of cliff avoidance (day 7 after birth), and negative geotaxis (day 8 after birth). The development of motor-sensory reflexes of the progeny (open field test) was evaluated on day 30 after birth. The open field apparatus consisted of an unobstructed field with walls preventing animal escape. The field is marked with black and white squares. The corners of each square had round holes. Each test animal was placed into the field for 3 min. An investigator recorded the number of lines crossed by the rat and how often the animal was rearing, grooming, defecating, and head dipping into the holes. The flip/rollover test measured the percentage of pups rolling onto their four paws within 30 s. The negative geotaxis test measured motor skills and cerebellar integration. Pups were placed on an inclined surface (45° angle, length 30 cm) with their heads down. The time (s) spent for a turn of 180° was recorded.

4.7. Statistical Analysis

All data obtained from experimental or control rats were included in the analysis. Results included male fertility, gonadotropic effects, pre- and post-implantation death, number of newborns, and offspring postnatal development. The results were analyzed using Statistica software, version 13 (TIBCO Software Inc., Santa Clara, CA, USA). One-way ANOVA, Student's t-test of significance, and test of the equality of continuous (the Kolmogorov–Smirnov test) were used for data analysis. The differences were considered statistically significant when the p-value was less than 0.05.

5. Conclusions

Preclinical studies presented in this manuscript demonstrated that CE has significant stimulatory effects on the male reproductive system, evidenced by an increase in the diameter of seminiferous tubules, spermatogenesis index, total number of spermatozoa and their viable forms, and serum testosterone levels. This study also evaluated the effect of CE treatment of male rats on fertility, pregnancy, and offspring development. No adverse effects were observed on pregnancy, evidenced by no change in the fertility and pregnancy indexes and embryonic pre- and post-implantation death. There was a nonsignificant decrease in pre- and post-implantation fetal death in groups where males were treated with higher doses of CE. The offspring development of pups born from CE-treated males was not different from control pups.

Author Contributions: Conceptualization, A.N.B., L.V.K. and E.Y.E.; methodology, L.V.K. and E.Y.E.; validation, A.N.B., M.V.B., O.S.K., L.V.K. and K.M.J.; formal analysis, A.N.B., M.V.B., V.A.M. and L.V.K.; investigation, A.N.B., M.V.B., O.S.K. and V.A.M.; writing—original draft preparation, L.V.K. and E.Y.E.; writing—review and editing, L.V.K., E.Y.E. and K.M.J.; visualization, E.Y.E., M.V.B. and K.M.J. All authors have read and agreed to the published version of the manuscript.

Funding: This research received no external funding.

Institutional Review Board Statement: All studies were conducted according to the "Guidelines for conducting preclinical studies of drugs" implemented by the Ministry of Public Health of the Russian Federation. The study protocols No 42 from 2 May 2021, No 43 from 3 March 2021, and No 59 from 11 August 2021 had been approved by the VILAR Ethical Committee on Animal Experimentation and carried out per the "European Convention for the Protection of Vertebrate Animals Used for Experimental and Other Scientific Purposes (ETS 123). Strasbourg, 1986".

Informed Consent Statement: Not applicable.

Data Availability Statement: Data are available upon reasonable request.

Conflicts of Interest: K.M.J. and E.Y.E. are Editors of this Special Issue. The authors declare no conflicts of interest.

References

1. Mann, U.; Shiff, B.; Patel, P. Reasons for worldwide decline in male fertility. *Curr. Opin. Urol.* **2020**, *30*, 296–301. [CrossRef] [PubMed]
2. Methorst, C.; Perrin, J.; Faix, A.; Huyghe, E. Infertilité masculine, environnement et mode de vie. *Progrès En Urol.* **2023**, *33*, 613–623. [CrossRef]
3. Perheentupa, A.; Toppari, J. Male fertility and semen quality are decreasing—Do we have the expertise to deal with this challenge? *Acta Obstet. Et Gynecol. Scand.* **2023**, *102*, 1606–1607. [CrossRef] [PubMed]
4. Ameratunga, D.; Gebeh, A.; Amoako, A. Obesity and male infertility. *Best. Pract. Res. Clin. Obstet. Gynaecol.* **2023**, *90*, 102393. [CrossRef] [PubMed]
5. Sharma, A.; Minhas, S.; Dhillo, W.S.; Jayasena, C.N. Male infertility due to testicular disorders. *J. Clin. Endocrinol. Metab.* **2021**, *106*, e442–e459. [CrossRef] [PubMed]
6. Karomatov, I.D.; Abduvokhidov, A.T. Medicinal herbs possessing spermatoprotective properties. *Biol. Integr. Med.* **2018**, *6*, 96–116.
7. Santos, H.O.; Howell, S.; Teixeira, F.J. Beyond tribulus (*Tribulus terrestris* L.): The effects of phytotherapics on testosterone, sperm and prostate parameters. *J. Ethnopharmacol.* **2019**, *235*, 392–405. [CrossRef] [PubMed]
8. Ramgir, S.S.; Renu, K.; Vellingiri, B.; George, A.; Tirupapuliyur, D.; Thiagarajan, P.; Valsala Gopalakrishnan, A. Phytomedicinal therapeutics for male infertility: Critical insights and scientific updates. *J. Nat. Med.* **2022**, *76*, 546–573. [CrossRef] [PubMed]
9. Gonzales, G.F. Ethnobiology and Ethnopharmacology of Lepidium meyenii (Maca), a Plant from the Peruvian Highlands. *Evid. Based Complement. Altern. Med.* **2012**, *2012*, 193496. [CrossRef] [PubMed]

10. Mahajan, G.K.; Mahajan, A.Y.; Mahajan, R.T. Efficacy of Aphrodisiac Plants towards Improvement in Semen Quality and Motility in Infertile Males. *J. Complement. Integr. Med.* **2012**, *9*, 1–12. [CrossRef] [PubMed]
11. Tahvilzadeh, M.; Hajimahmoodi, M.; Toliyat, T.; Karimi, M.; Rahimi, R. An evidence-based approach to medicinal plants for the treatment of sperm abnormalities in traditional Persian medicine. *Andrologia* **2016**, *48*, 860–879. [CrossRef] [PubMed]
12. Boroujeni, S.N.; Malamiri, F.A.; Bossaghzadeh, F.; Esmaeili, A.; Moudi, E. The most important medicinal plants affecting sperm and testosterone production: A systematic review. *JBRA Assist. Reprod.* **2022**, *26*, 522–530. [CrossRef] [PubMed]
13. Krepkova, L.V.; Babenko, A.N.; Lemyaseva, S.V.; Saybel, O.L.; Sherwin, C.M.; Enioutina, E.Y. Modulation of Hepatic Functions by Chicory (*Cichorium intybus* L.) Extract: Preclinical Study in Rats. *Pharmaceuticals* **2023**, *16*, 1471. [CrossRef] [PubMed]
14. Mehran, D.; Seyyed Mansour, S.; Marzieh Noroozi Tabrizi, N. Beneficial effects of *Cichorium intybus* L. extract on oxidative status and reproductive parameters in male Wistar rats: An experimental study. *Int. J. Reprod. Biomed.* **2019**, *17*, 425–434. [CrossRef]
15. Kondakova, L.I.; Kalashnikova, S.A.; Polyakova, L.V. Morphofunctional status of interstitial endocrinocytes (Leydig cells) with premature aging caused by dark deprivation. *J. Volgogr. State Med. Univ.* **2023**, *20*, 70–73. [CrossRef]
16. Kiss, P.; Tamas, A.; Lubics, A.; Szalai, M.; Szalontay, L.; Lengvari, I.; Reglodi, D. Development of neurological reflexes and motor coordination in rats neonatally treated with monosodium glutamate. *Neurotox. Res.* **2005**, *8*, 235–244. [CrossRef] [PubMed]
17. Abramova, O.; Ushakova, V.; Zorkina, Y.; Zubkov, E.; Storozheva, Z.; Morozova, A.; Chekhonin, V. The Behavior and Postnatal Development in Infant and Juvenile Rats after Ultrasound-Induced Chronic Prenatal Stress. *Front. Physiol.* **2021**, *12*, 659366. [CrossRef] [PubMed]
18. Dorostghoal, M.; Seyyednejad, S.M.; Nejad, M.N.T. *Cichorium intybus* L. extract ameliorates testicular oxidative stress induced by lead acetate in male rats. *Clin. Exp. Reprod. Med.* **2020**, *47*, 161–167. [CrossRef] [PubMed]
19. Eltamany, E.E.; Mosalam, E.M.; Mehanna, E.T.; Awad, B.M.; Mosaad, S.M.; Abdel-Kader, M.S.; Ibrahim, A.K.; Badr, J.M.; Goda, M.S. Potential Gonado-Protective Effect of Cichorium endivia and Its Major Phenolic Acids against Methotrexate-Induced Testicular Injury in Mice. *Biomedicines* **2022**, *10*, 1986. [CrossRef] [PubMed]
20. Koloko, B.L.; Bushra, I.; Wankeu-Nya, M.; Ngaha Njila, M.I.; Kenmogne, H.; Nyonseu Nzeubang, D.C.; Nzangueu, C.B.; Dimo, T.; Dongmo, A.B.; Massoma Lembe, D. In vivo effects of Rauvolfia vomitoria (Apocynaceae) ethanolic extract on sexual performance and reproductive activity in male rats. *Andrologia* **2020**, *52*, e13414. [CrossRef] [PubMed]
21. Yan, M.; Zhang, Z.; Liu, Y. Difference analysis of different parts of chicory based on HPLC fingerprint and multi-component content determination. *Chin. Herb. Med.* **2022**, *14*, 317–323. [CrossRef]
22. Roy-Choudhury, A.; Venkatakrishna-Bhatt, H. Spermatogenic inhibition by *Cichorium intybus* L. aqueous root suspension in mice. *Naturwissenschaften* **1983**, *70*, 365–366. [CrossRef] [PubMed]
23. Pizent, A.; Tariba, B.; Živković, T. Reproductive toxicity of metals in men. *Arh. Hig. Rada Toksikol.* **2012**, *63* (Suppl. S1), 35–46. [CrossRef]
24. Türk, E.; Ozan Tekeli, I.; Özkan, H.; Uyar, A.; Cellat, M.; Kuzu, M.; Yavas, I.; Alizadeh Yegani, A.; Yaman, T.; Güvenç, M. The protective effect of esculetin against aluminium chloride-induced reproductive toxicity in rats. *Andrologia* **2021**, *53*, e13930. [CrossRef] [PubMed]
25. Hashemi, M.; Azarnia, M.; Hajebrahimi, Z.; Nejad Ebrahimi, S. The effect of hydroalcoholic extract of *Cichorium intybus* leaf on aryl hydrocarbon receptor expression in the testis of Wistar rats exposed to cigarette smoke. *Avicenna J. Phytomed.* **2023**, *13*, 58–69. [CrossRef]
26. Liu, Z.J.; Liu, Y.H.; Huang, S.Y.; Zang, Z.J. Insights into the Regulation on Proliferation and Differentiation of Stem Leydig Cells. *Stem Cell Rev. Rep.* **2021**, *17*, 1521–1533. [CrossRef] [PubMed]
27. Liu, Y.; Liu, Y.; Chen, G.; Wang, H. Epigenetic programming of TBX2/CX43 mediates lower sperm quality in male offspring induced by prenatal dexamethasone exposure. *Toxicol. Sci.* **2023**, *192*, 178–193. [CrossRef] [PubMed]
28. Tuimah Alabedi, G.S.; Al-Baghdady, H.F.; Alahmer, M.A.; Bustani, G.S.; Al-Dhalimy, A.M.B. Effects of Ocimum tenuiflorum on Induced Testicular Degeneration by Filgrastim in Wistar Rats. *Arch. Razi Inst.* **2021**, *76*, 1555–1559. [CrossRef] [PubMed]
29. Kaltsas, A. Oxidative Stress and Male Infertility: The Protective Role of Antioxidants. *Medicina* **2023**, *59*, 1769. [CrossRef]
30. Barati, E.; Nikzad, H.; Karimian, M. Oxidative stress and male infertility: Current knowledge of pathophysiology and role of antioxidant therapy in disease management. *Cell Mol. Life Sci.* **2020**, *77*, 93–113. [CrossRef] [PubMed]
31. Abarikwu, S.O.; Onuah, C.L.; Singh, S.K. Plants in the management of male infertility. *Andrologia* **2020**, *52*, e13509. [CrossRef] [PubMed]
32. Safarnavadeh, T.; Rastegarpanah, M. Antioxidants and infertility treatment, the role of Satureja Khuzestanica: A mini-systematic review. *Iran. J. Reprod. Med.* **2011**, *9*, 61–70.
33. Yimam, M.; Lee, Y.-C.; Hyun, E.-J.; Jia, Q. Reproductive and Developmental Toxicity of Orally Administered Botanical Composition, UP446-Part III: Effects on Fertility and Early Embryonic Development to Implantation in Sprague Dawley Rats. *Birth Defects Res. Part. B Dev. Reprod. Toxicol.* **2015**, *104*, 166–176. [CrossRef] [PubMed]
34. Lee, H.W.; Lee, M.S.; Kim, T.H.; Alraek, T.; Zaslawski, C.; Kim, J.W.; Moon, D.G. Ginseng for erectile dysfunction. *Cochrane Database Syst. Rev.* **2021**, *4*, Cd012654. [CrossRef]
35. Salgado, R.M.; Marques-Silva, M.H.; Gonçalves, E.; Mathias, A.C.; Aguiar, J.G.; Wolff, P. Effect of oral administration of Tribulus terrestris extract on semen quality and body fat index of infertile men. *Andrologia* **2017**, *49*. [CrossRef] [PubMed]
36. Hsieh, C.-H.; Tsai, H.-C.; Hsu, G.-L.; Chen, C.-C.; Hsu, C.-Y. Herb formula enhances treatment of impotent patients after penile venous stripping: A randomised clinical trials. *Andrologia* **2016**, *48*, 754–760. [CrossRef] [PubMed]

37. Fahed, G.; Aoun, L.; Bou Zerdan, M.; Allam, S.; Bou Zerdan, M.; Bouferraa, Y.; Assi, H.I. Metabolic Syndrome: Updates on Pathophysiology and Management in 2021. *Int. J. Mol. Sci.* **2022**, *23*, 786. [CrossRef] [PubMed]
38. Saad, B. A Review of the Anti-Obesity Effects of Wild Edible Plants in the Mediterranean Diet and Their Active Compounds: From Traditional Uses to Action Mechanisms and Therapeutic Targets. *Int. J. Mol. Sci.* **2023**, *24*, 12641. [CrossRef] [PubMed]
39. Mironov, A.N. *Guidelines for Preclinical Studies of Drugs. Part 1*; Grif and K: Moscow, Russia, 2012.
40. European Convention for the Protection of Vertebrate Animals Used for Experimental and other Scientific Purposes (ETS 123). Strasbourg, 1986. Available online: https://rm.coe.int/168007a67b (accessed on 13 February 2024).
41. Bortnikova, V.V.; Krepkova, L.V.; Babenko, A.N.; Saybel, O.L.; Borovkova, M.V.; Kuzina, O.S.; Mizina, P.G.; Job, K.M.; Sherwin, C.M.; Enioutina, E.Y. A perspective botanical drug: Hepatoprotective activity of dry extract prepared from the aerial part of chicory plant (*Cichorium intybus* L.), ACCP annual conference abstract #119. *Clin. Pharmacol. Drug Dev.* **2021**, *10* (Suppl. S1), 100.

pharmaceuticals

Article

Profibrotic Inflammatory Cytokines and Growth Factors Are Predicted as the Key Targets of *Uncaria gambir* (Hunter) Roxb. in Keloids: An Epistatic and Molecular Simulation Approach

Sri Suciati Ningsih [1,2], Fadilah Fadilah [1,3], Sri Widia A. Jusman [4,5], Rahimi Syaidah [1,6,*] and Takashi Yashiro [7]

1 Doctoral Program in Biomedical Sciences, Faculty of Medicine, Universitas Indonesia, Jakarta 10430, Indonesia; sri.suciati11@ui.ac.id (S.S.N.); fadilah.msi@ui.ac.id (F.F.)
2 Faculty of Medicine, Universitas Muhammadiyah Prof. Dr. Hamka, Jakarta 12130, Indonesia
3 Department of Medical Chemistry, Faculty of Medicine, Universitas Indonesia, Jakarta 10430, Indonesia
4 Department of Biochemistry, Faculty of Medicine, Universitas Indonesia, Jakarta 10430, Indonesia; sriwidiaaj@gmail.com
5 Center of Hypoxia and Oxidative Stress Studies, Faculty of Medicine, Universitas Indonesia, Jakarta 10430, Indonesia
6 Department of Histology, Faculty of Medicine, Universitas Indonesia, Jakarta 10430, Indonesia
7 Department of Histology, Jichi Medical University School of Medicine, Tochigi 329-0498, Japan; tyashiro@jichi.ac.jp
* Correspondence: rahimisyaidah@ui.ac.id

Abstract: Keloid is characterized as the fibrotic tissue resulting from the increase of fibroblast activity. *Uncaria gambir* (Hunter) Roxb. possesses bioactive compounds that have potential as antifibrotic agents, while the mechanism of action in keloid has not yet been elucidated. The aim of this study was to investigate the interaction of gambir bioactive compounds with keloid target proteins using an epistatic and molecular simulation approach. The known bioactive compounds of gambir targets and keloid-related protein targets were screened using databases. The network was constructed and analyzed to obtain the core protein targets. The targets were enriched to describe the Gene Ontology (GO) and pathway related to the proteins. Eleven targets were defined as the main targets of gambir bioactive compounds related to keloid disease. Gambiriin C, Isogambirine, and Procyanidin B1 were identified as the most promising compounds with the highest binding energy to transforming growth factor beta 1 (TGFβ1), AKT serine/threonine kinase 1 (AKT1), and matrix metallopeptidase 1 (MMP1) as the target proteins. GO enrichment and pathway analysis found that gambir bioactive compounds may act on keloid-related target proteins to regulate cell proliferation, migration, transcription, and signal transduction activity via profibrotic cytokine and growth factor signaling pathways. This study provides a reference for potential targets, compounds, and pathways to explain the mechanism of gambir against keloid.

Keywords: gambir; keloid; target protein; molecular simulation

Citation: Ningsih, S.S.; Fadilah, F.; Jusman, S.W.A.; Syaidah, R.; Yashiro, T. Profibrotic Inflammatory Cytokines and Growth Factors Are Predicted as the Key Targets of *Uncaria gambir* (Hunter) Roxb. in Keloids: An Epistatic and Molecular Simulation Approach. *Pharmaceuticals* **2024**, *17*, 662. https://doi.org/10.3390/ph17060662

Academic Editors: Catherine Sherwin, Elena Y. Enioutina and Kathleen M. Job

Received: 17 April 2024
Revised: 3 May 2024
Accepted: 8 May 2024
Published: 21 May 2024

1. Introduction

Keloids display exophytic overgrowth beyond the site of injury. The latest demographic study of keloid incidence reported that the incidence of keloids is higher in pigmented-skin individuals, particularly in Africa (8.5–16%). Even though this disease may not directly result in fatality, the manifestation may cause cosmetic, physical, and physiological effects that consequently affect the patient's quality of life [1,2]. The pathomechanism of keloid has not been fully elucidated. Abnormality of the wound-healing process is addressed as the critical point of keloid formation. Robust inflammatory stimulation and over-sensitized fibroblasts driven by cytokines and growth factors during the wound-healing process contribute to excessive extracellular matrix (ECM) deposits in keloids. Over-sensitized fibroblasts are activated into myofibroblasts, which tend to have a higher level of proliferation, migration, and extracellular matrix synthesis capacity [3–5].

Several existing treatments for keloid, including surgery, steroid therapy, stem cell, radiation, and targeted therapy, are intended to inhibit the proliferation and activation of keloid fibroblasts. Unfortunately, none of these are considered a universal gold standard for keloid treatment due to the high recurrence rate, emergence of side effects, and requiring high cost and further study to reveal the effects in a clinical approach [2,6,7]. Thus, herb-based therapy is proposed as an option for an alternative way to treat keloid disease. Traditional herbal medicine possesses the characteristics of being multicomponent, multifunction, and multitarget; is of low toxicity; and has limited side effects, in general [8].

Gambir is an herbal medicine originating from Indonesia that has long been used by local residents as a traditional remedy. A majority of the phytochemical substances derived from gambir are categorized into the flavonoid, phenolic, and alkaloid groups [9]. Recent studies proved that the bioactive compounds of gambir have antibacterial, anticancer, anti-inflammation, as well as antifibrotic effects [10–13]. Desdiani et al. [14,15] found using in vivo study that gambir has antifibrotic effect against lung fibrosis through inhibition of nuclear factor kappa-B (NF-κB) and transforming growth factor receptor (TGF-βR). In line with these findings, Sriningsih [16] identified that gambir extract could inhibit the expression of tissue inhibitor matrix metalloproteinase (TIMP) and collagen-1 in rat liver fibrosis tissue. Keloid is defined as tissue fibrosis due to its effusive accumulation of ECM, particularly collagen [2]. Jusman et al. [17] have shown that some gambir bioactive compounds have potency to inhibit platelet-derived growth factor subunit A (PDGFA) as a target protein to reduce fibroblast proliferation through in silico study. Therefore, gambir is assumed to be a promising herb-based antifibrotic agent to deal with keloid disease.

Recent studies have highlighted the efficiency of bioinformatic analysis as a beneficial tool to explore the molecular mechanism of disease [18]; one form of this is epistatic study. Epistatic study is a beneficial tool to discover a new drug candidate for human disease by understanding the gene interaction and pathway that contribute to the disease risk. Furthermore, the researcher can identify potential targets that can disrupt the interaction and reduce the disease progression [19–21]. One branch of epistatic interaction study is network pharmacology, which can be used as an appropriate approach to analyze and model the interactions between drug–target networks [22]. To date, a comprehensive understanding of gambir's mechanism of action against fibrotic tissue, particularly keloid, is still lacking. The conventional experimental method to explore all the proteins included in the mechanism is time-consuming, expensive, and so forth [23]. Therefore, this bioinformatic approach is suggested as an efficient pathway to analyze the interactions between keloid-related proteins and the bioactive compounds of gambir. This study aims to investigate the bioactive compounds of gambir and their interaction with keloid target proteins using a network pharmacology and molecular simulation approach. The result of this study is expected to provide a scientific explanation of the mechanism of gambir as an antikeloid candidate.

2. Results

2.1. Screening for Uncaria Gambir Bioactive Compounds and Its Target Proteins

A total 74 bioactive compounds of *Uncaria gambir* (Hunter) Roxb. were identified from the literature study [9,17,24], with 5048 protein-specific targets based on SWISS target prediction. A total of 277 targets from 29 bioactive compounds were predicted to be targeted to keloid-related target proteins. The drug-likeness nature, pharmacokinetic properties, and toxicity of the compounds are shown in Table 1. The drug-likeness properties identified from this study were the molecular weight (Mw), octanol–water partition coefficients (Log P), hydrogen-bond acceptor, and donor (HBA and HBD). The pharmacokinetic parameters included were the gastrointestinal absorption (GI Abs) and cytochrome (CYP) inhibition. The toxicity of the compounds was described by the toxicity class (1–6) according to the globally harmonized system of classification for the labeling of chemicals (GHS). Classes 1–2 mean fatal if swallowed, Class 3 is toxic if swallowed, Class 4 is harmful if swallowed,

Class 5 may be harmful if swallowed, and Class 6 is non-toxic. All of the compounds were categorized in Classes 3 to 6.

Table 1. The drug-likeness nature, pharmacokinetics properties, and toxicity of *Uncaria gambir* bioactive compounds.

No	Molecule	Drug-Likeness				Pharmacokinetics		Predicted Toxicity Class
		Mw	Log P	HBA	HBD	GI Abs	CYP Inhibitor	
1	Catechol	110.11	0.94	2	2	High	No	3
2	Gambiriin C	562.52	1.84	11	9	Low	CYP3A4	5
3	Gambiriin A1	580.54	1.69	12	11	Low	CYP3A4	5
4	Gambiriin A3	580.54	1.45	12	11	Low	CYP3A4	5
5	Procyanidin B3	578.52	1.53	12	10	Low	CYP3A4	5
6	Procyanidin B1	578.52	1.53	12	10	Low	CYP3A4	5
7	Gambiriin A2	580.54	1.69	12	11	Low	CYP3A4	5
8	Procyanidin B2	578.52	1.53	12	10	Low	CYP3A4	5
9	Procyanidin B4	578.52	1.53	12	10	Low	CYP3A4	5
10	Ursolic acid	456.70	5.88	3	2	Low	No	4
11	Quercetin	302.24	1.23	7	5	High	CYP2D6CYP3A4CYP3A2	3
12	Quinic acid	192.17	1.75	6	5	Low	No	6
13	Kaempferol	286.24	1.58	6	4	High	CYP2D6CYP3A4CYP3A2	5
14	Protocatechuic acid	154.12	0.65	4	3	High	CYP3A4	4
15	Epicatechin gallate	442.37	1.25	10	7	Low	No	4
16	Dimeric proanthocyanidin	576.50	1.61	12	9	Low	CYP3A4	5
17	Gambirflavan D1	562.52	2.29	11	9	Low	CYP2C9 CYP3A4	5
18	Gambirflavan D2	562.52	2.29	11	9	Low	CYP2C9CYP3A4	5
19	Hyperoside	464.38	−0.25	12	8	Low	No	5
20	Isoquercitrin	464.38	−0.25	12	8	Low	No	5
21	Pyrocatechol	110.11	0.97	2	2	High	CYP3A4	3
22	Phloroglucinol	126.11	0.45	3	3	High	CYP3A4	3
23	4-methoxyphenol	124.14	1.41	2	1	High	No	4
24	4-allyl-2-methoxyphenol	164.20	2.25	2	1	High	CYP1A2	4
25	Gambirine	384.47	2.85	5	2	High	CYP2D6	3
26	Isogambirine	384.50	2.82	5	2	High	CYP2D6	3
27	Tetrahydroalstonine	352.43	2.67	4	1	High	CYP2D6	3
28	Dihydrocorynantheine	368.47	3.22	4	1	High	CYP2D6 CYP3A4	3
29	Uncariagambiriine	620.65	3.61	9	6	Low	CYP2C9	4

2.2. *Screening for Keloid-Related Target Proteins*

A total of 96 out of 695 keloid-related target proteins were identified after combining the 2 databases. The 96 genes were then imported into Cytoscape 3.9.1 to plot the keloid-related target network diagram. A total of 96 nodes and 100 edges were obtained using the Cytoscape 3.9.1 platform, with a high confidence score (0.98). The top 11 of the 96 targets were selected based on the degree, betweenness centrality (BC), and closeness centrality

(CC) score (Table 2). The keloid-related protein–protein interaction (PPI) network was visualized using GeneMANIA (Figure 1).

Table 2. Top 11 keloid-related core protein targets in the PPI network.

Gene	Gene Full Name	BC	CC	Degree
EP300	E1A-binding protein p300	0.19	0.43	12
AKT1	AKT serine/threonine kinase 1	0.12	0.44	10
STAT3	Signal transducer and activator of transcription 3	0.26	0.39	10
TGFB1	Transforming growth factor beta 1	0.11	0.44	8
VEGFA	Vascular endothelial growth factor A	0.17	0.43	7
EGFR	Epidermal growth factor receptor	0.18	0.44	6
CCND1	Cyclin D1	0.05	0.41	4
IGF1R	Insulin-like growth factor 1 receptor	0.02	0.39	3
TIMP1	TIMP metallopeptidase inhibitor 1	0.11	0.39	2
MMP1	Matrix metallopeptidase 1	0.14	0.33	1
PDGFA	Platelet-derived growth factor alpha	0.07	0.31	1

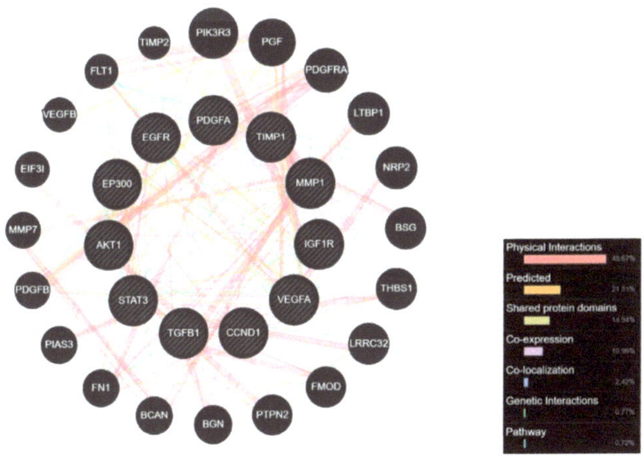

Figure 1. PPI network for the candidate targets. Black node indicates target protein and the correlation is represented as connecting colors.

2.3. *Interaction of Bioactive Compounds of Gambir on Keloid-Related Target Proteins*

A total of 277 targets from 29 bioactive compounds were predicted to be targeted to keloid-related target proteins. All of the gambir bioactive compounds' targets were merged with the keloid-related targets and keloid-related targets with a high degree value (HDV) to further discover the potential targets and mechanism (Figure 2A). Based on the diagram, there were 11 target proteins defined in the intersection area. All of these target proteins were defined as the main targets of gambir bioactive compounds in treating keloid disease. The drug–protein interaction (DPI) network of gambir's bioactive compounds targeted to keloid-related target proteins is shown in Figure 2B. The pink dots represent the keloid protein targets, the orange dots represent gambir bioactive compounds, and the connecting lines represent the compound–target interactions. Gambiriin A1, Procyanidin B1, Procyanidin B3, Gambiriin A2, Epicatechin gallate, Gambiriin A3, Gambiriin C, Isogambirine, Procyanidin B2, and Procyanidin B4 are the top 10 bioactive compounds of gambir with high degree values resulting from the DPI network analysis (Table S3, Supplementary).

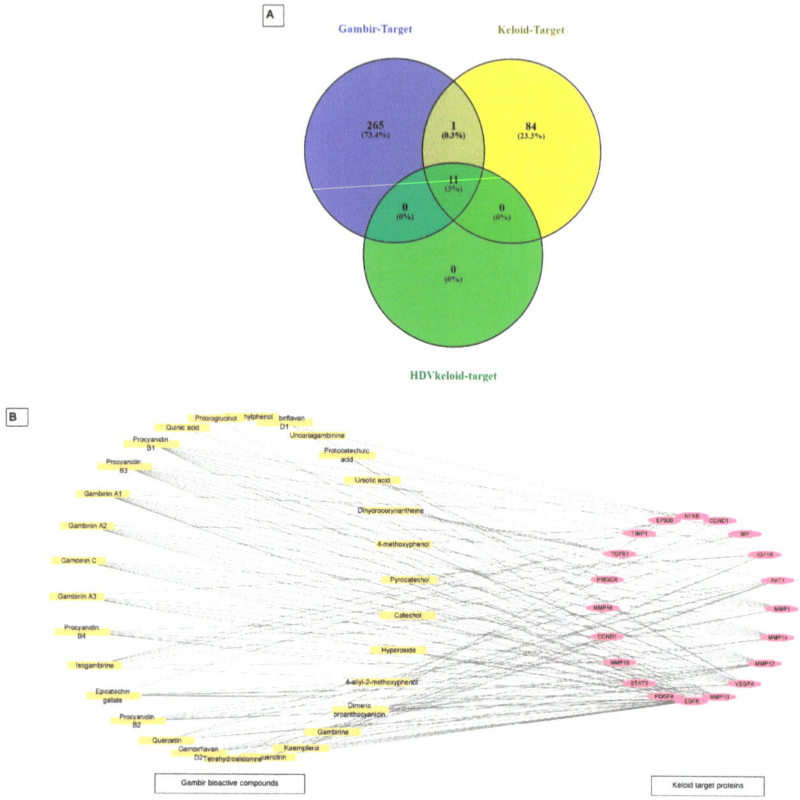

Figure 2. (**A**) Intersection Venn diagram between the predicted target proteins of gambir bioactive compounds, keloid-related target proteins, and high degree of connection values of keloid-related target proteins. (**B**) Compound–target network of gambir bioactive compounds targeted to keloid disease.

2.4. Gene Ontology (GO) and Pathway Enrichment Analysis

GO enrichment analysis of the 11 target proteins in the intersection area was performed using the DAVID database. The result discovered 111 biological processes (BPs), 12 cellular components (CCs), and 17 molecular functions (MFs). Table 3 shows the sorted BPs, CCs, and MFs by degree of significance, $p < 0.05$. The BP of the gambir compound–keloid–target is significantly enriched in the regulation of cell proliferation, transcription, protein phosphorylation, cell migration, apoptotic process, signal transduction, peptidyl-serine phosphorylation, and protein kinase B signaling. On the other hand, the MF is mainly enriched in identical protein and enzyme binding, growth factor and cytokine activity, protein (serine/threonine/tyrosine) kinase binding and activity, and protein homodimerization activity. The CC is primarily enriched in cytoplasm, nucleus, extracellular space, extracellular matrix, extracellular region, platelet alpha granule lumen, cell surface, collagen trimer, and secretory granule.

Table 3. GO analysis of core target proteins.

Category	Gene Function	Count	*p*-Value
BP	Positive regulation of cell proliferation	6	1.9×10^{-6}
BP	Positive regulation of transcription from RNA polymerase II promoter	6	1.0×10^{-4}
BP	Positive regulation of protein phosphorylation	5	1.7×10^{-6}
BP	Positive regulation of cell migration	5	3.9×10^{-6}
BP	Negative regulation of apoptotic process	5	5.8×10^{-5}
BP	Positive regulation of transcription, DNA-templated	5	2.1×10^{-4}
BP	Negative regulation of transcription from RNA polymerase II promoter	5	6.8×10^{-4}
BP	Signal transduction	5	1.8×10^{-3}
BP	Positive regulation of peptidyl-serine phosphorylation	4	8.5×10^{-6}
BP	Positive regulation of protein kinase B signaling	4	2.3×10^{-5}
MF	Identical protein binding	6	5.4×10^{-4}
MF	Enzyme binding	4	6.1×10^{-4}
MF	Growth factor activity	3	2.7×10^{-3}
MF	Cytokine activity	3	3.5×10^{-3}
MF	Protein kinase activity	3	1.3×10^{-2}
MF	Protein serine/threonine/tyrosine kinase activity	3	1.7×10^{-2}
MF	Protein kinase binding	3	2.4×10^{-2}
MF	Protein homodimerization activity	3	4.5×10^{-2}
CC	Cytoplasm	8	2.5×10^{-3}
CC	Nucleus	7	2.2×10^{-2}
CC	Extracellular space	5	7.1×10^{-3}
CC	Extracellular matrix	4	1.5×10^{-4}
CC	Extracellular region	4	6.1×10^{-2}
CC	Platelet alpha granule lumen	3	3.7×10^{-4}
CC	Cell surface	3	3.1×10^{-2}
CC	Collagen trimer	2	4.0×10^{-2}
CC	Secretory granule	2	4.2×10^{-2}

The pathway analysis obtained 211 hits from REACTOME and 146 hits from KEGG, respectively. The first five pathways were screened and sorted according to the adjusted $p < 0.05$, which most likely shared comparable signaling pathways. The top five signaling pathways discovered from REACTOME are signaling by interleukin (IL; IL-4 and IL-13), cytokine signaling in the immune system, transcriptional regulation of transcription factors or growth factors. Meanwhile, the AGE_RAGE signaling pathway in diabetic complication, pathway in cancer, HIF-1 signaling pathway, proteoglycan in cancer, FOXO signaling pathway are the top signaling pathways discovered from KEGG. The pathway prediction of the target proteins using KEGG is illustrated in Figure 3. This analysis showed results corresponding to the GO biological process and molecular function analyses. This indicates that the bioactive compounds of *Uncaria gambir* might treat keloid by acting on these pathways.

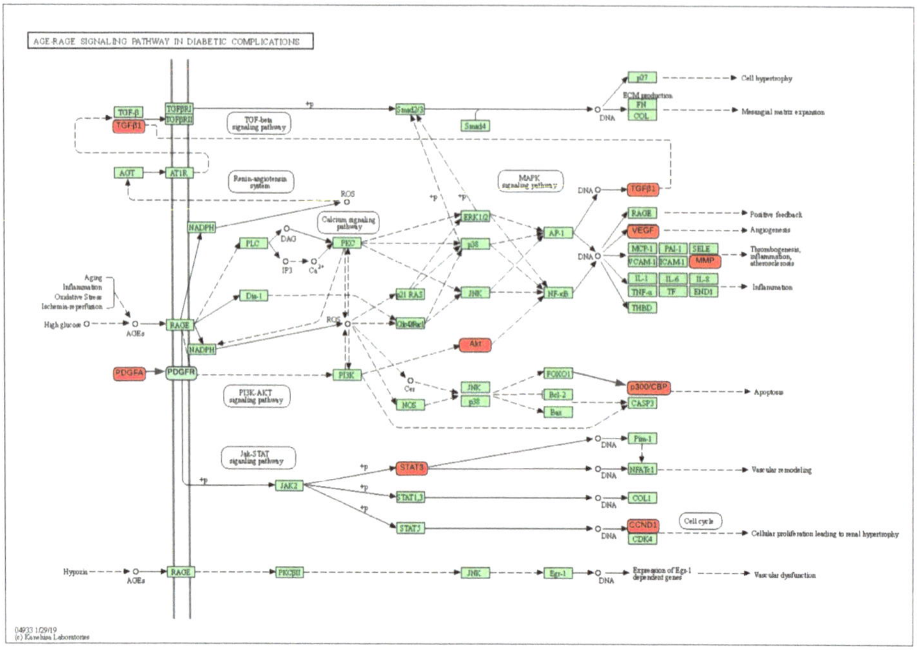

Figure 3. Pathway prediction of the target proteins using KEGG. The red nodes are potential target proteins of *Uncaria gambir*, while the green nodes are relevant targets in the pathway.

2.5. Molecular-Docking Analysis

Molecular docking was used to validate the interaction between the gambir compounds and targets. The top 10 gambir bioactive compounds with high degree values were docked with TGFβ1, AKT1, and MMP1. Some compounds had lower binding energy compared with TAC as the positive control, as shown in Table 4 and visualized in Figure 4. The lower the binding energy, the more stable the binding between the ligand and the protein [25]. It was assumed that the compounds may affect the keloid pathomechanism through these target proteins. Gambiriin C and TGFβ1, Isogambirine and AKT1, and Procyanidin B1 and MMP1 are the compound–protein complexes with the highest binding energy.

Table 4. Docking scores of *Uncaria gambir* bioactive compounds with target proteins.

Compound/Affinity (kcal/mol)	TGFβ1	AKT1	MMP1
Gambiriin A1	−4.47	−7.43	−5.32
Procyanidin B1	−6.76	−3.66	−9.54
Procyanidin B3	−6.56	−6.52	−7.49
Procyanidin B2	−6.03	−5.98	−8.38
Gambiriin A2	−5.53	−5.27	−5.99
Epicatechin gallate	−5.18	−7.79	−9.48
Gambiriin A3	−5.45	−7.68	−6.24
Gambiriin C	−6.90	−7.99	−8.46
Isogambirine	−6.02	−8.68	−8.44
Procyanidin B4	−6.62	−8.47	−8.84
TAC	−6.19	−8.88	−6.69

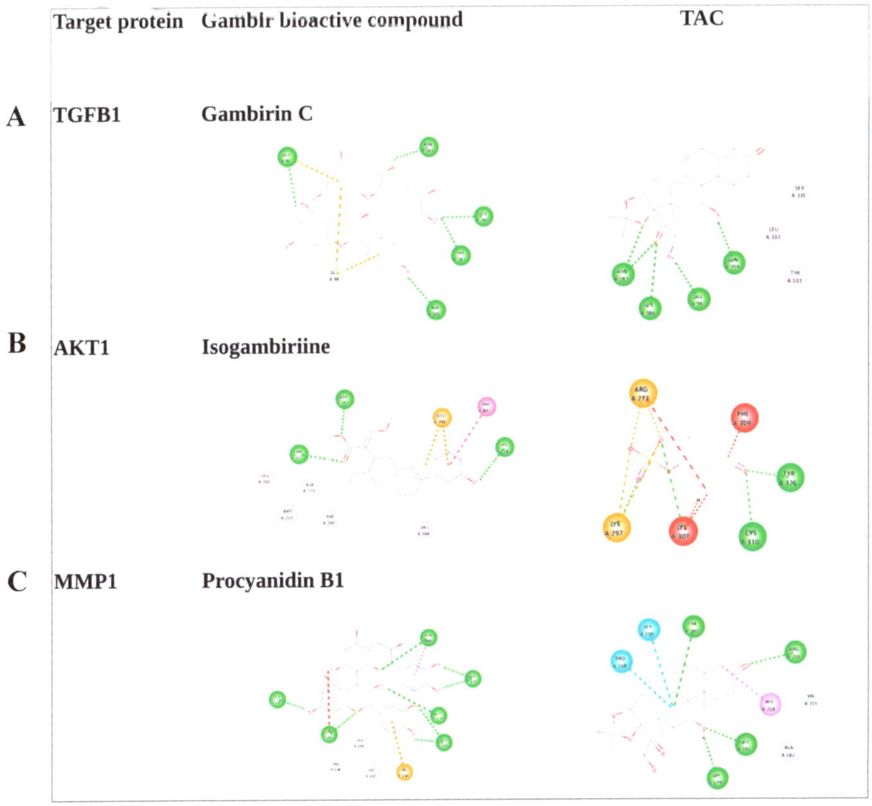

Figure 4. Three best molecular docking results: TGFB1 and Gambiriin C (**A**), AKT1 and Isogambirine (**B**), and MMP1 and ProcyanidinB1 (**C**).

3. Discussion

Keloid is defined as a skin fibrosis-associated disorder that is characterized by excessive growth of fibroblasts, leading to aberrant accumulation of extracellular matrix (ECM) [2]. Herbal-based therapy is expected as an alternative treatment with low toxicity and side effects in treating keloid. *Uncaria gambir* (Hunter) Roxb. is an original herbal medicine from Indonesia that has potential as an antifibrosis agent. This study first identified the bioactive compounds of gambir related to keloid target proteins through an epistatic interaction and molecular simulation approach. Network pharmacology is one of the branches of epistatic study that is considered the next paradigm in discovering the pharmacology of certain herbal compounds and their relationship to target genes of the disease. The relationship between herbs, disease, and molecular targets is discovered using a network basis that represents the action of the compound in the disease pathomechanism. Therefore, this method is considered the ideal approach for studying an herbal-based medicine that has multiple compounds and multiple targets [26,27].

This study found that there are 10 bioactive compounds of gambir with high degree values (cut-off degree value ≥ 5). Molecular-docking validation was conducted on these bioactive compounds and target proteins (TGFβ1, AKT1, and MMP1). Gambiriin C and TGFβ1, Isogambirine and AKT1, and Procyanidin B1 and MMP1 were identified as the compound–protein complexes with the highest binding energy (Table 4 and Figure 4). Therefore, Gambiriin C, Isogambirine, and Procyanidin B1 were proposed to be the most promising gambir compounds to treat keloid disease. All these compounds are classified as flavonoids, particularly chalcane-flavan dimers [28]. Flavonoids have a number of medicinal benefits, including antioxidant and anti-inflammatory properties [29]. In addition, these bioactive compounds have approved drug-likeness, pharmacokinetics, and toxicity properties as a drug candidate. Gambir's bioactive compounds show adverse properties to ideal categories, particularly molecular weight. In term of the pharmacokinetics properties, most of the compounds are highly absorbed in GI tracts and inhibit CYP3A4 enzyme. Most of the compounds are categorized in class 4 to 6 predicted toxicity classes, meaning that most of the compounds have middle to low toxic properties.

The keloid-related proteins were represented in the PPI network produced from the datamining of two databases. DisGeNet and GeneCards are sophisticated search engines that integrate and standardize data about disease-associated genes from multiple sources, including the scientific literature [30,31]. The other network was constructed by merging the previous PPI network and gambir–target network, resulting in the DPI network (Figure 2B). The networks were then analyzed to identify the most impactful proteins in the network based on three important values. The first value is the degree of a node; this referred to the number of edges between nodes in the network. The greater the degree, the more important the nodes in the network. The second is the BC; this represents the signal probability passed through a node. The higher the BC value, the more important the node. The third is the CC value, which reflects the network tightness. The tighter the network, the higher the efficiency [8]. Based on the analysis, 11 targets were identified as the main targets of gambir bioactive compounds related to keloid disease: EP300, AKT1, STAT3, TGFB1, VEGFA, EGFR, CCND1, IGF1R, TIMP1, MMP1, and PDGFA. Thus, it is speculated that the bioactive compounds of gambir may have pharmacological activity in keloid through these targets.

GO enrichment analysis of the 11 potential protein targets was performed to clarify the role of the gambir-targeted proteins in relation to the gene function. The biological process showed that regulation of cell proliferation, transcription, protein phosphorylation, cell migration, apoptotic process, signal transduction, peptidyl-serine phosphorylation, and protein kinase B signaling are the main aspects whereby gambir may play a crucial role in dealing with keloids. In line with this, the molecular function was mainly enriched in identical protein and enzyme binding, growth factor and cytokine activity, protein (serine/threonine/tyrosine) kinase activity, and protein homodimerization activity. Interestingly, the enrichment result shared the same main characteristic of keloid disease. The main characteristic of keloid is over-synthesis and accumulation of extracellular matrix (ECM) due to effusive fibroblast proliferation and differentiation. The fibroblast is the key player in tissue fibrosis, including keloid. The activation of keloid fibroblasts is stimulated by the paracrine effect of cytokines and growth factor in the keloid's surrounding microenvironment [2,4,32]. Dysregulation of cytokines and growth factor at any stage of the wound-healing process may lead to prolonged inflammation as a favorable condition for keloid formation [33].

In parallel with the cellular component enrichment, the protein targets were primarily enriched in cytoplasm, nucleus, extracellular space, extracellular matrix, extracellular region, platelet alpha granule lumen, cell surface, collagen trimer, and secretory granule. The highly proliferated fibroblast and its activation into a myofibroblast leads to excessive ECM synthesis and deposition, particularly collagen [34]. Keloid scars have a 20-fold increase in collagen production compared with normal skin [3]. Overproduction of ECM is closely related to prolonged inflammation in keloid pathogenesis. Keloid formation is driven by multiple cytokines, growth factors, and transcription factors [2,35]. The study by Nangole et al. [36] revealed that the high expression of proinflammatory cytokines in keloid impacts the sensitivity and increases the production of collagen on keloid fibroblasts. This is in accordance with the result of the pathway enrichment analysis from REACTOME that showed signaling by cytokine, transcription factor, and growth factor were predicted as the main pathways of gambir on keloid. Some of the cytokines and growth factors counted as main players in tissue fibrosis are interleukin-4 (IL-4), IL-13, PDGF, and TGF-β1 [37].

The closest pathway prediction was generated from KEGG, which showed TGFB1 as one of the frontline proteins in the pathway (Figure 3). TGF-β is the key activator of fibroblasts in response to fibrosis. TGF-β could be released from epithelial or endothelial cells, resident fibroblasts, platelets, and macrophages [38]. TGF-β initiates a downstream signaling cascade through activation of the Smad2/3 protein and then forms a complex protein with Smad4. This complex protein migrates to the nucleus as the regulator of ECM organization, fibroblast proliferation, and differentiation [38,39]. From the same group of growth factors, PDGF regulates fibroblast activity through the phosphatidylinositol3-kinase–AKT (PI3K/Akt) pathway [40]. The activation of the catalytic subunit of PI3K undergoes enzymatic function to catalyze phosphorylation of phosphatidylinositol 4,5-bisphosphate to phosphatidylinositol 3,4,5-trisphosphate. These triphosphate molecules activate the Akt/PKB protein to induce cell proliferation and inhibit apoptosis [41]. Most of growth factor signaling pathways are categorized as protein kinase receptors with homodimerization activity, including PDGF, EGF, VEGF, and TGF-β receptor [42]. This is in accordance with the result of the molecular function enrichment analysis.

The TGF-β pathway is associated with epithelial mesenchymal transition (EMT) activation in the keloid pathomechanism. This is a process whereby epithelial cells lose adhesion and acquire expression of a mesenchymal component and manifest the increase of cell migration. EMT plays an important role in fibroblasts differentiation into myofibroblasts. There are four common sources of myofibroblasts: fibrocytes, resident fibroblasts, endothelial cells, and epithelial cells [37]. EMT may be induced by epidermal growth factor (EGF) and EGFR via activation of Smad2/3 [43]. Another study proved that the EGF/EFGR signaling pathway promotes EMT mediated by STAT3 [44,45]. Research by Lee et al. [46] on STAT3 found signaling was the most significantly enriched Gene Ontology term in keloid fibroblast. Along with the activation of EMT, fibroblast differentiation and activation impact the imbalance of ECM remodeling.

Abnormal ECM reconstruction during wound healing contributes to keloid formation. Unlike normal scars, a decreased level of MMP1 and an increased level of TIMP1 are found in keloids that are related to tissue fibrosis [47]. MMP1 is one of the type of collagenase that catalyzes the cleave of types I and III collagens. Collagen I and III are highly expressed in keloid tissue [48,49]. Meanwhile, TIMP1 is the endogenous inhibitor of MMP1. The imbalance between the expression of MMP and TIMP leads to excessive collagen I and III synthesis and deposition in fibrotic tissue like keloid [47]. The expression of MMP and TIMP is regulated by TGF-β. The inhibition of TGF-β and the subsequent downstream signaling contribute to a more balanced MMP1/TIMP1 ratio and may be a promising therapeutic approach for keloid treatments [50].

This recent study revealed the multicomponent, multitarget, and multipathway mechanism of *Uncaria gambir* bioactive compounds against keloid through network interaction and molecular-docking simulation. EP300, AKT1, STAT3, TGFB1, VEGFA, EGFR, CCND1, IGFR, TIMP, MMP, and PDGFA are defined as the core proteins targeted by gambir's bioactive compounds through profibrotic cytokines and growth factor signaling pathways. On the other hand, other signaling pathways should not be ignored. Therefore, the other pathway enrichment analysis result is worthy of further study. In addition, further experimental research is required to analyze and validate the mechanism of gambir in keloid identified in this study.

4. Materials and Methods

4.1. Mining Databases of Gambir Bioactive Components and Target Protein

The bioactive compounds of *Uncaria gambir* were obtained from a literature study. The structure and canonical simplified molecular-input line-entry (SMILE) were accessed from PubChem (https://pubchem.ncbi.nlm.nih.gov) between 4–8 January 2023. The bioactive compounds that were predicted to be targeted to keloid-related target proteins were listed for further analysis. The data were then submitted to SwissADME (http://www.swissadme.ch/) on 14 July 2023 to predict the absorption, distribution, metabolism, and excretion

(ADME) parameters, pharmacokinetics properties, and drug-likeness nature. The Mw, HBA and HBD and Log P were utilized as parameters to consider the drug-likeness assessment. The Log P value was presented as the consensus the partition coefficient between n-octanol and water ($LogP_{o/w}$), which was generated from SwissADME [51]. The prediction of the toxicity profile of the compounds was analyzed using a toxicity database, Protox II (https://tox-new.charite.de/protox_II/) (accessed on 16 July 2023). Furthermore, SWISS target prediction (http://www.swisstargetprediction.ch/), searching for target proteins corresponding to each molecule with only human (*Homo sapiens*) genes, was set as data retrieval. The list of proteins was aligned using UniProt (http://www.uniprot.org/uploadlists/) to eliminate double-listed proteins (accessed on 20 June 2023).

The protein targets related to keloid were identified in the Gene Cards (https://www.genecards.org/) and DisGeNet (https://www.disgenet.org/) databases using "Keloid" as the keyword in the search engine column (accessed on 13 February 2023). The identified proteins were filtered to only *Homo sapiens* genes. We utilized a Venn script (https://bioinfogp.cnb.csic.es/tools/venny/) to identify keloid-related protein targets at the intersection of the databases [52]. This tool was also used for the gambir bioactive compound targets, keloid-related targets, and protein targets related to keloid with high degree values intersection lists.

4.2. Construction of Protein–Protein Interaction (PPI) and Drug–Protein Interaction (DPI) Network

The PPI and DPI networks were constructed, visualized, and analyzed using Cytoscape 3.9.1 software on 15 February 2023. The PPI network was constructed from the keloid-related protein list. The proteins were uploaded to the String database (https://string-db.org/) on 20 February 2023, with 0.98 as the high confidence score for protein interaction and *Homo sapiens* set as the only organism. STRING suggests a threshold of 0.15 to be considered as low confidence, 0.40 as medium confidence, and 0.90 as high confidence. The higher confidence score of the interaction reflects higher supporting evidence and reduced false positives. On the other hand, the higher confidence may reduce the sensitivity and potentially exclude valid interactions inadvertently [23,53].

Afterwards, the network was analyzed to discover the top rank of significance proteins based on the degree, betweenness centrality (BC), and closeness centrality (CC) scores. The network was then visualized using GeneMANIA (http://genemania.org). This website allows users to find genes likely to share functions based on the interaction [54]. The second network is drug–protein interaction (DPI). The network was created to visualize and analyze the interactions of the bioactive compounds of gambir with keloid-related target proteins. Furthermore, the networks were merged to determine a new network of compound–targets of gambir targeted to keloid disease. The screening of the key bioactive compounds was also subjected to this step. The bioactive compounds with high degree values were considered the key important compounds [55].

4.3. Gene Annotation (GO) and Pathway Enrichment Analyses

The core protein targets from the previous step were uploaded to perform enrichment analysis for Gene Ontology (GO), biological process (BP), cellular component (CC), and molecular function (MF), as well as the pathway. All of these were conducted to describe the gene set mechanism of action through the Database for Annotation, Visualization, and Integrated Discovery (DAVID, https://david.ncifcrf.gov/), REACTOME (https://reactome.org/), and Kyoto Encyclopedia of Genes and Genomes (KEGG) (https://www.genome.jp/kegg/). The list of genes was based on the adjusted p value of less than 0.05 as the cut-off value that indicates statistical significance [56,57]. All of these analysis were accessed between 20 June 2023 and 7 July 2023.

4.4. Molecular Docking

The interactions between the gambir bioactive compounds and target proteins were validated using molecular-docking analysis. The top 10 gambir bioactive compounds with HDVs were searched for and downloaded in SDF format for the 2D structure in PubChem (https://pubchem.ncbi.nlm.nih.gov/) on 25 July 2023. The 2D structures were then prepared and saved as pdb format using MarvinSketch 23.11 software. TGFB1, AKT1, and MMP1 were selected as the target proteins, considering that these proteins were in the up, middle, and downstream of the KEGG pathway prediction. Triamcinolone acetonide (TAC) was used as a positive control since this chemical has been widely used for keloid treatment due to its anti-inflammatory properties [58]. The pdb formats of the 3D structure were downloaded from the RCSB PDB (https://www.rcsb.org/) database on 28 July 2023. Moreover, 3KFD, 4GV1, and 1HFC were the PDB ID for TGFβ1, AKT1, and MMP1, respectively. All the protein and ligand structures were saved as pdbqt formats. Molecular docking between the gambir bioactive compounds and target proteins was conducted using AutoDockTools 1.5.6 software on 9 August 2023. The ligands were set as a rigid structure and positioned at the central of cavity, which was docked by the native ligand corresponding to each protein model. Afterwards, the grid box was adjusted for the x-, y-, and z-axis for each protein models and the grid box with the lowest binding energy was selected for further analysis. The Lamarckian Genetic Algorithm was employed for running the molecular-docking simulation. The absolute value of the docking score was identified as the binding affinity and stability between the compound and target. Discovery Studio 4.5. was used to visualize the result of the molecular-docking analyses on 15 August 2023 [59].

5. Conclusions

In conclusion, this study first predicted the interactions of the bioactive compounds of gambir with keloid target proteins through an epistatic interaction and molecular simulation approach. EP300, AKT1, STAT3, TGFB1, VEGFA, EGFR, CCND1, IGFR, TIMP, MMP, and PDGFA were defined as the core proteins targeted by gambir's bioactive compounds with high degree values. Gambiriin C and TGFβ1, Isogambirine and AKT1, and Procyanidin B1 and MMP1 were identified as the compound–protein complexes with the highest binding energy. GO enrichment and pathway analysis found that gambir's bioactive compounds may act on keloid-related target proteins to regulate cell proliferation, migration, transcription, and signal transduction activity via cytokine, transcription, and growth factor signaling pathways. This is proposed to be correlated to the dysregulation of cytokines and growth factors in prolonged inflammation as favorable conditions for keloid formation. This study provides a reference for potential targets and pathways to explain the molecular mechanism of gambir's bioactive compounds against keloid disease.

Supplementary Materials: The following supporting information can be downloaded at https://www.mdpi.com/article/10.3390/ph17060662/s1, Table S1. Keloid-related target proteins, Table S2. Gambir's bioactive compound target proteins. Table S3. Degree ranking of Gambir bioactive compound analysed by Cytoscape 3.9.1.

Author Contributions: Conceptualization, S.S.N. and F.F.; methodology, S.S.N. and F.F.; validation, F.F., S.W.A.J. and R.S.; formal analysis, S.S.N.; investigation, S.S.N.; funding acquisition, R.S. and T.Y.; writing—original draft preparation, S.S.N.; writing—review and editing, F.F., S.W.A.J., R.S. and T.Y.; visualization, S.S.N. and R.S.; supervision, F.F., S.W.A.J., R.S. and T.Y. All authors have read and agreed to the published version of the manuscript.

Funding: This study was funded by Universitas Indonesia (PUTI 2023 grant; grant number: NKB-400/UN2.RST/HKP.05.00/2023).

Institutional Review Board Statement: Not applicable.

Informed Consent Statement: Not applicable.

Data Availability Statement: All data are available in this manuscript.

Acknowledgments: The support from Universitas Indonesia, Centre or Education Services (Ministry of Education, Culture, Research, and Technology of the Republic of Indonesia), and Indonesia Endowment Funds for Education (LPDP) is gratefully acknowledged.

Conflicts of Interest: The authors declare no conflicts of interest.

References

1. Elsaie, M.L. Update on management of keloid and hypertrophic scars: A systemic review. *J. Cosmet. Dermatol.* **2021**, *20*, 2729–2738. [CrossRef] [PubMed]
2. Andrews, J.P.; Marttala, J.; Macarak, E.; Rosenbloom, J.; Uitto, J. Keloids: The paradigm of skin fibrosis—Pathomechanisms and treatment. *Matrix Biol.* **2016**, *51*, 37–46. [CrossRef] [PubMed]
3. Berman, B.; Maderal, A.; Raphael, B. Keloids and hypertrophic scars: Pathophysiology, classification, and treatment. *Dermatol. Surg.* **2017**, *43*, S3–S18. [CrossRef] [PubMed]
4. Ashcroft, K.J.; Syed, F.; Bayat, A. Site-specific keloid fibroblasts alter the behaviour of normal skin and normal scar fibroblasts through paracrine signalling. *PLoS ONE* **2013**, *8*, e75600. [CrossRef] [PubMed]
5. Ud-Din, S.; Bayat, A. Keloid scarring or disease: Unresolved quasi-neoplastic tendencies in the human skin. *Wound Repair Regen.* **2020**, *28*, 422–426. [CrossRef]
6. Ekstein, S.F.; Wyles, S.P.; Moran, S.L.; Meves, A. Keloids: A review of therapeutic management. *Int. J. Dermatol.* **2021**, *60*, 661–671. [CrossRef] [PubMed]
7. Naik, P.P. Novel targets and therapies for keloid. *Clin. Exp. Dermatol.* **2022**, *47*, 507–515. [CrossRef] [PubMed]
8. Kang, P.; Wu, Z.; Zhong, Y.; Wang, Z.; Zhou, C.; Huo, S.; Guo, H.; Li, S.; Xu, K.; Liu, L.; et al. A Network Pharmacology and Molecular Docking Strategy to Explore Potential Targets and Mechanisms Underlying the Effect of Curcumin on Osteonecrosis of the Femoral Head in Systemic Lupus Erythematosus. *BioMed Res. Int.* **2021**, *2021*, 5538643. [CrossRef] [PubMed]
9. Munggari, I.P.; Kurnia, D.; Deawati, Y.; Julaeha, E. Current Research of Phytochemical, Medicinal and Non-Medicinal Uses of *Uncaria gambir* Roxb.: A Review. *Molecules* **2022**, *27*, 6551. [CrossRef] [PubMed]
10. Dharsono, H.D.A.; Wibisono, L.; Hayati, A.T.; Apriyanti, E.; Satari, M.H.; Kurnia, D. Mode action prediction of catechin from *Uncaria gambir* Roxb. against UDP-N-acetylenolpyruvyl-glucosamine reductase (MurB enzyme) of Streptococcus mutans: In silico study. *J. Adv. Pharm. Technol. Res.* **2022**, *13*, 197–201. [CrossRef] [PubMed]
11. Syarifah, S. Anticancer activity of *Uncaria gambir* roxb on T47D breast cancer cells. *J. Phys.* **2019**, *1317*, 012106. [CrossRef]
12. Wardana, A.P.; Aminah, N.S.; Kristanti, A.N.; Zahrah, H.I.; Fahmi, M.Z.; Yuliati, A.; Suhaili; Choudhary, M.I. Anticancer Activity of Nano *Uncaria gambir*. 2022. Available online: https://www.researchsquare.com/article/rs-1497841/v1 (accessed on 19 September 2022).
13. Yimam, M.; Lee, Y.C.; Kim, T.W.; Moore, B.; Jiao, P.; Hong, M.; Kim, H.J.; Nam, J.B.; Kim, M.R.; Oh, J.S.; et al. Analgesic and anti-Inflammatory effect of UP3005, a botanical composition Containing two standardized extracts of *Uncaria gambir* and Morus alba. *Pharmacogn. Res.* **2015**, *7*, S39–S46. [CrossRef] [PubMed]
14. Desdiani, D.; Rengganis, I.; Djauzi, S.; Setiyono, A.; Sadikin, M.; Jusman, S.W.A.; Siregar, N.C.; Suradi, S.; Eyanoer, P.C.; Fadilah, F. In vitro assay and study interaction of *Uncaria gambir* (Hunter) Roxb. as anti-fibrotic activity against A549 cell line. *Pharmacogn. J.* **2020**, *12*, 1232–1240. [CrossRef]
15. Desdiani, D.; Rengganis, I.; Djauzi, S.; Setiyono, A.; Sadikin, M.; Jusman, S.W.A.; Siregar, N.C.; Suradi, S.; Eyanoer, P.C. Fibropreventive and Antifibrotic Effects of *Uncaria gambir* on Rats with Pulmonary Fibrosis. *Evid.-Based Complement. Altern. Med.* **2022**, *2022*, 6721958. [CrossRef] [PubMed]
16. Ningsih, S. Efek Hepatoprotektor Gambir (*Uncaria gambir* (Hunter) Roxb.) dalam Menghambat Pembentukan Pembentukan Kolagen dengan Menekan TiMP-1 *In Vivo*. Ph.D. Thesis, Universitas Indonesia, Kota Depok, Indonesia, 2015.
17. Jusman, S.W.A.; Amalia, M.F.; Paramita, R.; Ningsih, S.; Fadilah, F. Structure-based screening of inhibitor platelet-derived growth factor from ethanol extract of *Uncaria gambir* (Hunter) Roxb. as an antifibrotic in keloid fibroblast cells. *Appl. Pharm. Sci.* **2023**, *13*, 36–43. [CrossRef]
18. Wang, Q.; Zhong, Y.; Li, Z.; Zhu, D.; Lu, H.; Chen, P.; Li, C.; Peng, X.; Li, Q.; Zeng, K. Multitranscriptome analyses of keloid fibroblasts reveal the role of the HIF-1α/HOXC6/ERK axis in keloid development. *Burn. Trauma* **2022**, *10*, tkac013. [CrossRef] [PubMed]
19. Nagel, R.L. Epistasis and the genetics of human diseases. *Comptes Rendus Biol.* **2005**, *328*, 606–615. [CrossRef] [PubMed]
20. Quan, Y.; Liu, M.-Y.; Liu, Y.-M.; Zhu, L.-D.; Wu, Y.-S.; Luo, Z.-H.; Zhang, X.-Z.; Xu, S.-Z.; Yang, Q.-Y.; Zhang, H.-Y. Facilitating anti-cancer combinatorial drug discovery by targeting epistatic disease genes. *Molecules* **2018**, *23*, 736. [CrossRef] [PubMed]
21. Wilkins, J.F.; Cannataro, V.L.; Shuch, B.; Townsend, J.P. Analysis of mutation, selection, and epistasis: An informed approach to cancer clinical trials. *Oncotarget* **2018**, *9*, 22243–22253. [CrossRef] [PubMed]
22. Zhou, Y.; Lauschke, V.M. Pharmacogenomic network analysis of the gene-drug interaction landscape underlying drug disposition. *Comput. Struct. Biotechnol. J.* **2020**, *18*, 52–58. [CrossRef] [PubMed]
23. Ding, Z.; Kihara, D. Computational identification of protein-protein interactions in model plant proteomes. *Sci. Rep.* **2019**, *9*, 8740. [CrossRef] [PubMed]

24. Nur Sazwi, N.; Nalina, T.; Rahim, Z.H.A. Antioxidant and cytoprotective activities of Piper betle, Areca catechu, *Uncaria gambir* and betel quid with and without calcium hydroxide. *BMC Complement. Altern. Med.* **2013**, *13*, 351. [CrossRef] [PubMed]
25. Ye, J.; Li, L.; Hu, Z. Exploring the Molecular Mechanism of Action of Yinchen Wuling Powder for the Treatment of Hyperlipidemia, Using Network Pharmacology, Molecular Docking, and Molecular Dynamics Simulation. *BioMed Res. Int.* **2021**, *2021*, 9965906. [CrossRef] [PubMed]
26. Wang, Y.; Yang, S.H.; Zhong, K.; Jiang, T.; Zhang, M.; Kwan, H.Y.; Su, T. Network Pharmacology-Based Strategy for the Investigation of the Anti-Obesity Effects of an Ethanolic Extract of Zanthoxylum bungeanum Maxim. *Front. Pharmacol.* **2020**, *11*, 572387. [CrossRef] [PubMed]
27. Lu, Z.; Huang, M.; Lin, H.; Wang, G.; Li, H. Network pharmacology and molecular docking approach to elucidate the mechanisms of Liuwei Dihuang pill in diabetic osteoporosis. *J. Orthop. Surg. Res.* **2022**, *17*, 314. [CrossRef] [PubMed]
28. Taniguchi, S.; Kuroda, K.; Doi, K.-I.; Tanabe, M.; Shibata, T.; Yoshida, T.; Hatano, T. Revised structures of gambiriins A1, A2, B1, and B2, chalcane-flavan dimers from gambir (*Uncaria gambir* extract). *Chem. Pharm. Bull.* **2007**, *55*, 268–272. [CrossRef] [PubMed]
29. Ullah, A.; Munir, S.; Badshah, S.L.; Khan, N.; Ghani, L.; Poulson, B.G.; Emwas, A.-H.; Jaremko, M. Important Flavonoids and Their Role as a Therapeutic Agent. *Molecules* **2020**, *25*, 5243. [CrossRef] [PubMed]
30. Piñero, J.; Ramírez-Anguita, J.M.; Saüch-Pitarch, J.; Ronzano, F.; Centeno, E.; Sanz, F.; Furlong, L.I. The DisGeNET knowledge platform for disease genomics: 2019 update. *Nucleic Acids Res.* **2020**, *48*, D845–D855. [CrossRef] [PubMed]
31. Safran, M.; Dalah, I.; Alexander, J.; Rosen, N.; Stein, T.I.; Shmoish, M.; Nativ, N.; Bahir, I.; Doniger, T.; Krug, H.; et al. GeneCards Version 3: The human gene integrator. *Database* **2010**, *2010*, baq020. [CrossRef] [PubMed]
32. Macarak, E.J.; Wermuth, P.J.; Rosenbloom, J.; Uitto, J. Keloid disorder: Fibroblast differentiation and gene expression profile in fibrotic skin diseases. *Exp. Dermatol.* **2021**, *30*, 132–145. [CrossRef] [PubMed]
33. Wang, Z.-C.; Zhao, W.-Y.; Cao, Y.; Liu, Y.-Q.; Sun, Q.; Shi, P.; Cai, J.-Q.; Shen, X.Z.; Tan, W.-Q. The Roles of Inflammation in Keloid and Hypertrophic Scars. *Front Immunol.* **2020**, *11*, 603187. [CrossRef] [PubMed]
34. Mcginty, S.; Siddiqui, J.W. *Keloid*; StatPearls Publishing: St. Petersburg, FL, USA, 2022.
35. Lee, C.C.; Tsai, C.H.; Chen, C.H.; Yeh, Y.C.; Chung, W.H.; Chen, C.B. An updated review of the immunological mechanisms of keloid scars. *Front. Immunol.* **2023**, *14*, 1117630. [CrossRef] [PubMed]
36. Nangole, F.W.; Agak, G.W. Keloid pathophysiology: Fibroblast or inflammatory disorders?: Pathophysiology of Keloids. *JPRAS Open* **2019**, *22*, 44–54. [CrossRef] [PubMed]
37. Borthwick, L.A.; Wynn, T.A.; Fisher, A.J. Cytokine mediated tissue fibrosis. *Biochim. Biophys. Acta Mol. Basis Dis.* **2013**, *1832*, 1049–1060. [CrossRef] [PubMed]
38. Varmeh, S.; Egia, A.; McGrouther, D.; Tahan, S.R.; Bayat, A.; Pandolfi, P.P. Cellular Senescence as a Possible Mechanism for Halting Progression of Keloid Lesions. *Genes Cancer* **2011**, *2*, 1061–1066. [CrossRef] [PubMed]
39. Deng, C.-C.; Hu, Y.-F.; Zhu, D.-H.; Cheng, Q.; Gu, J.-J.; Feng, Q.-L.; Zhang, L.-X.; Xu, Y.-P.; Wang, D.; Rong, Z.; et al. Single-cell RNA-seq reveals fibroblast heterogeneity and increased mesenchymal fibroblasts in human fibrotic skin diseases. *Nat Commun.* **2021**, *12*, 1–16. [CrossRef] [PubMed]
40. Papadopoulos, N.; Lennartsson, J. The PDGF/PDGFR pathway as a drug target. *Mol. Aspects Med.* **2018**, *62*, 75–88. [CrossRef] [PubMed]
41. Klinkhammer, B.M.; Floege, J.; Boor, P. PDGF in organ fibrosis. *Mol. Aspects Med.* **2018**, *62*, 44–62. [CrossRef] [PubMed]
42. Dowling, C.M.; Kiely, P.A. Targeting protein Kinase C downstream of growth factor and adhesion signalling. *Cancers* **2015**, *7*, 1271–1291. [CrossRef] [PubMed]
43. Kim, J.; Kong, J.; Chang, H.; Kim, H.; Kim, A. EGF induces epithelial-mesenchymal transition through phosphor-Smad2/3-Snail signaling pathway in breast cancer cells. *Oncotarget* **2016**, *7*, 85021–85032. [CrossRef] [PubMed]
44. Lo, H.-W.; Hsu, S.-C.; Xia, W.; Cao, X.; Shih, J.-Y.; Wei, Y.; Abbruzzese, J.L.; Hortobagyi, G.N.; Hung, M.-C. Epidermal Growth Factor Receptor Cooperates with Signal Transducer and Activator of Transcription 3 to Induce Epithelial-Mesenchymal Transition in Cancer Cells via Up-regulation of TWIST Gene Expression. *Cancer Res.* **2008**, *23*, 9066–9076. [CrossRef] [PubMed]
45. Lee, Y.I.; Shim, J.E.; Kim, J.; Lee, W.J.; Kim, J.W.; Nam, K.H.; Lee, J.H. WNT5A drives interleukin-6-dependent epithelial–mesenchymal transition via the JAK/STAT pathway in keloid pathogenesis. *Burn. Trauma.* **2022**, *10*, tkac023. [CrossRef] [PubMed]
46. Lee, Y.S.; Liang, Y.C.; Wu, P.; Kulber, D.A.; Tanabe, K.; Chuong, C.M.; Ming, C.; Randall, W.; Tai-Lan, T. STAT3 Signaling Pathway is Implicated in Keloid Pathogenesis by Preliminary Transcriptome and Open Chromatin Analyses. *Physiol. Behav.* **2017**, *174*, 139–148. [CrossRef] [PubMed]
47. Xue, M.; Jackson, C.J. Extracellular Matrix Reorganization During Wound Healing and Its Impact on Abnormal Scarring. *Adv. Wound Care* **2015**, *4*, 119–136. [CrossRef] [PubMed]
48. Lee, D.E.; Trowbridge, R.M.; Ayoub, N.T.; Agrawal, D.K. High-mobility Group Box Protein-1, Matrix Metalloproteinases, and Vitamin D in Keloids and Hypertrophic Scars. *PRS Glob. Open* **2015**, *3*, e425. [CrossRef] [PubMed]
49. Wulandari, E.; Jusman, S.W.A.; Moenadjat, Y.; Jusuf, A.A.; Sadikin, M. Expressions of Collagen I and III in Hypoxic Keloid Tissue. *Kobe J. Med. Sci.* **2016**, *62*, 58–69.
50. Dohi, T.; Miyake, K.; Aoki, M.; Ogawa, R.; Akaishi, S.; Shimada, T.; Okada, T.; Hyakusoku, H. Tissue Inhibitor of Metalloproteinase-2 Suppresses Collagen Synthesis in Cultured Keloid Fibroblasts. *PRS Glob. Open* **2015**, *3*, e520. [CrossRef] [PubMed]

51. Daina, A.; Michielin, O.; Zoete, V. SwissADME: A free web tool to evaluate pharmacokinetics, druglikeness and medicinal chemistry friendliness of small molecules. *Sci. Rep.* **2017**, *7*, 42717. [CrossRef] [PubMed]
52. Venny, O.J. An Interactive Tool for Comparing Lists with Venn's Diagrams. Available online: https://methods.sagepub.com/reference/dictionary-of-statistics-methodology/n2067.xml (accessed on 14 February 2023).
53. Bozhilova, L.V.; Whitmore, A.V.; Wray, J.; Reinert, G.; Deane, C.M. Measuring rank robustness in scored protein interaction networks. *BMC Bioinform.* **2019**, *20*, 446. [CrossRef] [PubMed]
54. Franz, M.; Rodriguez, H.; Lopes, C.; Zuberi, K.; Montojo, J.; Bader, G.D.; Morris, Q. GeneMANIA update 2018. *Nucleic Acids Res.* **2018**, *46*, 60–64. [CrossRef] [PubMed]
55. Cui, Y.; Wang, H.; Wang, D.; Mi, J.; Chen, G.; Li, F.; Wang, Y.; Zhang, Y. Network Pharmacology Analysis on the Mechanism of Huangqi Sijunzi Decoction in Treating Cancer-Related Fatigue. *J. Healthc. Eng.* **2021**, *2021*, 9780677. [CrossRef] [PubMed]
56. Huang, D.W.; Sherman, B.T.; Lempicki, R.A. Systematic and integrative analysis of large gene lists using DAVID bioinformatics resources. *Lempicki RA. Nat. Protoc.* **2009**, *4*, 44–57. [CrossRef] [PubMed]
57. Fabregat, A.; Sidiropoulos, K.; Viteri, G.; Marin-Garcia, P.; Ping, P.; Stein, L.; D'eustachio, P.; Hermjakob, H. Reactome diagram viewer: Data structures and strategies to boost performance. *Bioinformatics* **2018**, *34*, 1208–1214. [CrossRef] [PubMed]
58. Coppola, M.M.; Salzillo, R.; Segreto, F.; Persichetti, P. Triamcinolone acetonide intralesional injection for the treatment of keloid scars: Patient selection and perspectives. *Clin. Cosmet. Investig. Dermatol.* **2018**, *11*, 387–396. [CrossRef] [PubMed]
59. Dong, Y.; Zhao, Q.; Wang, Y. Network pharmacology-based investigation of potential targets of astragalus membranaceous-angelica sinensis compound acting on diabetic nephropathy. *Sci. Rep.* **2021**, *11*, 19496. [CrossRef] [PubMed]

pharmaceuticals

Review

The Therapeutic Potential of Essential Oils in Managing Inflammatory Skin Conditions: A Scoping Review

Anouk E. W. K. Dontje [1], Catharina C. M. Schuiling-Veninga [2], Florence P. A. M. van Hunsel [2,3], Corine Ekhart [3], Fatih Demirci [4] and Herman J. Woerdenbag [1,*]

[1] Department of Pharmaceutical Technology and Biopharmacy, Groningen Research Institute of Pharmacy (GRIP), University of Groningen, Antonius Deusinglaan 1, 9713 AV Groningen, The Netherlands; anoukdontje@gmail.com
[2] Department of Pharmacotherapy, -Epidemiology and -Economics, Groningen Research Institute of Pharmacy (GRIP), University of Groningen, Antonius Deusinglaan 1, 9713 AV Groningen, The Netherlands; c.c.m.schuiling-veninga@rug.nl (C.C.M.S.-V.); f.vanhunsel@lareb.nl (F.P.A.M.v.H.)
[3] Netherlands Pharmacovigilance Centre Lareb, Goudsbloemvalei 7, 5237 MH 's-Hertogenbosch, The Netherlands; c.ekhart@lareb.nl
[4] Department of Pharmacognosy, Faculty of Pharmacy, Anadolu University, 26470 Eskisehir, Türkiye; demircif@gmail.com
* Correspondence: h.j.woerdenbag@rug.nl; Tel.: +31-6-31921365

Abstract: Conventional therapy is commonly used for the treatment of inflammatory skin conditions, but undesirable effects, such as erythema, dryness, skin thinning, and resistance to treatment, may cause poor patient compliance. Therefore, patients may seek complementary treatment with herbal plant products including essential oils (EOs). This scoping review aims to generate a broad overview of the EOs used to treat inflammatory skin conditions, namely, acne vulgaris, dermatitis and eczema, psoriasis, and rosacea, in a clinical setting. The quality, efficacy, and safety of various EOs, as well as the way in which they are prepared, are reviewed, and the potential, as well as the limitations, of EOs for the treatment of inflammatory skin conditions are discussed. Twenty-nine eligible studies (case studies, uncontrolled clinical studies, and randomized clinical studies) on the applications of EOs for inflammatory skin conditions were retrieved from scientific electronic databases (PubMed, Embase, Scopus, and the Cochrane Library). As an initial result, tea tree (*Melaleuca alternifolia*) oil emerged as the most studied EO. The clinical studies with tea tree oil gel for acne treatment showed an efficacy with fewer adverse reactions compared to conventional treatments. The uncontrolled studies indicated the potential efficacy of ajwain (*Trachyspermum ammi*) oil, eucalyptus (*Eucalyptus globulus*) oil, and cedarwood (*Cedrus libani*) oil in the treatment of acne, but further research is required to reach conclusive evidence. The placebo-controlled studies revealed the positive effects of kānuka (*Kunzea ericoides*) oil and frankincense (*Boswellia* spp.) oil in the treatment of psoriasis and eczema. The quality verification of the EO products was inconsistent, with some studies lacking analyses and transparency. The quality limitations of some studies included a small sample size, a short duration, and the absence of a control group. This present review underscores the need for extended, well-designed clinical studies to further assess the efficacy and safety of EOs for treating inflammatory skin conditions with products of assured quality and to further elucidate the mechanisms of action involved.

Keywords: acne vulgaris; case reports; clinical studies; dermatitis; eczema; efficacy; essential oils (EOs); psoriasis; rosacea; quality; tea tree oil (TTO)

Citation: Dontje, A.E.W.K.; Schuiling-Veninga, C.C.M.; van Hunsel, F.P.A.M.; Ekhart, C.; Demirci, F.; Woerdenbag, H.J. The Therapeutic Potential of Essential Oils in Managing Inflammatory Skin Conditions: A Scoping Review. *Pharmaceuticals* **2024**, *17*, 571. https://doi.org/10.3390/ph17050571

Academic Editors: Catherine Sherwin, Elena Y. Enioutina and Kathleen M. Job

Received: 4 April 2024
Revised: 23 April 2024
Accepted: 28 April 2024
Published: 29 April 2024

1. Introduction

As an introduction to this scoping review, we first (Section 1.1) provide general information about aromatherapy (the definition and history) and essential oils (EOs) (the definition, production methods, chemistry, and dermatological applications) followed by the aim of this study. Second (Section 1.2), we present the background information (the clinical picture, pathophysiology, and treatment options) of the inflammatory skin conditions this article focuses on: acne vulgaris, dermatitis and eczema, psoriasis, and rosacea.

1.1. Essential Oils and Aim of this Scoping Review

Among consumers and healthcare providers, there is an increasing interest in using essential oils (EOs) (also known as volatile oils, ethereal oils, or aetherolea) from plants for medicinal purposes [1,2]. The application of EOs for therapeutic purposes is known as (clinical) aromatherapy [3]. Aromatherapy comprises the inhalation, topical application, and enteral intake of EOs, involving, respectively, the olfactory system, the skin, and the digestive tract as the route through which an EO can exert its physiological and pharmacological effects [4]. Aromatherapy is used for the treatment and prevention of diseases and to obtain a positive effect on mood, emotions, and psychological well-being. The French perfumer chemist Rene-Maurice Gattefosse coined the term 'aromatherapy' in 1928. While working in his laboratory, he burned his hands and found that lavender EO helped the healing of the wounds with little scarring. Further significant steps in the development of aromatherapy were set by the physician Jean Valnet, who, in the 1960s, expanded aromatherapy to include wider medical applications. More recently and still active, Robert Tisserand is an important scientist and ambassador for the safe and therapeutic use of aromatherapy and EOs [3,5–8].

EOs are mostly volatile lipophilic liquids, which are, according to international definitions (including pharmacopoeias), obtained from aromatic plant material (leaves, flowers, fruits, and roots) mostly by hydrodistillation (or steam distillation), as well as by expression (in the case of *Citrus* spp.). The word 'essential' refers to the 'essence' of a plant (volatiles, odor, and flavor) captured in the EO. The extracts of aromatic plants that are obtained using organic solvents (known as concretes or absolutes) or using supercritical carbon dioxide are not considered to be true EOs, although they may be marketed as such. Their composition is different from EOs, both qualitatively and quantitatively, and, in addition to volatile (EO) constituents, they will contain a number of non-volatile compounds as well. Thus, their pharmacological and safety profiles may differ from EOs [3,5,6,9,10].

The constituents of EOs originate from three distinct biosynthetic pathways: the mevalonate pathway and the methyl–erythritol pathway leading to terpenes and terpenoids, respectively; and the shikimic acid pathway resulting in volatile phenylpropanes. The number of individual substances analyzed in EOs is generally large (>300), resulting in a great variation in their composition. EOs may contain one or a few main constituents. EOs typically consist of monoterpenes (C10), volatile sesquiterpenes (C15), and phenylpropane derivatives with a molecular mass up to around 300 Dalton. Based on their chemical structure, they are aliphatic or cyclic hydrocarbons, alcohols, aldehydes, ketones, acids, esters, or phenols [3,5,9,10]. EO-producing plants are concentrated in a distinct number of plant families. EOs exhibit various biological activities, including antibacterial, anti-inflammatory, and antifungal [3,5,6,9,10]. These specific properties make several EOs beneficial for the treatment of inflammatory skin conditions.

EOs are rarely applied undiluted onto the skin as such a direct application can cause severe irritation. Commonly, in practice, they are diluted with a carrier oil (oleum, vegetable oil, fixed oil, or fat), a cream base, or a gel. Usually, concentrations of 2–5% are used in practice, but strongly irritating EOs are applied in maximal dilutions of 0.5% [2,7,8,11]. This reduces the rate of evaporation of the EO and may increase the rate and depth of its penetration into the skin. Transdermal absorption may occur as well, resulting in systemic effects including possible acute and chronical adverse reactions. A hydrophilic base, such as a gel, may enhance the skin penetration compared to a lipophilic base. Additionally, a base may also enhance the therapeutic benefits based on its skin healing, moisturizing, soothing, and nourishing properties [8].

This present scoping review aims to generate a broad overview of EOs used in a clinical setting to treat inflammatory skin conditions such as acne vulgaris, dermatitis and eczema, psoriasis, and rosacea, in order to define their clinical potential. The focus is on the frame of the clinical studies, the safety aspects, and the quality of the EOs and the administered preparations thereof. First, in the next section, the relevant background information on the inflammatory skin conditions is provided.

1.2. Inflammatory Skin Conditions

Acne vulgaris is a common and persistent inflammatory skin condition of the hair follicle and sebaceous glands [12] mainly occurring in the age group of 12 to 24 years due to hormonal changes during puberty. The pathophysiological factors include an increased sebum production, the hyperkeratinization of the hair follicles, inflammatory factors, and bacterial overgrowth, primarily involving *Cutibacterium acnes* (formerly known as *Propionibacterium acnes*) [13,14]. Acne vulgaris is characterized by the persistent or recurring presence of comedones, pustules, and red papules on the skin of the face, upper limbs, and neck [12]. The treatment options for mild-to-moderate acne vulgaris include topical treatment with retinoids, benzoyl peroxide, and/or topical antibiotics. Often, erythema and dryness of the skin are experienced as undesirable effects, reducing adherence to these therapies [15].

Eczema is a form of dermatitis characterized by symptoms such as skin redness, swelling, scaling, oozing or weeping, and dryness. The most prevalent type is atopic eczema, a chronic inflammatory skin condition causing patients to experience a decrease in their quality of life. Exacerbations may cause emotional stress among patients. Various factors are involved in the development of the condition including a compromised skin barrier, the enhanced activity of immune cells in the skin, the composition of the skin microflora, and external factors, such as low environmental humidity [16]. Another form of dermatitis, seborrheic dermatitis, manifests in areas of the body with a high concentration of sebaceous glands, especially on the scalp. Consequently, the condition is prominently visible and requires treatment to improve the patient's quality of life [17,18]. Topical corticosteroids are frequently used in the management of dermatitis and eczema and are proven to be effective. However, extended use of these drugs can lead to undesirable effects, including skin thinning, stretch marks (striae), dilated blood vessels (telangiectasias), and reduced skin pigmentation [19]. This may cause poor patient compliance, leading to treatment failure [20].

Psoriasis is a persistent immune-mediated inflammatory skin condition [21]. The most prevalent form of psoriasis is (chronic) plaque psoriasis. It is characterized by erythematous scaly patches or plaques, commonly located on the extensor surfaces of the knees and elbows, as well as the scalp, but can also affect the intertriginous areas, such as the palms, soles, and nails [21,22]. Lesions may appear at sites where the skin experiences trauma or pressure with the concomitant risk of bacterial infection [23]. Most psoriasis patients experience a negative impact on their quality of life, with many reporting significant psychosocial distress [23]. The current treatment options for mild psoriasis include topical treatment with corticosteroids, vitamin D analogs, and keratolytics, as well as phototherapy [23]. These strategies aim to alleviate symptoms, enhance the quality of life, and curb the condition progression. However, adverse drug reactions, resistance to treatment, long-term safety concerns, and the high costs associated with certain therapies may restrict their utilization and negatively influence patient compliance [24].

Rosacea is a chronic inflammatory skin condition characterized by one or more primary features, including flushing (or transient facial redness), persistent central facial redness, inflammatory papules or pustules, and telangiectasia [14,25]. It mainly affects the centrofacial regions, including cheeks, chin, nose and forehead, and eyes. Rosacea may adversely affect the quality of life, including social and psychological well-being [26]. While a complete understanding of rosacea's pathogenesis remains elusive, there is evidence suggesting a complex etiology, involving genetic, immunological, and neurovascular factors, and various triggers, including pathogens, ultraviolet radiation, and dietary factors [27,28].

Due to the presence of these multiple contributing factors, the management of rosacea can be challenging [28].

Patients suffering from one of the above-mentioned inflammatory skin conditions may face disappointing results from the conventional treatment options and/or experience adverse drug reactions leading to premature termination of the therapy. If so, patients may be willing to try an alternative or complementary therapy, for instance, in the form of an EO, in the hope of better clinical outcomes and fewer adverse drug reactions [3,7–9,29–32]. In this context, it is worth mentioning that a rising global trend has been found in the use of complementary medicines among psoriatic patients, especially in semi-urban areas where such therapies are favored due to their accessibility and affordability, as well as their presumed effectiveness and safety [33].

2. Results

2.1. Scoping Review

A total of 2918 studies (covering all publication dates) were initially identified. After removing duplicates (n = 569), 2349 titles and abstracts were screened for the inclusion criteria. As a result, the full texts of 51 studies were sought for retrieval. Unfortunately, the full texts of four articles were unavailable and, therefore, excluded. A total of 47 studies were assessed for eligibility, and 28 were excluded for the reasons provided in Section 4.2. Based on the reference lists of the studies assessed for eligibility, ten additional studies were included. Consequently, a total of 29 studies were included in this scoping review. Sixteen of the eligible studies focus on acne, four on dermatitis, five on psoriasis, and one on rosacea. Additionally, three eligible clinical studies without specifics resulted from the search strategy. The PRISMA flow diagram of the study selection process is presented in Figure 1 [34]. The composition of the EO-containing preparations, as described in the respective references, is shown in Table S1 (Supplementary Materials).

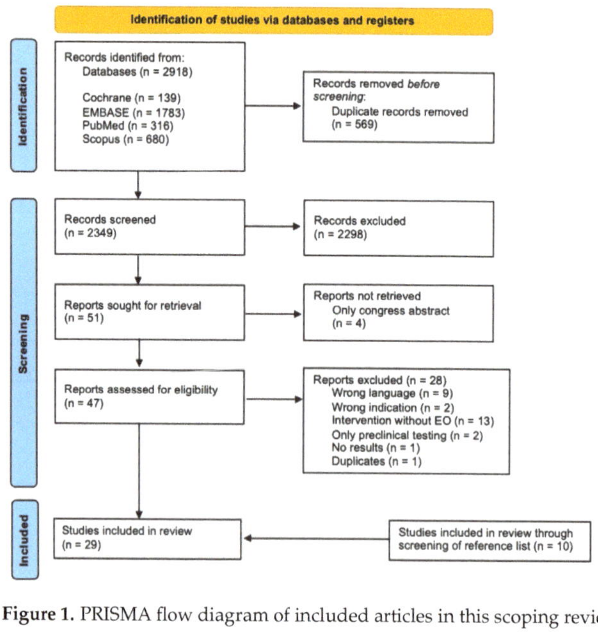

Figure 1. PRISMA flow diagram of included articles in this scoping review [34].

2.2. Acne

Table 1 gives an overview of the characteristics, main results, and limitations of the included studies focusing on acne. Table 2 gives an overview of the characteristics of the products used in the included studies focusing on acne to assess their quality. The studies cover a range of interventions, with tea tree (*Melaleuca alternifolia*) oil (TTO) as the primary EO used in the various formulations. The key findings include the superior effectiveness of benzoyl peroxide over TTO in reducing inflamed lesions, the positive outcomes of TTO in treating mild-to-moderate acne, the efficacy of cinnamon bark (*Cinnamomum verum*) oil in reducing acne lesions, the potential of cedarwood (*Cedrus libani*) oil in improving acne, and the antimicrobial effects of tea tree and lavender (*Lavandula* spp.) oils. The other studies evaluate the effectiveness of different formulations such as clindamycin–tretinoin, *Aloe vera* with African basil (*Ocimum gratissimum*) oil, Unani herbomineral cream, and the EO from copaiba (*Copaifera officinalis*). Overall, these studies indicate promising results for various EO-containing treatments in managing acne, with generally minimal ADRs (adverse drug reactions) reported in the studies. The studies are presented and discussed in order from the highest to lowest power of clinical evidence.

A double-blind, placebo-controlled study conducted by Enshaieh et al. aimed to assess the effectiveness of TTO in treating mild-to-moderate acne vulgaris in young patients. The study included 60 patients, divided into two groups receiving either a 5% TTO gel or a placebo gel. The TTO group experienced a significant reduction in acne lesions, total lesion count (TLC), and acne severity index (ASI) compared to the placebo group, and the TTO gel was found to be significantly more effective. Few ADRs were reported in both groups including minimal pruritus (five subjects; 8.3%) and a little burning sensation (three subjects; 5%). In the study, the origin of TTO was declared to be Melaleuca alternifolia (from Cinere Company, without any further specifications), while the physical and chemical properties of the commercial products containing TTO were stated to be regulated by an international standard [35]. Therefore, no additional analyses were performed by the authors on the purchased intervention and control products [36].

Kwon et al. conducted an 8-week, double-blind, randomized, controlled split-face trial with 34 participants, comparing the clinical efficacy, safety, and histopathological changes between 5% of *Lactobacillus*-fermented *Chamaecyparis obtusa* (LFCO) in cream and 5% of TTO in cream for treating acne vulgaris. The LFCO reduced inflammatory acne counts significantly after one week, while the TTO did so after four weeks. The LFCO also reduced non-inflammatory acne lesions and significantly decreased sebum levels. Additionally, the LFCO was more effective than the TTO in reducing the lesion counts. A significant difference between both groups in inflammatory lesion counts and acne grading was observed after two weeks and for non-inflammatory lesion counts after four weeks. In the TTO group, mild dryness (four subjects; 12.5%), mild erythema (six subjects; 18.8%), and desquamation (six subjects; 18.8%) were reported as ADRs. In the LFCO group, mild erythema (two subjects; 6.3%) and dryness (two subjects; 6.3%) were reported. The origin of the TTO was declared to be *Melaleuca alternifolia* (obtained by the steam distillation of leaves and terminal branches), while the LFCO originated from the needles (leaves) of *Chamaecyparis obtusa*, a type of cypress frequently found in Korea and Japan which is known as hinoki oil. Both intervention and control products were purchased from commercial sources. However, the production process was described and additional analyses for quality control were conducted such as ultra-performance liquid chromatography (UPLC) and high-resolution mass spectrometry analysis [37].

Da Silva et al. investigated the use of 1% of EOs from copaiba (*Copaifera langsdorffii*) in natrozol gel for the treatment of mild acne. The study, a double-blind, placebo-controlled clinical trial, involved ten volunteers with grade one (mild) acne lesions. The results showed a significant decrease in the extent of the area affected by acne in both the intervention and placebo groups, but the effect was more significant in the intervention-treated group. ADRs were not monitored or documented in this study. The intervention product was obtained from copaiba oil resin through steam distillation and used at a concentration of 1% in natrozol gel. Analyses, like high-resolution gas chromatography, were conducted on the EO for quality control, whereas the control was purchased without additional analyses [38].

The study conducted by Bassett et al. aimed to compare the efficacy and skin tolerance of a 5% TTO gel with a 5% benzoyl peroxide lotion for the treatment of mild (grade one) and moderate (grade two) acne. This prospective, single-blind study involved 124 patients divided into two groups receiving either TTO gel or benzoyl peroxide lotion. Both treatments effectively reduced the number of inflamed lesions. However, benzoyl peroxide was significantly more effective than TTO after one, two, and three months of treatment. TTO was better tolerated on the facial skin than benzoyl peroxide, and minimal ADRs were reported including skin dryness, pruritus, stinging, burning, and redness. The intervention and control products were purchased, and no additional analyses were conducted [39].

Ghovvati et al. investigated the safety and efficacy of a topical cinnamon bark EO (*Cinnamomum verum*) formulation for mild-to-moderate acne. An open-labelled, assessor-blind, uncontrolled clinical trial was conducted including 20 patients receiving 0.5% cinnamon gel. This gel reduced acne lesions, especially inflammatory ones, and lowered sebum content. Minor yet tolerable ADRs were reported including mild burning (13 subjects; 65%) and facial redness (11 subjects; 55%). Subsequently, the topical gel (an ethanolic carbomer gel) was prepared, and additional analyses for quality control, including the chemical quantification of the formulation, were conducted [40].

Talebi et al. evaluated the safety and efficacy of a topical ajwain (*Trachyspermum ammi*) EO formulation for treating facial acne through an open-label, uncontrolled, phase 2 clinical trial including twenty volunteers. The study's outcomes included a therapeutic efficacy assessment, a clinical evaluation, an assessment of patient satisfaction, the measurement of biophysical skin parameters, and the monitoring of ADRs. The ajwain gel showed a statistically significant reduction in acne lesions, especially non-inflammatory ones, as well as improvements in the skin characteristics. Local ADRs were monitored according to the authors, but none were reported in the article. The ajwain gel was extracted and prepared by the researchers and additional analyses for quality control were conducted by gas chromatography coupled with mass spectrometry (GC-MS) [41].

Malhi et al. aimed to evaluate the efficacy, tolerability, and acceptability of 200 mg/g TTO gel and a 7 mg/g TTO face wash for treating mild-to-moderate acne. A dual-center, open-label, phase II pilot study with fourteen participants was conducted. The TTO gel significantly reduced lesion counts and acne severity. Additionally, the adherence of the participants was high. They expressed satisfaction with the reduction in lesion counts. The TTO products were well tolerated with only mild local tolerability events including dryness, scaling, and peeling. The Australian TTO in both purchased products met the specifications of the British Pharmacopoeia monograph for TTO and both the ISO 4730:2004 and Australian 2782–2009 standards for 'Oil of *Melaleuca*, terpinen-4-ol type'. Furthermore, a visual determination of each product's minimum inhibitory concentrations (MIC) against *Cutibacterium acnes* after 48 h of anaerobic incubation was included in the study [42].

In the study of Hassan et al., the effect of eucalyptus (*Eucalyptus* spp.) oil in a fatty cream basis on the treatment of acne was investigated involving five patients. The study reported good results and improvements in the volunteers' acne conditions after the second week of treatment. Any ADRs were not evaluated. The constituents needed to prepare the eucalyptus oil cream, and the constituents were purchased and subsequently mixed without additional analyses [43].

Najafi-Taher et al. conducted a triple-blind, randomized clinical trial with 100 mild-to-moderate acne vulgaris patients. The aim was to evaluate the efficacy and safety of a TTO nano-emulsion (6%) containing adapalene (a topical retinoid) gel (0.1%) compared to a marketed adapalene gel. The TTO nano-emulsion in combination with adapalene gel was more effective than the marketed adapalene gel. The ADRs were mild and similar in both groups with dryness being the most common ADR. The TTO was purchased and subsequently manufactured into a nano-emulsion. The additional characterization of the products, and in vitro, ex vivo, and in vivo analyses were conducted [44,45].

Mazzarello et al. evaluated the efficacy of a cream containing propolis, TTO, and aloe vera (PTAC) for mild-to-moderate acne compared to a 3% erythromycin cream and a placebo. There were no specifications reported about the cream base. A double-blind, comparative study with 60 patients divided into three groups was conducted. The PTAC was more effective in reducing acne lesions, erythema, and sebum compared to the erythromycin cream. No ADRs were reported. The intervention and control products were purchased without conducting additional analyses [46].

Mazzarello et al. compared the anti-acne effectiveness of clindamycin–tretinoin with a cream containing *Myrtus communis* and *Origanum vulgare* EOs and tretinoin (MOTC). The study design was a comparative, randomized, single-center, single-blind study involving 60 patients. Both treatments improved the clinical parameters, including the number of comedones, papules, pustules, TLC, and ASI, with no significant differences between them. However, the MOTC had a better efficacy in reducing the papular erythema. No ADRs were documented. Both the intervention and control products were acquired from commercial sources without undergoing supplementary analyses [47].

Parveen et al. evaluated the effectiveness of an Unani herbomineral cream (UHC) for treating acne vulgaris in a controlled, randomized, single-blind clinical trial. The control and test groups each included 30 patients. UHC is a complex product containing several EOs in addition to other herbal products. The UHC demonstrated effectiveness in reducing acne lesions over 60 days compared to the control cream. The ADRs were not monitored or reported. The UHC was self-made by the researchers. According to the authors, the quality was assured on the basis of the descriptions given in the botanical sources and the classical Unani literature. No further analyses were reported [48].

Kim and Shin examined the effect of treating acne with a basic, weekly acne treatment (not specified) and a dermal application of a mixture of 3% TTO, 2% lavender (*Lavandula* spp., no further specification) oil, and jojoba (fixed) oil. The study was designed with a non-equivalent control group design with 60 participants divided into control and intervention groups. A significant reduction in the total number of *Cutibacterium acnes*, the sebum excretion rate, and non-inflammatory skin lesions was observed in the intervention group but not in the control group. In contrast, the number of acne lesions was significantly reduced in both groups. However, the reduction in the number of human skin pathogens did not significantly differ between both groups. The ADRs were not monitored or reported. The EOs used were permitted by the Korean Food & Drug Administration and assessed by the standards of the Korea Laboratory Accreditation Scheme. No additional analyses were reported [49].

Orafidiya et al. aimed to determine the effective concentration and base for a topical African basil (ocimum) (*Ocimum gratissimum*) oil formulation for managing acne vulgaris, compared to benzoyl peroxide. The clinical study with 126 subjects assessed the reduction in lesion counts and skin tolerance. The preparations containing ocimum oil in alcohol and a cetomacrogol base were the most effective in reducing the lesion counts. The reported ADRs in the intervention group were minimal and limited to a burning sensation, whereas no ADRs were reported in the placebo group. The intervention and control products were obtained from commercial sources without performing additional analyses [50].

Another study conducted by Orafidiya et al. aimed to investigate the synergistic effect of *Aloe vera* gel on the anti-acne properties of ocimum oil and compared them with clindamycin. The study included 84 participants. Ocimum oil lotion with aloe gel exhibited the most significant effects in reducing lesion counts. The higher the aloe gel content, the greater the product activity. The aloe gel-based preparations were the most active in resolving acne lesions. As many as 96% of the patients reported a mild stinging sensation on the skin and a mild skin irritation. Again, the intervention and control products were purchased without conducting additional analyses [51].

Hassoun et al. reported a case study discussing a 35-year-old woman with acne vulgaris. Cedarwood (*Juniperus virginiana*) oil was added to tretinoin cream, and the acne case was improved with no ADRs being reported. The commercial cedarwood oil was purchased and self-added to the tretinoin cream by the patient [52].

Table 1. Characteristics, main results, and limitations of the included studies focusing on acne. Details about the composition of the preparations are given in Table S1 (Supplementary Materials).

Author(s) (Publication Year; Country)	Study Design (n)	Intervention (n)	Control (n)	Outcome Measure(s)	Study Duration (Evaluation Period)	Main Results	Limitations
Enshaieh et al. (2007; Iran) [36]	Randomized, double-blind, and placebo-controlled study (60)	5% TTO [1] in carbomer gel (30)	Carbomer gel (30)	—Total lesion count —ASI [2] —Number of comedones, papules, and pustules —Monitoring ADRs [3]	45 days (baseline and every 15-day period)	—After treatment, a significant reduction in the mean TLC [4], ASI [2], and the numbers of comedones, pustules, and papules in the intervention group was observed but not in the control group (significant difference) —5 patients reported minimal pruritus, 3 patients reported a little burning sensation, and 1 patient reported minimal scaling (divided over the intervention and placebo groups)	—Short duration of study and follow-up time —Small sample size
Kwon et al. (2014; South Korea) [37]	Prospective double-blind, randomized, and controlled split-face trial (34)	5% *Lactobacillus*-fermented *Chamaecyparis obtusa* (LFCO) in cream (34)	5% TTO [1] in cream (34)	—Acne grade —(Non-) Inflammatory lesion count —Histopathology and immunohistochemistry of lesions —Patients' subjective assessment —Average size of sebaceous glands —Sebum secretion —Monitoring ADRs [3]	8 weeks (baseline; 1, 2, 4, and 8 weeks)	—A significant difference between both groups in inflammatory lesion counts and acne grading was observed after 2 weeks and for non-inflammatory lesion counts after 4 weeks —A significant reduction in the overall size of the sebaceous gland was observed on the lactobacillus side when compared to the baseline, but not on the tea tree oil side —In the tea tree oil group, 4 patients reported mild dryness and 6 reported mild erythema and desquamation —In the lactobacillus group, 2 patients reported mild dryness and 2 reported dryness	—Risk of cross-contamination —Lack of comparison to a control or placebo —Small sample size and all were Korean

Table 1. *Cont.*

Author(s) (Publication Year; Country)	Study Design (n)	Intervention (n)	Control (n)	Outcome Measure(s)	Study Duration (Evaluation Period)	Main Results	Limitations
Da Silva et al. (2012; Brazil) [38]	Double-blind and placebo-controlled clinical trial (10)	1% Copaiba essential oil in natrozol gel (10)	Natrozol gel (10)	—Photographs to determine the total area occupied by acne	21 days (baseline and weekly)	—After 21 days, a highly significant decrease in the extent of the area affected by acne was observed in both the placebo and intervention groups; however, the effect in the intervention group was greater —The results observed in the placebo group could not be explained, and aggravations occurred in most of the participants —The decrease in the surface area affected with acne in the intervention group can mostly be explained by the model	—Short duration of study and follow-up time —Small sample size —Only one outcome —No safety assessment —No demographics reported
Bassett et al. (1990; Australia) [39]	Prospective and single-blind comparative study (124)	5% TTO [1] in gel (61)	5% benzoyl peroxide in lotion (63)	—Severity of acne (counting technique) —(Non-)Inflammatory lesion count —Oiliness, erythema, scaling, pruritus, and dryness —Monitoring ADRs [3]	3 months (baseline and three times with monthly intervals)	—At the baseline, a greater facial erythema assessment was observed in the tea tree oil group compared to the benzoyl peroxide group —At 1, 2, and 3 months, benzoyl peroxide reduced a greater number of inflamed lesions compared to the tea tree oil group; however, the reduction in both groups was significant —There was not a significant reduction in non-inflamed lesions observed in both groups —79% of the benzoyl peroxide group reported ADRs [3], whereas 44% of the tea tree oil group reported ADRs [3] (a significant difference)	—Lack of control or placebo group

Table 1. *Cont.*

Author(s) (Publication Year; Country)	Study Design (n)	Intervention (n)	Control (n)	Outcome Measure(s)	Study Duration (Evaluation Period)	Main Results	Limitations
Ghovvati et al. (2019; Iran) [40]	Open-label, assessor-blind, and uncontrolled clinical trial (20)	0.5% cinnamon in gel (20)	NA	—(Non-)Inflammatory lesion count —Size and quantity of follicular fluorescence spots —Skin biophysical parameters —Monitoring ADRs [3]	45 days (baseline; 4 and 8 weeks)	—ADRs to 1% cinnamon in gel were observed in 6 subjects; therefore, the 0.5% cinnamon in gel was used in this trial —After 8 weeks, significant reductions in the non-inflammatory and inflammatory lesion counts, sebum content, and erythema index were observed compared to the baseline —Non-significant changes were observed for the skin hydration and melanin index —13 patients reported mild burning and 11 patients reported facial redness after using the cinnamon gel	—Lack of comparison to a control, placebo, or standard therapy —Short duration of study and follow-up time —Small sample size —No demographics reported
Talebi et al. (2020; Iran) [41]	Open-label, assessor-blind, and uncontrolled clinical trial (20)	1% (*w*/*w*) ajwain in gel (20)	NA	—Digital and fluorescence photography —Biophysical skin profile measurement (stratum corneum hydration, sebum content, TEWL [5], erythema index, melanin, and pH value) —TLC [4] —VAS [6] —Monitoring ADRs [3]	8 weeks (baseline; 4 and 8 weeks)	—After 8 weeks, a significant reduction in the total lesion count, non-inflammatory lesion count, and a mean decrease in the size and quantity of red spots was observed —After 8 weeks, the decreases in sebum and pH values were significant —No ADRs [3] were reported	—Lack of comparison to a control, placebo or standard therapy —Small sample size

Table 1. *Cont.*

Author(s) (Publication Year; Country)	Study Design (n)	Intervention (n)	Control (n)	Outcome Measure(s)	Study Duration (Evaluation Period)	Main Results	Limitations
Malhi et al. (2017; Australia) [42]	Uncontrolled, dual-center, and open-label phase II pilot study (14)	200 mg/g of TTO [1] gel and 7 mg/g of tea tree face wash (14)	NA	—IGA [7] score —TLC [4] —Skin oiliness —Frequency of ADRs [3] —Mean local tolerability score	12 weeks (baseline; 4, 8, and 12 weeks)	—After 4, 8, and 12 weeks, a significant reduction in the TLC [4], IGA [7] score, and facial oiliness score was observed —Adherence was high, and no serious adverse events were reported	—Lack of comparison to a control, placebo, or standard therapy —Short duration of study and follow-up time —Small sample size
Hassan et al. (2013; Saudi Arabia) [43]	Clinical trial (5)	Eucalyptus oil in cream (5)	NA	—Photographs —Outcomes not defined	10 days (monitored routinely)	—All patients showed good results after the second week of treatment	—Lack of comparison to a control, placebo, or standard therapy —Short duration of study and follow-up time —Small sample size —No specific outcomes reported —No safety assessment
Najafi-Taher et al. (2022; Iran) [44]	Triple-blind and randomized clinical trial (100)	TTO [1] nano-emulsion in adapalene gel (53)	Adapalene gel (47)	—Number of (non-)inflammatory lesions —TLC [4] —ASI [2] —Monitoring ADRs [3]	12 weeks (baseline; 4, 8, and 12 weeks)	—Number of (non-)inflammatory lesions, TLC [4], and ASI [2] showed a greater improvement in the intervention group compared to the positive control —Only mild ADRs [3] were reported in both groups, with dryness being the most common adverse effect	—Lack of comparison to a control or placebo

Table 1. *Cont.*

Author(s) (Publication Year; Country)	Study Design (n)	Intervention (n)	Control (n)	Outcome Measure(s)	Study Duration (Evaluation Period)	Main Results	Limitations
Mazzarello et al. (2018; Italy) [46]	Single-center, randomized, and double-blind comparative study (60)	—Group A: 20% propolis, 3% TTO [1], and 10% *Aloe vera* (PTAC) in cream (20)	—Group B: erythromycin cream (20; positive control) —Group C: vehicle (20; placebo)	—Cutaneous status —Macro-photography —Quantity of sebum —Skin surface pH —Cutaneous erythema index —Number of comedones, papules, and pustules —TLC [4] —ASI [2]	30 days (baseline; 15 and 30 days)	—All the clinical and instrumental values studied were statistically different from the placebo group —The sebometry, pH, and erythema index values were not significantly different statistically during the treatment in the three study groups —The intervention of group A was more effective in reducing ASI [2] and TLC [4] compared to the intervention of group B —The interventions of both groups A and B showed a significant reduction in the number of (non-)inflammatory lesions	—Short duration of study and follow-up time —No safety assessment
Mazzarello et al. (2020; Italy) [47]	Comparative randomized, single-center, and single-blind study (60)	3.74% *Myrtus communis* L. essential oil, 0.1% *Origanum vulgare* essential oil, and 0.025% tretinoin (MOTC) in cream (30)	1% clindamycin and 0.025% tretinoin (CTG) (30; cream)	—Amount of skin sebum, pH, erythema index, and TEWL [5] —Macro-photography —Number of comedones, papules, and pustules —TLC [4] —ASI [2]	30 days (baseline; 15 and 30 days)	—All the instrumental values studied were statistically different between the two groups; however, no sebometry and pH changes were observed in both groups —The MOTC intervention was better than the CTG control in reducing the popular erythema index —In the CTG control group, erythema of the inter-papular healthy skin significantly increases statistically —Both products improved clinical parameters, and no statistically significant differences were detected between the groups	—Lack of comparison to a placebo —Short duration of study and follow-up time —No safety assessment

Table 1. *Cont.*

Author(s) (Publication Year; Country)	Study Design (n)	Intervention (n)	Control (n)	Outcome Measure(s)	Study Duration (Evaluation Period)	Main Results	Limitations
Parveen et al. (2009; India) [48]	Controlled, randomized, and single-blind clinical trial (30)	Unani herbomineral in cream (20)	Vehicle of cream (10)	—IGA [7]	60 days (baseline; 15, 30, 45, and 60 days)	—The IGA [7] means show a very significant difference between the baseline and day 15, day 30, day 40, and day 60 after treatment, whereas very significant differences in the placebo group were observed between the baseline and days 45 and 60 —No significant difference in the IGA [7] was observed between the baseline and days 15 and 30 in the placebo group	—Lack of comparison to a standard therapy —No safety assessment —Low number of outcomes
Kim and Shin (2013; South Korea) [49]	Non-equivalent control group, pretest–post-test design (54)	A basic, weekly acne treatment and a dermal application of a mixture of 3% TTO [1] and 2% lavender oil in jojoba oil as the carrier (27)	Basic, weekly acne treatment (27)	—Acne-related characteristics —Number of P. acnes —Number of human skin pathogens —Number of acne lesions —Sebum secretion rates	4 weeks (baseline and weekly)	—A significant reduction in the total number of P. acnes, the sebum excretion rate, and non-inflammatory skin lesions was observed in the intervention group but not in the control group —The number of human skin pathogens showed no significant difference in both groups —The number of acne lesions was significantly reduced in both groups	—Short duration of study and follow-up time —Small sample size —No safety assessment

Table 1. *Cont.*

Author(s) (Publication Year; Country)	Study Design (n)	Intervention (n)	Control (n)	Outcome Measure(s)	Study Duration (Evaluation Period)	Main Results	Limitations
Orafidiya et al. (2002; Nigeria) [50]	Preliminary clinical tests (126; seven subjects per product)	*Ocimum gratissimum* leaf essential oil preparations (1% *v*/*v* polysorbate 80, cetomacrogol blend, and petrolatum base, or 50% *v*/*v* alcohol) (112)	—Reference: 10% benzoyl peroxide in lotion (7) —Placebo: 40% arachis oil in 1% *v*/*v* polysorbate 80 (7)	—Number of comedones, papules, and pustules (acne lesion count) —Number of days taken to achieve a 50% reduction in lesion count —Skin sensitivity —Patient acceptability —Monitoring ADRs [3]	4 weeks (baseline and weekly)	—The intervention products were significantly more effective in reducing lesions than the placebo —The effect of the reference treatment was gradual over the 9 days, being more pronounced in the later part of the treatment period —A burning sensation was the most reported adverse event within the intervention group —In the placebo group no adverse events were reported	—Short duration of study and follow-up time —Small sample size in the different treatment groups —No demographics reported
Orafidiya et al. (2004; Nigeria) [51]	Preliminary clinical investigation (84; 12 subjects per product)	*Ocimum gratissimum* leaf essential oil preparations (lotion in 25% and 50% of aqueous aloe gel or 100% of aloe gel) (48)	—Reference/positive control: 1% clindamycin solution (12) —Negative control: Neat aloe gel dispersed in 1% polysorbate 80 (12) —Placebo: 40% of arachis oil emulsion in 1% *v*/*v* polysorbate 80 (12)	—Number of comedones, papules, and pustules (acne lesion count) —Number of days taken to achieve a 50% reduction in lesion count —Skin sensitivity —Patient acceptability —Monitoring ADRs [3]	4 weeks (baseline and weekly)	—In the negative control group, minimal activity was observed —A greater reduction in the substant lesion counts was observed in the intervention group compared to the negative and positive control groups —The preparations containing a greater quantity of aloe vera showed greater improved outcomes —Stinging sensation on the skin was the most reported adverse event (96%), which was tolerable —Only mild skin irritation was reported within the intervention group	—Short duration of study and follow-up time —Small sample size in the different treatment groups —No demographics reported

Table 1. *Cont.*

Author(s) (Publication Year; Country)	Study Design (n)	Intervention (n)	Control (n)	Outcome Measure(s)	Study Duration (Evaluation Period)	Main Results	Limitations
Hassoun et al. (2016; United States) [52]	Case study (1)	Cedarwood oil tretinoin cream (1)	NA	NA	4 weeks (baseline and 4 weeks)	—After 4 weeks of treatment, the patients' faces were clear and had rare open and closed comedones on the chest with no papules	—Lack of comparison to a control, placebo, or standard therapy —Combination preparation —Only one case —Retrospective study —Uncontrolled

[1] TTO: tea tree oil. [2] ASI: acne severity index. [3] ADRs: adverse drug reactions. [4] TLC: total lesion count. [5] TEWL: transepidermal water loss. [6] VAS: visual analog scale.
[7] IGA: Investigator's Static Global Assessment. Clinical trial registration numbers: Ref. [37]: NCT01930565 and Ref. [42]: NCT 01657110. NA = not applicable.

Table 2. Characteristics of the products used in the included studies focusing on acne. Details about the composition of the preparations are given in Table S1 (Supplementary Materials).

Author(s) (Publication Year; Country)	Intervention (Origin)	Intervention: Self-Made or Purchased	Control	Control: Self-Made or Purchased	Analyses of the EO-Containing Product
Enshaieh et al. (2007; Iran) [36]	5% TTO [1] gel (*Melaleuca alternifolia*)	Purchased from Cinere Company	Carbomer gel	Purchased from Cinere Company	The component levels were established through gas chromatographic analysis in accordance with the international standard
Kwon et al. (2014; South Korea) [37]	5% *Lactobacillus*-fermented *Chamaecyparis obtusa* (LFCO) cream (fermentation of *C. obtusa* by *Lactobacillus fermentum*)	Manufactured and provided by BST Corporation	5% TTO in cream	Manufactured and provided by BST Corporation	—Bacterial strains and MIC [2] determination —RT-PCR [3] —Ultra-performance liquid chromatography and high-resolution mass spectrometry analysis

Table 2. *Cont.*

Author(s) (Publication Year; Country)	Intervention (Origin)	Intervention: Self-Made or Purchased	Control	Control: Self-Made or Purchased	Analyses of the EO-Containing Product
Da Silva et al. (2012; Brazil) [38]	1% copaiba essential oil (*Copaifera langsdorfii*) in natrozol gel	Self-extracted and self-made	Natrozol gel	Purchased	—Density and phytochemical profile —High-resolution gas chromatography analysis for identification of the EO [4] components
Bassett et al. (1990; Australia) [39]	5% TTO [1] gel (*Melaleuca alternifolia* tree)	Purchased	5% benzoyl peroxide lotion	Purchased	Not conducted
Ghovvati et al. (2019; Iran) [40]	0.5% cinnamon gel (*Cinnamomum verum* bark oil)	Self-conducted extraction and preparation of topical gel	NA	NA	—Evaluation of color, odor, consistency, homogeneity, pH, density, and viscosity —Chemical quantification of the formulation
Talebi et al. (2020; Iran) [41]	1% (*w*/*w*) ajwain gel (*Trachyspermum ammi* (ajwain fruits)	Self-extracted and self-made	NA	NA	—Physicochemical evaluation: stability and viscosity —Gas chromatography analysis for identification of the EO [4] components
Malhi et al. (2017; Australia) [42]	200 mg/g TTO [1] gel and 7 mg/g tea tree face wash (*Melaleuca alternifolia*)	Purchased from Thursday Plantation	NA	NA	—Visual in vitro evaluation of MIC [2] after 48 h of anaerobic incubation (repeated thrice)
Hassan et al. (2013; Saudi Arabia) [43]	Eucalyptus oil (*Eucalyptus amaldulensis*) in cream	Self-mixed all the purchased constituents	NA	NA	Not conducted
Najafi-Taher et al. (2022; Iran) [44]	TTO [1] nano-emulsion (*Melaleuca alternifolia*) containing adapalene gel	Self-made adapalene-loaded TTO [1] nano-emulsion	Adapalene gel	Purchased from Aburaihan pharmaceutical Co.	—Characterization of nano-emulsion: DLS [5] and zeta potential analysis, TEM [6], viscosity, pH, and stability —In vitro: antimicrobial activity —Ex vivo: drug permeation and skin distribution —In vivo: skin irritation, systemic absorption, biochemical parameters, and histopathological analysis

Table 2. *Cont.*

Author(s) (Publication Year; Country)	Intervention (Origin)	Intervention: Self-Made or Purchased	Control	Control: Self-Made or Purchased	Analyses of the EO-Containing Product
Mazzarello et al. (2018; Italy) [46]	—Group A: 20% propolis, 3% TTO [1], and 10% *Aloe vera* (enzymatic hydrolysis of the original plant glycosides, *Melaleuca alternifolia* and *Aloe vera*)	Purchased	—Group B: erythromycin cream (positive control) —Group C: vehicle (placebo)	Purchased by Humana Pharma International Spa	Not conducted
Mazzarello et al. (2020; Italy) [47]	3.74% *Myrtus communis* oil, 0.1% *Origanum vulgare* oil, and 0.025% tretinoin (MOTC)	Self-made	1% clindamycin and 0.025% tretinoin (CTG)	Purchased	—Stability —pH —PET [7] (challenge test) —Susceptible test to different antibiotics
Parveen et al. (2009; India) [48]	Unani herbomineral cream	Self-made	Vehicle cream	Not mentioned	Not conducted
Kim and Shin (2013; South Korea) [49]	A basic, weekly acne treatment and a dermal application of a mixture of 3% TTO [1], 2%lavender oil, and jojoba oil	Unknown (the EOs are permitted by the Korean Food & Drug Administration)	Basic, weekly acne treatment.	Unknown (the acne intervention program was created through collaboration with a dermatologist, a member of the family practice faculty, and an aromatherapist)	Not conducted
Orafidiya et al. (2002; Nigeria) [50]	*Ocimum gratissimum* leaf EO preparations	Purchased	— Reference/positive control: 1% benzoyl peroxide solution	Purchased	Not conducted
Orafidiya et al. (2004; Nigeria) [51]	*Ocimum gratissimum* leaf EO preparations	Purchased	— Reference/positive control: 1% clindamycin solution	Purchased	Not conducted
Hassoun et al. (2016; United States) [52]	Cedarwood oil (from *Juniperus virginiana*) mixed with tretinoin cream	Cedarwood oil was purchased and self-added to the tretinoin cream by the patient	Not conducted	NA	NA

[1] TTO: tea tree oil. [2] MIC: minimum inhibitory concentration. [3] RT-PCR: reverse transcription polymerase chain reaction. [4] EO: essential oil. [5] DLS: dynamic light scattering. [6] TEM: transmission electron microscopy. [7] PET: preservative efficacy testing. NA = not applicable.

2.3. Dermatitis and Eczema

Table 3 gives an overview of the characteristics, main results, and limitations of the included studies focusing on dermatitis and eczema. Table 4 gives an overview of the characteristics of the products used in the included studies focusing on dermatitis and eczema to assess their quality. The studies cover a range of interventions, with TTO, kānuka oil, and mixtures of EOs. The key findings of two case reports include the effectiveness of a mix of several EOs with a base shampoo to treat scalp dermatitis. The TTO gel and kānuka oil cream showed promising results in the subsequent treatment of facial seborrheic dermatitis and eczema, with minimal ADRs. The studies are discussed in order from the highest to lowest power of clinical evidence.

Behehsti Roy et al. aimed to assess the effectiveness of TTO gel in treating mild-to-moderate facial seborrheic dermatitis. The study used a double-blind design with block randomization for treatment allocation involving 54 patients. The results showed a relatively increased improvement in the TTO group, with 39% achieving a total cure after two weeks. No allergic reactions or inflammation were reported. The control and vehicle products were provided by Dr. Jahangir's Company, and the constituents were described in detail without additional analyses [53].

Shortt et al. investigated the use of 3% kānuka oil in an emollient cream base in treating moderate-to-severe eczema with a single-blind randomized controlled trial involving 80 participants. The results showed a significant improvement in the kānuka oil group, as evidenced by lower patient-oriented eczema measure (POEM) scores and a higher proportion of responders. The POEM score is a validated assessment measure derived from patient input and is used for monitoring the severity of atopic eczema. Furthermore, no significant differences in quality of life or safety issues were observed between the groups. In the kānuka oil group, 22 patients (53.7%) reported ADRs versus 15 (38.5%) in the control group. Three ADRs, including one case of transient stinging and two cases of exacerbated eczema, were determined to be related in the kānuka oil group. Two ADRs, both cases of exacerbated eczema, were reported in the vehicle control group. Hikurangi Bioactives Limited Partnership extracted the kānuka oil and Zealand Health Manufacturing compounded it into the study products. Both creams were produced following good nutraceutical manufacturing processes. No additional analyses were conducted, and the constituents were not reported [20].

De Valois reported a case study of a 72-year-old woman with severe scalp eczema experiencing extreme dryness, flaking, and itching. The initial treatments with olive oil and an antifungal shampoo (Nizoral, containing ketoconazole) were ineffective. An EO formula, including TTO, was applied as a shampoo and scalp soak. Over time, her condition improved considerably, with a complete clearance after seven months of daily treatment. The patient's hair grew back, and her scalp returned to a healthy state. No ADRs were reported. The patient herself mixed the purchased EO formulation with the base shampoo and scalp soak [54].

Allan reported a case study of a 38-year-old man with long-standing seborrheic dermatitis on his scalp and face. The conventional medications with hydrocortisone creams provided temporary relief, but the condition returned upon discontinuation. The patient tried anti-dandruff shampoos with limited success. An EO mixture, including geranium, palmarosa, laurel, tansy, and spike lavender, was applied in a shampoo and a cream. Within a few days, the dermatitis disappeared, and the scalp remained clear for several months with some occasional, minimal reoccurrence on the face. Furthermore, no ADRs were reported. A base shampoo and cream were purchased after which the patient mixed them with the EO mixture [55].

Table 3. Characteristics, main results and limitations of the included studies focusing on dermatitis and eczema. Details about the composition of the preparations are given in Table S1 (Supplementary Materials).

Author(s) (Publication Year; Country)	Study Design (n)	Intervention (n)	Control (n)	Outcome Measure(s)	Study Duration (Evaluation Period)	Main Results	Limitations
Behehsti Roy et al. (2014; Iran) [53]	Randomized, vehicle-controlled, double-blind design (54)	5% TTO [1] gel (27)	Vehicle gel (27)	—Severity of seborrheic dermatitis —Extent of itching, erythema, scaling, and greasy crusts score —Patient satisfaction —Monitoring ADRs [2]	4 weeks (baseline; 2 and 4 weeks)	—After 4 weeks, a significant decrease in the values of all parameters in the intervention group was observed, but there was no change in the vehicle group —After 4 weeks of treatment, 91% of the intervention group revealed a total cure —No allergic irritation or inflammation was reported	—Lack of comparison with standard therapy —Small sample size —Short duration
Shortt et al. (2022; New Zealand) [20]	Single-blind, parallel group, superiority, randomized controlled trial, in a community setting (80)	3% kānuka oil in cream (41)	Vehicle cream (39)	—POEM [3] —PO-SCORAD [4] —DLQI [5] —TSQM [6] —Photographs of eczema lesions —Monitoring ADRs [2], compliance, and concomitant medication use	6 weeks (baseline; 6 and 8 weeks)	—The mean POEM [3] showed a statistically significant improvement with a greater degree in the intervention group compared to the control group —More participants in the intervention group experienced a clinically significant improvement of their POEM [3] score compared to the control group —No statistical difference in the PO-SCORAD [4], DLQI [5], and TSQM [6] scores between groups was observed —22 ADRs [2] were reported by the intervention group compared to 15 in the control group (no serious ADRs [2])	—Odor of the intervention might lead to bias —Bias between pharmacists and dermatologists —Short duration

Table 3. *Cont.*

Author(s) (Publication Year; Country)	Study Design (n)	Intervention (n)	Control (n)	Outcome Measure(s)	Study Duration (Evaluation Period)	Main Results	Limitations
De Valois (2004; United Kingdom) [54]	Case study (1)	EO [7] formulation (base shampoo and scalp soak) (1)	NA	NA	7 months (baseline; 2, 3, and 7 months)	—At 2 months, the condition was improved considerably but had not disappeared —At 3 months, continued improvement was observed, but the condition was still lingering —At 7 months, the condition had completely disappeared	—Only one case —Retrospective study —Uncontrolled —Patient was non-adherent and was not applying the intervention as prescribed
Allan (2003; unknown) [55]	Case study (1)	Drops of EO [7] mixture (base shampoo) and a 2% dilution of the EO [7] mixture (aqueous-based cream) (1)	NA	NA	Number of weeks (few days, number of weeks, and number of months)	—Within a few days, the problem had completely gone —After stopping treatment for a number of months, the scalp had remained clear, but within the first weeks a tiny amount of dermatitis would reappear on his face —By using the cream once a week on his face, the areas affected by dermatitis remained clear	—Only one case —Retrospective study —Uncontrolled

[1] TTO: tea tree oil. [2] ADRs: adverse drug reactions. [3] POEM: patient-oriented eczema measure. [4] PO-SCORAD: patient-oriented scoring atopic dermatitis. [5] DLQI: dermatology life quality index. [6] TSQM: treatment satisfaction questionnaire for medication. [7] EO: essential oil. NA = not applicable.

Table 4. Product characteristics of the products used in the included studies focusing on dermatitis and eczema. Details about the composition of the preparations are given in Table S1 (Supplementary Materials).

Author(s) (Publication Year; Country)	Intervention (Origin)	Intervention: Self-Made or Purchased	Control	Control: Self-Made or Purchased	Analyses of the EO-Containing Product
Behehsti Roy et al. (2014; Iran) [53]	5% TTO [1] gel (*Melaleuca alternifolia*)	Purchased from Dr. Jahangir's Company	Vehicle gel	Purchased from Dr. Jahangir's Company	Not conducted
Shortt et al. (2022; New Zealand) [20]	3% kānuka oil cream (*Kunzea ericoides*)	Purchased	Vehicle cream	Not mentioned	Not conducted
De Valois (2004; United Kingdom) [54]	EO [2] formulation with base shampoo and scalp soak	Purchased	NA	NA	Not conducted
Allan (2003; unknown) [55]	Drops of EO [2] mixture, base shampoo, and a 2% dilution of the EO [2] mixture with an aqueous-based cream origin	Patient mixed 2–3 mL base shampoo with four drops of the EO [2] mixture	NA	NA	Not conducted

[1] TTO: tea tree oil. [2] EO: essential oil. NA = not applicable.

2.4. Psoriasis

Table 5 gives an overview of the characteristics, main results, and limitations of the included studies focusing on psoriasis. Table 6 gives an overview of the characteristics of the products used in the included studies focusing on psoriasis to assess their quality. The studies cover a range of interventions, with frankincense oil (from *Boswellia* spp.), Soratinex® products, ChP oleogel, and kānuka oil (from *Kunzea ericoides*). The key findings include improved Psoriasis Area and Severity Index (PASI) scores and other primary outcomes after the treatment with a *Boswellia*-based cream, Soratinex®, and ChP oleogel with a generally mild ADR profile. The studies are discussed in order from the highest to lowest power of clinical evidence.

The double-blind, randomized study conducted by Thomas et al. explored the efficacy of kānuka oil-containing formulations compared to a control formulation for treating psoriasis. The study involved 30 individuals with psoriasis covering up to 10% of the body surface. The patients applied either the test formulation (with kānuka oil) or the control formulation (without kānuka oil) to the affected areas twice daily for 8 weeks. The primary endpoint was the change in the PASI score, and the secondary endpoint was the improvement in pruritus. Both formulations showed significant improvements in the signs of psoriasis and pruritus, with no statistically significant difference between the test and control formulations. Only minor ADRs were observed, including itchiness, after applying the scalp lotion (four subjects; 15.2%). The preparation of the intervention and control products was outsourced, and no additional analyses were conducted [56].

Fadaei et al. evaluated the safety and efficacy of the intervention consisting of a cream combining frankincense oil and ethanolic extract from *Boswelia* spp., with bioactive flavonoids from a licorice root extract (*Glycyrrhiza glabra* aqueous extract) and pumpkin seed oil (*Cucurbita pepo*), while the control group received the vehicle cream for the treatment of plaque psoriasis. A randomized, triple-blind, vehicle-controlled study with 108 participants was conducted. After 4 weeks, the *Boswellia*-based cream group had notable improvements in the scores for the psoriasis area and severity index (PASI), dermatology life quality index (DLQI), body surface area (BSA), and physician's global assessment (PGA) compared to the control group. A significant portion of patients experienced PASI 50 and PASI 75 improvements. In the intervention group, two patients (4.2%) developed skin reactions including rash and severe itching and were withdrawn from the study. No other ADRs were reported. The researchers prepared both the intervention and control products with materials purchased from a local market in Teheran (Iran). Additionally, extensive analyses were conducted including the determination of the pH and the mechanical stability and microbial tests. Lastly, the constituents of each product were described in detail [33].

Kolahdooz et al. evaluated the efficacy of a topical herbal preparation called ChP oleogel on plaque psoriasis. ChP oleogel contains chamomile (*Matricaria recutita*) oil, pumpkin seed oil (*Cucurbita pepo*), and colloidal silicon dioxide. A randomized, intra-patient, double-blind, placebo-controlled trial with 40 patients was conducted. The ChP oleogel demonstrated significant improvements in the PASI, PGA, and patient satisfaction scores compared to the placebo, with minimal ADRs. Three patients (7.5%) reported itching and irritations, which were more severe on the side treated with the ChP oleogel. The intervention and control products were extracted and prepared by the researchers without conducting additional analyses [31].

Hercegova et al. investigated and described the efficacy and safety of Soratinex® skin-care products for the topical treatment of stable chronic plaque psoriasis in a non-controlled pilot study including 286 patients. After 8 weeks, a substantial number of patients had moderate-to-outstanding improvements, with some achieving a complete clearance or significant reductions in lesions. Temporary ADRs were reported including folliculitis (fifteen subjects; 6.0%) and contact dermatitis (seven subjects; 28%). The Soratinex® products were purchased, and no analyses were conducted, whereas the constituents were described in detail [57].

Table 5. Characteristics, main results, and limitations of the included studies focusing on psoriasis. Details about the composition of the preparations are given in Table S1 (Supplementary Materials).

Author(s) (Publication Year; Country)	Study Design (n)	Intervention (n)	Control (n)	Outcome Measure(s)	Study Duration (Evaluation Period)	Main Results	Limitations
Thomas et al. (2015; Australia) [56]	Randomized, active-controlled, double-blind design (30)	20% kānuka oil in ointment and/or scalp lotion (15)	The same as the test formulation, but without the kānuka oil component (15)	—PASI [1] —Pruritus (VAS [2] scoring) —Monitoring ADRs [3]	8 weeks (baseline; 2, 4, and 8 weeks)	—Two individuals from the test group and three from the control group did not respond to the treatment —After 8 weeks, both treatments showed significant improvements and the PASI [1] and VAS [2] scores decreased equally in the test group and control group (no significant difference between the groups) —Individuals treated with the test scalp lotion displayed a statistically comparable improvement rate compared to the control scalp lotion —No serious adverse events were reported; only 4 out of 26 individuals that used the scalp lotion reported itchiness in the beginning of the treatment	—Short-term follow-up —Control medication containing coal tar and salicylic acid —Short duration of the study
Fadaei et al. (2021; Iran) [33]	Randomized, triple-blind, vehicle-controlled, parallel group study (108)	Frankincense oil (plus other constituents) in cream (45)	Vehicle cream (54)	—Photos of skin lesions —Compliance —PASI [1] —PGA [4] —BSA [5] —DLQI [6] —Pruritus severity scale —Patient satisfaction —Monitoring ADRs [3]	4 weeks (baseline; 2 and 4 weeks)	—After 4 weeks of intervention, 53.19% of the patients in the intervention group and 2.44% in the vehicle group achieved a PASI [1] of 50% —Mean DLQI [6], PGA [4], and pruritus scores decreased in both groups over time —Mean BSA [5] score decreased significantly over time in the intervention group but not significantly in the vehicle group —After 4 weeks of intervention, the median patient satisfaction score was significantly higher in the intervention group compared to the vehicle group —2 patients reported skin reactions 24 h after exposure to the intervention	—Lack of comparison with a current topical treatment —Short duration of study and follow-up time

Table 5. *Cont.*

Author(s) (Publication Year; Country)	Study Design (n)	Intervention (n)	Control (n)	Outcome Measure(s)	Study Duration (Evaluation Period)	Main Results	Limitations
Kohladooz et al. (2018; Iran) [31]	Randomized, intra-patient, double-blind, placebo-controlled clinical trial (40)	Chamomile-pumpkin (ChP) in oleogel (40)	Vehicle (40; liquid paraffin)	—Erythema, scaling, and induration severity scores —PSI [7] —PGA [4] —Photographs of the lesions —Patient satisfaction —Monitoring ADRs [3]	4 weeks (baseline and 4 weeks)	—After 4 weeks, the PSI [7] score decline was significantly greater in the intervention group compared to the placebo group —After 4 weeks, the PGA [4] and overall patient satisfaction scores showed a significantly greater improvement in the intervention group compared to the placebo group —3 patients reported itching and irritation, which was more severe in the intervention group	—Lack of comparison with a current topical treatment —Risk of cross-contamination —Short duration of study and follow-up time —Small sample size
Hercegova et al. (2016; Italy) [57]	Non-controlled pilot study (251)	Soratinex® scalp and body cleansing gel; scalp and body ointment and skin conditioner (251)	NA	—PASI [1] —Photography analysis —Monitoring ADRs [3]	8 weeks (2 weeks before treatment; baseline; 1, 2, 4, 6, and 8 weeks)	—After 8 weeks, 13 individuals had no clinical improvements, 46 had a moderate improvement, 77 showed a good improvement, and 115 patients had an outstanding improvement —ADRs [3] were mild and temporary; however, 15 patients reported folliculitis and 7 patients reported contact dermatitis	—Lack of control group —Short duration of study and follow-up time —Small amount of outcome measures
Fioranelli et al. (2016; Italy) [58]	Non-controlled pilot study (26)	Soratinex® scalp and body cleansing gel; scalp and body ointment and skin conditioner (26)	NA	—PASI [1] —Photography analysis —Monitoring ADRs [3]	6 weeks (baseline; 1, 2, 3, 4, and 6 weeks (total time of observation was 8 weeks))	—After 6 weeks, 3 individuals had no clinical improvements, 6 showed a slight improvement, 9 showed a good response, and 5 achieved an excellent improvement —7 patients reported mild and transient itching and 1 patient with scalp psoriasis discontinued treatment because of folliculitis-like inflammation	—Lack of control group —Small sample size —Short duration of study and follow-up time —Small amount of outcome measures

[1] PASI: psoriasis area severity index. [2] VAS: visual analog scale. [3] ADRs: adverse drug reactions. [4] PGA: physician global assessment. [5] BSA: body surface area. [6] DLQI: dermatology life quality index. [7] PSI: psoriasis severity index. NA = not applicable.

Table 6. Product characteristics of the products used in the included studies focusing on psoriasis. Details about the composition of the preparations are given in Table S1 (Supplementary Materials).

Author(s) (Publication Year; Country)	Intervention (Origin)	Intervention: Self-Made or Purchased	Control	Control: Self-Made or Purchased	Analyses of the EO-containing Product
Thomas et al. (2015; Australia) [56]	20% kānuka oil (from *Kunzea ambigua*)	Prepared in the compounding pharmaceutical laboratory of the School of Pharmacy at the University of Tasmania	The same as the test formulation, but without the kānuka oil component	Prepared in the compounding pharmaceutical laboratory of the School of Pharmacy at the University of Tasmania	Not conducted
Fadaei et al. (2021; Iran) [33]	*Boswellia* spp. (the EO of frankincense and an ethanolic extract, the pulp of *Cucurbita pepo*, the and roots of *Glycyrrhiza glabra*)	Self-made (active products purchased from a local market in Teheran)	Vehicle cream	Self-made	—Organoleptic characteristics —Determination of pH —Mechanical stability —Temperature cycle test —Determination of viscosity —Microbial test —Total phenolic contents
Kohladooz et al. (2018; Iran) [31]	Chamomile-pumpkin (ChP) oleogel (*Matricaria chamomilla* and *Cucurbita pepo* seed)	Self-extracted and self-made (standard pumpkin seed oil was purchased from the Giah Essence Phytopharm Co.)	Vehicle (liquid paraffin)	Self-made	Not conducted
Hercegova et al. (2016; Italy) [57]	Soratinex® scalp and body cleansing gel; scalp and body ointment and skin conditioner	Purchased	NA	NA	Not conducted
Fioranelli et al. (2016; Italy) [58]	Soratinex® scalp and body cleansing gel; scalp and body ointment and skin conditioner	Purchased	NA	NA	Not conducted

NA = not applicable.

Fioranelli et al. investigated the efficacy and safety of Soratinex® skincare products in treating chronic plaque psoriasis in a non-controlled pilot study including 30 patients with mild-to-moderate psoriasis vulgaris. Five patients showed no clinical improvement, six had slight improvements, nine had a good response, and five showed an excellent improvement. Mild and transient itching without redness of the skin was reported (26.9%). Furthermore, one patient (3.8%) with scalp psoriasis dropped out due to the development of a folliculitis-like inflammation. The Soratinex® products were purchased, and no analyses were conducted, whereas the constituents were described in detail [58].

2.5. Rosacea

Table 7 gives an overview of the characteristics, main results, and limitations of the included studies focusing on rosacea. Table 8 gives an overview of the characteristics of the products used in the included studies focusing on rosacea to assess their quality.

The study conducted by Ebneyamin et al. aimed to evaluate the effectiveness and safety of a topical gel containing 2.5% of permethrin with TTO (no concentration mentioned) versus a placebo (with a carbomer gel base) in reducing *Demodex* mites and improving clinical symptoms in individuals with rosacea. The study was a randomized, double-blind, placebo-controlled clinical trial and included 47 patients with mild-to-moderate papulopustular rosacea. After five weeks, the test product was more effective than the placebo in reducing the mite density, and, after twelve weeks, the treatment side showed a significant reduction in mite density, as well as an improvement in the papules, pustules, burning, stinging, and dryness. However, no significant changes were observed in plaques, telangiectasia, flushing, or edema. The global assessments by patients and physicians both indicated a better improvement in the permethrin with the TTO group compared to the placebo group. The ADRs included burning, stinging, dryness, erosion, erythema, itching, scaling, and vesiculation, with no major allergic reactions. Nothing was reported about the origin of the intervention and control products, and no additional analyses were conducted [58].

Table 7. Characteristics, main results, and limitations of the included study focusing on rosacea. Details about the composition of the preparation are given in Table S1 (Supplementary Materials).

Author(s) (Publication Year; Country)	Study Design (n)	Intervention (n)	Control (n)	Outcome Measure(s)	Study Duration (Evaluation Period)	Main Results	Limitations
Ebneyamin et al. (2019; Iran) [59]	Randomized, double-blind, placebo-controlled, prospective clinical trial (35)	2.5% TTO [1] in permethrin gel (35)	Vehicle gel (35)	—SSSB [2] (mean Dd/cm^2 [3]) —Erythema, papule and pustules, flushing, telangiectasia, edema, plaque, and stinging were monitored via photographs —Monitoring ADRs [4]	12 weeks (baseline; 2, 5, 8, and 12 weeks)	—After 12 weeks, the mean Dd/cm2 [3] on the treatment side were significantly decreased compared to the placebo side —After 12 weeks, a significant improvement in the papules and pustules, burning, stinging, and dry appearance were observed on the treatment side and not on the placebo side —Plaques, telangiectasia, flushing, and edema did not change on both sides —Mild-to-moderate ADRs [4] were reported by most of the individuals on both sides of their face with skin dryness, erosion, burning, and stinging being prevalent	—Risk of cross-contamination —No demographics reported —Small sample size —No distinction between the effect of permethrin and TTO [1]

[1] TTO: tea tree oil. [2] SSSB: standard skin surface biopsy. [3] Dd/cm^2: Demodex density per cm^2. [4] ADRs: adverse drug reactions.

Table 8. Product characteristics of the product used in the included studies focusing on rosacea. Details about the composition of the preparation are given in Table S1 (Supplementary Materials).

Author(s) (Publication Year; Country)	Intervention (Origin)	Intervention: Self-Made or Purchased	Control	Control: Self-Made or Purchased	Analyses of the EO-Containing Product
Ebneyamin et al. (2019; Iran) [59]	2.5% permethrin with TTO [1] gel (*Melaleuca alternifolia*)	Not mentioned	Vehicle gel	Not mentioned	Not conducted

[1] TTO: tea tree oil.

3. Discussion

3.1. General Aspects

There is a growing interest in the use of topical treatments that are effective, easy to use, and generally have minor ADRs [1]. Therefore, this scoping review provides an extensive overview of the current knowledge regarding the efficacy, safety, product characteristics, and quality of topical treatments containing EOs used in a clinical setting to treat inflammatory skin conditions. The search strategy focused on the four most prevalent inflammatory skin conditions including acne, dermatitis and eczema, psoriasis, and rosacea. Overall, limited clinical studies on the application of EOs in the treatment of inflammatory skin conditions have been performed. Preclinical research on the inflammatory effects of EOs in in vitro models is more abundant [12], supporting the traditional use of EOs in the treatment of inflammatory skin processes and constructing a bridge to studies in humans.

3.2. Tea Tree Oil (TTO)

TTO stands out as the most extensively examined EO from this scoping review. Nine studies investigated the efficacy of treatments with TTO alone or in combination with other constituents to treat acne, dermatitis and eczema, psoriasis, and/or rosacea [36,39,42,44,46,47,49,53,54,59]. TTO is obtained by the steam distillation of the leaves and branches of *Melaleuca alternifolia*, a tree belonging to the Myrtaceae family [7]. The main component of TTO is terpinene-4-ol. *M. alternifolia* exhibits distinct oil chemotypes characterized by varying percentages of terpinen-4-ol, 1,8-cineole, and terpinolene [60]. The in vitro anti-inflammatory, antibacterial, antiviral, and antifungal properties of TTO make it an interesting treatment option for inflammatory skin conditions [12,60]. The antibacterial, antiviral, and antifungal properties have been ascribed to terpinene-4-ol, whereas the anti-inflammatory effect has been attributed to other terpenoids [60].

Comparing the acne-related assessment outcomes after the use of 5% TTO gel with 5% of benzoyl peroxide, a better symptom reduction was found with benzoyl peroxide by comparison [38]. Nevertheless, the TTO gel had substantially fewer ADRs compared to the 5% benzoyl peroxide, and the TTO gel significantly reduced acne-related assessment outcomes compared to the placebo [36,39]. The efficacy of a 5% TTO gel has also been reported for the treatment of facial seborrheic dermatitis by significantly reducing the scores for itching, erythema, scaling, and greasy crusts and the scoring of patient satisfaction, compared to a placebo group and compared to the baseline values [53]. Additionally, a 20% TTO gel and a 0.7% TTO face wash showed a significant reduction in the total lesion count (TLC) and Investigator's Static Global Assessment (IGA) score after 8 weeks, compared to the baseline, demonstrating the efficacy of TTO to treat acne [42].

Furthermore, this present scoping review showed the potential of TTO to enhance the effects of conventional acne treatments such as adapalene gel [44]. This study showed a relatively better improvement in the number of (non-)inflammatory lesions, TLC, and ASI after treatment with a TTO nano-emulsion containing adapalene gel compared to a marketed adapalene gel. Additionally, a combination product containing tea tree, lavender, and jojoba oil was tested to treat acne and a 2.5% permethrin with TTO gel to treat rosacea [49,59]. It remains a challenge however, to differentiate the individual contribution of each constituent in a combination product. The absence in the study design of a focus on the separate effects of each constituent makes it unclear how TTO specifically influences the observed therapeutic effects and ADRs.

Based on the combined results, it seems plausible that patients suffering from ADRs from the standard acne treatment may consider switching to a 5% TTO gel, which is still effective but has fewer ADRs. Additionally, the individuals who experience poor results with a conventional acne treatment may consider enhancing their treatment by combining it with TTO to achieve better outcomes and acceptability.

3.3. Placebo-Controlled Clinical Studies

Six studies were retrieved in this scoping review that solely compared the intervention to a placebo (vehicle) [20,31,33,38,48,56]. Placebo controls are interventions employed in clinical studies that lack the active components of the experimental treatment [61]. Placebos are considered instruments, serving as research tools that help discover the genuine effectiveness and mode of action of 'authentic' medications [62]. The objective of using placebo control interventions is to establish a baseline for evaluating the efficacy of the active interventions, allowing a comparison of their effects [61]. The goal is to have an equitable assessment of the drug's superiority compared to a placebo and of the drug's non-inferiority when compared to another drug [62]. The use of a placebo control product strengthens a clinical trial.

Three studies prepared an EO and other constituents in a hydrophilic cream base [20,33,48]. Although the constituents of the cream base varied between studies, the emollient and moisturizing properties remained consistent. Moreover, an indifferent cream base itself is not expected to elicit ADRs, which makes the safety assessment of the active treatment valid, because any ADRs can be principally attributed to an active ingredient. However, Shortt et al. reported as many as fifteen ADRs after treatment with the placebo cream base in their trial investigating the efficacy of kānuka oil in the treatment of moderate-to-severe eczema, with 80 participants [20]. Since no information regarding the components of the cream base was provided, the cause for the observed ADRs remains undetermined. Shortt et al. attributed the improvement of the disease state in the placebo group to the emollient and moisturizing properties of the cream base. Furthermore, the restoration of the hydration state of the skin to normal was attributed to the cream base [20].

Regarding the effectiveness of the aforementioned EOs in combination with the cream base [20,33,48], a randomized controlled trial using 3% kānuka oil cream to treat eczema showed no significant difference in the Patient Oriented SCOring Atopic Dermatitis (PO-SCORAD), Dermatology Life Quality Index (DLQI), and Treatment Satisfaction Questionnaire for Medication (TSQM) between the intervention and placebo group suggesting that the effect of the 3% kānuka oil was restricted to diminishing the frequency of symptoms, rather than reducing their overall severity [19]. On the contrary, the Unani herbomineral cream (UHC) significantly improved the IGA in acne patients [48].

Additionally, a previous placebo-controlled, double-blind, randomized trial showed that a topical cream based on *Boswellia serrata* oil (frankincense) and an ethanolic extract of Boswellia was an effective anti-inflammatory solution for reducing scales and erythema in psoriatic patients [63]. The oleogum resin, obtained by tapping *Boswellia* trees, is steam distilled, yielding the EO, which is also known as frankincense oil or olibanum. Typically, α-pinene, α-phellandrene, limonene, β-myrcene, β-pinene, p-cymene, and β-caryophyllene are the main constituents [10]. The promising results of a topical cream based on *Boswellia serrata* oil aligns with the findings of a subsequent clinical trial, where a $\geq$50% reduction in the PASI score was seen in 53.19% of patients, and a $\geq$75% reduction in the PASI score was noted in 21.28% of the patients after using the *Boswellia* cream [33]. The frankincense properties can be linked to the active biological compounds of the *Boswellia* cream, including boswellic acids, diterpenoids, and triterpenoids (contained in the ethanolic extract). Furthermore, *Boswellia* cream contained pumpkin oil possessing antiseptic, anti-eczematous, antidermatitic, antitoxic, and antipyretic properties [33]. Boswellic acid has anti-inflammatory properties, but would not be present in the EO because its molecular mass is relatively high.

Another randomized clinical trial retrieved from the search strategy showed the positive effects of a combination of chamomile (*Matricaria chamomilla*) oil with pumpkin (*Cucurbita pepo*) seed oil. A significant enhancement in various psoriasis-related factors was found in comparison to the placebo group, which was treated with liquid paraffin [31]. Bisabolol and chamazulene, the main components of the chamomile EO, possess anti-inflammatory properties [3].

Additionally, two other studies comparing an EO product with a vehicle to investigate the efficacy and safety of the EO product, used natrozol gel and ointment/lotion to treat acne and psoriasis, respectively [38,56]. A highly significant decrease in the extent of the area affected by acne in both the intervention group treated with 1% copaiba EO in natrozol gel and the placebo group treated with only natrozol gel was observed showing the potential to treat mild acne [38]. Copaiba oil is obtained via the hydrodistillation of copaiba balsam, an oleoresin from *Copaifera officinalis*. The EO contains many sesquiterpenes, among which β-caryophyllene is the most abundant [10]. In contrast, the kānuka oil-containing ointment and lotion showed no significant differences after treatment when comparing the control and treatment groups. This aligns with previous studies that have concluded that there is no compelling reason to consider the kānuka oil as an alternative for psoriasis treatment [56]. Kānuka oil comes from the leaves and twigs of *Kunzea ericoides*. It contains monoterpenes with α-pinene, 1,8-cineole, and α-terpineol as main components [10].

3.4. Clinical Studies without Comparison to a Control, Placebo, or Standard Therapy

In this scoping review, seven studies were identified that conducted research without comparison with a control, placebo, or standard therapy, called uncontrolled studies/trials [40,41,43,52,55,57,58,64]. Uncontrolled studies are known for yielding higher mean effect estimates than controlled studies, potentially inflating expectations regarding the intervention. This design carries a risk of inherent bias, and its results are generally considered less reliable than those of randomized controlled studies. Additionally, using this design in cases of spontaneously resolving conditions can further exaggerate the perceived effect [64]. However, uncontrolled studies can give insights into the potential efficacy of a new drug compound.

Of those seven uncontrolled studies, four were specifically centered on treating acne, each employing distinct products [40,41,43,52]. Analyzing the results of the uncontrolled studies, a clinical trial investigated the efficacy and safety of a 1% (*w*/*w*) ajwain gel showed improvements in the acne-related parameters without reported ADRs, possibly indicating the safety of the product. The observed effect can be assigned to the anti-inflammatory, antimicrobial, and anti-oxidant effects of *Trachyspermum ammi* fruits, the origin of ajwain (or ajowan) EO, described in in vitro investigations [41]. Ajwain EO contains p-cymene, γ-terpinene, thymol, and carvacrol as its main constituents [64]. Comparing the 1% ajwain gel with a 0.5% cinnamon bark gel, several distinctions could be observed [40,41]. Cinnamaldehyde is the main constituent of the EO from cinnamon bark [7]. The application of cinnamon gel led to a notable reduction in the size of the fluorescence spots, while ajwain gel was effective in decreasing both the size and the number of these spots. However, the alterations in the skin's biophysical profile following the application of ajwain and cinnamon gel were comparable. Both formulations significantly reduced the non-inflammatory and inflammatory lesion counts, the sebum content, and the erythema index compared to the baseline. Regarding safety, the use of ajwain gel resulted in no (reported) ADRs, while thirteen patients reported mild burning and eleven patients reported facial redness after using the cinnamon gel. Additionally, another uncontrolled trial showed positive results in all patients after the second week of treatment with eucalyptus oil cream in the treatment of acne vulgaris [43]. Although the results of the uncontrolled trial look promising, the study design is unreliable. The trial included only five participants who were observed over ten days, while the primary and/or secondary outcomes were not defined, and no safety assessment was conducted. Comparable limitations exist for the case study that describes the additional value of cedarwood oil combined with tretinoin to treat acne [52]. Therefore, additional research is required to assess the potential of eucalyptus oil and cedarwood oil in the treatment of acne.

Regarding the treatment of stable chronic plaque psoriasis with combination products including EOs (Soratinex®), two uncontrolled pilot studies were conducted in a Hungarian (251 patients) and Polish (30 patients) population [57,58]. Following the treatment period of 6 to 8 weeks, 46% of Hungarian patients and 17% of Polish patients showed a 75–100%

reduction in the PASI scores. However, in both patient populations, mild and temporary itching was reported, with folliculitis proving to be a recurring ADR in both preliminary studies. The combination of different EOs in the Soratinex® products makes it impossible to identify the contribution of individual EOs. Despite this obvious limitation, these studies may serve as the foundation for an extended investigation into these products for the treatment of stable chronic plaque psoriasis, which should involve comparisons with placebos and/or standard therapy, longer study durations, and a broader spectrum of endpoints or outcomes.

Finally, one case study showed the disappearance of the patients' seborrheic dermatitis in a matter of days after being treated with shampoo and an aqueous-based cream containing an EO mixture [55]. While the combination of EOs demonstrates promising effects, a single case retrospectively examined is not conclusive. Therefore, further extensive research is required.

3.5. Clinical Studies with Comparison to Standard Therapy

One study conducted a clinical trial comparing MOTC cream, which served as the intervention, and CTG cream, which acted as the positive control [47]. The MOTC cream contained two EOs: from myrtle (*Myrtus communis*) and from oregano (*Origanum vulgare*); the CTG cream contained 1% clindamycin. Additionally, both creams contained 0.025% tretinoin (a retinoid). Due to the absence of a placebo, this trial can only draw conclusions regarding the efficacy and safety of the intervention compared to the already established treatment (the positive control). Overall, both products improved the clinical parameters at each assessment time, and no statistically significant differences were observed in the inter-group comparison. The MOTC cream proved significantly more effective than the CTG in reducing the papular erythema index. Furthermore, erythema in the healthy inter-papular skin area increased significantly only in the skin treated with the CTG. In conclusion, this clinical trial suggests that MOTC cream holds promise as a potential alternative to antibiotics in formulations with retinoids. However, determining the specific contributions of the two EOs versus the low concentration of tretinoin, or any potential synergistic effects, remains challenging. Furthermore, there were no reference data available because of the absence of a placebo, and the clinical trial's reliance on a small sample size amplified the inter-individual variability.

3.6. Clinical Studies with Comparison to a Placebo, Positive Control, and Negative Control

Orafidiya et al. conducted two consecutive clinical studies [50,51]. The first trial aimed to clinically establish the ideal concentration of African basil (*Ocimum gratissimum*) oil and the most suitable base for the effective treatment of acne vulgaris, comparing it with a reference drug product (clindamycin) and a placebo. The second trial aimed to assess the impact of *Aloe vera* leaf gel on the anti-acne properties of ocimum oil, as well as to compare the effectiveness of both agents individually and in combination with a positive control (1% clindamycin solution), a negative control (neat aloe gel dispersed in 1% polysorbate 80), and a placebo. A negative control outcome is an outcome that exhibits similar potential sources of bias as the primary outcome but lacks a plausible connection to the treatment under investigation. Adding a negative control to the clinical trial serves as an approach to detect and reduce bias [65]. Preparations containing ocimum oil, particularly at concentrations of 2% and 5% in alcohol and in cetomacrogol blend bases, have demonstrated a superior effectiveness and a quicker reduction in lesion counts compared to the positive control. Additionally, a favorable effect of *Aloe vera* leaf gel was found by observing increasing improvements in acne lesions with increasing *Aloe vera* content in the preparations.

3.7. Reported ADRs

Overall, the clinical studies revealed that ADRs were more frequently reported in the group receiving the EO-containing intervention than in the placebo group. However, the number of reported ADRs was higher in patients receiving the standardized (conventional) treatment compared to the EO-containing intervention group. The most reported ADRs, after using an EO-containing gel to treat the acne or rosacea, were dryness of the skin, mild burning, and erythema, which typically disappeared within 30 min after the application [36,37,40,44,50,51]. The clinical studies involving EO-containing products treating psoriasis primarily reported itching and folliculitis as ADRs [31,56–58]. Notably, nine out of the thirty-one studies, including five case studies, did not monitor nor record ADRs, creating a knowledge gap regarding the product's tolerability [38,42,43,46–49,52,54,55]. Furthermore, a few studies mentioned that only minor or no serious ADRs were reported without specifying details [20,33,41,53]. The studies involving TTO products reported ADRs consistent with those reported for the EO products, including dryness, erythema, and a burning sensation [37,39,44,59]. No severe ADRs were reported, and only a small number of patients withdrew from the trial due to ADRs without any improvement of the disease. In conclusion, the EO-containing treatment comes with ADRs, but there is an improvement in tolerability compared to standardized treatments.

3.8. The Quality of the EO Products

Concerning the quality of the EO products, most clinical studies acquired the EO products from commercial sources, while no further quality evaluation analyses were performed [20,36,39,40,43,44,49–52,54,57–59]. Therefore, the identity and quality of these products has not been established and cannot be guaranteed. Nonetheless, it is possible that the authors obtained quality assessments from the manufacturers; however, these were not mentioned. A comparison of the outcomes of repeated studies is therefore difficult or even impossible. Often the authors stated from which manufacturer the EO products were purchased, allowing the possibility of research depending on the transparency of the specific manufacturer. In contrast, six clinical studies prepared the EO products themselves and conducted several analyses to identify the substituents and to control quality and stability [33,38,40,41,44,47]. Additionally, two clinical studies acquired their EO products externally but conducted independent analyses [37,56]. The execution of the analyses with concomitant transparent documentation yields a higher quality of study, because the EO products are well described. Furthermore, in several clinical studies, the EO products were prepared by the investigators, but they did not carry out any subsequent analyses, resulting in uncertainties related to the quality of the final products [31,43,48,55].

What is important for preclinical and clinical research on herbal products and for their use in practice and patient care is their characterization, as well as the quality validation. Unfortunately, these aspects are regularly neglected or underestimated. Missing details about the source material, preparation method, the chemical composition of a product (qualitative and quantitative), its principal constituents, contents, and possible standardization should be considered as a major limitation in the scientific communication, as well as in conveying information about a product to the healthcare provider and the user [3,5,6,9,10,66].

Most EOs are obtained by the hydrodistillation of fresh or dried plant material. This implies that only volatile constituents are found in the product, with limits regarding molecular mass and polarity. The EOs obtained by expression (e.g., from *Citrus* fruits) may contain (furano)coumarines. Also available are extracts produced with non-polar solvents like n-hexane. These products may be marketed as such but are not real EOs (according to the definition). They are actually of a lower quality and are generally cheaper. In general, the production method will strongly influence the composition and quality of the product. In addition, the place where the EO is produced and where the plants were growing (the latitude, soil, sunlight, and rainfall) affect the composition of the EO [3,5,6,9,10,66].

It is very important to know exactly which source and plant species (and part) was used to produce the EO. Possible adulterations and contaminations must be identified to avoid fraud and low quality, as well as toxic products. The identity of the plant species must be determined and confirmed by professionals. This leads to the correct Latin binomial species name and author. Synonyms and homonyms easily lead to confusion.

Finally, mistakes with the source plant may possibly lead to the occurrence of ADRs during use [3,5,6,9,10,66].

The chemical composition of an EO must be reported, at least regarding the main constituents and their contents, as this usually relates to the safety and bioactivity. Gas chromatography (CG-FID) and gas chromatography coupled with mass spectrometry (GC-MS) are common analytical techniques to determine this, combined with a reference library [3,5,6,9,10,66].

For a number of pharmaceutically used EOs, more than one species is allowed according to the monographs of the European Pharmacopoeia (Ph. Eur.) and the European Medicines Agency (EMA) [67]. For instance, Eucalyptus oil (Eucalypti aetheroleum) for application in the therapeutic areas of pain and inflammation and coughs and the cold can be obtained from *Eucalyptus globulus* Labill., *Eucalyptus polybractea* R.T. Baker, and *Eucalyptus smithii* R.T. Baker.

Intraspecies variation may lead to differences in the composition of EOs. Examples of the potential causes for fluctuations are environmental, including the growing conditions, and the development stage of the plant at the time of harvesting. The Ph. Eur. sets the upper and lower limits for a number of the main constituents for EOs, of which a monograph is included. Furthermore, several species of chemotypes exist (e.g., *Thymus vulgaris* ct. geraniol, linalool, thujanol-4, and carvacrol are distinguished), yielding considerably different EO compositions, both regarding the principal constituents and contents. Concomitantly, this may result in different profiles of biological activities [3,5,6,9,10,66].

Finally, analytical data should prove that the EOs were stored properly and that the shelf life was not exceeded. The decomposition of the EO constituents, which are often oxidation products (especially if the EO constituents contain double bonds) under the influence of elevated temperatures and light has been described in the literature [8]. This leads to the inferior quality of a product upon aging and may be the cause of ADRs associated with their use. A well-known example is oxidation products of terpinene-4-ol in improperly stored or old tea tree oil [68].

To guarantee the quality and associated biological activity and safety, it is preferable that pharmaceutical grade EOs (complying to pharmacopoeia requirements) should be used for therapeutic purposes.

3.9. Limitations of the Clinical Studies

As already mentioned, some studies lack the comparison with a placebo and/or standardized treatment. Additionally, in three clinical studies, the patients had to apply the intervention and placebo on two different parts of the body suffering from the disease [31,37,59]. This approach may increase the risk of cross-contamination and confusing the tubes. The advantage is that inter-individual differences are ruled out. Only five clinical studies included 100 or more eligible participants [33,39,44,50,57]. An appropriate large sample size of a clinical trial is necessary to give it statistical power and to detect clinically relevant differences between the intervention and placebo groups. A clinical trial involving a limited number of participants is more susceptible to variability and bears a significant risk of failing to show the effectiveness of a given intervention even when it is genuinely present [69]. Moreover, the duration of the clinical studies ranged from 10 days to 7 months, with the majority lasting between 4 and 8 weeks. A short study duration has the consequence of not examining the longer-term effects and ADRs. Additionally, when an intervention, a placebo, or a positive control requires more time to elicit effects, this may remain unnoticed. On the other hand, shorter trial durations can enhance patient participation, and one could argue whether an intervention that does not yield significant improvements within a few weeks is suitable for clinical practice. The time needed to see an effect of the treatment also concurs with the nature of the ailment that is treated. Finally, for only two studies [37,42] clinical trial registration numbers were retrieved from ClinicalTrials.gov. Although (pre)registration of clinical trials should be common practice nowadays, providing access to information that can be used for further analyses [70], it is known that a substantial portion of trials are published without a registration number [71].

3.10. Strengths and Limitations of this Scoping Review

The main strength of this scoping review is the comprehensive broad overview of the conducted clinical studies with topical treatments containing EOs used for inflammatory skin disease, together with a critical assessment of the information about the characteristics, quality, efficacy, and safety of the EO products used. This targeted approach highlights knowledge gaps and opportunities for further studies, including the need for more research identifying the EO product constituents or enhancing transparency in their reporting. The need for clinical studies with larger sample sizes and extended study durations has become clear from our scoping review. Our work also has several limitations. For example, four eligible articles were excluded because the authors of the current review only had access to a congress abstract providing very limited data. Nonetheless, this information could have provided further insights into the comprehensive picture of EO products. Finally, the data quality obtained from the literature and the databases utilized in this scoping review could be compromised by inconsistencies due to the absence of critical information, such as the origin and quality of the EOs.

3.11. Future Perspectives

This scoping review yielded insights into the future prospects and limitations regarding the utilization of EO-containing products for treating acne, dermatitis and eczema, psoriasis, and/or rosacea. In addition, the protocols of three clinical studies were found to be registered in the Iranian Registry of Clinical Trials [72–74], but the results have not (yet) been published. Taken together, the findings so far indicate that good quality research on pharmaceutical grade EO-containing products remains valuable, with promising results anticipated.

4. Materials and Methods

4.1. Search Strategy

This scoping review was performed following the Preferred Reporting Items for Systematic Reviews and Meta-Analyses (PRISMA) Extensions for Scoping Reviews (PRISMA-Scr) [34]. A systematic search was conducted by using four global electronic databases, PubMed, Embase, the Cochrane Library, and Scopus, from 28 September to 13 October 2023. Clinical studies and case reports investigating the efficacy and safety of EOs used to treat acne, dermatitis and eczema, psoriasis, and/or rosacea were included. Only articles written in Dutch or English, without any publication date limits, were included. The search strategies, individualized for each electronic database, used are provided in Table S2 (Supplementary Materials). This study was registered at the Open Science Framework (OSF), https://osf.io, on 25 January 2024.

4.2. Study Selection

Initially, the title and abstract were screened and studies were considered to be eligible for inclusion if they met one of the following inclusion criteria:

1. Clinical studies, case studies, and randomized controlled studies making use of a product containing an EO or multiple EOs to treat acne, dermatitis and eczema, psoriasis, and/or rosacea.
2. Reported efficacy and safety outcomes after the use of the intervention, control, and/or placebo.

Studies were excluded if they met any of the following exclusion criteria:

1. The studies were conducted with in vitro or in vivo models only.
2. The article was a review or clinical trial protocol.
3. The article's full text was not available.

4. Articles that reported an inflammatory skin condition caused by the use of a product containing an EO.
5. Articles that made use of fixed plant-derived oils (triacyl glycerides) only.

4.3. Data Extraction

The articles were selected and duplicates were removed using the EndNote20 software [75]. Upon the inclusion of the studies in this study, the data were extracted into a Microsoft Word and Excel file. The extracted study characteristics of interest included the following: the study objective, study design, type of intervention, control and/or placebo, number of participants and their demographics, indication, concentration and dosage of the products, primary and secondary outcomes, efficacy and safety results reported, intervention and control constituents, origin, effects, preparation and self-made or purchased, and additional analyses conducted on the intervention and control products.

The data extraction was conducted by a single researcher (A.E.W.K.D.). To decrease the potential for errors and the risk of missing relevant clinical studies, a randomly taken sample of ten included and ten excluded articles was assessed by another researcher (C.E.).

5. Conclusions

This scoping review provides a broad overview of the current knowledge regarding the product characteristics, quality, efficacy, and safety of topical treatments with EOs for inflammatory skin conditions in humans. Overall, the clinical evidence for the efficacy of EOs to treat these conditions is sparse and incommensurate. The clinical studies were classified as limited regarding the sample size and trial duration, while research on the longer-term effects in a broad population is required. Furthermore, most studies did not specify the characteristics of the EO products used, leaving a knowledge gap in the quality of the EO products and their conclusive mode of action. Thus, extended placebo-controlled clinical studies with larger groups of eligible patients and a longer study duration are necessary to assess the promising potential of EO products to treat inflammatory skin conditions.

Supplementary Materials: The following supporting information can be downloaded at https://www.mdpi.com/article/10.3390/ph17050571/s1. Table S1: composition of the preparations as described in the corresponding references; and Table S2: search strategies used for each electronic database.

Author Contributions: Conceptualization, A.E.W.K.D., C.C.M.S.-V., F.P.A.M.v.H., C.E., F.D. and H.J.W.; methodology, A.E.W.K.D., F.P.A.M.v.H. and C.E.; investigation, A.E.W.K.D. and H.J.W.; writing—original draft preparation, A.E.W.K.D. and H.J.W.; writing—review and editing, A.E.W.K.D., C.C.M.S.-V., F.P.A.M.v.H., C.E., F.D. and H.J.W.; and supervision, H.J.W. All authors have read and agreed to the published version of the manuscript.

Funding: This research received no external funding.

Institutional Review Board Statement: Not applicable.

Informed Consent Statement: Not applicable.

Data Availability Statement: Requests to access the datasets may be directed to the first author.

Conflicts of Interest: The authors declare no conflicts of interest.

References

1. Malik, S. *Essential Oil Research: Trends in Biosynthesis, Analytics, Industrial Applications and Biotechnological Production*; Springer: Cham, Switzerland, 2019.
2. Manion, C.R.; Widder, R.M. Essentials of essential oils. *Am. J. Health-Syst. Pharm.* **2017**, *74*, e153–e162. [CrossRef] [PubMed]
3. Price, S.P.; Price, L.; Price, P. *Aromatherapy for Health Professionals*, 5th ed.; Elsevier Limited: Amsterdam, The Netherlands, 2021.
4. Koyama, S.; Heinbockel, T. The effects of essential oils and terpenes in relation to their routes of intake and application. *Int. J. Mol. Sci.* **2020**, *21*, 1558. [CrossRef] [PubMed]

5. Başer, K.H.C.; Buchbauer, G. *Handbook of Essential Oils: Science, Technology, and Applications*, 3rd ed; CRC Press/Taylor & Francis: Boca Raton, FL, USA, 2020.
6. Heinrich, M.B.; Rieto-Garcia, J.; Gibbons, S.; Williamson, E.M. *Fundamentals of Pharmacognosy and Phytotherapy*, 4th ed.; Elsevier Limited: Amsterdam, The Netherlands, 2023.
7. Rhind, J.P. *Essential Oils. A Comprehensive Handbook for Aromatic Therapy*, 3rd ed.; Singing Dragon: London, UK; Philadelphia, PA, USA, 2020.
8. Tisserand, R.; Young, R. *Essential Oil Safety*, 2nd ed.; Churchill Livingstone: Edingburgh, UK, 2014.
9. Başer, K.H.C.; Demirci, F. Chemistry of essential oils. Chapter 4. In *Flavours and Fragrances*; Berger, R.G., Ed.; Springer: Berlin/Heidelberg, Germany, 2007; pp. 43–86. [CrossRef]
10. De Sousa, D.P.; Damasceno, R.O.S.; Amorati, R.; Elshabrawy, H.A.; De Castro, R.D.; Bezerra, D.P.; Nunes, V.R.V.; Gomes, R.C.; Lima, T.C. *Essential oils*: Chemistry and pharmacological activities. *Biomolecules* **2023**, *13*, 1144. [CrossRef] [PubMed]
11. Orchard, A.; Sandasi, M.; Kamatou, G.; Viljoen, A.; Van Vuuren, S. The in vitro antimicrobial activity and chemometric modelling of 59 commercial essential oils against pathogens of dermatological relevance. *Chem. Biodivers.* **2017**, *14*, e16218. [CrossRef] [PubMed]
12. Bungau, A.F.; Radu, A.F.; Bungau, S.G.; Vesa, C.M.; Tit, D.M.; Purza, A.L.; Endres, L.M. Emerging insights into the applicability of essential oils in the management of acne vulgaris. *Molecules* **2023**, *28*, 6395. [CrossRef]
13. Eichenfield, D.Z.; Sprague, J.; Eichenfield, L.F. Management of acne vulgaris: A review. *JAMA* **2021**, *326*, 2055–2067. [CrossRef] [PubMed]
14. Picardo, M.; Eichenfield, L.F.; Tan, J. Acne and rosacea. *Dermatol. Ther.* **2017**, *7* (Suppl. 1), 43–52. [CrossRef] [PubMed]
15. Agnew, T.; Leach, M.; Segal, L. The clinical impact and cost-effectiveness of essential oils and aromatherapy for the treatment of acne vulgaris: A protocol for a randomized controlled trial. *J. Alternat. Complement. Med.* **2014**, *20*, 399–405. [CrossRef]
16. Chovatiya, R. Atopic dermatitis (eczema). *JAMA* **2023**, *329*, 268. [CrossRef]
17. Clark, G.W.; Pope, S.M.; Jaboori, K.A. Diagnosis and treatment of seborrheic dermatitis. *Am. Fam. Physician* **2015**, *91*, 185–190. [PubMed]
18. Naldi, L.; Diphoorn, J. Seborrhoeic dermatitis of the scalp. *BMJ Clin. Evid.* **2015**, *2015*, 1713. [PubMed] [PubMed Central]
19. Jirabundansuk, P.; Ophaswongse, S.; Udompataikul, M. Comparative trial of moisturizer containing spent grain wax, *Butyrospermum parkii* extract, *Argania spinosa* kernel oil vs. 1% hydrocortisone cream in the treatment of childhood atopic dermatitis. *J. Med. Assoc. Thai.* **2014**, *97*, 820–826. [PubMed]
20. Shortt, N.; Martin, A.; Kerse, K.; Shortt, G.; Vakalalabure, I.; Barker, L.; Singer, J.; Black, B.; Liu, A.; Eathorne, A.; et al. Efficacy of a 3% kānuka oil cream for the treatment of moderate-to-severe eczema: A single blind randomised vehicle-controlled trial. *EClinicalMedicine* **2022**, *51*, 101561. [CrossRef]
21. Armstrong, A.W.; Read, C. Pathophysiology, clinical presentation, and treatment of psoriasis: A review. *JAMA* **2020**, *323*, 1945–1960. [CrossRef]
22. Reich, K. Approach to managing patients with nail psoriasis. *J. Eur. Acad. Dermatol. Venereol.* **2009**, *23* (Suppl. 1), 15–21. [CrossRef]
23. Griffiths, C.E.M.; Armstrong, A.W.; Gudjonsson, J.E.; Barker, J. Psoriasis. *Lancet* **2021**, *397*, 1301–1315. [CrossRef]
24. Lee, H.J.; Kim, M. Challenges and future trends in the treatment of psoriasis. *Int. J. Mol. Sci.* **2023**, *24*, 13313. [CrossRef]
25. Two, A.M.; Wu, W.; Gallo, R.L.; Hata, T.R. Rosacea: Part I. Introduction, categorization, histology, pathogenesis, and risk factors. *J. Am. Acad. Dermatol.* **2015**, *72*, 749–758. [CrossRef]
26. Van Zuuren, E.J.; Arents, B.W.M.; Van der Linden, M.M.D.; Vermeulen, S.; Fedorowicz, Z.; Tan, J. Rosacea: New concepts in classification and treatment. *Am. J. Clin. Dermatol.* **2021**, *22*, 457–465. [CrossRef]
27. Searle, T.; Al-Niaimi, F.; Ali, F.R. Rosacea. *Br. J. Hosp. Med.* **2021**, *82*, 1–8. [CrossRef]
28. Ahn, C.S.; Huang, W.W. Rosacea pathogenesis. *Dermatol. Clin.* **2018**, *36*, 81–86. [CrossRef] [PubMed]
29. Zhao, H.; Ren, S.; Yang, H.; Tang, S.; Guo, C.; Liu, M.; Tao, Q.; Ming, T.; Xu, H. *Peppermint* essential oil: Its phytochemistry, biological activity, pharmacological effect and application. *Biomed. Pharmacother.* **2022**, *154*, 113559. [CrossRef] [PubMed]
30. Rai, V.K.; Sinha, P.; Yadav, K.S.; Shukla, A.; Saxena, A.; Bawankule, D.U.; Tandon, S.; Khan, F.; Chanotiya, C.S.; Yadav, N.P. Anti-psoriatic effect of *Lavandula angustifolia* essential oil and its major components linalool and linalyl acetate. *J. Ethnopharmacol.* **2020**, *261*, 113127. [CrossRef] [PubMed]
31. Kolahdooz, S.; Karimi, M.; Esmaili, N.; Zargaran, A.; Kordafshari, G.; Mozafari, N.; Hossein Ayati, M. Evaluation of the efficacy of a topical chamomile-pumpkin oleogel for the treatment of plaque psoriasis: An intra-patient, double-blind, randomized clinical trial. *Biomed. Res. Ther.* **2018**, *5*, 2811–2819. [CrossRef]
32. Lin, Y.K.; See, L.C.; Huang, Y.H.; Chang, Y.C.; Tsou, T.C.; Lin, T.Y.; Lin, N.L. Efficacy and safety of indigo naturalis extract in oil (Lindioil) in treating nail psoriasis: A randomized, observer-blind, vehicle-controlled trial. *Phytomedicine* **2014**, *21*, 1015–1020. [CrossRef]
33. Fadaei, F.; Ayati, M.H.; Firooz, A.; Younespour, S.; Abouali, M.; Tabarrai, M.; Shirbeigi, L. Efficacy of a topical herbal cream containing frankincense oil, pumpkin oil and licorice aqueous extract in patients with mild-to-moderate plaque psoriasis: A randomized clinical trial. *Res. J. Pharmacogn* **2022**, *9*, 89–101. [CrossRef]
34. Shamseer, L.; Moher, D.; Clarke, M.; Ghersi, D.; Liberati, A.; Petticrew, M.; Shekelle, P.; Stewart, L.A.; PRISMA-P Group. Preferred reporting items for systematic review and meta-analysis protocols (PRISMA-P) 2015: Elaboration and explanation. *BMJ* **2015**, *350*, g7647. [CrossRef] [PubMed]

35. *ISO 4730:2017*; Essential oil of Melaleuca, Terpinen-4-ol Type (Tea Tree Oil). International Organization for Standardization (ISO): Geneva, Switzerland, 2017.
36. Enshaieh, S.; Jooya, A.; Siadat, A.H.; Iraji, F. The efficacy of 5% topical tea tree oil gel in mild to moderate acne vulgaris: A randomized, double-blind placebo-controlled study. *Ind. J. Dermatol Venereol. Leprol.* **2007**, *73*, 22–25. [CrossRef] [PubMed]
37. Kwon, H.H.; Yoon, J.Y.; Park, S.Y.; Min, S.; Suh, D.H. Comparison of clinical and histological effects between lactobacillus-fermented *Chamaecyparis obtusa* and tea tree oil for the treatment of acne: An eight-week double-blind randomized controlled split-face study. *Dermatology* **2014**, *229*, 102–109. [CrossRef]
38. Da Silva, A.G.; Puziol Pde, F.; Leitao, R.N.; Gomes, T.R.; Scherer, R.; Martins, M.L.; Cavalcanti, A.S.; Cavalcanti, L.C. Application of the essential oil from copaiba (*Copaifera langsdori* Desf.) for acne vulgaris: A double-blind, placebo-controlled clinical trial. *Altern. Med. Rev.* **2012**, *17*, 69–75. [PubMed]
39. Bassett, I.B.; Pannowitz, D.L.; Barnetson, R.S. A comparative study of tea-tree oil versus benzoylperoxide in the treatment of acne. *Med. J. Australia* **1990**, *153*, 455–458. [CrossRef] [PubMed]
40. Ghovvati, M.; Afshari, G.K.; Nasrollahi, S.A.; Firooz, A.; Samadi, A.; Karimi, M.; Talebi, Z.; Kolahdooz, S.; Vazirian, M. Efficacy of topical cinnamon gel for the treatment of facial acne vulgaris: A preliminary study. *Biomed. Res. Ther.* **2019**, *6*, 2958–2965. [CrossRef]
41. Talebi, Z.; Afshari, G.K.; Nasrollahi, S.A.; Firooz, A.; Ghovvati, M.; Samadi, A.; Karimi, M.; Kolahdooz, S.; Vazirian, M. Potential of *Trachyspermum ammi* (Ajwain) gel for treatment of facial acne vulgaris: A pilot study with skin biophysical profile assessment and red fluorescence photography. *Res. J. Pharmacogn.* **2020**, *7*, 61–69. [CrossRef]
42. Malhi, H.K.; Tu, J.; Riley, T.V.; Kumarasinghe, S.P.; Hammer, K.A. Tea tree oil gel for mild to moderate acne; a 12 week uncontrolled, open-label phase II pilot study. *Australas. J. Dermatol.* **2017**, *58*, 205–210. [CrossRef] [PubMed]
43. Hassan, K.A.M.; Eltayb, N. Eucalyptus oil as a treatment for acne. *Pharmanest* **2013**, *4*, 557–566.
44. Najafi-Taher, R.; Jafarzadeh Kohneloo, A.; Eslami Farsani, V.; Mehdizade Rayeni, N.; Moghimi, H.R.; Ehsani, A.; Amani, A. A topical gel of tea tree oil nanoemulsion containing adapalene versus adapalene marketed gel in patients with acne vulgaris: A randomized clinical trial. *Arch. Dermatol. Res.* **2022**, *314*, 673–679. [CrossRef] [PubMed]
45. Najafi-Taher, R.; Ghaemi, B.; Amani, A. Delivery of adapalene using a novel topical gel based on tea tree oil nano-emulsion: Permeation, antibacterial and safety assessments. *Eur. J. Pharm. Sci.* **2018**, *120*, 142–151. [CrossRef] [PubMed]
46. Mazzarello, V.; Donadu, M.G.; Ferrari, M.; Piga, G.; Usai, D.; Zanetti, S.; Sotgiu, M.A. Treatment of acne with a combination of propolis, tea tree oil, and *Aloe vera* compared to erythromycin cream: Two double-blind investigations. *Clin. Pharmacol.* **2018**, *10*, 175–181. [CrossRef] [PubMed]
47. Mazzarello, V.; Gavini, E.; Rassu, G.; Donadu, M.G.; Usai, D.; Piu, G.; Pomponi, V.; Sucato, F.; Zanetti, S.; Montesu, M.A. Clinical assessment of new topical cream containing two essential oils combined with tretinoin in the treatment of acne. *Clin. Cosmet. Investigat. Dermatol.* **2020**, *13*, 233–239. [CrossRef] [PubMed]
48. Parveen, S.; Zafar, S.; Qureshi, M.; Bano, H. Clinical trial of Unani herbomineral cream to evaluate its topical effects on acne vulgaris. *Ind. J. Tradit. Knowl.* **2009**, *8*, 431–436.
49. Kim, B.Y.; Shin, B.S. Antimicrobial and improvement effects of tea tree and lavender oils on acne lesions. *J. Converg. Informat. Technol.* **2013**, *8*, 339–345.
50. Orafidiya, L.O.; Agbani, E.O.; Oyedele, A.O.; Babalola, O.O.; Onayemi, O. Preliminary clinical tests on topical preparations of *Ocimum gratissimum* Linn leaf essential oil for the treatment of acne vulgaris. *Clin. Drug Investig.* **2002**, *22*, 313–319. [CrossRef]
51. Orafidiya, L.O.; Agbani, E.O.; Oyedele, A.O.; Babalola, O.O.; Onayemi, O.; Aiyedun, F.F. The effect of aloe vera gel on the anti-acne properties of the essential oil of *Ocimum gratissimum* Linn leaf—A preliminary clinical investigation. *Int. J. Aromather.* **2004**, *14*, 15–21. [CrossRef]
52. Hassoun, L.A.; Ornelas, J.N.; Sivamani, R.K. Cedarwood oil as complementary treatment in refractory acne. *J. Alternat. Complement. Med.* **2016**, *22*, 252–253. [CrossRef] [PubMed]
53. Beheshti Roy, A.; Tavakoli-Far, B.; Fallah Huseini, H.; Tousi, P.; Shafigh, N.; Rahimzadeh, M. Efficacy of *Melaleuca alternifolia* essential oil in the treatment of facial seborrheic dermatitis: A double-blind, randomized, placebo-controlled clinical trial. *J. Med. Plants* **2014**, *13*, 26–32.
54. De Valois, B. Using essential oils to treat scalp eczema. *Int. J.Aromather.* **2004**, *14*, 45–47. [CrossRef]
55. Allan, R. Seborrhoeic dermatitis. *Int. J. Aromather.* **2003**, *13*, 47–48. [CrossRef]
56. Thomas, J.; Narkowicz, C.K.; Jacobson, G.A.; Peterson, G.M. Safety and efficacy of kunzea oil-containing formulations for the management of psoriasis: A randomized, controlled trial. *J. Clin. Pharm. Ther.* **2015**, *40*, 566–572. [CrossRef] [PubMed]
57. Hercogova, J.; Fioranelli, M.; Gianfaldoni, S.; Chokoeva, A.A.; Tchernev, G.; Wollina, U.; Tirant, M.; Novotny, F.; Roccia, M.G.; Maximov, G.K.; et al. Dr Michaels® (Soratinex®) product for the topical treatment of psoriasis: A Hungarian/Czech and Slovak study. *J. Biol. Reg. Homeostat. Agents* **2016**, *30*, 43–47.
58. Fioranelli, M.; Gianfaldoni, H.J.S.; Chokoeva, A.; Tchernev, G.; Wollina, U.; Tirant, M.; Novotni, F.; Roccia, M.G.; Maximov, G.K.; França, K. Clinical evaluation of the effectiveness of Dr Michaels® (also branded as Soratinex®) products in the topical treatment of patients with plaque psoriasis. *J Biol. Reg. Homeostat. Agents* **2016**, *30*, 29–34.
59. Ebneyamin, E.; Mansouri, P.; Rajabi, M.; Qomi, M.; Asgharian, R.; Azizian, Z. The efficacy and safety of permethrin 2.5% with tea tree oil gel on rosacea treatment: A double-blind, controlled clinical trial. *J. Cosmet. Dermatol.* **2019**, *19*, 1426–1431. [CrossRef]

60. Nascimento, T.; Gomes, D.; Simoes, R.; Maria Da Graca, M. Tea tree oil: Properties and the therapeutic approach to acne—A review. *Antioxidants* **2023**, *12*, 1264. [CrossRef]
61. Howick, J.; Hoffmann, T. How placebo characteristics can influence estimates of intervention effects in trials. *CMAJ* **2018**, *190*, E908–E911. [CrossRef]
62. Barrett, J.E.; Page, C.P.; Michel, M.C. *Concepts and Principles of Pharmacology—100 Years of the Handbook of Experimental Pharmacology*; Springer Nature: Cham, Switzerland, 2019.
63. Togni, S.; Maramaldi, G.; Di Pierro, F.; Biondi, M. A cosmeceutical formulation based on boswellic acids for the treatment of erythematous eczema and psoriasis. *Clin. Cosmet. Investigat. Dermatol.* **2014**, *7*, 321–327. [CrossRef]
64. Nair, B. Clinical trial designs. *Ind. Dermatol. Online J.* **2019**, *10*, 193–201. [CrossRef]
65. Arnold, B.F.; Ercumen, A. Negative control outcomes: A tool to detect bias in randomized trials. *JAMA* **2016**, *316*, 2597–2598. [CrossRef]
66. Sticher, O.; Heilmann, J.; Zündorf, I. *Hänsel/Sticher Pharmakognosie Phytopharmazie*, 10th ed.; Wissenschaftliche Verlagsgesellschaft: Stuttgart, Germany, 2015.
67. European Medicines Agency (EMA). *Community Herbal Monograph on Eucalyptus Globulus Labill., Eucalyptus Polybractea R.T. Baker and/or Eucalyptus Smithii R.T. Baker, Aetheroleum*; EMA: Amsterdam, The Netherlands, 2014. Available online: https://www.ema.europa.eu/en/documents/herbal-monograph/final-community-herbal-monograph-eucalyptus-globulus-labill-eucalyptus-polybractea-rt-baker-andor-eucalyptus-smithii-rt-baker-aetheroleum_en.pdf (accessed on 28 March 2024).
68. Bekhof, A.S.M.W.; Van Hunsel, F.P.A.M.; Van de Koppel, S.; Woerdenbag, H.J. Safety assessment and adverse drug reaction reporting of tea tree oil (*Melaleuca aetheroleum*). *Phytother. Res.* **2023**, *37*, 1309–1318. [CrossRef]
69. Evans, C.H.; Ildstad, S.T. *Institute of Medicine (US) Committee on Strategies for Small-Number-Participant Clinical Research Trials*; National Academies Press: Washington, DC, USA, 2001.
70. Tse, T.; Fain, K.M.; Zarin, D.A. How to avoid common problems when using ClinicalTrials.gov in research: 10 issues to consider. *BMJ* **2018**, *361*, k1452. [CrossRef]
71. Van de Wetering, F.T.; Scholten, R.J.P.M.; Haring, T.; Clarke, M.; Hooft, L. Trial registration numbers are underreported in biomedical publications. *PLoS ONE* **2012**, *7*, e49599. [CrossRef]
72. Saeedi, M. Effect of Lavander Essential Oil in Comparison with Tretinoin on Acne. Trial Registry Record 22 February 2018. Available online: https://trialsearch.who.int/Trial2.aspx?TrialID=IRCT2014072110203N3 (accessed on 2 April 2024).
73. Rashidipour, M. Compare the Effectiveness of Betamethasone and Lavender and Peppermint in Reducing the Severity of Symptoms in Patients with Eczema and Psoriasis. Trial Registry Record 17 August 2020. Available online: https://trialsearch.who.int/Trial2.aspx?TrialID=IRCT20100420003760N4 (accessed on 2 April 2024).
74. Soltani, R. Evaluation of the Effectiveness of *Berberis integerrima* and Thyme Essential Oil in the Treatment of Acne. Trial Registry Record 29 November 2021. Available online: https://trialsearch.who.int/Trial2.aspx?TrialID=IRCT20150721023282N21 (accessed on 2 April 2024).
75. The EndNote Team. *EndNote, Version EndNote X9*; Clarivate: Philadelphia, PA, USA, 2013.

pharmaceuticals

Review

Unveiling the Potential of *Ent*-Kaurane Diterpenoids: Multifaceted Natural Products for Drug Discovery

Shadrack Kibet [1,2], Njogu M. Kimani [1,3,*], Syombua S. Mwanza [1,2], Cynthia M. Mudalungu [2,4], Cleydson B. R. Santos [5,6] and Chrysantus M. Tanga [2,*]

1 Department of Physical Sciences, University of Embu, Embu P.O. Box 6-60100, Kenya; skibet@icipe.org (S.K.); smwanza@icipe.org (S.S.M.)
2 International Centre of Insects Physiology and Ecology, Nairobi P.O. Box 30772-00100, Kenya; cmudalungu@icipe.org
3 Natural Product Chemistry and Computational Drug Discovery Laboratory, Embu P.O. Box 6-60100, Kenya
4 School of Chemistry and Material Science, The Technical University of Kenya, Nairobi P.O. Box 52428-00200, Kenya
5 Graduate Program in Medicinal Chemistry and Molecular Modelling, Health Science Institute, Federal University of Pará, Belém 66075-110, Brazil; breno@unifap.br
6 Laboratory of Modelling and Computational Chemistry, Department of Biological and Health Sciences, Federal University of Amapá, Macapá 68902-280, Brazil
* Correspondence: njogu.mark@embuni.ac.ke (N.M.K.); ctanga@icipe.org (C.M.T.); Tel.: +254-728132596 (N.M.K.); +254-702729931 (C.M.T.)

Abstract: Natural products hold immense potential for drug discovery, yet many remain unexplored in vast libraries and databases. In an attempt to fill this gap and meet the growing demand for effective drugs, this study delves into the promising world of *ent*-kaurane diterpenoids, a class of natural products with huge therapeutic potential. With a dataset of 570 *ent*-kaurane diterpenoids obtained from the literature, we conducted an in silico analysis, evaluating their physicochemical, pharmacokinetic, and toxicological properties with a focus on their therapeutic implications. Notably, these natural compounds exhibit drug-like properties, aligning closely with those of FDA-approved drugs, indicating a high potential for drug development. The ranges of the physicochemical parameters were as follows: molecular weights—288.47 to 626.82 g/mol; number of heavy atoms—21 to 44; the number of hydrogen bond donors and acceptors—0 to 8 and 1 to 11, respectively; the number of rotatable bonds—0 to 11; fraction Csp3—0.65 to 1; and TPSA—20.23 to 189.53 Å^2. Additionally, the majority of these molecules display favorable safety profiles, with only 0.70%, 1.40%, 0.70%, and 46.49% exhibiting mutagenic, tumorigenic, reproduction-enhancing, and irritant properties, respectively. Importantly, *ent*-kaurane diterpenoids exhibit promising biopharmaceutical properties. Their average lipophilicity is optimal for drug absorption, while over 99% are water-soluble, facilitating delivery. Further, 96.5% and 28.20% of these molecules exhibited intestinal and brain bioavailability, expanding their therapeutic reach. The predicted pharmacological activities of these compounds encompass a diverse range, including anticancer, immunosuppressant, chemoprotective, anti-hepatic, hepatoprotectant, anti-inflammation, antihyperthyroidism, and anti-hepatitis activities. This multi-targeted profile highlights *ent*-kaurane diterpenoids as highly promising candidates for further drug discovery endeavors.

Keywords: *ent*-kauranes; natural products; diterpenoids; ADMET properties; drug-likeness; pharmacokinetics

Citation: Kibet, S.; Kimani, N.M.; Mwanza, S.S.; Mudalungu, C.M.; Santos, C.B.R.; Tanga, C.M. Unveiling the Potential of *Ent*-Kaurane Diterpenoids: Multifaceted Natural Products for Drug Discovery. *Pharmaceuticals* **2024**, *17*, 510. https://doi.org/10.3390/ph17040510

Academic Editors: Catherine Sherwin, Elena Y. Enioutina and Kathleen M. Job

Received: 15 March 2024
Revised: 29 March 2024
Accepted: 2 April 2024
Published: 16 April 2024

1. Introduction

Natural products have for a long time been used as nutraceuticals [1–3]. The search for natural products continues to grow due to their unique and vast chemical and biological properties. These properties have been subjected to natural selection and evolutionary processes, shaping their utility over hundreds of thousands of years. Consequently, they display a great variety of biological and therapeutic potentials spanning anti-tumor, antimicrobial, antiviral, antitripanosomal, α-Glucosidase inhibitory activity, and immunosuppressive actions to the inhibition of vascular smooth muscle contraction [4–12]. More than one-third of the drugs so far approved by the United States' Food and Drug Administration (FDA) are either derived from natural product precursors or are purely natural products [13–15].

Many of the natural products with therapeutic potential have been isolated from various sources. Nonetheless, their progression towards clinical utilization has often been met by significant impediments, attributable to multifaceted obstacles. These challenges include stringent regulatory guidelines governing experimental tests, especially when dealing with human subjects [16]. The conventional process of drug development is also laborious and financially stretched. For instance, a single drug requires 8–12 years of research and approximately USD 2.7 billion to be developed [17]. However, there is a very high attrition and failure rate (80–90%) of potential drugs in drug discovery pipelines, leading to huge financial losses [18]. To circumvent these, several in silico approaches have been brought upfront to determine the drug-likeness of a molecule. These approaches have linked the reduced likelihood of attrition of a potential drug to the control of physicochemical and ADMET properties [19–25].

In the existing libraries of natural products, there is proof that resources and labor-intensive approaches have been employed to isolate and characterize bioactive compounds [26]. Some of these compounds possess several bioactivities [27–29] and yet are relegated to natural product databases because of the high possibility of their failures if pursued in the classical drug discovery pipelines. Previous in silico studies on compounds isolated from diverse genera have shown that these compounds have great potential but are underexplored [30–32]. One particular class of vastly bioactive set of compounds that have been isolated from a diverse source is the *ent*-kaurane diterpenoids.

Ent-kaurane diterpenoids are an important class of natural products derived majorly from *Jungermania* species of liverworts and higher plants of the genus Isodon [5–7,33,34] in addition to other minor sources such as corn silk [35] and genus Chelonopsis [9]. Structurally, these molecules are constituted by a perhydrophenanthrene subunit (rings A, B and C) and a cyclopentane, ring D. *Ent*-kauranes differ from kauranes by the inversion of carbon configurations at C-5, C-9, and C-10 [36].

Their history dates back to the year 1961 after the discovery of *ent*-kaurene from the leaf essential oil of the New Zealand kauri [5]. These biomolecules have been reported to cause cell cycle arrest and apoptosis while exhibiting moderate-to-low toxicities on normal cell lines. Therefore, they have been the center of focus in the continuous search for active biomolecules. The objective of this study was to review the existing literature on *ent*-kaurane diterpenoids with a focus on phytochemistry. Further, the study involves an extensive investigation using in silico approaches to evaluate the compounds' drug-like properties, with specificity on absorptivity, distribution, metabolism, excretion, and toxicity (ADMET). Additionally, bioactivity scores, biological potentials, and macromolecular targets of a selected subset are determined in silico.

2. Results

2.1. Bioactivity of Ent-Kaurane Diterpenoids

This review utilized a dataset of 570 *ent*-kaurane diterpenoids accessed from the literature (Supplementary Information S1). These molecules have diverse bioactivities including anti-cancer and the inhibition of NO production (Figure 1, Supplementary Information S2 and S3). Figure 1 presents the number of molecules demonstrating different bioactivities, expressed as a percentage of the total molecules ($n = 570$).

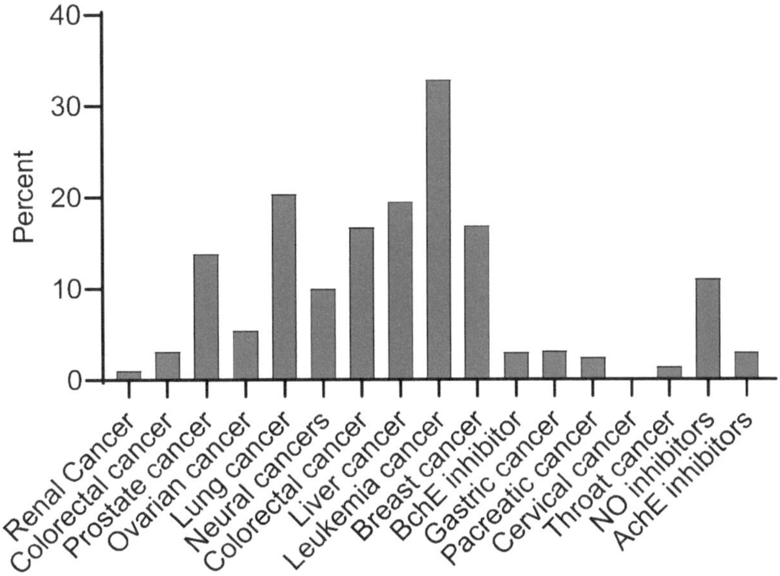

Figure 1. A bar graph showing the percentage of molecules exhibiting various bioactivities.

2.2. Physicochemical Properties of Ent-Kaurane Diterpenoids

The physicochemical properties were similar to those of FDA-approved drugs, as shown by the scatter plot in Figure 2. The considered properties included the molecular weights, the number of heavy atoms, the number of aromatic heavy atoms, fraction Csp3, the number of rotatable bonds, the number of hydrogen bond acceptors and donors, topological polar surface (TPSA), and molar refractivity (MR). Based on this initial screening, the distribution of the physicochemical parameters of the *ent*-kaurane diterpenoids (blue colored data points) was within the chemical spaces of the FDA-approved drugs (red colored data points).

To gain a more detailed understanding of the distribution of these physicochemical properties of *ent*-kaurane diterpenoids, individual physicochemical parameters were analyzed. The molecular weights varied from 288.47 to 626.82 g/mol. The median molecular weight was 366.45, whereas the mean was 382.72 g/mol (Figure 3a). In contrast, the FDA-approved drugs utilized for comparison had molecular weights varying from 60.06 to 972.66, a median of 278.32, and a mean of 302.30 (Figure 3b). The mean tally of heavy atoms among the scrutinized *ent*-kaurane diterpenoids stood at 27.37, exhibiting a notable diversity, and the minimum number of heavy atoms was 21, while the maximum number of heavy atoms was 44 (Figure 3c). The FDA-approved drugs used for comparison, on the other hand, displayed an average number of heavy atoms of 20.99, spanning from 3 to 68 (Figure 3d).

The mean tally of the number of hydrogen bond donors was 2.54 while that of FDA-approved drugs was 1.24 (Figure 3g,h). It is worth noting that some FDA-approved drugs exhibited anomalously higher quantum of hydrogen bond donors, reaching a zenith of 13 in comparison to the maximum value of 8 recorded for the sampled *ent*-kauranes. The number of hydrogen bond acceptors for the examined *ent*-kaurane diterpenoids displayed a range of 1 to 11 (Figure 3e) while that of FDA-approved drugs exhibited a broader range of 0 to 19 (Figure 3f). The mean number of hydrogen bond acceptors was 5.50, while that of FDA-approved drugs was 4.26, and the median values for *ent*-kauranes and FDA-approved drugs were 6 and 4, respectively. The number of rotatable bonds exhibited a span of 0 to a maximum of 11, with an average of 2.06 and a median of 2 (Figure 3i). On the other hand, among the FDA-approved drugs, the range extended from 0 to 24, with an average of 4.71

and a median of 4 (Figure 3j). The variation in fraction Csp3 values among the scrutinized *ent*-kaurane diterpenoids and FDA-endorsed pharmaceuticals exhibited extensive ranges, i.e., 0.65 to 1 (Figure 3k) and 0.00 to 1 (Figure 3l), respectively. The mean of this parameter for the surveyed *ent*-kaurane diterpenoids was 0.84, in stark contrast to the value of 0.41 for FDA-approved drugs. The median fraction Csp3 value observed for the sampled *ent*-kaurane diterpenoids was notably elevated at 0.85, compared to the corresponding value of 0.38 delineated for FDA-approved drugs. The mean TPSA observed among the sampled *ent*-kaurane diterpenoids in this study was 91.19 Å^2, whereas the corresponding TPSA value for FDA-approved drugs was slightly lower at 76.65 Å^2. The ranges were recorded at 20.23 to 189.53 Å^2 for *ent*-kauranes (Figure 3m) and 0 to 379.82 Å^2 for FDA-approved drugs (Figure 3n). The median TPSA values were 94.06 Å^2 for *ent*-kauranes and 67.40 Å^2 for FDA-approved drugs.

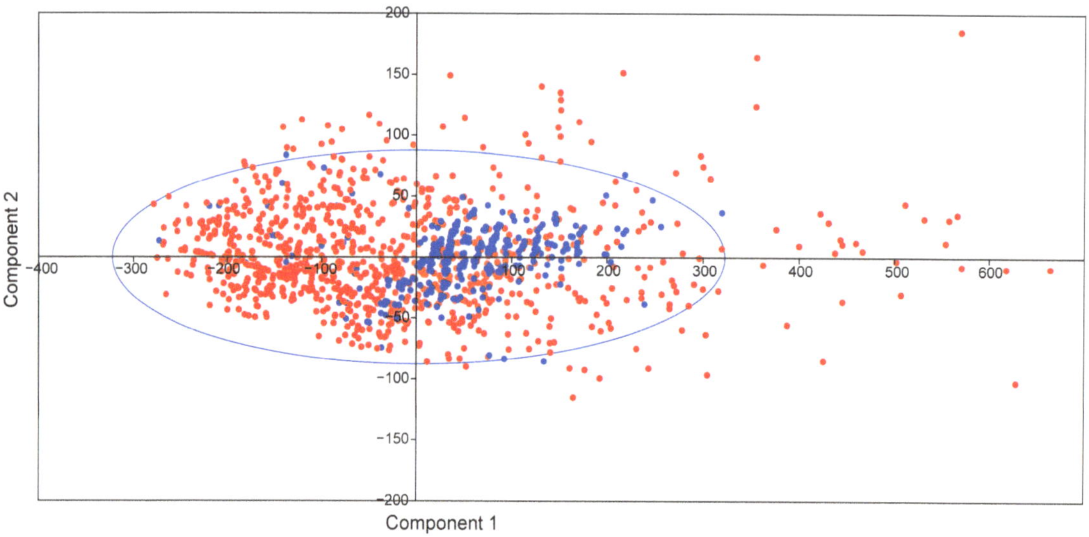

Figure 2. The scatter (PCA) representation of the physicochemical parameters of *ent*-kaurane diterpenoids (blue-colored data points) in comparison to the FDA-approved drugs (red-colored data points).

2.3. Lipophilicity and Water Solubility of Ent-Kaurane Diterpenoids

The lipophilicity values spanned from −1.09 to a maximum of 7.58 with an average of 2.21. The distribution plot (Figure 4a) shows that most of these compounds possessed lipophilicities of ≤5, whereas water solubilities ranged from −10.44 to −0.4300 with an average of −3.46 according to the Ali approach. According to ESOL and SILICOS-IT approaches, the ranges were −8.85 to −2.01 and −7.77 to 0.86, and the means were −3.29 and −2.81, respectively (Figure 4b).

2.4. Pharmacokinetic Properties

Of the sampled molecules, 96.5% had high gastro-intestinal (GI) absorption, whereas the remaining subset was classified to possess low GI absorption. Only 28.20% of the molecules were predicted as blood–brain barrier (BBB) permeant. A majority of these molecules, i.e., 86.34%, were flagged as P-glycoprotein (P-gp) substrates. Further, a bigger subset did not inhibit the CYP1A2, CYP2C19, CYP2C9, CYP2D6, and CYP3A4 isoforms (Figure 5).

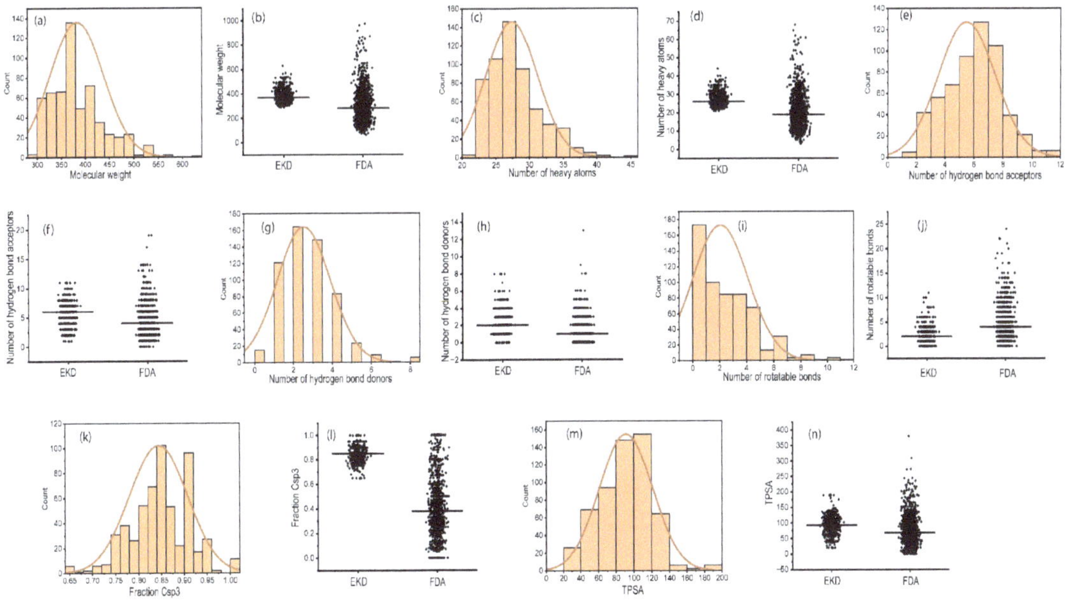

Figure 3. (**a**,**c**,**e**,**g**,**i**,**k**,**m**) Distribution plots showing a characteristic distribution of various physicochemical properties of sampled *ent*-kaurane diterpenoids. (**b**,**d**,**f**,**h**,**j**,**l**,**n**) Data distribution plots of various physicochemical properties of *ent*-kaurane diterpenoids in comparison to those of FDA-approved drugs.

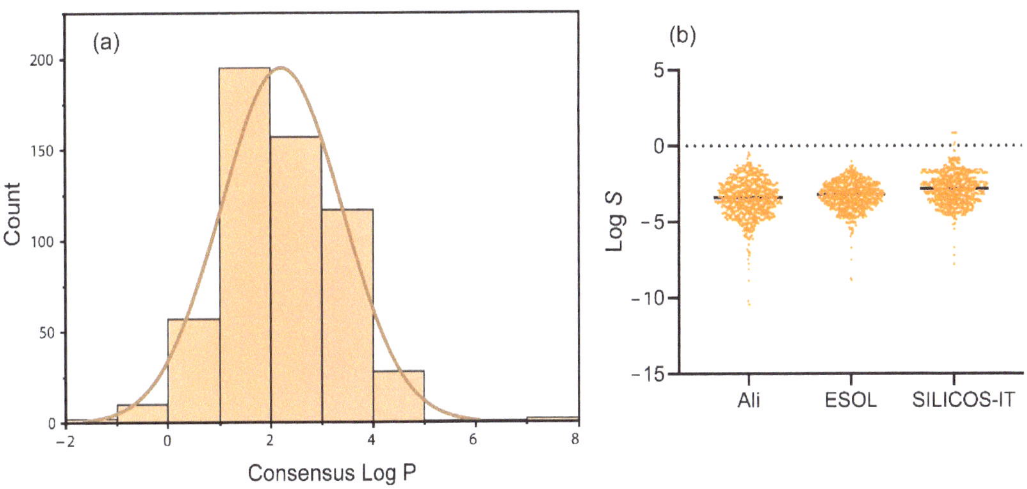

Figure 4. The lipophilicities (**a**) and water solubilities (**b**) of *ent*-kaurane diterpenoids.

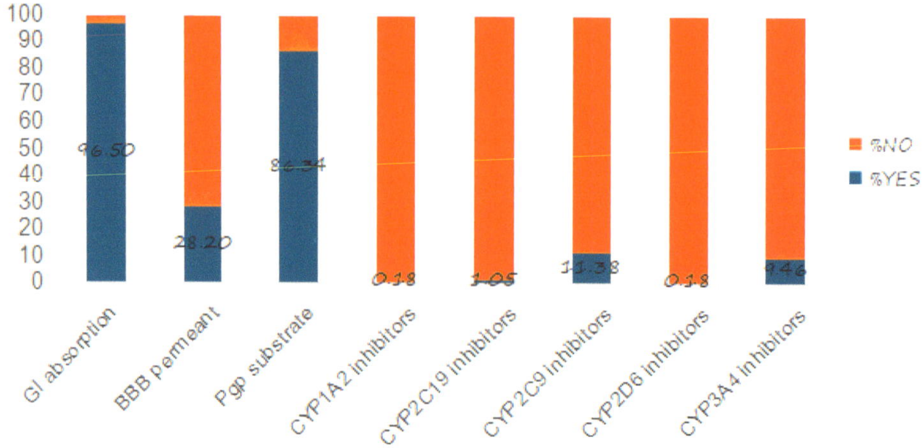

Figure 5. Stacked percentage column graph showing different pharmacokinetic properties of *ent*-kaurane diterpenoids.

2.5. Toxicological Properties

The findings (Figure 6a) showed that the majority of the sampled compounds, accounting for 99.12%, do not exhibit mutagenic properties. A small fraction, constituting 0.70% of the compounds, was identified as highly mutagenic, while a further 0.18% exhibited low mutagenicity. In terms of tumorigenicity, 98.42% of the compounds displayed no tumorigenic potential, while 1.4% and 0.18% of the compounds exhibited high and low tumorigenic potentials, respectively. The determination of the reproductive effects revealed that 92.28% of the compounds have no discernible impact on reproduction, whereas 7.02% and 0.70% of the compounds were associated with low and high reproductive effects, respectively. Investigation of irritant properties revealed that a significant subset, 46.49% of the compounds, displayed high irritant properties, while the other subset was either devoid of irritant properties (52.36%) or had low irritant properties (1.05%).

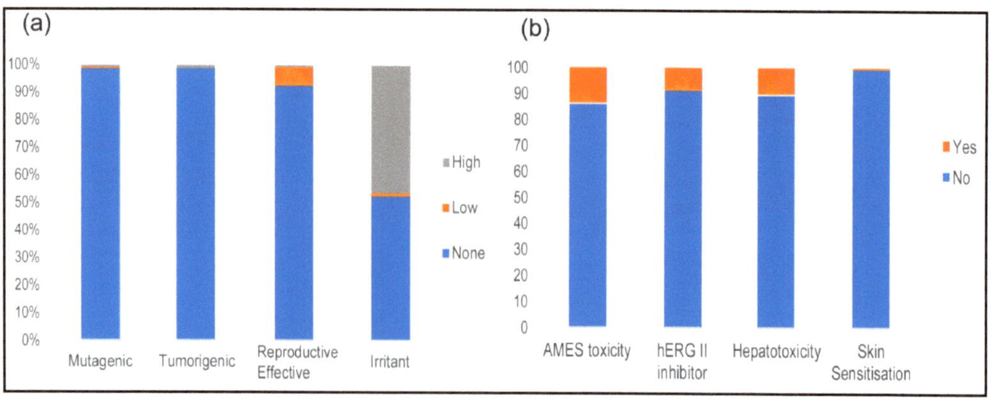

Figure 6. The toxicological properties of *ent*-kaurane diterpenoids: (**a**) stacked bar graphs showing the percent of mutagenic, tumorigenic, reproduction-enhancing, and irritant molecules determined using the DataWarrior and (**b**) stacked bar graphs showing the AMES toxicity, hERG II inhibition, hepatotoxicity, and skin sensitization properties determined using pKCSM.

AMES, hERG II inhibition, and hepatotoxicity determination using pKCSM revealed that a significant portion of these molecules are not toxic. Only 13.87%, 8.77%, 10.18%, and 0.35% were, in this respective order, flagged as AMES toxic, hERG II inhibitors, hepatotoxic, and skin sensitizers (Figure 6b). Not a single molecule was flagged as an hERG I inhibitor.

2.6. Synthetic Accessibility, PAINS, BRENK, and Lead-likeness

The synthetic accessibility scores for most of the studied *ent*-kauranes ranged from 5.0 to 7.5 (Figure 7a). Not a single *ent*-kaurane studied was flagged as PAINS. Approximately 64% of the examined compounds displayed a single BRENK alert, indicating the presence of a fragment possibly associated with unfavorable characteristics. Furthermore, about 5% of the molecules had two BRENK alerts and about 2% of the molecules had three BRENK alerts, suggesting a higher level of complexity in terms of potential undesired attributes. As shown in Figure 7b, about 74% of the studied *ent*-kauranes violated one rule of lead-likeness and about 5% violated two rules and about 1% violated three rules.

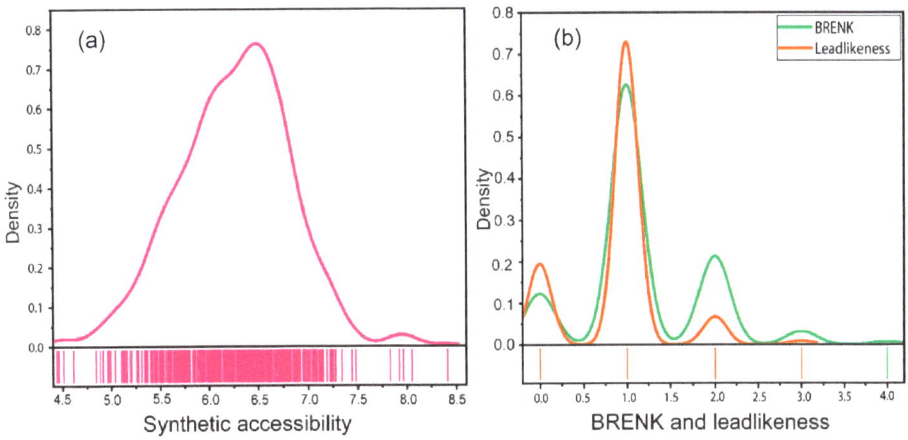

Figure 7. The distribution and rug plots showing the medicinal chemistry properties of *ent*-kaurane diterpenoids: (**a**) the synthetic accessibility and (**b**) BRENK and lead-likeness.

2.7. Bioactivity Scores and Macromolecular Targets of Selected Molecules

Six *ent*-kaurane diterpenoid molecules were selected for further investigation based on their adherence to drug-likeness criteria, specifically, the absence of any violations and demonstrated non-toxicity. These were 11β-hydroxy-*ent*-16-kauren-15-one (23) isolated from Jungermania tetragona, 16R-3α,11β-dihydroxy-ent-9(11)-kauren-15-one (87) and 16S-3α,11β-dihydroxy-*ent*-9(11)-kauren-15-one (88) isolated from *Jungermania* sp., *Ent*-7α-acetoxy-16β,18-dihydroxy-kaurane (219) isolated from *Sideris congesta*, Coetsanoic acid (332) isolated from *Isodon albopilosus*, and acid (545) isolated from *Siegesbeckia pubescens* (Figure 8).

As shown in Table 1, these molecules showed activity for the GPCR ligands and as ion channel modulators, nuclear receptor ligands, protease inhibitors, and enzyme inhibitors, and moderate activity as kinase inhibitors.

The further prediction of pharmacological activities of these representative molecules using PASS online revealed that *ent*-kaurane diterpenoids have immense potential biological activities including antineoplastic, antileukemic, apoptosis induction, immunosuppressant, chemoprotective, anti-hepatic, and hepatoprotectant activities, among others (Table 2).

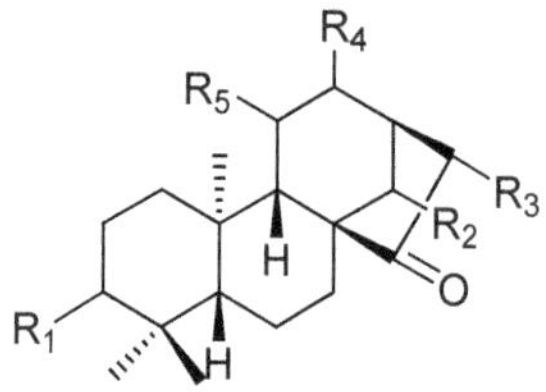

	R_1	R_2	R_3	R_4	R_5
23.	ß-OH	H	ß-Me	H	ß-OH
87.	a-OH	H	a-Me	H	ß-OH
88.	ß-OH	H	a-Me	H	ß-OH
332.	H	ß-OH	ß-OH	a-OH	H

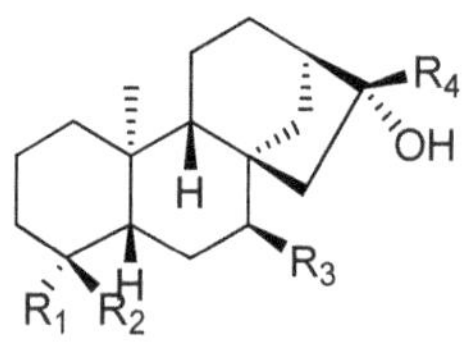

	R_1	R_2	R_3	R_4
219.	Me	MeOH	ß-OAC	Me
545.	COOH	Me	H	MeOH

Figure 8. Selected drug-like *ent*-kaurane diterpenoids.

Table 1. Bioactivity scores of drug-like *ent*-kaurane diterpenoid compounds against targets.

S/N	Compound	GPCR Ligand	Ion Channel Modulator	Kinase Inhibitor	Nuclear Receptor Ligand	Protease Inhibitor	Enzyme Inhibitor
1	23	0.43	0.36	−0.42	0.72	0.28	0.69
2	87	0.43	0.36	−0.42	0.72	0.28	0.69
3	88	0.43	0.36	−0.42	0.72	0.28	0.69
4	219	0.28	0.25	−0.23	0.79	0.31	0.53
5	332	0.19	0.19	−0.18	0.64	0.21	0.57
6	545	0.37	0.20	−0.19	0.62	0.20	0.53

Table 2. Probability of pharmacological activity of the selected *ent*-kaurane diterpenoids.

Activity	Probability of Pharmacological Activity (Pa)			
	Compounds 23, 87, and 88	Compound 219	Compound 332	Compound 545
Antineoplastic	0.946	0.957	0.969	0.712
Acylcarnitine hydrolase inhibitor	0.888	0.845	0.863	NA
Testosterone 17beta-dehydrogenase (NADP+) inhibitor	0.874	0.827	0.846	0.780
Apoptosis agonist	0.836	0.729	0.735	NA
Alkylacetylglycerophosphatase inhibitor	0.824	0.757	0.785	NA
Alkenylglycerophosphocholine hydrolase inhibitor	0.824	0.746	0.782	0.780
CYP2J substrate	0.815	0.832	0.849	0.702
Phosphatase inhibitor	0.780	NA	NA	NA
Antineoplastic (lung cancer)	0.777	0.858	0.899	NA
Caspase 8 stimulant	0.754	0.701	0.723	0.761
Oxidoreductase inhibitor	0.754	NA	NA	NA
Antinociceptive	0.742	NA	NA	NA
Caspase 3 stimulant	0.746	NA	NA	NA
Transcription factor NF kappa B stimulant	0.738	0.713	0.725	0.746
Transcription factor stimulant	0.738	0.713	0.725	0.746
Polarization stimulant	0.732	0.748	NA	NA
Antileukemic	0.731	NA	0.759	NA
CYP3A4 inducer	0.733	NA	NA	NA
Gluconate 2-dehydrogenase (acceptor) inhibitor	0.750	0.763	NA	NA
CYP2J2 substrate	0.740	NA	NA	NA
CYP3A inducer	0.720	NA	NA	NA
Myc inhibitor	0.711	NA	NA	NA
Glyceryl-ether monooxygenase inhibitor	0.711	NA	NA	NA
Immunosuppressant	0.701	NA	NA	NA
Antineoplastic (breast cancer)	NA	NA	0.740	NA
DNA polymerase I inhibitor	NA	NA	NA	0.716
Chemoprotective	NA	NA	NA	0.879
Hepatoprotectant	NA	NA	NA	0.879
Hepatic disorder treatment	NA	NA	NA	0.942

Values are Pa scores, while NA represents not active (Pa < 0.7).

Macromolecular target prediction using the SwissTargetPrediction indicated that these molecules could also target enzymes associated with metabolic diseases (HSD11B1), could be aromatase inhibitors (CYP19A1), and exhibited anti-hepatitis and antihyperthyroidism (SHBG) activities, among others (Figure 9).

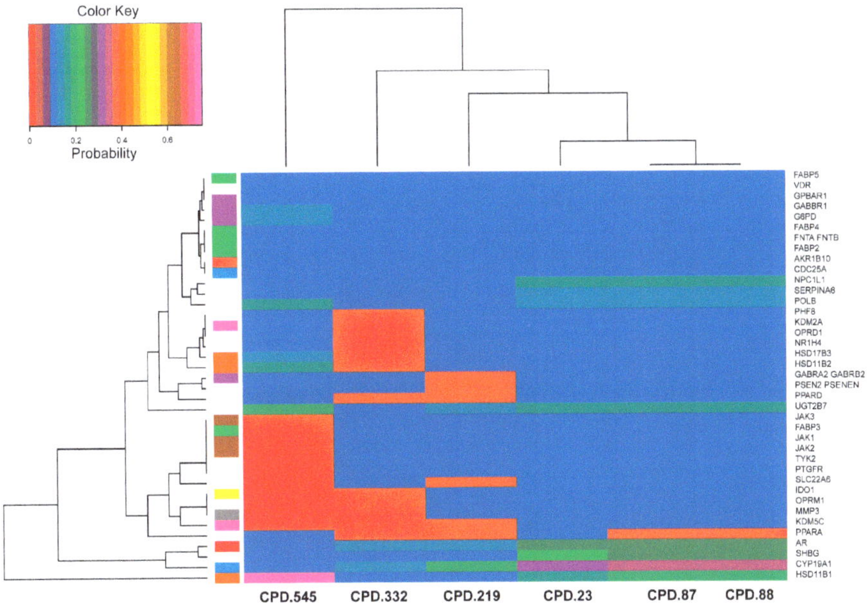

Figure 9. A heat map showing the macromolecular targets of selected *ent*-kaurane diterpenoids.

3. Discussion

3.1. Sources and Bioactivity of Ent-Kaurane Diterpenoids

The genesis of discovery of *ent*-kaurane diterpenoids can be traced back to the year 1961, when *ent*-kaurene was isolated from the leaf essential oil of *Agathis,* commonly known as the New Zealand Kauri pine [5]. This molecule was assigned the name "*ent*-kaurene" due to its negative optical rotation and enantiomeric nature, with "*ent*" denoting its enantiomeric status. Since then, a vast number of *ent*-kauranes with diverse bioactivities have been isolated and characterized, predominantly derived from plants of the *Isodon* family among the higher plants and also the *Jungermania* species of liverworts [5,37]. Synthetically and semi-synthetically, various other *ent*-kaurane diterpenoids have been accessed [38–41].

Biologically, a relatively higher number of sampled molecules have activities against leukemia and lung cancer, suggesting a potentially higher responsiveness of these cancer types to this class of molecules. Bioactivities against NO production and AchE and BchE inhibition were also found to be prevalent, further asserting the versatility and wider spectrum of bioactivities of this class of molecules. The widely accepted mechanism of action of these diterpenoids is the Michael addition of soft nucleophiles such as thiols and protein sulfihydryl (SH) groups onto the α,β-unsaturated ketone moiety, leading to the deactivation of SH enzymes or SH coenzymes and the accumulation of Reactive Oxygen Species (ROS) [37,42]. The deactivation of SH enzymes or SH coenzymes causes the retardation of intracellular redox homeostasis, while the accumulation of ROS, on the other hand, leads to apoptosis since high levels of ROS cause oxidative damage to tumor cells [37]. However, it is important to note that the bioactivity results presented are based on in vitro tests and translating these findings into effective and safe treatments for human use requires in-depth, laborious, and resource-intensive research, necessitating the use of computational chemistry as a filtration step. Further, these in vitro tests are often targeted to few specific targets, and this calls for polypharmacology prognostication. However, the pharmacological potential of a molecule is affected by several factors including physicochemical, pharmacokinetic, and toxicological properties.

3.2. Physicochemical Properties

Molecular weight is an important physicochemical parameter that is considered in drug discovery as it directly affects the diffusion of molecules across cell membranes [43]. The Lipinski tenet, positing that an ideal molecular weight for effective absorption and distribution of a biomolecule should fall below 500 g/mol, serves as a foundational principle in drug designing [19]. Most *ent*-kauranes studied complied with this tenet, boasting molecular weights below 500 g/mol. However, a subset of these molecules deviated from this requirement, surpassing the mark. Notably, quite a number of FDA-approved drugs, a benchmark of pharmaceutical excellence, surpassed this mark by a bigger margin (max = 972.66 g/mol) as compared to the *ent*-kaurane diterpenoids (max = 626.82 g/mol). This divergence of FDA-approved drugs from Lipinski's prescribed limit of molecular weight, yet being bioavailable molecules, suggests a multifaceted interplay with other molecular parameters. This beckons the need to unravel other complexities underlying successful drug absorption and distribution beyond the canons of Lipinski.

The number of heavy atoms refers to the collective count of non-hydrogen atoms within the chemical structure of a molecule. They typically include carbon, nitrogen, oxygen, sulfur, and other elements within the higher atomic masses. This physicochemical parameter wields a direct influence on ligand efficiency (LE), a metric calculated by dividing the binding free energy by the count of heavy atoms [44]. The relationship between ligand efficiency and drug potency is that ligand efficiency is a measurement of the binding energy per atom of a ligand to its binding partner such as an enzyme or receptor proteins, and therefore, a heightened LE postulates an elevated drug potency [44]. Based on the means, this study elicited that the sampled *ent*-kaurane diterpenoids generally had a higher number of heavy atoms than the FDA-approved drugs. However, certain FDA-approved drugs surpassed the heavy atom count of some sampled *ent*-kaurane diterpenoids, peaking at 68. This observation suggests that *ent*-kaurane diterpenoids, akin to FDA-approved therapeutics, could exhibit commendable ligand efficiencies if progressed towards drug development.

The quantitation of the numbers of hydrogen bond donors and acceptors stands as a pivotal physicochemical parameter in the prognostication of the oral bioavailability of a drug candidate [45]. By virtue of the influence of these parameters on the mechanisms of passive diffusion across cell membranes, they hold a discernible impact on the processes of adsorption and distribution of pharmaceutical agents. According to the tenets of Lipinski and Veber, a favorable number of hydrogen bond donors is not more than five, and the violation of this rule may indicate potential issues with bioavailability [19,46]. Some *ent*-kaurane diterpenoids sampled for this study violated this rule, and similar violations were also observed for chemotherapeutics already approved by the FDA. This underscores the fact that intricacies of drug development extend beyond the confines of a single parameter, and that those *ent*-kaurane diterpenoids violating this criterion should not be swiftly dismissed as they might harbor latent bioactivities. Alex et al. [47] highlights that more hydrogen bond donors than acceptors may engender deleterious effects on the intricate equilibrium of the drug's membrane partitioning and permeability. However, this requisite is just a factor to consider in drug designing, and as such, several drugs violating this criterion are in the market such as acetaminophen, ibuprofen, aspirin, caffeine [48], and morphine [49].

The number of rotatable bonds assume a pivotal role in influencing biochemical and physicochemical characteristics of a therapeutic molecule. An excess of the number of rotatable bonds, above a threshold of nine, culminates in compromised oral bioavailability due to hindered diffusion through cell membranes [50,51]. This, in turn, often leads to diminished binding efficiency with the intended target, thereby undermining therapeutic potency. As outlined by Bryant et al. [52], molecules characterized by excessive flexibility may not conform to the criteria of drug-likeness. In this study, a substantial proportion of the investigated *ent*-kaurane diterpenoids exhibited a tally of rotatable bonds below the threshold of nine. Nonetheless, it is worth pointing out that a subset of these molecules displayed counts exceeding nine. However, within the domain of FDA-approved drugs, certain drugs showcased counts of rotatable bonds as high as 24, and yet they were qualified as potent therapeutics.

Fraction Csp3 is the ratio of sp^3-hybridized carbons to the total carbon count of the molecule. This physicochemical parameter determines the carbon saturation of a molecule and characterizes the spatial structure of molecules. The empirical evidence showcases that the heightened saturation as quantified by the fraction of carbon atoms with sp^3 hybridization (Csp3) correlates with an augmented rate of favorable clinical outcomes of pharmaceutical agents. This is because highly saturated molecules are more likely to be metabolized and eliminated from the body [53]. This phenomenon is conceivably associated with an elevation in solubility properties, and it has actually been previously used as a solubility predictor [54]. A suitable value of this physicochemical parameter for a drug-like molecule should be at least 0.42; however, just about 82% of marketed drugs meet this criterion [53]. The results emanating from this study impart a noteworthy implication that the assessed *ent*-kaurane diterpenoids exhibited a discernibly heightened state of saturation as opposed to the already approved drugs by the FDA. Evidently, in light of the stipulated threshold criterion (fraction Csp3 of ≥ 0.42), a considerably large number of the investigated *ent*-kaurane diterpenoids presented superior solubility and consequently superior drug-like properties in contrast to the majority of FDA-approved drugs.

The Topological Polar Surface Area (TPSA) of a molecule is defined as the sum of the contributions to the molecular surface area of polar atoms such as nitrogen, oxygen, and their attached hydrogens. This parameter has been shown to have a strong positive correlation with passive molecular transport through membranes and is advantageous as it does not require the generation of 3D structures [55]. It estimates the ability of a drug-like molecule to permeate cell membranes, and consequently, it has been used to study the intestinal absorption and blood–brain barrier penetration of therapeutic molecules [56]. As noted by Verber et al. [46], the TPSA of a suitable drug should be less than 140 Å^2. A bigger subset of sampled *ent*-kaurane diterpenoids possessed a figure lower than 140 Å^2, implying that this subset could be bioavailable. Remarkably, certain FDA-approved pharmaceutical agents exhibited TPSA values exceeding 140 Å^2, thereby contravening the established criterion (TPSA < 140 Å^2). This observation implies that solely relying on the TPSA metric might not be definitive for disqualifying prospective therapeutic agents, and that other parameters ought to be considered.

3.3. Lipophilicity and Water Solubilities

The lipophilicity and water solubility influences the bioavailability of a drug candidate. Lipophilicity, i.e., the *n*-octanol/water partition coefficient ($\log P_{o/w}$), is a measure of a compound's capacity to dissolve in fats or lipids. This parameter wields significant control over molecular transportation across membranes, impacts binding to plasma proteins and target receptors, and thus serves as a cornerstone for predicting the biological efficacy of potential drugs. It is generally believed that drug molecules must be generally lipophilic to have good absorption [57]; however, the optimal lipophilicity for a drug-like molecule depends on the intended use and the target protein [58]. A compound that is too lipophilic may have poor solubility and bioavailability, while a compound that is too hydrophilic may have poor membrane permeability [59]. Lipophilicity exceeding five is often linked with undesired drug characteristics including limited water solubility, tissue accumulation, rapid metabolic turnover, and strong plasma protein binding [60–62]. Moreover, the literature indicates that compounds with moderate lipophilicity, oscillating around two, often show optimal abilities to reach molecular targets [60]. The mean of lipophilicities of the *ent*-kaurane diterpenoids studied was 2.21, suggesting that these compounds display promise as prospective candidates for drug design and research.

To predict water solubility, SwissADME incorporates two topological approaches, i.e., the ESOL model [63] and the Ali model [64], and one fragmental approach developed by SILICOS-IT. However, the Ali model has a stronger positive correlation for the predicted water solubility with the experimental water solubility of a compound (R^2 = 0.81), as compared to SILICOS-IT (R^2 = 0.75) and the ESOL model (R^2 = 0.69) [50]. Based on the solubility classification criteria provided by Daina et al. [50], i.e., insoluble $< -10 <$ poorly $< -6 <$ moderately $< -4 <$ soluble $< -2 <$ very $< 0 <$ highly, the solubility of the *ent*-kaurane diterpenoids analyzed ranged from highly soluble to insoluble based on the Ali approach and highly soluble to poorly soluble based on SILICOS-IT and ESOL approaches. Only 0.35% of the compounds were labeled insoluble by the Ali approach. However, empirical evidence suggests that the target log S range of -1 to -5 for most drugs reflects a compromise desired to achieve aqueous solubility and, at the same time, hydrophobicity needed for a drug molecule to cross a membrane [65]. Arguably, a bigger subset of *ent*-kauranes studied were concentrated within this range, inferring that these compounds are amenable to crossing cell membranes and getting absorbed.

3.4. Pharmacokinetic Properties

Bioavailability is further influenced by pharmacokinetic properties including GI absorption, BBB permeability, P-gp substrates, and the inhibition of main cytochromes. The human GI absorption is quantified as the fraction of a given dose that has reached the portal vein. The extent of absorption by intestinal villi and microvilli determines how much of the administered drug enters the bloodstream. It is a multifaceted parameter influenced by several factors including the physicochemical state of the substance, GI physiology, formulation, and other biopharmaceutical factors [66]. Of the sampled molecules, 96.5% had high GI absorption, suggesting the high bioavailability of these molecules through the intestines.

The blood–brain barrier (BBB) serves as a semipermeable and selective barrier, preventing the entry of unwanted external substances, and thereby maintaining the homeostatic balance of the central nervous system (CNS) [67]. The permeability of this membrane is maintained at extremely low levels, thus making the delivery of drugs to the brain very difficult [68]. The in silico determination of BBB permeability can help predict the performance of drugs in the CNS [69]. A small subset of *ent*-kaurane diterpenoids (28.20%) was predicted to be BBB permeants, suggesting that *ent*-kaurane diterpenoids are largely non-bioavailable to the brain. Nevertheless, this may not pose a significant challenge since several techniques have been devised to enable the delivery of non-BBB permeant drugs to the brain. These methods encompass the utilization of nanotechnology to encapsulate drugs within BBB-permeant nanoparticles, the use of ultrasound and microbubbles to disrupt the BBB, intranasal drug delivery, efflux transporters inhibition, and direct injections into the brain [70].

P-glycoprotein (P-gp) is a transmembrane protein that plays a crucial role in drug transport and efflux in various tissues, including the GI and the BBB [71]. This protein effluxes those drug substrates that it binds from enterocytes into the GI lumen, thereby limiting their bioavailability and efficacy [72]. Common drugs that are known to be P-gp substrates include vinblastine, indinavir, fostemsavir, mitapivat, etoposide, ritonavir, and digoxin [43]. The overexpression of the MDR1 gene responsible for the synthesis of this protein has been associated with the multidrug resistance of tumor cells [71]. Since this protein is substrate specific, it is imperative to determine if potential drug-like molecules can bind to it, as it helps in the prognostication of possible dosage for administration. A large number of molecules (86.34%) were found to be substrates of P-gp. This implies that a significant subset of these drugs is potentially recognized and effluxed from their targets by P-gp. This recognition will consequently lead to the reduced concentration of the active ingredients and bioavailability, particularly in the GI tract and across the BBB, thereby influencing their therapeutic efficacy in vivo. This result affirms the observed low levels of BBB permeability of the *ent*-kauranes. Interestingly, the GI absorption of these molecules was very high; overall, 96.50% of the studied molecules were flagged to have a high GI absorption. This is in tandem with reports that this protein is only localized to the apical membranes of the small intestines [71]. Therefore, other regions of the small intestines could serve as the alternative regions of absorption of these molecules, and hence, the observed high GI absorptivity of the studied molecules. These results underscore the importance of understanding the substrate–P-gp interactions and the possible ways of evading the binding or liberating the drug substrate from this protein, with a view of ensuring their successful therapeutic outcomes.

Understanding how molecules interact with cytochrome P450 (CYP) is pivotal in the realm of drug development and metabolism. Inhibition of these isoforms is a significant contributor to pharmacokinetics-related interactions between co-administered drugs. When one drug inhibits the activity of these enzymes, it can lead to alterations in the metabolism of the other drugs, potentially leading to their accumulation or production of other metabolites that differ from the original drug, which may be toxic [73]. Using in vitro bioluminescent assays, several P450 cytochrome inhibitors have been determined, and it became apparent that some compounds affect different CYP isoforms while others are selective to specific isoenzymes [74]. A significant number of *ent*-kaurane diterpenoids are the non-inhibitors of P450 cytochromes; thus, these molecules might have a lower likelihood of interfering with metabolism should they be co-administered with other therapeutics and therefore leading to lesser chances of causing toxicities.

3.5. Toxicological Properties

Computational toxicology evaluation is an important aspect in the early stages of drug discovery as it helps to identify potentially hazardous compounds. The upfront elimination of molecules with undesirable toxicological properties could help reduce the attrition and failure rates of drug candidates evaluated in drug discovery pipelines [75]. With regard to the studied toxicological endpoints, a significant number of *ent*-kaurane diterpenoids have minimal tumorigenic and mutagenic potentials, underscoring the promising safety profile of the compounds. These results, combined with the bioactivities of these molecules, substantiate the hypothesis that *ent*-kaurane diterpenoids have a great potential as candidates for further exploration and research in the domain of drug discovery.

3.6. Medicinal Chemistry: Synthetic Accessibility, PAINS, BRENK, and Lead-likeness

Synthetic accessibility (SA) refers to the ease with which a molecule can be synthesized. It is an important factor to consider when profiling compounds for drug discovery, as an intention to synthesize them may arise at later stages. The SA is normally expressed on a scale of 1 to 10, where a lower score indicates that a molecule is easier to synthesize, while a higher score suggests that synthesis might be more challenging [50]. Majority of the studied *ent*-kaurane diterpenoids could therefore be classified as moderately challenging to synthesize (SA: 5.0–7.5), and this could be attributed to their structural complexity or presence of certain functional groups that may require intricate synthetic steps. This augments the need to come up with novel reaction sequences or unique synthetic strategies to overcome synthetic challenges.

PAINS (Pan Assay Interference Compounds) are molecules that contain substructures showing potent responses in assays, regardless of the protein target. PAINS help identify potentially problematic fragments that may produce false positive responses in in silico assays [76]. Not a single studied *ent*-kaurane was flagged as a PAIN compound, suggesting that their interaction with various protein targets in in silico assays is less susceptible to generating misleading positive responses. The non-inclusion of the studied *ent*-kauranes in the PAINS category underscores the favorable prospect of utilizing these compounds in in silico assays without substantial concerns regarding the generation of false-positive results.

On the other hand, BRENK alerts identify fragments of compounds that could be toxic, chemically reactive, or metabolically unstable, thus helping in identifying compounds that may have undesirable properties [76]. However, in-depth analysis revealed that the main motif that played a pivotal role in generating the observed heightened BRENK alerts (up to three) was the presence of Michael acceptors. This same motif is paradoxically the very motif that has been determined to confer cytotoxic and anticancer potential to these molecules.

Lead-likeness is a concept that focusses on identifying compounds that are suitable for optimization in drug discovery based on their physicochemical properties [77,78]. Approximately 74% of the compounds exhibited non-compliance with one lead-likeness rule, while around 5% of the compounds demonstrated non-compliance with two rules. Additionally, approximately 1% of the *ent*-kauranes violated three lead-likeness rules. The main physicochemical property of *ent*-kauranes leading to the heightened violation of the rules for lead-likeness was their molecular weights being higher than 350 Da. This means that a significant portion of these molecules are heavier than the recommended weight for lead-likeness and that these molecules could pose challenges during drug optimization processes.

3.7. Macromolecular Targets of Selected Molecules

Using Molinspiration cheminformatics, the bioactivity scores of these six molecules were predicted. This model encompasses various drug targets including G protein-coupled receptor (GPCR) ligands, kinase inhibitors, ion channel modulators, enzymes, and nuclear receptors. A higher bioactivity score indicates an increased probability of a compound exhibiting a biological activity. Consequently, a molecule with a bioactivity score exceeding 0.00 is deemed likely to possess biological activity, scores within the range of −0.50 to 0.00 are considered moderately active, and scores below −0.50 are presumed to indicate inactivity [79]. Importantly, the better the bioactivity score, the higher the possibility that the compound will be an active drug. The results showed that *ent*-kaurane diterpenoids exhibits activity for the GPCR ligands, as ion channel modulators, nuclear receptor ligands, protease inhibitors, and enzyme inhibitors, and have moderate activity as kinase inhibitors. Further prediction of pharmacological activities of these representative molecules using PASS online revealed that *ent*-kaurane diterpenoids have immense potential biological activities including antineoplastic, antileukemic, apoptosis induction, immunosuppressant, chemoprotective, anti-hepatic, and hepatoprotectant activities. If Pa score of a molecule is >0.7 on a specific target, it is expected that that molecule will show a high activity against that target [80]. Molecules displaying such potential are sought after, particularly for the management of chronic diseases and disorders. For example, aromatase inhibitors have been shown to be an effective and safer group of drugs for the first-line endocrine therapy of breast cancer [81], while HSD11B1 inhibitors are being explored as a potential strategy for managing conditions such as metabolic syndrome, diabetes, obesity, and inflammatory diseases [82]. Despite compounds 23, 87, and 88 being stereoisomers, they show different probabilities for different targets. The subtle difference in the spatial arrangement of their functional groups can influence their shape, flexibility, electronic properties, solvation, and other factors. These factors, in turn, can significantly impact how each epimer positions itself interacts with and fits into the binding pockets of the protein targets. This ultimately affects the overall binding probability.

4. Materials and Methods

4.1. Accessing Ent-Kaurane Diterpenoids and FDA-Approved Drugs

The words "*ent*-kaurane diterpenoids" were searched in the published literature such as Google Scholar, Web of Science, Science Direct, Pubmed, and Sci-Finder. The range used was customized to span from the year 1960 to 2023. The relevant and readable papers published in peer-reviewed journals and libraries such as Wiley, Elsevier, American Chemical Society, The Royal Society of Chemistry, etc. were downloaded and reviewed for the natural *ent*-kaurane diterpenoids, filtering out the synthetic and semi-synthetic analogues. To remove duplicates and repetitions, one compound from the dereplicated compounds was picked for this study. The chemical structures of *ent*-kauranes, as reported by the authors, were drawn using a licensed Chemdraw (Professional-2016). The structures were then converted to simplified molecular input line entry system (SMILES) to enable downstream analyses. The physicochemical properties of 1040 drug molecules approved by the United States' Food and Drug Administration (FDA) were downloaded from the Enamine Bioactive Libraries "https://enamine.net/compound-libraries/bioactive-libraries (accessed on 28 September 2023)".

4.2. *Physicochemical and ADME Properties of Ent-Kaurane Diterpenoids*

The SwissADME (http://www.swissadme.ch/, accessed on 7 October 2023), a free online tool, was used to determine the physicochemical properties of the *ent*-kauranes and to predict their pharmacokinetic, lipophilicity, water solubility, and drug-likeness properties [50]. In batches of 100, the SMILES of the compounds were pasted in the "Enter list of SMILES here:" in the SwissADME webpage. The "Run!" icon was clicked, and the analyses were allowed to finish after which the data were exported into Excel in a CSV format. The Excel files for each batch of molecules were then matched.

4.3. *Toxicological Properties of Ent-Kaurane Diterpenoids*

The mutagenic, tumorigenic, reproduction-enhancing, and irritant properties were predicted using DataWarrior: an open-source program for data visualization and analysis with chemical intelligence (https://openmolecules.org/datawarrior/, accessed on 10 October 2023). AMES toxicity, hERG I and II inhibition, hepatotoxicity, and skin sensitization toxicities were predicted using the pKCSM web server (https://biosig.lab.uq.edu.au/pkcsm/, accessed on 10th October 2023). In pKCSM, SMILES for all the molecules were submitted singly for toxicity prediction, and the results were recorded in an Excel spreadsheet.

4.4. *Selection of Molecules and Prediction of Their Macromolecular Targets*

Molecules were chosen for further analysis by evaluating their physicochemical properties according to the rules set forth by Lipinski, Veber, Ghose, Muegge, and Egan. The Lipinski rule posits that a molecule is likely to be poorly absorbed if HBD > 5, HBA > 10, MW > 500 Da, and log P > 5 [19]. Ghose delineates drug-like attributes within the ranges of 0.4 < log P > 5.6, 160 < MW > 480, molar refractivity (MR) 40 < MR > 130, and a total atom count (TOC) 20 < TOC > 70 [83]. Veber's rule introduces the concept that desirable oral bioavailability is attainable if a molecule exhibits an RTB of $\leq$10 and a TPSA of $\leq$ 140 Å^2 [46]. Egan criteria posit that a promising oral drug candidate should manifest $-1.0 \leq \log P \leq 5.8$ and TPSA $\leq$ 130 Å^2. On the other hand, the Muegge criteria stipulate that a drug-like molecule should comply to the following: 200 < MW > 600 Da, −2 < XLogP > 5, TPSA < 150 Å^2, RTB < 15, and HBD $\leq$ 5 [84]. *Ent*-kaurane diterpenoid molecules that did not violate these rules and that were not toxic were further scrutinized. The toxicological endpoints considered were hepatotoxicity, skin sensitization, AMES toxicity, tumorigenicity, mutagenicity, hERG I and II inhibitors, irritants, reproductive effectiveness, and BRENK alerts. The chosen molecules underwent the predictive analysis of their bioactivity scores, pharmacological activities, and most probable molecular targets, facilitated by the Molinspiration cheminformatics, PASS online, and SwissTargetPrediction websites. The visualization of data was accomplished by using software tools, including OriginPro (2023b), GraphPad (8.0.1.244), Past (4.06b), and R-vegan (2.6-4).

5. Conclusions

This study conducted a review of 570 natural bioactive *ent*-kaurane diterpenoids and the pharmacological effects of their physicochemical properties. The findings indicated that a substantial subset of these molecules demonstrates promising drug-like characteristics. The studied physicochemical parameters of the *ent*-kauranes fell within the ranges of the corresponding physicochemical parameters of the so far FDA-approved drugs, suggesting their potential suitability for drug development. While some compounds exhibited BRENK alerts and poor lead-likeness potential, none were marked as PAINS. Further, the majority of these diterpenoids do not strongly inhibit key cytochrome enzymes, suggesting a lower likelihood of interfering with drug metabolism and reducing the risk of toxic interactions when co-administered with other therapeutics. The observation that a significant subset of these molecules is GI permeant and is particularly promising for the development of drugs for oral administration. However, the low BBB permeability of a significant portion necessitates specialized delivery approaches to the brain cells. Synthetically, the majority of these compounds were classified as moderately challenging to synthesize, and this calls for better synthetic approaches for these compounds. The toxicity studies revealed that the majority of these compounds are not toxic. The curated six compounds demonstrated a diverse potential for the treatment of different cancers, hepatic disorders, and metabolic diseases. These findings underscore the potential of ent-kaurane diterpenoids as viable leads in drug discovery. This warrants further exploration towards the development of novel and efficacious pharmaceutical interventions, contributing to the achievement of Sustainable Development Goal (SDG) 3.

Supplementary Materials: The following supporting information can be downloaded at: https://www.mdpi.com/article/10.3390/ph17040510/s1, Supplementary Information S1: Chemical structures of *ent*-kaurane diterpenoids, Supplementary Information S2: Sources and bioactivities of *ent*-kaurane diterpenoids, and Supplementary Information S3: Bioactivities and molecular descriptors of *ent*-kaurane diterpenoids.

Author Contributions: Conceptualization, S.K., N.M.K. and C.M.M.; methodology, S.K., N.M.K., C.M.M. and S.S.M.; validation, S.K., N.M.K., C.M.M., C.M.T. and C.B.R.S.; formal analysis, S.K. and N.M.K.; investigation, S.K. and N.M.K.; data curation, S.K., S.S.M., N.M.K. and C.M.M.; writing—original draft preparation, S.K.; writing—review and editing, N.M.K., S.S.M., C.M.M., C.B.R.S. and C.M.T.; visualization, S.K.; supervision, N.M.K., C.M.M. and C.M.T.; funding acquisition, C.M.T. All authors have read and agreed to the published version of the manuscript.

Funding: The authors gratefully acknowledge the financial support for this research from the following organizations and agencies: Australian Centre for International Agricultural Research (ACIAR) (ProteinAfrica; Grant No: LS/2020/154); the Rockefeller Foundation (WAVE-IN; Grant No: 2021 FOD 030); Bill & Melinda Gates Foundation (INV-032416); Horizon Europe (NESTLER Project: 101060762 & INNOECOFOOD Project: 101136739]; the Curt Bergfors Foundation Food Planet Prize Award; Norwegian Agency for Development Cooperation, the Section for research, innovation, and higher education (grant number: RAF–3058 KEN–18/0005) (CAP–Africa); the Swedish International Development Cooperation Agency (SIDA); the Swiss Agency for Development and Cooperation (SDC); the Australian Centre for International Agricultural Research (ACIAR); the Norwegian Agency for Development Cooperation (NORAD); the German Federal Ministry for Economic Cooperation and Development (BMZ); and the Government of the Republic of Kenya. The funders had no role in study design, data collection and analysis, decision to publish, or preparation of the manuscript. The views expressed herein do not necessarily reflect the official opinion of the funders.

Data Availability Statement: Data are contained within the article and Supplementary Materials.

Conflicts of Interest: The authors declare no conflicts of interest.

References

1. Malik, S.; Brudzyńska, P.; Khan, M.R.; Sytar, O.; Makhzoum, A.; Sionkowska, A. Natural Plant-Derived Compounds in Food and Cosmetics: A Paradigm of Shikonin and Its Derivatives. *Materials* **2023**, *16*, 4377. [CrossRef]
2. Newman, D.J.; Phil, D. Natural products and drug discovery. *Natl. Sci. Rev.* **2022**, *9*, nwac206. [CrossRef] [PubMed]
3. Dzobo, K. The role of natural products as sources of therapeutic agents for innovative drug discovery. *Compr. Pharmacol.* **2022**, *408*, 408–422. [CrossRef]
4. Sorokina, M.; Steinbeck, C. Review on natural products databases: Where to find data in 2020. *J. Cheminformat.* **2020**, *12*, 1–51. [CrossRef] [PubMed]
5. Zhao, X.; Li, W.; Wang, J.; Ma, D. A Convergent Route to *ent*-Kaurane Diterpenoids: Total Synthesis of Lungshengenin D and 1α,6α-Diacetoxy-*ent*-kaura-9(11),16-dien-12,15-dione. *J. Am. Chem. Soc.* **2017**, *139*, 2932–2935. [CrossRef]

6. Yang, J.; Wang, W.-G.; Wu, H.-Y.; Du, X.; Li, X.-N.; Li, Y.; Pu, J.-X.; Sun, H.-D. Bioactive Enmein-Type *ent*-Kaurane Diterpenoids from Isodon phyllostachys. *J. Nat. Prod.* **2015**, *79*, 132–140. [CrossRef]
7. Zhao, X.; Cacherat, B.; Hu, Q.; Ma, D. Natural Product Reports Recent advances in the synthesis of ent-kaurane diterpenoids. 2022, 39, 119–138. *39*. [CrossRef]
8. Lee, J.E.; Thuy, N.T.T.; Lee, Y.; Cho, N.; Yoo, H.M. An Antiproliferative ent-Kaurane Diterpene Isolated from the Roots of Mallotus japonicus Induced Apoptosis in Leukemic Cells. *Nat. Prod. Commun.* **2020**, *15*, 1934578X19897496. [CrossRef]
9. Deng, Z.; Chen, J.; Geng, C. Bioorganic Chemistry α -glucosidase inhibitory activity. *Bioorg. Chem.* **2020**, *95*, 103571.
10. Kimani, N.M.; Backhaus, S.; Matasyoh, J.C.; Kaiser, M.; Herrmann, F.C.; Schmidt, T.J.; Langer, K. Preparation of sesquiterpene lactone-loaded PLA nanoparticles and evaluation of their antitrypanosomal activity. *Molecules* **2019**, *24*, 2110. [CrossRef]
11. Kimani, N.M.; Matasyoh, J.C.; Kaiser, M.; Brun, R.; Schmidt, T.J. Antiprotozoal sesquiterpene lactones and other constituents from Tarchonanthus camphoratus and Schkuhria pinnata. *J. Nat. Prod.* **2018**, *81*, 124–130. [CrossRef]
12. Kimani, N.M.; Ochieng, C.O.; Ogutu, M.D.; Yamo, K.O.; Onyango, J.O.; Santos, C.B.R. Inhibition Kinetics and Theoretical Studies on Zanthoxylum chalybeum Engl. Dual Inhibitors of α-Glucosidase and α-Amylase. *J. Xenobiotics* **2023**, *13*, 102–120. [CrossRef] [PubMed]
13. Newman, D.J.; Cragg, G.M. Natural products as sources of new drugs over the nearly four decades from 01/1981 to 09/2019. *J. Nat. Prod.* **2020**, *83*, 770–803. [CrossRef]
14. Newman, D.J.; Cragg, G.M. Natural products as sources of new drugs over the 30 years from 1981 to 2010. *J. Nat. Prod.* **2012**, *75*, 311–335. [CrossRef]
15. Newman, D.J.; Cragg, G.M. Natural products as sources of new drugs from 1981 to 2014. *J. Nat. Prod.* **2016**, *79*, 629–661. [CrossRef]
16. Parveen, A.; Parveen, B.; Parveen, R.; Ahmad, S. Challenges and guidelines for clinical trial of herbal drugs. *J. Pharm. Bioallied Sci.* **2015**, *7*, 329.
17. Cui, W.; Aouidate, A.; Wang, S.; Yu, Q.; Li, Y.; Yuan, S. Discovering Anti-Cancer Drugs via Computational Methods. *Front. Pharmacol.* **2020**, *11*, 542271. [CrossRef]
18. Hingorani, A.D.; Kuan, V.; Finan, C.; Kruger, F.A.; Gaulton, A.; Chopade, S.; Sofat, R.; MacAllister, R.J.; Overington, J.P.; Hemingway, H.; et al. Improving the odds of drug development success through human genomics: Modelling study. *Sci. Rep.* **2019**, *9*, 18911. [CrossRef] [PubMed]
19. Lipinski, C.A.; Lombardo, F.; Dominy, B.W.; Feeney, P.J. Experimental and computational approaches to estimate solubility and permeability in drug discovery and development settings. *Adv. Drug Deliv. Rev.* **1997**, *23*, 3–25. [CrossRef]
20. Leeson, P.D.; Springthorpe, B. The influence of drug-like concepts on decision-making in medicinal chemistry. *Nat. Rev. Drug Discov.* **2007**, *6*, 881–890. [CrossRef]
21. Gleeson, M.P. Generation of a set of simple, interpretable ADMET rules of thumb. *J. Med. Chem.* **2008**, *51*, 817–834. [CrossRef]
22. Hughes, J.D.; Blagg, J.; Price, D.A.; Bailey, S.; DeCrescenzo, G.A.; Devraj, R.V.; Ellsworth, E.; Fobian, Y.M.; Gibbs, M.E.; Gilles, R.W.; et al. Physiochemical drug properties associated with in vivo toxicological outcomes. *Bioorg. Med. Chem. Lett.* **2008**, *18*, 4872–4875. [CrossRef] [PubMed]
23. Peters, J.; Schnider, P.; Mattei, P.; Kansy, M. Pharmacological promiscuity: Dependence on compound properties and target specificity in a set of recent Roche compounds. *ChemMedChem Chem. Enabling Drug Discov.* **2009**, *4*, 680–686. [CrossRef] [PubMed]
24. Gleeson, M.P.; Hersey, A.; Montanari, D.; Overington, J. Probing the links between in vitro potency, ADMET and physicochemical parameters. *Nat. Rev. Drug Discov.* **2011**, *10*, 197–208. [CrossRef] [PubMed]
25. Luker, T.; Alcaraz, L.; Chohan, K.K.; Blomberg, N.; Brown, D.S.; Butlin, R.J.; Elebring, T.; Griffin, A.M.; Guile, S.; St-Gallay, S.; et al. Strategies to improve in vivo toxicology outcomes for basic candidate drug molecules. *Bioorg. Med. Chem. Lett.* **2011**, *21*, 5673–5679. [CrossRef] [PubMed]
26. Bucar, F.; Wube, A.; Schmid, M. Natural product isolation–how to get from biological material to pure compounds. *Nat. Prod. Rep.* **2013**, *30*, 525–545. [CrossRef]
27. Pham, J.V.; Yilma, M.A.; Feliz, A.; Majid, M.T.; Maffetone, N.; Walker, J.R.; Kim, E.; Cho, H.J.; Reynolds, J.M.; Song, M.C.; et al. A review of the microbial production of bioactive natural products and biologics. *Front. Microbiol.* **2019**, *10*, 1404. [CrossRef] [PubMed]
28. Brinkmann, S.; Spohn, M.S.; Schäberle, T.F. Bioactive natural products from Bacteroidetes. *Nat. Prod. Rep.* **2022**, *39*, 1045–1065. [CrossRef] [PubMed]
29. Liang, X.-T. *Medicinal Chemistry of Bioactive Natural Products*; Wiley Online Library: Hoboken, NJ, USA, 2006.
30. Ojuka, P.; Kimani, N.M.; Apollo, S.; Nyariki, J.; Ramos, R.S.; Santos, C.B.R. Phytochemistry of plants in the genus Vepris: A review and in silico analysis of their ADMET properties. *S. Afr. J. Bot.* **2023**, *157*, 106–114. [CrossRef]
31. Wekesa, E.N.; Kimani, N.M.; Kituyi, S.N.; Omosa, L.K.; Santos, C.B.R. Therapeutic potential of the genus Zanthoxylum phytochemicals: A theoretical ADME/Tox analysis. *S. Afr. J. Bot.* **2023**, *162*, 129–141. [CrossRef]
32. Simoben, C.V.; Qaseem, A.; Moumbock, A.F.A.; Telukunta, K.K.; Günther, S.; Sippl, W.; Ntie-Kang, F. Pharmacoinformatic Investigation of Medicinal Plants from East Africa. *Mol. Inform.* **2020**, *39*, 2000163. [CrossRef]
33. Sun, H.D.; Xu, Y.L.; Jiang, B. Diterpenoids from Isodon species. *Nat. Prod. Rep.* **2001**, *23*, 673–698. [CrossRef] [PubMed]
34. Xing, H.; An, L.; Song, Z.; Li, S.; Wang, H.; Wang, C.; Zhang, J.; Tuerhong, M.; Abudukeremu, M.; Li, D.; et al. *Anti-Inflammatory ent -Kaurane Diterpenoids from Isodon serra. no. Table 2*; American Chemical Society and American Society of Pharmacognosy: Washington, DC, USA, 2019; pp. 2–11. [CrossRef]

35. Qi, X.; Zhang, Y.; Zhao, P.; Zhou, L.; Wang, X.; Huang, X. ent -Kaurane Diterpenoids with Neuroprotective Properties from Corn Silk (*Zea mays*). *J. Nat. Prod.* **2017**, *7*, 1225–1234. [CrossRef]
36. García, P.A.; De Oliveira, A.B.; Batista, R. Occurrence, Biological Activities and Synthesis of Kaurane Diterpenes and their Glycosides. *Molecules* **2007**, *12*, 455–483. [CrossRef]
37. Sun, Y.; Qiao, Y.; Liu, Y.; Zhou, J.; Wang, X.; Zheng, H.; Xu, Z.; Zhang, J.; Zhou, Y.; Qian, L.; et al. Redox Biology ent -Kaurane diterpenoids induce apoptosis and ferroptosis through targeting redox resetting to overcome cisplatin resistance. *Redox Biol.* **2021**, *43*, 101977. [CrossRef] [PubMed]
38. Zhao, X.H.; Meng, L.L.; Liu, X.T.; Shu, P.F.; Yuan, C.; An, X.T.; Jia, T.X.; Yang, Q.Q.; Zhen, X.; Fan, C.A. Asymmetric Divergent Synthesis of ent-Kaurane-, ent-Atisane-, ent-Beyerane-, ent-Trachylobane-, and ent-Gibberellane-type Diterpenoids. *J. Am. Chem. Soc.* **2023**, *145*, 311–321. [CrossRef] [PubMed]
39. Wang, J.; Hong, B.; Hu, D.; Kadonaga, Y.; Tang, R.; Lei, X. Protecting-Group-Free Syntheses of ent-Kaurane Diterpenoids: [3+2+1] Cycloaddition/Cycloalkenylation Approach. *J. Am. Chem. Soc.* **2020**, *142*, 2238–2243. [CrossRef] [PubMed]
40. Cherney, E.C.; Green, J.C.; Baran, P.S. Synthesis of ent-Kaurane and Beyerane Diterpenoids via Controlled Fragmentations of Overbred Intermediates. *Angew. Chem. Int. Ed. Engl.* **2013**, *52*, 9019–9022. [CrossRef]
41. Hu, Y.; Li, X.N.; Ma, Z.J.; Puno, P.T.; Zhao, Y.; Zhao, Y.; Xiao, Y.Z.; Zhang, W.; Liu, J.P. Synthesis of Novel ent-Kaurane-Type Diterpenoid Derivatives Effective for Highly Aggressive Tumor Cells. *Molecules* **2018**, *23*, 3216. [CrossRef] [PubMed]
42. Lin, Z.; Guo, Y.; Gao, Y.; Wang, S.; Wang, X.; Xie, Z.; Niu, H.; Chang, W.; Liu, L.; Yuan, H.; et al. ent-kaurane diterpenoids from Chinese liverworts and their antitumor activities through Michael addition as detected in situ by a fluorescence probe. *J. Med. Chem.* **2015**, *58*, 3944–3956. [CrossRef]
43. Elmeliegy, M.; Vourvahis, M.; Guo, C.; Wang, D.D. Effect of P-glycoprotein (P-gp) inducers on exposure of P-gp substrates: Review of clinical drug–drug interaction studies. *Clin. Pharmacokinet.* **2020**, *59*, 699–714. [CrossRef]
44. Murray, C.W.; Erlanson, D.A.; Hopkins, A.L.; Keserü, G.M.; Leeson, P.D.; Rees, D.C.; Reynolds, C.H.; Richmond, N.J. Validity of Ligand Efficiency Metrics. *ACS Med. Chem. Lett.* **2014**, *5*, 616–618. [CrossRef] [PubMed]
45. Coimbra, J.T.S.; Feghali, R.; Ribeiro, R.P.; Ramos, M.J.; Fernandes, P.A. The importance of intramolecular hydrogen bonds on the translocation of the small drug piracetam through a lipid bilayer. *RSC Adv.* **2020**, *11*, 899–908. [CrossRef] [PubMed]
46. Veber, D.F.; Johnson, S.R.; Cheng, H.-Y.; Smith, B.R.; Ward, K.W.; Kopple, K.D. Molecular properties that influence the oral bioavailability of drug candidates. *J. Med. Chem.* **2002**, *45*, 2615–2623. [CrossRef] [PubMed]
47. Alex, A.; Millan, D.S.; Perez, M.; Wakenhut, F.; Whitlock, G.A. Intramolecular hydrogen bonding to improve membrane permeability and absorption in beyond rule of five chemical space. *Medchemcomm* **2011**, *2*, 669–674. [CrossRef]
48. Gu, J.; Gui, Y.; Chen, L.; Yuan, G.; Lu, H.Z.; Xu, X. Use of Natural Products as Chemical Library for Drug Discovery and Network Pharmacology. *PLoS ONE* **2013**, *8*, e62839. [CrossRef] [PubMed]
49. Kenny, P.W. Hydrogen-Bond Donors in Drug Design. *J. Med. Chem.* **2022**, *65*, 14261–14275. [CrossRef]
50. Daina, A.; Michielin, O.; Zoete, V. SwissADME: A free web tool to evaluate pharmacokinetics, drug-likeness and medicinal chemistry friendliness of small molecules. *Sci. Rep.* **2017**, *7*, 42717. [CrossRef] [PubMed]
51. Bojarska, J.; Remko, M.; Breza, M.; Madura, I.D.; Kaczmarek, K.; Zabrocki, J.; Wolf, W.M. A Supramolecular Approach to Structure-Based Design with A Focus on Synthons Hierarchy in Ornithine-Derived Ligands: Review, Synthesis, Experimental and in Silico Studies. *Molecules* **2020**, *25*, 1135. [CrossRef] [PubMed]
52. Bryant, M.J.; Black, S.N.; Blade, H.; Docherty, R.; Maloney, A.G.P.; Taylor, S.C. The CSD Drug Subset: The Changing Chemistry and Crystallography of Small Molecule Pharmaceuticals. *J. Pharm. Sci.* **2019**, *108*, 1655–1662. [CrossRef]
53. Wei, W.; Cherukupalli, S.; Jing, L.; Liu, X.; Zhan, P. Fsp3: A new parameter for drug-likeness. *Drug Discov. Today* **2020**, *25*, 1839–1845. [CrossRef]
54. Yan, A.; Gasteiger, J. Prediction of aqueous solubility of organic compounds based on a 3D structure representation. *J. Chem. Inf. Comput. Sci.* **2003**, *43*, 429–434. [CrossRef] [PubMed]
55. Ertl, P.; Rohde, B.; Selzer, P. Fast Calculation of Molecular Polar Surface Area as a Sum of Fragment-Based Contributions and Its Application to the Prediction of Drug Transport Properties. *J. Med. Chem.* **2000**, *43*, 3714–3717. [CrossRef] [PubMed]
56. Prasanna, S.; Doerksen, R.J. Topological Polar Surface Area: A Useful Descriptor in 2D-QSAR. *Curr. Med. Chem.* **2009**, *16*, 21. [CrossRef] [PubMed]
57. Zupančič, O.; Bernkop-Schnürch, A. Lipophilic peptide character–What oral barriers fear the most. *J. Control. Release* **2017**, *255*, 242–257. [CrossRef] [PubMed]
58. Young, R.J.; Flitsch, S.L.; Grigalunas, M.; Leeson, P.D.; Quinn, R.J.; Turner, N.J.; Waldmann, H. The time and place for nature in drug discovery. *JACS Au* **2022**, *2*, 2400–2416. [CrossRef] [PubMed]
59. Wardecki, D.; Dołowy, M.; Bober-Majnusz, K. Assessment of Lipophilicity Parameters of Antimicrobial and Immunosuppressive Compounds. *Molecules* **2023**, *28*, 2820. [CrossRef] [PubMed]
60. Tsaioun, K.; Blaauboer, B.J.; Hartung, T. Evidence-based absorption, distribution, metabolism, excretion (ADME) and its interplay with alternative toxicity methods. *ALTEX-Alternatives Anim. Exp.* **2016**, *33*, 343–358. [CrossRef] [PubMed]
61. Kathuria, H.; Handral, H.K.; Cha, S.; Nguyen, D.T.P.; Cai, J.; Cao, T.; Wu, C.; Kang, L. Enhancement of skin delivery of drugs using proposome depends on drug lipophilicity. *Pharmaceutics* **2021**, *13*, 1457. [CrossRef] [PubMed]
62. Mahgoub, R.E.; Atatreh, N.; Ghattas, M.A. Using filters in virtual screening: A comprehensive guide to minimize errors and maximize efficiency. *Annu. Rep. Med. Chem.* **2022**, *59*, 99–136. [CrossRef]

63. Delaney, J.S. ESOL: Estimating aqueous solubility directly from molecular structure. *J. Chem. Inf. Comput. Sci.* **2004**, *44*, 1000–1005. [CrossRef]
64. Ali, J.; Camilleri, P.; Brown, M.B.; Hutt, A.J.; Kirton, S.B. Revisiting the general solubility equation: In silico prediction of aqueous solubility incorporating the effect of topographical polar surface area. *J. Chem. Inf. Model.* **2012**, *52*, 420–428. [CrossRef] [PubMed]
65. Jorgensen, W.L.; Duffy, E.M. Prediction of drug solubility from structure. *Adv. Drug Deliv. Rev.* **2002**, *54*, 355–366. [CrossRef] [PubMed]
66. Sjögren, E.; Thorn, H.; Tannergren, C. In silico modeling of gastrointestinal drug absorption: Predictive performance of three physiologically based absorption models. *Mol. Pharm.* **2016**, *13*, 1763–1778. [CrossRef] [PubMed]
67. Kumar, R.; Sharma, A.; Alexiou, A.; Bilgrami, A.L.; Kamal, M.A.; Ashraf, G.M. DeePred-BBB: A blood brain barrier permeability prediction model with improved accuracy. *Front. Neurosci.* **2022**, *16*, 858126. [CrossRef] [PubMed]
68. Fu, B.M.; Zhao, Z.; Zhu, D. Blood-Brain Barrier (BBB) permeability and transport measurement in vitro and in vivo. *Permeability Barrier Methods Protoc.* **2021**, *2367*, 105–122. [CrossRef]
69. Geldenhuys, W.J.; Mohammad, A.S.; Adkins, C.E.; Lockman, P.R. Molecular determinants of blood–brain barrier permeation. *Ther. Deliv.* **2015**, *6*, 961–971. [CrossRef] [PubMed]
70. Bors, L.A.; Erdő, F. Overcoming the blood–brain barrier. challenges and tricks for CNS drug delivery. *Sci. Pharm.* **2019**, *87*, 6. [CrossRef]
71. Hunter, J.; Hirst, B.H. Intestinal secretion of drugs. The role of P-glycoprotein and related drug efflux systems in limiting oral drug absorption. *Adv. Drug Deliv. Rev.* **1997**, *25*, 129–157. [CrossRef]
72. Mai, Y.; Dou, L.; Yao, Z.; Madla, C.M.; Gavins, F.K.H.; Taherali, F.; Yin, H.; Orlu, M.; Murdan, S.; Basit, A.W. Quantification of P-Glycoprotein in the gastrointestinal tract of humans and rodents: Methodology, gut region, sex, and species matter. *Mol. Pharm.* **2021**, *18*, 1895–1904. [CrossRef]
73. Kirchmair, J.; Göller, A.H.; Lang, D.; Kunze, J.; Testa, B.; Wilson, I.D.; Glen, R.C.; Schneider, G. Predicting drug metabolism: Experiment and/or computation? *Nat. Rev. Drug Discov.* **2015**, *14*, 387–404. [CrossRef]
74. Veith, H.; Southall, N.; Huang, R.; James, T.; Fayne, D.; Artemenko, N.; Shen, M.; Inglese, J.; Austin, C.P.; Lloyd, D.G. Comprehensive characterization of cytochrome P450 isozyme selectivity across chemical libraries. *Nat. Biotechnol.* **2009**, *27*, 1050–1055. [CrossRef] [PubMed]
75. Hughes, J.; Rees, S.; Kalindjian, S.; Philpott, K. Principles of early drug discovery. *Br. J. Pharmacol.* **2011**, *162*, 1239–1249. [CrossRef] [PubMed]
76. Ononamadu, C.; Ibrahim, A. Molecular docking and prediction of ADME/drug-likeness properties of potentially active antidiabetic compounds isolated from aqueous-methanol extracts of Gymnema sylvestre and Combretum micranthum. *BioTechnologia* **2021**, *102*, 85–99. [CrossRef] [PubMed]
77. Polinsky, A. Lead-likeness and drug-likeness. In *The Practice of Medicinal Chemistry*; Elsevier: Amsterdam, The Netherlands, 2008; pp. 244–254.
78. Hann, M.M.; Oprea, T.I. Pursuing the leadlikeness concept in pharmaceutical research. *Curr. Opin. Chem. Biol.* **2004**, *8*, 255–263. [CrossRef] [PubMed]
79. Unnisa, A.; Abouzied, A.S.; Baratam, A.; Lakshmi, K.N.V.C.; Hussain, T.; Kunduru, R.D.; Banu, H.; Fatima, S.B.; Hussian, A.; Selvarajan, K.K. Design, synthesis, characterization, computational study and in-vitro antioxidant and anti-inflammatory activities of few novel 6-aryl substituted pyrimidine azo dyes. *Arab. J. Chem.* **2020**, *13*, 8638–8649. [CrossRef]
80. Emon, N.U.; Alam, S.; Rudra, S.; Riya, S.R.; Paul, A.; Hossen, S.M.M.; Kulsum, U.; Ganguly, A. Antidepressant, anxiolytic, antipyretic, and thrombolytic profiling of methanol extract of the aerial part of Piper nigrum: In vivo, in vitro, and in silico approaches. *Food Sci. Nutr.* **2021**, *9*, 833–846. [CrossRef]
81. Czajka-Oraniec, I.; Simpson, E.R. Aromatase research and its clinical significance. *Endokrynol. Pol.* **2010**, *61*, 126–134. [PubMed]
82. Kupczyk, D.; Bilski, R.; Kozakiewicz, M.; Studzińska, R.; Kędziora-Kornatowska, K.; Kosmalski, T.; Pedrycz-Wieczorska, A.; Głowacka, M. 11β-HSD As a new target in pharmacotherapy of metabolic diseases. *Int. J. Mol. Sci.* **2022**, *23*, 8984. [CrossRef] [PubMed]
83. Ghose, A.K.; Viswanadhan, V.N.; Wendoloski, J.J. A knowledge-based approach in designing combinatorial or medicinal chemistry libraries for drug discovery. 1. A qualitative and quantitative characterization of known drug databases. *J. Comb. Chem.* **1999**, *1*, 55–68. [CrossRef]
84. Muegge, I.; Heald, S.L.; Brittelli, D. Simple selection criteria for drug-like chemical matter. *J. Med. Chem.* **2001**, *44*, 1841–1846. [CrossRef]

pharmaceuticals

Article

Proportion of Over-The-Counter Medicines Containing a Plant Component and Those with Synthetic Substances Administered among Children in a Bulgarian Population

Bozhidarka Hadzhieva [1,*,†] and Valentina Petkova-Dimitrova [2,†]

1 Medical College, Medical University of Plovdiv, 15a Vasil Aprilov Blvd., 4000 Plovdiv, Bulgaria
2 Department of Social Pharmacy, Faculty of Pharmacy, Medical University of Sofia, 2 Dunav St., 1000 Sofia, Bulgaria; vpetkova@pharmfac.mu-sofia.bg
* Correspondence: bozhidarka.hadzhieva@mu-plovdiv.bg; Tel.: +359-32-200-908
† These authors contributed equally to this work.

Abstract: Over-the-counter medicines are intended to influence a number of symptoms and also to cure some human diseases without having to see the doctor. These medicines are used for self-medication and parents also give them to their children. The following fall within the scope of over-the-counter medicines: analgesics, antipyretics, antihistamines, decongestants, gastroprotectors, anti-cough medicines, and others. Their composition also includes one or a combination of medicinal plants. In addition to synthetic substances, some nonprescription medicines contain plant substances and their derivatives. Medicinal plants and their extracted derivatives are applicable in the therapies of a number of diseases. Considering the fact that over-the-counter medicines can be used among children from birth, the subject of our study is those whose composition includes biologically active plant substances. Within this study, we have established the number of nonprescription medicines containing a plant substance individually or in combination with another substance of the same kind and/or other substances, which have been included in a list published on the website of the Bulgarian Drug Agency. The objective of our study is to present the percentage of OTC medicines containing a plant substance intended to affect the symptoms of upper respiratory tract diseases and pain, which are used among children during different periods of their development. Some of these medicines also contain substances such as antihistamines (pheniramine maleate) and decongestants (pseudoephedrine, phenylephrine hydrochloride, dimetidine) that can cause various unwanted side effects. Considering the aforementioned aspects and also the peculiarities of childhood, we recommend that self-treatment be conducted only after consulting a health specialist.

Keywords: herbal medicinal products; over-the-counter medicines; children; diseases; childhood age

Citation: Hadzhieva, B.; Petkova-Dimitrova, V. Proportion of Over-The-Counter Medicines Containing a Plant Component and Those with Synthetic Substances Administered among Children in a Bulgarian Population. *Pharmaceuticals* **2024**, *17*, 192. https://doi.org/10.3390/ph17020192

Academic Editors: Daniela De Vita, Catherine Sherwin, Elena Y. Enioutina and Kathleen M. Job

Received: 24 October 2023
Revised: 26 January 2024
Accepted: 28 January 2024
Published: 31 January 2024

1. Introduction

Various historical sources such as written documents, monuments, and some preserved medicines serve as evidence that medicinal plants have been used since ancient times [1,2].

The use of medicinal plants like *Aloe vera* L., *Senna alexandrina* Mill., *Thymus vulgaris* L., *Foenicumum vulgare* L., *Allium sativum* L., and others in the treatment of a number of diseases was described in the Ebers Papyrus, which was written around 1500 BC and contains about 800 prescriptions and 700 plant types [3]. Some of the oldest civilizations of the Chinese, the Egyptians, the Romans, and the ancient Slavs knew a number of medicinal plants and used them for thousands of years. They passed their experience on to other peoples through their folklore and traditions [4]. The medicinal plants common yarrow (*Achillea millefolium* L.) and *chamomile* (*Matricaria chamomilla* L.), which have been written into the European Pharmacopeia, have been used since the time of the Neanderthals and so have poplar buds (*Populus spec.* L.) [5–7].

The knowledge about medicinal plants over the past centuries has become scarce. They have been used on the grounds of the accumulated empirical experience over the centuries. The use of herbal medicines has increased over the past years and nowadays, about 80% of the world population continues to use them as part of primary healthcare [8,9]. According to the World Health Organization (WHO), this trend observed even in developed countries is related to the increase and extension of the scope of use of traditional medicines [10]. Some authors believe that the use of medicinal plants could be examined with reference to the following aspects—phytotherapy, nonprescription medicines, and traditional herbal medicines [11,12].

Herbal treatment/phytotherapy is a method of treatment and prophylaxis of diseases by applying medicinal plants, as in different countries, both traditional medicines and standardized herbal extract are used [9,13]. Herbal treatment is based on the empirical knowledge of medicinal plants, while phytotherapy is a scientifically substantiated medical practice and, thus, is distinguished from the more traditional approaches [14].

In order to classify a plant as a drug, it must contain a biologically active substance in its morphological parts. There are a number of plants whose active compounds and therapeutic properties have been scientifically established as a result of in-depth studies, which allows researchers to regard these plants as medicinal plants [15]. The term "herbal drugs" denotes plants or plant parts that have been converted into phytopharmaceuticals by means of simple processes which include collection, drying, and storage [16].

The medicinal value of such medicinal plants depends on the presence of the biologically active ingredient/s with bioactive properties. Studies have been conducted and a number of biologically active substances/ingredients have been identified in plant materials of land and marine origin [17].

Surveys have been performed worldwide in order to establish the composition of medicinal plants and their efficiency. As a result of these surveys, herbal medicines have been developed and produced in order to be used for various indications and by people of different ages [15]. At present, the extraction of bioactive compounds and the synthesis of their analogs is an effective approach for developing herbal products [18].

The use of medicinal plants among children, which is included in some mothers' "caring" practices, is based on traditions passed on from generation to generation that guarantee good health and the cure of diseases [19]. It has been stated in the existing scientific literature that pediatricians integrate complementary/alternative medical therapy into their conventional therapy for a number of diseases [20,21].

In addition, pharmacists can recommend a medicine sold without a doctor's prescription that contains a plant substance that can be applied among children in case of a certain disease. No consultation with a medical specialist is required for nonprescription medicines [22]. They can be purchased without the supervision of a medical specialist. Nonprescription medicines or over-the-counter medicines are those determined by the Food and Drug Administration (FDA) to be safe and effective to be used without a doctor's prescription [23].

In the European Union, there is a complex regulatory framework for traditional herbal medicinal products. It is based on the principle that the marketing authorization issued by the competent authorities is analogous to that required for the marketing of medicinal products. The requirements and procedures for obtaining such marketing authorization are set out in regulations, directives, and scientific guidelines.

Herbal medicinal products fall within the scope of the amended European Directive 2001/83/EC, which requires that any application for authorization to place a medicinal product on the market must be accompanied by documentation containing data on the results of physicochemical, biological, and microbiological tests, as well as pharmacological, toxicological, and clinical tests of the product, which prove its quality, harmlessness, and efficacy.

The amended Directive 2001/83 EC as Directive 2004/24 EC establishes a simplified registration procedure. This procedure should only be acceptable if the herbal medicinal product can be demonstrated to have a medicinal use of sufficient duration within a community. Medical use outside the community should only be taken into account if the medicinal product has been used within the community for a period of a specified duration [24,25].

Today, the member states of the European Union use this directive as a guideline for registering herbal medicines for self-treatment. Registration of these herbal medicines requires evidence of a well-established tradition and that they are safe enough to be marketed as over-the-counter (OTC) medicines. Herbal medicinal products can only be offered in pharmacies under the supervision of a pharmacist and after receiving registration under a full or simplified procedure depending on their classification, i.e., such as over-the-counter drugs and those that must be prescribed by a healthcare professional [26].

In addition to their use for prophylactic purposes, nonprescription medicines are also included in the treatment of a number of conditions such as headaches, ordinary colds, musculoskeletal pains, allergies, nicotine addiction, acids, and others [27].

The composition of some over-the-counter medicines includes plant substances such as: marshmallow (*Althaea officinalis* L.); common mallow (*Malva sylvestris* L.); ribwort plantain (*Plantago lanceolata* L.); Icelandic moos (*Cetraria islandica* (L.) Ach; etc., which mainly have an emollient effect and soothe irritation in case of inflammation of the upper respiratory tract. For example, on the pharmaceutical market in Bulgaria, there are over-the-counter medicines such as: Mucoplant Spitzwegerich Hustcnsaft 5 g/100 g syrup; Tussavit 7.53 g/7.53 g/100 g syrup; and Expectorans No 5, syrup, whose composition includes some of the aforementioned plant raw materials. Other biologically active substances help to extract the secretion that covers the bronchial walls and bronchioles. Plant raw materials having an expectorant effect include the following: primrose (*Primula veris* L.); licorice (*Glycyrrhiza glabra* L.); senega (*Polygala senega* L.); mullet (*Verbascum phlomoides* L.); and soapwort (*Saponaria officinalis* L.). They mainly contain triterpene saponins. The expectorant medicinal plants include cinnamon (*Cinnamomum zeylanicum* Blume); fennel (*Foeniculum vulgare* Mill.); and ginger (*Zingiber officinale* Roscoe) [28,29].

OTC medicines intended to treat pain among children contain substances such as: paracetamol, acetylsalicylic acid, caffeine, propyphenazone, and codeine phosphate (trade name of the Aceffein and Caffetin Forte tablets). Due to the presence of substances such as caffeine and codeine phosphate as well as acetylsalicylic acid in these and other OTC drugs, they can be applied among children over 12 years of age (according to the brief description of the product).

These medicines are used for self-treatment and thus a number of benefits are obtained both medicinally and economically. We need to point out that self-treatment with over-the-counter medicines may have serious consequences when an inappropriate medicine has been used or improper dosage has been applied [30]. Self-treatment with over-the-counter medicines poses a number of risks, mainly among pediatric and geriatric patients. Over-the-counter medicines have the potential to provide faster access to healthcare, but their improper use poses a number of risks [31]. Incorrect self-diagnosis and usage as well as an improper dosage may lead to unwanted side effects, medicinal interactions, and/or unwanted reactions [32]. Therefore, the role of the pharmacist is very important for reducing the risk of any potential unwanted medicinal reactions and also for improving the patients' results [33].

The purpose of our study is to establish what percentage of the medicines registered as nonprescription medicines are applied among children and contain a plant substance(s) at the same time. We also aimed to establish the presence or the absence of any dependence between the composition of the over-the-counter medicines and the age of the pediatric patients. We would also like to present medicinal plants and their extracted derivatives that are most commonly contained in medicines used for self-treatment.

2. Results

An analysis of the list of over-the-counter medicines made in 2020 has shown that out of 999 medicines in total, 198 are applied among children and contain a plant-based active substance.

As a result of the conducted analysis of the registered over-the-counter medicines containing a plant-based active substance, we have established that these medicines are prescribed to children aged 0+ to 18 years old. Depending on the separate periods of the child's development, we have grouped the different ages from the table of over-the-counter medicines and have obtained the following result: the over-the-counter medicines containing a plant-based active substance that can be used for breastfeeding babies are 2 in number; those applied in early childhood—21; those applied during the pre-school period—49; those applied during the school period to children aged 7–10 years old—7; those applied to children aged 11–14 years old—100; and those applied in the period of adolescence—19.

The grouping based on the content of a plant substance/derivative/synthetic substance of these 198 nonprescription medicines that can be applied among the pediatric population has been illustrated in Figure 1.

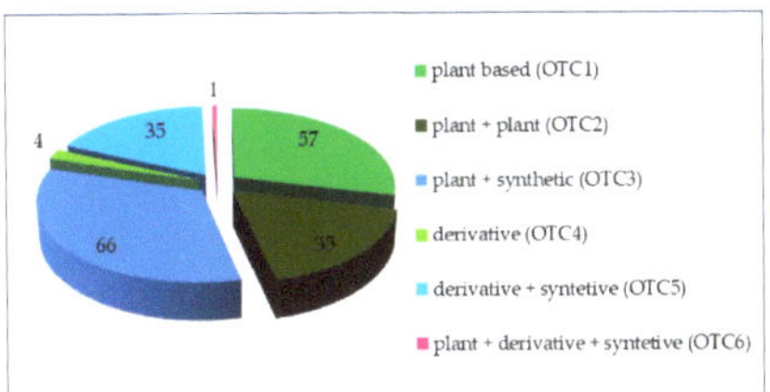

Figure 1. Grouping of plant-based OTCs by active substance.

Our study has shown that the nonprescription medicines containing the combination of a plant + derivative + syntetive (OTC6) are intended to be applied among children in the secondary school age (Schp, middle). This group is only one in number, owing to which it cannot be expressed in percentage on the graph.

The analyzed medicines are intended to be applied for various diseases, for example, respiratory infections, gastrointestinal problems (acids, meteorism, and others), hepatic diseases (hepatoprotector), pain, edema, trauma, and others.

We have applied statistical analyses to these over-the-counter medicines containing a plant component. We have conducted this study taking into account the most common symptoms typical of childhood, namely, diseases of the upper respiratory tract and pain.

For the purposes of our analysis, we examined each children's age group as follows: breastfeeding babies by the 28th day (BB by the 28th day); breastfeeding babies by the 12th month (BB by the 12th month); early childhood (Ech); pre-school period (PSchp); school period (Schp), which includes early school age (Schp, early) and secondary school age (Schp, middle); and adolescence (Adul). We grouped the over-the-counter medicines (OTC) containing a plant component in the following way: OTC1—containing only a plant component; OTC2—containing a combination of plant components; OTC3—containing a combination of a plant substance + a synthetic substance; OTC4—containing a derivative; OTC5—containing a combination of a derivative + a synthetic substance; OTC6—containing a combination of a plant substance + a derivative + a synthetic substance. We have excluded OTC4 and OTC6 because with reference to OTC4, there are no such medicines to be applied among children in case of the studied symptoms, and in the OTC6 group, only one medicine has been registered.

2.1. Upper Respiratory Tract

The two-dimensional division between the "age groups" and "OTC type" variables has shown the following (Figure 2):

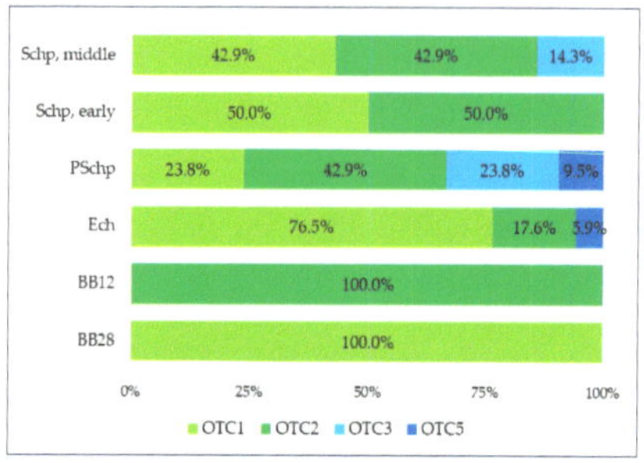

Figure 2. Respiratory tract—distribution of OTCs across age groups.

- over-the-counter medicines containing only a plant component (OTC1) and over-the-counter medicines containing a combination of a plant substance + a synthetic substance (OTC3) entirely dominate the lowest age groups such as breastfeeding babies by the 28th day (BB28) and breastfeeding babies by the 12th month (BB12);
- three types of OTCs are applied in the Ech group, of which those that dominate are over-the-counter medicines containing only a plant component (OTC1) at 76.5%, and over-the-counter medicines containing a combination of a derivative + a synthetic substance (OTC5) have the smallest share (5.9%);
- in the fourth age group (PSchp), there are four types of OTCs, the largest share (42.9%) of which is over-the-counter medicines containing a combination of a plant components (OTC2) and the smallest share (9.5%) of which is over-the-counter medicines containing a combination of a derivative + a synthetic substance (OTC5);
- in the school period, which includes the early school age (Schp early) group, two types are present—over-the-counter medicines containing only a plant component (OTC1) and over-the-counter medicines containing a combination of a plant components (OTC2), which have equal shares (50% each);
- in the last school period age group that includes the secondary school age (Schp, middle), there are three types of OTC, wherein over-the-counter medicines containing only a plant component (OTC1) and over-the-counter medicines containing a combination of a plant components (OTC2) have equal shares (42.9% each), and the smallest share is comprises over-the-counter medicines containing a combination of a plant substance + a synthetic substance (OTC3) (14.3%).

The analysis has shown that with reference to the diseases of the upper respiratory tract, there are no medicines of types over-the-counter medicines containing a derivative (OTC4) and over-the-counter medicines containing a combination of a plant + a derivative + a syntetive (OTC6).

If we examine the two-dimensional division of medicines from different groups in the aforementioned age groups, we will establish the following (Figure 3):

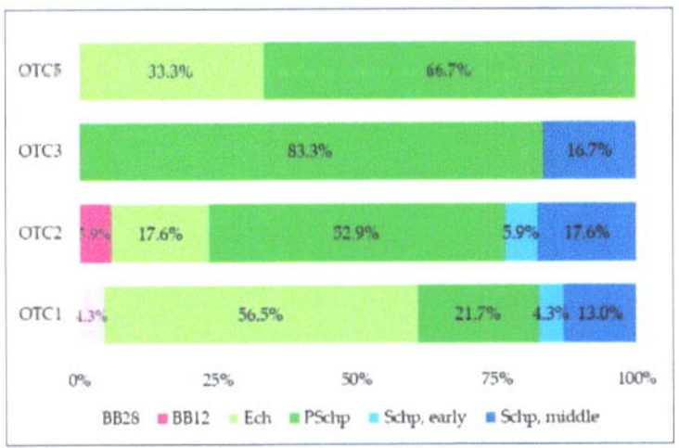

Figure 3. Respiratory tract—share of the age groups within the scope of OTCs.

- in the first group of over-the-counter medicines containing only a plant component (OTC1), there are medicines for five of all age groups (with the exception of breastfeeding babies by the 12th month (BB12)), but over half of them (56.5%) are intended for children in the pre-school period (PSchp);
- there is a similar distribution in the over-the-counter medicines containing a combination of a plant component (OTC2) group where the medicines intended for children in the pre-school period (PSchp) dominate (52.9%), as in this group there are also medicines intended for the youngest children—breastfeeding babies by the 12th month (BB12);
- in the over-the-counter medicines containing a combination of a plant substance + a synthetic substance (OTC3) group, over 80% of all medicines are intended for children in the pre-school period (PSchp) and 16.7% are intended for children in the secondary school period (Schp, middle);
- over-the-counter medicines containing a combination of a derivative + a synthetic substance (OTC5) are divided in a 33% to 66% proportion in two age groups—early childhood (Ech) and pre-school period (PSchp).

On the grounds of the two-dimensional division, an χ^2 test has been prepared in order to check the presence of any dependence between the two variables. The formulated hypotheses are as follows:

$\mathbf{H_0}$ *There is no dependence between the number of OTCs of different types and the age groups in which they are offered.*

$\mathbf{H_1}$ *We expect some dependence between the number of OTCs of different types and the age groups in which they are offered.*

The result from the check of the zero hypothesis has shown that we have to accept it as being correct.

(Pearson chi-square = 16.284, df = 15, p = 0.363).

2.2. Pain

Sixteen medicines in total have been observed in this category as fifteen of them belong to the over-the-counter medicines containing a combination of a plant substance + a synthetic substance (OTC3) group, and one is from the over-the-counter medicines containing only a plant component (OTC1) group. The medicines for pain relief were intended for three age groups—Schp early, Schp middle, and Adul. In two of them (Adul and Schp middle), all of the medicines are from the OTC3 group, whereas in the Schp early group, they are equally divided between OTC1 and OTC3 (Figure 4).

The development of a child is an incessant process that starts from the child's birth and continues until the time the child becomes mature. It is characterized by morphological and functional changes of the organs and the systems, maturity of the immune-biological reactivity and improvement of the intellect. Every age in a person's life is distinguished by its own features and anatomic and physiological peculiarities of adaptation of reactivity, motor activity, and nervous and psychological development.

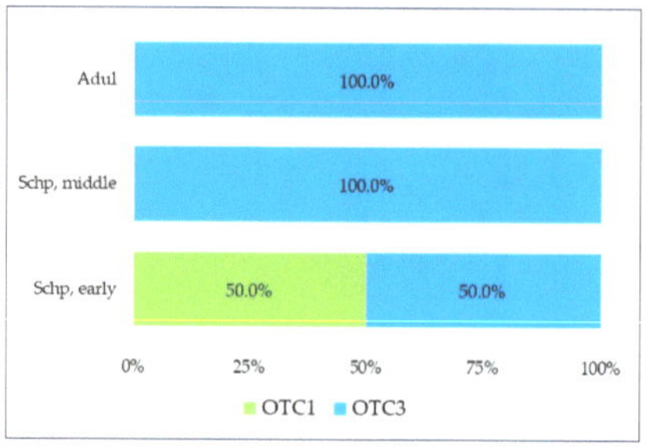

Figure 4. Pain—distribution of OTCs across age groups.

As commented above, OTC1 medicines are entirely intended for the Schp small age group. In the OTC3 group, the division includes a dominant share (68.8%) of the medicines intended for children in the Schp middle group, 25% for children in the Adul group, and 6.3% for the children in the Schp early group (Figure 5).

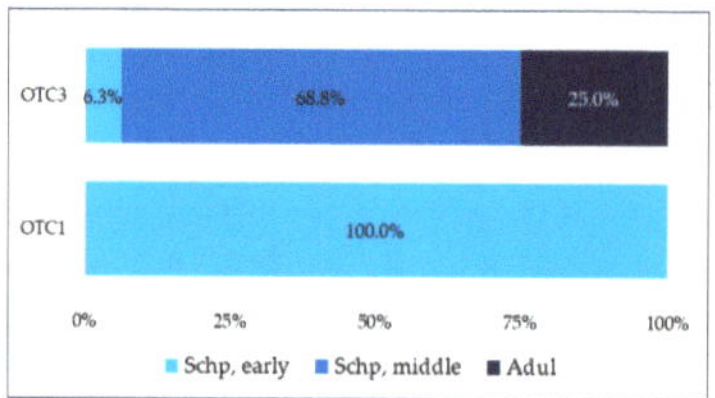

Figure 5. Pain—share of the age groups within the scope of OTCs.

Considering the fact that the immune system is not completely developed in younger children, children are much more susceptible to viral infections, colds, and influenza [34]. Premature babies are also very susceptible to infections [35]. Children have colds much more frequently, 6–8 times a year, compared to adults who usually have a cold 4–6 times a year [36].

The reasons for a cold among children are different; in most cases, it is caused by viruses, but bacteria can also trigger its emergence. A usual cold lasts for a short time. In most cases, the symptoms reach their peak on the third day and disappear within a week, although the cough may still be present [37]. Nonprescription medicines are also used to influence the cold symptoms, in addition to synthetic substances like paracetamol, dimethidine, and derivatives—pseudoephedrine, and phenylephrine hydrochloride, which are present both individually or in combination—these medicines contain extracts of a number of medicinal plants.

The results from our study have undoubtedly shown that among the youngest pediatric patients, over-the-counter medicines intended to influence the symptoms related to the upper respiratory tract contain mainly a plant component. We have established that among the groups examined by us that are applied to pediatric patients, over-the-counter medicines containing only a plant component (OTC1) and over-the-counter medicines containing a combination of a plant components (OTC2), whose compositions contain plants and their extracted derivatives, are represented mainly by the following plant raw materials: *Tymus vulgaris* L., herba; *Hedera helix* L., folium; *Cetraria islandica* (L.) Ach., tallus; *Althaea officinalis* L., radix or folium; *Primula officinalis* L., radix; and some rare plants such as *Glaucium flavum* Crantz (Glaucine hydrobromide) and *Pelargonium sidoides* DC. Table 1 shows the studied OTC1 and OTC2, with their commercial and international names, their contents of active substances, the symptoms for which they are intended, and the age groups for which they can be applied.

Table 1. Registered nonprescription medicines containing plant raw materials announced on the official website of the Bulgarian Drug Agency.

№	Freely Chosen Name	Medicinal Form and Quantity of the Active Substance in a Dose Unit	INN	ATC Code	Content	Use among Pediatric Patients	Plant-Based OTC Depending on the Active Substance	Use of OTC in the Period of (in Accordance with the Age Differentiation among the Pediatric Population)	Therapeutic Indications
1.	Bronchicum	100 mg compressed lozenges × 20; × 50	Thyme fluid extract	R05CA00	Each tablet contains: ✔ *Thymi herba extractum siccum* equivalent to 100 mg *Thymi herba extractum fluidum* (1: 2–2.5)	Over 4 years of age	OTC1	Pre-school period	Upper respiratory tract
2.	Bronchicum Elixir S	5.0 g/2.5 g/100 g syrup—130 g	Thymi herbae tincture//Grindelii herbae tincture/Quebrachi corticis tincture/Primulae radicis tincture/Pimpinellae radicis tincture	R05CA10	100 mL of the syrup contains: ✔ *Thymus vulgaris/zygis* L., *herba* (1:2–2.5) (liquid extract from a blade of thymes)—5.0 g; ✔ *Primula veris/elatior* L., *radix* (1:2–2.5)—2.5 g.	Over 4 years of age	OTC2	Pre-school period	Upper respiratory tract, cough
3.	Broncholytin	5.75 mg/4.6 mg/5 ml syrup × 125 g	Glaucine bromide/Basilici oil/Ephedrine hydrochloride	R05FA02	B 5 mL of the syrup contains: ✔ *Glaucine hydrobromide*—5.75 mg; ✔ *Eephedrine hydrochloride*—4.6 mg.	Over 3 years of age	OTC2	Pre-school period	Upper respiratory tract, cough
4.	Bronchostop	59.5 mg pastilles × 20; × 40	Plant medicinal product	R05CA	1 pastille contains: 59.5 mg *Thymus vulg./Thymus zyg.* L.) dry extract from blades (7–13:1)	Over 12 years of age	OTC1	School period (middle school age)	Upper respiratory tract, throat
5.	Bronchostop	0.77 g/0.66 g/5 ml—syrup × 150 ml	Plant medicinal product	R05CA10	5 ml (approximately 5.7 g) of syrup contains: ✔ 0.77 g *Thymus vulg./Thymus zyg.* dry extract from blades (1:2–2.5 ✔ *Althaea off.*, (liquid extract from roots (1:20)	Over 4 years of age	OTC2	Pre-school period	Upper respiratory tract, cough
6.	Bronchostop Duo	51.1 mg/4.5 mg pastilles × 10; × 20; × 30; × 40	Plant medicinal product	R05CA	1 pastille contains: ✔ 51.1 mg *Thymus vulg./Thymus zyg.*) (7–13:1) water extract); ✔ 4.5 *Althaea off.* (7–9:1)	Over 6 years of age	OTC2	Pre-school period	Upper respiratory tract, cough
7.	Bronchostop Sine	0.12 g/1.28 g/15 ml oral solution—100 ml; × 120 ml; × 150 ml; × 200 ml	Plant medicinal product	R05CA10	15 ml (=15.45 g) of the solution contains: ✔ 0.12 g *Thymus vulg. Thymus zyg.* dry extract from blades (7–13:1). ✔ *Althaea off.*, liquid extract from the roots (1:12–14)	Over 2 years of age (not recommended for children under 2 years of age)	OTC2	Early childhood	Upper respiratory tract, cough
8.	Bronchoton	4.6 mg/5.75 mg/5 ml syrup × 125 g	Glaucine hydrochloride/Ephedrine hydrochloride/Basilici oil	R05FA02	5 ml of syrup contains: ✔ *Ephedrine hydrochloride*—4.6 mg. ✔ *Glaucine hydrobromide*—5.75 mg.	Over 3 years of age	OTC2	Pre-school period	Upper respiratory tract, cough
9.	Carmolis	Oral drops, solution/cutaneous solution/inhalation vapor, solution—20 ml; × 40 ml, × 80 ml; × 160 ml	Anise oil/Clove oil/Citronella oil/Lavander oil/Lemon oil/Spirit of lemon balm/Menthol racemic/Nutmeg oil/Sage oil/Spiciae aetheroleum/Thyme oil	Plant medicinal product	100 g Carmolis contains: ✔ *Laevomentholum*—1.72000 g. ✔ *Thymi aetheroleum*—0.00172 g; ✔ *Anisi aetheroleum*—0.01548 g; ✔ *Cinn.cassiae aetheroleum*—0.17716 g; ✔ *Caryophylli floris aetheroleum*—0.17716 g; ✔ *Limonis aetheroleum*—0.01118 g; ✔ *Lavandulae aetheroleum*—0.17716 g; ✔ *Spicae aetheroleum*—0.17716 g; ✔ *Citronellae aetheroleum*—0.01720 g; ✔ *Salviae aetheroleum*—0.03526 g; ✔ *Myristicae aetheroleumi* 0.07052 g ✔ *Melissae spiritus*/1:5/	Not recommended for children under 12 years of age	OTC2	School period (middle school age)	Upper respiratory tract, cough

Table 1. *Cont.*

№	Freely Chosen Name	Medicinal Form and Quantity of the Active Substance in a Dose Unit	INN	ATC Code	Content	Use among Pediatric Patients	Plant-Based OTC Depending on the Active Substance	Use of OTC in the Period of (in Accordance with the Age Differentiation among the Pediatric Population)	Therapeutic Indications
10.	Cefabronchin	50 g/21 g/100 g oral drops, solution × 20 ml, × 50 ml, × 100 ml	Plant medicinal product		100 g of drops contains: ✔ *Thymi herba extractum fluidum* (1:2–3) 50 g *Extractum fluidum compositum* (1:3–4) 21 g: ✔ *Lichen islandicus;* ✔ *Saponariae rubrae radix;* ✔ *Pimpinellae radix;* ✔ *Eucalypti folium;* ✔ *Foeniculi amari fructus* (1:1:1:1:1) et 1 pars ✔ *Anisi stellati fructus*	Over 4 years of age	OTC2	Pre-school period	Upper respiratory tract, cough
11.	Hedelix	0.8 g/100 ml syrup	Hederae helicis folium extractum spissum	R05CA12	100 ml of syrup contains: 0.8 g *Hederae helicis folium extractum spissum* with a proportion of the active substance and the extract (2.2–2.9: 1).	Yes 0 +	OTC1	Breastfeeding period	Upper respiratory tract, cough
12.	Hedespan	7 mg/ml syrup ×100 ml	Plant medicinal product	R05CA 0	1 ml contains: 7 mg extr. siccum *Hedera helix* L., *folium*	Over 2 years of age	OTC1	Early childhood	Upper respiratory tract, cough
13.	Herbion iceland Moss	6 mg/ml syrup × 150 ml	Plant medicinal product		1 ml of syrup contains: 6 mg *Cetraria islandica* (L.) Ach, *tallus* (16–18:1)	Yes (for children aged 4–6 after being diagnosed)	OTC1	Pre-school period	Upper respiratory tract, cough
14.	Herbion Ivy	7 mg/ml syrup × 150 ml	Plant medicinal product	R05CA 12	1 ml of syrup contains: 7 mg *Hederae helicis folium extractum spirituosum siccum* (5–7.5:1)	Over 2 years of age (contraindicated for children under 2 years of age)	OTC1	Early childhood	Upper respiratory tract, cough
15.	Herbion Ivy	lozengez × 8; × 16; × 24; × 32; × 40	Plant medicinal product	R05CA 12	1 tablet for sucking contains: 35 mg *Hedera helix* L., *folium extractum siccum* (5–7.5:1)	Over 6 years of age	OTC1	Pre-school period	Upper respiratory tract, cough
16.	Hustagil Thyme Cough Syrup	syrup × 150 ml	Thyme fluid extract	R05CA	6 g (= 5 ml) contains medicinal substance: 480 mg *Extr. Thymi fluidum* (DAB) standardized over min. 0.03% Tymol	Over 1 year of age	OTC1	Early childhood	Upper respiratory tract, cough
17.	Ivitus	7 mg/ml oral solution— × 100 ml; × 150 ml; × 200 ml	Expetorants	R05CA 0	1 ml of solution contains: *Hedera helix* L. folium (5–8:1)	Over 2 years of age	OTC1	Early childhood	Upper respiratory tract, cough
18.	Mucohelix	syrup × 100 ml	Hederae helicis folii extractium siccum	R05CA12	1 ml of syrup contains: 8.25 mg *Hederae helicis folium extractum siccum*	Over 2 years of age	OTC1	Early childhood	Upper respiratory tract, cough
19.	Mucoplant Spitzwegerich Hustensaft	syrup 5 g/100 g × 100 ml; × 250 ml	Plant medicinal product	R05FB02	1 g (0.8 ml) of syrup contains: 50 mg *Plantaginis lanceolatae folium extractum fluidum* (*Plantago lanceolata* L.) (1:1)	Over 2 years of age	OTC1	Early childhood	Upper respiratory tract, cough
20.	Mucoplant Anisol	Capsules 100 mg × 30	Anise oil/Anisi aetheroleum	R05CA	1 capsule contains: *Anisi stellati aetheroleum*—100 mg	Over 12 years of age	OTC1	School period (middle school age)	Upper respiratory tract, cough
21.	Mucoplant Cough Syrup Ivy	154 mg/100 ml syrup × 100 ml; × 200 ml; × 250 ml	Ivy leaf dry extract (*Hedera helix* L.) Extraction solvent: Ethanol	R05C	Each ml contains:1.54 mg *Hedera helix* L. (DER 4–8:1)	Over 2 years of age (contraindicated for children under 2 years of age owing to a risk of deterioration of the respective symptoms)	OTC1	Early childhood	Upper respiratory tract, cough
22.	Pinosol	nasal drops, solution 10 ml	Pine oil/Eucalyptus oil/Tocopherol acetate/Thymol/Guaizulene/Peppermint oil	R01AX00	Medicines contain: ✔ *Scots pine, oil*—375.2 mg; ✔ *Hot mint, oil*—100 mg; ✔ *Eucalyptus oil*—50 mg; ✔ *Alpha-tocopheryl acetate*—170 mg; ✔ *Thymol*—3.2 mg; ✔ *Guaiazulene*—2.0 mg. in 10 g solution. 1 mL = 25 gutt	Over 6 years of age for inhalation among children over 12 years of age	OTC2	Pre-school period	Upper respiratory tract, inflammation of the nasal and nasopharyngeal mucous membrane

Table 1. *Cont.*

№	Freely Chosen Name	Medicinal Form and Quantity of the Active Substance in a Dose Unit	INN	ATC Code	Content	Use among Pediatric Patients	Plant-Based OTC Depending on the Active Substance	Use of OTC in the Period of (in Accordance with the Age Differentiation among the Pediatric Population)	Therapeutic Indications
23.	Prospan	20 mg/ml oral drops, solution × 20 ml	Hedera helix extract	R05FB00	1 ml of solution contains: ✔ 20 mg *Hedera helix folium extractum siccum* (5–7.5:1)	Over 1 year of age	OTC1	Early childhood	Upper respiratory tract, cough
24.	Prospan	65 mg eff. tablets × 10; × 20	Hedera helix extract	R05FB00	1 effervescent tablet contains: 65 mg *Hedera helix folium extractum siccum* (5–7.5:1)	Over 12 years of age (children over 6 years of age take $\frac{1}{2}$ of an effervescent tablet 2 times a day)	OTC1	Pre-school period	Upper respiratory tract, cough
25.	Prospan	26 mg lozenges × 10; × 20	Hedera helix extract	R05CA	1 tablet for sucking contains: 26 mg *Hedera helix folium extractum siccum* (5–7.5): 1)	Over 6 years of age	OTC1	Pre-school period	Upper respiratory tract, cough
26.	Prospan	7 mg/ml syrup × 5 ml; × 100 ml; × 200 ml	Hedera helix extract	R05FB00	1 ml of syrup contains: 7 mg *Hedera helix folium extractum siccum* (5–7.5:1)	Over 1 year of age. For children under 1 year of age it must be prescribed by a doctor	OTC1	Early childhood	Upper respiratory tract, cough
27.	Prospan Liquid	7 mg/ml oral liquid—5 ml × 21	Hedera helix extract	R05FB00	1 ml of syrup contains: 7 mg *Hedera helix folium extractum siccum* (5–7.5:1)	Over 6 years of age	OTC1	Pre-school period	Upper respiratory tract, cough
28.	Sinupret	syrup × 50 ml, × 100 ml, × 200 ml, × 500 ml	Plant medicinal product	R05CA10	100 g of syrup contains: extract (1:11) from: ✔ *Gentianae radix;* ✔ *Primulae flos calycibus;* ✔ *Verbenae herba;* ✔ *Rumicis herba;* ✔ *Sambuci flos* (1:3:3:3:3)	Over 2 years of age	OTC2	Early childhood	Upper respiratory tract, inflammation of the paranasal sinuses
29.	Sinupret	coated tablets × 50; × 100; × 200; × 500	Rumicis herbae pulvis/Sambuci flos pulvis/Gentianae radix pulvis/Primulae flos pulvis/Verbenae herbae pulvis	R05CA10	1 coated tablet contains: ✔ *Gentianae radix pulv.*—6 mg; ✔ *Primulae flos cum calycibus pulv.*—18 mg; ✔ *Rumicis herba pulv.*—18 mg; ✔ *Sambuci flos pulv.*—18 mg; ✔ *Verbenae herba pulv.*—18 mg.	Over 6 years of age (not recommended for children under 6 years of age owing to the lack of sufficient evidence)	OTC2	School period (early school age)	Upper respiratory tract, inflammation of the paranasal sinuses
30.	Sinupret Forte	coated tablets × 20; × 50; × 100; × 500	Rumicis herbae pulvis/Sambuci flos pulvis/Gentianae radicis pulvis/Primulae flos pulvis/Verbenae herbae pulvis	R05CA10	1 coated tablet contains: ✔ *Gentianae radix pulv.*—12 mg; ✔ *Primulae flos cum calycibus pulv.*—36 mg; ✔ *Rumicis herba pulv.*—36 mg; ✔ *Sambuci flos pulv.*—36 mg; ✔ *Verbenae herba pulv.*—36 mg	Not recommended for children under 12 years of age owing to the lack of sufficient data	OTC2	School period (middle school age)	Upper respiratory tract, inflammation of the paranasal sinuses
31.	Tavipec	150 mg gastro-resistant capsules, soft × 20; × 30	Spicae aetheroleum	R05CA00	1 capsule contains: *Spicae aetheroleum*—150 mg	Over 12 years of age	OTC1	School period (middle school age)	Upper respiratory tract, expectorant
32.	Tuspan	7 mg/ml syrup × 120 ml	Ivy leaf dry extract	R05CA12	1 ml of syrup contains: 7 mg *extract from Hedera helix* L. (5–7.5:1)	Over 2 years of age (not recommended for children under 2 years of age owing to their oversensitivity to the active substance)	OTC1	Early childhood	Upper respiratory tract, expectorant

Table 1. *Cont.*

№	Freely Chosen Name	Medicinal Form and Quantity of the Active Substance in a Dose Unit	INN	ATC Code	Content	Use among Pediatric Patients	Plant-Based OTC Depending on the Active Substance	Use of OTC in the Period of (in Accordance with the Age Differentiation among the Pediatric Population)	Therapeutic Indications
33.	Tussavit	7.53 g/7.53 g/100 g syrup 125 g; 250 g	Thymi folium extr./Plantaginis folium	R05CA00	100 g of syrup contains: ✔ 7.53 g *Thymi vulgaris herba/Thymi zygis herba extractum fluidum* (1:1); ✔ 7.53 g *Plantaginis lanceolatae folium extractum fluidum* (1:1)	Over 2 years of age (not recommended for children under 2 years of age owing to the content of alcohol)	OTC2	Early childhood	Upper respiratory tract, cough
34.	Umckalor	20 mg film-coated tablets × 15; × 30	Plant medicinal product	R05	1 coated tablet contains: 20 mg. dried *liquid extract from Pelargonii sidoidi radix* (1:8–10) (EPs 7630)	Over 6 years of age	OTC1	School period (early school age)	Respiratory tract, acute infections, bronchitis, sinusitis
35.	Umckalor	8 g/10 g oral drops, solution × 20 ml; 50 ml; × 100 ml	Pelargonii sidoidi radicis extractum liquidum	R05	10 g (= 9.75 ml) contains *Pelargonii sidoidi radix extr. fliudum* (1:8–10) (EPs 7630)	Over 1 year of age	OTC1	Early childhood	Respiratory tract, acute infections, bronchitis, sinusitis

3. Discussion

Medicinal plants having a mitigating effect and relieving irritation in case of inflammation of the upper respiratory tract include the following: marshmallow (*Althaea officinalis* L.); common mallow (*Malva sylvestris* L.); ribwort plantain (*Plantago lanceolata L.*); Icelandic moos (*Cetraria islandica* (L.) Ach); coltsfoot (*Tussilago farfara* L.) and others. The effectiveness of (*Althaea officinalis* L.) for coughs has been proven. The blossom of (*Malva sylvestris* L.) contains anthocyanins and mucilage. The mucilage is contained in all parts of the plant and the softening effect on the respiratory tract is due to the presence of this substance [38]. The most important bioactive compounds contained in the leaves of *P. lanceolata* L. are catalpol, aucubin, acteoside, and verbascoside. These compounds are responsible for the anti-inflammatory, antioxidant, antineoplastic, and hepatoprotective effects of the plant [39].

Other traditional plants characterized by mucolytic and antiseptic properties are thyme (*Thymus vulgaris* L.) and garlic (*Allium sativum* L.) [40,41]. The anti-inflammatory effect of extracts of *Tymus vulgaris* L. and *Hedera helix* L. has been studied in a lipopolysaccharide (LPS)-induced model of acute pulmonary inflammation in a rat [42]. The extract of *H. helix* is contained in a number of medicines that can also be applied for children from birth. Its anti-inflammatory, anti-bacterial, antifungal, and anthelmintic properties have been established. A conducted study has described that the simultaneous application of an extract of *H. helix* and Oseltamivir leads to a decrease in the pulmonary inflammation of mice infected with type A influenza virus (PR8). When used perorally, the extract of *H. helix*, whose activity is due to the presence of hederasaponin F, leads to an increased antiviral activity of Oseltamivir, which when applied individually provides insufficient defense against the PRS infection [43].

The medicinal plant *thyme* and its extract are applied perorally for coughs resulting from a cold, bronchitis, laryngitis, and gastrointestinal inflammations, and are also applied locally in the treatment of small wounds and mouth cavity diseases. The plant material contains an ethereal oil whose composition varies depending on the chemotype. The main components of the ethereal oil of *T. vulgaris* L. are: tymol and carvacrol. According to the conducted studies and the scientific sources, these isomeric monoterpenes (tymol, carvacrol) are responsible for the antiseptic, antitussive, and expectorant properties of thyme to a large extent [44].

The stalks of *T. vulgaris* L. and *Tymus zygis* L. are among the most widely used plant materials in the pharmaceutic industry [45]. In the literature, there are descriptions of the activity of cineole and myrtol and also of combined preparations containing primrose, which have manifested good activity during the treatment of sinusitis and bronchitis—some of the most common respiratory infections [46]. Medicines based on medicinal plants are used owing to their antitussive and expectorant effects. Antitussive medicines affect centrally the focus of the cough in the brain or peripherally affect receptors in the respiratory tract.

The use of herbal medicines among children may also pose a number of risks which, on the one hand, arise from the multi-component composition of the plant material and also from the lack of any evidence guaranteeing their safety [47,48]. The continuous use of the so-called traditional plant-based medicines is to be regarded as a guarantee for their safety and efficiency, but their multi-component compositions and the differences in the standardization of various plant materials impede the clinical testing of them. In the composition of the OTC medicines, including those tested by us, there are substances such as paracetamol (acetaminophen), antihistamines (pheniramine maleate), and decongestants (pseudoephedrine, phenylephrine hydrochloride, dimethidine), which lead to a more frequent manifestation of unwanted reactions [49].

Shefrin and Goldman have indicated in their study that the existing evidence related to the application of the over-the-counter medicines in case of infections of the upper respiratory tract is insufficient. In addition, they have also stated that the manifestations of unwanted medicinal reactions resulting from the use of nonprescription medicines are most commonly caused by improper dosage, uncontrolled swallowing, or an inappropriate medicine [50].

Paracetamol, also known as acetaminophen, is a medicine applied individually or in combination with other substances. It has been used since 1955 and is one of the most common medicines for reducing the body temperature (antipyretic) and relieving pain [51]. In medical practice, paracetamol is also a first-line medicine for pain. Based on data contained in the medical literature, paracetamol is safe to be applied from birth and does not cause any hepatic damages when used in accordance with the existing recommendations. Single intakes exceeding the recommended dose ten times are potentially toxic [52]. Conducted studies have described the probability that a chronic use of paracetamol may increase the risk of allergic reactions or asthma among children [53]. The evidence on paracetamol-induced disorders in neurological development is still insufficient [54].

The current study has shown that in the period of breastfeeding (BB12 and BB28) as well as in early childhood (Ech), the composition of the over-the-counter medicines contains primarily substances individually or in combination—as shown in Figure 2. As can be seen from the graph, over-the-counter medicines containing a derivative (OTC4) and OTC6 have not been detected. We could explain their absence with their composition, which comprises a derivative (OTC4) or the combination of a plant + derivative + synthetic substance (OTC6). The presence of a derivative and/or a synthetic substance leads to an increased frequency of the manifestation of unwanted medicinal effects. Another similar study has emphasized that the use of over-the-counter medicines containing antihistamines and decongestants is related to unwanted effects resulting from overdosing and improper use. The American Food and Drug Administration has approved these medicines among adult patients, but with reference to pediatric patients, they have not been tested sufficiently to ensure their safety and efficiency. Owing to this, the FDA has recommended that the content indicated on the label of these medicines be reviewed and also that the use of these medicines among children under 2 years of age be ceased.

Pseudoephedrine and phenylephrine hydrochloride are substances that are present in the composition of medicines used to treat nasal congestion (clogged nose), cold, influenza, and allergies.

Pseudoephedrine (PSE) as a stereoisomer of ephedrine and the medicines containing it, when administered in hid doses, trigger physical symptoms such as reduced appetite, dryness in the mouth, palpitation, and motor symptoms (for example, disruption of gait and balance, postural instability, generalized dystonia, psychomotor retardation, and others) [55]. When applied among pediatric patients, PSE, even in therapeutic doses, may cause the emergence of dizziness, increased heart rate, excitement, and sleeplessness [56,57]. Within the European Union, over-the-counter medicines containing pseudoephedrine can be found on the pharmaceutical market under various tradenames. Owing to considerations related to the safety of the use of medicines containing pseudoephedrine, in early 2023, the Pharmacovigilance Risk Assessment Committee (PRAC) of the European Medicines Agency (EMA) started reviewing these medicines [58].

A study carried out within the period 2003–2006 in Germany has described that self-medication among children and adolescents is increasingly spreading and that this is valid for families with a higher socio-economic status. The use of flu and cold medications, as well as aspirin, among pediatric patients poses potential risks [59]. In general, the rational use of the appropriate OTC drug will result in fewer adverse effects and may be beneficial.

Our study has confirmed that substances like paracetamol, pheniramin maleate, and decongestants are contained in OTCs applied among children in the pre-school and the school periods of their development. The purpose of our subsequent study will be to check N0 again (the zero hypothesis) by comparing the other nosological units in which OTCs containing a plant substance are applied.

4. Materials and Methods

4.1. A Documentary Analysis of the List of Medicines Registered as Nonprescription Medicines

The list of the over-the-counter medicines was made in 2020 and published on the website of the Bulgarian Drug Agency. The list includes medicines whose permission for use has not expired, although they can be sold until the exhaustion of the available quantity, but no more than a year past the expiry date of the permission for use, which is in accordance with the pharmaceutical legislation of the country.

We have analyzed these medicines based on their active substance(s), indications for use, and age groups. We have distinguished those with a plant component applied among pediatric patients.

4.2. Statistical Analysis

Cross-tabulation and chi-square test.

We used the Pearson's chi-square test (Fisher, 1922; Pearson, 1900) to examine whether there is a relationship between two variables in a cross-table. The purpose of cross-tabulation is to show in a tabular format the relationship between two variables. The purpose of a chi-square test of independence is to determine whether the observed values for the cells deviate significantly from the corresponding expected values for those cells.

Cross-tabulation displays the two variables—age groups (v1) and OTCs (v2)—in a series of rows and columns. The two cross-tables have six rows (v1) and four columns (v2) (v2 has non-zero frequencies for OTC1, OTC2, OTC3, and OTC5). The cross-tabulation table produced using IBM SPSS v.26 contains the number of cases that fall into each combination. We can also look at the percentages within the age groups by looking at the rows. This tells us, for example, that of those within the Ech age group, 76.5% are OTC1, 17.6% are OTC2, and 5.9% are OTC5.

The Pearson's chi-square (χ^2) uses the following equation:

$$\chi^2 = \sum \frac{\left(observed_{ij} - expected_{ij}\right)^2}{expected_{ij}}$$

in which i represents the rows in the cross-table and j represents the columns.

Expected frequencies for each of the cells in the table are calculated following the equation below:

$$E_{ij} = \frac{row\ total_i \times column\ total_j}{n}$$

where n is simply the total number of observations.

The x^2 statistic can then be checked against a distribution with known properties. The degrees of freedom of these are calculated as (r − 1)(c − 1), in which r is the number of rows and c is the number of columns. We used SPSS, and this simply produces an estimate of the precise probability of obtaining a chi-square statistic. If the significance value is small enough (conventionally, Sig. must be less than 0.05), then we reject the hypothesis that the variables are independent and gain confidence in the hypothesis that they are in some way related.

Correlation describes the relationship between variables. We assess that relationship (or association) in terms of a 'correlation coefficient', which measures the way in which the 'values' in one variable (in our case, age groups) change in relation to 'values' in a second variable (in our case, OTCs). A positive correlation coefficient occurs when values change in the same direction. A negative correlation exists when values change in opposite directions. We used Spearman's correlation test (at least one of the variables was not parametric).

During the preparation of the statistical analyses, we used abbreviations for nonprescription medicines and the separate periods of the development of the child/age groups, as indicated in Abbreviations.

5. Conclusions

Our study has shown a limited-type diversity of the plant substances contained in nonprescription medicines applied among children. Some nonprescription medicines contain pseudoephedrine, whose safety is currently being examined by the European Drug Agency. As a result, it is recommended that the Bulgarian Drug Agency, in its capacity as a control body for medicines in Bulgaria, reviews the over-the-counter medicines containing pseudoephedrine which are applied among children.

When developing herbal medicines for children, it is necessary to use all of the available resources, integrate the scientific strategies for clinical assessment, and also encourage ethnobotanical studies. Further studying and extending the scope of clinical tests of herbal medicines by applying the latest techniques are necessary, as well as assessments of the bioequivalence of the entire extract. The concept of good clinical practice (GCP) shall focus on the safety and the efficiency of phytopharmaceuticals as a whole and in particular of the phytopharmaceuticals applied among pediatric patients. On the other hand, good pharmacy practice obliges the pharmacist to inform the parents of the rational use of nonprescription medicines and the possible manifestation of unwanted effects and the potential related interactions.

Author Contributions: B.H. and V.P.-D. conceptualized the study, designed the experiments, performed investigations, interpreted the results, performed the statistical analysis, and wrote the main manuscript; V.P.-D. software and revised the manuscript. All authors have read and agreed to the published version of the manuscript.

Funding: This research received no external funding.

Institutional Review Board Statement: Not applicable.

Informed Consent Statement: Not applicable.

Data Availability Statement: Data are contained within the article.

Conflicts of Interest: The authors declare no conflicts of interest.

Abbreviations

OTC1	Over-the-counter medicines containing only a plant component
OTC2	Over-the-counter medicines containing a combination of plant components
OTC3	Over-the-counter medicines containing a combination of a plant substance + a synthetic substance
OTC4	Over-the-counter medicines containing a derivative
OTC5	Over-the-counter medicines containing a combination of a derivative + a synthetic substance
OTC6	Over-the-counter medicines containing a combination of a plant substance + a derivative + a synthetic substance
BB12	Breastfeeding babies by the 28th day
BB28	Breastfeeding babies by the 12th month
Ech	Early childhood
PSchp	Pre-school period
Schp, early	School period which includes the early school age
Schp, middle	School period which includes the secondary school age
Adul	Adolescence

References

1. Petrovska, B.B. Historical review of medicinal plants usage. *Pharmacogn. Rev.* **2012**, *6*, 1–5. [CrossRef]
2. Dias, D.A.; Urban, S.; Roessner, U. A Historical Overview of Natural Products in Drug Discovery. *Metabolites* **2012**, *2*, 303–336. [CrossRef]
3. Aboelsoud, N.H. Herbal medicine in ancient Egypt. *J. Med. Plants Res.* **2010**, *4*, 82–86.
4. Šantić, Ž.; Pravdić, N.; Bevanda, M.; Galić, K. The historical use of medicinal plants in traditional and scientific medicine. *Psychiatr. Danub.* **2017**, *29*, 787–792.

5. Hardy, K.; Buckley, S.; Collins, M.J.; Estalrrich, A.; Brothwell, D.; Copeland, L.; García-Tabernero, A.; García-Vargas, S.; de la Rasilla, M.; Lalueza-Fox, C.; et al. Neanderthal medics? Evidence for food, cooking, and medicinal plants entrapped in dental calculus. *Naturwissenschafte* **2012**, *99*, 617–626. [CrossRef]
6. Weyrich, L.S.; Duchene, S.; Soubrier, J.; Arriola, A.; Llamas, B.; Breen, J.; Morris, A.G.; Alt, K.W.; Caramelli, D.; Dresely, V.; et al. Neanderthal behaviour, diet, and disease inferred from ancient DNA in dental calculus. *Nature* **2017**, *544*, 357–361. [CrossRef]
7. Kuchta, K.; Cameron, S. Tradition to Pathogenesis: A Novel Hypothesis for Elucidating the Pathogenesis of Diseases Based on the Traditional use of Medicinal Plants. *Front. Pharmacol.* **2021**, *12*, 70507. [CrossRef]
8. Ekor, M. The growing use of herbal medicines: Issues relating to adverse reactions and challenges in monitoring safety. *Front. Pharmacol.* **2014**, *4*, 177. [CrossRef]
9. Miraldi, E.; Baini, G. Medicinal plants and health in human history: From empirical use to modern phytotherapy. *J. Siena Acad. Sci.* **2019**, *10*, 7–12. [CrossRef]
10. Eddouks, M.; Chattopadhyay, D.; De Feo, V.; Cho, W.C. Medicinal Plants in the Prevention and Treatment of Chronic Diseases. *Evid. Based Complement. Altern. Med.* **2012**, *2012*, 1–2. [CrossRef]
11. Ernst, E. Herbal medicine: Buy one, get two free. *Postgrad. Med. J.* **2007**, *83*, 615–616. [CrossRef]
12. Mohamed, I.; Shuid, A.; Borhanuddin, B.; Fozi, N. The Application of Phytomedicine in Modern Drug. *Internet J. Herbal. Plant Med.* **2012**, *1*, 1–9.
13. Firenzuoli, F.; Gori, L. Herbal medicine today: Clinical and research issues. *Evid. Based Complement. Altern. Med.* **2007**, *4*, 37–40. [CrossRef]
14. Gupta, R.C.; Lall, R.; Srivastava, A. *Nutraceuticals: Efficacy, Safety and Toxicity*, 2nd ed.; Gupta, R.C., Ed.; Academic Press: Cambridge, MA, USA, 2021; p. 1396.
15. Sofowora, A.; Ogunbodede, E.; Onayade, A. The role and place of medicinal plants in the strategies for disease prevention. *Afr. J. Tradit. Complement. Altern. Med.* **2013**, *10*, 210–229. [CrossRef]
16. Sachan, A.K.; Vishnoi, G.; Kumar, R. Need of standardization of herbal medicines in Modern era. *Int. J. Phytomedicine* **2016**, *8*, 300–307. [CrossRef]
17. Pan, S.Y.; Zhou, S.F.; Gao, S.H.; Yu, Z.L.; Zhang, S.F.; Tang, M.K.; Sun, J.N.; Ma, D.L.; Han, Y.F.; Fong, W.F.; et al. New Perspectives on How to Discover Drugs from Herbal Medicines: CAM's Outstanding Contribution to Modern Therapeutics. *Evid.-Based Complement. Altern. Med.* **2013**, *2013*, 627375. [CrossRef]
18. Ahmed, E.; Arshad, M.N.; Khan, M.Z.; Amjad, M.; Sadaf, H.M.; Riaz, I.; Sabir, S.; Ahmad, N.; Saboon. Secondary metabolites and their multidimensional prospective in plant life. *J. Pharmacogn. Phytochem.* **2017**, *6*, 205–214.
19. Freire, C.J.; Barbosa, L.R.; Costa, J.G.; Santos, R.; Santos, A.F. Phytotherapy in pediatrics: The production of knowledge and practices in Primary Care. *Rev. Bras. Enferm.* **2018**, *71*, 637–645. [CrossRef]
20. Cohen, M.H.; Kemper, K.J.; Stevens, L.; Hashimoto, D.; Gilmour, J. Pediatric use of complementary therapies: Ethical and policy choices. *Pediatrics* **2005**, *116*, e568–e575. [CrossRef]
21. Cohen, M.H.; Kemper, K.J. Complementary Therapies in Pediatrics: A Legal Perspective. *Pediatrics* **2005**, *115*, 774–780. [CrossRef]
22. Catlin, J.R.; Brass, E.P. The Effectiveness of Nonprescription Drug Labels in the United States: Insights from Recent Research and Opportunities for the Future. *Pharmacy* **2018**, *6*, 119. [CrossRef]
23. El-Khatib, F.M.; Yafi, N.R.; Yafi, F.A. Over-the-Counter supplements and men's health. In *Effects of Lifestyle on Men's Health*; Academic Press: Cambridge, MA, USA, 2019; pp. 281–300. [CrossRef]
24. European Union. Directive 2004/24/EC of the European Parliament and of the Council of 31 March 2004 amending, as Regards Traditional Herbal Medicinal Products, Directive 2001/83/EC on the Community Code Relating to Medicinal Products for Human Use. Available online: https://eur-lex.europa.eu/eli/dir/2004/24/oj (accessed on 1 December 2020).
25. Minghetti, P.; Franzè, S.; Zaccara, V.; Raso, F.; Morazzoni, P. Innovation in Phytotherapy: Is a New Regulation the Feasible Perspective in Europe? *Planta Med.* **2016**, *82*, 591–595. [CrossRef]
26. Bilia, A.R. Herbal medicinal products versus botanical-food supplements in the European market: State of art and perspectives. *Nat. Prod. Commun.* **2015**, *10*, 125–131. [CrossRef]
27. Sansgiry, S.S.; Bhansali, A.H.; Bapat, S.S.; Xu, Q. Abuse of Over-the-Counter Medicines: A Pharmacist's Perspective. *Integr. Pharm. Res. Pract.* **2017**, *6*, 1–6. [CrossRef]
28. Kulevanova, S. Modern herbal medicine. In *Phytotherapy*; Max Zeller Söhne AG: Romanshorn, Switzerland, 2014; p. 584.
29. Wijesundara, N.M.; Sekhon-Loodu, S.; Rupasinghe, H.V. Phytochemical-rich medicinal plant extracts suppress bacterial antigens-induced inflammation in human tonsil epithelial cells. *PeerJ* **2017**, *5*, e3469. [CrossRef]
30. Sherazi, B.A.; Mahmood, K.T.; Amin, F.; Zaka, M.; Riaz, M.; Javed, A. Prevalence and Measure of Self Medication: A Review. *J. Pharm. Sci. Res.* **2012**, *4*, 1774–1778.
31. Marathe, P.A.; Kamat, S.K.; Tripathi, R.K.; Raut, S.B.; Khatri, N.P. Over-the-counter medicines: Global perspective and Indian scenario. *J. Postgrad. Med.* **2020**, *66*, 28–34. [CrossRef]
32. Sánchez-Sánchez, E.; Fernández-Cerezo, F.L.; Díaz-Jimenez, J.; Rosety-Rodriguez, M.; Díaz, A.J.; Ordonez, F.J.; Rosety, M.Á.; Rosety, I. Consumption of over-the-Counter Drugs: Prevalence and Type of Drugs. *Int. J. Environ. Res. Public Health* **2021**, *18*, 5530. [CrossRef]
33. Dalton, K.; Byrne, S. Role of the pharmacist in reducing healthcare costs: Current insights. *Integr. Pharm. Res. Pract.* **2017**, *6*, 37–46. [CrossRef]

34. Olin, A.; Henckel, E.; Chen, Y.; Lakshmikanth, T.; Pou, C.; Mikes, J.; Gustafsson, A.; Bernhardsson, A.K.; Zhang, C.; Bohlin, K.; et al. Stereotypic Immune System Development in Newborn Children. *Cell* **2018**, *174*, 1277–1292.e14. [CrossRef]
35. Kollmann, T.R.; Kampmann, B.; Mazmanian, S.K.; Marchant, A.; Levy, O. Protecting the Newborn and Young Infant from Infectious Diseases: Lessons from Immune Ontogeny. *Immunity* **2017**, *46*, 350–363. [CrossRef]
36. Worrall, G. Common cold. *Can. Fam. Physician* **2011**, *57*, 1289–1290.
37. Arroll, B. Common cold. *BMJ Clin. Evid.* **2011**, *2011*, 1510. [PubMed]
38. Delfan, B.; Kazemeini, H.; Bahmani, M. Identifying Effective Medicinal Plants for Cold in Lorestan Province, West of Iran. *J. Evid. Based Complement. Altern. Med.* **2015**, *20*, 173–179. [CrossRef]
39. Abate, L.; Bachheti, R.; Tadesse, M.; Bachheti, A. Ethnobotanical Uses, Chemical Constituents, and Application of Plantago lanceolata L. *J. Chem.* **2022**, *2022*, 1532031. [CrossRef]
40. Chitra, S.; Sebareze, L. Antibacterial Activity of Thymus Vulgaris L. (Thyme) From Leaf Extract—A Medicinal Plant. *Int. J. Ecol. Dev.* **2011**, *20*, 60–68.
41. Lissiman, E.; Bhasale, A.L.; Cohen, M. Garlic for the common cold. *Cochrane Database Syst. Rev.* **2014**, *11*, CD006206. [CrossRef]
42. Csikós, E.; Csekő, K.; Ashraf, A.R.; Kemény, Á.; Kereskai, L.; Kocsis, B.; Böszörményi, A.; Helyes, Z.; Horváth, G. Effects of *Thymus vulgaris* L., *Cinnamomum verum* J.Presl and *Cymbopogon nardus* (L.) Rendle Essential Oils in the Endotoxin-induced Acute Airway Inflammation. *Molecules* **2020**, *25*, 3553. [CrossRef]
43. Hong, E.-H.; Song, J.-H.; Shim, A.; Lee, B.-R.; Kwon, B.-E.; Song, H.-H.; Kim, Y.-J.; Chang, S.-Y.; Jeong, H.G.; Kim, J.G.; et al. Coadministration of Hedera helix L. Extract Enabled Mice to Overcome Insufficient Protection against Influenza A/PR/8 Virus Infection under Suboptimal Treatment with Oseltamivir. *PLoS ONE* **2015**, *10*, e0131089. [CrossRef]
44. Fecka, I.; Turek, S. Determination of polyphenolic compounds in commercial herbal drugs and spices from Lamiaceae: Thyme, wild thyme and sweet marjoram by chromatographic techniques. *Food Chem.* **2008**, *108*, 1039–1053. [CrossRef]
45. Kowalczyk, A.; Przychodna, M.; Sopata, S.; Bodalska, A.; Fecka, I. Thymol and Thyme Essential Oil—New Insights into Selected Therapeutic Applications. *Molecules* **2020**, *25*, 4125. [CrossRef]
46. Anheyer, D.; Cramer, H.; Lauche, R.; Saha, F.J.; Dobos, G. Herbal Medicine in Children with Respiratory Tract Infection: Systematic Review and Meta-Analysis. *Acad. Pediatr.* **2018**, *18*, 8–19. [CrossRef]
47. Polat, S.; Gürol, A. Safety of Herbal Medicines in Children. *Altern. Med.* **2020**. [CrossRef]
48. Snodgrass, W.R. Herbal products: Risks and benefits of use in children. *Curr. Thera Res.* **2001**, *62*, 724–737. [CrossRef]
49. Lokker, N.; Sanders, L.; Perrin, E.M.; Kumar, D.; Finkle, J.; Franco, V.; Choi, L.; Johnston, P.E.; Rothman, R.L. Parental Misinterpretations of over-the-Counter Pediatric Cough and Cold Medication Labels. *Pediatrics* **2009**, *123*, 1464–1471. [CrossRef]
50. Shefrin, A.E.; Goldman, R.D. Use of over-the-counter cough and cold medications in children. *Can. Fam. Physician* **2009**, *55*, 1081–1083.
51. Tittarelli, R.; Pellegrini, M.; Scarpellini, M.G.; Marinelli, E.; Bruti, V.; Di Luca, N.M.; Busardo, F.P.; Zaami, S. Hepatotoxicity of paracetamol and related fatalities. *Eur. Rev. Med. Pharmacol. Sci.* **2017**, *21*, 95–101.
52. Cranswick, N.; Coghlan, D. Paracetamol Efficacy and Safety in Children: The First 40 Years. *Am. J. Ther.* **2000**, *7*, 135–141. [CrossRef]
53. Lowe, A.J.; Carlin, J.B.; Bennett, C.M.; Hosking, C.S.; Allen, K.J.; Robertson, C.F.; Axelrad, C.; Abramson, M.J.; Hill, D.J.; Dharmage, S.C. Paracetamol use in early life and asthma: Prospective birth cohort study. *BMJ* **2010**, *341*, c4616. [CrossRef]
54. Cendejas-Hernandez, J.; Sarafian, J.T.; Lawton, V.G.; Palkar, A.; Anderson, L.G.; Larivière, V.; Parker, W. Paracetamol (acetaminophen) use in infants and children was never shown to be safe for neurodevelopment: A systematic review with citation tracking. *Eur. J. Pediatr.* **2022**, *181*, 1835–1857. [CrossRef]
55. Schifano, F.; Chiappini, S.; Miuli, A.; Mosca, A.; Santovito, M.C.; Corkery, J.M.; Guirguis, A.; Pettorruso, M.; Di Giannantonio, M.; Martinotti, G. Focus on Over-the-Counter Drugs' Misuse: A Systematic Review on Antihistamines, Cough Medicines, and Decongestants. *Front. Psychiatry* **2021**, *12*, 657397. [CrossRef]
56. Piątek, A.; Koziarska-Rościszewska, M.; Zawilska, J.B. Recreational use of over-the counter drugs: The doping of the brain. *Alcohol. Drug Addict.* **2015**, *28*, 65–77. [CrossRef]
57. Głowacka, K.; Wiela-Hojeńska, A. Pseudoephedrine-Benefits and Risks. *Int. J. Mol. Sci.* **2021**, *22*, 5146. [CrossRef]
58. European Medicines Agency. Available online: https://www.ema.europa.eu/en/news/prac-starts-safety-review-pseudoephedrine-containing-medicines (accessed on 7 April 2023).
59. Du, Y.; Knopf, H. Self-medication among children and adolescents in Germany: Results of the National Health Survey for Children and Adolescents (KiGGS). *Br. J. Clin. Pharmacol.* **2009**, *68*, 599–608. [CrossRef]

pharmaceuticals

MDPI

Article

In Vitro Screening of Antimicrobial and Anti-Coagulant Activities, ADME Profiling, and Molecular Docking Study of *Citrus limon* L. and *Citrus paradisi* L. Cold-Pressed Volatile Oils

Assia Hamdi [1], Mabrouk Horchani [2], Hichem Ben Jannet [2], Mejdi Snoussi [3,4,*], Emira Noumi [3,4], Nouha Bouali [3,4], Adel Kadri [5,6], Flavio Polito [7], Vincenzo De Feo [7,*] and Hayet Edziri [8]

1. Laboratory of Chemical, Pharmaceutical and Pharmacological Development of Drugs, Faculty of Pharmacy, University of Monastir, Monastir 5000, Tunisia; hamdiessia@gmail.com
2. Laboratory of Heterocyclic Chemistry, Natural Products and Reactivity, Medicinal Chemistry and Natural Products (LR11ES39), Department of Chemistry, Faculty of Science of Monastir, University of Monastir, Avenue of Environment, Monastir 5019, Tunisia; horchani.mabrouk@gmail.com (M.H.); hichem.bjannet@gmail.com (H.B.J.)
3. Department of Biology, College of Science, University of Ha'il, Hail 2440, Saudi Arabia; eb.noumi@uoh.edu.sa (E.N.); nouhabouali82@gmail.com (N.B.)
4. Medical and Diagnostic Research Centre, University of Ha'il, Hail 55473, Saudi Arabia
5. College of Science and Arts in Baljurashi, Al Baha University, Al Baha 65527, Saudi Arabia; lukadel@yahoo.fr
6. Laboratory of Plant Biotechnology Applied to Crop Improvement, Faculty of Sciences of Sfax, University of Sfax, Sfax 3000, Tunisia
7. Department of Pharmacy, University of Salerno, Via Giovanni Paolo II, 132, 84084 Fisciano, Italy; fpolito@unisa.it
8. Laboratory of Transmissible Diseases and Biologically Active Substances, Faculty of Pharmacy, Monastir 5000, Tunisia; jaziri_hayet@yahoo.fr

* Correspondence: m.snoussi@uoh.edu.sa or snmejdi@yahoo.fr (M.S.); defeo@unisa.it (V.D.F.)

Citation: Hamdi, A.; Horchani, M.; Jannet, H.B.; Snoussi, M.; Noumi, E.; Bouali, N.; Kadri, A.; Polito, F.; De Feo, V.; Edziri, H. In Vitro Screening of Antimicrobial and Anti-Coagulant Activities, ADME Profiling, and Molecular Docking Study of *Citrus limon* L. and *Citrus paradisi* L. Cold-Pressed Volatile Oils. *Pharmaceuticals* **2023**, *16*, 1669. https://doi.org/10.3390/ph16121669

Academic Editors: Elena Y. Enioutina, Kathleen M. Job and Catherine Sherwin

Received: 23 October 2023
Revised: 26 November 2023
Accepted: 28 November 2023
Published: 30 November 2023

Abstract: *Citrus*, which belongs to the Rutaceae family, is a very widespread genus in the Mediterranean Basin. In Tunisia, various parts of these spontaneous or cultivated plants are used in common dishes or in traditional medicine. The purpose of this work was to investigate *C. limon* and *C. paradisi* essential oil (EO). The samples were studied for their chemical composition using SPME/MS, as well as their antibacterial and antifungal activities. Prothrombin time (PT) and activated partial thromboplastin time (aPTT) methods were used to evaluate the anticoagulant potentialities. The obtained results show that both essential oils are rich in monoterpenes hydrocarbons, whereby limonene is the main compound in *C. paradisi* EO (86.8%) and *C. limon* EO (60.6%). Moreover, *C. paradisi* EO contains β-pinene (13.3%), sabinene (2.2%) and α-pinene (2.1%). The antibacterial assay of the essential oils showed important bactericidal and fungicidal effects against all strains tested. In fact, the MICs values of *C. limon* EO ranged from 0.625 to 2.5 mg/mL against all Gram-positive and Gram-negative bacteria, and from 6.25 to 12.5 mg/mL for *Candida* spp. strains, while *C. paradisi* EO was more active against all bacteria with low MICs values ranging from 0.192 to 0.786 mg/mL, and about 1.5 mg/mL against *Candida* species. Both tested *Citrus* EOs exhibited interesting anticoagulant activities as compared to heparin. The molecular docking approach was used to study the binding affinity and molecular interactions of all identified compounds with active sites of cytidine deaminase from *Klebsiella pneumoniae* (PDB: 6K63) and the C (30) carotenoid dehydrosqualene synthase from *Staphylococcus aureus* (PDB: 2ZCQ). The obtained results show that limonene had the highest binding score of -4.6 kcal.mol^{-1} with 6K63 enzyme, and -6.7 kcal.mol^{-1} with 2ZCQ receptor. The ADME profiling of the major constituents confirmed their important pharmacokinetic and drug-like properties. Hence, the obtained results highlight the potential use of both *C. limon* and *C. paradisi* essential oils as sources of bioactive compounds with antibacterial, antifungal, and anti-coagulant activities.

Keywords: *Citrus* species; essential oils; cold press; antibacterial; anti-coagulant; docking study; ADME

1. Introduction

Many serious health problems, such as heart and cardiovascular diseases, the emergence of nosocomial infections, and multidrug resistance in microorganisms, impact daily human life. Plant-derived molecules are promising alternatives used to counteract the effects of such human diseases [1,2]. As coagulation and thrombosis are among the major causes of atherosclerosis and cardiovascular diseases, numerous methods of treating or preventing thrombosis have been explored [3]. It is well documented that blood coagulation is directly associated with cardiovascular diseases via many factors, such as platelet activation and factor VIII level. Several commercial anticoagulant drugs have shown limited applicability because of their narrow therapeutic range. Their application doses can be considered unsafe as a result of their potential interactions with other drugs. Thus, due to interference with different medicines and certain negative effects, efforts are still being made to find new safe candidates for use as anticoagulants [3,4].

Plant essential oils are among the main sources of biological molecules considered promising, such as anticoagulant and antimicrobial agents. Different factors are implicated in the complexity of the chemical composition of citrus essential oils, such as genotype–cultivar [5], harvest year [6], harvest date, maturity of the species [7] and the extraction system [8]. This variability leads, in turn, to the different biological effects correlated with the major and minor compounds presented in these volatile oils. These studies have revealed that the fruits of three cultivar citrus species showed differences in terms of their biometrics and physico-chemical characteristics. The flavonoid contents also varied from one cultivar species to another. A study has demonstrated that these chemical compounds were similar but varied between areas [5]. Moreover, a great variability in the essential oil composition of *Citrus bergamia*, Risso was registered over thirty-five years, and this can be explained by several factor, such as the production year, the plant age, the microclimate, the cultivar, the techniques of agronomy, the harvest date of fruits, and the conditions and duration of storage [6]. Previous work has shown that cold-pressing, hydrodistillation and microwave-accelerated distillation can be used to extract essential oils, and these affect citrus fruits' fragrance, yield and chemical composition [8].

Essential oil compounds can directly influence hemostasis or modify the antithrombotic action. They have antiplatelet and fibrinolytic or thrombin-inhibiting effects, induced by modifying prostaglandin levels, inhibiting cyclo-oxygenase, inhibiting platelet activating factor, etc. [4]. Volatile oil components are also known for their strong antimicrobial activity against bacteria, yeasts, and viruses.

Citrus is among the most famous fruits, cultivated today in all Mediterranean regions. Fresh or dried, Citrus compounds are used in foods, flavors, refreshing drinks, pastries, and confectionery [9]. They are known as a potential source of bioactive natural molecules, such as phenolic compounds, minerals, citric acid, ascorbic acid, and terpenoids. Several works have shown their possible uses as antioxidant, anti-inflammatory, antipathogenic and anticancer substances [10]. They are also used as natural preservatives that preserve food from different oxidative or microbial alterations [11]. Some citrus extracts, such as aqueous extracts, essential oils and juice, have already been studied for their anticoagulant activity [3,12]. They are endowed with important broad-spectrum activities [13], and have revealed great potential in their use against bacteria and fungi [14,15]. *C. medica* (citron), *C. limon* (lemon), *C. reticulata* (mandarin, tangerine), *C. aurantium* (sour orange), *C. sinensis* (sweet orange), *C. clementina* (clementine) and *C. paradise* (grapefruit) are some of the citrus species cultivated around the world [16].

Tunisia is a country that produces cultivated or adapted citrus species. In 2019, the total production level of these plants in Tunisia was 393.3 thousand tones, divided between 135.0 thousand tons of oranges, 94.7 thousand tons of tangerines, 54.3 thousand tons of lemons and limes, and 109.3 thousand tons of grapefruits [17]. Different organs of these species are already widely used in traditional medicine, as well as for culinary and in economic purposes. The literature shows wide investigations into Tunisian citrus species [18,19].

New works have focused on in vitro experiments via the biological activity approach coupled to the computational approach, which combines molecular docking and ADMET prediction to estimate the biological importance of certain compounds present in essential oil [20–22]. Thus, the goal of the present research is to study the chemical composition, as well as the antibacterial and antifungal potentialities, of essential oils of *C. paradisi* L. and *C. limon* L. against multidrug-resistant bacteria and yeasts, and to determine their anticoagulant activities. In addition to the ADME analysis, a molecular docking investigation was undertaken to estimate the molecular interactions and binding affinities of all identified compounds with the target enzymes involved in antibacterial activities.

2. Results

2.1. Chemical Composition of Essential Oils

The characterization of volatile oils was carried out by GC-SPME. Twenty-two and twenty components were identified in C. limon and C. paradise, representing 99.9% and 98.9% of the total identified compounds, respectively (Table 1). These compositions show that C. limon volatile oil was rich in monoterpene hydrocarbons (93.3%), followed by oxygenated monoterpenes (4.8%). In addition, C. paradisi EO was dominated by limonene (60.6%), β-pinene (13.3%) and γ-terpinene (11%). However, limonene, with a prevalence of 86.8%, was the main compound in C. paradisi EO. The obtained chromatograms are listed in Supplementary Material SM1.

2.2. Antibacterial Activity

The obtained results are summarized in Table 2. *C. limon* and *C. paradisi* EOs were found to be active against all tested microorganisms to different degrees. Interestingly, *C. limon* seems to have been more active against Gram-negative bacteria as compared to *C. paradisi* essential oil. The obtained minimal inhibitory concentrations (MICs) ranged between 3.84 and 12.5 mg/mL for both essential oils.

Moreover, the two tested essential oils derived from *C. limon* and *C. paradisi* exhibited bactericidal effects against imipenem-resistant *Acinetobacter baumannii, Klebsiella pneumoniae, Pseudomonas aeruginosa* and *Escherichia coli*. Similarly, the minimal bactericidal concentration values (MBCs) varied between 1.25 and 2.5 mg/mL for *C. limon* EO, and between 0.192 and 1.536 mg/mL for *C. paradisi* EO.

Our results also show that *C. limon* was active against Gram-positive bacteria such as methicillin-resistant *S. aureus* strains (MRSA-3 and MRSA-126), as well as *Enterococcus faecalis* ATCC 29212 and *E. faecium* (CI234). These MIC values were lower than those of the essential oil of *C. limon*, and ranged between 0.192 and 0.786 mg/mL. The MBC/MIC ratio was less than 4; therefore, the essential oils studied showed bactericidal effects against the bacterial strains tested [23].

2.3. Antifungal Activity

The results of the anticandidal activity are summarized in Table 3. *C. paradisi* EO exhibited significant antifungal activities against *C. albicans, C. krusei, C. parapsilosis* and *C. glabrata*, with the lowest MIC values (1.2 mg/mL), while the same *Candida* species were killed when using 2.4 mg/mL of *C. paradisi* EO.

Furthermore, the essential oil of *C. limon* showed moderate anticandidal activities, with MIC values varying from 6.25 to 12.5 mg/mL, and MFC values of about 12.5 mg/mL against all tested *Candida* species. The tested essential oils exhibited fungicidal activities against all tested yeast strains (MFC/MIC value < 4) [24].

Table 1. Chemical compositions (%) of *C. limon* and *C. paradisi* volatile oils determined by SPME/MS.

Composition	RI	EOL	EOP
α-Thujene	933	0.4	
α-Pinene	941	2.1	0.5
Camphene	955	0.1	
Sabinene	977	2.2	0.2
β-Pinene	982	13.3	0.2
Myrcene	993	1.9	0.5
Octanal	1003		0.2
δ-3-Carene	1013		0.1
α-Terpinene	1020	0.2	
p-Cymene	1028	0.9	0.2
Limonene	1032	60.6	86.8
(E)-β-ocimene	1052	0.1	
γ-Terpinene	1063	11.0	
Terpinolene	1090	0.5	
Linalool	1101		0.4
Cis-p-menth-2-en-1-ol	1123		0.8
Cis-limonene oxide	1136		1.9
Trans-limonene oxide	1140		2.4
Citronellal	1155	0.1	
α-Terpineol	1191	0.2	
Decanal	1206		0.3
Trans-carveol	1219		1
Cis-carveol	1230		0.8
Neral	1241	1.2	
Carvone	1244		1.4
Geranial	1271	2.0	
Linalyl acetate	1259		0.8
Neryl acetate	1365	0.7	
Geranyl acetate	1383	0.6	0.2
Caryophyllene oxide	1582		0.1
Nootkatone	1809		0.2
Cis-α-bergamotene	1416	0.1	
β-Caryophyllene	1419	0.4	
Trans-α-bergamotene	1437	0.5	
β-Bisabolene	1508	0.8	
Monoterpene hydrocarbons (%)		93.3	88.4
Oxygenated monoterpenes (%)		4.8	9.7
Sesquiterpene hydrocarbons (%)		1.8	0.0
Oxygenated sesquiterpenes (%)		0.0	0.3
Non-terpene derivatives (%)		0.0	0.5
Total identified compound (%)		99.9	98.9

RI: Retention Index; EOL: *C. limon* essential oil; EOP: *C. paradisi* essential oil.

Table 2. Antibacterial activity of *C. limon* and *C. paradisi* essential oils determined by disc diffusion and microdilution assays.

Tested Microorganisms	*C. limon* Essential Oil			*C. paradisi* Essential Oil			Ciprofloxacin		
	MIC *	MBC **	MBC/MIC Ratio	MIC	MBC	MBC/MIC Ratio	MIC	MBC	MBC/MIC Ratio
Pseudomonas aeruginosa BLSE 2	2.5	2.5	1	0.768	0.768	1	0.125	>0.125	-
Pseudomonas aeruginosa BLSE13	2.5	2.5	1	0.768	0.768	1	0.125	>0.125	-
Pseudomonas aeruginosa IMP24	2.5	2.5	1	0.768	0.768	1	0.125	>0.125	-
Pseudomonas aeruginosa ATCC 27853	2.5	2.5	1	0.768	0.768	1	0.125	>0.125	-
Escherichia coli ATCC 25922	1.25	2.5	2	0.384	0.384	1	0.062	0.062	1
Klebsiella pneumoniae ATCC 13883	0.625	1.25	2	0.192	0.192	1	0.125	>0.125	-
Acinetobacter baumannii ATCC 19606	2.5	2.5	1	0.192	0.192	1	0.031	0.125	4
Enterococcu faecalis ATCC 29212	1.25	2.5	2	0.384	0.384	1	0.125	>0.125	-
Enterococcus faecium CI234	1.25	2.5	2	0.384	0.384	1	0.125	>0.125	-
Staphylococcus aureus ATCC 25923	0.625	1.25	2	0.384	0.768	2	0.031	0.125	4
Staphylococcus aureus MRSA-3	1.25	2.5	2	0.384	0.768	2	0.031	0.125	4
Staphylococcus aureus MRSA-126	1.25	2.5	2	0.384	0.768	2	0.031	0.125	4
Bacilus cereus ATCC 11778	1.25	2.5	2	0.768	1.536	2	0.002	0.062	31
Bacilus subtilis ATCC 14579	1.25	2.5	2	0.768	0.768	1	0.002	0.062	31

MIC *: minimal inhibitory concentration expressed in mg/mL; MBC **: minimal bactericidal concentration expressed in mg/mL.

Table 3. Anti-*Candida* spp. activity (mg/mL) of *C. limon* and *C. paradisi* essential oils using microdilution assays. MIC and MFC values expressed in mg/mL.

Candida Species	*C. limon* EO		MFC/MIC Ratio	*C. paradisi* EO		MFC/MIC Ratio	Amphotericin B
	MIC	MFC		MIC	MFC		MIC
C. glabrata ATCC 90030	6.25	12.5	2	1.2	2.4	2	0.5
C. albicans ATCC 90028	6.25	12.5	2	1.2	2.4	2	0.5
C. parapsilosis ATCC 22019	6.25	12.5	2	1.2	2.4	2	0.5
C. krusei ATCC 6258	12.5	12.5	1	1.2	2.4	2	0.5

2.4. Determination of Anticoagulant Activity

The anticoagulant activities of both essential oils were calculated using prothrombin time (PT) and activated partial thromboplastin time (aPTT) estimations. The results are summarized in Table 4. In fact, our results show that *C. limon* and *C. paradisi* EOs possessed the same prothrombin prolongation times, estimated at 80.00 ± 1.67 s and 82.21 ± 2.65 s, respectively.

Table 4. Anticoagulant activities of *C. limon and C. paradisi* essential oils.

Essential Oil/Control	PT(s)	aPTT(s)
C. paradisi EO	82.21 ± 2.65	180.00 ± 1.20
C. limon EO	80.00 ± 1.67	38.50 ± 2.05
Normal saline	15.00 ± 2.87	34.40 ± 1.54
Heparin	40.80 ± 4.71	120.50 ± 1.18

However, *C. paradisi* EO showed the highest aPTT of about 180.00 ± 1.20 s. This value is higher than the aPTT obtained with heparin (120.50 ± 1.18 s), which was the positive control.

2.5. Molecular Docking Studies

Klebsiella pneumoniae is a Gram-negative nosocomial pathogen responsible for various types of healthcare-associated infections, such as urinary tract infections, sepsis, and bacteremia [25]. On the other hand, *S. aureus* (Gram-positive bacterium) is an opportunistic pathogen responsible for nosocomial infections and human disorders [26].

In light of the above facts and based on previous works, we can infer the importance of docking studies for determining antibacterial activity [27,28]. Molecular docking studies have been performed to explore the interactions via binding between the components of the samples biologically tested for their antibacterial potency and the active sites of the cytidine deaminase from *K. pneumoniae* (PDB ID: 6K63) on one side and *S. aureus* dehydrosqualene synthase (PDB ID: 2ZCQ) on the other side.

The results (Table 5) are laid out as the docking score (kcal/mol) of a ligand onto a target enzyme next to the interaction mechanisms (Van der Waals, H-bond, and hydrophobic interactions). Interestingly, a high degree of negativity in the binding affinity values suggests greater effectivity, and that the tested compound could be used in controlling the tested bacteria.

Table 5. Docking binding energies (kcal/mol) of promising antibacterial agents.

Compound	Free Binding Energy of Pdb: 6K63 (kcal/mol)	Free Binding Energy of Pdb: 2ZCQ (kcal/mol)
α-Pinene	−4.4	−5.7
Sabinene	−4.1	−6.2
β-Pinene	−4.1	−5.9
Limonene	−4.6	−6.7
γ-Terpinene	−4.3	−6.8
Geranial	−4.1	−6.9
Ciprofloxacin (Standard)	−4.2	−6.7

Table 6 suggests the ligands and receptors bind with interaction residues. Overall, in the context of the cytidine deaminase from *K. pneumoniae*, most of the compounds showed significant results, especially limonene (having the lowest free binding energy value, −4.6 kcal/mol).

Table 6. The ligand- and receptor-binding interaction patterns.

Ligand	Docking Results of Pdb 6K63: Interacting Amino Acids (Types of Interactions)	Docking Results of Pdb 2ZCQ: Interacting Amino Acids (Types of Interactions)
α-Pinene	His182 (b,c); Phe184 (4b); Pro210 (2a)	Phe22 (4b); Tyr41 (b); Ala134 (2a); Val137 (a); Leu164 (a)
Sabinene	His182 (4b); Phe184 (b); His208 (2b); Pro210 (a)	Phe22 (2b); Phe26 (2b); Val137 (2a); Leu141 (2a); Leu164 (a)
β-Pinene	His182 (3b,c); Ala204 (a); His208 (b); Pro210 (2a)	Phe22 (4b); Ala134 (a); Val137 (a); Leu164 (a)
Limonene	His182 (3b); Phe184 (2b); Cys202 (a); Ala204 (a); His208 (b); Pro210 (2a)	Phe22 (2b); Phe26 (b); Tyr41 (2b); Cys44 (a); Val137 (2a); Leu164 (a)
γ-Terpinene	His182 (b,c); Phe184 (2b); Cys202 (a); Ala204 (a); Pro210 (2a); Lys265 (a)	Met15 (a); Phe22 (b); Phe26 (b); Val37 (a); Tyr41 (b); Ala134 (a); Val137 (2a); Leu141 (2a); Leu164 (a)
Geranial	His182 (b,c); Cys202 (a); Ala204 (a); His208 (2b); Pro210 (a)	Met15 (a); Phe22 (2b); Phe26 (2b); Val37 (2a); Ile40 (a); Tyr41 (2b); Val137 (a); Gly138 (d); Leu141 (2a); Ala157 (e); Leu164 (a)
Ciprofloxacin (Standard)	Thr174 (d); His182 (f); His208 (d,f,g)	Phe22 (2f); Phe26 (b); Val37 (a); Tyr41 (b); Val133 (g); Ala134 (b); Val137 (2c); Leu141 (a); Gly161 (d)

Na: a = alkyl; N = number of alkyl interactions; Nb: b = Pi–alkyl; N = number of Pi–alkyl interactions; Nc: c = Pi–Sigma; N = number of Pi–Sigma interactions; Nd: d = carbon–hydrogen bond; N = number of carbon–hydrogen bonds; Ne: e = conventional hydrogen bond; N = number of conventional hydrogen bonds; Nf: f = Pi–Pi; N = number of Pi–Pi interactions; Ng: g = halogen; N = number of halogen interactions.

Since the chain skeleton forming this molecule is devoid of heteroatoms, the formation of hydrogen bonds is impossible (Figure 1A,B,B′). The inhibition force of the target enzyme is perceptible through the strength of hydrophobic interactions (alkyl and Pi–alkyl interactions) formed with the residues His182, Phe184, Cys202, Ala204, His208 and Pro210. This significance is proven by the binding energy values of limonene, α-pinene and γ-terpinene, which exceed those of the standard docked ligand (ciproflo–acin), as Table 5 displays. However, α-pinene was found to be the second most active compound, with −4.4 kcal/mol, showing two alkyl interactions with Pro210, in addition to five Pi–alkyl interactions with His182 and Phe184 and Pi–Sigma with His182.

On the other hand, as the tabulated data show, γ-terpinene (−4.3 kcal/mol) is considered the third most active compound, exhibiting five alkyl interactions with residues Cys202, Ala204, Pro210 and Lys265, in addition to three Pi–alkyl interactions with His182 and Phe184 and a Pi–Sigma integration with His182. Sabinene, β-pinene and geranial compounds with binding energy values of −4.1 kcal/mol were found to be moderately active molecules compared to other compounds.

Regarding *S. aureus*'s dehydrosqualene synthase–ligand complex, the obtained results show that geranial at −6.9 kcal/mol was the most potent compound, followed by γ-terpinene (−6.8 kcal/mol) then limonene (−6.7 kcal/mol), compared to other docked ligands in the standard (Ciprofloxacin). As shown in Figure 2C,D,D′, geranial is involved in a conventional hydrogen bond with Ala157 through its hydroxyl group, in addition to some hydrophobic interactions (alkyl and Pi–alkyl) with a sequence of amino acids—Met15, Phe22, Phe26, Val37, Ile40, Tyr41, Val137, Leu141 and Leu164—in addition to a carbon–hydrogen bond with Gly138. Further, the potential enzyme-inhibiting action of γ-terpinene is perceivable through its several hydrophobic interactions with more or less the same residues as geranial, while α-pinene (−5.7 kcal/mol) was found to be the least active compound, although it engaged in multiple hydrophobic interactions as detailed in Table 5.

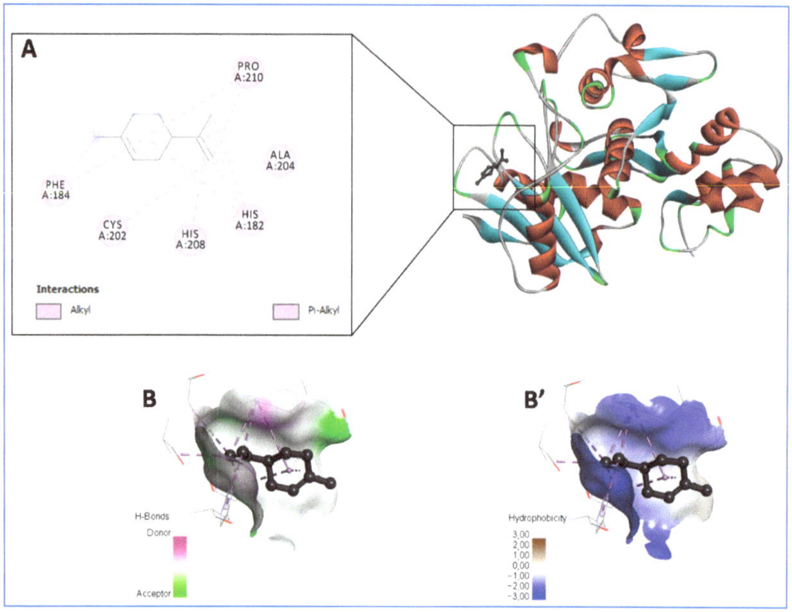

Figure 1. Representation of the best docked compounds bound to the pocket region of cytidine deaminase from *Klebsiella pneumoniae* (PDB ID: 6K63). Micrographs of the pocket region with hydrogen bond (**B**) and hydrophobicity illustrations (**B′**), and a corresponding 2D diagram of interactions (**A**).

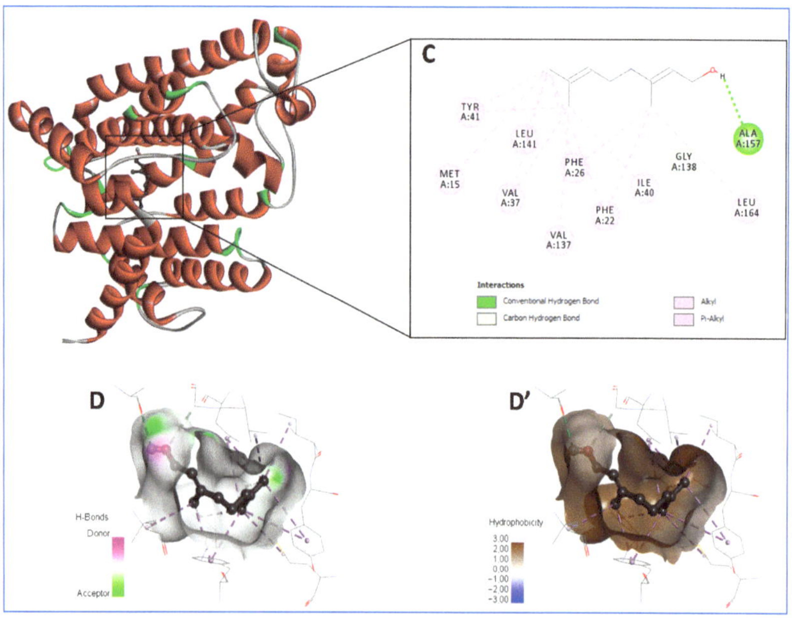

Figure 2. A representation of the best-docked compounds bound to the pocket region of *Staphylococcus aureus* dehydrosqualene synthase (PDB ID: 2ZCQ). Micrographs of the pocket region with hydrogen bond (**D**) and hydrophobicity illustrations (**D′**), and the corresponding 2D diagram of interactions (**C**).

2.6. Predictive ADME Analysis

The ADME (absorption, distribution, metabolism, and excretion) properties of the six predominant constituents of the tested *Citrus* EOs were studied, including their pharmacokinetic and drug-like properties, using Swiss ADME online server (http://www.swissadme.ch/, accessed on 7 August 2023). Indeed, the tested compounds (Table 7) were found to adhere to Lipinski's rule, and also share topological polar surface area (TPSA) values below 30 Å2, thus exhibiting good brain penetration in addition to good lipophilicity behavior, which is expressed by their consensus Log Po/w in the range 2.74–3.44. Their bioavailability score of 0.55 displays their greater drug-like properties.

Table 7. Physicochemical properties, pharmacokinetics, drug-likeness, and lipophilicity of four selected compounds, according to Swiss ADME online server.

Entry	α-Pinene	Sabinene	β-Pinene	Limonene	γ-Terpinene	Geranial
GI absorption	Low	Low	Low	Low	Low	High
BBB permeant	Yes	Yes	Yes	Yes	Yes	Yes
P–gp substrate	No	No	No	No	No	No
CYP1A2 inhibitor	No	No	No	No	No	No
CYP2C19 inhibitor	No	No	No	No	No	No
CYP2C9 inhibitor	Yes	No	Yes	Yes	No	No
CYP2D6 inhibitor	No	No	No	No	No	No
CYP3A4 inhibitor	No	No	No	No	No	No
Log Kp (cm/s) [a]	−3.95	−4.94	−4.18	−3.89	−3.94	−4.71
Lipinski	Yes	Yes	Yes	Yes	Yes	Yes
TPSA (Å^2)	00.00	00.00	00.00	00.00	00.00	20.23
Consensus Log *Po*/w	3.44	3.25	3.42	3.37	3.35	2.74
Bioavailability Score	0.55	0.55	0.55	0.55	0.55	0.55

a: skin permeation.

As shown in the tabulated data, all compounds achieved low gastrointestinal absorption (GI) and easily passed the blood–brain barrier (BBB), meaning they could bind to specific receptors. Furthermore, the study's components interacted the most with isoenzymes of the Cytochrome P (CYP) family, demonstrating their greater effectiveness and insignificant toxicity. Moreover, in their radar plots (Figure 3), all tested compounds were entirely within the pink zone, confirming their greater drug-likeness along with a good bioavailability profile. Besides this, in the boiled egg graph (Figure 4), the compounds A (α-pinene), B (sabinene), C (β-pinene), D (limonene), E (γ-terpinene) and F (geranial) all appear in the yellow region (yolk), with a red point confirming their high capacity for brain penetration, with "BB" acting as a non-substrate of P–gp.

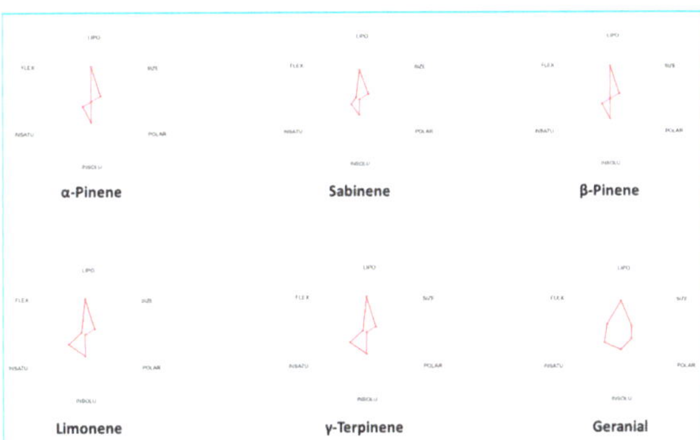

Figure 3. Bioavailability radar of the selected phytoconstituants.

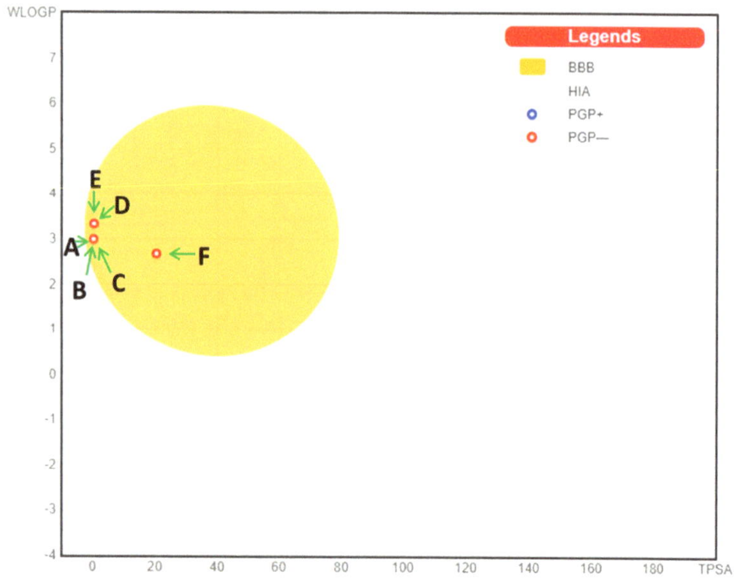

Figure 4. Boiled-egg graph of the selected phytoconstituants: A—α-Pinene, B—Sabinene, C—β-Pinene, D—Limonene, E—γ-Terpinene and F—Geranial.

3. Discussion

In this work, we have studied the chemical compositions and antimicrobial and anticoagulant activities of two *Cirus* plant species: *C. limon* and *C. paradisi*. Our results reveal the identification of two different chemotypes: *C. limon* (limonene/β-pinene chemotype; 606/13.3%) and *C. paradisi* (Limonene 86.6%). A literature survey has indicated that the volatile oil of *C. limon* collected from the Cap Bon, Tunisia contained limonene (39.74%) and β-pinene (25.44%) [11], while *C. limon* EO from Menzel Bouzelfa (Northeast Tunisia) was rich in limonene (37.63–69.71%), β-pinene (0.63–31.49%), γ-terpinene (0.04–9.96%), and *p*-cymene (0.23–9.84%) [29]. Previous studies on cultivated species *C. limon* collected from northeastern India indicated that the major compounds were limonene (55.40%) and neral (10.39%), followed by trans-verbenol (6.43%) and decanal (3.25%) [30]. Limonene (52.77%), geranyl acetate (9.92%), and trans-limonene oxide (7.13%) were found to be the major components of *C. limon* EO from Picos City, state of Piaui, Brazil [31].

Using Gas Chromatography–Mass Spectrometry, essential oils of *C. limon* and *C. paradisi* purchased from Ravetllat Aromatics (Barcelona, Spain) showed limonene (69.9%), followed by β-pinene (11.2%) and γ-terpinene (8.21%), and limonene (96.2%) and myrcene (1.5%), as their main compounds, respectively [32].

Moreover, *C. paradisi* EO from Kukeng, Yunlin County, southern Taiwan, obtained by hydro-distillation and cold-pressing, showed limonene at contents of 96.06% and 92.83%, respectively [33]. D-limonene (75.05%) and β-myrcene (7.25%) were the major components of *C. paradisi* EO purchased from Onilegogoro market, Mushin, Lagos, West Nigeria [34,35]. In addition, *C paradisi* EO obtained via cold-pressing extraction by the company Frutech International Corporation de México S.A. showed limonene as its major compound (area = 94.4%) [36].

Overall, the results of previous studies on *C. limon* and *C. paradisi* EOs from various countries and regions show that, in most cases, limonene (monoterpene hydrocarbon) was the major compound, which results agree with our findings on the characteristics of citrus. A small variability has been recorded in the compositions of minor components. This variability can be explained by the differences in environmental conditions, such as temperature, rainfall and soil composition.

The investigation of the antibacterial effects against a wide range of bacteria showed that *C. paradisi* EO was more active than *C. limon* EO. This important antibacterial activity of EOP may be explained by its richness in limonene (86.8%) and oxygenated monoterpenes (9.7%) compared to EOL, comprising 60.6% limonene and 4.8% oxygenated monoterpenes.

Concerning the antibacterial activities of the obtained citrus EOs, our results show that *C. limon* and *C. paradisi* EOs were active against Gram-positive and Gram-negative bacteria to different degrees. Previous reports on *C. limon* EO show that it was active against Gram-positive bacteria, with MIC and MBC values against *S. aureus* of about 0.023 mg/L and 0.011 mg/L, respectively [37]. Using both disc diffusion (inhibition zone determination—IZ) and microdilution (MIC and MBC value determination) assays, Ben Hsouna and colleagues [11] reported that *C. limon* EO was active against *Bacillus subtilis* ATCC 6633 (IZ = 19 mm; MIC = 0.625 mg/mL), *B. cereus* ATCC 14579 (IZ= 24 mm; MIC = 1.25 mg/mL), *S. aureus* ATCC 25923 (IZ = 22 mm; MIC = 0.078 mg/mL), *S. epidermis* ATCC 12228 (IZ = 16 mm; MIC = 1.25 mg/mL), *E. faecalis* ATCC 29212 (IZ = 15 mm; MIC = 0.625 mg/mL), *Listeria monocytogenes* (IZ = 26 mm; MIC = 0.039 mg/mL), *Salmonella enterica* ATCC 43972 (IZ = 18 mm; MIC = 0.625 mg/mL), *E. coli* ATCC 25922 (IZ = 15 mm; MIC = 1.25 mg/mL), and *P. aeruginosa* ATCC 9027 (IZ = 14 mm; MIC = 2.5 mg/mL).

As essential oil is a mixture of large numbers of compounds belonging to various chemical classes; its antimicrobial activity may be related to the cumulative effects of major and/or minor components. Therefore, its antibacterial mechanism of action can be affected by several pathways on various cell organelles, such as the cell membrane and mitochondria, which may provoke cell death [38]. Its potentiality is highly correlated with the stability of its compounds, their volatility, their lipophilicity, and also their hydrophobicity in the wells. In our present study, although both EOL and EOP had the same major compound, limonene (60.6%, 86.8%), and the bacterial response was different, Gram-negative bacteria were found to be more resistant than Gram-positive bacteria. This variability in results has also been seen in previous studies, which showed that positive bacteria were more affected by EOs [38].

Limonene, the dominant compound in both *C. limon* and *C. paradisi* EOs, is well known to exhibit antibacterial effects [39]. Previous works have highlighted that oxygenated monoterpene such as alcohol and phenols had stronger bacterial inhibition effects than hydrocarbons, which may explain our findings [40].

In this study, we have also shown the anticandidal activities of *C. limon* and *C. paradisi* EOs tested against *C. glabrata* ATCC 90030, *C. albicans* ATCC 90028, *C. parapsilosis* ATCC 22019, and *C. krusei* ATCC 6258 using microdilution assays. Our findings show that the tested citrus EOs were active at high concentrations (MICs and MFCs values) as compared to bacterial strains. Previous reports have indicated that *C. limon* EO inhibited *Candida* species and dermatophytes. For instance, *C. tropicalis* (IZ = 23.61 mm, MIC = 0.017 mg/mL, MFC = 0.011 mg/mL), *Rhizopus nigricans* (14.15 mm) and *Aspergillus flavus* (MIC = 0.058 mg/L, MBC = 0.023 mg/mL) were active against EOL [41]. Similarly, *C. limon* EO prevented the growth of *A. niger* CTM 10099 (IZ= 26 mm; MIC = 0.625 mg/mL), *A. flavus* (IZ = 26 mm; MIC = 0.312 mg/mL), *A. nidulans* (IZ = 20 mm; MIC = 0.625 mg/mL), *A. fumigatus* (IZ = 18 mm; MIC = 0.625 mg/mL), *Fusarium graminearum* ISPAVE 271 (IZ = 20 mm; MIC = 0.625 mg/mL), *F. oxysporum* (CTM10402) (IZ = 18 mm; MIC = 0.625 mg/mL), *F. culmorum* ISPAVE 21w (IZ = 21 mm; MIC = 0.312 mg/mL) and *Alternaria alternata* CTM 10230 (IZ = 17 mm; MIC = 1.25 mg/mL) [11].

Recently, it has been shown that *C. limon* EO obtained from flowers exhibited antifungal activity against *Fusarium* sp. (MIC = 0.625 mg/mL) and *Aspergillus* sp. (MIC = 1.25 mg/mL) [11]. At the concentration of 0.94%, EOL and EOP totally inhibited the growth of dermatophytes *A. flavus*, *A. niger*, *Penicillium chrysogenum* and *P. verrucosum* [41]. EOP also exhibited a wide inhibitory effect on some fungi cultures. For instance, *C. albicans* was effective against EOP at 5, 10 and 20 μg/mL, with inhibition percentages 51.9, 70.1 and 123%, respectively [36].

As the major component of both oils was limonene, this substance is probably responsible for the antifungal proprieties of the oils. *R*-(+)-limonene and *S*-(−)-limonene have been reported to inhibit, respectively, *C. albicans* ATCC 90028 (MIC = 0.31 mg/mL, MFC = 0.62 mg/mL; MIC = 0.31 mg/mL, MFC = 0.62 mg/mL), *C. glabrata* ATCC 90030 (MIC = 0.31 mg/mL, MFC = 1.25 mg/mL; MIC = 0.62 mg/mL, MFC = 1.25 mg/mL), *C. parapsilosis* ATCC 22019 (MIC = 0.31 mg/mL, MFC = 1.25 mg/mL; MIC = 0.31 mg/mL, MFC = 1.25 mg/mL) and *C. krusei* ATCC 6258 (MIC = 0.07 mg/mL, MFC = 0.62 mg/mL; MIC = 0.15 mg/mL, MFC = 0.31 mg/mL) [42]. Limonene has been documented to possess antifungal effects. It induces damage in ADN and in the membrane of fungi, and induces apoptosis [43]. This compound can inhibit *C. albicans* with an MIC value of about 300 µg/mL and an MFC value of about 400 µg/mL. Limonene reduced the secretion of proteinases (73%) and phospholipases (53%), as well as adhesion (91%) and biofilm formation (87%) in *C. albicans* [44]. These important antifungal capacities of both volatile oils may be related to their main component (Limonene) or to the other chemical compounds present, such as pinene and myrcene.

The anticoagulant potentialities of the volatile oils show that *C. paradisi* EO is more active than *C. limon* EO. The complex relation between inflammation and coagulation makes these processes interdependent, showing a substantial impact on each other. The coagulation system can be activated by inflammation reactions. In natural defense systems, coagulation pathways may amplify the inflammatory response and thus prevent catastrophic events [45]. Previous reports have shown that monoterpenes exhibit anticoagulant activities by affecting the hemostasis process. They can reduce collagen-induced platelet aggregation, induce antithrombotic reactions and block the P2Y12 platelet receptor [46,47]. Citrus caused the inactivation of thrombin and a decrease in the concentration of fibrinogen. The inhibition of platelet aggregation caused by citrus was also registered in rabbits [48]. Thus, the components may intervene in any anticoagulant process, such as via the inhibition of platelet activation, and/or modify the adhesiveness of collagen and fibrinogen. The oils may also induce the S-sulhydration of platelet proteins [49]. However, there are no clear mechanisms of the anticoagulant effects of these two varieties of essential oils.

4. Materials and Methods

4.1. Sample Preparation

In this study, *C. paradisi* and *C. lemon* essential oils were purchased from Bio-orient, Tunisia. *C. limon* and *C. paradisi* were collected on 11 April 2022 from Hammamet; they had grown in sandy soil, without fertilization and human intervention via irrigation. They were sampled at the mature period of 5 years, showing yellow and orange colors, respectively.

The fresh *C. limon* and *C. paradisi* were washed and then peeled separately. After drying the peels at room temperature, the white inner membranes were eliminated. A sugarcane juice presser, from Taiwan, was used to press almost three kilograms of each species. The obtained juice was centrifuged at 6000 rpm for 30 min. Then, excess water was removed using anhydrous sodium sulfate.

4.2. GC–EIMS Analysis

GC-EIMS analyses of each cultivar were carried out using a Varian CP-3800 gas chromatograph equipped with a DB-5 capillary column (30 m × 0.25 mm; coating thickness 0.25 µm) and a Varian Saturn 2000 ion trap mass detector. Analytical conditions: injector and transfer line temperatures 220 and 240 °C, respectively; oven temperature programmed from 60 to 240 °C at 3 °C/min; carrier gas helium at 1 mL/min. Essential oils were injected at 0.2 mL (10% hexane solution), with a split ratio of 1:30; SPME employed an injector temperature of 250 °C, with splitless injection. The identification of the components was based on comparisons of the retention times with those of standard samples, comparing their linear retention indices relative to the series of n-hydrocarbons, and using computer matching against commercial (NIST 2000 and Adams 2007) and home-made library mass spectra composed of pure ingredients and constituents of known oils, along with data on MS from the literature [50]. Volatile compounds were assembled into classes of monoterpene hydrocarbons, oxygenated monoterpenes, oxygenated sesquiterpenes, sesquiterpene hydrocarbons and other compounds. Three repeated injections were performed in order to verify the data obtained from SPME and GC-MS.

4.3. Antimicrobial Activity

4.3.1. Microbial Strains

The essentials oils were tested against *Pseudomonas aeruginosa* imipenem-resistant and methicillin-resistant *S. aureus* (MRSA), *Bacillus cereus* ATCC 14579, *B. cereus* ATCC 11778, *E. faecium* CI234, *E. faecalis* ATCC 29212, *K. pneumoniae* ATCC 13883, *A. baumannii* ATCC 19606, *E. coli* ATCC 25922, *S. aureus* ATCC 25923, *C. krusei* ATCC 6258, *C. albicans* ATCC 90028, *C. glabrata* ATCC 90030, and *C. parapsilosis* ATCC 22019. All the above species were kindly provided by the Laboratory of Microbiology, Hospital of Fattouma Bourguiba, Monastir.

4.3.2. Microdilution Method

This technique was used to estimate the minimum inhibitory concentration (MIC) and minimal bactericidal (MBC), as previously described [51,52].

The volatile oils were dissolved in dimethyl sulfoxide (DMSO, 10%) and physiological water. The tested oils were diluted to the highest concentration (50 mg/mL) and serial dilutions were prepared. A volume of 100 µL of brain–heart broth (BHI Broth, Sigma-Aldrich, Steinheim, Germany) was added into the 96-well plates with the bacteria. Then, 20 µL of the overnight culture was adjusted to 0.5 McFarland turbidity. The plates were incubated for 24 h at 37 °C [49].

The MIC represents the lowest concentration of essential oil that could prevent any growth visible to the eye after 24 h of incubation at 37 °C. In addition, the MBC presents the weakest concentration of essential oil that could prevent any growth visible to the eye. The MBC/MIC ratio allowed us to determine the bactericidal and bacteriostatic profiles of the tested essential oils. If this ratio was greater than 4, the essential oil had a bacteriostatic effect, and the effect was bactericidal when this was lessthan or equal to 4 [23,35].

4.4. Anticoagulant Activity

In order to determine the prothrombin time (PT) and activated partial thromboplastin time (aPTT), we used assay kits for the determination of PT, thrombin time (TT) and activated partial thromboplastin time (APTT)—SINNOWA Medical Science & Technology Co., Ltd. (Nanjing, Jiangsu, China). The activity was evaluated according to the protocol described by [53,54]. Human blood was collected from the Laboratory of Hematology of Fattouma Bourguiba Hospital, Monastir. Then, it was anticoagulated using 3.8% tri-sodium citrate (Sigma-Aldrich, Steinheim, Germany) in a polypropylene container. Immediately after, it was centrifuged for 15 min.

The plasma was separated, pooled, and stored at 4 °C until its use. In total, 50 µL of the essential oil was mixed with 100 µL of plasma and incubated for 5 min at 37 °C. A volume of 200 µL of PT assay reagent (rabbit brain extract and calcium chloride), pre-warmed to 37 °C for 15 min, was added. The clotting time was determined using a coagulometer (RT-2204C Medical expo). For aPTT tests, plasma (100 µL) was mixed with 50 µL of each sample and 100 of aPTT reagent, and thereafter incubated at 37 °C for 2 min. A volume of 50 µL of calcium chloride (0.25 mM) (Sigma-Aldrich, Steinheim, Germany) was added, and the clotting time was measured using a coagulometer. Normal saline was used as the negative control, and heparin (1 IU/mL) was used as the positive control. The tests were performed in triplicate.

4.5. Molecular Docking Study

Molecular docking studies were carried out using the Auto Dock 4.2 program package [49]. ACD (3D viewer) 2017.2.1 software (http://www.filefacts.com/acd3d-viewer-freeware-info, accessed on 15 May 2023). was used to perform the optimization of all the geometries of the compounds. We obtained "the crystal structure of cytidine deaminase from *K pneumoniae*" (PDB: 6K63) with grid box parameters of 30 (x-dimension) × 30 (y-dimension)

× 30 (z-dimension) Å along with the x, y and z values of 38.321, −75.601 and −9.572, respectively, and "the crystal structure of the C (30) carotenoid dehydrosqualene synthase from *S. aureus* complexed with bisphosphonate BPH-652" (PDB: 2ZCQ) [55] with grid box parameters of 30 (x-dimension) × 30 (y-dimension) × 30 (z-dimension) Å and x, y and z values of 15.285, 54.913 and 41.662, respectively, for antibacterial activity assessment from the RSCB protein data bank. During the preparation of the receptor input file, water molecules were erased and the missing hydrogen and Gasteiger charges were added to the system. The corresponding ligand and protein files (PDBQT) were prepared using AutoDock Tools.

After this, the pre-calculation of the grid maps was performed using Auto Grid to save time during docking. The visualizations and analyses of interactions and images depicting the results of the in silico analysis were constructed using the software BIOVIA Discovery Studio Visualizer 2017R2 (https://www.3dsbiovia.com/products/collaborative-science/biovia-discovery-studio/, accessed on 22 October 2023).

4.6. ADME properties

The pharmacokinetic and drug-likeness properties of the predominant constituents of the volatile oils of two varieties of citrus were estimated using ADME (absorption, distribution, metabolism and excretion) descriptors via a SwissADME online server (http://www.swissadme.ch/, accessed on 22 October 2023).

5. Conclusions

The chemical compositions of *C. limon* EO and *C. paradisi* EO, as analyzed by gas chromatography coupled to mass spectrometry, reveal that *C. paradisi* EO possessed a higher concentration of limonene than *C. limon* EO. In fact, β-pinene was found at a high concentration (13.3%) in *C. limon* EO as compared to *C. paradisi* EO (0.2%). The in vitro effectiveness of these essential oils as natural antimicrobial and anticoagulant agents was tested. In silico docking simulations were performed to investigate the modes of action of the major constituents of cold-pressed volatile oils against some bacterial stains. The results suggest these oils could be used as natural antimicrobial and anticoagulant agents. Further studies will be needed to more deeply understand the compounds' mechanisms of action on bacteria and *Candida* species.

Supplementary Materials: The following supporting information can be downloaded at: https://www.mdpi.com/article/10.3390/ph16121669/s1. SM1. Chromatograms obtained for both *C. limon* and *C. paradisi* obtained by using by SPME/MS technique.

Author Contributions: Conceptualization, E.N., H.E., A.H., M.S. and V.D.F.; methodology, A.H., M.H., H.B.J. and N.B.; software, M.H., A.H., F.P. and E.N.; writing—original draft preparation, A.H., A.K., F.P., A.H. and H.E.; writing—review and editing, H.E., A.H., M.H., A.K. and V.D.F.; supervision, E.N., M.S. and V.D.F. All authors have read and agreed to the published version of the manuscript.

Funding: This research has been funded by Scientific Research Deanship at University of Ha'il—Saudi Arabia through project number MDR-22 021.

Institutional Review Board Statement: Not applicable.

Informed Consent Statement: Not applicable.

Data Availability Statement: All data are presented in the manuscript.

Acknowledgments: This research has been funded by Scientific Research Deanship at University of Ha'il—Saudi Arabia through project number MDR-22 021.

Conflicts of Interest: The authors declare no conflict of interest.

References

1. Okoye, C.O.; Okeke, E.S.; Ezeorba, T.P.C.; Chukwudozie, K.I.; Chiejina, C.O.; Fomena Temgoua, N.S. Microbial and Bio-based Preservatives: Recent Advances in Antimicrobial Compounds. In *Microbes for Natural Food Additives*; Springer: Singapore, 2023; pp. 53–74.
2. Snoussi, M.; Noumi, E.; Trabelsi, N.; Flamini, G.; Papetti, A.; De Feo, V. *Mentha spicata* essential oil: Chemical composition, antioxidant and antibacterial activities against planktonic and biofilm cultures of *Vibrio* spp. strains. *Molecules* **2015**, *20*, 14402–14424. [CrossRef]
3. Leite, P.M.; Miranda, A.P.N.; Gomes, I.; Rodrigues, M.L.; Amorim, J.M.; de Lima, G.; Duarte, R.C.F.; Fuly, A.L.; Faraco, A.A.G.; das Graças Carvalho, M.; et al. Anticoagulant and antiplatelet activity of aqueous extracts of *Citrus sinensis* and *Lippia alba*: Interactions and potential for the development of antithrombotics. *Blood Coagul. Fibrinolysis* **2022**, *33*, 457–462. [CrossRef]
4. Alves-Silva, J.M.; Zuzarte, M.; Girão, H. The role of essential oils and their main compounds in the management of cardiovascular disease risk factors. *Molecules* **2021**, *26*, 3506. [CrossRef]
5. Maria, G.A.; Riccardo, N. *Citrus bergamia,* Risso: The peel, the juice and the seed oil of the bergamot fruit of Reggio Calabria (South Italy). *Emir. J. Food Agric.* **2020**, *32*, 522–532. [CrossRef]
6. Gioffrè, G.; Ursino, D.; Labate, M.L.C.; Giuffrè, A.M. The peel essential oil composition of bergamot fruit (*Citrus bergamia,* Risso) of Reggio Calabria (Italy): A review. *Emir. J. Food Agric.* **2020**, *32*, 835–845. [CrossRef]
7. Rowshan, V.; Najafian, S. Changes of peel essential oil composition of *Citrus aurantium* L. during fruit maturation in Iran. *J. Essent. Oil-Bear. Plants* **2015**, *18*, 1006–1012. [CrossRef]
8. Ferhat, M.-A.; Boukhatem, M.N.; Hazzit, M.; Meklati, B.Y.; Chemat, F. Cold pressing, hydrodistillation and microwave dry distillation of citrus essential oil from Algeria: A comparative study. *Electron. J. Biol.* **2016**, *1*, 30–41.
9. Pasdaran, A.; Hamedi, A.; Shiehzadeh, S.; Hamedi, A. A review of citrus plants as functional foods and dietary supplements for human health, with an emphasis on meta-analyses, clinical trials, and their chemical composition. *Clin. Nutr. ESPEN* **2023**, *54*, 311–336. [CrossRef] [PubMed]
10. Liu, S.; Lou, Y.; Li, Y.; Zhang, J.; Li, P.; Yang, B.; Gu, Q. Review of phytochemical and nutritional characteristics and food applications of *Citrus* L. fruits. *Front. Nutr.* **2022**, *9*, 968604. [CrossRef] [PubMed]
11. Ben Hsouna, A.; Ben Halima, N.; Smaoui, S.; Hamdi, N. *Citrus lemon* essential oil: Chemical composition, antioxidant and antimicrobial activities with its preservative effect against *Listeria monocytogenes* inoculated in minced beef meat. *Lipids Health Dis.* **2017**, *16*, 146. [CrossRef] [PubMed]
12. Mallick, N.; Alam Khan, R.; Riaz, A.; Afroz, S. Anticoagulant, antiplatelet and antianemic effects of *Citrus paradisi* (grape fruit) juice in rabbits. *Pharm. Pharmacol.* **2016**, *7*, 397–406. [CrossRef]
13. Ceccato-Antonini, S.R.; Shirahigue, L.D.; Varano, A.; da Silva, B.N.; Brianti, C.S.; de Azevedo, F.A. *Citrus* essential oil: Would it be feasible as antimicrobial in the bioethanol industry? *Biotechnol. Lett.* **2023**, *45*, 1–12. [CrossRef] [PubMed]
14. Meryem, S.; Mohamed, D.; Nour-eddine, C.; Faouzi, E. Chemical composition, antibacterial and antioxidant properties of three Moroccan *citrus* peel essential oils. *Sci. Afr.* **2023**, *20*, e01592. [CrossRef]
15. Lahiri, D.; Nag, M.; Dey, A.; Pandit, S.; Joshi, S.; Upadhye, V.J.; Ray, R.R. *Citrus* Essential Oils: A Treasure Trove of Antibiofilm Agent. *Appl. Biochem. Biotechnol.* **2022**, *194*, 4625–4638. [CrossRef] [PubMed]
16. Favela-Hernández, J.M.J.; González-Santiago, O.; Ramírez-Cabrera, M.A.; Esquivel-Ferriño, P.C.; Camacho-Corona, M.D.R. Chemistry and Pharmacology of *Citrus sinensis*. *Molecules* **2016**, *21*, 247. [CrossRef] [PubMed]
17. FAO. Citrus Fruit Statistical Compendium 2020. In *Citrus Fruit. Fresh and Processed*; 0002-9440; FAO: Rome, Italy, 2020; Available online: https://www.fao.org/3/cb6492en/cb6492en.pdf (accessed on 1 April 2020).
18. Makni, M.; Jemai, R.; Kriaa, W.; Chtourou, Y.; Fetoui, H. *Citrus limon* from Tunisia: Phytochemical and physicochemical properties and biological activities. *BioMed Res. Int.* **2018**, *2018*, 6251546. [CrossRef] [PubMed]
19. Maaroufi, Z.; Cojean, S.; Loiseau, P.M.; Yahyaoui, M.; Agnely, F.; Abderraba, M.; Mekhloufi, G. In vitro antileishmanial potentialities of essential oils from *Citrus limon* and *Pistacia lentiscus* harvested in Tunisia. *Parasitol. Res.* **2021**, *120*, 1455–1469. [CrossRef]
20. Kandsi, F.; Elbouzidi, A.; Lafdil, F.Z.; Meskali, N.; Azghar, A.; Addi, M.; Hano, C.; Maleb, A.; Gseyra, N. Antibacterial and antioxidant activity of *Dysphania ambrosioides* (L.) mosyakin and clemants essential oils: Experimental and computational approaches. *Antibiotics* **2022**, *11*, 482. [CrossRef]
21. Alminderej, F.; Bakari, S.; Almundarij, T.I.; Snoussi, M.; Aouadi, K.; Kadri, A. Antioxidant activities of a new chemotype of *Piper cubeba* L. fruit essential oil (Methyl eugenol/Eugenol): In Silico molecular docking and ADMET studies. *Plants* **2020**, *9*, 1534. [CrossRef]
22. Noumi, E.; Ahmad, I.; Adnan, M.; Merghni, A.; Patel, H.; Haddaji, N.; Bouali, N.; Alabbosh, K.F.; Ghannay, S.; Aouadi, K. GC/MS Profiling, antibacterial, anti-quorum sensing, and antibiofilm properties of *Anethum graveolens* L. essential oil: Molecular docking study and In-silico ADME profiling. *Plants* **2023**, *12*, 1997. [CrossRef]
23. Edziri, H.; Ammar, S.; Souad, L.; Mahjoub, M.; Mastouri, M.; Aouni, M.; Mighri, Z.; Verschaeve, L. In vitro evaluation of antimicrobial and antioxidant activities of some Tunisian vegetables. *S. Afr. J. Bot.* **2012**, *78*, 252–256. [CrossRef]
24. Ghannay, S.; Aouadi, K.; Kadri, A.; Snoussi, M. GC-MS profiling, vibriocidal, antioxidant, antibiofilm, and anti-quorum sensing properties of *Carum carvi* L. essential oil: In vitro and in silico approaches. *Plants* **2022**, *11*, 1072. [CrossRef] [PubMed]

25. Liu, W.; Shang, F.; Chen, Y.; Lan, J.; Wang, L.; Chen, J.; Gao, P.; Ha, N.-C.; Quan, C.; Nam, K.H.; et al. Biochemical and structural analysis of the *Klebsiella pneumoniae* cytidine deaminase CDA. *Biochem. Biophys. Res. Commun.* **2019**, *519*, 280–286. [CrossRef] [PubMed]
26. Muñoz-Silvestre, A.; Penadés, M.; Selva, L.; Pérez-Fuentes, S.; Moreno-Grua, E.; García-Quirós, A.; Pascual, J.J.; Arnau-Bonachera, A.; Barragán, A.; Corpa, J.M. Pathogenesis of intradermal staphylococcal infections: Rabbit experimental approach to natural *Staphylococcus aureus* skin infections. *Am. J. Pathol.* **2020**, *190*, 1188–1210. [CrossRef]
27. Horchani, M.; Hajlaoui, A.; Harrath, A.H.; Mansour, L.; Ben Jannet, H.; Romdhane, A. New pyrazolo-triazolo-pyrimidine derivatives as antibacterial agents: Design and synthesis, molecular docking and DFT studies. *J. Mol. Struct.* **2020**, *1199*, 127007. [CrossRef]
28. Horchani, M.; Edziri, H.; Harrath, A.H.; Jannet, H.B.; Romdhane, A. Access to new Schiff bases tethered with pyrazolopyrimidinone as antibacterial agents: Design and synthesis, molecular docking and DFT analysis. *J. Mol. Struct.* **2022**, *1248*, 131523. [CrossRef]
29. Bourgou, S.; Rahali, F.Z.; Ourghemmi, I.; Saïdani Tounsi, M. Changes of peel essential oil composition of four Tunisian *Citrus* during fruit maturation. *Sci. World J.* **2012**, *2012*, 528593. [CrossRef] [PubMed]
30. Paw, M.; Begum, T.; Gogoi, R.; Pandey, S.K.; Lal, M. Chemical composition of *Citrus limon* L. Burmf peel essential oil from north east India. *J. Essent. Oil-Bear. Plants* **2020**, *23*, 337–344. [CrossRef]
31. Lopes Campêlo, L.M.; Moura Gonçalves, F.C.; Feitosa, C.M.; de Freitas, R.M. Antioxidant activity of *Citrus limon* essential oil in mouse hippocampus. *Pharm. Biol.* **2011**, *49*, 709–715. [CrossRef]
32. Viuda-Martos, M.; Ruiz-Navajas, Y.; Fernández-López, J.; Pérez-Álvarez, J.A. Chemical composition of mandarin (*C. reticulata* L.), grapefruit (*C. paradisi* L.), lemon (*C. limon* L.) and orange (*C. sinensis* L.) essential oils. *J. Essent. Oil-Bear. Plants* **2009**, *12*, 236–243. [CrossRef]
33. Ou, M.-C.; Liu, Y.-H.; Sun, Y.-W.; Chan, C.-F. The composition, antioxidant and antibacterial activities of cold-pressed and distilled essential oils of *Citrus paradisi* and *Citrus grandis* (L.) Osbeck. *Evid.-Based Complement. Altern. Med.* **2015**, *2015*, 804091. [CrossRef]
34. Okunowo, W.O.; Oyedeji, O.; Afolabi, L.O.; Matanmi, E. Essential Oil of Grape Fruit (Citrus paradisi) Peels and Its Antimicrobial Activities. *Am. J. Plant Sci.* **2013**, *4*, 34556. [CrossRef]
35. Edziri, H.; Jaziri, R.; Chehab, H.; Verschaeve, L.; Flamini, G.; Boujnah, D.; Hammami, M.; Aouni, M.; Mastouri, M. A comparative study on chemical composition, antibiofilm and biological activities of leaves extracts of four Tunisian olive cultivars. *Heliyon* **2019**, *5*, e01604. [CrossRef]
36. Delgado, A.J.M.; Velázquez, U.C.; González, J.G.B.; Montes, A.C.; Villarreal, S.M.L.; García, L.E.V.; Casas, R.M.S.; Luis, O.E.R. Evaluation of the essential oil of *Citrus paradisi* as an alternative treatment against *Candida albicans*. *Open J. Stomatol.* **2020**, *10*, 258. [CrossRef]
37. Akarca, G.; Sevik, R. Biological activities of *Citrus limon* L. and *Citrus sinensis* L. peel essential oils. *J. Essent. Oil-Bear. Plants* **2021**, *24*, 1415–1427. [CrossRef]
38. Trombetta, D.; Castelli, F.; Sarpietro, M.G.; Venuti, V.; Cristani, M.; Daniele, C.; Saija, A.; Mazzanti, G.; Bisignano, G. Mechanisms of antibacterial action of three monoterpenes. *Antimicrob. Agents Chemother.* **2005**, *49*, 2474–2478. [CrossRef]
39. Hąc-Wydro, K.; Flasiński, M.; Romańczuk, K. Essential oils as food eco-preservatives: Model system studies on the effect of temperature on limonene antibacterial activity. *Food Chem.* **2017**, *235*, 127–135. [CrossRef]
40. Bassolé, I.H.N.; Juliani, H.R. Essential oils in combination and their antimicrobial properties. *Molecules* **2012**, *17*, 3989–4006. [CrossRef]
41. Viuda-Martos, M.; Ruiz-Navajas, Y.; Fernández-López, J.; Pérez-Álvarez, J. Antifungal activity of lemon (*Citrus lemon* L.), mandarin (*Citrus reticulata* L.), grapefruit (*Citrus paradisi* L.) and orange (*Citrus sinensis* L.) essential oils. *Food Control* **2008**, *19*, 1130–1138. [CrossRef]
42. Hamdi, A.; Majouli, K.; Flamini, G.; Marzouk, B.; Marzouk, Z.; Heyden, Y. Antioxidant and anticandidal activities of the Tunisian *Haplophyllum tuberculatum* (Forssk.) A. Juss. essential oils. *S. Afr. J. Bot.* **2017**, *112*, 210–214. [CrossRef]
43. Thakre, A.; Zore, G.; Kodgire, S.; Kazi, R.; Mulange, S.; Patil, R.; Shelar, A.; Santhakumari, B.; Kulkarni, M.; Kharat, K. Limonene inhibits *Candida albicans* growth by inducing apoptosis. *Med. Mycol. J.* **2018**, *56*, 565–578.
44. Ahmedi, S.; Pant, P.; Raj, N.; Manzoor, N. Limonene inhibits virulence associated traits in *Candida albicans*: In-Vitro and in-silico studies. *Phytomed. Plus.* **2022**, *2*, 100285. [CrossRef]
45. D'Angelo, G. Inflammation and coagulation: A "continuum" between coagulation activation and prothrombotic state. *J. Blood Disord.* **2015**, *2*, 1023.
46. Li, L.-Z.; Gao, P.-Y.; Song, S.-J.; Yuan, Y.-Q.; Liu, C.-T.; Huang, X.-X.; Liu, Q.-B. Monoterpenes and flavones from the leaves of *Crataegus pinnatifida* with anticoagulant activities. *J. Funct. Foods* **2015**, *12*, 237–245. [CrossRef]
47. Ksenofontov, A.A.; Bocharov, P.S.; Antina, E.V.; Shevchenko, O.G.; Samorodov, A.V.; Gilfanov, I.R.; Pavelyev, R.S.; Ostolopovskaya, O.V.; Startseva, V.A.; Fedyunina, I.V.; et al. Thioterpenoids as potential antithrombotic drugs: Molecular docking, antiaggregant, anticoagulant and antioxidant activities. *Biomolecules* **2022**, *12*, 1599. [CrossRef]
48. Riaz, A.; Khan, R.A.; Mirza, T.; Mustansir, T.; Ahmed, M. In vitro/in vivo effect of *Citrus limon* (L. Burm. f.) juice on blood parameters, coagulation and anticoagulation factors in rabbits. *Pak. J. Pharm. Sci.* **2014**, *27*, 907–915.
49. Edziri, H.; Mastouri, M.; Mahjoub, M.A.; Mighri, Z.; Mahjoub, A.; Verschaeve, L. Antibacterial, antifungal and cytotoxic activities of two flavonoids from *Retama raetam* flowers. *Molecules* **2012**, *17*, 7284–7293. [CrossRef]

50. Joulain, D.; König, W.A. The atlas of spectral data of sesquiterpene hydrocarbons. *Phytochemistry* **1999**, *52*, 1385–1986. [CrossRef]
51. Ghannay, S.; Aouadi, K.; Kadri, A.; Snoussi, M. In vitro and in silico screening of anti-*Vibrio* spp., antibiofilm, antioxidant and anti-quorum sensing activities of *Cuminum cyminum* L. volatile oil. *Plants* **2022**, *11*, 2236. [CrossRef]
52. Snoussi, M.; Ahmad, I.; Aljohani, A.M.; Patel, H.; Abdulhakeem, M.A.; Alhazmi, Y.S.; Tepe, B.; Adnan, M.; Siddiqui, A.J.; Sarikurkcu, C. Phytochemical analysis, antioxidant, and antimicrobial activities of *Ducrosia flabellifolia*: A combined experimental and computational approaches. *Antioxidants* **2022**, *11*, 2174. [CrossRef]
53. Czaikoski, P.G.; Menaldo, D.L.; Marcussi, S.; Baseggio, A.L.; Fuly, A.L.; Paula, R.C.; Quadros, A.U.; Romao, P.R.; Buschini, M.L.; Cunha, F.Q. Anticoagulant and fibrinogenolytic properties of the venom of *Polybia occidentalis* social wasp. *Blood Coagul Fibrinolysis* **2010**, *21*, 653–659. [CrossRef]
54. Edziri, H.; Guerrab, M.; Anthonissen, R.; Mastouri, M.; Verschaeve, L. Phytochemical screening, antioxidant, anticoagulant and in vitro toxic and genotoxic properties of aerial parts extracts of *Fumaria officinalis* L. growing in Tunisia. *S. Afr. J. Bot.* **2020**, *130*, 268–273. [CrossRef]
55. Liu, C.I.; Liu, G.Y.; Song, Y.; Yin, F.; Hensler, M.E.; Jeng, W.Y.; Nizet, V.; Wang, A.H.; Oldfield, E. A cholesterol biosynthesis inhibitor blocks *Staphylococcus aureus* virulence. *Science* **2008**, *319*, 1391–1394. [CrossRef]

pharmaceuticals MDPI

Article

Modulation of Hepatic Functions by Chicory (*Cichorium intybus* L.) Extract: Preclinical Study in Rats †

Lubov V. Krepkova [1], Alexandra N. Babenko [1], Svetlana V. Lemyaseva [1], Olga L. Saybel [1], Catherine M. Sherwin [2,3] and Elena Y. Enioutina [3,*]

1 All-Russian Institute of Medicinal and Aromatic Plants (VILAR), Moscow 113628, Russia
2 Boonshoft School of Medicine, Wright State University, Dayton Children's Hospital, Dayton, OH 45435, USA; catherine.sherwin85@gmail.com
3 Division of Clinical Pharmacology, Department of Pediatrics, School of Medicine, University of Utah, Salt Lake City, UT 84108, USA
* Correspondence: elena.enioutina@hsc.utah.edu

† The results of the hepatoprotective activity of the chicory extract described in this manuscript were presented at the American College of Clinical Pharmacology annual meeting on 15 September 2021.

Abstract: The liver is important in detoxifying organisms from xenobiotics, supporting immune functions, and metabolizing lipids and glucose. In addition, a growing number of drug-induced liver injuries and diseases associated with liver dysfunction make the development of phytodrugs targeting multiple liver functions particularly crucial. Therefore, we investigated the effects of a novel chicory extract prepared from aerial parts of the wild *Cichorium intybus* L. plant (CE) on liver enzymes and on lipid and glucose metabolism in rats with acute liver injury or hyperlipidemia. A single subcutaneous injection of mercury chloride induced an acute liver injury. Hyperlipidemia was induced by a single intraperitoneal injection of Tween-80 or by feeding rats with cholesterol and mercazolil for 28 days. Under varying regimens, the experimental rats received 100 mg/kg b.w. or 500 mg/kg b.w. of CE. CE treatment ameliorated acute liver injury by reducing liver enzyme activity, bilirubin, glucose, and lipid levels. Treatment of hyperlipidemic rats with CE effectively reduced serum lipid and glucose levels. The data obtained in this study suggest that chicory-based phytodrugs may be used to effectively treat acute liver injury and for the prophylaxis or treatment of diseases such as hyperlipidemia, type 2 diabetes, and metabolic syndrome. Clinical trials are needed to prove the effectiveness of chicory extract in human patients.

Keywords: chicory; *Cichorium intybus* L.; multi-targeting properties; hypolipidemic; hypoglycemic; hepatoprotective

Citation: Krepkova, L.V.; Babenko, A.N.; Lemyaseva, S.V.; Saybel, O.L.; Sherwin, C.M.; Enioutina, E.Y. Modulation of Hepatic Functions by Chicory (*Cichorium intybus* L.) Extract: Preclinical Study in Rats. *Pharmaceuticals* **2023**, *16*, 1471. https://doi.org/10.3390/ph16101471

Academic Editors: Daniela De Vita and Chung-Yi Chen

Received: 8 June 2023
Revised: 26 September 2023
Accepted: 3 October 2023
Published: 16 October 2023

1. Introduction

The liver is a critical organ supporting multiple functions, including nutrient metabolism, xenobiotic compound detoxification, immune and endocrine functions, and lipid and cholesterol homeostasis [1]. Dysregulation of lipid metabolism usually manifests in increased levels of triglycerides and total cholesterol and low levels of high-density lipoprotein (HDL), which is one of the hallmarks of metabolic syndrome [2]. Obesity, elevated fasting glucose levels, and high blood pressure are other diagnostic criteria for metabolic syndrome. Since the 1990s, when Dr. Reaven introduced this syndrome to the medical community, the number of people with metabolic syndrome has increased significantly [2]. According to the NIH National Heart, Lung, and Blood Institute, "1 in 3 adults have metabolic syndrome" in the U.S. [3]. The pathophysiology of the syndrome is not well understood. It appears that increased calorie uptake, low physical activity, and, potentially, genetic factors may lead to chronic inflammation, insulin resistance, and alterations of the renin–angiotensinogen system [2]. The downstream effects lead to the development of dyslipidemia, type 2 diabetes, hypertension, and cardiovascular diseases.

A recent systematic analysis of the relationship between metabolic syndrome and liver function revealed an increased risk (49 86%) of developing liver-associated diseases such as hepatic fibrosis, acute liver failure, and cirrhosis [4]. Patients' extensive use of drugs, herbal remedies, and dietary supplements in the modern world could also significantly affect liver functions, leading to Drug-Induced Liver Injury (DILI) [5]. Most liver injuries associated with prescription or non-prescription drugs are due to an acetaminophen (paracetamol) overdose. An overdose of acetaminophen may lead to acute liver failure and death. The excessive use of medicinal herbs and dietary supplements may also cause DILI [6]. The basic mechanisms leading to DILI are associated with the cytolysis of hepatocytes and induced inflammation by recruited immune cells [7,8]. Tyrosine kinase inhibitors, for example, Crizotinib, exhibit liver toxicity. This side effect of chemotherapeutic drugs is well known, and patients are carefully monitored for possible liver injury. However, the concomitant uncontrolled use of medicinal herbs with prescription drugs may potentially enhance liver distress [9,10]. Therefore, pharmacologists must develop effective medicines for the prophylaxis and treatment of liver dysfunction.

Nowadays, patients prefer to use herbal medicines and natural products to support their well-being. It has been reported that several constituents isolated from medicinal plants have hepatoprotective properties [5]. Among them are phenolic components (e.g., salvianolic acid, resveratrol, and curcumin), flavonoids (e.g., hesperetin, quercetin, and luteolin), and terpenoids (e.g., ginsenosides and betulin). The phenolic compounds present in the leaves of chicory (*Cichorium intybus* L., *C. intybus*) have multiple health benefits, including hepatoprotective, antioxidant, antidiabetic, and antimicrobial properties [11]. In addition, chicory is a part of a multi-component phytodrug (Liv-52) marketed by the Himalaya Drug Company since 1955 as a phytodrug intended to treat various liver diseases [12–14].

The chicory plant contains vitamins (e.g., vitamins C and A, thiamin, riboflavin, niacin, and pantothenic acid), minerals (e.g., Ca, Mg, Fe, P, K), and amino acids (e.g., tryptophan, leucine, isoleucine, valine, and arginine) [11,15]. Extracts from the aerial part of chicory demonstrated antioxidant and antimicrobial properties [16]. Methanolic and aqueous extracts of the aerial part showed broad-spectrum antimicrobial (e.g., *Staphylococcus* spp., *Pseudomonas aeruginosa*, and *Klebsiella pneumoniae*) and antifungal (e.g., *Candida albicans*) activity. The plant roots contain high amounts of inulin, a water-soluble polysaccharide (40–60%). Inulin may regulate low-density lipoprotein and triglyceride levels and support the intestinal microbiome [15]. Therefore, chicory-based drugs may represent a promising approach for preventing acute liver injury by hepatotoxic drugs and for the prophylaxis of metabolic-syndrome-associated diseases.

A few years ago, the All-Russian Institute of Medicinal and Aromatic Plants (VILAR) developed a novel highly purified extract from the aerial part of wild chicory collected during the flowering stage (CE). The ultimate goal was to obtain an extract with the highest concentration of polyphenolic constituents. The extraction of phenolic compounds is usually performed using 60–80% ethanol or methanol [16–18]. CE was obtained via the triple extraction of dried plant material with 70% v/v ethyl alcohol. Our initial study determined that this extraction method provides ~9.2–9.3% w/w of phenolic constituents calculated as chicoric acid (CA) [19]. The same study reported that CE possesses hepatoprotective activity in the model of acute hepatitis induced by tetrachloromethane (CCl4). A preclinical analysis of the extract demonstrated its low toxicity following oral and intraperitoneal administration [20].

The main objective of this study was to investigate whether CE improves liver functions by normalizing lipid and glucose metabolism in experimental animal models of hyperlipidemia. We also confirmed previous observations that CE can effectively prevent acute liver injury.

2. Results

2.1. Chemical Composition of CE

Content analysis of the extract showed that oxycoumarins, derivatives of hydroxycinnamic acids, and flavonoids represented the main phenolic compounds in CE. More than 20 compounds were identified in the extract (Supplemental Table S1). The CE's predominant compounds were cichoriin (1.44 ± 0.05% *w*/*w*), esculetin (0.44 ± 0.14% *w*/*w*), CA (2.90 ± 0.09% *w*/*w*), chlorogenic acid (1.77 ± 0.06% *w*/*w*), and caftaric acid (0.20 ± 0.01% *w*/*w*) (Supplemental Figure S1). The study extract contained 9.20 + 0.46% *w*/*w* of phenolic constituents, calculated as CA (Figure 1).

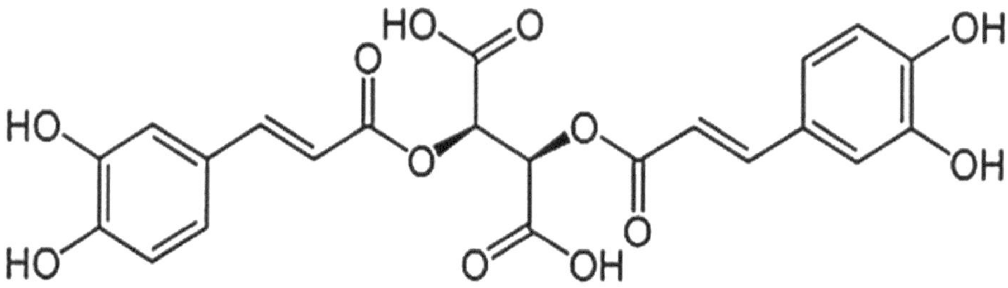

Figure 1. Chicoric acid.

2.2. Hepatoprotective Properties of CE

The hepatotoxic effect of the subcutaneous (SQ) administration of $HgCl_2$ was evidenced by a decrease in body weight; an increase in the relative liver weight; increased activity of γ-glutamyl transferase (GGT), alkaline phosphatase (ALP), aspartate aminotransferase (AST), and alanine aminotransferase (ALT); and destruction of lipid and glucose metabolism compared to the untreated control (Table 1). Serum levels of total proteins, triglyceride, total cholesterol, total bilirubin, and glucose significantly increased in the $HgCl_2$-treated group compared with the untreated control. The body weight in the $HgCl_2$-treated group dropped by 15% on day 10 after treatment initiation compared to the untreated control group and recovered to almost the body weight of naïve controls by day 21. The relative liver weight in rats receiving SQ $HgCl_2$ increased by ~30% compared to that in the untreated control group on day 21 after treatment initiation ($p < 0.05$).

The body weights of animals receiving $HgCl_2$ treatment followed by treatment with CE at doses of 100 mg/kg per body weight (mg/kg) or 500 mg/kg also fell by 11% and 8% on day 10 compared to the untreated control and recovered to weights comparable to those of the untreated controls on day 21 after treatment initiation. The relative liver weight of animals receiving CE was higher than the relative liver weight of untreated control animals but significantly lower than that of rats receiving $HgCl_2$ only (Table 1).

The administration of CE in doses of 100 and 500 mg/kg to $HgCl_2$-treated animals significantly reduced serum levels of GGT and ALT, but a statistically significant reduction in ALP and AST was observed only in animals receiving 500 mg/kg of CE (Table 1). Rats with acute liver injury treated with either 100 mg/kg or 500 mg/kg of CE also demonstrated a significant reduction in the levels of triglyceride, total cholesterol, total bilirubin, and glucose compared to $HgCl_2$-treated animals ($p < 0.05$) (Table 1).

Table 1. The effect of CE on body weight, relative liver weight, and biochemical serum profile of rats with acute liver injury.

Biomarker (Mean ± SD)	Treatment Groups [a]			
	Untreated Control	$HgCl_2$-Treated	$HgCl_2$-Treated + CE 100 mg/kg	$HgCl_2$-Treated + CE 500 mg/kg
Body weight on day 10 after experiment initiation (% of initial body weight)	131.6 ± 1.7	112.4 ± 2.4 *	117.1 ± 2.6	120.7 ± 2.9 *
Body weight on day 21 after experiment initiation (% of initial body weight)	147.5 ± 2.5	140.1 ± 1.9	144.9 ± 1.1	145.9 ± 2.0
Relative liver weight	3.93 ± 0.13	5.12 ± 0.15 *	4.53 ± 0.16 #	4.16 ± 0.06 #
Total protein, g/L	74.7 ± 1.0	83.7 ± 1.1 *	75.3 ± 0.7 #	76.3 ± 0.9 #
Glucose, mmol/L	7.04 ± 0.17	9.01 ± 0.16 *	7.2 ± 0.14 #	7.5 ± 0.13 #
Total cholesterol, mmol/L	1.72 ± 0.04	2.80 ± 0.08 *	2.1 ± 0.08 #	1.8 ± 0.05 #
Triglycerides, mmol/L	0.98 ± 0.11	1.55 ± 0.12 *	1.2 ± 0.15 #	1.2 ± 0.15 #
Total bilirubin, mmol/L	4.9 ± 0.2	7.8 ± 0.1 *	4.6 ± 0.1 #	4.8 ± 0.1 #
γ-glutamyl transferase (GGT), U/L	6.5 ± 0.7	11.0 ± 04 *	9.0 ± 0.5 #	8.7 ± 0.7 #
Alkaline phosphatase (ALP), U/L	784.0 ± 28.4	1005 ± 44.2 *	971.0 ± 80.4	897.6 ± 57.0 #
Aspartate aminotransferase (AST), U/L	136.8 ± 4.2	175.1 ± 4.4 *	155 ± 10.5	151.1 ± 7.1 #
Alanine aminotransferase (ALT), U/L	89.3 ± 3.7	126.3 ± 4.1 *	90.0 ± 5.4 #	80.9 ± 1.6 #

[a]—Hepatoprotective activity of CE was evaluated at 21 days after $HgCl_2$-induced liver damage; *—Significantly different compared with control, $p < 0.05$; #—Significantly different compared with $HgCl_2$-treated group, $p < 0.05$.

2.3. *Hypolipidemic and Hypoglycemic Effects of CE on the Tween-80 Model of Hyperlipidemia in Rats*

A single intraperitoneal (i.p.) administration of Tween-80 caused a significant increase in the levels of LDL (44%), triglycerides (40%), and glucose (14%) and a decrease in the levels of HDL (22%) in the serum of Tween-80-treated rats compared to naïve controls (Table 2). Total cholesterol levels increased by ~13%, but the differences were not statistically significant.

Table 2. Effect of CE on the serum biochemical profile of rats treated with a single i.p. injection of Tween-80.

Biomarkers (Mean ± SD)	Treatment Groups [a]			
	Untreated Control	Tween-80-Treated	Tween-80-Treated + CE 100 mg/kg	Tween-80-Treated + CE 500 mg/kg
Total cholesterol, mmol/L	1.56 ± 0.09	1.83 ± 0.10	1.62 ± 0.08	1.74 ± 0.05
High-density lipoproteins (HDL), mmol/L	0.73 ± 0.03	0.57 ± 0.03 *	0.65 ± 0.04	0.67 ± 0.03 #
Low-density lipoproteins (LDL), mmol/L	0.58 ± 0.04	0.84 ± 0.03 *	0.57 ± 0.02 #	0.62 ± 0.04 #
Triglycerides, mmol/L	0.68 ± 0.03	0.95 ± 0.04 *	0.60 ± 0.07 #	0.65 ± 0.06 #
Glucose, mmol/L	5.23 ± 0.21	5.95 ± 0.13 *	4.76 ± 0.17 #	4.47 ± 0.15 #

[a]—Hypolipidemic and hypoglycemic activities of CE were evaluated 8 h post Tween-80 administration; *—Significantly different compared with control, $p < 0.05$; #—Significantly different compared with Tween-80-treated group, $p < 0.05$.

The prophylactic administration of CE at doses of 100 and 500 mg/kg for 14 days before the Tween-80 injection significantly reduced the levels of LDL by 32% and 26%, triglycerides by 37% and 32%, and glucose by 20% and 25%, respectively, compared to those of Tween-80-treated rats (Table 2). CE pretreatment also increased the serum HDL levels in rats by 14% (100 mg/kg) and 18% (500 mg/kg) compared to those in Tween-80-treated rats ($p < 0.05$, Table 2).

2.4. Hypolipidemic and Hypoglycemic Effects of CE on the Model of Alimentary Hyperlipidemia

The administration of cholesterol–mercazolil to experimental rats resulted in a statistically significant increase in the total cholesterol and triglyceride levels compared to those of the untreated control (Table 3). Rats with alimentary hyperlipidemia demonstrated a slight increase in HDL, LDL, and glucose levels, but the differences were not statistically significant. Animals receiving cholesterol–mercazolil gained weight slightly faster than the untreated control group, but the differences were not statistically significant. Based on our observations, rats on the high-cholesterol diet gained significantly more weight than did untreated control animals 80–90 days after transfer to the high-cholesterol diet.

Table 3. Effect of CE on body weight and serum biochemical profile of rats with alimentary hyperlipidemia.

Biomarkers (Mean ± SD)	Treatment Groups [a]			
	Untreated Control	Cholesterol–Mercazolil Treatment	Cholesterol–Mercazolil Treatment + CE 100 mg/kg	Cholesterol–Mercazolil Treatment + CE 500 mg/kg
Body weight on day 29 after experiment initiation (% of initial body weight)	119.4 ± 1.9	123.1 ± 2.4	119.2 ± 1.7	115.0 ± 1.5 #
Total cholesterol, mmol/L	1.65 ± 0.08	1.82 ± 0.04 *	1.56 ± 0.07 #	1.53 ± 0.05 #
High-density lipoproteins (HDL), mmol/L	0.80 ± 0.04	0.93 ± 0.03	0.83 ± 0.02	0.77 ± 0.03
Low-density lipoproteins (LDL), mmol/L	0.55 ± 0.03	0.53 ± 0.05	0.38 ± 0.04 #	0.39 ± 0.03 #
Triglycerides, mmol/L	0.76 ± 0.06	0.99 ± 0.08 *	0.69 ± 0.04 #	0.78 ± 0.02 #
Glucose, mmol/L	4.80 ± 0.14	5.04 ± 0.13	5.01 ± 0.17	5.14 ± 0.18

[a]—Hypolipidemic activities of CE were evaluated 29 days after cholesterol–mercazolil administration with or without CE treatment; *—Significantly different compared with control, $p < 0.05$; #—Significantly different compared with the alimentary hyperlipidemia group, $p < 0.05$.

The oral administration of CE to rats with alimentary hyperlipidemia at doses of 100 mg/kg and 500 mg/kg significantly reduced the serum levels of triglycerides by 30% and 21%, respectively ($p < 0.05$); reduced the levels of LDL by 28% and 26%, respectively; and moderately reduced the levels of total cholesterol by 14% and 16%, respectively, compared to those in animals with alimentary hyperlipidemia (Table 3). Additionally, animals treated with 500 mg/kg of CE had low body weight on day 28 of treatment initiation compared to rats with alimentary hyperlipidemia, and the differences were statistically significant (Table 3).

The liver histology of the control rats is presented in Figure 2A. The histological evaluation of livers from rats receiving the cholesterol–mercazolil treatment revealed that the treatment resulted in hyaline-droplet degeneration of hepatocytes (Figure 2B). Treatment of these rats with CE 100 mg/kg and 500 mg/kg led to a more normal liver appearance (Figure 2C,D). The liver capsule consists of densely packed connective tissue fibers. The hepatic beams are radially oriented, the lobules are formed correctly, the hepatocytes have a pale eosinophilic cytoplasm, and the nuclei are preserved. The architectonics of the vessels are normal. The endothelium of the vessels of the portal tract is not changed; the bile ducts are lined with cuboidal epithelium.

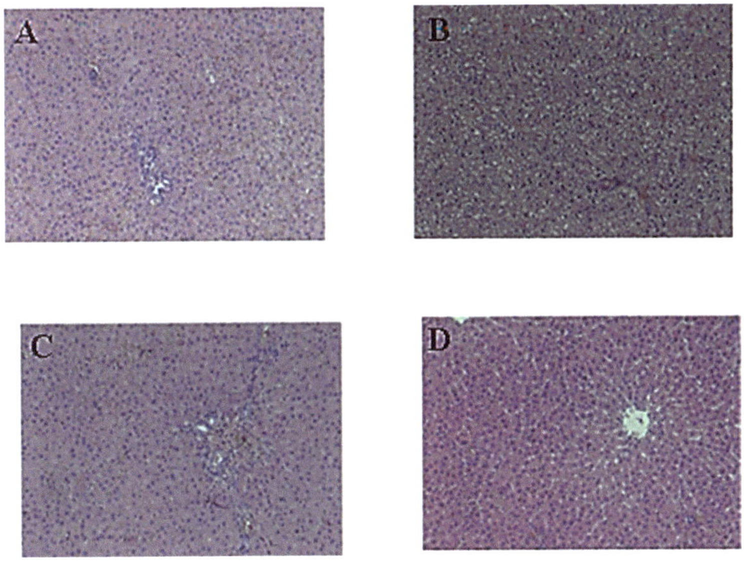

Figure 2. Effect of CE on the liver structure: (**A**) liver histology of untreated control rats; (**B**) liver histology of rats 29 days after cholesterol–mercazolil treatment; (**C**) liver histology 29 days after cholesterol–mercazolil treatment and 100 mg/kg CE; (**D**) liver histology 29 days after cholesterol–mercazolil treatment and 500 mg/kg CE. Hematoxylin and eosin staining, magnification ×100.

3. Discussion

This study supports previously published observations that CE demonstrates hepatoprotective properties. Previously, we showed that CE improves the liver function of rats with acute liver injury induced by SQ injection of CCl_4 [19]. The current study confirmed the hepatoprotective properties of CE in another model: acute intoxication with $HgCl_2$.

The study results demonstrate that treatment of rats with CE restored body weight and reduced relative liver weight, total cholesterol levels, triglycerides, glucose, and hepatic enzymes in the model of acute liver injury. *C. intybus* is a known plant with hepatoprotective properties [21,22]. For example, chicory syrup treatment decreased lipid peroxidation and improved liver histology in weanling rats exposed to deltamethrin [23]. The treatment of rats with obstructive cholestasis with 70% ethanolic extract of chicory reduced bilirubin and liver enzyme (ALT, AST, and ALP) levels [24]. Additionally, this treatment significantly decreased serum levels of TNFα and nitric oxide. Chicory extract administered to rats with thioacetamide-induced liver cirrhosis was able to normalize serum liver enzyme activity, albumin, and bilirubin levels [25]. This treatment reduced oxidative stress levels and IL-6 production by regulating AMP-activated protein kinase signaling. 6-Gingerol, a main constituent of ginger, attenuated liver injury induced by a well-known hepatocarcinogen, diethylnitrosamine [26]. The authors ascribe the hepatoprotective properties of 6-gingerol to its ability to reduce oxidative stress and TNFα protein levels.

Hepatoprotective compounds can be classified based on their mechanisms of action: antioxidants, compounds capable of regenerating hepatocytic membranes, and stimulators of regeneration of hepatic parenchyma [27]. The mechanisms of chicory's hepatoprotective properties can be mainly attributed to its antioxidant activity. The hepatoprotective effects of chicory extracts have been attributed to the presence of phenolic compounds, specifically, chicoric acid, and its antioxidant and anti-inflammatory properties [19,28]. The hepatoprotective effects of another polyphenolic compound, kaempferol, are also ascribed to its antioxidant and anti-inflammatory properties [29,30].

The presented data showed CE's pronounced hypolipidemic effect on two hyperlipidemia models induced by single i.p. Tween-80 administration or oral administration of cholesterol and mercazolil for 28 days. Currently, various experimental models of hyperlipidemia are used to study the hypolipidemic properties of drug candidates. One such model is experimental hypercholesterolemia induced by feeding animals a diet with excess cholesterol and simultaneous treatment with a drug interfering with thyroid peroxidase (e.g., mercazolil). The metabolism of lipoproteins in rodents (e.g., mice and rats) is different to that in humans. Rodents lack cholesteryl ester transfer protein, which is critical in human lipoprotein metabolism [31]. Inadequate enzyme activity may lead to increased levels of HDL and LDL. The absence of cholesteryl ester transfer protein explains the difficulties with the induction of hyperlipidemia in rats. It has been demonstrated that hypothyroid animals have increased LDL and very-low-density lipoproteins [32]. Triiodothyronine (T3) regulates hepatic cholesterol metabolism, specifically, cholesterol 7-alpha-hydroxylase, an enzyme involved in bile acid synthesis [33]. This explains the use of mercazolil in the rodent models of hyperlipidemia. The use of the "mercazolil model" has another advantage: it models conditions of hyperlipidemia in patients with hypothyroidism and suggests that the test drug would be effective in this category of patients.

Interestingly, the administration of CE to healthy rats with normal lipid levels for 90 days significantly decreased serum levels of low-density lipoproteins and glucose (data not shown). Keshk et al. reported that whole chicory plant powder administered to hyperlipidemic rats reduced total cholesterol, HDL, LDL, ALT, and AST levels [34]. The authors concluded that chicory and other herbal medicines could be an inexpensive alternative for treating dyslipidemia in humans.

Our study also found that CE reduced serum glucose levels in hyperlipidemic rats. Several studies have demonstrated the effectiveness of chicory extracts in animal models of type 2 diabetes. For example, one week of oral treatment with 80% ethanol/water extract of *C. intybus* in diabetic mice induced by nicotinamide–streptozotocin resulted in significantly reduced serum glucose levels [35]. Chicory extract enriched for caffeoylquinic acid ameliorated dyslipidemia and hyperglycemia by potentially reducing oxidative stress in rats fed a high-cholesterol/fructose diet [36]. A recent study demonstrated that chicory extract and a mixture of chicoric and chlorogenic acids improved glucose tolerance and normalized glucose levels in streptozotocin-treated diabetic rats [28]. It has been reported that extracts from dandelion and burdock enriched with chicoric and chlorogenic acids cause insulin resistance in rats on a high-fructose diet (experimental model of metabolic syndrome) [29].

The ability of chicory extracts to treat diabetes can be attributed to their antioxidant properties [30]. Indeed, both chicoric and chlorogenic acids demonstrated significant antioxidant properties, but only chicory extract significantly reduced glucose levels in streptozotocin-treated diabetic rats [30]. Therefore, the antidiabetic properties of chicory cannot be entirely attributed to the antioxidant activity of its bioactive compounds.

The anti-inflammatory activities of the bioactive compounds present in chicory extract may potentiate the hypoglycemic activity of the extract. White adipose tissues are a major source of inflammatory cytokines (e.g., TNFα, IL1, IL6, and others) and play a critical role in the development of type 2 diabetes [37].

Chicory extract also decreased serum glucose levels and normalized glucose tolerance test results in mice fed a high-fat diet for 6 weeks [38]. The authors suggest that one of the potential mechanisms of the hypoglycemic effects of chicory extract is its ability to reduce serum IL1β levels through inhibition of NLRP3 inflammasome activation. Furthermore, the caffeic acid moiety (e.g., caffeoylquinic, chlorogenic, 3-caffeoylquinic, caffeic, and quinic acids) is responsible for the hypoglycemic effect by reducing the activities of glucose-6-phosphatase and phosphoenolpyruvate carboxykinase, enzymes regulating glycogenesis [39].

The number of people with metabolic syndrome is rapidly increasing, and as a result, we see a significant increase in the number of patients with type 2 diabetes and cardiovascular diseases [2]. It has been believed that abdominal obesity is one of the earliest symptoms of metabolic syndrome [40]. The next stage of metabolic syndrome is the development of hepatic and pancreatic steatosis [40]. Increased lipid and glucose levels are biomarkers of metabolic syndrome [2]. Another key biomarker of metabolic syndrome is the development of insulin resistance [40]. Our data and the above studies demonstrate that chicory or chicory bioactive compounds possess hypolipidemic and hypoglycemic properties that may reduce insulin resistance. Therefore, chicory-based phytodrugs may be used to prevent and treat metabolic syndrome.

A recent publication by Pouille et al. demonstrated that, similarly to the aerial part of chicory, its roots possess anti-inflammatory, antioxidant, hypolipidemic, and hypoglycemic properties [41]. The authors attributed the observed chicory root extract activity to the presence of fructose. Chlorogenic acids and sesquiterpene lactones found at smaller concentrations in the root extract significantly suppressed IL1β and IL8 production by U937-differentiated macrophages. Chlorogenic acids are esters formed between caffeic acid and the 3-hydroxyl of L-quinic acid, and they include 4-O-caffeoylquinic acid and 5-O-caffeoylquinic acid [42]. These bioactive compounds were also identified in CE. This might suggest that chlorogenic acids are one of the bioactive compounds affecting inflammatory cytokine production by immune cells.

Interestingly, bioactive compounds from chicory demonstrated beneficial effects on other organ functions. For example, CA showed neuroprotective properties in the mouse model of Parkinson's disease via dopaminergic neuron survival and suppression of glial-mediated neuroinflammation [43]. Additionally, the treatment of mice with CA reduced IFN-γ and IL17 protein expression in the serum, striatum, spleen, and colon. CA also attenuated renal tubular damage in obese mice by reducing mitochondrial damage and oxidative stress [44]. The same study showed that treating obese mice with CA reduced body weight and lipid and glucose levels—symptoms associated with metabolic syndrome in humans [44].

In summary, chicory and its bioactive compounds have multiple beneficial effects on liver, brain, and kidney functions. In this study, CE demonstrated simultaneously hepatoprotective, hypolipidemic, and hypoglycemic properties (Figure 3). CE may help treat acute xenobiotic-induced liver injury (Figure 3). CE can also be used as a hypoglycemic and hypolipidemic phytodrug (Figure 3). Based on the dysregulation of lipid and carbohydrate metabolism in patients with metabolic syndrome, chicory extracts should effectively prevent and treat metabolic syndrome (Figure 3). Based on the reported potential mechanisms responsible for the hepatoprotective, hypolipidemic, and hypoglycemic properties of chicory plant, the potential mechanisms of CE's effects on liver functions are likely to be its antioxidant and anti-inflammatory properties. Our research group is conducting experiments to confirm this statement. Unfortunately, little is known about the effects of chicory extracts on human organisms. Therefore, it is imperative that clinical trials are designed to evaluate chicory extracts and determine their efficacy and toxicity in humans.

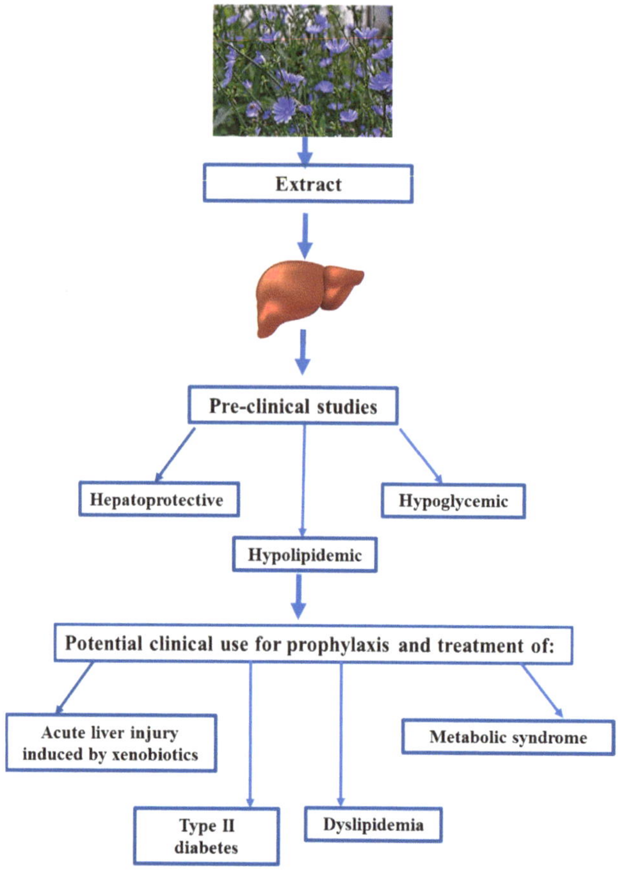

Figure 3. Preclinical properties of chicory and potential clinical use.

4. Materials and Methods

4.1. *Phytodrug*

The highly purified dry extract (CE) was obtained from the aerial part of wild chicory during the flowering stage. CE was developed at the All-Russian Research Institute of Medicinal and Aromatic Plants (VILAR). The aerial part of the chicory (*C. intybus*) was harvested in the Ryazan region in 2020–2021 according to the VILAR recommendations [45] and the International Standard for Sustainable Wild Collection of Medicinal and Aromatic Plants [46].

The extract was obtained by threefold extraction of dried plant material with 70% v/v ethyl alcohol at 50 ± 5 °C. After extraction, the liquid components were separated from the solid biomass via vacuum filtration at 50 ± 5 °C. The aqueous–alcoholic extract was concentrated, treated with dichloroethane (Chemical Point UG, Oberhaching, Germany) to separate aqueous part of extract, and dried. The resulting dry extract was crushed, sieved, and used for the phenolic compound profiling and for the evaluation of hepatoprotective, hypolipidemic and hypoglycemic properties of CE.

4.2. *Profiling of Polyphenolic Compounds Present in CE*

Polyphenolic compounds were identified in a similar way to that described by Chawech et al., with some modifications [19,47]. Briefly, polyphenolic compounds from CE were profiled using an LCMS-8040 high-performance liquid chromatography (HPLC) system

(Shimadzu, Kyoto, Japan), including a Nexera HPLC chromatograph and triple quadrupole detector with an electrospray ionization source (liquid chromatography with tandem mass spectrometry, LC-MS/MS). The compounds were separated on a Luna 5 μm C18 100 Å (250 × 4.6 mm) column (Phenomenex, Torrance, CA, USA). The mobile phases (A and B) comprised 0.2% formic acid solution (A) and acetonitrile (B), respectively. The elution program was set as follows: 0–20 min, linear gradient from 10% eluent B; 20–30 min, linear gradient from 10 to 25% eluent B; 30–40 min, linear gradient from 40% eluent B; 40–44 min, linear gradient from 60% eluent B; 44–48 min, linear gradient from 80% eluent B; 48–60 min, linear gradient from 10% eluent B. The flow rate was maintained at 1 mL/min. The CE (0.01 g) was first dissolved in 25 mL of ethyl alcohol 70% (*w*/*v*). The extract filtrate (10 μL) was injected into the HPLC to separate phenolic compounds. Peaks were identified in negative and positive ionization modes. The mass spectra were obtained in the mass-to-charge range of 100–1000. Data were analyzed using LabSolutions (Shimadzu, Version 5.3).

4.3. Quantification of Total and Dominant Polyphenols in CE

The detailed protocol of quantification of the total and dominant polyphenols was described by Thomas et al. [19]. The total content of phenolic compounds was determined using a UV-1800 spectrophotometer (Shimadzu, Japan) at a wavelength of 327 nm. The content of phenolic compounds was calculated as CA.

The quantification of the dominant polyphenolic compounds was performed using a Prominence-I LC-2030C 3D HPLC system (Shimadzu, Japan) connected to a photodiode array detector. The column and analysis conditions were the same as those applied in the liquid chromatography–mass spectrometry (LC-MS/MS) analysis, with a 10 μL injection volume of samples. Peak identification was performed at 330 nm. Data analysis was achieved using LabSolutions (Version 5.73). Each dominant compound was quantified by constructing a standard curve with different external standard concentrations, including cichoriin, esculetin, chicoric acid, chlorogenic acid, and caftaric acid.

4.4. Animals

The study of CE's hepatoprotective and hypolipidemic effects was carried out per the "Guidelines for conducting preclinical studies of drugs" implemented by the Ministry of Public Health of the Russian Federation [27]. The study protocol was approved by the VILAR Ethical Committee on Animal Experimentation and carried out per the "European Convention for the Protection of Vertebrate Animals Used for Experimental and Other Scientific Purposes (ETS 123). Strasbourg, 1986" [48,49].

Wistar male rats were obtained from the animal nursery "Andreevka", a branch of FSBIS of the Scientific Center of Biomedical Technologies of the Medical and Biological Agency, Moscow, Russia. Animals were housed in groups of 4–5 rats in a plastic cage. Animals were kept under controlled environmental conditions of light (12 h light cycle), temperature (20–22 °C), and humidity (40–60%) with free access to standard chow for laboratory rats (Laboratorkorm LLC, Moscow, Russia) and water.

Rats were lightly anesthetized with isoflurane using a drop jar method to reduce stress following short procedures (e.g., a blood draw). At the end of each experiment, anesthetized by isoflurane, animals were euthanized by CO_2 inhalation at a chamber replacement range (CRR) of 30% [50].

4.5. Analysis of CE's Hepatoprotective Effect on the Model of Acute Liver Injury in Rats

The hepatoprotective activity of CE was studied in a model of acute liver injury induced by a single SQ injection of mercury chloride ($HgCl_2$, 3 mg/kg) into male rats [50]. Male rats were randomly assigned to four groups (10 rats/group). Rats receiving a single SQ saline injection were used as an untreated control. Animals receiving a single SQ injection of $HgCl_2$, with 3 mg/kg H_2O orally 60 min before and 20 days after $HgCl_2$ treatment, were used as positive controls for liver injury. The CE stock solutions were prepared daily by dissolving the dry extract in tap water. CE was administered orally by gavage in 100 and 500 mg/kg doses 60 min before $HgCl_2$ administration and for 20 days following the treatment. On day 21, all animals were weighed and anesthetized with isoflurane, and peripheral blood was collected (~1.0 mL) from the lateral tail vein.

The collected blood was spun down at 1000 g for 15 min at room temperature, and serum was collected. Several biochemical parameters were analyzed using a URIT-8030 Automated Chemistry Analyzer (China Medial Devices, North Andover, MA, USA): total proteins, triglyceride, total cholesterol, total bilirubin, glucose, γ-glutamyl transferase (GGT), alkaline phosphatase (ALP), aspartate aminotransferase (AST), and alanine aminotransferase (ALT).

4.6. Analysis of CE's Hypolipidemic Effect on the Model of Hyperlipidemia Caused by a Single Intraperitoneal Injection of Tween-80

Hyperlipidemia was induced by a single i.p. administration of Tween-80 [27,51]. The experiment was conducted on 32 Wistar male rats with an initial body weight of 400–500 g. The experimental animals were randomly assigned to four groups of 8 rats per group. Animals receiving i.p. saline and oral tap water were used as a naïve control (group 1); animals receiving a single i.p. injection of Tween-80 (Chemical Point UG, Germany) at a dose of 200 mg/100 g of body weight and tap water orally were used as a positive control (group 2, hyperlipidemia model); and group 3 and 4 rats were treated with CE for 14 days prior to the i.p. Tween-80 injections. The CE was administered by gavage at 100 and 500 mg/kg doses. The CE solutions were prepared daily by dissolving the dry extract in tap water. Eight hours after Tween-80 administration, peripheral blood samples were collected from the tail vein of isoflurane-anesthetized rats. Serum was obtained by centrifugation of blood samples, and biochemical parameters were analyzed (total cholesterol, LDL HDL, triglycerides, and glucose) using a URIT-8030 Automated Chemistry Analyzer (China Medial Devices, Beijing, China).

4.7. Study of the Lipid-Lowering Effect on a Model of Alimentary Hyperlipidemia

Alimentary hyperlipidemia in rats was induced by daily intragastric administration (by gavage) of cholesterol and mercazolil for 28 days [52]. Thirty-two male rats were randomly assigned to four groups of eight rats per group. Group 1 received daily tap water by gavage and was used as a naïve control; group 2 received daily cholesterol (Chemical Point UG, Germany) and mercazolil (Akrikhin, Moscow, Russia) for 28 days by gavage and was used as a positive control; and groups 3 and 4, in addition to the daily administration of cholesterol and mercazolil, were also treated with CE at doses of 100 and 500 mg/kg, respectively, 1 h prior to cholesterol–mercazolil administration for 28 days. CE solutions were prepared fresh prior to administration by dissolving dry extract in tap water. Cholesterol–mercazolil solution was prepared from 30 mg of cholesterol and 1 mg of mercazolil per 100 g of body weight, mixed with warm vegetable oil, and cooled down for animal treatment.

On day 29 after treatment initiation, rats were weighed, and peripheral blood samples were collected from the tail vein of anesthetized rats. The serum was obtained by $1000\times g$ centrifugation for 15 min. Serum samples were analyzed for total cholesterol, LDL, HDL, triglyceride, and glucose levels using a URIT-8030 Automated Chemistry Analyzer (China Medial Devices, China).

Then, the animals were euthanized by CO_2 inhalation. Livers were collected, and the relative liver weight was calculated using the following formula: Relative liver weight = [liver weight/body weight] $\times$ 100.

The livers from five rats in each group were fixed in 10% formalin; histological sections were then made, stained with hematoxylin and eosin, and examined using a light microscope at a magnification of $\times 100$.

4.8. Statistical Analysis

All data obtained from experimental and control animals were included in the analysis. Statistical analysis of the obtained results was conducted using TIBCO Statistica, version 13 (TIBCO Software Inc., Palo Alto, CA, USA). The difference between the control and experimental groups was considered statistically significant at $p < 0.05$.

5. Conclusions

This study demonstrated that chicory (*Cichorium intybus* L.) extract made from aerial parts of the plant possesses simultaneously hepatoprotective, hypolipidemic, and hypoglycemic properties. The hepatoprotective properties of CE previously reported in the liver injury model induced by CCl_4 were confirmed using the rat model of acute liver injury induced by heavy metals. Animals exposed to $HgCl_2$ and treated with CE showed reduced serum levels of GGT, ALT, ALP, AST, triglyceride, and total cholesterol. The treatment with CE reduced levels of lipids—specifically, HDL, LDL, triglycerides, and total cholesterol—and glucose in hyperlipidemic rats. To our knowledge, this is the first demonstration of single extract that can alter multiple liver functions.

The hepatoprotective, hypolipidemic, and hypoglycemic properties of CE were investigated in models of acute liver injury and hyperlipidemia in rats and cannot be generalized to humans. Clinical studies are needed to confirm these findings. The exact mechanisms by which CE supports liver function are unknown. Our group is currently conducting experiments to shed light on the mechanisms responsible for the extract's activities.

Supplementary Materials: The following supporting information can be downloaded at: https://www.mdpi.com/article/10.3390/ph16101471/s1, Figure S1: HPLC chromatogram of polyphenolic compounds of chicory extract (330 nm); Table S1: Phenolic compounds identified in CE.

Author Contributions: Conceptualization, L.V.K., O.L.S., E.Y.E. and C.M.S.; methodology, L.V.K. and E.Y.E.; validation, A.N.B., S.V.L. and L.V.K.; formal analysis, A.N.B., S.V.L. and L.V.K.; investigation, A.N.B., S.V.L. and O.L.S.; writing—original draft preparation, L.V.K. and E.Y.E.; writing—review and editing, L.V.K., E.Y.E. and C.M.S.; visualization, E.Y.E. and C.M.S. All authors have read and agreed to the published version of the manuscript.

Funding: This research received no external funding.

Institutional Review Board Statement: The study of CE's hepatoprotective and hypolipidemic effects was carried out in accordance with "Guidelines for conducting preclinical studies of drugs" implemented by the Ministry of Public Health of the Russian Federation. The study protocols were approved by the VILAR Ethical Committee on Animal Experimentation: Protocol No. 27, dated 18 May 2020, "Study of the hepatoprotective properties of dry wild chicory herb extract on mature Wistar rats"; Protocol No. 45, dated 13 April 2021 "Study of the lipid-lowering effect of dry wild chicory herb extract on rats—a twin model"; and Protocol No. 47, dated 19 April 2021 "Study of the lipid-lowering effect of wild chicory herb dry extract on a cholesterol model".

Informed Consent Statement: Not applicable.

Data Availability Statement: Data is contained within the article and supplementary material.

Acknowledgments: The photo "Blue flowers of chicory on the background of the summer landscape" is a free download from Shutterstock, Stock Photo ID: 696808174. Photo contributor: Shutova Elena.

Conflicts of Interest: C.M.S. and E.Y.E. are Editors of this Special Issue. All other authors declare no conflicts of interest.

References

1. Trefts, E.; Gannon, M.; Wasserman, D.H. The liver. *Curr. Biol.* **2017**, *27*, R1147–R1151. [CrossRef]
2. Fahed, G.; Aoun, L.; Bou Zerdan, M.; Allam, S.; Bou Zerdan, M.; Bouferraa, Y.; Assi, H.I. Metabolic Syndrome: Updates on Pathophysiology and Management in 2021. *Int. J. Mol. Sci.* **2022**, *23*, 786. [CrossRef] [PubMed]
3. NIH National Heart, Lung and Blood Institute. Metabolic Syndrome. Available online: https://www.nhlbi.nih.gov/health/metabolic-syndrome (accessed on 26 March 2023).

4. Ren, H.; Wang, J.; Gao, Y.; Yang, F.; Huang, W. Metabolic syndrome and liver-related events: A systematic review and meta-analysis. *BMC Endocr. Disord.* **2019**, *19*, 40. [CrossRef] [PubMed]
5. Sun, Y.K.; Zhang, Y.F.; Xie, L.; Rong, F.; Zhu, X.Y.; Xie, J.; Zhou, H.; Xu, T. Progress in the treatment of drug-induced liver injury with natural products. *Pharmacol. Res.* **2022**, *183*, 106361. [CrossRef] [PubMed]
6. Enioutina, E.Y.; Job, K.M.; Sherwin, C.M.T. Why we need to pay attention to toxicity associated with herbal medicines. *Br. J. Clin. Pharmacol.* **2020**, *86*, 1793–1794. [CrossRef]
7. Yuan, L.; Kaplowitz, N. Mechanisms of drug-induced liver injury. *Clin. Liver Dis.* **2013**, *17*, 507–518. [CrossRef]
8. Umbaugh, D.S.; Jaeschke, H. Biomarkers of drug-induced liver injury: A mechanistic perspective through acetaminophen hepatotoxicity. *Expert. Rev. Gastroenterol. Hepatol.* **2021**, *15*, 363–375. [CrossRef] [PubMed]
9. Revol, B.; Gautier-Veyret, E.; Arrivé, C.; Fouilhé Sam-Laï, N.; McLeer-Florin, A.; Pluchart, H.; Pinsolle, J.; Toffart, A.C. Pharmacokinetic herb-drug interaction between ginger and crizotinib. *Br. J. Clin. Pharmacol.* **2020**, *86*, 1892–1893. [CrossRef]
10. Laube, R.; Liu, K. An unwanted complement: Rare case of potential liver injury induced by an interaction between ginseng and atorvastatin. *Br. J. Clin. Pharmacol.* **2019**, *85*, 1612–1613. [CrossRef]
11. Perović, J.; Tumbas Šaponjac, V.; Kojić, J.; Krulj, J.; Moreno, D.A.; García-Viguera, C.; Bodroža-Solarov, M.; Ilić, N. Chicory (*Cichorium intybus* L.) as a food ingredient—Nutritional composition, bioactivity, safety, and health claims: A review. *Food Chem.* **2021**, *336*, 127676. [CrossRef]
12. Sama, S.K.; Krishnamurthy, L.; Ramachandran, K.; Lal, K. Efficacy of an indigenous compound preparation (Liv-52) in acute viral hepatitis-a double blind study. *Indian. J. Med. Res.* **1976**, *64*, 738–742.
13. Saxena, A.; Garg, N.K. Effect of Liv-52 on hepatic enzymes. *Indian. J. Exp. Biol.* **1979**, *17*, 662–664.
14. Thabrew, M.I.; Emerole, G.O.; Subbarao, V.V. Effect of Liv-52 on carbon tetrachloride-induced changes in hepatic microsomal drug-metabolizing enzymes of the rat. *Toxicol. Lett.* **1982**, *14*, 183–188. [CrossRef]
15. Janda, K.; Gutowska, I.; Geszke-Moritz, M.; Jakubczyk, K. The Common Cichory (*Cichorium intybus* L.) as a Source of Extracts with Health-Promoting Properties—A Review. *Molecules* **2021**, *26*, 1814. [CrossRef] [PubMed]
16. Jasim, R.; Antioxidant, Antimicrobial Activities and Phytochemical Constituents of *Cichorium intybus* L. Aerial Parts. *Int. J. Bot.* **2018**, *14*, 24–29. [CrossRef]
17. Zanoni, F.; Primiterra, M.; Angeli, N.; Zoccatelli, G. Microencapsulation by spray-drying of polyphenols extracted from red chicory and red cabbage: Effects on stability and color properties. *Food Chem.* **2020**, *307*, 125535. [CrossRef]
18. Cova, C.M.; Boffa, L.; Pistocchi, M.; Giorgini, S.; Luque, R.; Cravotto, G. Technology and Process Design for Phenols Recovery from Industrial Chicory (*Chicorium intybus*) Leftovers. *Molecules* **2019**, *24*, 2681. [CrossRef] [PubMed]
19. Saybel, O.L.; Rendyuk, T.D.; Dargaeva, T.D.; Lupanova, I.A.; Ferubko, E.V.; Kurmanova, E.N.; Martynchik, I.A. Phenolic Compounds and Hepatoprotective Activity of Chicory Herb Extract. *Drug Dev. Regist.* **2021**, *10*, 36–45. [CrossRef]
20. Kuzina, O.S.; Borovkova, M.V.; Lemyaseva, S.V.; Saybel, O.L. Toxicity of dry extract of *Chicorium intybus* L. following single administration. *Bull. Med. Sci.* **2019**, *1*, 29–32.
21. Krepkova, L.V.; Babenko, A.N.; Saybel, O.L.; Lupanova, I.A.; Kuzina, O.S.; Job, K.M.; Sherwin, C.M.; Enioutina, E.Y. Valuable Hepatoprotective Plants—How Can We Optimize Waste Free Uses of Such Highly Versatile Resources? *Front. Pharmacol.* **2021**, *12*, 738504. [CrossRef]
22. Ignat, M.V.; Coldea, T.E.; Salanță, L.C.; Mudura, E. Plants of the Spontaneous Flora with Beneficial Action in the Management of Diabetes, Hepatic Disorders, and Cardiovascular Disease. *Plants* **2021**, *10*, 216. [CrossRef]
23. Mohafrash, S.M.M.; Mossa, A.H. Herbal syrup from chicory and artichoke leaves ameliorate liver damage induced by deltamethrin in weanling male rats. *Environ. Sci. Pollut. Res. Int.* **2020**, *27*, 7672–7682. [CrossRef] [PubMed]
24. Moloudi, M.R.; Hassanzadeh, K.; Abdi, M.; Zandi, F.; Rahimi, K.; Izadpanah, E. Hepatoprotective effect of the hydroalcoholic extract of Cichorium intybus in a rat model of obstructive cholestasis. *Arab. J. Gastroenterol.* **2021**, *22*, 34–39. [CrossRef]
25. Keshk, W.A.; Soliman, N.A.; Ali, D.A.; Elseady, W.S. Mechanistic evaluation of AMPK/SIRT1/FXR signaling axis, inflammation, and redox status in thioacetamide induced liver cirrhosis: The role of *Cichorium intybus* linn (chicory)-supplemented diet. *J. Food Biochem.* **2019**, *43*, e12938. [CrossRef] [PubMed]
26. Alsahli, M.A.; Almatroodi, S.A.; Almatroudi, A.; Khan, A.A.; Anwar, S.; Almutary, A.G.; Alrumaihi, F.; Rahmani, A.H. 6-Gingerol, a Major Ingredient of Ginger Attenuates Diethylnitrosamine-Induced Liver Injury in Rats through the Modulation of Oxidative Stress and Anti-Inflammatory Activity. *Mediators Inflamm.* **2021**, *2021*, 6661937. [CrossRef]
27. Mironov, A.N. *Guidelines for Preclinical Studies of Drugs. Part 1*; Grif and K: Moscow, Russia, 2012; pp. 80–93.
28. Iqbal, Y.; Ponnampalam, E.N.; Suleria, H.A.R.; Cottrell, J.J.; Dunshea, F.R. LC-ESI/QTOF-MS Profiling of Chicory and Lucerne Polyphenols and Their Antioxidant Activities. *Antioxidants* **2021**, *10*, 932. [CrossRef] [PubMed]
29. Alkandahri, M.Y.; Pamungkas, B.T.; Oktoba, Z.; Shafirany, M.Z.; Sulastri, L.; Arfania, M.; Anggraeny, E.N.; Pratiwi, A.; Astuti, F.D.; Indriyani; et al. Hepatoprotective Effect of Kaempferol: A Review of the Dietary Sources, Bioavailability, Mechanisms of Action, and Safety. *Adv. Pharmacol. Pharm. Sci.* **2023**, *2023*, 1387665. [CrossRef]
30. Mahdi, T.; Hossein, A. Changes in Kaempferol content of Chicory (*Cichorium intybus* L.) under water deficit stresses and planting densities. *J. Med. Plants Res.* **2014**, *8*, 30–35. [CrossRef]
31. Inazu, A.; Brown, M.L.; Hesler, C.B.; Agellon, L.B.; Koizumi, J.; Takata, K.; Maruhama, Y.; Mabuchi, H.; Tall, A.R. Increased high-density lipoprotein levels caused by a common cholesteryl-ester transfer protein gene mutation. *N. Engl. J. Med.* **1990**, *323*, 1234–1238. [CrossRef]

32. Pedrelli, M.; Pramfalk, C.; Parini, P. Thyroid hormones and thyroid hormone receptors: Effects of thyromimetics on reverse cholesterol transport. *World J. Gastroenterol.* **2010**, *16*, 5958–5964. [CrossRef] [PubMed]
33. Gullberg, H.; Rudling, M.; Forrest, D.; Angelin, B.; Vennström, B. Thyroid hormone receptor beta-deficient mice show complete loss of the normal cholesterol 7alpha-hydroxylase (CYP7A) response to thyroid hormone but display enhanced resistance to dietary cholesterol. *Mol. Endocrinol.* **2000**, *14*, 1739–1749. [CrossRef]
34. Keshk, W.A.; Noeman, S.A. Impact of Chicory-Supplemented Diet on HMG-CoA Reductase, Acetyl-CoA Carboxylase, Visfatin and Antioxidant Status in Triton WR-1339-Induced Hyperlipidemia. *J. Food Biochem.* **2015**, *39*, 164–172. [CrossRef]
35. AbouZid, S.F.; Ahmed, O.M.; Ahmed, R.R.; Mahmoud, A.; Abdella, E.; Ashour, M.B. Antihyperglycemic effect of crude extracts of some Egyptian plants and algae. *J. Med. Food* **2014**, *17*, 400–406. [CrossRef]
36. Jurgoński, A.; Juśkiewicz, J.; Zduńczyk, Z.; Król, B. Caffeoylquinic acid-rich extract from chicory seeds improves glycemia, atherogenic index, and antioxidant status in rats. *Nutrition* **2012**, *28*, 300–306. [CrossRef]
37. Tsalamandris, S.; Antonopoulos, A.S.; Oikonomou, E.; Papamikroulis, G.A.; Vogiatzi, G.; Papaioannou, S.; Deftereos, S.; Tousoulis, D. The Role of Inflammation in Diabetes: Current Concepts and Future Perspectives. *Eur. Cardiol.* **2019**, *14*, 50–59. [CrossRef]
38. Shim, D.W.; Han, J.W.; Ji, Y.E.; Shin, W.Y.; Koppula, S.; Kim, M.K.; Kim, T.K.; Park, P.J.; Kang, T.B.; Lee, K.H. Cichorium intybus Linn. Extract Prevents Type 2 Diabetes Through Inhibition of NLRP3 Inflammasome Activation. *J. Med. Food* **2016**, *19*, 310–317. [CrossRef]
39. Jackson, K.M.P.; Rathinasabapathy, T.; Esposito, D.; Komarnytsky, S. Structural constraints and importance of caffeic acid moiety for anti-hyperglycemic effects of caffeoylquinic acids from chicory. *Mol. Nutr. Food Res.* **2017**, *61*, 1601118. [CrossRef]
40. Bokarev, I.N. The metabolic syndrome. *Klin. Med.* **2014**, *92*, 71–76.
41. Pouille, C.L.; Ouaza, S.; Roels, E.; Behra, J.; Tourret, M.; Molinié, R.; Fontaine, J.-X.; Mathiron, D.; Gagneul, D.; Taminiau, B.; et al. Chicory: Understanding the Effects and Effectors of This Functional Food. *Nutrients* **2022**, *14*, 957. [CrossRef] [PubMed]
42. Clifford, M.N.; Johnston, K.L.; Knight, S.; Kuhnert, N. Hierarchical scheme for LC-MSn identification of chlorogenic acids. *J. Agric. Food Chem.* **2003**, *51*, 2900–2911. [CrossRef] [PubMed]
43. Wang, N.; Li, R.; Feng, B.; Cheng, Y.; Guo, Y.; Qian, H. Chicoric Acid Prevents Neuroinflammation and Neurodegeneration in a Mouse Parkinson's Disease Model: Immune Response and Transcriptome Profile of the Spleen and Colon. *Int. J. Mol. Sci.* **2022**, *23*, 2031. [CrossRef] [PubMed]
44. Ding, X.-Q.; Jian, T.-Y.; Gai, Y.-N.; Niu, G.-T.; Liu, Y.; Meng, X.-H.; Li, J.; Lyu, H.; Ren, B.-R.; Chen, J. Chicoric Acid Attenuated Renal Tubular Injury in HFD-Induced Chronic Kidney Disease Mice through the Promotion of Mitophagy via the Nrf2/PINK/Parkin Pathway. *J. Agric. Food Chem.* **2022**, *70*, 2923–2935. [CrossRef] [PubMed]
45. All-Russian Research Institute of Medicinal and Aromatic Plants. *Wild Medicinal Plants in Russia: Collection, Drying, Preparation of Raw Materials (Collection, Drying, Preparation of Raw Materials)*; FGBNU All-Russian Research Institute of Medicinal and Aromatic Plants (FGBNU VILAR): Moscow, Russia, 2015; Volume 344.
46. Medicinal Plant Specialist Group Species Survival Commission IUCN—The World Conservation Union. International Standard for Sustainable Wild Collection of Medicinal and Aromatic Plants (ISSC-MAP). Available online: https://static1.squarespace.com/static/5bec424b297114f64cb908d8/t/6256dca1510d52627bf4bda3/1649859747671/ISSC-MAP_Version1_0.pdf (accessed on 12 April 2023).
47. Chawech, R.; Pesnel, S.; Haddada, M.B.; Gauvin-Bialecki, A.; Morel, A.L. Polyphenol Characterization of the Aqueous Extract from *Hubertia ambavilla* L. (Asteraceae) by HPLC-DAD-ESI-MS(n) and Assessment of Its Antioxidant Activity. *Chem. Biodivers.* **2022**, *19*, e202200217. [CrossRef]
48. European Convention for the Protection of Vertebrate Animals Used for Experimental and Other Scientific Purposes (ETS 123). Strasbourg. 1986. Available online: https://rm.coe.int/168007a67b (accessed on 31 March 2023).
49. Boivin, G.P.; Hickman, D.L.; Creamer-Hente, M.A.; Pritchett-Corning, K.R.; Bratcher, N.A. Review of CO_2 as a Euthanasia Agent for Laboratory Rats and Mice. *J. Am. Assoc. Lab. Anim. Sci.* **2017**, *56*, 491–499.
50. Dobyan, D.C.; Bulger, R.E. Partial protection by chlorpromazine in mercuric chloride-induced acute renal failure in rats. *Lab. Invest.* **1984**, *50*, 578–586. [PubMed]
51. Khodko, S.V.; Makarova, M.N.; Selezneva, A.I.; Saveliev, S.A.; Makarov, V.G.; Malinin, V.V. Effectiveness and mechanisms of action of Lys-Glu-Trp peptide on the model of hyperlipidemia caused by administration of Tween-80. *Atheroscler. Dyslipidemia* **2016**, *1*, 40–47.
52. Polyakov, L.M.; Lushnikova, E.L.; Nepomnyashikh, L.M.; Russkikh, G.S.; Pichugin, V.I.; Yujik, E.I. Indicators of lipid metabolism and protein composition of blood plasma lipoproteins in hypothyroid rats with experimental hypercholesterolemia. *Fundam. Res.* **2014**, *10*, 342–345.

pharmaceuticals

MDPI

Article

Quality, Safety and Biological Studies on *Campylanthus glaber* Aerial Parts

Katelene Lima [1], Maryam Malmir [1], Sérgio P. Camões [1], Kamrul Hasan [1], Samuel Gomes [2], Isabel Moreira da Silva [1], Maria Eduardo Figueira [1], Joana P. Miranda [1], Rita Serrano [1], Maria Paula Duarte [3] and Olga Silva [1,*]

[1] Research Institute for Medicines (iMed.ULisboa), Faculty of Pharmacy, Universidade de Lisboa, 1649-003 Lisbon, Portugal; k.lima@edu.ulisboa.pt (K.L.); m.malmir@edu.ulisboa.pt (M.M.); sergiocamoes@edu.ulisboa.pt (S.P.C.); mdkamrul@edu.ulisboa.pt (K.H.); icsilva@ff.ulisboa.pt (I.M.d.S.); efigueira@ff.ulisboa.pt (M.E.F.); jmiranda@ff.ulisboa.pt (J.P.M.); rserrano@edu.ulisboa.pt (R.S.)

[2] Instituto Nacional de Investigação e Desenvolvimento Agrário (INIDA), São Jorge dos Orgãos, Santiago CP 84, Cabo Verde; samuel.gomes@inida.gov.cv

[3] The Mechanical Engineering and Resource Sustainability Center (MEtRICs), Nova School of Science and Technology, Universidade Nova de Lisboa, 2829-516 Caparica, Portugal; mpcd@fct.unl.pt

* Correspondence: osilva@edu.ulisboa.pt; Tel.: +35-12-1794-6400

Abstract: In Cabo Verde, several endemic species are used in traditional medicine. However, no scientific studies have been conducted on the quality, efficacy, and safety of most of these plants. This study focused on establishing the botanical and chemical identification parameters required for a quality monograph of *Campylanthus glaber* Benth. aerial parts, a medicinal plant of Cabo Verde traditionally used to treat fever and muscular pain. In addition, in vitro antioxidant and antihyperglycemic activity, cytotoxicity, and genotoxicity were assessed for this medicinal plant. Optical microscopy, LC/UV-DAD-ESI/MS, and colorimetric assays were used for botanical, chemical, and biological studies, respectively. Cytotoxicity was assessed by the MTT assay with HepG2 cells, and genotoxicity by the Ames test. Microscopically, the xeromorphic leaf of *C. glaber* presents a thick cuticle (13.6–25.5 μm), thick-walled epidermal cells, anomocytic-type stomata, glandular trichomes (stalk length = 49.4–120.8 μm), and idioblasts containing calcium oxalate microcrystals. The chemical screening of aqueous and hydroethanolic extracts of this medicinal plant revealed the presence of organic acids, iridoids, phenylethanoids, and flavonoids as the main classes of marker compounds, with malic acid, citric acid, and verbascoside being the main marker compounds identified. Both extracts showed similar LC/UV-DAD/ESI-MS qualitative profiles and DPPH radical scavenger activity (IC_{50} = 130.9 ± 1.4; 134.3 ± 3.1 μg/mL). The hydroethanolic extract inhibited both α-amylase and α-glucosidase enzymes in a dose-dependent manner. Both extracts showed no cytotoxicity (up to 1000 μg/mL) by the MTT assay and no genotoxic potential with or without metabolic activation up to 5 mg /plate. The results obtained are an important contribution to the monographic quality assessment of *C. glaber* aerial parts and suggest that this medicinal plant may be safe and potentially used as an herbal drug raw material for pharmaceutical purposes.

Keywords: antioxidant; antihyperglycemic; *Campylanthus glaber*; herbal drug; herbal medicine; quality control; safety; verbascoside

Citation: Lima, K.; Malmir, M.; Camões, S.P.; Hasan, K.; Gomes, S.; Moreira da Silva, I.; Figueira, M.E.; Miranda, J.P.; Serrano, R.; Duarte, M.P.; et al. Quality, Safety and Biological Studies on *Campylanthus glaber* Aerial Parts. *Pharmaceuticals* **2023**, *16*, 1373. https://doi.org/10.3390/ph16101373

Academic Editors: Elena Y. Enioutina, Kathleen M. Job and Catherine Sherwin

Received: 9 September 2023
Revised: 22 September 2023
Accepted: 24 September 2023
Published: 28 September 2023

1. Introduction

Campylanthus glaber Benth. is a species endemic to the Cabo Verde archipelago that belongs to *Plantaginaceae* Juss., a highly heteromorphic family containing 107 genera and around 2000 species [1]. The genus *Campylanthus* Roth was taxonomically controversial for several years and was for a long time included in the family *Scrophulariaceae* Juss. and in the tribes *Digitaleae* and *Veroniceae* [2]. However, after molecular phylogenetic analysis, the genus was identified as related to *Globularia* Tourn ex L. and included in the *Plantaginaceae* family [3].

The genus *Campylanthus* includes 18 species with a wide distribution; 16 species occur from northeast Africa to southern Arabia and Pakistan, and the two other species (*Campylanthus salsaloides* (L.f.) Roth and *Campylanthus glaber*) are restricted to Macaronesia (Canary Islands and Cabo Verde Islands, respectively) [3,4]. In Cabo Verde, the species is distributed across the islands of Santo Antão, São Vicente, São Nicolau, Brava, Fogo, and Santiago, where it grows on cliffs and rocky and sandy slopes [4,5].

Campylanthus glaber (Figure 1) is a shrub that is moderately branched, decumbent, or ascending to erect and grows up to 1 m high. The branches are puberulent to hirsute and leafy, with persistent leaf bases in older parts. The leaves are linear and narrowly oblong to spathulate, 2–5 cm long and 0.1–0.9 cm wide, more or less succulent, glabrous to hirsute, with apex acute to obtuse, and entire margin [5].

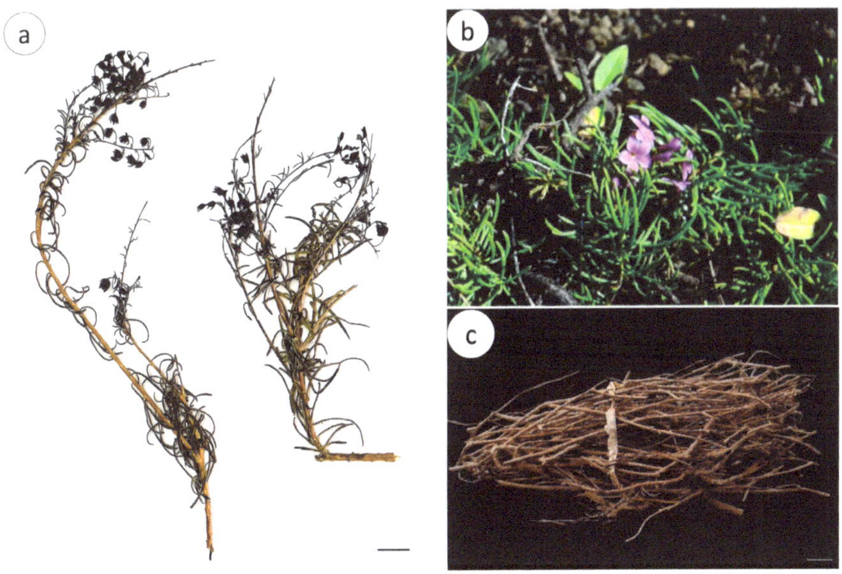

Figure 1. Macroscopic characteristics of *Campylanthus glaber* aerial parts; (**a**) *C. glaber* dried aerial parts; (**b**) *C. glaber* flowering branch; (**c**) Bunch of dried aerial parts of *C. glaber* (alecrim-bravo) sold in Santiago Island market (Praia market); scale bars: 1 cm. Photographies by Katelene Lima (**a**,**b**) and Maria Cristina Duarte (**c**).

According to Plants of the World Online, *Campylanthus glaber* is the currently accepted name for this species. *Campylanthus glaber* is a highly variable species, and for this reason, several morphologically different populations of this species were frequently described as distinct species, subspecies, and varieties. However, they are currently recognized as synonyms. Nowadays, *Campylanthus benthamii* Webb, *Campylanthus benthamii* var. *glaber* (Benth.) Webb, *Campylanthus benthamii* var. *hirsutus* Webb, *Campylanthus glaber var. puberulus Cout.*, *Campylanthus glaber var. pumilus Pett.*, *Campylanthus glaber* subsp. *spathulatus* (A.Chev.) Brochmann, N.Kilian, Lobin & Rustan., and *Campylanthus spathulatus* A.Chev. are considered homotypic and heterotypic synonyms of *C. glaber* [1].

C. glaber's chemical composition is sparsely studied. Ronsted and Jensen (2002) [2] analyzed fresh aerial parts of *C. glaber* ethanolic extracts and identified, by NMR and comparison with literature data, two main classes of compounds: iridoid glucosides (aucubin, erigeroside, gardoside, monomellithoside, melittoside, geniposidic acid, and 8-epilogonic acid) and caffeoyl phenylethanoid glycosides (salidroside and lavandulifolioside). In

Campylanthus salsaloides, fresh aerial parts ethanolic extract similar compounds (erigeroside, aucubin, gardoside, monomellithoside, geniposidic acid, lavandulifolioside), were identified in addition to mussaenosidic acid, mannitol, and sorbitol, [2].

Aerial parts of *C. glaber*, commonly known as "alecrim-brabo", are used in Cabo Verde to treat muscular pain [6], headache and menstrual problems [7], fever, flu, and congestion [8], and the whole plant is also used as food, animal feed (pasture), and wood fuel [8].

The estimated percentage of the African population's reliance on traditional forms of medicine to satisfy their healthcare needs is still extremely high [9]. In Cabo Verde, traditional medicine plays an important role in the health system of the country since rural communities still have limited access to conventional medicine [10,11].

While in Africa traditional medicines and herbal medicines continue to be widely used, the world is gradually turning back to herbal medicines to treat multiple diseases and ailments with more affordable costs and a greater degree of safety (less side effects) compared to conventional drugs [12].

Plants are an extensive source of natural products [13] with broad pharmacological potential [14]. Over millions of years, plant secondary metabolites have evolved and acquired a unique chemical diversity, which subsequently led to a variety of biological activities and drug-like properties [15]. Therefore, even after all the advances in drug development and the globalization of modern medicine, plants and herbal medicines continue to be one of the most important raw materials for medicines and continue to play a central role in healthcare systems around the world [16].

C. glaber is listed as an endangered (EN) species on the International Union for the Conservation of Nature's (IUCN) Red List of Threatened Species and is likely to be critically endangered. The species is included in the protected areas [17,18]. However, more strategies for its conservation are of crucial importance. The cultivation and valorization of medicinal plants as raw materials for pharmaceuticals [19] are some strategies that could be explored. Hence, with the present study, we aimed to obtain quality, efficacy, and safety data on *C. glaber* aerial parts, useful to allow its appropriate use as an herbal medicine according to official monographic quality parameters for herbal products.

2. Results

2.1. Botanical Quality Monographic Studies

2.1.1. Macroscopic Characterization

C. glaber dried aerial parts (Figure 1a–c) are characterized by the presence of dried and fragmented leaves and stems with variable lengths.

Macroscopically, the *C. glaber* stem is dark brown, cylindrical, decumbent to erect, moderately branched, with longitudinal striation, alternate nodes, and rarely hirsute branch nodes (Figure 2a). The *C. glaber* stem presents three distinct regions: the periderm, cork, and vascular cylinder (Figure 2b). The dried leaf is dark brown, linear to narrowly obovate, 1–5 cm long and 3–10 mm wide, with an acute apex, tubular base, revolute margin forming a longitudinal groove covered by trichomes (Figure 2c,d), and an indistinct venation pattern.

2.1.2. Microscopic Characterization

A microscopy examination of the *C. glaber* stem, leaf, and aerial parts powdered drug was carried out by light optical microscopy. The quantitative analysis of the different anatomical features identified in both the leaf and stem is presented in Table 1.

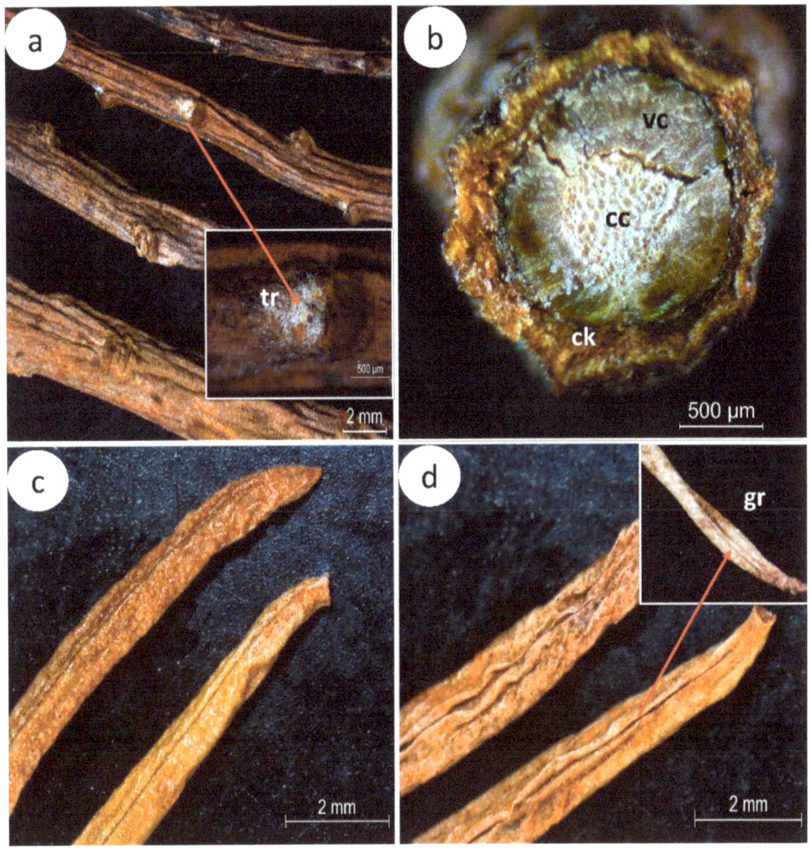

Figure 2. Macroscopic characteristics of *Campylanthus glaber*, aerial parts: (**a**) general aspect of the stem branches with the presence of trichomes (arrow) in the younger branch nodes; (**b**) cross-section section of the stem branch with details of the cork region and vascular cylinder; (**c**) leaf abaxial view; (**d**) leaf adaxial view with detail of groove (arrow) formed by revolute margin covered by trichomes. Abbreviations: cc: central cylinder; ck: cork; vc: vascular cylinder; tr: trichomes.

Table 1. Quantitative anatomical features of the *C. glaber* stem and leaf.

Anatomical Parameters	Min–Max	Mean	±SD
	Stem		
Cork (no. of cell layers)	3–7	4	1
Sclereid cell wall thickness (µm)	3.3–10.2	6.8	2.1
Xylem vessel area (µm^2)	82.1–324.1	208	74
Central cylinder cell area (µm^2)	770.9–4340.5	2304	1024
	Leaf		
Cuticule thickness (µm)	13.7–25.6	19.2	3.3
Pallissade parenchyma thickness (µm)	154–323	254.7	34.2
Epidermal cell length (µm)	22.1–55.4	36.4	7.9
Epidermal cell width (µm)	13.6–38.5	24.8	5.8
Stomata length (µm)	31.3–46.6	38.4	3.8
Stomata width (µm)	25.9–38.6	32.4	3.2
Stomata index	-	4.3	1.2

Table 1. *Cont.*

Anatomical Parameters	Min–Max	Mean	±SD
Idioblast area (μm^2)	73.1–96.8	88.7	6.5
Thrichome stalk length (μm)	49.4–120.7	77.1	16.6

Max: maximum; Min: minimum; SD: standard deviation.

Stem

In cross-sections, the stem shows a typically cylindrical format (Figures 2b and 3a), organized into the periderm, cork, and vascular cylinder (Figure 3a) from outside to inside. In the periderm, the phellem region of about 4–7 rows of quadrangular-shape cork cells (Figure 3b, Table 1), followed by a parenchyma region (Figure 3a), is below a one-layer epidermis covered with a striate cuticle. The cortex region is characterized by the presence of a circular layer of grouped sclereids (sclerenchyma) with thick walls (3.28–10.17 μm) (Figure 3a–c, Table 1) surrounding the vascular cylinder, mainly occupied by a broad xylem with 2–8 rows of vessels (82.1–324.1 μm^2) (Figure 3a–e, Table 1), a narrow phloem (Figure 3a–d), and a central cylinder with large (770.9–4340.5 μm^2) thick-walled cells (Figure 3f, Table 1). Few trichomes were observed; however, they are rarely present (Figure 3g).

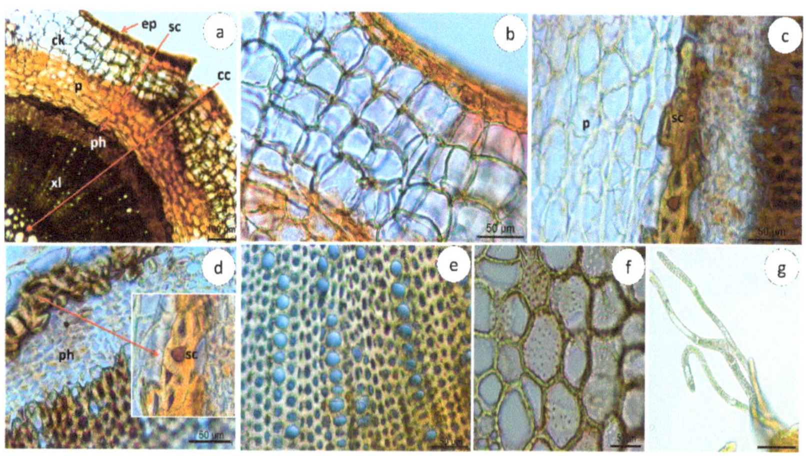

Figure 3. Microscopic characteristics of the *Campylanthus glaber* stem cross-section. (**a**) General aspect of the epidermis (arrow (ep)), cork, parenchyma, sclerenchyma (arrow (sc)), phloem, xylem, and central cylinder (arow(cc)) (from outside to inside). Details of (**b**) cork with four layers of quadrangular-shape cells; (**c**) parenchyma and groups of sclereids; (**d**) groups of sclereids forming a ring around the phloem; (**e**) xylem vessels organized in 2–8 cells; (**f**) central cylinder large thick-walled cells; (**g**) trichomes located in the epidermis. Abbreviations: cc: central cylinder; ck: cork; ep: epidermis; p: parenchyma; ph: phloem; sc: sclereids; xl: xylem. Scale bars: (**a**) = 100 μm; (**b–g**) = 50 μm.

Leaf

C. glaber leaf shows a circular shape in cross-section, with revolute margins forming a longitudinal groove over the upper surface. The leaf is characterized as monofacial since the epidermis consists of one single layer of epidermis covered by a thick striated cuticle (13.7–25.6 μm) (Table 1), continuous from the upper to the lower surface (Figure 4a). Stomata inserted around the cylindrical mesophyll and glandular trichomes (Figure 4a,b), restricted to the groove formed by the leaf revolute margins, were observed.

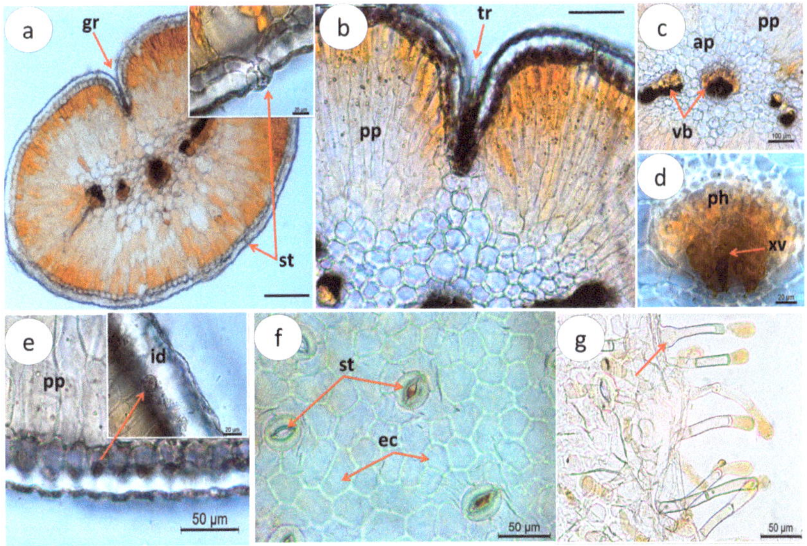

Figure 4. Microscopic characteristics of *Campylanthus glaber* leaf. (**a**) Cross-section of the midrib showing the cylindrical mesophyll with detail of stomata (arrow (st)) and groove (arrow (gr)); (**b**) detail of trichome (arrow) located in the groove formed by the curved margins and palisade parenchyma; (**c**) vascular bundles (arrows) embedded in the aquifer parenchyma; (**d**) xylem vessels (arrow) and phloem; (**e**) idioblasts (arrow) with calcium oxalate microcrystals; (**f**) epidermal cells (arrows (ep)) and anomocytic-type stomata (arrows (st)); (**g**) trichomes located on the leaf margins with detail of trichomes with swollen base (arrow). Abbreviations: ap: aquifer parenchyma; ec: epidermal cells; gr: groove; id: idioblast; pp: palisade parenchyma; ph: phloem; st: stomata; vb: vascular bundle; xv: xylem vessel. Scale bars: (**a**) = 200 µm; (**b**,**c**) = 100 µm; (**d**) = 20 µm; (**e**–**g**) = 50 µm.

C. glaber cylindrical mesophyll is differentiated into a strongly developed layer of palisade parenchyma organized in a tightly packed thick multilayer (154–323µm) of 3–5 columnar cells arranged perpendicularly pointing towards the center (Figure 4a,b, Table 1) and water-storage parenchyma (aquifer parenchyma), consisting of 3–4 layers of large, thick-walled cells located in the central part of the mesophyll (Figure 4c).

The leaf vascularization pattern, observed after a cross-section, revealed the presence of a large central bundle and a variable number of small lateral vascular bundles embedded in the aquifer parenchyma (Figure 4c). The xylem, organized in rows of 2–4 vessels (Figure 4d), is oriented towards the upper surface, with angular collenchyma occurring around the largest bundle (Figure 4d). Calcium oxalate microcrystals (sands) grouped in idioblasts dispersed in the epidermis were also observed (Figure 4e).

Paradermal sections revealed rectangular to polygonal epidermis cells with variable length (22.1–55.4 µm), anomocytic-type stomata (subsidiary cells like epidermal cells) (Figure 4f), and multicellular, uniseriate capitate glandular trichomes, constituted by a bicellular to multicellular pedicel with one or two cells and a unicellular secretory head. The trichomes distinctively swollen bases were also observed (Figure 4g).

Powdered Herbal Drug

The powder drug is dark brown and is characterized by the presence of typical structures of both leaf and stem. The most common structures observed are isolated anomocytic stomata, idioblasts with microcrystals, sclereids, fragmented leaf epidermal cells with stomata and clustered crystals, glandular (Figure 5a) and protective trichomes (Figure 5b), pitted vessels (Figure 5c), and the stem central cylinder (Figure 5d).

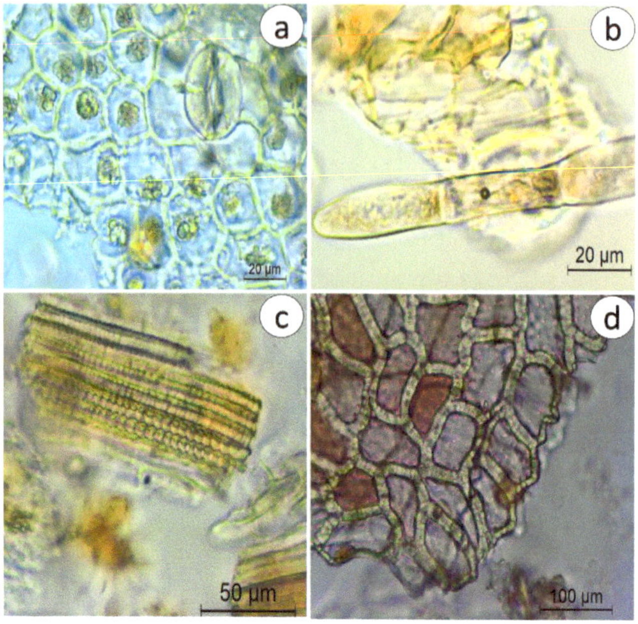

Figure 5. Microscopic characteristics of *C. glaber* aerial part powder. (**a**) Fragmented leaf epidermal cells with stomata and idioblasts with microcrystals; (**b**) protective trichome; (**c**) fragment of pitted vessels; (**d**) fragment of the stem central cylinder.

2.2. *Chemical Characterization*

2.2.1. Drug–Extract Ratio

The drug–water extract (CgAE) ratio was 4.39:1 and the drug-70% ethanol extract (CgEE) ratio was 2.89:1. The yield for CgAE was found to be 22.75% and 34.48% for CgEE.

2.2.2. LC-UV/DAD Fingerprinting

The liquid chromatography coupled with ultraviolet photodiode array (LC-UV/DAD) profiles obtained for CgAE and CgEE are presented in Figure 6. Observation of the chromatographic characteristics (UV spectra and retention times) permitted the tentative identification of the 16 major peaks as organic acids (Figure 6a,b), iridoid glucosides (Figure 6c–e,g), caffeoyl phenylethanoids glycosides (Figure 6f,j–p), flavonoids (Figure 6h,k) and an unknown compound (Figure 6i).

2.2.3. LC-UV-ESI/MS-MS Chemical Profile

The identity of the main marker compounds detected in *C. glaber* extracts was tentatively made through the comparison of retention times (t_r), maximum wavelengths (λ_{max}), pseudo-molecular ion ([M-H], and corresponding fragment ions (MSn) with those of reference standards and of published literature data (Table 2).

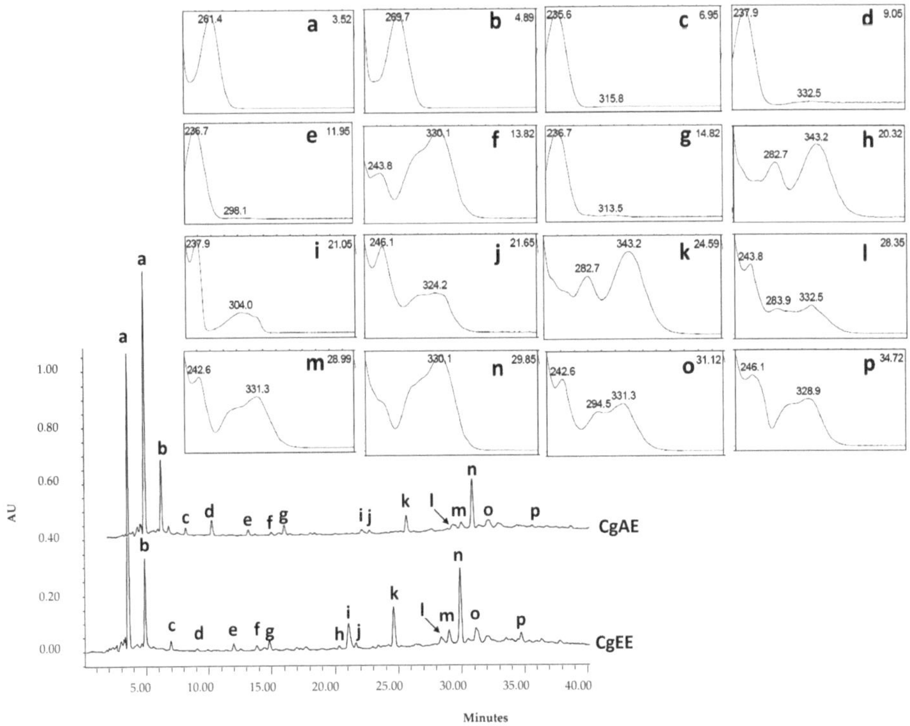

Figure 6. LC/UV-DAD profile of CgAE and CgE with UV spectra and retention times of the main marker classes of compounds identified: organic acids (peaks (**a**,**b**)), iridoid glucosides (peaks (**c**–**e**,**g**)), caffeoyl phenylethanoids glycosides ((**f**,**j**,**l**–**p**)) flavonoids (peaks (**h**,**k**)), and an unknown compound (**i**). Abbreviations: CgAE: *Campylanthus glaber* aqueous extract; CgEE: *Campylanthus glaber* ethanolic extract.

Table 2. HPLC-UV-ESI/MS-MS identification of *C. glaber* aerial parts main marker compounds.

Peak	t_r (min)	UVλ_{max} (nm)	[M-H]$^-$	MS-MS Fragment Ions *m/z* (Relative Abundance)	Proposed Compound	Class
a	3.52	261	133	133 (88); 115 (100); 71(40); 73 (18)	Malic acid	Organic acid
b	4.89	269	191	191(45); 111(100); 87(38); 85 (27)	Citric acid	Organic acid
c	6.95	234	373	123 (100); 193(75); 149 (48)	Gardoside	Iridoid
d	9.05	238	373	123 (100); 149 (80)	Geniposidic acid *	Iridoid
e	11.95	235	375	169 (100); 89 (65); 151 (59); 213(50)	8-Epiloganic acid	Iridoid
f	13.82	244; 330	487	179 (100); 135(13); 161 (12); 341 (5)	Cistanoside derivative	Phenylethanoid glycoside
g	14.82	236	451	243(100); 101(50)	Iridoid derivative	Iridoid
h	20.32	283; 343	667	351 (100); 113 (12)	Unknown	Flavonoid
i	21.05	238; 304	453	89 (100); 159 (90)	Unknown	Unknown
j	21.65	246; 283sh; 324	639	639 (100); 621(33); 161(26); 179 (23); 451 (22)	β-Hydroxyverbascoside isomer	Phenylethanoid glycoside
k	24.59	283; 343	667	351 (100); 315 (28); 113 (25)	Unknown	Flavonoid
l	28.35	244; 284sh; 332	637	637 (100); 251 (70); 62(63); 623 (25)	Unknown	Phenylethanoid glycoside

Table 2. *Cont.*

Peak	t_r (min)	UVλ_{max} (nm)	[M-H]$^-$	MS-MS Fragment Ions *m/z* (Relative Abundance)	Proposed Compound	Class
m	28.99	331	755	755 (100); 161 (22); 593 (12)	Lavandulifolioside	Phenylethanoid glycoside
n	29.85	330	623	623 (100); 161 (28); 461 (12); 135 (3)	Verbascoside	Phenylethanoid glycoside
o	31.12	331	623	623 (100); 161 (28); 461 (12); 135 (3)	*cis*-Verbascoside	Phenylethanoid glycoside
p	34.72	328	623	623 (100); 161 (28); 461 (12); 135 (3)	Isoverbascoside	Phenylethanoid glycoside

* Identified with reference standard; [M-H]$^-$—negative mass electrospray ionization mode; MS/MS—mass spectrometry; m/z—mass-/charge ratio; t_r—retention time; UV λ_{max}—wavelength of maximum absorbance.

Peak **a** with λ_{max}: 261 nm, precursor ion [M-H]$^-$ at m/z 133, and characteristic fragment at m/z 115 corresponding to [M-H-H_2O]$^-$ was proposed as malic acid. Peak **b** with λ_{max}: 269 nm, precursor ion [M-H]$^-$ at m/z 191, and characteristic fragment at m/z 111 corresponding to [M-H-CO_2-2H_2O]$^-$ was proposed as citric acid [20,21].

The losses of H_2O (18 Da), CO_2 (44 Da), and glucosyl moiety (Glc,162 Da) were detected frequently in iridoids. Peak **c** with λ_{max}: 234 and peak **d** with λ_{max}: 238 and precursor ions [M-H]$^-$ at m/z 373 and characteristic fragment at m/z 149 corresponding to [M-Glc-CO_2-H_2O-H]$^-$ were proposed as gardoside and geniposidic acid, respectively [22,23]. The geniposidic acid identity was also confirmed by co-chromatography with a reference standard [22,23].

Peak **e** with λ_{max}: 235, precursor ion [M-H]$^-$ at m/z 375 and characteristic fragment at m/z 169 and m/z 151 corresponding to [M-Glc-CO_2-H]$^-$ and [M-Glc-CO_2-H_2O-H]$^-$, respectively, was proposed as 8-epiloganic acid [23,24].

In phenylethanoid glycosides, the frequent neutral losses are rhamnose (162 Da) and caffeoyl moiety (146 Da). In addition, fragments at m/z 179 and 161 are also detected frequently, as they are produced by caffeic acid and glucose. Peak **f** with a λ_{max}: 244, 330; precursor ion [M-H]$^-$ at 487; and characteristic fragment at m/z 341 corresponding to [M-caff-H]$^-$ was proposed as a cistanoside isomer.

Peak **j** with λ_{max}: 246, 283sh, 324 nm; precursor ion [M-H]$^-$ at m/z 639; and characteristic fragment at m/z 621, corresponding to [M-H-H_2O]$^-$ and the fragments m/z 161 and 179, belonging to the caffeoyl moiety, were proposed as a β-hydroxyverbascoside isomer.

Peak **m** with λ_{max}: 330, precursor ion [M-H]$^-$ at m/z 755, and characteristic fragment at m/z 593, corresponding to [M-H-rhamnose]$^-$, was proposed as lavandulifolioside [25].

Peaks **n**, **o**, and **p** with a λ_{max}: 330, 331, and 328 nm, respectively; precursor ion [M-H]$^-$ at m/z 623; characteristic fragment at m/z 461, corresponding to [M-H-Glc]$^-$; and the fragments m/z 161 and 135 belonging to the caffeoyl moiety were proposed as verbascoside, *cis*-verbascoside, and isoverbascoside, respectively [23,26].

Additionally, three other iridoid glucosides, with precursor ions [M-H]$^-$ at m/z 361, 345, and 523 and characteristic fragments at m/z 407, 391, and 593, respectively, corresponding to [M+HCOOH]$^-$ [23,27], were detected only by LC-UV-ESI/MS-MS. These compounds were proposed as melitoside, aucubin, and monomelitoside, respectively. Aucubin's identity was also confirmed by co-chromatography with an authentic reference standard.

2.2.4. Quantification of Secondary Metabolites

The results of the total polyphenolic content (TPC), total flavonoid content (TFC), and total iridoid content (TIC) of CgAE and CgEE are presented in Table 3. CgEE exhibited a higher content of TPC (148.1$\pm$ 9.5 mg GAE/g) and TFC (75.8 $\pm$ 0.2 CE/g) when compared to CgAE (131.3 $\pm$ 3.9 mg GAE/g, 71.0 $\pm$ 0.6 CE/g, respectively). CgEE exhibited a slightly higher value of TIC compared to CgAE (6.1 $\pm$ 1.3 and 4.9 $\pm$ 0.6 mg Au/g, respectively), butHowever, with no statistical significance (p value: 0.1074).

Table 3. DER, total phenols, flavonoids, and iridoid contents of *C. glaber* aerial part extracts.

Plant Extracts	DER	TPC (mg GAE/g)	TFC (mg CE/g)	TIC (mg AuE/g)
CgAE	4.39:1	131.3 ^{b} ± 3.9	71.0 ^{b} ± 0.6	4.9 ^{a} ± 0.6
CgEE	2.89:1	148.1 ^{a} ± 9.5	75.8 ^{a} ± 0.2	6.1 ^{a} ± 1.3

CgAE: *Campylanthus glaber* aqueous extract; CgEE: *Campylanthus glaber* ethanolic extract; DER: drug–extract ratio; TPC: total polyphenolic content; TFC: total flavonoid content; TIC: total iridoid content; GAE: gallic acid equivalents; CE: catechin equivalents; AuE: aucubin equivalents. In each column, different letters denote significant differences ($p < 0.05$).

Overall, CgEE exhibited a higher yield, drug–extract ratio (DER), and higher content of the main classes of secondary metabolites quantified.

2.3. *In Vitro Biological Studies*

2.3.1. In Vitro Antioxidant Activity

The results of the evaluation of CgAE and CgEE antioxidant potential by the CUPRAC (cupric-reducing antioxidant capacity), FRAP (ferric-reducing antioxidant power), and DPPH (2,2-diphenyl-1-picrylhydrazyl) assays are presented in Table 4.

Table 4. CUPRAC, FRAP, and DPPH radical scavenging capacity of *C. glaber* aerial part extracts.

Samples	CUPRAC (µg AA/g)	FRAP (µg AA/g)	DPPH• IC_{50} (µg/mL)
CgAE	197.9 ^{b} ± 2.6	109.8 ^{a} ± 3.2	130.9 ^{a} ± 1.4
CgEE	203.8 ^{a} ± 1.8	104.0 ^{a} ± 3.9	134.3 ^{a} ± 3.1
Ascorbic acid	-	-	17.3 ± 0.3

CgAE: *Campylanthus glaber* aqueous extract; CgEE: *Campylanthus glaber* ethanolic extract; CUPRAC: cupric-reducing antioxidant capacity; FRAP: ferric-reducing antioxidant power; DPPH•: 2,2-diphenyl-1-picrylhydrazyl radical; AA: ascorbic acid; IC_{50}: half maximal inhibitory concentration. In each column, different letters denote significant differences ($p < 0.05$).

The obtained CUPRAC values ranged from 197.9 ± 2.6 to 203.8 ± 1.8 µg/g for both tested extracts, with CgEE presenting significantly (p value: 0.017) higher reducing ability than CgAE. For the FRAP assay, CgAE (109.8 ± 3.2 µg/g) displayed slightly higher reducing capacity than CgEE (104.0a ± 3.9 µg/g); however, there was no statistical significance (p value: 0.058).

Obtained results for the DPPH radical scavenge assay showed that CgE with an IC_{50} value of 134.3 ± 1.4 µg/mL and CgA with an IC_{50} value of 130.9 ± 3.1 µg/mL had similar antioxidant potential (p value: 0.092) but were lower when compared to ascorbic acid used as a reference standard (IC_{50} = 17.3 ± µg/mL). Both extracts showed DPPH radical-scavenging activity in a dose-dependent manner.

2.3.2. In Vitro Enzymatic Inhibition of Diabetes Type 2-Related Enzymes

The inhibitory activity of *C. glaber* aerial part extracts against α-amylase and α-glucosidase, two important enzymes related to the management of postprandial serum glucose levels in diabetes type 2, was investigated, and the results are depicted in Table 5.

Both CgAE and CgEE exhibited low inhibition activity against α-amylase (IC_{50}: 7.21 ± 0.23 and 5.77 ± 0.11 mg/mL, respectively) when compared to the positive control acarbose (IC_{50}: 0.011 ± 0.001 mg/mL). Regarding the α-glucosidase enzyme, only CgEE was able to inhibit this enzyme in the range of the tested concentrations. The inhibition potential (IC_{50}: 827.9 ± 11.2 µg/mL), however, was moderate when compared to the positive control, acarbose (IC_{50}: 350.3 ± 15.4 µg/mL). Both extracts inhibited the α-amylase enzyme in a concentration-dependent manner, while only the CgEE was able to inhibit the activity of the α-glucosidase enzyme.

Table 5. *C. glaber* aerial part extract inhibitory enzymatic activity against α-amylase and α-glucosidase enzymes.

Samples	α-Amylase IC_{50} (mg/mL)	α-Glucosidase IC_{50} (μg/mL)
CgAE	7.21 ^{c} ± 0.23	nd
CgEE	5.77 ^{b} ± 0.10	827.9 ^{b} ± 11.2
Acarbose	0.011 ^{a} ± 0.001	350.3 ^{a} ± 15.4

CgAE: *Campylanthus glaber* aqueous extract; CgEE: *Campylanthus glaber* ethanolic extract; IC_{50}: The half maximal inhibitory concentration. In each column different letters denote significant differences ($p < 0.05$); nd: not defined.

2.4. Safety Assessment

2.4.1. In Vitro Genotoxic/Mutagenic Potential

The genotoxic potential of CgAE and CgEE was evaluated by the Ames test. The criteria to consider a compound/substance mutagenic in the Ames test are the observation of a reproducible and significant increase (2–3 fold) in the number of revertant colonies per plate in at least one of the tester strains and a dose–response relationship between the concentrations evaluated [28–30].

Based on these criteria, the obtained results (Tables 6 and 7) showed that CgAE and CgEE do not exhibit mutagenic/genotoxic potential, since none of these extracts induced an increase in the number of revertant colonies when compared to the negative control for any of the tester strains (TA98, TA100, TA102, TA1535, and TA1537), neither in the absence (Table 6) nor in the presence of metabolic activation (Table 7) (assay performed only for CgEE given the chemical similarities outlined in the previous section). Negative control values were according to the historical control data. As expected, the positive controls were able to meet the criteria of increasing more than twofold the mutation frequency when compared with the negative controls. The cytotoxicity evaluated in terms of a decrease in bacterial lawn background, a significant reduction in the number of revertant colonies, and/or the presence of microcolonies was not observed for any of the extracts at any of the tested concentrations.

Table 6. Genotoxic potential of *C. glaber* aerial part extracted by the Ames test without metabolic activation.

CgAE (μg/Plate)	Revertant Colonies per Plate (Mean ± SD) without Metabolic Activation				
	TA98	TA100	TA102	TA1535	TA1537
0	26 ± 4	148 ± 6	361 ± 9	20 ± 4	28 ±5
250	26 ± 4	167 ± 20	358 ± 24	14 ± 1	31 ± 9
625	25 ± 6	166 ± 22	388 ± 17	16 ± 5	26 ± 6
1250	26 ± 2	154 ± 15	365 ± 20	22 ± 5	27 ± 6
2500	25 ± 2	162 ± 13	377 ± 19	16 ± 2	21 ± 1
3750	28 ± 2	170 ± 61	384 ± 21	20 ± 6	30 ± 2
5000	26 ± 2	178 ± 5	406 ± 35	14 ± 3	27 ± 8
CgEE	Revertant colonies per plate (mean ± SD) without metabolic activation				
(μg/plate)	TA98	TA100	TA102	TA1535	TA1537
0	26 ± 5	196 ± 5	344 ± 5	13 ± 3	25 ± 3
250	25 ± 5	179 ± 22	364 ± 5	14 ± 3	25 ± 3
625	25 ± 7	192 ± 22	361 ± 7	14 ± 1	28 ± 3
1250	26 ± 6	199 ± 6	347 ± 6	12 ± 1	26 ± 3
2500	29 ± 8	204 ± 8	391 ± 8	14 ± 3	21 ± 5
3750	28 ± 5	213 ± 22	388 ± 5	20 ± 7	25 ± 8
5000	30 ± 3	221 ± 6	388 ± 3	11 ± 1	24 ± 4
PC	(1) 488 ± 30 *	(2) 1048 ± 43 *	(3) 881 ± 26 *	(2) 827 ± 13 *	(4) 1354 ± 5 *

CgAE: *Campylanthus glaber* aqueous extract; CgEE: *Campylanthus glaber* ethanolic extract; PC (positive control); SD (standard deviation); (1)—2-nitrofluorene; (2)—sodium azide; (3)—*tert*-butyl hydroperoxide; (4)—9-aminoacridine. * These values are similar to those obtained by Malmir et al. (2023) [31] and Malu et al. (2022) [32], since this study was performed simultaneously.

Table 7. Genotoxic potential of CgEE tested with *Salmonella* Typhimurium strains TA98, TA100, TA102, TA1535, and 1537 with metabolic activation.

CgEE (µg/Plate)	Revertant Colonies per Plate (Mean ± SD) with Metabolic Activation				
	TA98	**TA100**	**TA102**	**TA1535**	**TA1537**
0	47 ± 4	157 ± 6	172 ± 2	11 ± 2	12 ± 1
625	61 ± 7	146 ± 7	180 ± 35	12 ± 2	16 ± 3
1250	65 ± 4	167 ± 18	200 ± 11	16 ± 1	14 ± 3
2500	50 ± 6	175 ± 16	205 ± 3	16 ± 1	15 ± 2
5000	37 ± 3	162 ± 3	180 ± 35	12 ± 1	15 ± 4
PC	(1) 832 ± 35 *	(2) 947 ± 148 *	(1) 732 ± 12 *	(1) 266 ± 1 *	(1) 306 ± 50 *

CgAE: *Campylanthus glaber* aqueous extract; CgEE: *Campylanthus glaber* ethanolic extract; PC (positive control); SD (standard deviation); (1)—2-aminoanthracene; (2)—benzo(a)pyrene. * These values are similar to those obtained by Malmir et al. (2023) [31] and Malu et al. (2022) [32], since this study was performed simultaneously.

2.4.2. In Vitro Assessment of Cytotoxicity

The cytotoxicity of the *C. glaber* aerial part extracts was evaluated by the methylthiazolyldiphenyl-tetrazolium bromide (MTT) assay on HepG2 (a human liver cell line). Results expressed as cell viability percentage data are presented in Figure 7.

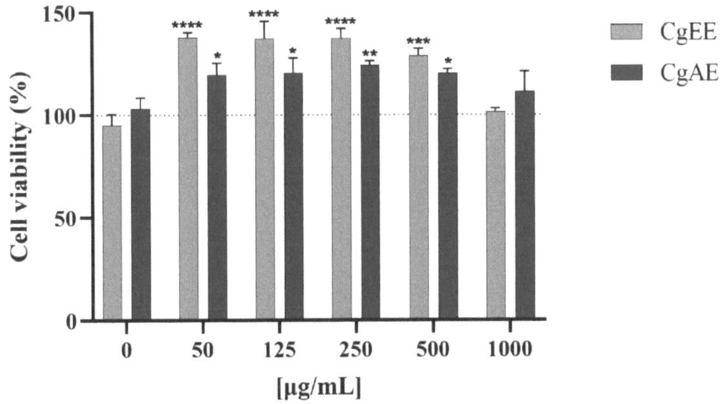

Figure 7. Viability of HepG2 after incubation (48 h) with CgAE and CgEE extracts assessed by MTT reduction assay. Data arpresented as percentage of solvent control (dashed line) and mean ± standard deviation; n = 2–3. * $p < 0.05$; ** $p < 0.01$; *** $p < 0.001$; **** $p < 0.0001$.

Neither CgAE nor CgEE cause cell death at any of the concentrations tested (50, 125, 250, 500, and 1000 µg/mL). On the other hand, an increase in the viability/proliferation of HepG2 was observed for both extracts at concentrations up to 1000 µg/mL when compared to the negative control (0 µg/mL). CgAE induced up to an approximately 24% increase in cell viability/proliferation, while CgEE induced an approximately 37% increase in viability/proliferation.

3. Discussion

There is an increasing demand for medicinal plants used as herbal drugs in traditional medicine worldwide. Therefore, the determination of botanical parameters of medicinal plants together with their chemical profiles is essential step in setting standards to determine the quality and authenticity of plant raw materials used as herbal drugs. This study focused on establishing macro- and micro-morphological parameters, phytochemical profiles, preclinical safety, and the pharmacological potential of *Campylanthus glaber* aerial parts.

The observed macroscopic and microscopic morphological characteristics of *C. glaber* leaf, stem, and aerial parts powder allowed identification of the most useful features for botanical monographic quality identification of this medicinal plant as an herbal drug.

Macroscopic characteristics observed for *C. glaber* leaf morphology, such as linear to narrowly obovate shape, length and width (1–5 cm long and 3–10 mm wide), and acute apex, agree with the data reported by Brochman et al. (1994) and Hjertson (2003) [4,5] for this plant part. However, features like revolute margins were noticed for the first time in *C. glaber*, although already reported by Hjertson (2003) for *Campylanthus anisotrichus*, a species of the same botanical genus.

The present study is original and concerns the first microscopic characterization of *Campylanthus* species as herbal medicines, in particular *Campylanthus glaber* leaf and stem. In fact, apart from some studies on seed, pollen, and calix indumentum scanning electron microscopy [4,33], no studies regarding the micromorphology of these plant parts were found concerning other *Campylanthus* species. Therefore, the obtained results are considered fundamental for the identification of this medicinal plant (*C. glaber* aerial parts) as raw material for pharmaceutical purposes and for providing new elements that can facilitate the correct identification of other species of the same botanical genus.

The most distinctive elements for the quality control are the leaf cylindrical shape in cross-section, the presence of strongly developed palisade parenchyma, the centrally located vascular bundles, the rectangular and polygonal thick-walled epidermal cells, the anomocytic type of stomata, glandular trichomes with a swollen base, and idioblasts with calcium oxalate crystals. Trichomes with swollen bases already described in the leaves of *C. antonii*, *C. junceus*, *C. pungens*, *C. ramosissimus*, and *C. yemenensis* [4] were observed for the first time in *C. glaber* leaf.

Concerning the stem microscopic characteristics, the cork layer with 3–7 rows of quadrangular-shape cells, thick-walled grouped sclereids surrounding the vascular cylinder with narrow phloem, broad xylem, and thick-walled central cylinder cells are the most distinctive features.

The macro- and microscopy examination of *C. glaber* leaf revealed xeromorphic morphological and anatomical adaptations. In fact, according to Hjertson 2003, most *Campylanthus* species show quite obvious xerophytic adaptations, and in *C. glaber* leaves, this is confirmed by the presence of small and narrow cylindrical leaves, succulence, thick cuticles, thick-walled epidermal cells, mesophyll mainly occupied by highly developed palisade parenchyma, and trichomes confined to a protected groove.

All of these traits can be related to the species adaptation to an habitat that constantly suffers from water stress, such as the Cabo Verde archipelago [34]. The thickening of the cuticle increases the resistance to water loss through the leaf surface [35], the cylindrical, small, narrow leaf reduces the surface area to volume ratio, minimizing excessive leaf heating and consequently reducing transpiration [36], and the succulence is due to the presence of water storage tissue. Another important xeromorphic adaptation is the trichomes, confined to a protected area formed by the revolute margins. According to Crang et al. (2018) [37], plants with trichomes located in crypts (grooves), an area of high trichome density, form a kind of water vapor pocket that significantly reduces water loss through transpiration. In this study, the aqueous extract prepared by infusion simulated the traditional herbal preparation used in Cabo Verde, and to provide a more stable preparation, a 70% hydroethanolic extract was obtained by maceration, a common method of preparation used to obtain total extracts from plant raw materials, as it allows obtaining extracts with a more representative composition of the secondary metabolites present in the plant material. In fact, the extraction yield depends on the extraction method and the solvent used for extraction. The use of aqueous mixtures containing ethanol, methanol, acetone, and ethyl acetate provides good results in the extraction of natural products from plant matrices; however, ethanol is recognized as a good solvent for polyphenol extraction and is safe for human consumption [11,38].

The analysis of our results showed that the hydroethanolic extracts had slightly higher extraction yields and DERs than the aqueous extract, proving that the mixture of water and ethanol (30:70 v/v, T = 22 °C) was more efficient in extracting the phenolic compounds than water (T = 95 °C). Nevertheless, since the majority of the main marker compounds (organic acids, iridoids, and phenylethanoid glycosides) are also soluble or partially soluble in water, the differences observed were not particularly pronounced, as observed in LC-UV/DAD fingerprinting and quantification of marker compounds (Figure 6, Table 3).

Phytochemical investigation of *C. glaber* aerial part extracts enabled the tentative identification of compounds belonging to organic acids, iridoid glycosides, phenylethanoid glycosides, and flavonoids. Based on their MS and MS/MS spectral data in negative ion mode together with relevant literature data and the use of authentic standards (co-chromatography), fourteen compounds, namely, malic acid (a), citric acid (b), gardoside (c), geniposidic acid (d), 8-epiloganic acid (e), cistanoside isomer (f), β-hydroxyverbascoside isomer (j), lavandulifolioside (m), verbascoside (n), cis-verbascoside (o), and isoverbascoside (p), in addition to the compounds monomelitoside, aucubin, and melitoside, were identified as major marker compounds of *C. glaber* extracts.

Iridoid glycosides and phenylethanoid glycosides have been previously reported in the *Campylanthus* genus [2,39], where they present important chemotaxonomy values. The presence of aucubin, gardoside, lavandulifolioside, and melittoside shows the chemotaxonomic relationship of *Campylanthus* with *Plantago* L. [2,40]. Although chemotaxonomy studies *on Campylanthus* have been documented, detailed phytochemical studies of other *Campylanthus* species are scarce. According to Ronsted and Jensen (2002) [2], the chemical profiles of *C. glaber* and *C. salsaloides* differ only by the presence of 8-epiloganic acid and salidroside in *C. glaber* and mussaenosidic acid in *C. salsoloides*. Salidroside, as well as erigeroside, previously detected in both species, were not detected in the present study. On the other hand, this is the first report of the phenylethanoid glycosides *β*-hydroxyverbascoside isomer, verbascoside, cis-verbascoside, and isoverbascoside, as well as the organic acids citric acid and malic acid, in *C. glaber*.

Regarding the quantification results of the main marker secondary metabolites, phenolic compounds, namely, phenylethanoid glycosides, are the main chemical classes of *C. glaber* aerial part extracts. Although iridoid glucosides are present in significantly smaller amounts in both extracts, they may still contribute to the biological potential of these extracts, as in studies related to the correlation of chemical composition and biological studies of other Plantaginaceae species, namely, the *Plantago* genus, both phenylethanoids and iridoids are referred to as the major classes of chemical compounds responsible for their pharmacological activities [41,42].

The severity of many chronic diseases, such as diabetes mellitus, chronic inflammation, cardiovascular disease, or age-related neurodegenerative disorders, is influenced by the abundance of reactive oxygen species (ROS) and other free radicals in the body. The ability of antioxidants to scavenge ROS and other free radicals [43] can delay the progression of many diseases by minimizing redox imbalances and counteracting the oxidative damage to tissues and biological macromolecules, such as lipids, proteins, and DNA [42,44].

C. glaber aerial part extracts presented in vitro antioxidant potential in three different ways: CUPRAC, FRAP, and DPPH radical scavenging ability. Although both extracts showed similar antioxidant activity in the FRAP and DPPH assays, CgEE displayed slightly higher antioxidant potential in the CUPRAC assay, which may be related to a higher amount of phenolic compounds displayed by CgEE compared to CgAE.

The antioxidant activity displayed by both extracts may be mainly due to the presence of phenylethanoids and flavonoids, since phenolic compounds, particularly flavonoids, can directly scavenge free radicals by donating electrons or hydrogen atoms. The presence of an OH group in their structure is the most significant determinant of electron-donating activity [43,45]. Concerning the iridoids, although they have been reported to have great anti-inflammatory potential, they appear to contribute less to the antioxidant activity of *C. glaber* extracts compared to the other phenolic compounds, as their chemical structure has a low number of OH groups, making them poor donors of hydrogen [24]. In this study, citric and malic acids were the main organic acids present in *C. glaber* extracts.

Previous studies have shown that organic acids' effective antioxidant potential is due to their chelation capacity, which can inactivate reduced cations [46]. It has been reported that organic acids are able to decrease reactive oxygen species and increase the bioavailability of phenolic compounds. Hence, it is possible to suppose a synergistic effect of malic and citric acid and the phenolic compounds present in *C. glaber*'s antioxidant potential.

The potential of *C. glaber* aerial part extracts to inhibit enzymes related to diabetes type 2 was also investigated. Diabetes mellitus is a metabolic disorder characterized by chronic hyperglycemia [47,48]. One of the most common approaches to controlling postprandial hyperglycemia is the inhibition of key enzymes such as α-amylase and α-glucosidase, responsible for the breakdown of carbohydrate and polysaccharides into monosaccharides [49]. The inhibition of the activity of these enzymes helps decrease the rate of carbohydrate digestion, decreasing the rate of absorption of monosaccharides, thereby lowering postprandial serum glucose levels. CgEE exhibited higher enzymatic inhibition potential than CgAE. The observed differences between these two extracts may be related to the small differences observed in their quantitative chemical profiles. Although both extracts presented similar qualitative chemical profiles, CgEE exhibited a higher amount of phenolic compounds (flavonoids and phenylethanoid glycosides).

The phenylethanoid glycoside verbascoside (peak n in Figure 6), identified as the third major marker compound of these extracts, has been linked to the management of diabetes in studies with other medicinal plants. In fact, verbascoside and its isomers have shown inhibition potential against α-amylase and α-glucosidase enzymes [47,50]. In addition, a study by Gali et al. (2020) [51] found a dose-dependent protective effect of verbascoside against oxidative stress in clonal and human pancreatic β-cells, where dysfunction and failure are linked to the development of diabetes, therefore revealing the antioxidant potential of verbascoside as an important mechanism of action in diabetes management. Iridoid glucosides identified in *C. glaber* aerial part extracts, such as aucubin [52,53] and geniposidic acid [54], have also been associated with the management of diabetes and diabetes complications.

Acarbose, as an inhibitor of both α-amylase and α-glucosidase, is widely used to treat diabetes mellitus, but its clinical use is associated with side effects such as abdominal discomfort, bloating, diarrhea, and nausea. In addition, the use of acarbose is still limited in some developing countries due to its high cost [55]. The search for naturally abundant and safe sources of inhibitors of α-amylase and α-glucosidase is therefore of great relevance as a complementary/alternative treatment for diabetes type 2 [56].

Although the inhibitory potential of *C. glaber* aerial part extracts on both α-amylase and α-glucosidase enzymes was lower than that of acarbose, the obtained results showed that this medicinal plant is a natural source of natural products capable of inhibiting the activity of both enzymes in a dose-dependent manner.

Medicinal plants are often assumed to be safe, even though this is not always true [57,58], as several studies are reporting the mutagenic potential of medicinal plants that have been used for many years [29,59,60], raising safety and economic concerns [61].

The Ames test and the cell proliferation assay (MTT assay) are recently being widely used in in vitro toxicology and genetic toxicology to predict the toxicity and genotoxic potential of plant extracts as preclinical safety assays on herbal drug production and to support the safe use of plants [29,61]. The Ames test uses Salmonella enterica Serovar Typhimurium LT-2 strains with mutations in the genes involved in histidine biosynthesis [30,62]. The histidine auxotrophic strains (his-) are able to detect gene mutations, specifically frameshift mutations and base pair substitutions [29]. The MTT assay is based on the ability of viable cells to reduce the MTT reagent, a yellow water-soluble tetrazolium salt, into purple formazan crystals through the succinate dehydrogenase system. The amount of purple formazan crystals produced is directly proportional to the number of viable cells in culture [63].

Results from the Ames assay showed that, tested up to the highest dose (5 mg per plate), *C. glaber* extracts did not induce a significant increase in the number of histidine revertant colonies over the negative control values obtained for tester strains TA 98, TA 100, TA 102, TA 1535, and TA 1537, neither in the presence nor in the absence of metabolic activation (Aroclor 1254-induced rat liver S9). In addition, the MTT assay results showed that *C. glaber* extracts did not induce cytotoxicity up to the highest dose tested (1000 μg/mL) in HepG2 cells when compared to the negative control, suggesting that neither CgAE nor CgEE may have toxic or genotoxic potential. Based on the obtained results, the use of *C. glaber* aerial parts in traditional medicine may pose no toxic or genotoxic risks for human consumption; however, further in vivo toxicity studies are an important future step to complete the safety profile of this medicinal plant.

4. Materials and Methods

4.1. Chemicals, Reference Items, and Reagents

α-Amylase from porcine pancreas, α-glucosidase from *Sacharomyces cerevisiae*, α-MEM, 2-aminoanthracene, 2-nitrofluorene, 2,2-diphenyl-1-picrylhydrazyl (DPPH), 2,4,6-tris(2-pyridyl)-s-triazine (TPTZ), 3,5-dinitrosalicylic acid, 4-nitrophenyl-α-D-glucopyranoside (NPG), 9-aminoacridine, aluminum chloride, benzo(a)pyrene, D-biotin, D-(+)-glucose monohydrate, glucose-6-phosphate, (+)-catechin, dimethyl sulfoxide, neocuproine, nicotinamide adenine dinucleotide phosphate, methylthiazolyldiphenyl-tetrazolium bromide (MTT), soluble potato starch, and *tert*-butyl hydroperoxide were purchased from Sigma-Aldrich (St. Louis, MO, USA). Ammonium sodium phosphate dibasic tetrahydrate, dipotassium hydrogen phosphate anhydrous, and sodium chloride were purchased from Fluka (Seelze, Germany). Bacto™ agar was obtained from Becton Dickinson & Co (Sparks, MD, USA). Acetic acid, ascorbic acid, citric acid monohydrate, disodium hydrogen phosphate dihydrate, hydrochloric acid, sodium acetate trihydrate, and sodium dihydrogen phosphate monohydrate were purchased from Panreac (Barcelona, Spain). Acetonitrile, Folin–Ciocalteu reagent, iron(III) chloride hexahydrate, L-histidine monohydrochloride monohydrate, methanol sodium carbonate, sodium hydroxide, and sodium nitrite were purchased from Merck (Darmstadt, Germany). Geniposidic acid was acquired from BLD Pharmatech GmbH (Kaiserslauterm, Germany). 4-Dimethylaminobenzaldehyde was acquired from Thermo Fisher Scientific™ (Waltham, MA, USA). Acarbose and gallic acid were purchased from AlfaAesar (Karlsruhe, Germany). Ethanol was purchased from Carlo Erba Reagents (Val-de-Reuil, France. Ammonium acetate, copper (II) chloride dihydrate, and iron sulfate heptahydrate were purchased from Riedel-de Haën (Seelze, Germany); magnesium sulfate heptahydrate was purchased from LabChem Inc (Zelienople, PA, USA); nutrient broth n° 2 was purchased from Oxoid (Basingstoke, UK); and sodium azide was purchased from J.T. Baker Chemical Company (Phillipsburg, NJ, USA). Aucubin was acquired from Extrasynthese (Genay, France). Formic acid (99–100%) was from VWR (Radnor, PA, USA). Fetal bovine serum was purchased from FBS, Gibco®-Thermo Fisher ScientificTM (Waltham, MA, USA). Non-essential amino acids (NEAA) and sodium pyruvate were purchased from PAN Biotech (Aidenbach, Germany). Aroclor 1254-induced rat liver S9 was purchased from Trinova Biochem (GmbH, Giessen, Germany). A Milli-Q water purification system (Millipore, Molsheim, France) was used to obtain ultra-pure water.

4.2. Plant Material Collection and Processing

C. glaber aerial parts were collected at the Natural Park of Serra Malagueta, Santiago Island, Cabo Verde Archipelago, between April 2016 and May 2018. Botanical identification was performed by Samuel Gomes, and a voucher specimen (022016KL) has been preserved at the Herbarium of INIDA, Santiago, Cabo Verde. The fresh aerial parts were dried in the shade for one week.

4.3. Preparation of Extracts

The dried aerial parts of *C. glaber* were extracted with hot water (water extract, CgAE) and 70% ethanol (hydroethanolic extract, CgEE). CgAE was prepared through the infusion method by adding 200 mL of boiling ultra-pure water (95 °C) to 3 g of dried plant material.

After 5 min of infusion and cooling, the extract was filtered, freeze-dried (Heto, LyoLab 3000), and stored. To prepare the CgEE, the dried plant material was previously ground into a homogenous powder using a grinder. This extract (1:10—1 part of the plant powder to 10 parts of solvent) was prepared by the maceration method at room temperature under agitation for 72 h. After filtration, the extract was evaporated under reduced pressure and a temperature of 38 ± 1 °C, freeze-dried (Heto, LyoLab 3000), and stored.

4.4. Botanical Characterization

4.4.1. Macroscopic Evaluation

Macroscopic analyses were executed according to the methods of the European Pharmacopoeia (10th edition, 2019) [64]. The plant material was analyzed by naked eye and with an Olympus SZ61 stereomicroscope (Leica Microsystems Ltd., Heerbrugg, Switzerland) coupled with a Leica MC170 HD digital camera controlled by Leica Application Suite (LAS) Version 4.8.0 software (Leica Microsystems Ltd., Heerbrugg, Switzerland).

4.4.2. Microscopic Evaluation

Microscopic analyses of dried leaves, stems, and aerial part powders were analyzed according to the European Pharmacopoeia (10th edition, 2019) [64]. An Olympus SZ61 stereo microscope coupled with a Leica MC170 HD digital camera for image capture was used. Image analysis was executed using Leica Application Suite (LAS) Version 4.8.0 software. Leaf (midrib) and stem microscopic analysis, freehand cross-section, and paradermal sections were analyzed. The samples were hydrated in distilled water and clarified with chloral hydrate (60%). The stoma index was determined using the following equation:

$$SI = \frac{St \times 100}{St + Ep}$$

where SI is the stomata index, St is the number of stomata, and Ep is the number of epidermal cells.

The dried powdered aerial parts of *C. glaber* were analyzed by placing small amounts of powder on a slide and observed under the microscope. Samples were mounted in chloral hydrate (60%). Characteristic structures and cell contents were observed.

All macro- and microscopic characterization results were expressed as mean ± standard deviation.

4.5. Chromatographic Conditions

The LC-UV/DAD analysis was performed with a Liquid Chromatograph Waters Alliance 2690 Separations Module (Waters Corporation, Milford, MA, USA) coupled with a Diode Array Detector (Water 966 PDA; Waters Corporation, Milford, MA, USA). The chromatograms were recorded at a maximum absorbance of each band (MaxPlot) between 210 and 450 nm, and Waters Millennium® 32 Chromatography Software (Waters Corporation, Milford, MA, USA) was used for data analysis. A Purospher STAR RP-18 endcapped column (4 × 250 mm, 5 μm) with pre-column (4 × 250 mm, 5 μm) from Merck (Darmstadt, Germany) was used, and as mobile phase, a linear gradient of water (0.1% formic acid) (solvent A) and acetonitrile) (solvent B) (*v*/*v*) was used: 0 min, 5% A, 95% B; 12 min, 89% A, 11% B; 40 min, 0% A, 100% B. The flow rate used was 1 mL/min, and the column temperature was 25 ± 5 °C.

For LC-MS/ESI, the analysis was undertaken with an HPLC (Waters Alliance 2695), coupled with a photodiode array detector and an autosampler (Waters PDA 2996), in tandem with a triple quadrupole mass spectrometer (Micromass® Quatro MicroTM API, Waters®, Ireland) and an electrospray ionization source (ESI) functioning in negative mode. A LiChrospher 100 RP-18 (5 μm) 250 × 4 mm column with a respective pre-column (Merck, Germany) was used. Water + 0.1% formic acid (solvent A) and methanol (solvent B) (*v*/*v*) were used as the mobile phase with a linear gradient: 0 min, 95% A, 5% B; 20 min, 80% A, 20% B; 60 min, 50% A, 50% B; 90 min, 0% A, 100% B. Acquired data were analyzed using

MassLynx™ V4.1 software (Waters®, Ireland). The injection volume was 20 µL, the flow rate used was 0.3 µL/min, and the column temperature was 25 ± 5 °C.

All samples were prepared in 50% methanol at concentrations of 10 mg/mL for LC/UV-DAD analysis and at concentrations of 30 mg/mL for LC-MS/ESI analysis. The standards were prepared at concentrations of 1 mg/mL.

The identification of compounds was made based on a comparison of UV–Vis, retention time, and mass spectral data with those of standards injected in co-chromatography and/or with literature data.

4.6. *Quantification of Main Classes of Secondary Metabolites*

4.6.1. Total Phenolic Content

Total phenolic content was estimated using the Folin–Ciocalteu colorimetric method described by Loebler et al. (2020) [65]. The absorbance was spectrophotometrically recorded at 765 nm (SPEKOL 1500, Analytik, Jena, Germany). Total phenolics amount was calculated using a gallic acid calibration curve (concentration range: 100–700 µg/mL; linear regression equation: $y = 0.0896x + 0.0281$; $R^2 = 0.9986$), and the results were presented as mg of gallic acid equivalents per g of dry extract (mg GAE/g).

4.6.2. Flavonoid Content

Flavonoid content was estimated according to the method described by [66]. The absorbance was spectrophotometrically recorded at 510 nm (SPEKOL 1500, Analytik, Jena, Germany). The amounts of flavonoids were calculated using a catechin calibration curve (concentration range: 18–290 µg/mL; linear regression equation: $y = 0.0032x + 0.0029$, $R^2 = 0.9991$), and the results are presented as mg of catechin equivalents per g of dry extract (mg CE/g).

4.6.3. Iridoid Content

Iridoid content was determined according to the method described by Niziol-Lukaszewska et al. (2017) [67]. The absorbance was spectrophotometrically recorded at 540 nm (Hitachi, U–2000, Tokyo, Japan). The amounts of iridoids were calculated using an aucubin calibration curve (concentration range: 10–200 µg/mL; linear regression equation: $y = 0.0014x + 0.0119$, $R^2 = 0.9906$) and expressed as mg of aucubin equivalents per g of dry extract (mg Au/g).

4.7. *Antioxidant Capacity*

4.7.1. CUPRAC Assay

The assay was performed following the method described by [68] with slight modifications. In a test tube, 1 mL of the following solutions were mixed: copper (II) chloride dehydrate (10 mM), ammonium acetate (1 M), and neocuproine in ethanol (7.5 mM). Then, 300 µL of extracts in appropriate dilutions were added to the previous mixture and water up to the final volume of 4.1 mL. After 1 h at room temperature, absorbance was spectrophotometrically recorded at 450 nm (SPEKOL 1500, Analytik, Jena, Germany). A calibration curve of ascorbic acid (concentration range: 2–45 µg/mL; linear regression equation: $y = 0.025x + 0.057$, $R^2 = 0.9966$) was used, and the results were expressed as µg of ascorbic acid equivalents per g of dry extract (µg AAE/g).

4.7.2. FRAP Assay

The assay was performed according to the procedure described by [69] with minor modifications. In test tubes, 100 µL of extracts of appropriate dilutions were mixed with 3 mL of freshly prepared and pre-warmed (37 °C) FRAP reagent (0.25 M sodium acetate buffer, pH 3.6, 10 mM TPTZ solution in 40 mM HCl, and 20 mM $FeCl_3$. $6H_2O$ at a ratio of 10:1:1). After incubation (4 min, 37 °C), the absorbance of the mixture was spectrophotometrically recorded at 593 nm (SPEKOL 1500, Analytik, Jena, Germany). A calibration curve of ascorbic acid (concentration range: 25–125 µg/mL; linear regression equation:

y = 0.2692x + 0.0871, R^2 = 0.9941) was used, and the results were presented as μg of ascorbic acid equivalents per g of dry extract (μg AAE/g).

4.7.3. DPPH Radical Scavenging Assay

The ability of the samples to scavenge the DPPH radical was evaluated according to the method described by [70]. In test tubes, 500 μL of extract dilutions were mixed with 3 mL of freshly prepared DPPH solution (24 mg/L in ethanol). After 30 min of incubation in the dark at room temperature, the absorbance was measured at 517 nm (SPEKOL 1500, Analytik, Jena, Germany). Ascorbic acid was used as a positive reference. The scavenging activity was measured as the decrease in absorbance of the samples versus the DPPH standard solution. Results were expressed as inhibitory concentrations (IC_{50} values), representing the sample concentration required to scavenge 50% of the DPPH free radicals. The percentage of DPPH radical scavenging activity was calculated according to the formula:

$$\text{Inhibition}(\%) = \left[\frac{\text{AbsControl} - \text{AbsSample}}{\text{AbsControl}}\right] \times 100$$

4.8. Enzymatic Inhibition

4.8.1. α-Amylase Inhibition Assay

The inhibition of the α-amylase enzyme was determined according to the method described by [71] with some modifications. Briefly, reaction mixtures containing 100 μL of Type VI-B porcine pancreatic α-amylase (0.5 mg/mL in 100 mM sodium phosphate buffer, containing 6.7 mM sodium chloride, pH 6.7) and 100 μL of extracts of appropriate dilutions were preincubated in test tubes at 37 °C for 10 min. Then, 100 μL of 1% starch (*w*/*v*, previously suspended in 100 mM sodium phosphate buffer, containing 6.7 mM sodium chloride, pH 6.7, and boiled for 10 min) was added. After 10 min at 37 °C, 200 μL of DNS reagent (consisting of 20 mL of 96 mM DNS, 8 mL of 5.315 M sodium potassium tartrate tetrahydrate in 2 M NaOH, and 12 mL of distilled water) was added. The reaction mixtures were heated at 100 °C for 15 min to stop the reaction, then cooled to room temperature and diluted with 2 mL of distilled water. The intensity of the redish color was spectrophotometrically measured at 520 nm (SPEKOL 1500, Analytik, Jena, Germany). The reaction mixture without the extracts was used as a negative control, and the reaction mixtures without α-amylase were used as samples' blanks. Increasing concentrations of acarbose (10–125 μg/mL) were used as positive controls. The results were presented as the concentration in the reaction mixture that reduced the enzyme activity by 50% (IC_{50}). The enzyme inhibitory rate was calculated according to the following formula:

$$\text{Inhibition}(\%) = \frac{(\text{AbsSample} - \text{AbsSampleblank}) \times 100}{\text{AbsNegativecontrol}}$$

4.8.2. α-Glucosidase Inhibition Assay

The α-glucosidase enzyme inhibition was determined according to the colorimetric method described by [72], with some modifications. Reaction mixtures containing 5 μL of α-glucosidase (6.25 U/mL in phosphate buffer (pH 6.9, 0.1 M)), 125 μL of phosphate buffer (pH 6.9, 0.1 M), and 20 μL of the plant extracts at different concentrations were prepared in a 96-well microplate (Greiner Bio-One, Rainbach im Mühlkreis, Austria) and incubated for 15 min at 37 °C. The reaction was started by adding 20 μL of substrate solution (p-nitrophenyl-*α*-*D*-glucopyranoside, 2.75 mM in phosphate buffer (pH 6.9, 0.1 M)), and the plates were incubated for an additional 15 min at 37 °C. The reaction was stopped by the addition of 80 μL of 0.2 M Na_2CO_3. The absorbance of the wells was measured in a microplate reader (FLUOstar® Omega Plate Reader, BMG 264 Labtech, Ortenberg, Germany) at 405 nm. The reaction mixture without the extracts was used as a negative control, and reaction mixtures without α-glucosidase were used as samples' blanks. Increasing concentrations of acarbose (1–12 mg/mL) were used as positive controls. The results were expressed as the concentration in the reaction mixture that reduced the enzyme activity by 50% (IC_{50}). The enzyme inhibitory rate was calculated as follows:

$$\text{Inhibition}(\%) = \frac{(\text{AbsSample} - \text{AbsSampleblank}) \times 100}{\text{AbsNegativecontrol}}$$

4.9. Safety Assessment

4.9.1. In Vitro Assessment of Genotoxicity/Mutagenicity

The genotoxicity/mutagenicity potential of *C. glaber* extracts was evaluated by the Ames test, through the direct plate incorporation method described by Maron and Ames (1983) [30] and Mortelmans and Zeiger (2000) [62] and according to OECD No. 471 and ICH S2 (R1) guidelines [73,74]. The assay was performed with and without metabolic activation using the *Salmonella enterica* serovar Typhimurium (His^-) tester strains TA98, TA100, TA102, and TA1535, provided by the Genetic Department of the Nova Medical School of the Universidade NOVA de Lisboa (Portugal) (received from Professor B.N. Ames (Berkeley, CA, USA)) and TA1537 (ATCC, NUMBER: 29630™ (LOT: 7405375)). Briefly, 200 µL of appropriate dilutions of the extracts in 30% DMSO (0–5 mg/plate), 100 µL of each tester strain (inoculated in nutrient broth medium and incubated in an orbital incubator for 12–16 h, 37 °C, 210 rpm in the dark, and kept at 4 °C until use) and 500 µL of phosphate buffer (0.1 M, pH 7.4) (assay without metabolic activation), or S9 mix (10%, *v/v* rat liver S9, 0.4 M $MgCl_2$, 1.65 M KCl, 1 M glucose-6-phosphate, 0.1 M NADP in 0.1 M sodium phosphate buffer (pH 7.4) prepared fresh and kept on ice during the experiment) (assay with metabolic activation) were mixed with 2 mL of top agar (45 °C) supplemented with biotin (0.05 mM) and histidine (0.05 mM) and plated into minimal glucose agar medium (1.5% Bacto-Difco agar and 2% glucose in Vogel-Bonner medium). After 48 h of incubation at 37 °C, manual counting of revertant colonies (His+) was performed.

Three independent experiments were performed for each assay, and the results were presented as the mean number of revertant colonies (His+) and the standard deviation (mean ± SD). The positive controls in the assay without metabolic activation were sodium azide (1.5 µg/plate for TA100 and TA1535), 2-nitrofluorene (5 µg/plate for TA98), 9-aminoacridine (100 µg/plate for TA1537), and tert-butyl hydroperoxide (50 µg/plate for TA102). The positive controls in the assay with metabolic activation were 2-aminoathracene (2 µg/plate for TA98 and 10 µg/plate for TA102, TA1535, and TA1537) and benzo(a)pyrene (5 µg/plate for TA100) in the assay with metabolic activation.

4.9.2. In Vitro Assessment of Cytotoxicity

The cytotoxicity of the *C. glaber* extracts was evaluated by the MTT reduction assay [75] on the human liver cell line HepG2 (ATCC Cat. No. HB-8065, Middlesex, UK), according to [31]. Briefly, 48 h after inoculation, the HepG2 culture medium was replaced by fresh medium with CgAE and CgEE (9:1) at final concentrations ranging from 50 to 1000 µg/mL. After 48 h, the MTT assay was performed. The data were expressed as a percentage relative to the solvent control. Four replicates of each sample were performed, n = 2–3. The % cell viability was calculated according to the following formula:

$$\text{Cellviability}(\%) = \left({}^{\text{Abs1}}/{}_{\text{Abs0}}\right) \times 100$$

where Abs1 is the absorbance of extract-treated cells and Abs0 is the absorbance of solvent control-treated cells.

4.10. Data Analysis

Statistical analysis was performed with STATISTICA version 7.0 (StatSoft Inc., Tulsa, OK, USA). The quantification of secondary metabolites, antioxidant activity, and inhibition of enzymes was tested by the Student t-test. Regression analyses were carried out using EXCEL (Microsoft Corporation, USA). Cytotoxicity data was analyzed with a two-way

ANOVA and graphs plotted using GraphPad Prism® software (version 9.0.0.121, GraphPad Software, San Diego, CA, USA). Results are presented as mean ± standard deviation; $p < 0.05$ was considered significant.

5. Conclusions

This study is the first report on micromorphology features, in vitro biological studies (antioxidant and antihyperglycemic potential), and the pre-clinical safety of *C. glaber* aerial parts used as an herbal drug in Cabo Verde. The characteristic micromorphological features identified together with the phytochemical profile are important for the quality control of this medicinal plant as they allow its correct identification and can be included in official quality monographs, which allow its pharmaceutical use as an herbal medicinal product or as part of herbal preparations for medicinal purposes. Our results showed that *C. glaber* aerial parts are a source of natural products with antioxidant and antihyperglycemic potential and possibly with multiple therapeutic and economic values. Furthermore, the data gathered in this study can serve as an incentive for the development of conservation strategies for this species, as it is a source of valuable natural products.

Future perspectives will include anti-inflammatory activity studies, according to its traditional use, and the isolation of selected promising compounds, to better understand the undelaying mechanisms of action of this medicinal plant.

Author Contributions: Conceptualization, K.L., M.M. and O.S.; Data curation, K.L., M.M., S.P.C., J.P.M. and M.P.D.; Formal analysis, K.L., M.M., J.P.M. and M.P.D.; Funding acquisition, M.P.D. and O.S.; Investigation, K.L., M.M., S.P.C., J.P.M. and O.S.; Methodology, K.L., M.M., S.P.C., K.H., S.G., J.P.M., M.P.D. and O.S.; Project administration, O.S.; Resources, S.G., M.E.F., M.P.D. and O.S.; Software, K.L., M.M., S.P.C., K.H. and M.P.D.; Supervision, M.E.F., M.P.D. and O.S.; Validation, K.L. and M.M.; Visualization, K.L., M.M., S.P.C., K.H. and S.G.; Writing—original draft, K.L.; Writing—review and editing, M.M., S.P.C., I.M.d.S., M.E.F., J.P.M., R.S., M.P.D. and O.S.; Plant collection and identification, K.L. and S.G. All authors have read and agreed to the published version of the manuscript.

Funding: This research was funded by the Foundation for Science and Technology (FCT, Portugal) through national funds to iMed.ULisboa (UIDP/04138/2020) and to the Mechanical Engineering and Resource Sustainability Center-MEtRICs unit, which is funded by national funds from FCT/MCTES (UIDB/04077/2020 and UIDP/04077/2020).

Institutional Review Board Statement: Not applicable.

Informed Consent Statement: Not applicable.

Data Availability Statement: Data is contained within the article.

Acknowledgments: The authors gratefully acknowledge the Natural Park of Serra Malagueta and INIDA for making available all the experimental plant materials and Maria Cristina Duarte (Centre for Ecology, Evolution and Environmental Changes (cE3c); Faculdade de Ciências, Universidade de Lisboa) for providing the photography of *C. glaber* species in natural habitat.

Conflicts of Interest: The authors declare no conflict of interest.

References

1. POWO Plantaginaceae Juss. | Plants of the World Online | Kew Science. Available online: https://powo.science.kew.org/taxon/urn:lsid:ipni.org:names:30001136-2 (accessed on 21 August 2023).
2. Rønsted, N.; Jensen, S.R. Iridoid Glucosides and Caffeoyl Phenylethanoid Glycosides from *Campylanthus salsaloides* and *Campylanthus glaber*. *Biochem. Syst. Ecol.* **2002**, *30*, 1091–1095. [CrossRef]
3. Thiv, M.; Thulin, M.; Hjertson, M.; Kropf, M.; Linder, H.P. Evidence for a Vicariant Origin of Macaronesian-Eritreo/Arabian Disjunctions in *Campylanthus* Roth (Plantaginaceae). *Mol. Phylogenet. Evol.* **2010**, *54*, 607–616. [CrossRef] [PubMed]
4. Hjertson, M. Revision of the Disjunct Genus *Campylanthus* (Scrophulariaceae). *Edinb. J. Bot.* **2003**, *60*, 131–174. [CrossRef]
5. Brochmann, C.; Rustan, Ø.H.; Lobin, W.; Kilian, N. The Endemic Vascular Plants of the Cape Verde Islands, W Africa. *Sommerfeltia* **1997**, *24*, 1–363. [CrossRef]
6. Gomes, A.; Vasconcelos, T.; Almeida, M.H. Plantas Na Medicina Tradicional de Cabo Verde. In Proceedings of the Workshop Plantas Medicinais e Fitoterapêuticas nos Trópicos, Instituto de Investigação Científica Tropical/Centro Científico e Cultural de Macau, Lisboa, Portugal, 29–31 October 2008; pp. 1–13.

7. Gomes, S. Plantas Endémicas Medicinais de Cabo Verde. Available online: http://portaldoconhecimento.gov.cv/handle/10961/3838 (accessed on 11 January 2020).
8. Roque, S.; Duarte, I.; Graziani, P.; Nascimento, M.; Ramos, N. *Usos Medicinais e Tradicionais Da Flora Endémica, Indígena e Exótica Do Monte Gordo*; Projecto Áreas Protegidas CVI/02/G31/A/1G/99/2006; Ministério do Ambiente e Agricultura: São Nicolau, Cabo Verde, 2008.
9. WHO. *WHO Global Report on Traditional and Complementary Medicine 2019*; WHO: Geneva, Switzerland, 2019.
10. Essoh, A.; Liberal, Â.; Fernandes, Â.; Dias, M.I.; Pereira, C.; Mandim, F.; Moldão-Martins, M.; Cravo, P.; Duarte, M.P.; Moura, M.; et al. Evaluation of the Polyphenolic Composition and Bioactivities of Three Native Cabo Verde Medicinal Plants. *Pharmaceuticals* **2022**, *15*, 1162. [CrossRef] [PubMed]
11. Romeiras, M.M.; Essoh, A.P.; Catarino, S.; Silva, J.; Lima, K.; Varela, E.; Moura, M.; Gomes, I.; Duarte, M.P.C.; Duarte, M.P.C. Diversity and Biological Activities of Medicinal Plants of Santiago Island (Cabo Verde). *Heliyon* **2023**, *9*, e14651. [CrossRef] [PubMed]
12. De Moura Sperotto, N.D.; Steffens, L.; Veríssimo, R.M.; Henn, J.G.; Péres, V.F.; Vianna, P.; Chies, J.A.B.; Roehe, A.; Saffi, J.; Moura, D.J. Wound Healing and Anti-Inflammatory Activities Induced by a *Plantago australis* Hydroethanolic Extract Standardized in Verbascoside. *J. Ethnopharmacol.* **2018**, *225*, 178–188. [CrossRef]
13. Sripahco, T.; Khruengsai, S.; Charoensup, R.; Tovaranonte, J.; Pripdeevech, P. Chemical Composition, Antioxidant, and Antimicrobial Activity of *Elsholtzia beddomei* C. B. Clarke Ex Hook. f. Essential Oil. *Sci. Rep.* **2022**, *12*, 2225. [CrossRef]
14. Fritzen, M.; Dutra, R.; Crivelli, S.; Farmacognosia, I.; Cabral, S.; Farias, P.; Paes, R.; Linhares, G. (Eds.) *1ª Edição*; SESES: Rio de Janeiro, Brazil, 2016; ISBN 2013206534.
15. Rabizadeh, F.; Mirian, M.S.; Doosti, R.; Kiani-Anbouhi, R.; Eftekhari, E. Phytochemical Classification of Medicinal Plants Used in the Treatment of Kidney Disease Based on Traditional Persian Medicine. *Evid. Based Complement. Alternat. Med.* **2022**, *2022*, 8022599. [CrossRef]
16. Jain, C.; Khatana, S.; Vijayvergia, R. Bioactivity of Secondary Metabolites of Various Plants: A Review. *Int. J. Pharm. Sci. Res.* **2019**, *10*, 494–504. [CrossRef]
17. Catarino, S.; Duarte, M.C.; Romeiras, M.M. *Campylanthus glaber*. *IUCN Red List Threat. Species* **2017**, *2017*, e.T107423655A107468087. [CrossRef]
18. Romeiras, M.M.; Catarino, S.; Gomes, I.; Fernandes, C.; Costa, J.C.; Caujapé-Castells, J.; Duarte, M.C. IUCN Red List Assessment of the Cape Verde Endemic Flora: Towards a Global Strategy for Plant Conservation in Macaronesia. *Bot. J. Linn. Soc.* **2016**, *180*, 413–425. [CrossRef]
19. Moyo, M.; Aremu, A.O.; Van Staden, J. Medicinal Plants: An Invaluable, Dwindling Resource in Sub-Saharan Africa. *J. Ethnopharmacol.* **2015**, *174*, 595–606. [CrossRef]
20. Tahir, N.I.; Shaari, K.; Abas, F.; Ahmad Parveez, G.K.; Hashim, A.T.; Ramli, U.S. Identification of Oil Palm (*Elaeis guineensis*) Spear Leaf Metabolites Using Mass Spectrometry and Neutral Loss Analysis. *J. Oil Palm Res.* **2013**, *25*, 72–83.
21. Fernández-Fernández, R.; López-Martínez, J.C.; Romero-González, R.; Martínez-Vidal, J.L.; Alarcón Flores, M.I.; Garrido Frenich, A. Simple LC-MS Determination of Citric and Malic Acids in Fruits and Vegetables. *Chromatographia* **2010**, *72*, 55–62. [CrossRef]
22. Fu, Z.; Xue, R.; Li, Z.; Chen, M.; Sun, Z.; Hu, Y.; Huang, C. Fragmentation Patterns Study of Iridoid Glycosides in Fructus Gardeniae by HPLC-Q/TOF-MS/MS. *Biomed. Chromatogr.* **2014**, *28*, 1795–1807. [CrossRef] [PubMed]
23. Gao, H.; Liu, Z.; Song, F.; Xing, J.; Zheng, Z.; Liu, S. A Strategy for Identification and Structural Characterization of Compounds from Plantago Asiatica L. by Liquid Chromatography-Mass Spectrometry Combined with Ion Mobility Spectrometry. *Molecules* **2022**, *27*, 4302. [CrossRef]
24. Kucharska, A.Z.; Fecka, I. Identification of Iridoids in Edible Honeysuckle Berries (*Lonicera caerulea* L. Var. *kamtschatica* Sevast.) by UPLC-ESI-QTOF-MS/MS. *Molecules* **2016**, *21*, 1157. [CrossRef]
25. Yang, L.; He, J. *Lagopsis supina* Extract and Its Fractions Exert Prophylactic Effects against Blood Stasis in Rats via Anti-Coagulation, Anti-Platelet Activation and Anti-Fibrinolysis and Chemical Characterization by UHPLC-QTOF-MS/MS. *Biomed. Pharmacother.* **2020**, *132*, 110899. [CrossRef]
26. Liao, X.; Hong, Y.; Chen, Z. Identification and Quantification of the Bioactive Components in *Osmanthus fragrans* Roots by HPLC-MS/MS. *J. Pharm. Anal.* **2021**, *11*, 299–307. [CrossRef]
27. Dimaki, V.D.; Zeliou, K.; Nakka, F.; Stavreli, M.; Bakratsas, I.; Papaioannou, L.; Iatrou, G.; Lamari, F.N. Characterization of *Sideritis clandestina* Subsp. *peloponnesiaca* Polar Glycosides and Phytochemical Comparison to Other Mountain Tea Populations. *Molecules* **2022**, *27*, 7613. [CrossRef] [PubMed]
28. Kelber, O.; Wegener, T.; Steinhoff, B.; Staiger, C.; Wiesner, J.; Knöss, W.; Kraft, K. Assessment of Genotoxicity of Herbal Medicinal Products: Application of the "Bracketing and Matrixing" Concept Using the Example of *Valerianae radix* (Valerian Root). *Phytomedicine* **2014**, *21*, 1124–1129. [CrossRef] [PubMed]
29. Da Silva Dantas, F.G.; de Castilho, P.F.; de Almeida-Apolonio, A.A.; de Araújo, R.P.; de Oliveira, K.M.P. Mutagenic Potential of Medicinal Plants Evaluated by the Ames *Salmonella*/Microsome Assay: A Systematic Review. *Mutat. Res. Mutat. Res.* **2020**, *786*, 108338. [CrossRef] [PubMed]
30. Maron, D.M.; Ames, B.N. Revised Methods for the *Salmonella* Mutagenicity Test. *Mutat. Res. Mutagen. Relat. Subj.* **1983**, *113*, 173–215. [CrossRef] [PubMed]

31. Malmir, M.; Lima, K.; Póvoas Camões, S.; Manageiro, V.; Duarte, M.P.; Paiva Miranda, J.; Serrano, R.; da Silva, I.M.; Silva Lima, B.; Caniça, M.; et al. Identification of Marker Compounds and In Vitro Toxicity Evaluation of Two Portuguese *Asphodelus* Leaf Extracts. *Molecules* **2023**, *28*, 2372. [CrossRef]
32. Malú, Q.; Lima, K.; Malmir, M.; Pinto, R.; da Silva, I.M.; Catarino, L.; Duarte, M.P.; Serrano, R.; Rocha, J.; Lima, B.S.; et al. Contribution to the Preclinical Safety Assessment of *Lannea velutina* and *Sorindeia juglandifolia* Leaves. *Plants* **2023**, *12*, 130. [CrossRef]
33. Kilian, A.N.; Hein, P.; Bahah, S.O.; Kilian, N.; Hein, P.; Bahah, S.O.; Kilian, A.N.; Hein, P.; Bahah, S.O.; Kilian, N.; et al. A New Species of *Campylanthus* (*Scrophulariaceae*) from Ras Fartak, Al-Mahra, and Notes on Other Species of the Genus in Yemen. *Willdenowia* **2002**, *32*, 271–279. [CrossRef]
34. Kummerow, J. *Comparative Anatomy of Sclerophylls of Mediterranean Climatic Areas*; Springer: Berlin/Heidelberg, Germany, 1973; pp. 157–167.
35. Simioni, P.F.; Eisenlohr, P.V.; Pessoa, M.J.G.; da Silva, I.V. Elucidating Adaptive Strategies from Leaf Anatomy: Do Amazonian Savannas Present Xeromorphic Characteristics? *Flora* **2017**, *226*, 38–46. [CrossRef]
36. Abd Elhalim, M.E.; Abo-Alatta, O.K.; Habib, S.A.; Abd Elbar, O.H. The Anatomical Features of the Desert Halophytes *Zygophyllum album* L.F. and *Nitraria retusa* (Forssk.) Asch. *Ann. Agric. Sci.* **2016**, *61*, 97–104. [CrossRef]
37. Crang, R.; Lyons-Sobaski, S.; Wise, R. Leaves. In *Plant Anatomy*; Springer: Cham, Switzerland, 2018; pp. 395–441. [CrossRef]
38. Do, Q.D.; Angkawijaya, A.E.; Tran-Nguyen, P.L.; Huynh, L.H.; Soetaredjo, F.E.; Ismadji, S.; Ju, Y.H. Effect of Extraction Solvent on Total Phenol Content, Total Flavonoid Content, and Antioxidant Activity of *Limnophila aromatica*. *J. Food Drug Anal.* **2014**, *22*, 296–302. [CrossRef]
39. Kooiman, P. The Occurrence of Iridoid Glycosides in the Scrophulariaceae. *Acta Bot. Neerl.* **1975**, *24*, 459–468. [CrossRef]
40. Albach, D.C.; Meudt, H.M.; Oxelman, B. Piecing Together the "New" Plantaginaceae. *Am. J. Bot.* **2005**, *92*, 297–315. [CrossRef]
41. Gonda, S.; Nguyen, N.M.; Batta, G.; Gyémánt, G.; Máthé, C.; Vasas, G. Determination of Phenylethanoid Glycosides and Iridoid Glycosides from Therapeutically Used Plantago Species by CE-MEKC. *Electrophoresis* **2013**, *34*, 2577–2584. [CrossRef]
42. Gonçalves, S.; Romano, A. The Medicinal Potential of Plants from the Genus *Plantago* (Plantaginaceae). *Ind. Crops Prod.* **2016**, *83*, 213–226. [CrossRef]
43. Apak, R.; Capanoglu, E.; Shahidi, F. *Measurment of Antioxidant Activity and Capacity: Recent Trends and Applications*; Apak, R., Capanoglu, E., Shahidi, F., Eds.; Wiley: Oxford, UK, 2018; ISBN 9781119135357.
44. Atoui, A.; Mansouri, A.; Boskou, G.; Kefalas, P. Tea and Herbal Infusions: Their Antioxidant Activity and Phenolic Profile. *Food Chem.* **2005**, *89*, 27–36. [CrossRef]
45. Bartwal, A.; Mall, R.; Lohani, P.; Guru, S.K.; Arora, S. Role of Secondary Metabolites and Brassinosteroids in Plant Defense against Environmental Stresses. *J. Plant Growth Regul.* **2013**, *32*, 216–232. [CrossRef]
46. Zhang, D.; Nie, S.; Xie, M.; Hu, J. Antioxidant and Antibacterial Capabilities of Phenolic Compounds and Organic Acids from *Camellia oleifera* Cake. *Food Sci. Biotechnol.* **2020**, *29*, 17–25. [CrossRef] [PubMed]
47. Deb, P.K.; Khound, P.; Bhattacharjee, S.; Choudhury, P.; Sarma, H.; Devi, R.; Sarkar, B. Variation in Chemical Constituents, In-Vitro Bioactivity and Toxicity Profile among Different Parts of *Clerodendrum glandulosum* Lindl. (*C. colebrookianum* Walp.). *S. Afr. J. Bot.* **2021**, *140*, 50–61. [CrossRef]
48. Quazi, A.; Patwekar, M.; Patwekar, F.; Alghamdi, S.; Rajab, B.S.; Babalghith, A.O.; Islam, F. In Vitro Alpha-Amylase Enzyme Assay of Hydroalcoholic Polyherbal Extract: Proof of Concept for the Development of Polyherbal Teabag Formulation for the Treatment of Diabetes. *Evid.-Based Complement. Altern. Med.* **2022**, *2022*, 1577957. [CrossRef]
49. Somtimuang, C.; Olatunji, O.J.; Ovatlarnporn, C. Evaluation of In Vitro α-Amylase and α-Glucosidase Inhibitory Potentials of 14 Medicinal Plants Constituted in Thai Folk Antidiabetic Formularies. *Chem. Biodivers.* **2018**, *15*, e1800025. [CrossRef]
50. Yin, Z.; Zhang, W.; Feng, F.; Zhang, Y.; Kang, W. α-Glucosidase Inhibitors Isolated from Medicinal Plants. *Food Sci. Hum. Wellness* **2014**, *3*, 136–174. [CrossRef]
51. Galli, A.; Marciani, P.; Marku, A.; Ghislanzoni, S.; Bertuzzi, F.; Rossi, R.; Di Giancamillo, A.; Castagna, M.; Perego, C. Verbascoside Protects Pancreatic β-Cells against ER-Stress. *Biomedicines* **2020**, *8*, 582. [CrossRef] [PubMed]
52. Jin, L.; Xue, H.Y.; Jin, L.J.; Li, S.Y.; Xu, Y.P. Antioxidant and Pancreas-Protective Effect of Aucubin on Rats with Streptozotocin-Induced Diabetes. *Eur. J. Pharmacol.* **2008**, *582*, 162–167. [CrossRef] [PubMed]
53. Ma, B.; Zhu, Z.; Zhang, J.; Ren, C.; Zhang, Q. Aucubin Alleviates Diabetic Nephropathy by Inhibiting NF-KB Activation and Inducing SIRT1/SIRT3-FOXO3a Signaling Pathway in High-Fat Diet/Streptozotocin-Induced Diabetic Mice. *J. Funct. Foods* **2020**, *64*, 103702. [CrossRef]
54. Zhang, X.; Wang, L.; Zheng, Z.; Pi, Z.; Liu, Z.; Song, F. Online Microdialysis-Ultra Performance Liquid Chromatography–Mass Spectrometry Method for Comparative Pharmacokinetic Investigation on Iridoids from *Gardenia jasminoides* Ellis in Rats with Different Progressions of Type 2 Diabetic Complications. *J. Pharm. Biomed. Anal.* **2017**, *140*, 146–154. [CrossRef]
55. Thengyai, S.; Thiantongin, P.; Sontimuang, C.; Ovatlarnporn, C.; Puttarak, P. α-Glucosidase and α-Amylase Inhibitory Activities of Medicinal Plants in Thai Antidiabetic Recipes and Bioactive Compounds from *Vitex glabrata* R. Br. Stem Bark. *J. Herb. Med.* **2020**, *19*, 100302. [CrossRef]
56. Nguyen, V.B.; Nguyen, Q.V.; Nguyen, A.D.; Wang, S.L. Screening and Evaluation of α-Glucosidase Inhibitors from Indigenous Medicinal Plants in Dak Lak Province, Vietnam. *Res. Chem. Intermed.* **2017**, *43*, 3599–3612. [CrossRef]

57. Verschaeve, L. Genotoxicity and Antigenotoxicity Studies of Traditional Medicinal Plants: How Informative and Accurate Are the Results? *Nat. Prod. Commun.* **2015**, *10*, 1489–1493. [CrossRef]
58. Aydin, A.; Aktay, G.; Yesilada, E. A Guidance Manual for the Toxicity Assessment of Traditional Herbal Medicines. *Nat. Prod. Commun.* **2016**, *11*, 1763–1773. [CrossRef]
59. Bardoloi, A.; Soren, A.D. Genotoxicity Induced by Medicinal Plants. *Bull. Natl. Res. Cent.* **2022**, *46*, 119. [CrossRef]
60. Zhou, J.; Ouedraogo, M.; Qu, F.; Duez, P. Potential Genotoxicity of Traditional Chinese Medicinal Plants and Phytochemicals: An Overview. *Phyther. Res.* **2013**, *27*, 1745–1755. [CrossRef] [PubMed]
61. Sponchiado, G.; Adam, M.L.; Silva, C.D.; Silva Soley, B.; De Mello-Sampayo, C.; Cabrini, D.A.; Correr, C.J.; Otuki, M.F. Quantitative Genotoxicity Assays for Analysis of Medicinal Plants: A Systematic Review. *J. Ethnopharmacol.* **2016**, *178*, 289–296. [CrossRef] [PubMed]
62. Mortelmans, K.; Zeiger, E. The Ames *Salmonella*/Microsome Mutagenicity Assay. *Mutat. Res. Fundam. Mol. Mech. Mutagen.* **2000**, *455*, 29–60. [CrossRef] [PubMed]
63. Shoemaker, M.; Cohen, I.; Campbell, M. Reduction of MTT by Aqueous Herbal Extracts in the Absence of Cells. *J. Ethnopharmacol.* **2004**, *93*, 381–384. [CrossRef]
64. European Directorate for the Quality of Medicines & Healthcare. *European Pharmacopoeia*, 10th ed.; Newsroom: Strasbourg, France, 2019.
65. Loebler, M.; Sánchez, C.; Maurício, E.M.; Diogo, E.; Santos, M.; Vasilenko, P.; Cruz, A.S.; Mendes, B.; Gonçalves, M.; Duarte, M.P. Potential Application of Propolis Extracts to Control the Growth of *Stemphylium vesicarium* in 'Rocha' pear. *Appl. Sci.* **2020**, *10*, 1990. [CrossRef]
66. Barros, L.; Carvalho, A.M.; Morais, J.S.; Ferreira, I.C.F.R. Strawberry-Tree, Blackthorn and Rose Fruits: Detailed Characterisation in Nutrients and Phytochemicals with Antioxidant Properties. *Food Chem.* **2010**, *120*, 247–254. [CrossRef]
67. Nizioł-Lukaszewska, Z.; Wasilewski, T.; Bujak, T.; Osika, P. Iridoids from *Cornus mas* L. and Their Potential as Innovative Ingredients in Cosmetics. *Polish J. Chem. Technol.* **2017**, *19*, 122–127. [CrossRef]
68. Apak, R.; Güçlü, K.; Özyürek, M.; Karademir, S.E. Novel Total Antioxidant Capacity Index for Dietary Polyphenols and Vitamins C and E, Using Their Cupric Ion Reducing Capability in the Presence of Neocuproine: CUPRAC Method. *J. Agric. Food Chem.* **2004**, *52*, 7970–7981. [CrossRef]
69. Lima, K.; Silva, O.; Figueira, M.E.; Pires, C.; Cruz, D.; Gomes, S.; Maurício, E.M.; Duarte, M.P. Influence of the In Vitro Gastrointestinal Digestion on the Antioxidant Activity of *Artemisia gorgonum* Webb and *Hyptis pectinata* (L.) Poit. Infusions from Cape Verde. *Food Res. Int.* **2019**, *115*, 150–159. [CrossRef]
70. Miceli, N.; Trovato, A.; Dugo, P.; Cacciola, F.; Donato, P.; Marino, A.; Bellinghieri, V.; La Barbera, T.M.; Güvenç, A.; Taviano, M.F. Comparative Analysis of Flavonoid Profile, Antioxidant and Antimicrobial Activity of the Berries of *Juniperus communis* L. Var. *communis* and *Juniperus communis* L. Var. *Saxatilis* Pall. from Turkey. *J. Agric. Food Chem.* **2009**, *57*, 6570–6577. [CrossRef]
71. Ferron, L.; Colombo, R.; Mannucci, B.; Papetti, A. A New Italian Purple Corn Variety (Moradyn) Byproduct Extract: Antiglycative and Hypoglycemic In Vitro Activities and Preliminary Bioaccessibility Studies. *Molecules* **2020**, *25*, 1958. [CrossRef] [PubMed]
72. Rouzbehan, S.; Moein, S.; Homaei, A.; Moein, M.R. Kinetics of α-Glucosidase Inhibition by Different Fractions of Three Species of Labiatae Extracts: A New Diabetes Treatment Model. *Pharm. Biol.* **2017**, *55*, 1483–1488. [CrossRef] [PubMed]
73. OECD. *Test No. 471: Bacterial Reverse Mutation Test, OECD Guidelines for the Testing of Chemicals, Section 4;* OECD Publishing: Paris, France, 1997. Available online: http://www.oecd-ilibrary.org/environment/test-no-471-bacterial-reverse-mutation-test_9789264071247-en (accessed on 14 September 2021).
74. ICH International Conference on Harmonization (ICH). *Consensus Guideline S2(R1) Guidance on Genotoxicity Testing and Data Interpretation for Pharmaceuticals Intended for Human Use. Step 4 Version of November 2011*; ICH Guideline; ICH: Geneva, Switzerland, 2011.
75. Santos, J.M.; Camões, S.P.; Filipe, E.; Cipriano, M.; Barcia, R.N.; Filipe, M.; Teixeira, M.; Simões, S.; Gaspar, M.; Mosqueira, D.; et al. Three-Dimensional Spheroid Cell Culture of Umbilical Cord Tissue-Derived Mesenchymal Stromal Cells Leads to Enhanced Paracrine Induction of Wound Healing. *Stem Cell Res. Ther.* **2015**, *6*, 90. [CrossRef] [PubMed]

pharmaceuticals

MDPI

Article

Galangal–Cinnamon Spice Mixture Blocks the Coronavirus Infection Pathway through Inhibition of SARS-CoV-2 M^{Pro}, Three HCoV-229E Targets; Quantum-Chemical Calculations Support In Vitro Evaluation

Doaa G. El-Hosari [1,*], Wesam M. Hussein [1], Marwa O. Elgendy [2,3,*], Sara O. Elgendy [4], Ahmed R. N. Ibrahim [5], Alzhraa M. Fahmy [6], Afnan Hassan [7], Fatma Alzahraa Mokhtar [8], Modather F. Hussein [9,10], Mohamed E. A. Abdelrahim [11] and Eman G. Haggag [1]

1 Pharmacognosy Department, Faculty of Pharmacy, Helwan University, Cairo 11795, Egypt; ph.wesam95@gmail.com (W.M.H.); eman.g.haggag@pharm.helwan.edu.eg (E.G.H.)
2 Department of Clinical Pharmacy, Beni-Suef University Hospitals, Faculty of Medicine, Beni-Suef University, Beni-Suef 62521, Egypt
3 Department of Clinical Pharmacy, Faculty of Pharmacy, Nahda University (NUB), Beni-Suef 62513, Egypt
4 Clinical and Chemical Pathology Department, Faculty of Medicine, Beni-Suef University, Beni-Suef 62521, Egypt; drsaraosama88@med.bsu.edu.eg
5 Department of Clinical Pharmacy, College of Pharmacy, King Khalid University, Abha 61421, Saudi Arabia; aribrahim@kku.edu.sa
6 Tropical Medicine and Infectious Diseases Department, Faculty of Medicine, Beni-Suef University, Beni-Suef 62521, Egypt; alzhraamohamed@med.bsu.edu.eg
7 Biomedical Sciences Program, University of Science and Technology, Zewail City of Science and Technology, Cairo 12578, Egypt; t-afhassan@zewailcity.edu.eg
8 Department of Pharmacognosy, Faculty of Pharmacy, El Saleheya El Gadida University, El Saleheya El Gadida 44813, Egypt; fatma.mokhtar@sgu.edu.eg
9 Chemistry Department, Collage of Science, Jouf University, P.O. Box 2014, Sakaka 72388, Saudi Arabia; mfhussin@ju.edu.sa
10 Chemistry Department, Faculty of Science, Al-Azhar University, Asyut Branch, Assiut 71524, Egypt
11 Clinical Pharmacy Department, Faculty of Pharmacy, Beni-Suef University, Beni-Suef 62521, Egypt; mohamed.abdelrahim@pharm.bsu.edu.eg
* Correspondence: doaa.elhosari@pharm.helwan.edu.eg (D.G.E.-H.); marwa.elgendy@nub.edu.eg (M.O.E.)

Citation: El-Hosari, D.G.; Hussein, W.M.; Elgendy, M.O.; Elgendy, S.O.; Ibrahim, A.R.N.; Fahmy, A.M.; Hassan, A.; Mokhtar, F.A.; Hussein, M.F.; Abdelrahim, M.E.A.; et al. Galangal–Cinnamon Spice Mixture Blocks the Coronavirus Infection Pathway through Inhibition of SARS-CoV-2 M^{Pro}, Three HCoV-229E Targets; Quantum-Chemical Calculations Support In Vitro Evaluation. *Pharmaceuticals* **2023**, *16*, 1378. https://doi.org/10.3390/ph16101378

Academic Editors: Catherine Sherwin, Elena Y. Enioutina and Kathleen M. Job

Received: 29 June 2023
Revised: 17 September 2023
Accepted: 19 September 2023
Published: 28 September 2023

Abstract: Natural products such as domestic herbal drugs which are easily accessible and cost-effective can be used as a complementary treatment in mild and moderate COVID-19 cases. This study aimed to detect and describe the efficiency of phenolics detected in the galangal–cinnamon mixture in the inhibition of SARS-CoV-2's different protein targets. The potential antiviral effect of galangal–cinnamon aqueous extract (GCAE) against Low Pathogenic HCoV-229E was assessed using cytopathic effect inhibition assay and the crystal violet method. Low Pathogenic HCoV-229E was used as it is safer for in vitro laboratory experimentation and due to the conformation and the binding pockets similarity between HCoV-229E and SARS-CoV-2 M^{Pro}. The GCAE showed a significant antiviral effect against HCoV-229E (IC_{50} 15.083 μg/mL). Twelve phenolic compounds were detected in the extract with ellagic, cinnamic, and gallic acids being the major identified phenolic acids, while rutin was the major identified flavonoid glycoside. Quantum-chemical calculations were made to find molecular properties using the DFT/B3LYP method with 6-311++G(2d,2p) basis set. Quantum-chemical values such as EHOMO, ELUMO, energy gap, ionization potential, chemical hardness, softness, and electronegativity values were calculated and discussed. Phenolic compounds detected by HPLC-DAD-UV in the GCAE were docked into the active site of 3 HCoV-229E targets (PDB IDs. 2ZU2, 6U7G, 7VN9, and 6WTT) to find the potential inhibitors that block the Coronavirus infection pathways from quantum and docking data for these compounds. There are good adaptations between the theoretical and experimental results showing that rutin has the highest activity against Low Pathogenic HCoV-229E in the GCAE extract.

Keywords: galangal–cinnamon aqueous extract; SARS-CoV-2 M^{Pro}; antiviral assay; phenolic compounds; quantum-chemical methods

1. Introduction

The whole world has faced the coronavirus pandemic. This virus has infected millions of people and killed thousands [1]. It causes severe respiratory issues and multi-organ failure, where the mortality rate increases if the patient has a comorbid illness or is elderly [2,3]. At present, we do not have any available and affordable specific treatment for COVID-19. Consequently, the easiest way to avoid coronavirus is to prevent the possible causes and boost the body's immune response by eating nutritious meals with proper dietary consumption, such as fruits, vegetables, proteins, spices, and nuts [4,5].

Spices can be used to make herbal drinks that also serve as medicinal drinks, as they contain phytoconstituents that can minimize cell damage and reduce inflammation [6]. Because of the simplicity and ease of serving instant drinks, such as domestic herbal tea bags, they are currently in high demand among the general public. Recently, using herbal plants is favorable due to their fewer side effects and natural origin compared to drugs of chemical origin; they have anti-inflammatory, antipyretic, and antimicrobial properties, and they have secondary metabolites such as polyphenols, flavonoids, tannins, alkaloids, lignins, coumarins, stilbenes, and terpenoids [7,8]. Flavors and sweeteners could be added to herbal tea drinks to improve their taste and make them more appealing. As a result, we have decided to assess the consequences of using herbal tea in coronavirus patients with moderate illness and explore its effectiveness.

The application of virtual computational studies is considered the first obligatory step in the drug discovery field. The computational tools are time-saving, economically valuable, and are of high need in highly infectious diseases. The computational studies include molecular docking [9], molecular dynamics [10], quantum studies [11], and pharmacology networking [12]. These tools are able to discover new medical applications of existing drugs or natural products. The determination of possible pathways or involved genes can be performed through these virtual computational tools [13].

In this study, we selected galangal and cinnamon to be used as a mixture. According to recent studies, these two herbs are among some herbal plants that exert an antiviral effect on the Coronavirus family members [14]. The galangal (*Alpinia officinarum* Hance) (lesser galangal) rhizome belongs to the family Zingiberaceae, and cinnamon (*Cinnamomum verum* J.Presl) (Ceylon cinnamon) bark belongs to the family Lauraceae. In silico investigations have stated that these two herbs can inhibit the activity of Coronaviruses as they have various effective constituents such as flavonoids, essential oils, and terpenoids [15,16]. This research aims to evaluate the inhibitory and antiviral efficacy of a galangal–cinnamon mixture on the Coronavirus family and discover which of its major phenolic constituents contribute to these effects.

2. Results

2.1. Antiviral Effect of the Galangal–Cinnamon Aqueous Extract (GCAE) on Low Pathogenic Coronavirus (229E)

The galangal–cinnamon aqueous extract (GCAE) was tested to examine its inhibitory effect on Low Pathogenic Coronavirus HCoV-229E compared to remdesivir as a standard antiviral drug, using the cytopathic effect (CPE) inhibition assay and the crystal violet method [17,18]. The antiviral activities of the extract and the remdesivir standard were determined using a concentration range from 0.1 to 1000 µg/mL (10-fold dilutions). The development of the cytopathic effect was monitored by light microscopy and the 50% inhibitory concentration (IC_{50}) results were determined for both (see Table 1 and Figure 1).

Table 1. The antiviral activity of GCAE compared to remdesivir against HcoV-229E.

	The 50% Inhibitory Concentration (IC_{50}) μg/mL
GCAE	15.083
Remdesivir	8.76

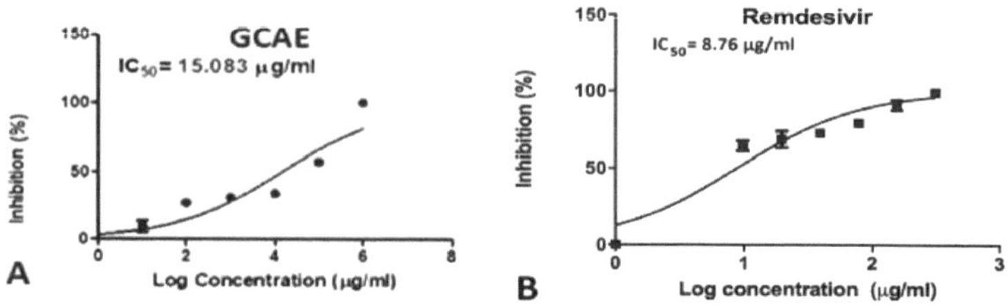

Figure 1. Inhibitory effects of GCAE (**A**) and remdesivir (**B**) on HCoV-229E. The IC_{50} value for each is inserted in each plot.

2.2. HPLC-UV Analysis of Phenolic Compounds in GCAE, Galangal Aqueous Extract (GAE), and Cinnamon Aqueous Extract (CAE)

HPLC-DAD-UV analysis was performed for the galangal–cinnamon extract (GCAE) and for cinnamon (CAE) and galangal (GAE) extracts individually at the same conditions against 19 phenolic standards to evaluate the effect of admixing and the major flavonoids and phenolic acids in the galangal–cinnamon mixture (Table 2, Figure 2). HPLC-DAD chromatograms of cinnamon and galangal extracts individually are illustrated in Figure 3

Table 2. HPLC-DAD analysis results of GCAE compared to GAE and CAE.

Cpd No.	RT (min)	Concentration (μg/g)			
		Phenolic Compounds	GCAE	CAE	GAE
1	3.32	Gallic acid	871.34	570.91	607.15
2	4.131	Chlorogenic acid	386.20	338.86	366.10
3	4.51	Catechin	140.10	1145.88	133.45
4	5.98	Methyl gallate	94.78	202.50	61.67
5	5.92	Coffeic acid	6.26	0.00	23.61
6	6.46	Syringic acid	68.35	51.77	48.43
7	6.67	Pyro catechol	0.00	0.00	0.00
8	7.76	Rutin	1293.35	123.13	2442.36
9	8.62	Ellagic acid	4057.01	64.08	7244.25
10	8.95	Coumaric acid	79.59	7.86	80.72
11	9.63	Vanillin	0.00	0.00	24.00
12	10.14	Ferulic acid	0.00	45.14	82.58
13	10.43	Naringenin	0.00	164.60	66.57
14	12.23	Daidzein	0.00	29.76	107.54
15	12.72	Quercetin	153.88	72.55	215.67
16	14.01	Cinnamic acid	1789.61	2153.55	63.39
17	14.49	Apigenin	0.00	0.00	7.77
18	15.00	Kaempferol	454.72	352.05	0.00
19	15.58	Hesperetin	0.00	0.00	20.81

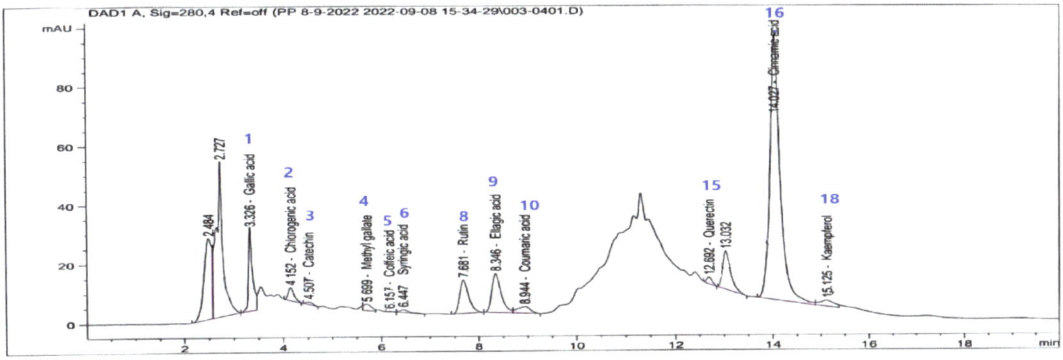

Figure 2. HPLC-DAD chromatogram of GCAE.

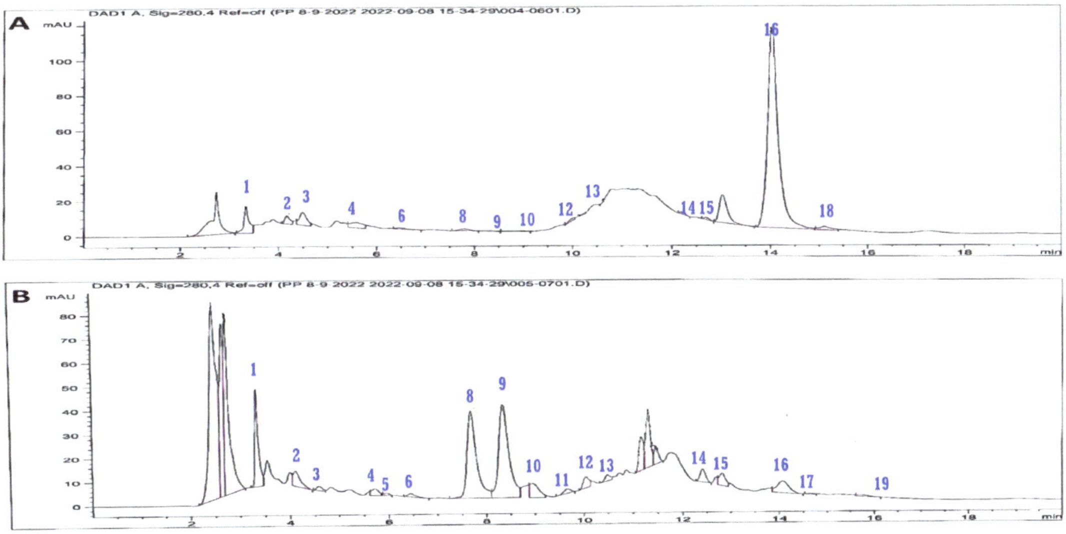

Figure 3. HPLC-DAD chromatograms of (**A**) CAE, (**B**) GAE.

2.3. Quantum-Chemical Calculations

Quantum-chemical calculations of the major detected phenolics in GCAE were made to find molecular properties. Quantum-chemical values such as EHOMO, ELUMO, energy gap (ΔE), ionization potential (I), chemical hardness (η), softness (σ), electronegativity (X), and hydrophobicity were calculated and listed in Table 3 using density functional theory (DFT), which predicts the molecular reactivity descriptors by Equations (1)–(8). Frontier molecular orbitals (HOMOs, LUMOs) of the GCAE detected phenolic compounds and the molecular electrostatic potential (MEP) surface are represented in Figure 4.

Table 3. Calculated quantum-chemical parameters of the detected phenolic compounds using the B3LYP/6-311++G(2d,2p) method.

Phenolic Cpds	ELUMO	EHOMO	ΔE	A	I	X	η	σ	ω
Rutin	−0.18509	−0.19474	0.00965	0.18509	0.19474	0.189915	0.004825	207.2539	7.475172
Chlorogenic acid	−0.17956	−0.20162	0.02206	0.17956	0.20162	0.19059	0.01103	90.66183	3.29325
Quercetin	−0.16462	−0.27037	0.10575	0.16462	0.27037	0.217495	0.052875	18.91253	0.89464
Kaempferol	−0.16468	−0.27157	0.10689	0.16468	0.27157	0.218125	0.053445	18.71082	0.890233
Coffeic acid	−0.17679	−0.28741	0.11062	0.17679	0.28741	0.2321	0.05531	18.07991	0.973972
Ellagic acid	−0.16152	−0.27310	0.11158	0.16152	0.2731	0.21731	0.05579	17.92436	0.846453
Coumaric acid	−0.17712	−0.29902	0.1219	0.17712	0.29902	0.23807	0.06095	16.40689	0.929899
Syringic acid	−0.15418	−0.28435	0.13017	0.15418	0.28435	0.219265	0.065085	15.36452	0.738682
Cinnamic acid	−0.18398	−0.31745	0.13347	0.18398	0.31745	0.250715	0.066735	14.98464	0.941905
Gallic acid	−0.15421	−0.28885	0.13464	0.15421	0.28885	0.22153	0.06732	14.85443	0.728989
Methyl gallate	−0.15393	−0.28880	0.13487	0.15393	0.2888	0.221365	0.067435	14.82909	0.726662
Catechin	−0.13643	−0.28986	0.15343	0.13643	0.28986	0.213145	0.076715	13.03526	0.592202

ELUMO energy of the lowest unoccupied molecular orbital, EHOMO energy of the highest occupied molecular orbital, ΔE HOMO–LUMO energy gap, A electron affinity, I ionization potential, X electronegativity, η chemical hardness, σ chemical softness, ω global electrophilicity.

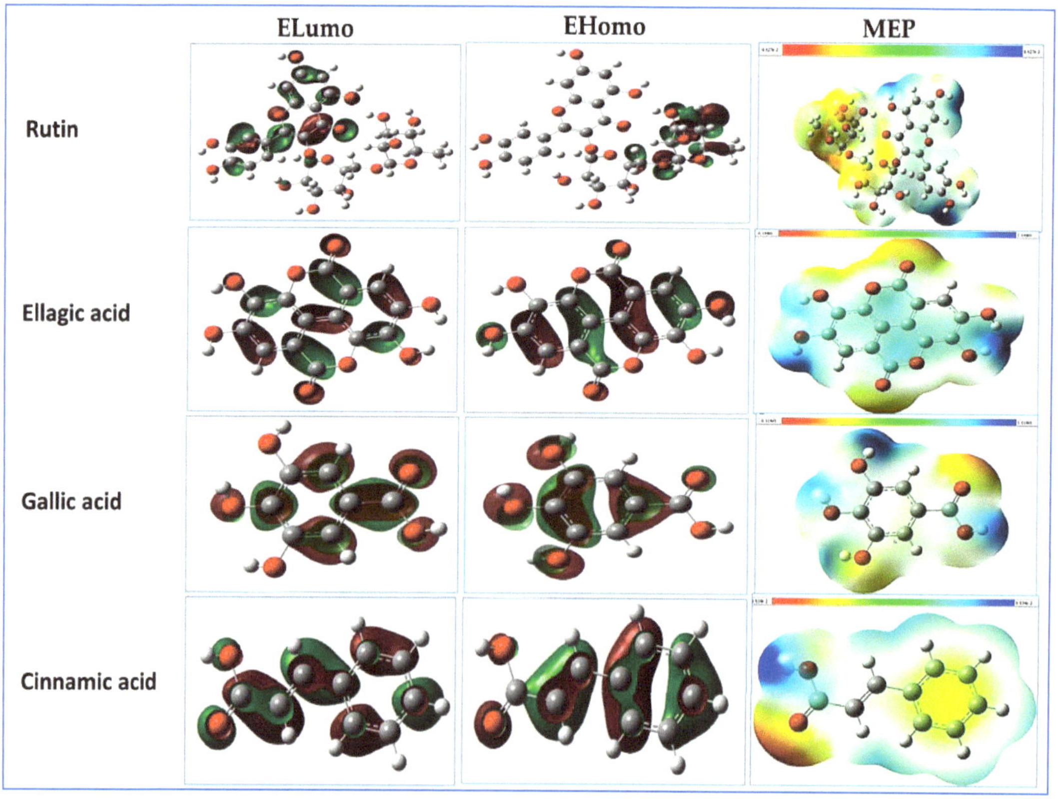

Figure 4. Frontier molecular orbitals (HOMOs, LUMOs) and molecular electrostatic potential (MEP) surface of the rutin, ellagic, gallic, and cinnamic acids by using the DFT/B3LYP/6-311++G(2d,2p) method.

The frontier molecular orbitals (FMO) of the detected phenolic compounds show that ELUMO and EHOMO represent the capacity of a compound to receive or donate electrons, respectively. DFT-based parameters have been calculated to estimate the reactivity of the detected compounds, where the reactivities of these compounds are arranged according to their activity. The highest active molecule was rutin with the lowest ΔE value and ionization potential. It is noted in this table that the energy gap between EHOMO and ELUMO of most bioactive molecules varies between 0.1 to 0.17, except for rutin and chlorogenic acid, which have higher activity of 0.00965 and 0.02206, respectively, and this is caused by the presence of a large number of (OH) phenolic groups in these two molecules. The hardness values of the phenolic compounds were calculated and are presented in Table 3; these range from 0.01 to 0.07 eV, except rutin, which has a value of 0.0048 eV, and this means that rutin is the softest and most active compound. The softness values of most phenolic compounds vary between 13 and 18 eV, except rutin and chlorogenic acid, which have the highest values. Overall, the activity of the galangal–cinnamon spice mixture can be predicted by its softness value, which is a whole number. Therefore, the activity of the mixture can be predicted by the following: Firstly, by collecting the experimental concentrations of each and dividing each one of them by the total, then multiplying by resulting the percentage of each component in relation to the total of 12 detected phenolic compounds. The next step involves multiplying each of these values by its softness value to produce a valuable effectiveness, then the effectiveness of each component is divided by the total to produce the quantum relative concentration. According to the hypothesis, softness values, and experimental concentrations, rutin shows the highest quantum relative concentration (61.95%), compared to the other phenolic compounds detected in the galangal–cinnamon aqueous extract. The data presented in Table 3 show a high reactivity characteristic of bioactive compounds that resulted from the presence of (OH) phenolic groups, which have a lone pair of electrons that act as a nucleophile and can interact with soft acceptor molecules (electrophile) as the coronavirus protein.

The EHOMO and ELUMO maps of the major molecules are shown in Figure 4 and the rest of the molecules are presented in Figure S1 in the supplementary file. The ELUMO and EHOMO map shows anti-bonding and bonding characteristics, from which it can be seen that the electron densities of the FMOs are more concentrated on the six-membered ring and attached by OH groups. These regions are assumed to be chemically active, in accordance with the frontier molecular orbital theory.

Electrostatic potential (ESP) suggests the molecules' electrophilic and nucleophilic nature, and it is an important tool to study the compounds reactivity nature. The maps of ESP at the surface are expressed by 17 distinct colors. The blue color stands for the highest amount of the positive region where the nucleophilic reaction occurs, and the reddish region indicates the negative region where the electrophilic reaction takes place, while zero potential is represented by the green color. The molecular electrostatic potential (ESP) of the bioactive molecules is shown in Figures 4 and S1. Most of the electron density is localized on the OH phenolic groups (active site), which act as nucleophiles. The ESPs show that the oxygen atoms of the hydroxyl group provide favorable sites for hard–hard interactions (Figures 4 and S1) between the nucleophile and the electrophile, which are active sites for electrophilic attacks. Accordingly, rutin has negative electrostatic potential as the highest active molecule compared to the others.

Quantum-chemical methods play an essential role in the molecular reactivity or stability determination. Reported researches revealed that FMO theory is effective in predicting interactive centers of molecules [19]. The methods used depend on measuring HOMO–LUMO energy gap (ΔE) and MEP and using DFT calculations [20]. MEP is utilized to outline the electrostatic interaction between a molecule and an atom.

2.4. Molecular Docking Studies

To find the potential target for GCAE phenolic extracts, a molecular docking study was carried out on three HCoV-229E targets: M^{pro}, RBD and spike glycoprotein, in addition to SARS-CoV-2 M^{pro}. The predicted binding energies of the 12 phenolic compounds in addition to remdesivir (positive control) on 2ZU2, 6U7G, 7VN9, and 6WTT active pockets are listed in Table 4. Rutin possesses the highest binding affinity among all GCAE extracts against the three targets, confirming our findings in quantum-chemical calculations that rutin is the most reactive compound.

Table 4. Docking ΔG scores of 12 phenolic compounds and remdesivir on 2ZU2, 6U7G, 7VN9, and 6WTT active pockets.

Cpd	ΔG (Kcal/mol)			
	2ZU2	6U7G	7VN9	6WTT
Remdesivir	−8.7640	−6.7442	−6.8270	−8.5391
Rutin	−7.6667	−7.0607	−6.7486	−8.5519
Chlorogenic acid	−5.9897	−5.3078	−5.0056	−6.8119
Quercetin	−5.7422	−5.1478	−4.9061	−6.1569
Kaempferol	−5.5863	−4.9378	−4.9439	−6.1614
Caffeic acid	−4.4261	−4.2180	−4.1875	−4.8618
Ellagic acid	−5.1831	−4.7615	−4.7619	−5.9172
Coumaric acid	−4.4789	−4.1064	−4.2298	−4.7411
Syringic acid	−4.7306	−4.4892	−4.6226	−5.1851
Cinnamic acid	−4.2583	−4.1707	−4.1572	−4.6575
Gallic acid	−4.3674	−3.9848	−4.0322	−4.5764
Methyl gallate	−4.4899	−4.2326	−4.3924	−4.8474
Catechin	−5.6074	−5.1583	−5.1000	−6.1628

Rutin was able to bind with HCoV-229E M^{pro} with a ΔG of −7.6667 Kcal/mol, which is approaching remdesivir's binding affinity (−8.7640 Kcal/mol). Moreover, rutin was able to form a large number of interactions with the M^{pro} pocket including nine H-bonds, a pi–pi, pi–anion, and pi–alkyl interactions with 10 different residues, as shown in Figure 5. Some of these residues are the same ones which interact with remdesivir, like Gly 142, ILE 164, and GLU 165. In addition to these residues, rutin was able to interact with M^{pro} catalytic dyad residues (HIS41/CYS144), two main reported residues for M^{pro} inhibition [21]. The remaining 11 phenolic extracts also reported good binding affinities but less than rutin towards inhibiting M^{pro} ($-4.2583 < \Delta G < -5.9897$) (Figures 4 and S2).

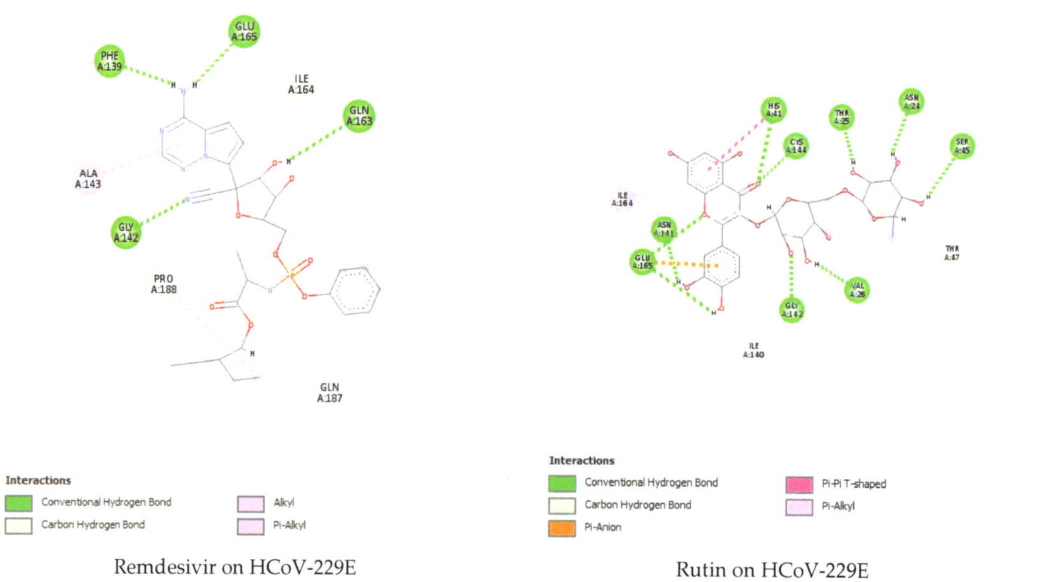

Figure 5. *Cont.*

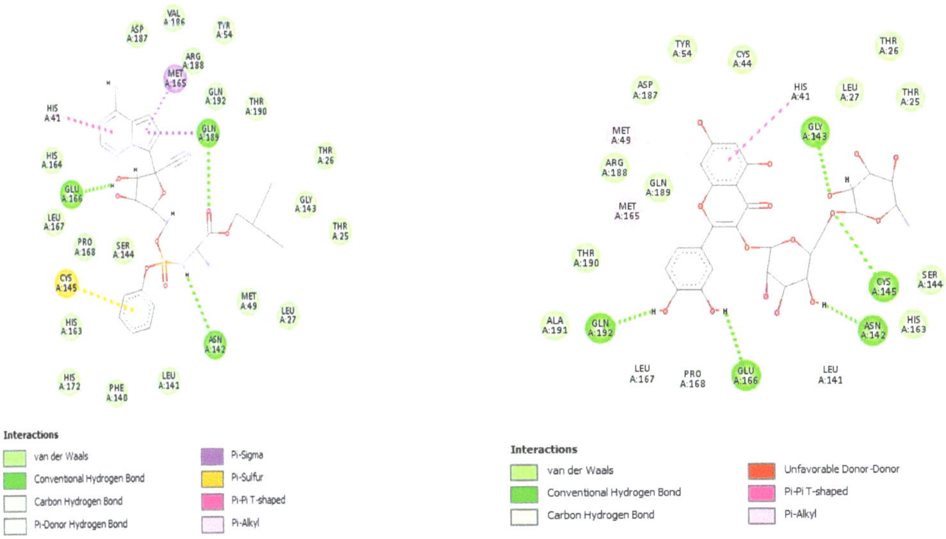

Remdesivir on SARS-CoV-2 Rutin on SARS-CoV-2

Figure 5. Two-dimensional interactions rutin (best hit) and remdesivir (positive control) docked on HCoV-229E and SARS-CoV-2 main protease.

For HCoV-229E RBD Class V, rutin reported a better binding score towards its active pocket than remdesivir's results ($\Delta G = -7.0607$ and -6.7442, respectively) (Table 4). It also binds to the RBD pocket with four H-bonds and two pi–pi stacking interactions, which is better than remdesivir, which forms only two H-bonds with RBD active residues (Figure S3). Likewise is the case with spike glycoprotein: Rutin was able to bind to spike glycoprotein with a very stable binding energy (−6.7486 Kcal/mol). It interacts with the same residues as remdesivir, like TYR 354, TYR 406, and ARG 350 (Figure S4). Like M^{pro}, all other GCAE phenolic extracts were able to block RBD and spike glycoprotein but with lower affinities (Figures S3 and S4). The second-best phenolic compound that was able to bind to the three targets is chlorogenic acid. This also confirms QC calculations where chlorogenic acid is reported to be the second most soft phenolic derivative due to the presence of a large number of (OH) groups.

The galangal–cinnamon spice mixture was also tested for its capability to block the Coronavirus infection pathway through the inhibition of SARS-CoV-2 M^{pro}, where they were docked against PDB ID 6WTT. The binding energies shown in Table 4 present similar energies for all compounds to those of HCoV-229E M^{pro}. This brings us to the 2D interactions of the best hit (rutin) and positive control (remdesivir) on the SARS-CoV-2 M^{pro} pocket and compare them to those of HCoV-229E M^{pro} (Figure 5). As shown in Figure 5, the key interactions are reserved in the four complexes, especially the catalytic dyad HIS 41/CYS 145, where rutin was also able to form five H-bonds with SARS-CoV-2 M^{pro} in addition to pi–pi stacking interaction. These very similar binding affinities and interactions prove our postulate that, despite the low (48%) homologs identity between SARS-CoV-2 and HCoV-229E (M^{pro}), the active pockets of both are of identical sequence, and hence, any detected hit on the less virulent one can also inhibit the SARS-CoV-2 protease.

3. Discussion

The COVID-19 pandemic is a serious global health concern, and finding new and effective ways to deal with its risks is critical. Natural products have become potential therapeutic alternatives for treating several diseases, such as viral infections, due to their innately high tolerance in the human body [22]. Galangal is very useful for its uses in food and medicine. It can be used for treating hemorrhoids, abdominal discomfort, abnormal menstruation, inflammation, metastatic breast cancer, and as an anti-aging agent [23]. Cinnamon has been used in cooking since centuries past and has a wide variety of culinary applications. It is a widely used spice that has been proven to be helpful in promoting health, owing to its specific properties. These characteristics could be beneficial in the treatment of a vast range of diseases, including cardiovascular disease, cancer, diabetes, and neurological issues. Cinnamon's properties and antioxidant activities are responsible for its medicinal benefits [24].

The galangal–cinnamon aqueous extract (GCAE) was tested to examine its inhibitory effect on Low Pathogenic Coronavirus HCoV-229E compared to remdesivir as a standard antiviral drug, using the cytopathic effect (CPE) inhibition assay and the crystal violet method. Given that the SARS-CoV-2 virus is fatal and cannot be assessed safely and easily in the laboratories, we chose the less pathogenic HCoV-229E to assess the extract's inhibitory activity. The identity of SARS-CoV-2's and HCoV-229E's main protease (M^{pro}) homologs is just about 48% according to the amino acid sequence alignment, with the binding sites being almost identical. This similarity remains true with respect to the conformation and binding pocket of the M^{pro} enzyme in both viruses [25]. The GCAE showed significant antiviral activity with IC_{50} equal to 15.083 µg/mL, almost half the antiviral potency of remdesivir (IC_{50}, 8.76 µg/mL). Remdesivir is an antiviral drug with potent broad-spectrum in vitro and in vivo antiviral activity against the COVID family [26,27].

HPLC-DAD-UV analysis of (GCAE), (CAE), and (GAE) revealed that ellagic, cinnamic, and gallic acids are the major identified phenolic acids in GCAE in concentrations of 4057.01, 1789.61, 871.34 µg/g, respectively, while rutin is the major flavonoid glycoside identified in a concentration of 1293.35 µg/g. Other phenolic compounds were not detected in GCAE, although they were detected in GAE or CAE individually. This may refer to the mixing effect, which could oxidize or reduce or form other chemical modifications such as chelation or precipitation due to compound–compound interactions and the mixture preparation technique.

We build the hypothesis at the expense of calculating the quantum relative concentration for each detected phenolic compound of the GCAE. Collecting the experimental concentrations of each compound and dividing each one of them by the total, then multiplying by 100, results in the percentage of each component in relation to the total of 12 detected phenolics. Multiplying each of these values by its softness value produces a valuable effectiveness, then the effectiveness of each component is divided by the total to produce the quantum relative concentration. According to the hypothesis, softness values, and experimental concentrations, rutin shows the highest quantum relative concentration (61.95%) compared to the other phenolic compounds detected in the galangal–cinnamon aqueous extract (Table 5).

Molecular docking was applied to predict the specific target of these detected phenolic compounds in the GCAE. Virtual screening on three potential targets HCoV-229E revealed that rutin is the main component responsible for GCAE inhibitory activity. Rutin possesses a very high affinity towards inhibiting M^{pro}, spike glycoprotein, and RBD [28,29]. These three main targets are essential for the entry and replications of SARS-CoV-2 via RBD blockage inhibiting RBD-hACE2 interaction and also inhibiting the viral main protease, which is involved in the viral replication. Therefore, identifying a natural product that can block these three targets at the same time is a win–win situation.

Table 5. The calculated activity of each detected phenolic compound in the GCAE using the softness value.

	Chemical Softness (σ)	Experimental Concentration μg/g	Experimental Concentration %	Activity	Activity %
Rutin	207.2539	1293.35	13.76609	2853.07515	61.95381
Chlorogenic acid	90.66183	386.2	4.110614	372.675792	8.092561
Quercetin	18.91253	153.88	1.6378 59	30.9760645	0.672637
Kaempferol	18.71082	454.72	4.839923	90.5589357	1.966464
Coffeic acid	18.07991	6.26	0.06663	1.2046615	0.026159
Ellagic acid	17.92436	4057.01	43.18178	774.005717	16.80734
Coumaric acid	16.40689	79.59	0.847136	13.8988607	0.30181
Syringic acid	15.36452	68.35	0.7275	11.1776871	0.242721
Cinnamic acid	14.98464	1789.61	19.04815	285.429689	6.198034
Gallic acid	14.85443	871.34	9.27432	137.76474	2.991527
Methyl gallate	14.82909	94.78	1.008814	14.9597949	0.324848
Catechin	13.03526	140.1	1.491189	19.4380308	0.422092

Phenolic compounds in natural medicinal plants offer various beneficial health effects such as antioxidant [30], anti-microbial [31], anti-inflammatory [32], as well as anti-carcinogenic effects. In addition to their proven role here as significant antivirals by the in silico studies carried out, phenolic compounds that are prominent in GCAE have been proved in the literature to exert other activities useful to assess COVID patients in recovery. Ellagic acid has antioxidant and anti-inflammatory effects that are considered as cofactors in the speed recovery of COVID patients [33]. Moreover, cinnamic acid modulates inflammatory cytokines in adipose tissue, the liver, the hypothalamus, and decreases TNF-α in serum [34]. Gallic acid is known for its strong free radical scavenging activities and anti-inflammatory properties; it has also shown immunomodulatory effects, as supported by a decrease in the inflammation cytokines and an increase of anti-inflammatory cytokines [35]. Additionally reported data stated that rutin has an immune regulatory effect, which can regulate cytokines and immune-related signaling pathways and cause a strong enhancement of antibody levels, increase immunoglobulin levels, and restore the functioning of leucocytes [36].

4. Materials and Methods

4.1. Collection of Medicinal Plants

Dried rhizomes of galangal and barks of cinnamon were purchased from a local spice shop in Cairo, Egypt, and identified by Prof. Loutfy M. Hassan, professor of Flora and Plant Ecology, Botany Department, Faculty of Science, Helwan University, Cairo, Egypt. A sample of each herb was assigned a voucher number, 28-Aof-3/2021 for galangal and 36-Cve-1/2021 for cinnamon, and kept in the herbarium of the Faculty of Pharmacy, Pharmacognosy Department, Helwan University, Cairo, Egypt. Powders of each sample were prepared by grinding to a suitable particle size and were stored in glass jars at room temperature in a dark, dry place until investigation. Pharmacognostic and microbiological quality control tests were carried out for the powders for safety and quality assurance.

4.2. Preparation of the Herbal Extracts

For the preparation of the galangal–cinnamon mixture aqueous extract, we followed the optimized easy-to-use at-home extraction protocol [37] to imitate the effect of domestic herbal mixture infusion. The herbal mixture (2.5 g galangal + 2.5 g cinnamon powders) was emptied into a 500 mL flask and extracted with de-ionized boiling water (250 mL), mixed well by manual rotation for 5 s, covered, and allowed to brew for 6–10 min. It was then filtered with Whatman No.1 filter paper, and the filtrate was concentrated and lyophilized to obtain the dry crude extract (325 mg). The galangal–cinnamon aqueous extract (GCAE) was stored in the dark at 4 °C for further investigation. Using the same procedure, galangal and cinnamon extracts were prepared separately starting with 2.5 g powder for each, yielding 117 mg galangal (GAE) and 93 mg cinnamon (CAE) aqueous extracts.

4.3. Antiviral Assay Using Low Pathogenic Coronavirus (229E)

The cytopathic effect (CPE) inhibition assay and the crystal violet method were applied to pinpoint the potential antiviral effect of GCAE against Low Pathogenic Coronavirus (229E) compared to remdesivir as a standard antiviral drug [38]. Coronavirus (229E) and Vero E6 cells were offered by Nawah-Scientific, Egypt. Vero E6 cells were grown in DMEM medium supplemented with 10% fetal bovine serum (Grand Island, NY, USA) and 0.1% antibiotic/antimycotic solution (Gibco BRL Thermo Fisher Scientific Inc., Waltham, MA, USA). The method, in brief, is as follows: Vero E6 cells at a density of 2×10^4 cells/well were bedded into a 96-well culture plate one day before infection. The next day, the culture medium was eliminated, and the cells were rinsed with phosphate-buffered saline (PBS). The infectivity of the Coronavirus was determined by employing the crystal violet method, which screened CPE and helped in the calculation of the percentage of cell viability. Virus suspension 229E (0.1 mL) containing cell culture infectious dose 50% CCID 50 (1.0×10^4) of virus stock was put on Vero E6 cells, as this selected dose gave the desired CPEs after two days of infection. Mediums (0.01 mL) each containing the GCAE and remdesivir concentrations were added to the cells. The antiviral activity of each sample was determined using a concentration range of 0.1–1000 µg/mL (10-fold dilutions). Control cells were used in the experiment (virus-infected, non-drug-treated cells) for virus controls and non-infected, non-drug-treated cells for cell controls. For 72 h, the culture plates were incubated at 37 °C in 5% carbon dioxide. The development of the CPE was tracked by light microscopy. After washing with PBS, the cell monolayers were fixed and stained with a 0.03% crystal violet solution in 2% ethanol and 10% formalin. The optical density of each well, after washing and drying, was quantified spectrophotometrically at 570/630 nm. The samples' antiviral activities percentage was calculated according to Pauwels et al., 1988 [18] using the following equation:

$$\text{Antiviral activity} = [\text{MOD of cell controls} - \text{MOD of virus controls} \\ (\text{MOD sample} - \text{MOD of virus controls})] \times 100\%.$$

$$\text{MOD} = \text{Mean Optical Density}.$$

The 50% CPE inhibitory dose (IC_{50}) was calculated based on these results. The 50% inhibitory concentration (IC_{50}) results were determined using Graph pad prism software version 8 (Graph-Pad Software, San Diego, CA, USA).

4.4. High-Performance Liquid Chromatography–Ultraviolet Analysis (HPLC-UV)

Phenolic compounds determination of the GCAE and of GAE and CAE separately were analyzed by the HPLC-DAD-UV technique, and separation was carried out on Eclipse C18 column on Agilent 1260 instrument. Phenolic compounds standards were purchased from Sigma Aldrich Merck, Darmstadt, Germany, Merck. Water (A) and 0.05% trifluoroacetic acid in acetonitrile (B) constituted the mobile phase at a flow rate of 0.9 mL/min. The elution was performed as follows: 0 min (82% A); 0–5 min. (80% A); 5–8 min. (60% A); 8–12 min. (60% A); 12–15 min. (82% A); 15–16 min. (82% A); and 16–20 (82%A) in a linear gradient. The multi-wavelength detector was monitored at 280 nm using a Diod array detector. The volume of injection for each of the sample solutions was 5 µL, and the column temperature was maintained at 40 °C.

4.5. Quantum-Chemical Calculations

Quantum-chemical calculations of the detected compounds were made to find molecular properties using the Gauss View 06 and Gaussian 09 program package [39,40]. EHOMO and ELUMO analysis, molecular structure, and MEP (Molecular Electrostatic Potential) of detected compounds were determined by using Becke–3–Lee Yang Parr (B3LYP) [41] using the DFT/B3LYP method with 6-311++G(d,p) basis set, and their 3D plots were verified with density functional theory (DFT) methods with 6-311++G(d,p) in the ground state. From the data obtained from the gauss view, the theoretical values for EHOMO, ELUMO, ΔE, electron affinity, ionization potential, softness, hardness, electronegativity, and hydrophobicity were calculated according to Oyewole et al., 2020 [42]. The quantum-chemical descriptors were calculated using Equations (1)–(8). Both physical and chemical properties of the molecules are intimately interrelated to the energy gap (ΔE, Equation (1)) [43,44]. One of the essential parameters of chemical reactivity is the ionization potential (Equation (2)). A high value of ionization potential demonstrates strong stability and low chemical activity, while a low value predicts the high activity of compounds [43]. In chemistry, the terms "hardness (η)" and "softness (σ)" are frequently employed to describe the stability of molecules. The concept of chemical hardness (Equation (3)), first used by Pearson in the 1960s, is the resistance of chemical species to electron cloud deformation or polarization [45]. Therefore, chemical hardness could be used to predict the stability of the molecules. A compound is referred to as hard if it has a significant energy gap, and as soft otherwise [46]. Accordingly, active molecules possess high softness and low hardness values (Equation (4)). Further, the chemical potential (μ) was calculated according to Equation (5). The electronegativity (χ) is considered as the negative value of μ (Equation (6)). In general, a compound with decreased electronegativity possesses a robust ability to donate electrons, resulting in more activity than a compound with a high electronegativity value. The susceptibility of the compound to accept electrons or electron density is indicated by the electronegativity as well [47] (Equation (7)). The electron affinity (A) can be considered as the negative value of E_{LUMO} [48]. Another important reactivity indicator for comparing compounds' potential to donate electrons is the global electrophilicity indicator (ω, Equation (8)) [49]. A strong electrophile has a significant electrophilicity value, whereas a strong nucleophile has a low electrophilicity value [50].

Equations:

$$\Delta E = \text{ELUMO} - \text{EHOMO} \tag{1}$$

$$I = -\text{EHOMO} \tag{2}$$

$$\eta = (1 - A)/2 \tag{3}$$

$$\sigma = 1/2\eta \tag{4}$$

$$\mu = -\chi \cong (\text{EHOMO} + \text{ELUMO})/2 \tag{5}$$

$$\chi = (I + A)/2 \tag{6}$$

$$A = -\text{ELUMO} \tag{7}$$

$$\omega = \mu 2/2\eta \tag{8}$$

All methods were carried out in accordance with relevant guidelines.

4.6. Molecular Docking Studies

Twelve phenolic compounds detected by HPLC-DAD-UV in the GCAE were tested in silico against 3 different targets of HCoV-229E in addition to the SARS-CoV-2 main protease to find out a potent target for them. Four crystal structures were chosen and procured from the PDB (Protein Data Bank), https://www.rcsb.org/, namely (accessed on 10 March 2023), PDB ID. 2ZU2 for HCoV-229E M^{pro}, PDB ID. 6U7G for HCoV-229E RBD

Class V, PDB ID. 7VN9 for HCoV-229E spike protein receptor-binding domain, and PDB ID. 6WTT for SARS-CoV-2 M^{pro}. Only the needed chains were kept and the receptor structures were prepared using Auto Dock Vina, where polar hydrogens were added and energy was minimized utilizing the prepare_receptor4.py command of the ADT. The receptors pockets were chosen for docking according to those reported in literature [51,52].

For the phenolic compound's chemical structures, a test set of the previously minimized structured obtained from QM step using the DFT was used and converted to PDBQT format via AutoDockTools (ADT, v1.5.6). Moreover, remdesivir was docked on the same target pockets as a positive control. The search engine used was the Lamarckian genetic algorithm with local search, with 100 runs and a population size of 150. To evaluate the docking results, ten conformers of the ligands were considered. Eventually, the conformer with the minimal binding free energy was evaluated and 2D interaction figures were generated via BIOVA Discovery Studio visualizer 2021.

5. Conclusions

The whole world has faced the Coronavirus pandemic, where hospitals were filled with critical cases and mild cases were sent home with the government routine protocol therapy and were remotely monitored. This study was designed to evaluate the effectiveness of some domestic herbs on COVID-19 and shed the light on the myth of whether they actually help or not. The galangal–cinnamon aqueous extract exerts a significant antiviral effect against HCoV-229E with IC_{50} equal to 15.083 μg/mL, almost half the antiviral potency of remdesivir. Among the twelve phenolic compounds detected in the mixture's aqueous extract, it was found that rutin showed the highest activity against HCoV-229E M^{pro}, RBD, spike glycoproteins, and SARS-CoV-2 M^{pro} when tested in silico.

From these findings, we conclude that this mixture with the same ratio can offer a domestic herbal tea to help mild COVID-19 patients to safely manage their manifestations.

Supplementary Materials: The following supporting information can be downloaded at: https://www.mdpi.com/article/10.3390/ph16101378/s1, Figure S1: Frontier molecular orbitals (HOMOs, LUMOs) and Molecular electrostatic potential (MEP) surface of all detected phenolic compounds by using DFT/B3LYP/6-311++G(2d,2p) method; Figure S2: 2D interactions 12 phenolic compounds of GCAE and Remdesivir docked on HCoV-229E M^{pro} (PDB ID: 2ZU2); Figure S3: 2D interactions 12 phenolic compounds of GCAE and Remdesivir docked on HCoV-229E RBD Class V (PDB ID: 6U7G); Figure S4: 2D interactions 12 phenolic compounds of GCAE and Remdesivir docked on HCoV-229E spike protein (PDB ID: 7VN9); Figure S5: 2D interactions 12 phenolic compounds of GCAE and Remdesivir docked on SARS-CoV-2 M^{pro} (PDB ID: 6WTT).

Author Contributions: Conceptualization, D.G.E.-H., E.G.H. and M.E.A.A.; methodology, W.M.H. and M.O.E.; formal analysis, W.M.H., M.O.E., S.O.E., A.R.N.I., A.M.F., F.A.M., A.H. and M.F.H.; investigation, W.M.H., M.O.E., S.O.E., A.R.N.I., A.M.F., F.A.M. and M.F.H.; resources, all authors; data curation, all authors; writing—original draft preparation, D.G.E.-H. and M.O.E.; writing—review and editing, all authors; visualization, all authors; supervision, all authors; project administration, all authors. All authors have read and agreed to the published version of the manuscript.

Funding: This research was funded by the Deanship of Scientific Research at King Khalid University through a large group Research Project under grant number (RGP2/145/44).

Institutional Review Board Statement: Not applicable.

Informed Consent Statement: Not applicable.

Data Availability Statement: Data are contained within the article and supplementary information file.

Acknowledgments: The King Khalid University Deanship of Scientific Research funded this work through a large group Research Project with grant number RGP2/145/44, for which the authors express their gratitude.

Conflicts of Interest: The authors declare no conflict of interest.

Abbreviations

(ΔE) EHOMO-ELUMO energy gap, (A) Electron affinity, (CAE) Cinnamon Aqueous Extract, (CCID 50). cell culture infectious dose 50%, (DFT) Density Function Theory, (EHOMO) Energy of the Highest Occupied Molecular Orbital, (ELUMO) Energy of the Lowest Unoccupied Molecular Orbital, (ESP) Electrostatic potential, (GAE) Galangal Aqueous Extract, (GCAE) Galangal–Cinnamon Aqueous Extract, (I) Ionization potential, (MEP) Molecular Electrostatic Potential, (PDB) Protein Data Bank, (X) Electronegativity, (η) Chemical hardness, (σ) Chemical softness, (ω) Global electrophilicity.

References

1. Dhawan, M.; Choudhary, O.P.; Saied, A.A. Russo-ukrainian war amid the COVID-19 pandemic: Global impact and containment strategy. *Int. J. Surg.* **2022**, *102*, 106675. [CrossRef]
2. Hui, D.S.; Azhar, E.I.; Madani, T.A.; Ntoumi, F.; Kock, R.; Dar, O.; Ippolito, G.; Mchugh, T.D.; Memish, Z.A.; Drosten, C. The continuing 2019-ncov epidemic threat of novel coronaviruses to global health—The latest 2019 novel coronavirus outbreak in wuhan, china. *Int. J. Infect. Dis.* **2020**, *91*, 264–266. [CrossRef] [PubMed]
3. Kumar, M.; Taki, K.; Gahlot, R.; Sharma, A.; Dhangar, K. A chronicle of SARS-CoV-2: Part-i-epidemiology, diagnosis, prognosis, transmission and treatment. *Sci. Total Environ.* **2020**, *734*, 139278. [CrossRef] [PubMed]
4. Elgendy, M.O.; El-Gendy, A.O.; Abdelrahim, M.E. Public awareness in egypt about COVID-19 spread in the early phase of the pandemic. *Patient Educ. Couns.* **2020**, *103*, 2598–2601. [CrossRef]
5. Losso, J.N.; Losso, M.N.; Toc, M.; Inungu, J.N.; Finley, J.W. The young age and plant-based diet hypothesis for low SARS-CoV-2 infection and COVID-19 pandemic in sub-saharan africa. *Plant Foods Hum. Nutr.* **2021**, *76*, 270–280. [CrossRef]
6. Purwidiani, N.; Kristiastuti, D.; Handajani, S.; Romadhoni, I.F.; Afifah, C.A.N.; Sutiadiningsih, A. Making instant spiced coffee drink to prevent COVID-19. In Proceedings of the International Joint Conference on Science and Engineering 2021 (IJCSE 2021), Online, 14 October 2021; Atlantis Press: Paris, France, 2021; pp. 40–45.
7. El-Hawary, S.S.; El-Hefnawy, H.M.; Osman, S.M.; Mostafa, E.S.; Mokhtar, F.; El-Raey, M. Chemical profile of two *Jasminum sambac* L. (ait) cultivars cultivated in egypt-their mediated silver nanoparticles synthesis and selective cytotoxicity. *Int. J. Appl. Pharm.* **2019**, *11*, 154–164. [CrossRef]
8. Hamed, E.M.; Ibrahim, A.R.N.; Meabed, M.H.; Khalaf, A.M.; El Demerdash, D.M.; Elgendy, M.O.; Saeed, H.; Salem, H.F.; Rabea, H. The Outcomes and Adverse Drug Patterns of Immunomodulators and Thrombopoietin Receptor Agonists in Primary Immune Thrombocytopenia Egyptian Patients with Hemorrhage Comorbidity. *Pharmaceuticals* **2023**, *16*, 868. [CrossRef]
9. El-Hawary, S.S.; El-Hefnawy, H.M.; El-Raey, M.A.; Mokhtar, F.A.; Osman, S.M. *Jasminum azoricum* L. Leaves: Hplc-pda/ms/ms profiling and in-vitro cytotoxicity supported by molecular docking. *Nat. Prod. Res.* **2021**, *35*, 5518–5520. [CrossRef] [PubMed]
10. Peele, K.A.; Durthi, C.P.; Srihansa, T.; Krupanidhi, S.; Ayyagari, V.S.; Babu, D.J.; Indira, M.; Reddy, A.R.; Venkateswarulu, T. Molecular docking and dynamic simulations for antiviral compounds against SARS-CoV-2: A computational study. *Inform. Med. Unlocked* **2020**, *19*, 100345. [CrossRef]
11. KUMER, A.; Sarker, M.N.; Sunanda, P. The theoretical investigation of homo, lumo, thermophysical properties and qsar study of some aromatic carboxylic acids using hyperchem programming. *Int. J. Chem. Technol.* **2019**, *3*, 26–37. [CrossRef]
12. Ahmed, S.R.; Al-Sanea, M.M.; Mostafa, E.M.; Qasim, S.; Abelyan, N.; Mokhtar, F.A. A network pharmacology analysis of cytotoxic triterpenes isolated from euphorbia abyssinica latex supported by drug-likeness and admet studies. *ACS Omega* **2022**, *7*, 17713–17722. [CrossRef] [PubMed]
13. Mohammed, M.H.H.; Hamed, A.N.E.; Elhabal, S.F.; Mokhtar, F.A.; Abdelmohsen, U.R.; Fouad, M.A.; Kamel, M.S. Chemical composition and anti-proliferative activities of hyophorbe lagenicaulis aerial parts and their biogenic nanoparticles supported by network pharmacology study. *S. Afr. J. Bot.* **2023**, *156*, 398–410. [CrossRef]
14. Ketabchi, S.; Papari Moghadamfard, M. Medicinal plants effective in the prevention and control of coronaviruses. *Complement. Med. J.* **2021**, *10*, 296–307. [CrossRef]
15. Prasanth, D.; Murahari, M.; Chandramohan, V.; Panda, S.P.; Atmakuri, L.R.; Guntupalli, C. In silico identification of potential inhibitors from cinnamon against main protease and spike glycoprotein of SARS CoV-2. *J. Biomol. Struct. Dyn.* **2021**, *39*, 4618–4632. [CrossRef] [PubMed]
16. Ou, R.; Lin, L.; Zhao, M.; Xie, Z. Action mechanisms and interaction of two key xanthine oxidase inhibitors in galangal: Combination of in vitro and in silico molecular docking studies. *Int. J. Biol. Macromol.* **2020**, *162*, 1526–1535. [CrossRef]
17. Vichai, V.; Kirtikara, K. Sulforhodamine b colorimetric assay for cytotoxicity screening. *Nat. Protoc.* **2006**, *1*, 1112–1116. [CrossRef]
18. Pauwels, R.; Balzarini, J.; Baba, M.; Snoeck, R.; Schols, D.; Herdewijn, P.; Desmyter, J.; De Clercq, E. Rapid and automated tetrazolium-based colorimetric assay for the detection of anti-hiv compounds. *J. Virol. Methods* **1988**, *20*, 309–321. [CrossRef]
19. Khaled, K.; Al-Qahtani, M. The inhibitive effect of some tetrazole derivatives towards al corrosion in acid solution: Chemical, electrochemical and theoretical studies. *Mater. Chem. Phys.* **2009**, *113*, 150–158. [CrossRef]
20. Bhattacharjee, D.; Devi, T.K.; Dabrowski, R.; Bhattacharjee, A. Birefringence, polarizability order parameters and dft calculations in the nematic phase of two bent-core liquid crystals and their correlation. *J. Mol. Liq.* **2018**, *272*, 239–252. [CrossRef]

21. Hassan, A.; Arafa, R.K. On the search for COVID-19 therapeutics: Identification of potential SARS-CoV-2 main protease inhibitors by virtual screening, pharmacophore modeling and molecular dynamics. *J. Biomol. Struct. Dyn.* **2022**, *40*, 7815–7828. [CrossRef]
22. Elgendy, M.O.; Saeed, H.; Abou-Taleb, H.A. Assessment of educated people awareness level and sources about COVID-19. *IJCMR* **2023**, *1*, 19–27. [CrossRef]
23. Das, G.; Patra, J.K.; Gonçalves, S.; Romano, A.; Gutiérrez-Grijalva, E.P.; Heredia, J.B.; Talukdar, A.D.; Shome, S.; Shin, H.-S. Galangal, the multipotent super spices: A comprehensive review. *Trends Food Sci. Technol.* **2020**, *101*, 50–62. [CrossRef]
24. da Silva, M.L.T.; Bernardo, M.A.S.; Singh, J.; de Mesquita, M.F. Beneficial uses of cinnamon in health and diseases: An interdisciplinary approach. In *The Role of Functional Food Security in Global Health*; Elsevier: Amsterdam, The Netherlands, 2019; pp. 565–576.
25. Carvalho, A.A.; dos Santos, L.R.; de Freitas, J.S.; de Sousa, R.P.; de Farias, R.R.S.; Júnior, G.M.V.; Rai, M.; Chaves, M.H. First report of flavonoids from leaves of machaerium acutifolium by di-esi-ms/ms. *Arab. J. Chem.* **2022**, *15*, 103765. [CrossRef]
26. Agostini, M.L.; Andres, E.L.; Sims, A.C.; Graham, R.L.; Sheahan, T.P.; Lu, X.; Smith, E.C.; Case, J.B.; Feng, J.Y.; Jordan, R. Coronavirus susceptibility to the antiviral remdesivir (gs-5734) is mediated by the viral polymerase and the proofreading exoribonuclease. *mBio* **2018**, *9*, e00221-18. [CrossRef]
27. Murphy, B.; Perron, M.; Murakami, E.; Bauer, K.; Park, Y.; Eckstrand, C.; Liepnieks, M.; Pedersen, N.C. The nucleoside analog gs-441524 strongly inhibits feline infectious peritonitis (fip) virus in tissue culture and experimental cat infection studies. *Vet. Microbiol.* **2018**, *219*, 226–233. [CrossRef]
28. Rahman, F.; Tabrez, S.; Ali, R.; Alqahtani, A.S.; Ahmed, M.Z.; Rub, A. Molecular docking analysis of rutin reveals possible inhibition of SARS-CoV-2 vital proteins. *J. Tradit. Complement. Med.* **2021**, *11*, 173–179. [CrossRef]
29. Deetanya, P.; Hengphasatporn, K.; Wilasluck, P.; Shigeta, Y.; Rungrotmongkol, T.; Wangkanont, K. Interaction of 8-anilinonaphthalene-1-sulfonate with SARS-CoV-2 main protease and its application as a fluorescent probe for inhibitor identification. *Comput. Struct. Biotechnol. J.* **2021**, *19*, 3364–3371. [CrossRef]
30. El-Hawary, S.S.; El-Hefnawy, H.M.; Osman, S.M.; El-Raey, M.A.; Mokhtar Ali, F.A. Phenolic profiling of different *Jasminum* species cultivated in egypt and their antioxidant activity. *Nat. Prod. Res.* **2021**, *35*, 4663–4668. [CrossRef]
31. Ajaiyeoba, E.; Fadare, D. Antimicrobial potential of extracts and fractions of the african walnut–tetracarpidium conophorum. *Afr. J. Biotechnol.* **2006**, *5*, 2322–2325.
32. Owoyele, B.V.; Adebukola, O.M.; Funmilayo, A.A.; Soladoye, A.O. Anti-inflammatory activities of ethanolic extract of carica papaya leaves. *Inflammopharmacology* **2008**, *16*, 168–173. [CrossRef] [PubMed]
33. Ding, Y.; Zhang, B.; Zhou, K.; Chen, M.; Wang, M.; Jia, Y.; Song, Y.; Li, Y.; Wen, A. Dietary ellagic acid improves oxidant-induced endothelial dysfunction and atherosclerosis: Role of nrf2 activation. *Int. J. Cardiol.* **2014**, *175*, 508–514. [CrossRef] [PubMed]
34. Lee, A.G.; Kang, S.; Im, S.; Pak, Y.K. Cinnamic acid attenuates peripheral and hypothalamic inflammation in high-fat diet-induced obese mice. *Pharmaceutics* **2022**, *14*, 1675. [CrossRef]
35. Liu, S.; Li, J.; Feng, L.H. Gallic acid regulates immune response in a mouse model of rheumatoid arthritis. *Immun. Inflamm. Dis.* **2023**, *11*, e782. [CrossRef] [PubMed]
36. Luo, M.; Sui, Y.; Tian, R.; Lu, N. Formation of a bovine serum albumin diligand complex with rutin for the suppression of heme toxicity. *Biophys. Chem.* **2020**, *258*, 106327. [CrossRef] [PubMed]
37. Cao-Ngoc, P.; Leclercq, L.; Rossi, J.-C.; Hertzog, J.; Tixier, A.-S.; Chemat, F.; Nasreddine, R.; Al Hamoui Dit Banni, G.; Nehmé, R.; Schmitt-Kopplin, P. Water-based extraction of bioactive principles from blackcurrant leaves and chrysanthellum americanum: A comparative study. *Foods* **2020**, *9*, 1478. [CrossRef]
38. Houghton, P.; Fang, R.; Techatanawat, I.; Steventon, G.; Hylands, P.J.; Lee, C. The sulphorhodamine (srb) assay and other approaches to testing plant extracts and derived compounds for activities related to reputed anticancer activity. *Methods* **2007**, *42*, 377–387. [CrossRef]
39. Ogliaro, F.; Bearpark, M.; Heyd, J.; Brothers, E.; Kudin, K.; Staroverov, V.; Kobayashi, R.; Normand, J.; Raghavachari, K.; Rendell, A. *Gaussian 09, Revision a. 02*; Gaussian. Inc.: Wallingford, CT, USA, 2009.
40. Janjua, M.R.S.A. All-small-molecule organic solar cells with high fill factor and enhanced open-circuit voltage with 18.25% pce: Physical insights from quantum chemical calculations. *Spectrochim. Acta Part A Mol. Biomol. Spectrosc.* **2022**, *279*, 121487. [CrossRef]
41. Tirado-Rives, J.; Jorgensen, W.L. Performance of b3lyp density functional methods for a large set of organic molecules. *J. Chem. Theory Comput.* **2008**, *4*, 297–306. [CrossRef]
42. Oyewole, R.O.; Oyebamiji, A.K.; Semire, B. Theoretical calculations of molecular descriptors for anticancer activities of 1, 2, 3-triazole-pyrimidine derivatives against gastric cancer cell line (mgc-803): Dft, qsar and docking approaches. *Heliyon* **2020**, *6*, e03926. [CrossRef]
43. Obot, I.; Obi-Egbedi, N.; Eseola, A. Anticorrosion potential of 2-mesityl-1h-imidazo [4, 5-f][1, 10] phenanthroline on mild steel in sulfuric acid solution: Experimental and theoretical study. *Ind. Eng. Chem. Res.* **2011**, *50*, 2098–2110. [CrossRef]
44. Obot, I.; Obi-Egbedi, N.; Ebenso, E.; Afolabi, A.; Oguzie, E.E. Experimental, quantum chemical calculations, and molecular dynamic simulations insight into the corrosion inhibition properties of 2-(6-methylpyridin-2-yl) oxazolo [5, 4-f][1, 10] phenanthroline on mild steel. *Res. Chem. Intermed.* **2013**, *39*, 1927–1948. [CrossRef]
45. Rauk, A. *Orbital Interaction Theory of Organic Chemistry*; John Wiley & Sons: Hoboken, NJ, USA, 2004.
46. Pearson, R.G. The principle of maximum hardness. *Acc. Chem. Res.* **1993**, *26*, 250–255. [CrossRef]

47. Özalp, A.; Kökbudak, Z.; Saracoglu, M.; Kandemirli, F.; Ilhan, I.Ö.; Vurdu, C.D. Synthesis and theoretical study of the novel 2-oxopyrimidin-1 (2h)-yl-amides derivative. *Chem. Sci. Rev. Lett.* **2015**, *4*, 719–728.
48. Pearson, R.G. Hard and soft acids and bases—The evolution of a chemical concept. *Coord. Chem. Rev.* **1990**, *100*, 403–425. [CrossRef]
49. Chattaraj, P.K.; Roy, D.R. Update 1 of: Electrophilicity index. *Chem. Rev.* **2007**, *107*, PR46–PR74. [CrossRef]
50. Ebenso, E.E.; Kabanda, M.M.; Arslan, T.; Saracoglu, M.; Kandemirli, F.; Murulana, L.C.; Singh, A.K.; Shukla, S.K.; Hammouti, B.; Khaled, K. Quantum chemical investigations on quinoline derivatives as effective corrosion inhibitors for mild steel in acidic medium. *Int. J. Electrochem. Sci.* **2012**, *7*, 5643–5676. [CrossRef]
51. Shahhamzehei, N.; Abdelfatah, S.; Efferth, T. In silico and in vitro identification of pan-coronaviral main protease inhibitors from a large natural product library. *Pharmaceuticals* **2022**, *15*, 308. [CrossRef]
52. Fuochi, V.; Floresta, G.; Emma, R.; Patamia, V.; Caruso, M.; Zagni, C.; Ronchi, F.; Ronchi, C.; Drago, F.; Rescifina, A. Heparan sulfate and enoxaparin interact at the interface of the spike protein of hcov-229e but not with hcov-oc43. *Viruses* **2023**, *15*, 663. [CrossRef]

pharmaceuticals

MDPI

Article

Synergistic Antihyperglycemic and Antihyperlipidemic Effect of Polyherbal and Allopolyherbal Formulation

Yahya Alhamhoom [1], Syed Sagheer Ahmed [2,*], Rupesh Kumar M. [3], MD. Salahuddin [4], Bharathi D. R. [2], Mohammed Muqtader Ahmed [5], Syeda Ayesha Farhana [6] and Mohamed Rahamathulla [1,*]

1 Department of Pharmaceutics, College of Pharmacy, King Khalid University, Al Faraa, Abha 62223, Saudi Arabia; ysalhamhoom@kku.edu.sa
2 Department of Pharmacology, Sri Adichunchanagiri College of Pharmacy, Adichunchanagiri University, BG Nagara, Mandya 571448, India; rambha.eesh@gmail.com
3 Department of Pharmacology, Alameen College of Pharmacy, Bengalore 560027, India; manirupeshkumar@yahoo.in
4 Department of Chemistry, Alameen College of Pharmacy, Bengalore 560027, India; rcsalahuddin@alameenpharmacy.edu
5 Department of Pharmaceutics, College of Pharmacy, Prince Sattam Bin Abdul Aziz University, Al Kharj 11942, Saudi Arabia; muqtadernano@psau.edu.sa
6 Department of Pharmaceutics, Unaizah College of Pharmacy, Qassim University, Unaizah 51911, Saudi Arabia; a.farhana@qu.edu.sa
* Correspondence: sysaha6835@gmail.com (S.S.A.); rahapharm@gmail.com (M.R.)

Abstract: Polyherbal formulation (PHF) enhances therapeutic efficacy and minimizes side effects by reducing individual herb dosages. Allopolyherbal formulation (APHF) combines polyherbal extracts with allopathic medication, effectively reducing the latter's required dose and mitigating associated adverse effects. The current study intends to assess the anti-diabetic effects of PHF and APHF *in-vivo*. Dried raw powders of *Cassia auriculata* leaf, *Centella asiatica* leaf, and *Zingiber officinale* rhizome were extracted by cold maceration process using 70% ethanol. These extracts were combined in three different ratios to make PHF. PHF was subjected to qualitative and quantitative phytochemical investigations. APHF has been prepared by combining a potent ratio of PHF with metformin in three different ratios. The compatibility of APHF has been confirmed by differential scanning calorimetry (DSC). In vivo activity was also evaluated in streptozotocin-induced diabetic albino rats. PHF (3 different ratios at a dose of 200–400 mg/kg b.w), APHF (combination of PHF and metformin in 3 different ratios, 200 + 22.5, 200 + 45, and 200 + 67.5 mg/kg b.w), and metformin (90 mg/kg b.w) were administered to albino rats for 21 consecutive days. Blood glucose levels were estimated on the 1st, 7th, 14th, and 21st days of treatment. On the 21st day, blood was collected by cardiac puncture for biochemical analysis. The liver and pancreas were isolated and subjected to histopathological analysis. PHF and APHF showed significant anti-diabetic and antihyperlipidemic efficacy. In comparison to PHF, APHF had the most promising action. The current study demonstrated that PHF and APHF are safe and efficacious drugs in the treatment of diabetes mellitus as they help to replace or lower the dose of metformin, thereby decreasing the risks of metformin.

Keywords: allopolyherbal; diabetes; polyherbal; streptozotocin; rat; in vivo

Citation: Alhamhoom, Y.; Ahmed, S.S.; M., R.K.; Salahuddin, M.; D. R., B.; Ahmed, M.M.; Farhana, S.A.; Rahamathulla, M. Synergistic Antihyperglycemic and Antihyperlipidemic Effect of Polyherbal and Allopolyherbal Formulation. *Pharmaceuticals* **2023**, *16*, 1368. https://doi.org/10.3390/ph16101368

Academic Editors: Catherine Sherwin, Elena Y. Enioutina and Kathleen M. Job

Received: 18 August 2023
Revised: 12 September 2023
Accepted: 21 September 2023
Published: 27 September 2023

1. Introduction

Diabetes mellitus (DM) is a metabolic disorder characterized by disturbances in glucose, protein, and lipid metabolism. It is caused by either a lack of insulin secretion (T1DM) or a decreased sensitivity of the tissues to insulin (T2DM). In 2021, the worldwide prevalence of diabetes among individuals aged 20 to 79 stood at 537 million, with projections indicating an anticipated increase to 783 million by the year 2045 [1]. Diabetes canbe managed with exercise, dietary restrictions, insulin injections, and the use of oral hypoglycemic medicines [2].

Herbal remedies have risen in popularity in recent years due to their safety, efficacy, and affordability when compared to synthetic therapies. Polyherbal formulations (PHF) are made up of two or more herbs. The concept of polyherbalism appeared in Ayurvedic literature (Sharangdhar Samhita) in1300 AD. A polyherbal composition boosts medicinal efficacy while limiting side effects by lowering the concentration of individual herbs in a mixture [3]. Allopolyherbal formulation (APHF) is a polyherbal formulation combined with an allopathic drug [4]. The major goal of combining allopathic drugs and herbs is to reduce the adverse effects of allopathic drugs. Most allopathic drugs have one or more side effects. As a consequence, combining polyherbs with allopathic therapy removes or reduces the unfavorable effects of allopathic medications. Allopolyherbal formulations are much more efficient and effective in the case of chronic or long-term diseases or issues [5].

Metformin is a member of the biguanideclass of oral hypoglycemic agents that operates by reducing hepatic gluconeogenesis and increasing tissue insulin sensitivity. Metformin side effects include nausea, vomiting, metallic taste, diarrhea, anorexia, and a variety of other gastrointestinal issues. Biguanides may increase the risk of lactic acidosis in those who have a history of alcoholism, kidney disease, liver disease, cardiovascular disease, chronic cardiopulmonary disease, pregnancy, and breastfeeding. By reducing the dose of metformin, such side effects can be reduced or avoided. However, lowering the dose of metformin is still a difficult approach, but it may help to mitigate the unfavorable effects as much as possible [6]. Incorporating a minimal dose of metformin into allopolyherbal formulation (APHF) results in a remarkably potent reduction in blood glucose levels, equivalent to the impact achieved by higher doses of metformin when administered on its own. The primary advantages of this research proposal lie in the potential to mitigate unwanted side effects and reduce the required dosage of allopathic medication, particularly metformin, by substituting it with PHF or APHF.

Cassia auriculata L. (CAr), often known as "Tanner's Cassia" (Ceasalpinaceae), is a medicinal plant found across India [7]. CAr leaves have long been used to treat ulcers, liver problems, jaundice, diabetes, and leprosy. It also possesses antispasmodic, antiviral, and antidiarrheal properties [8,9]. *Centella asiatica* (CAs) is a common Indian herb (Umbelliferae family). It has historically been used to treat a wide range of CNS disorders, such as schizophrenia, cognitive impairment, and epilepsy. It is also used to treat asthma, leprosy, jaundice, hepatitis, diarrhea, syphilis, and smallpox [10,11]. Ginger, or *Zingiber officinale* (ZO), is an underground rhizome of the Zingiberaceae family [12]. It is a nutritional supplement that is used to treat a wide range of diseases, including asthma, cough, indigestion, anorexia, and constipation [13].

Cassia auriculata, *Centella asiatica*, and *Zingiber officinale* have all been reported to lower blood glucose levels [14–16]. Despite the fact that each of these plants has potent anti-diabetic potential on its own, there is no conclusive evidence that the polyherbal formulation (a combination of *Cassia auriculata*, *Centella asiatica*, and *Zingiber officinale*) and the allopolyherbal formulation (a combination of polyherbal formulation and metformin) have a synergistic anti-diabetic effect.

Hence, the goal of the current investigation is to evaluate the antihyperglycemic and antihyperlipidemic effects of polyherbal and allopolyherbal formulations in streptozotocin-induced diabetic rats.

2. Results and Discussions

2.1. Phytochemical Analysis of Polyherbal Formulation (PHF)

Phytochemical analysis showed the presence of carbohydrates, proteins, alkaloids, glycosides, phenolic compounds, flavonoids, tannins, sterols, saponins, and terpenoids in PHF.

2.2. Quantitative Estimation of Total Phenolic, Flavonoid, and Tannins Content in PHF

2.2.1. Total Phenolic Content

The total phenolic content (TPC) of gallic acid and PHF was 968.42 ± 2.34 and 756.98 ± 3 ± 1.21 mg GAE/g of dry extract, respectively. PHF contains a high concentration of phenolic components.

2.2.2. Total Flavonoid Content

Catechin and PHF had a total flavonoid content (TFC) of 976.48 ± 3.714 and 464.18 ± 4.32 mg CAE/g of dry extract, respectively. It indicates a high level of flavonoid content in PHF.

2.2.3. Total Tannin Content

Catechin and PHF exhibited a total tannin content (TTC) of 477.26 ± 3.65 and 103.51 ± 4.84 mg CAE/g of dry extract, respectively. The quantity of tannins is lower in PHF.

2.3. Compatibility Study by Differential Scanning Calorimetry (DSC)

The DSC findings on metformin, polyherbal extract, and allopolyherbal formulation within the firstweek of their preparation are presented in Table 1 and Figures 1–3. The DSC curves show that there is no overlapping, interference, or significant change in the peaks between metformin and extracts. As a result, metformin may be compatible with plant extracts.

Table 1. DSC data of polyherbal extract and allopolyherbal formulation.

SL. NO	MATERIALS	PEAK (°C)	ONSET (°C)	ENDSET (°C)	HEAT (mJ)
1	Metformin (Figure 1)	244.2	234.7	251.4	−2.0
2	Polyherbal extract (Figure 2)	128.5	117.1	142.2	−607.5
3	Allopolyherbal formulation (Polyherbal + metformin) (Figure 3)	132.4 224.4	124.7 225.7	103.5 232.1	−299.7 −608.5

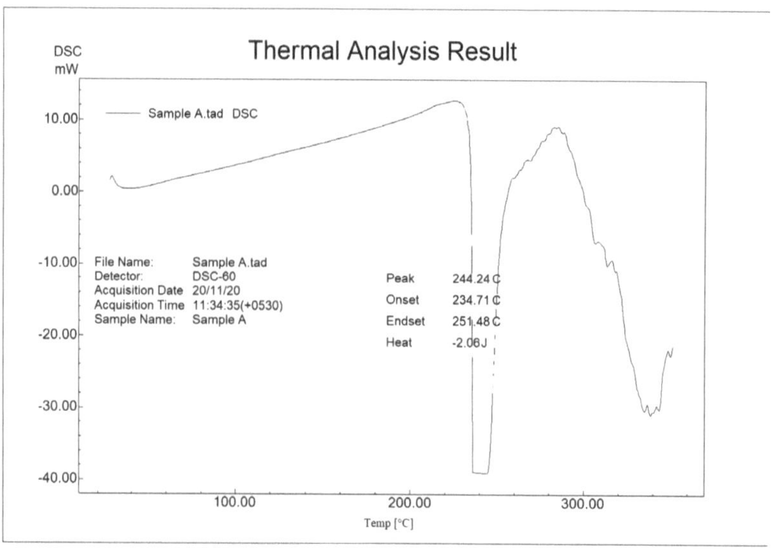

Figure 1. DSC curve of metformin.

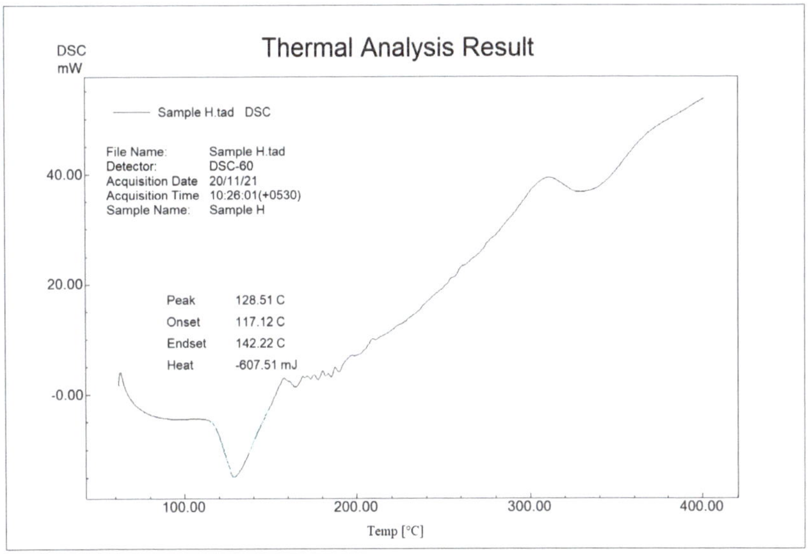

Figure 2. DSC curve of polyherbal extract.

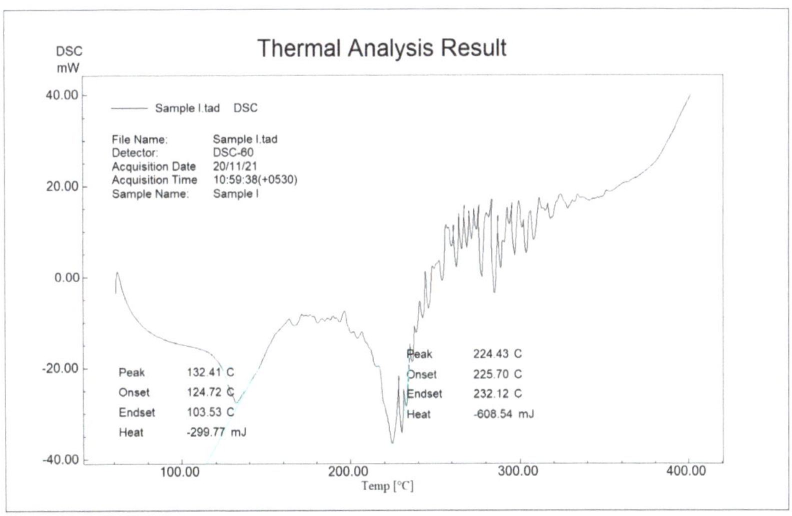

Figure 3. DSC curve of allopolyherbal extract.

2.4. Acute Toxicity Study of Polyherbal Formulation (PHF)

PHF did not show any drug-induced physical symptoms of toxicity, and no fatalities were recorded up to the dose of 2000 mg/kg body weight.

2.5. In Vivo Antidiabetic and Antihyperlipidemic Activity

Group I rats were considered normal and were simply given a vehicle (2.5% acacia arabica). Freshly prepared streptozotocin at a dosage of 55 mg/kg b.w was delivered intraperitoneally into group II and deemed as diabetic control.

Polyherbal formulations A, B, and C (PHF A, PHF B, and PHF C) were developed by combining CAr, CAs, and ZO in the following ratios: 1:1:1, 2:21, and 2:1:2. PHF A wasgiven to groups III and IV at doses of 200 mg/kg b.w. and 400 mg/kg b.w., respectively. PHF B was given to groups V and VI at doses of 200 and 400 mg/kg b.w., respectively. PHF C was administered to rats in groups VII (200 mg/kg b.w.) and VIII (400 mg/kg b.w.).

APHF wasmade by mixing PHF B (which is thought to be more significant than PHF A and C) with metformin in three distinct ratios. Groups IX, X, and XI received APHF A (PHF 200 mg/kg b.w + metformin 22.5 mg/kg b.w), APHF B (PHF 200 mg/kg b.w + metformin 45mg/kg b.w), and APHF C (PHF 200 mg/kg b.w + metformin 67.5mg/kg b.w). Group XII wasgiven a standard medication metformin at a dose of 90 mg/kg b.w.

All diabetic rats were given treatment for 21 consecutive days by oral approach. Variations in blood glucose levels and body weight were noted on the 1st, 7th, 14th, and 21st days of therapy. Total cholesterol (TC), triglycerides (TG), low density lipoproteins (LDL), very lowdensity lipoproteins (VLDL), highdensity lipoproteins (HDL), serum glutamate oxaloacetate transaminase (SGOT), serum glutamate pyruvate transaminase (SGPT), alkaline phosphatase (ALP), glycated hemoglobin (HbA1c), serum urea, creatinine, total protein, albumin, and total and differential white blood cell (WBC) count wereestimated on 21st day of treatment. The results are presented in Tables 2–7 and Figures 4–7.

From a mechanistic perspective, the notable antidiabetic activity observed in this study can be ascribed to several pivotal factors. The sustained decrease in blood glucose levels over the course of treatment signifies enhanced glycemic control. It potentially arises from increased insulin secretion, restoration of beta cells within the pancreatic islets, improved glucose utilization by peripheral tissues, and inhibition of alpha-amylase and alpha-glucosidase enzymes. Additionally, the positive alterations in lipid profile parameters, such as decreased total cholesterol (TC), triglycerides (TG), LDL, and VLDL, along with an increase in HDL, suggest a potential mechanism for the formulation's lipid-lowering effects. The normalization of liver enzyme levels (SGOT, SGPT, and ALP) reflects its hepatoprotective properties, while the reduction in HbA1c underscores its ability to manage long-term glucose regulation. Moreover, the maintenance of kidney function markers (serum urea and creatinine) and the preservation of total protein, albumin, and white blood cell counts indicate the formulation's systemic and renoprotective influence. These comprehensive findings collectively support the polyherbal formulation's multifaceted mechanisms for effectively managing diabetes and its associated complications.

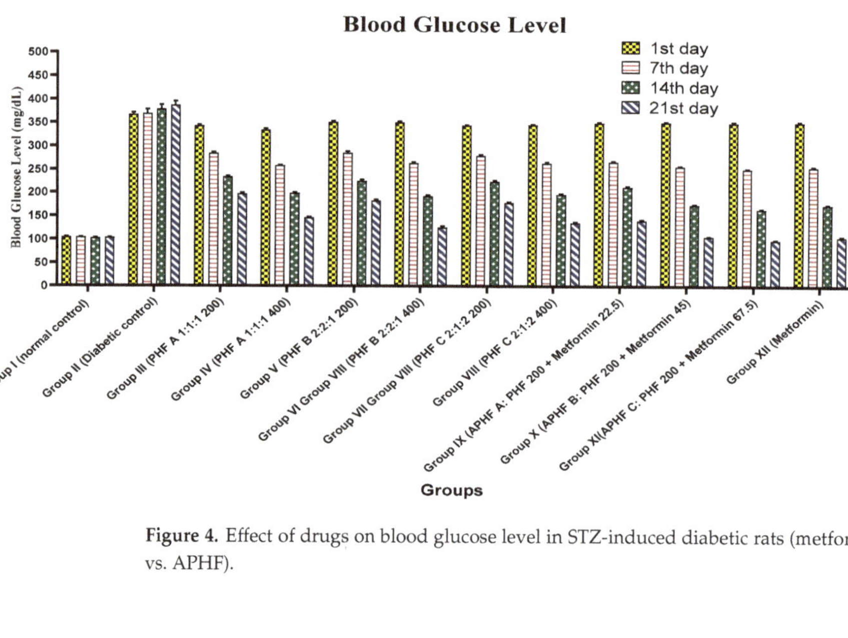

Figure 4. Effect of drugs on blood glucose level in STZ-induced diabetic rats (metformin vs. PHF vs. APHF).

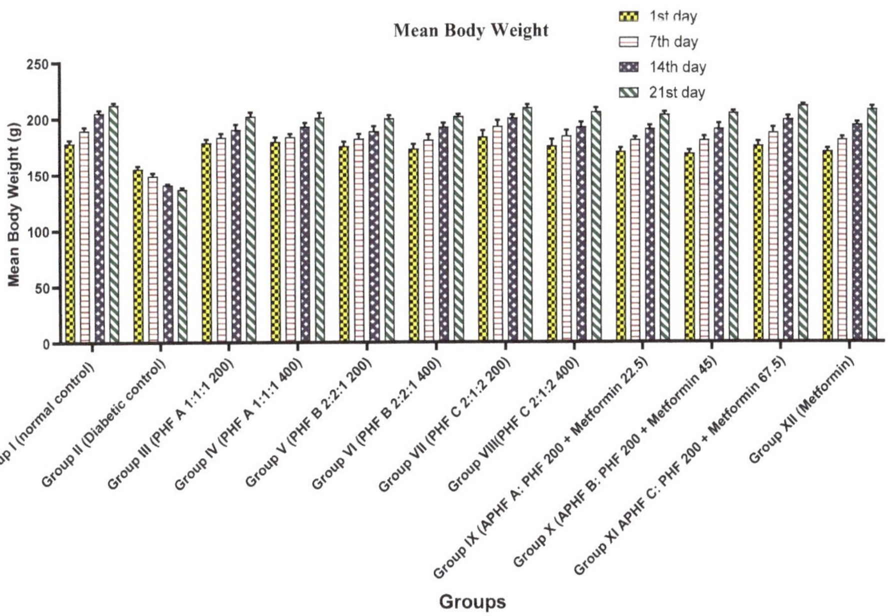

Figure 5. Effect of drugs on body weight (g) in STZ-induced diabetic rats (metformin vs. PHF vs. APHF).

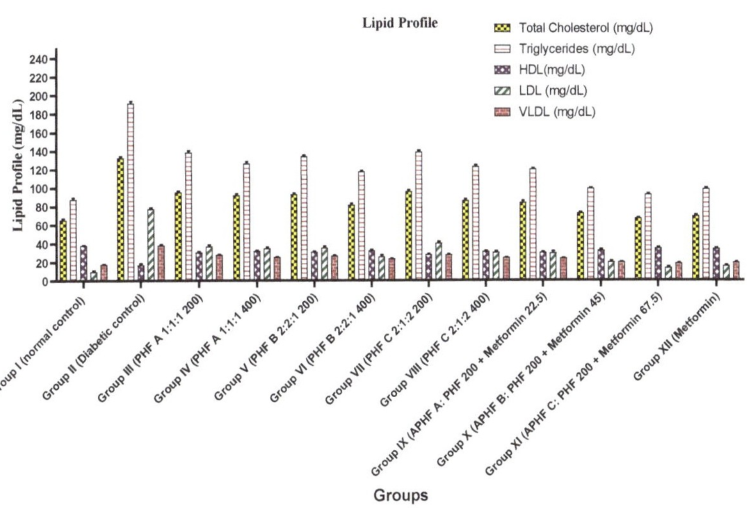

Figure 6. Effect of drugs on lipid profile in STZ-induced diabetic rats (metformin vs. PHF vs. APHF).

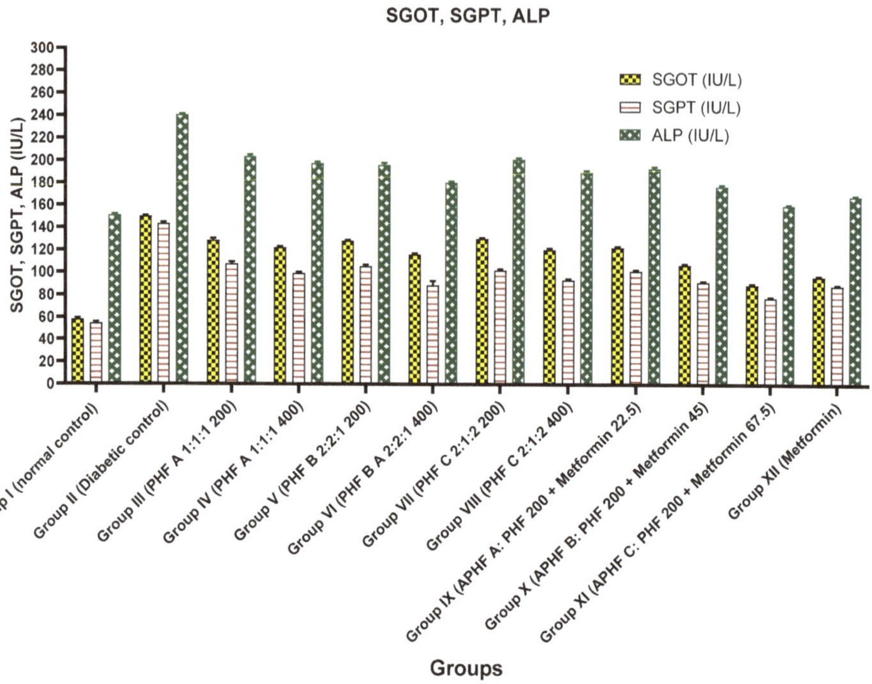

Figure 7. Effect of drugs on SGPT, SGOT, and ALP levels in STZ-induced diabetic rats (metformin vs. PHF vs. APHF).

Table 2. Effect of drugs on blood glucose level in STZ-induced diabetic rats (metformin vs. PHF vs. APHF).

Group	Blood Glucose Levels (mg/dL) (Mean ± SEM)			
	1st Day	**7th Day**	**14th Day**	**21st Day**
Group I (Normal control)	103.8 ± 1.6	103.6 ± 0.7	102.0 ± 0.9	103.0 ± 1.0
Group II (Diabetic control)	366.6 ± 4.6	368.8 ± 9.5	378.3 ± 9.2	386.6 ± 8.8
Group III (PHF A 1:1:1 200)	342.5 ± 2.6 *	284.5 ± 2.1 ***	233.8 ± 2.1 ***	196.6 ± 2.4 ***
Group IV (PHF A 1:1:1 400)	333.6 ± 3.0 *	258.1 ± 1 ***	198.5 ± 1.8 ***	146.0 ± 2.0 ***
Group V (PHF B 2:2:1 200)	351.0 ± 2.5 *	285.0 ± 3.5 ***	225.0 ± 3.2 ***	182.1 ± 2.8 ***
Group VI (PHF B 2:2:1 400)	350.1 ± 2.4 *	263.5 ± 2.07 ***	191.8 ± 2.9 ***	125.3 ± 3.2 ***
Group VII (PHF C 2:1:2 200)	343.5 ± 1.7 *	279.1 ± 2.7 ***	224.5 ± 2.0 ***	178.0 ± 2.3 ***
Group VIII (PHF C 2:1:2 400)	345.0 ± 1.7 *	263.5 ± 2.1 ***	195.8 ± 2.8 ***	135.5 ± 2.1 ***
Group IX APHF A	349.6 ± 1.8 *	266.3 ± 2.0 ***	212.6 ± 1.8 ***	140.3 ± 2.2 ***
Group X APHF B	351 ± 1.1 *	256.1 ± 1.3 ***	174.1 ± 1.3 ***	105.8 ± 0.9 ***
Group XI APHF C	349.3 ± 2.2 *	250.8 ± 1.4 ***	164.3 ± 1.5 ***	98.3 ± 1.3 ***
Group XII (Metformin)	350.8 ± 1.7 *	255.5 ± 1.1 ***	173.8 ± 1.49 ***	105.3 ± 1.4 ***

Values are expressed as mean ± SEM, (n = 6); $p < 0.05$ (*), $p < 0.001$ (***) compared to diabetic animals (two-way ANOVA followed by a Dunnett's *t*-test). *p*-values < 0.05 were considered statistically significant.

Table 3. Effect of drugs on body weight (g) in STZ-induced diabetic rats (metformin vs. PHF vs. APHF).

Group	Mean Body Weight (g) (Mean ± SEM)			
	1st Day	7th Day	14th Day	21st Day
Group I (Normal control)	178.1 ± 2.7	189.5 ± 2.7	205 ± 2.6 ***	212 ± 2.0 ***
Group II (Diabetic control)	155.1 ± 2.6	149 ± 2.3	140.5 ± 0.8 ***	136.5 ± 1.5 ***
Group III (PHF A 1:1:1 200)	178.3 ± 3.0 ***	183.3 ± 3.3 ***	190 ± 4.6 ***	201.8 ± 3.7 ***
Group IV (PHF A 1:1:1 400)	179.1 ± 4.1 ***	183.5 ± 2.8 ***	192.5 ± 3.5 ***	200.8 ± 4.1 ***
Group V (PHF B 2:2:1 200)	175 ± 4.2 **	181.6 ± 4.3 ***	188.5 ± 4.3 ***	199.6 ± 2.9 ***
Group VI (PHF B 2:2:1 400)	172.5 ± 4.4 **	180.8 ± 4.8 ***	192.1 ± 3.6 ***	201.6 ± 1.8 ***
Group VII (PHF C 2:1:2 200)	183.1 ± 5.8 ***	192.5 ± 5.4 ***	200.1 ± 2.8 ***	209.1 ± 3.0 ***
Group VIII (PHF C 2:1:2 400)	175 ± 6.1 **	184.1 ± 5.0 ***	192 ± 4.4 ***	205.5 ± 3.6 ***
Group IX APHF A	170 ± 3.6 **	180.5 ± 2.8 ***	190.3 ± 3.0 ***	203 ± 2.5 ***
Group X APHF B	168.3 ± 3.0 **	180.3 ± 3.4 ***	190.5 ± 4.6 ***	204.3 ± 2.0 ***
Group XI APHF C	175 ± 4.2 **	187 ± 4.6 ***	198.5 ± 3.4 ***	211 ± 1.3 ***
Group XII (Metformin)	170 ± 2.8 *	180.8 ± 2.5 ***	193.6 ± 2.7 ***	207.5 ± 2.8 ***

Values are expressed as mean ± SEM, (n = 6); $p < 0.05$ (*), $p < 0.01$ (**), $p < 0.001$ (***) compared to diabetic animals (two-way ANOVA followed by a Dunnett's t-test). p-values < 0.05 were considered statistically significant.

Table 4. Effect of drugs on lipid profile in STZ-induced diabetic rats (metformin vs. PHF vs. APHF).

Group	Lipid Profile (mg/dL)				
	TC	TG	HDL	LDL	VLDL
Group I (Normal control)	65.3 ± 1.5 ***	87.6 ± 1.7 ***	38 ± 0.3 ***	9.8 ± 1.1 ***	17.5 ± 0.3 ***
Group II (Diabetic control)	132.8 ± 1.3 ***	191.6 ± 2.0 ***	17.1 ± 1.1 ***	77.3 ± 1.2 ***	38.3 ± 0.4 ***
Group III (PHF A 1:1:1 200)	95.3 ± 1.3 ***	138.6 ± 1.6 ***	30.6 ± 0.4 ***	36.9 ± 1.3 ***	27.7 ± 0.3 ***
Group IV (PHF A 1:1:1 400)	91.8 ± 1.3 ***	126.1 ± 1.9 ***	32 ± 0.3 ***	34.6 ± 1.1 ***	25.2 ± 0.3 ***
Group V (PHF B 2:2:1 200)	93 ± 0.9 ***	134 ± 1.3 ***	30.8 ± 0.6 ***	35.3 ± 1.4 ***	26.8 ± 0.2 ***
Group VI (PHF B 2:2:1 400)	81.6 ± 1.3 ***	117.6 ± 0.7 ***	32.3 ± 0.5 ***	25.8 ± 1.8 ***	23.5 ± 0.1 ***
Group VII (PHF C 2:1:2200)	96 ± 1.2 ***	139 ± 1.3 ***	28 ± 0.6 ***	40.2 ± 1.3 ***	27.8 ± 0.2 ***
Group VIII (PHF C 2:1:2400)	86.1 ± 1.1 ***	122.8 ± 1.4 ***	31.3 ± 0.4 ***	30.2 ± 0.8 ***	24.5 ± 0.2 ***
Group IX APHF A	83.8 ± 1.6 ***	120 ± 0.9 ***	30.1 ± 0.4 ***	29.6 ± 1.8 ***	24 ± 0.1 ***
Group XAPHF B	72.3 ± 0.8 ***	99 ± 0.5 ***	32.5 ± 1.0 ***	20.0 ± 1.0 ***	19.8 ± 0.1 ***
Group XI APHF C	66.8 ± 0.6 ***	92.5 ± 0.7 ***	34.6 ± 0.7 ***	13.6 ± 1.0 ***	18.5 ± 0.1 ***
Group XII (Metformin)	69.5 ± 0.9 ***	98.3 ± 0.8 ***	34.1 ± 0.7 ***	15.6 ± 1.0 ***	19.6 ± 0.1 ***

Values are expressed as mean ± SEM, (n = 6); $p < 0.001$ (***) compared to diabetic animals (two-way ANOVA followed by a Dunnett's t-test). p-values < 0.05 were considered statistically significant.

Table 5. Effect of drugs on SGPT, SGOT andALP levels in STZ-induced diabetic rats (metformin vs. PHF vs. APHF).

Group	SGOT Level (IU/L)	SGPT Level (IU/L)	ALP Level (IU/L)
Group I (Normal control)	58 ± 1.2	54.3 ± 1.5	150.3 ± 1.3
Group II (Diabetic control)	149.8 ± 0.7	143.1 ± 1.2	240.3 ± 0.8
Group III (PHF A 1:1:1 200)	128.3 ± 1.9 ***	107.1 ± 2.0 ***	203.1 ± 1.8 ***
Group IV (PHF A 1:1:1 400)	121.8 ± 1.2 ***	99.2 ± 0.8 ***	197.1 ± 1.4 ***
Group V (PHF B 2:2:1 200)	128.1 ± 0.7 ***	105.3 ± 1.4 ***	195.8 ± 1.9 ***
Group VI (PHF B 2:2:1 400)	115.8 ± 1.1 ***	88.3 ± 4.1 ***	179.8 ± 0.9 ***
Group VII (PHF C 2:1:2 200)	129.8 ± 1.0 ***	102 ± 1.0 ***	200.8 ± 1.3 ***
Group VIII (PHF C 2:1:2 400)	120.3 ± 1.3 ***	93.1 ± 1.2 ***	189.6 ± 1.4 ***
Group IX APHF A	122.3 ± 1.1 ***	101.5 ± 0.9 ***	192.8 ± 1.7 ***
Group X APHF B	106.8 ± 1.1 ***	91.6 ± 0.6 ***	176.5 ± 1.6 ***
Group XI APHF C	89 ± 1.1 ***	77.5 ± 0.7 ***	159.8 ± 0.7 ***
Group XII (Metformin)	96.4 ± 0.9 ***	88.3 ± 1.0 ***	168 ± 0.9 ***

Values are expressed as mean ± SEM, (n = 6); $p < 0.001$ (***) compared to diabetic animals (two-way ANOVA followed by a Dunnett's *t*-test). *p*-values < 0.05 were considered statistically significant.

Table 6. Effect of drugs on leucocyte indices in STZ-induced diabetic rats (metformin vs. PHF vs. APHF).

Group	Leucocytes 10^3/Cumm	Neutrophils (%)	Lymphocytes (%)	Monocytes (%)	Eosinophils (%)
Group I (Normal control)	10.0 ± 0.1	61.1 ± 0.4	33.1 ± 0.6	4.1 ± 0.3	1.5 ± 0.4
Group II (Diabetic control)	5.2 ± 0.1	63.8 ± 0.5	29.8 ± 0.7	4.5 ± 0.4	1.8 ± 0.3
Group III (PHF A 1:1:1 200)	6.7 ± 0.1 ns	62 ± 0.8 ns	32 ± 0.6 *	4.3 ± 0.3 ns	1.6 ± 0.3 ns
Group IV (PHF A 1:1:1 400)	7.8 ± 0.1 **	62 ± 0.9 ns	32.5 ± 0.8 **	4.3 ± 0.3 ns	1.1 ± 0.3 ns
Group V (PHF B 2:2:1 200)	6.4 ± 0.1 ns	62.1 ± 0.7 ns	32.1 ± 0.7 *	4.1 ± 0.4 ns	1.5 ± 0.5 ns
Group VI (PHF B 2:2:1 400)	7.7 ± 0.1 **	61.5 ± 0.6 *	32.5 ± 0.7 **	4.3 ± 0.3 ns	1.6 ± 0.4 ns
Group VII (PHF C 2:1:2 200)	6.5 ± 0.0 ns	62.1 ± 0.8 ns	32.3 ± 0.9 **	4.1 ± 0.3 ns	1.3 ± 0.4 ns
Group VIII (PHF C 2:1:2 400)	7.9 ± 0.0 **	61.5 ± 0.4 *	33.3 ± 0.7 ***	4.1 ± 0.4 ns	1 ± 0.4 ns
Group IX APHF A	6.8 ± 0.0 ns	61.1 ± 0.4 **	34 ± 0.2 ***	4.1 ± 0.4 ns	0.6 ± 0.2 ns
Group X APHF B	7.1 ± 0.0	62.1 ± 0.4 ns	32.5 ± 0.6 ***	4.1 ± 0.5 ns	1.1 ± 0.4 ns
Group XI APHF C	7.9 ± 0.1 **	62.5 ± 0.7 ns	32 ± 0.6 ***	4 ± 0.5 ns	1.5 ± 0.4 ns
Group XII (Metformin)	8.0 ± 0.0 ***	62.3 ± 0.9 ns	32 ± 0.6 *	4.1 ± 0.4 ns	1.5 ± 0.4 ns

Values are expressed as mean ± SEM, (n = 6); $p < 0.05$ (*), $p < 0.01$ (**), $p < 0.001$ (***), ns (non-significant) compared to diabetic animals (two-way ANOVA followed by a Dunnett's *t*-test). *p*-values < 0.05 were considered statistically significant.

Table 7. Effect of drugs on HbA1c, serum urea, creatinine, total protein, and albumin in STZ-induced diabetic rats (metformin vs. PHF vs. APHF).

Group	HbA1c (%)	Urea (mg/dL)	Creatinine (mg/dL)	Total Protein (g/dL)	Albumin (mg/dL)
Group I (Normal control)	5.2 ± 0.0	29.3 ± 1.1	0.8 ± 0.0	7.3 ± 0.1	5.4 ± 0.0
Group II (Diabetic control)	15.0 ± 0.3	47.3 ± 0.6	2.0 ± 0.0	4.5 ± 0.0	2.9 ± 0.0
Group III (PHF A 1:1:1 200)	8.4 ± 0.0 ***	36.3 ± 1.0 ***	1.1 ± 0.0 ns	6.1 ± 0.0 *	3.7 ± 0.0 ns
Group IV (PHF A 1:1:1 400)	6.7 ± 0.0 ***	36.3 ± 0.8 ***	0.9 ± 0.0 ns	6.5 ± 0.0 **	4.0 ± 0.0 ns
Group V (PHF B 2:2:1 200)	7.9 ± 0.0 ***	38.1 ± 0.5 ***	1.2 ± 0.0 ns	6.2 ± 0.0 *	4.0 ± 0.4 ns
Group VI (PHF B 2:2:1 400)	5.9 ± 0.1 ***	34.1 ± 1.0 ***	1.1 ± 0.0 ns	6.4 ± 0.0 **	4.1 ± 0.0 ns
Group VII (PHF C 2:1:2 200)	7.8 ± 0.0 ***	38.6 ± 0.8 ***	1.2 ± 0.0 ns	5.8 ± 0.0 ns	3.8 ± 0.0 ns
Group VIII (PHF C 2:1:2 400)	6.3 ± 0.0 ***	32.3 ± 0.6 ***	1.0 ± 0.0 ns	6.1 ± 0.0 *	4.0 ± 0.0 ns
Group IX APHF A	6.5 ± 0.0 ***	33.1 ± 0.9 ***	1.0 ± 0.0 ns	6.1 ± 0.0 *	4.1 ± 0.0 ns
Group X APHF B	5.3 ± 0.0 ***	34.5 ± 0.7 ***	0.9 ± 0.0 ns	6.3 ± 0.0 **	4.4 ± 0.0 *
Group XI APHF C	5.0 ± 0.0 ***	29.8 ± 1.0 ***	0.8 ± 0.0 ns	6.8 ± 0.0 ***	4.8 ± 0.0 **
Group XII (Metformin)	5.2 ± 0.0 ***	30.3 ± 0.8 ***	0.9 ± 0.0 ns	6.7 ± 0.0 **	4.6 ± 0.1 *

Values are expressed as mean ± SEM, (n = 6); $p < 0.05$ (*), $p < 0.01$ (**), $p < 0.001$ (***), ns (non-significant) compared to diabetic animals (two-way ANOVA followed by a Dunnett's *t*-test). *p*-values < 0.05 were considered statistically significant.

2.5.1. Effect on Blood Glucose Level

Table 2 and Figure 4 show the effects of PHF (A, B, and C), APHF (A, B, and C), and metformin on blood sugar levels in streptozotocin-induced diabetic rats. Blood glucose levels were determined in normal and diabetic rats on the 1st, 7th, 14th, and 21st days of therapy. Untreated diabetic rats had much higher glucose levels than control rats. Oral treatment of PHF A, B, and C at 200 and 400 mg/kg b.w, APHF A, B, and C, and the standard medicine metformin at 90 mg/kg b.w resulted in a substantial reduction in blood glucose levels ($p < 0.05$) in a dose- and time-dependent manner. APHF was the most active of the test samples, followed by PHF. Among all PHFs, PHF B had the most noticeable outcomes, while among APHFs, APHF C had the most prominent activity. As compared to metformin, APHF C was considerably more effective in lowering blood glucose levels.

2.5.2. Effect on Bodyweight

Table 3 and Figure 5 show the differences in body weight between treatment groups. From day 1 to day 21, the diabetes control group's body weight was dramatically lowered. Nonetheless, it is worth noting that the animals' body weight was greatly restored after treatment with PHF, APHF, and metformin in a time- and dose-dependent manner.

2.5.3. Effect on Lipid Profile

Table 4 and Figure 6 illustrate the effects of PHF (A, B, and C), APHF (A, B, and C), and metformin on the lipid profile in streptozotocin-induced diabetic rats. On the 21st day, diabetic control rats had significantly higher levels of TC, TG, LDL, VLDL, and lower levels of HDL. Similar changes in the lipid profile were avoided in the treatment groups and brought closer to normal dosage dependently. Metformin produced the best outcomes, followed by APHF and finally PHF. PHF B produced the most notable outcomes among all PHF, while APHF C produced the most notableactivity. Nonetheless, it is worth noting that the improvements in lipid profile are greater in APHF C than metformin.

2.5.4. Effect on SGOT, SGPT, and ALP Levels

Table 5 and Figure 7 show the levels of blood enzymes such as SGOT, SGPT, and ALP in diabetic rats treated with PHF, APHF, and metformin. When diabetic control rats were compared to normal rats, the activity of these enzymes was dramatically elevated. On the 21st day of therapy, diabetic rats were given various doses of PHF, APHF, and metformin, and blood enzymes were considerably reduced in a dose-dependent manner.

The sequence of drug potency is APHF C > metformin > APHF B> APHFA > PHF B> PHF C > PHF A.

2.5.5. Effect on Total and Differential White Blood Cell Count

The total and differential WBC counts of rats treated with PHF, APHF, and metformin were compared to those of normal and diabetic control groups of rats to determine the capacity of the medications to maintain normal WBC counts, and the findings are shown in Table 6.

Diabetic control rats had a significantly lower total leucocyte count. However, in the therapy group, the fall in WBC count was avoided. The WBC count was greater in all treatment groups when compared to the diabetes control group. Metformin improved WBC count recovery more than APHF and PHF. There were no significant differences in differential WBC count; however, the proportion of lymphocytes was reduced in diabetic control rats and prevented in treatment groups.

2.5.6. Effect on HbA1c, Urea, Creatinine, Total Protein, and Albumin

Table 7 shows the effects of PHF (A, B, and C), APHF (A, B, and C), and metformin on HbA1c, urea, creatinine, total protein, and albumin. Diabetic rats' serum contained significantly higher levels of urea, creatinine, and HbA1c, as well as lower levels of total protein and albumin. Serum urea level and HbA1c% decreased significantly in the therapy group. Serum creatinine levels are also reduced, but not dramatically. Total protein and albumin levels in the serum of the treated rat group increased as well, although these variations were not statistically significant.

PHF at 400 mg/kg b.w, metformin, and APHF exhibit a substantial rise in total protein (A, B, and C). Albumin levels increased significantly withAPHF B, C, and metformin.

2.5.7. Histopathological Studies of Liver Cells

Normal control rats had a normal liver histoarchitecture. The hepatic parenchyma and sinusoids seemed normal, with normal Kupffer cell distribution. The livers of diabetic rats displayed necrotic changes, dilatation of the liver sinusoids, Kupffer cell activation, and cytoplasmic vacuolization of hepatocytes. Periportal inflammation, periportal infiltration, pykontic nuclei, and periportal fatty infiltration were also seen. Diabetic rats given metformin, PHF, or APHF had various degrees of augmentation. The liver of the metformin-treated group exhibited mild degenerative changes, moderate hepatic sinusoid dilatation, mild periportal inflammation, and a slightly greater number of Kupffer cells. The treated group's liver histoarchitecture was more or less normal, with only minimal necrotic alterations and degeneration (Figure 8).

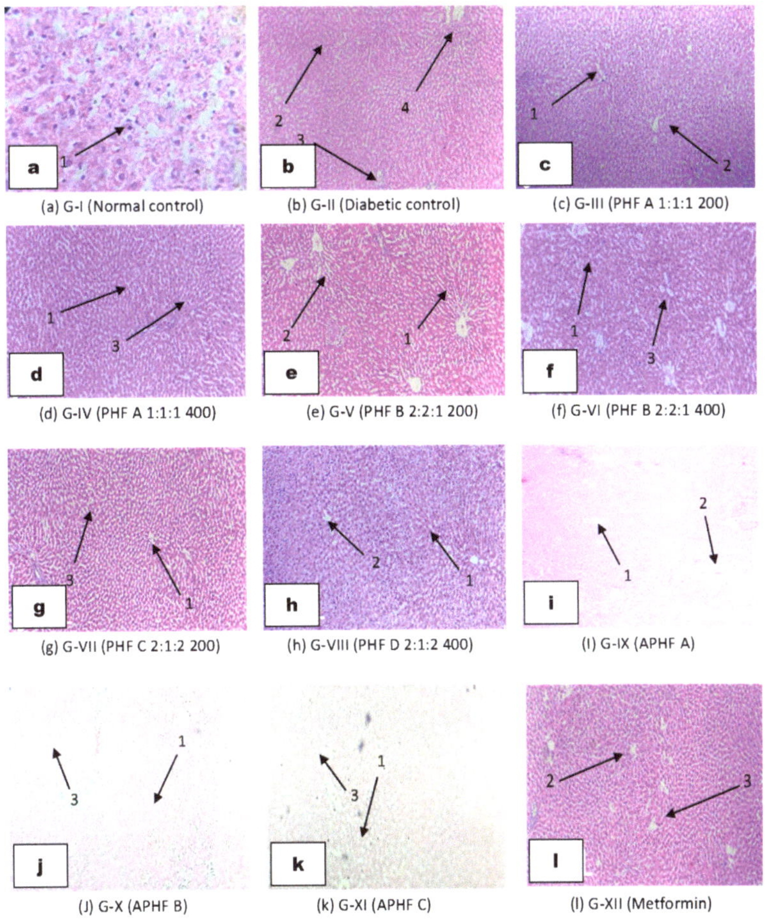

Figure 8. The liver section of histology. (**a**) G-I (normal control), (**b**) G-II (diabetic control), (**c**) G-III (PHF A 1:1:1 200), (**d**) G-IV (PHF A 1:1:1 400), (**e**) G-V (PHF B 2:2:1 200), (**f**) G-VI (PHF B 2:2:1 400), (**g**) G-VII (PHF C 2:1:2 200), (**h**) G-VIII (PHF C 2:1:2 400), (**i**) G-IX (APHF A), (**j**) G-X (APHF B), (**k**) G-XI (APHF C), (**l**) G-XII (metformin),where 1: normal hepatocyte, 2: pykontic nuclei, 3: mild periportal inflammation, 4: periportal fatty infiltration.

2.5.8. Histopathological Studies of Pancreatic Cells

Normal control rats' pancreases had normal histological architecture in the form of an acinar structure with normal beta cell islets. The number of Langerhans islets in the diabetic control group's pancreases was significantly reduced. Beta cell depletion, dilated islets, acini shrinkage, and vacuolar degeneration were all seen. Pancreatic cell recovery and improvement were found in the PHF-, APHF-, and metformin-treated groups. PHF-treated rats' pancreas revealed a moderate restoration of IL cells with fewnecrotic alterations. The pancreas of the APHF-treated group seemed normal, with restored islets and fewnecrotic alterations. The metformin-treated group showed restoration of islets to normal size, with normal acinar cells and fewnecrotic alterations (Figure 9).

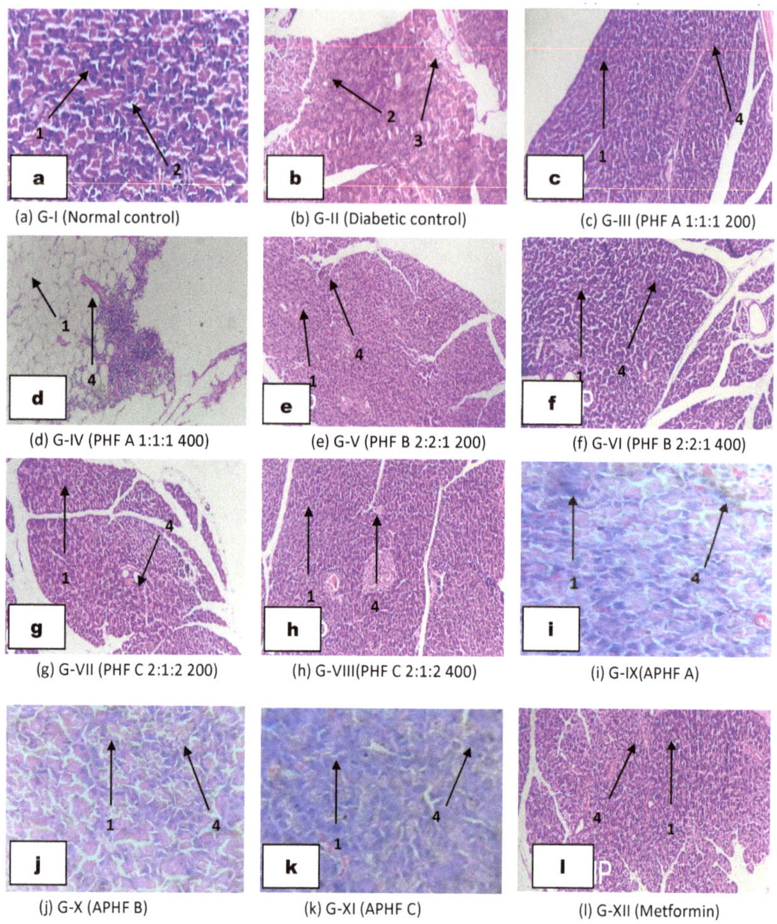

Figure 9. The pancreas section of histology. (**a**) G-I (normal control), (**b**) G-II (diabetic control), (**c**) G-III (PHF A 1:1:1 200), (**d**) G-IV (PHF A 1:1:1 400), (**e**) G-V (PHF B 2:2:1 200), (**f**) G-VI (PHF B 2:2:1 400), (**g**) G-VII (PHF2:1:2 200), (**h**) G-VIII (PHF C 2:1:2 400), (**i**) G-IX (APHF A), (**j**) G-X (APHF B), (**k**) G-XI (APHF C), (**l**) G-XII (metformin), where 1: beta cells islets, 2: depletion of beta cells, 3: deleted islets, 4: formation of islets.

3. Materials and Methods

3.1. Chemicals and Reagents

Streptozotocin and metformin were acquired from Yarrow Chem Products, Mumbai, Maharashtra, India. The remaining chemicals and reagents were of analyticalgrade.

3.2. Plant Material

Leaves of *Cassia auriculata* (CAr), *Centella asiatica* (CAs), and *Zingiber officinale* (ZO) rhizomes were obtained around Nagamangala Taluk, Mandya District, Karnataka, India. Plant samples were certified at the Foundation for Revitalisation of Local Health Traditions herbarium in Bangalore, India (FRLHT Acc. No. of plants is 5551, 5552, and 5553 for CAs, CAr, and ZO, respectively). The plant's components were thoroughly cleaned, shade dried, and pulverized to get a coarse powder. Powders were kept in an airtight container in a sterile environment for later usage.

3.3. Preparation of Extract

The cold maceration method was followed to extract dried powders of CAr, CAs, and ZO using 70% ethanol [17,18].

3.4. Preparation of Polyherbal and Allopolyherbal Formulations

Polyherbal formulations were developed by combining CAr, CAs, and ZO in three distinct ratios: 1:1:1 (PHF A), 2:2:1 (PHF B), and 2:1:2 (PHF C), and were given to rats at doses of 200 and 400 mg/kg body weight. The APHF formulation was produced by combining a potent polyherbal formulation (PHF B) with metformin.

The following are the APHF specifics:

APHF A: PHF B (200 mg/kg b.w) + 25% of metformin standard dose (22.5 mg/kg b.w)
APHF B: PHF B (200 mg/kg b.w) + 50% of metformin standard dose (45 mg/kg b.w)
APHF C: PHF B (200 mg/kg b.w) + 75% of metformin standard dose (67.5 mg/kg b.w)

3.5. Preliminary Phytochemical Investigation of Polyherbal Formulation

Qualitative phytochemical analysis of polyherbal formulations was carried out using standard procedures [19,20].

3.6. Quantitative Estimation of Total Phenolic, Flavonoid, and Tannin Content

The pathophysiology of many acute and chronic disorders is influenced by oxidative stress. Free radicals and other reactive oxygen species (ROS) have been linked to the pathophysiology of a variety of diseases, including diabetes. Antioxidants such as phenols, flavonoids, and tannins scavenge free radicals such as peroxide, hydroperoxide, and lipid peroxyl, which delay or prevent oxidative damage to the target molecule [21,22].

3.6.1. Estimation of Total Phenolic Content

The total phenolic content of PHF was determined using the Folin–Ciocâlteu (FC) reagent. The PHF was combined in a specific volume with FC reagent (10 times prediluted). Later, 1.6 mL of a 7.5% *w*/*v* sodium carbonate solution was added. The solution was stirred for 1 h before being incubated at room temperature. The absorbance at 765 nm was measured using a UV–visible spectrophotometer (Shimadzu UV-1700, PharmaSpec (Metro Manila, Philippines). A calibration curve for the standard solution (gallic acid) was created [23,24].

3.6.2. Estimation of Total Flavonoid Content

The total flavonoid content was determined colorimetrically using the aluminum chloride procedure. A known volume of the PHF or catechin was mixed with distilled water (1.25 mL) in a test tube, and a 5% sodium nitrite solution (75 µL) was added. Following that, 150 µL of a 10% aluminum chloride solution was added and left to rest for 5 min before adding 1 M sodium hydroxide (0.5 mL). The absorbance at 510 nm was measured immediately using a UV–visible spectrophotometer. The findings were expressed in milligrams of (+)-catechin equivalent per gram of extract. The calibration curve ofcatechin (standard reference drug) was drawn [25,26].

3.6.3. Estimation of Total Tannin Content

The vanillin–HCl procedure wasused to determine the total tannin content.

First, 250 µL of PHF was treated with 2250 µL of reagent combination (4:1 ratio of 4% vanillin and 8% concentrated HCl produced in methanol). For around 20 min, the resulting mixture was incubated at room temperature. At 500 nm, the absorbance was measured. The calibration curve was created using various concentrations of catechin (20–100 µg/mL), and the total tannin value was reported as mg catechin equivalents (CAE)/g dry extract [24].

3.7. Compatibility Study of APHF by Differential Scanning Calorimetry (DSC)

A compatibility study is one of the most vital areas of ensuring the stability of an allopolyherbal formulation and revealing potential interactions that may arise between the components in a mixture [27]. An in-depth understanding of the physical interactions between the components in a formulation is feasible with a thermal (differential scanning calorimetry) approach [28]. The compatibility of metformin with polyherbal extract wasinvestigated using DSC. This study looked for any potential physical interactions between the extract and metformin once they weremixed.

The samples were analyzed using Shimadzu heat-flux DSC in the temperature range of 0 °C to 600 °C, with a heating rate of 6 K/min and in an environment of flowing nitrogen [29].

3.8. InVivo Antidiabetic Activity

3.8.1. Experimental Animals

Albino rats weighing around 160–200 g and aged 3 to 4 months were obtained from Vaarunya Biolabs Pvt. Ltd., Bengaluru, India (CPCSEA Registration No. 2076/PO/RcBiBt/S/19/C PCSEA), Bengaluru, India. Rats were housed in spacious polyacrylic cages under typical husbandry conditions (25 °C temperature, 60–70% relative humidity, and a 12-h light/dark cycle). They were fed regular rat pellets and had unlimited access to drinking water. Experiments were carried out with the approval of Institutional Animal Ethical Committee (IAEC) of Sri Adichunchanagiri, College of Pharmacy, India (IAEC Approval No. SACCP-IAEC/2021-02/49 and SACCP-IAEC/2022-01/58).

3.8.2. Acute Toxicity Study of Polyherbal Formulation

Individually, all of the extracts employed in the development of the polyherbal formulation were shown to be safe [14,30,31]. As a result, an acute toxicity study using a limit test at one dose level of 2000 mg/kg body weight with six rats (three rats per step) for 14 days in each step was performed for the polyherbal extract (made by mixing equal proportions of CAr, CAs, and ZO).

3.8.3. Induction of Diabetes

To induce diabetes in overnight starved rats, a single intraperitoneal injection of freshly prepared STZ (55 mg/Kg b.w, Yarow Chem Products, Mumbai, Maharashtra, India) in 0.1 M citrate buffer (pH 4.5, Sisco Research Laboratories Pvt. Ltd., Taloja, Maharashtra, India) was employed. To prevent STZ-induced hypoglycemic death, the rats were given a 20% glucose solution to drink for 24 h. Diabetes was diagnosed one week after the STZ injection, and rats with fasting blood glucose levels of greater than 200 mg/dL were chosen for the investigation [32,33].

3.8.4. Experimental Design

The rats (n = 72) were divided into twelve groups, each comprising six rats. The test compounds were suspended in distilled water (dH_2O) in a vehicle containing 2.5% acacia suspension (Yarow Chem Products, Mumbai, Maharashtra, India) and administered orally once a day for 21 days to all rats. The anti-diabetic effects of individual extracts, PHF, and metformin were first tested. Based on the results, a very effective PHF ratio was chosen for the development of APHF. The antidiabetic activity of APHF was tested later.

Rats were grouped as follows:

Group I: Served as a normal control (2.5% acacia suspension b.w, p.o)
Group II: Served as a diabetic control (Streptozotocin 55 mg/kg b.w, i.p)
Group III: Treatment with PHF A—1:1:1 (200 mg/kg b.w, p.o)
Group IV: Treatment with PHF A—1:1:1 (400 mg/kg b.w, p.o)
Group V: Treatment with PHF B—2:2:1 (200 mg/kg b.w, p.o)
Group VI: Treatment with PHF B—2:2:1 (400 mg/kg b.w, p.o)
Group VII: Treatment with PHF C—2:1:2 (200 mg/kg b.w, p.o)

Group VIII: Treatment with PHF C—2:1:2 (400 mg/kg b.w, p.o)
Group IX: APHF A (200 mg/kg PHF B+22.5 mg/kg metformin b.w, p.o)
Group X: APHF B (200 mg/kg PHF B+45 mg/kg metformin b.w, p.o)
Group XI: APHF C (200 mg/kg PHF B+67.5 mg/kg metformin b.w, p.o
Group XII: Treatment with metformin (90 mg/kg b.w, p.o)

3.8.5. Body Weight (b.w) Analysis

The b.w of each rat was measured using an animal weighing balance (Docbel Industries, New Delhi, India) at 7-day intervals from the start to the completion of the experiment (i.e., the 1st, 7th, 14th, and 21st days).

3.8.6. Blood Glucose Level

Metformin, PHF, and APHF were administered to diabetic rats for 21 days. Blood samples were taken by rupturing the tail vein, and blood glucose was determined on the 1st, 7th, 14th, and 21st days of therapy using an On Call Plus glucometer (ACON Biotech (Hangzhou) Co., Ltd., West Lake District, Hangzhou, China).

3.8.7. Biochemical Analysis

The rats were sacrificed under anesthetic conditions (ketamine hydrochloride, 80 mg/kg b.w, intraperitoneally) at the end of the experiment (on the 21st day). Blood samples were collected through cardiac puncture and analyzed in accordance with previously reported procedures [34–36]. Lipid profiles such as total cholesterol (TC), triglycerides (TG), high-density lipoprotein (HDL), low-density lipoprotein (LDL), and very low-density lipoprotein (VLDL) were assessed. Serum glutamate oxaloacetate transaminase (SGOT), serum glutamate pyruvate transaminase (SGPT), alkaline phosphatase (ALP), glycated hemoglobin (Hb1Ac), urea, creatinine, total protein, albumin, and total count and differential count of leucocyte were also estimated.

3.8.8. Histopathological Analysis

The pancreas and liver were excised, rinsed constantly with phosphate buffered saline (1 PBS, pH 7.4), preserved in a 10% formalin solution, and embedded in paraffin blocks. Five micrometer thick slices were cut on a semi-automated rotator microtome and stained with hematoxylin and eosin. An inverted biological microscope (FM-BM-B200, Fison Instruments Ltd., Glasgow G2 4JR, UK) was used to image the sections [37].

3.8.9. Statistical Analysis

Results were presented as mean SEM, and statistical differences between groups were established using analysis of variance (ANOVA, GraphPad Prism version 8.0.2, San Diego, CA, USA). Statistical significance was defined as p-values less than 0.05.

4. Conclusions

The biguanide class of drugs (metformin) has been linked to a variety of side effects, including metallic taste, nausea, vomiting, diarrhea, anorexia, and lactic acidosis. The dose of marketed metformin used by patients is greater when compared to other allopathic hypoglycemic medications. The suggested research has the potential to minimize unwanted side effects and/or decrease the dose of allopathic medicine, specifically metformin, by substituting it with a polyherbal formulation (PHF) and/or an allopolyherbal formulation (APHF). PHF and APHF both showed synergistic anti-diabetic efficacy. The anti-diabetic impact of APHF is stronger than that of PHF.

In comparison to metformin alone at higher doses, APHF and a relatively low dose of metformin together produce an extremely potent hypoglycemic effect. As a result, the current study shows that PHF and APHF are safe and effective medications in the treatment of diabetes mellitus because they serve to replace or reduce the dose of metformin, hence lowering metformin hazards. Further research is needed to confirm the safety and efficacy of APHF in human volunteers, followed by its formulation into an acceptable dosage form that piques the interest of patients.

Author Contributions: Conceptualization, S.S.A., Y.A. and R.K.M.; methodology, S.S.A., M.S. and R.K.M.; software, S.A.F. and R.K.M.; validation, M.R.,Y.A. and R.K.M.; formal analysis, S.S.A., M.M.A. and R.K.M.; investigation, S.S.A. and R.K.M.; resources, B.D.R. and R.K.M.; data curation, S.S.A., M.S. and M.R.; writing—original draft preparation, S.S.A. and R.K.M.; writing—review and editing, Y.A., M.R. and B.D.R.; visualization, S.A.F. and M.R.; supervision, B.D.R. and R.K.M.; project administration, B.D.R. and R.K.M.; funding acquisition, M.R. All authors have read and agreed to the published version of the manuscript.

Funding: The authors extend their appreciation to the Deanship of Scientific Research at King Khalid University, Saudi Arabia, for funding this work through the Large Program (Grant number RGP-2/264/44).

Institutional Review Board Statement: All procedures used in the current studies were performed according to the guidelines of the committee for the purpose of supervision and experimentation on animals (CPCSEA). The study was approved by the Institutional Animal Ethical Committee of Sri Adichunchanagiri College of Pharmacy (377/PO/ReBi/S/01/CPCSEA). All efforts were made to minimize animal suffering and reduce the number of animals used according to the 3R rule.

Informed Consent Statement: Not applicable.

Data Availability Statement: Data that support the findings of this study are available from the corresponding author upon reasonable request.

Acknowledgments: The authors extend their appreciation to the Deanship of Scientific Research at King Khalid University, Saudi Arabia, for funding this work through the Large Program (Grant number RGP-2/264/44). Part of this research was supported by the statutory activity of the Sri Adichunchanagiri College of Pharmacy, Adichunchanagiri University, India.

Conflicts of Interest: The authors declare that they have no conflict of interest.

References

1. Motevalli, S.; Salahshour, H.M.; Bailey, R.P. The mediating role of cognitive flexibility in the relationship between cognitive emotion regulation strategies and mindfulness in patients with type 2 diabetes. *J. Affect. Disord.* **2023**, *339*, 676–682. [CrossRef] [PubMed]
2. Bnouham, M.; Ziyyat, A.; Mekhfi, H.; Tahri, A.; Legssyer, A. Medicinal plants with potential antidiabetic activity—A review of ten years of herbal medicine research (1990–2000). *Int. J. Diabetes Metab.* **2006**, *14*, 1–25. [CrossRef]
3. Petchi, R.R.; Vijaya, C.; Parasuraman, S. Antidiabetic activity of Polyherbal Formulation in Streptozotocin—Nicotinamide induced diabetic wistar rats. *J. Tradit. Complement. Med.* **2014**, *4*, 108–117. [CrossRef] [PubMed]
4. Bisht, L.; Ram, V. Allopolyherbal Formulations and their Strategies. *J. Phytochem. Biochem.* **2017**, *1*, 101.
5. Kumar, R.; Arora, V.; Ram, V.; Bhandari, A.; Vyas, P. Hypoglycemic and hypolipidemic effect of Allopolyherbal formulations in streptozotocin induced diabetes mellitus in rats. *Int. J. Diabetes Mellit.* **2015**, *3*, 45–50. [CrossRef]
6. DeRuiter, J. Overview of the Antidiabetic Agents. *Endocr. Pharmacother. Modul.* **2003**, *3*, 45–50.
7. Kalaivani, A.; Umamaheswari, A.; Vinayagam, A.; Kalaivani, K. Anti-hyperglycemic and antioxidant properties of *Cassia auriculata* leaves and flowers on alloxan induced diabetic rats. *Pharmacologyonline* **2008**, *1*, 204–217.
8. Pari, L.; Latha, M. Effect of *Cassia auriculata* flowers on blood sugar levels, serum and tissue lipids in streptozotocin diabetic rats. *Singapore. Med. J.* **2002**, *43*, 617–621.
9. Thangavelu, L.; Kumar, R.; Arivarasu, L.; Aravindan, M. Cytotoxic Effect and Antibacterial Activity of Ethanolic Extract of *Cassia auriculata*. *J. Pharm. Res. Int.* **2021**, *33*, 456–461.
10. Somchit, M.N.; Sulaiman, M.R.; Zuraini, A.; Samsuddin, L.; Somchit, N.; Israf, D.A.; Moin, S. Antinociceptive and antiinflammatory effects of *Centella asiatica*. *Indian. J. Pharmacol.* **2004**, *36*, 377.
11. Arora, D.; Kumar, M.; Dubey, S.D. *Centella asiatica*-A Review of it's Medicinal Uses and Pharmacological Effects. *J. Nat. Remedies.* **2002**, *2*, 143–149.
12. Akhani, S.P.; Vishwakarma, S.L.; Goyal, R.K. Anti-diabetic activity of *Zingiber officinale* in streptozotocin-induced type I diabetic rats. *J. Pharm. Pharmacol.* **2004**, *56*, 101–105. [CrossRef] [PubMed]
13. Grzanna, R.; Lindmark, L.; Frondoza, C.G. Ginger—An Herbal Medicinal Product with Broad Anti-Inflammatory Actions. *J. Med. Food.* **2005**, *8*, 125–132. [CrossRef] [PubMed]
14. Gupta, S.; Sharma, S.B.; Bansal, S.K.; Prabhu, K.M. Antihyperglycemic and hypolipidemic activity of aqueous extract of *Cassia auriculata* L. leaves in experimental diabetes. *J. Ethnopharmacol.* **2009**, *123*, 499–503. [CrossRef] [PubMed]

15. Kabir, A.U.; Samad, M.B.; D'Costa, N.M.; Akhter, F.; Ahmed, A.; Hannan, J.M. Anti- hyperglycemic activity of *Centella asiatica* is partly mediated by carbohydrase inhibition and glucose-fiber binding. *BMC. Complement. Med.* **2014**, *14*, 31. [CrossRef]
16. Ahmed, S.S.; Kumar, M.R. Elucidation of Antidiabetic Mechanism of *Centella asiatica* and *Zingiber officinale*-An In-vitro and In-vivo approach. *J. Res. Pharm.* **2023**, *27*, 420–431.
17. Weli, A.M.; Al-Salmi, S.; Al Hoqani, H.; Hossain, M.A. Biological and phytochemical studies of different leaves extracts of *Pteropyrum scoparium*. Beni-Suef. *Univ. J. Basic. Appl. Sci.* **2018**, *7*, 481–486.
18. Asha, L.; Londonkar, R.L.; Bankalgi, S.K. Standardization of extraction process for *Rumex vesicarius* L. *Int. J. Res. Sci. Eng.* **2014**, *5*, 1061–1064.
19. Kokate, C.K.; Purohit, A.P.; Gokhle, S.B. Khandelwal. In *Practical Pharmacognosy*; Nirali Publications: Pune, India, 2005; pp. 140–143.
20. Kokate, C.K.; Purohit, A.P.; Gokhle, S.B. *Practical Pharmacognosy*; Nirali Prakashan: Pune, India, 2005; pp. 108–111.
21. Mahdi-Pour, B.; Jothy, S.L.; Latha, L.Y.; Chen, Y.; Sasidharan, S. Antioxidant activity of methanol extracts of different parts of *Lantana camara*. *Asian Pac. J. Trop Biomed.* **2012**, *2*, 960–965. [CrossRef]
22. Saeed, N.; Khan, M.R.; Shabbir, M. Antioxidant activity, total phenolic and total flavonoid contents of whole plant extracts *Torilis leptophylla* L. *BMC Complement. Altern. Med.* **2012**, *12*, 1–12. [CrossRef]
23. Singleton, V.L.; Rossi, J.A. Colorimetry of total phenolics with phosphomolybdic-phosphotungstic acid reagents. *Am. J. Enol. Vitic.* **1965**, *16*, 144–158. [CrossRef]
24. Annegowda, H.V.; Bhat, R.; Tze, L.M.; Karim, A.A.; Mansor, S.M. The free radical scavenging and antioxidant activities of pod and seed extract of *Clitoria fairchildiana* (Howard)-an underutilized legume. *J. Food Sci. Technol.* **2013**, *50*, 535–541. [CrossRef] [PubMed]
25. Sakanaka, S.; Tachibana, Y.; Okada, Y. Preparation and antioxidant properties of extracts of *Japanese persimmon* leaf tea (kakinoha-cha). *Food Chem.* **2005**, *89*, 569–575. [CrossRef]
26. Burns, R.E. Method for estimation of tannin in grain sorghum. *Agron. J.* **1971**, *63*, 511–512. [CrossRef]
27. Aigner, Z.; Heinrich, R.; Sipos, E.; Farkas, G.; Ciurba, A.; Berkesi, O.; Szabó-Revesz, P. Compatibility studies of aceclofenac with retard tablet excipients by means of thermal and FT-IR spectroscopic methods. *J. Therm. Anal. Calorim.* **2011**, *104*, 265–271. [CrossRef]
28. de Andrade, F.H.; de Araujo Batista, R.S.; Melo, T.B.; Fernandes, F.H.; Macedo, R.O.; de Souza, F.S.; Wanderley, A.G. Characterization and compatibility of dry extract from *Annona muricata* L. and pharmaceutical excipients. *J. Therm. Anal. Calorim.* **2019**, *143*, 237–246. [CrossRef]
29. Costa, R.S.D.; Negrão, C.A.; Camelo, S.R.; Ribeiro-Costa, R.M.; Barbosa, W.L.; Costa, C.E.; Júnior, J.O. Investigation of thermal behavior of *Heliotropium indicum* L. lyophilized extract by TG and DSC. *J. Therm. Anal. Calorim.* **2013**, *111*, 1959–1964. [CrossRef]
30. Sasikala, S.; Lakshminarasaiah, S.; Naidu, M.D. Antidiabetic activity of *Centella asiatica* on streptozotocin induced diabetic male albino rats. *World. J. Pharm. Sci.* **2015**, *3*, 1701–1705.
31. John, A.O. Ojewole. Analgesic, Antiinflammatory and Hypoglycaemic Effects of Ethanol Extract of *Zingiber officinale* (Roscoe) Rhizomes (Zingiberaceae) in Mice and Rats. *Phyther. Res.* **2006**, *20*, 764–772.
32. Manik, S.; Gauttam, V.; Kalia, A.N. Anti-diabetic and antihyperlipidemic effect of allopolyherbal formulation in OGTT and STZ-induced diabetic rat model. *Indian. J. Exp. Biol.* **2013**, *51*, 702–708.
33. Nagaraja, S.; Ahmed, S.S.; Bharathi, D.R.; Goudanavar, P.; Fattepur, S.; Meravanige, G.; Shariff, A.; Shiroorkar, P.N.; Habeebuddin, M.; Telsang, M. Green Synthesis and Characterization of Silver Nanoparticles of *Psidium guajava* Leaf Extract and Evaluation for Its Antidiabetic Activity. *Molecules* **2022**, *27*, 4336. [CrossRef] [PubMed]
34. Tang, K.S. The current and future perspectives of zinc oxide nanoparticles in the treatment of DM. *Life Sci.* **2019**, *239*, 117011. [CrossRef] [PubMed]
35. Parasuraman, S.; Raveendran, R.; Kesavan, R. Blood sample collection in small laboratory animals. *J. Pharmacol. Pharmacother.* **2010**, *1*, 87. [PubMed]
36. Prabhu, S.; Vinodhini, S.; Elanchezhiyan, C.; Rajeswari, D. Evaluation of antidiabetic activity of biologically synthesized silver nanoparticles using *Pouteria sapota* in streptozotocin-induced diabetic rats. *J. Diabetes* **2018**, *10*, 28–42. [CrossRef] [PubMed]
37. Madić, V.; Petrović, A.; Jušković, M.; Jugović, D.; Djordjević, L.; Stojanović, G.; Vasiljević, P. Polyherbal mixture ameliorates hyperglycemia, hyperlipidemia and histopathological changes of pancreas, kidney and liver in a rat model of type 1 diabetes. *J. Ethnopharmacol.* **2021**, *265*, 113210. [CrossRef] [PubMed]

pharmaceuticals

Review

Multitargeted Herbal Prescription So Shiho Tang: A Scoping Review on Biomarkers for the Evaluation of Therapeutic Effects

Nguyen Khoi Song Tran [1], Ji Hwan Lee [1], Myong Jin Lee [1], Jun Yeon Park [2,*] and Ki Sung Kang [1,*]

[1] College of Korean Medicine, Gachon University, Seongnam 13120, Republic of Korea; kauri87@gachon.ac.kr (N.K.S.T.); kleert26@gmail.com (J.H.L.); myongene@naver.com (M.J.L.)
[2] Department of Food Science and Biotechnology, Kyonggi University, Suwon 16227, Republic of Korea
* Correspondence: rhemf@kgu.ac.kr (J.Y.P.); kkang@gachon.ac.kr (K.S.K.)

Abstract: Alternative medicines, especially herbal remedies, have been employed to treat infections and metabolism-related chronic inflammation because their safety and multidimensional therapeutic potential outweigh those of synthetic drugs. So Shiho Tang (SSHT), a well-known Oriental prescription (Xiao Chai Hu Tang in Chinese) composed of seven herbs, is traditionally prescribed to treat various viral infections and chronic metabolic disorders in Asia with or without the support of other natural medicines. To provide a general background on how SSHT is used as a medicinal alternative, we conducted a scoping review using the PubMed database system. Among the 453 articles, 76 studies used aqueous extracts of SSHT alone. This result included seven clinical studies and 69 basic studies: cell-based, animal-based, and ex vivo studies. The in vitro and clinical reports mainly focus on hepatic infection and hepatocarcinoma, and the documentation of in vivo tests of SSHT presents a wide range of effects on cancer, fibrosis, inflammation, and several metabolic disorder symptoms. Additionally, among the seven clinical records, two reverse-effect case studies were reported in middle-aged patients. In brief, this systematic review provides general knowledge on the natural remedy SSHT and its potential in phytotherapeutic primary health care.

Keywords: So Shiho Tang; chronic inflammation; systemic; herbal medicine; multitarget; biomarker

Citation: Tran, N.K.S.; Lee, J.H.; Lee, M.J.; Park, J.Y.; Kang, K.S. Multitargeted Herbal Prescription So Shiho Tang: A Scoping Review on Biomarkers for the Evaluation of Therapeutic Effects. *Pharmaceuticals* **2023**, *16*, 1371. https://doi.org/10.3390/ph16101371

Academic Editors: Catherine Sherwin, Elena Y. Enioutina and Kathleen M. Job

Received: 24 August 2023
Revised: 21 September 2023
Accepted: 26 September 2023
Published: 27 September 2023

1. Introduction

Abnormal biological functions of certain organelles can lead to many pathological conditions. As a common pathological condition, chronic inflammation is a therapeutic target for diseases, including infectious diseases, cancers, fibrosis, certain metabolic disorders, and vice versa [1–3]. Immune responses to external infections or dramatic internal metabolic shifts depend on various mechanisms [2,4]. Specifically, inflammatory cytokines, such as interleukin 2 (IL-2), interferon γ (IFN-γ), and tumor necrosis factor α (TNF-α) secreted by T helper cell 1 (Th1), participate in type 1 inflammation in response to cellular stimuli. Th2 cells secrete IL-4, IL-5, IL-10, IL-13, and tumor growth factor β (TGFβ) in type 2 immunity in response to body allergies and extracellular stimuli [5,6]. Therefore, etiopathology is a premise for chronic disease prevention and treatment.

A multidimensional medicinal approach has been successfully implemented using herbal medicines [7,8]. There are two major advantages of natural-origin therapies as alternatives: they are multitarget and naturally affordable. Unintended effects are the most observed concern in the pharmaceutical industry. Severe side effects can result in abnormal metabolism, permanent damage, and lethality [9]. For instance, antimicrobial studies have demonstrated that antibiotic resistance is the first consideration for pathogenic and anti-inflammatory drugs [10]. Some anti-allergy drugs, such as antihistamines, decongestants, antileukotriene agents, and corticosteroids, have been shown to lead to undesirable outcomes, including arrhythmia, vomiting, anxiety, neuropsychiatric disorders, nasal dryness, and irritation [11–15]. Thus, herbal remedies have been employed as substitutes and complementary medicines along with long-term synthetic drug medications. Traditional Chinese medicine (TCM) also plays a critical role in the complementary treatment of certain infectious diseases and cancers [16]. Phytotherapy has been developed to determine the appropriate use of multitargeted TCM, which can promote advantages and prevent possible risks [17].

So Shiho Tang (SSHT), or Xiao Chai Hu Tang in Chinese, has been an Oriental herbal medicine famous for fever, stomatitis, and gastrointestinal disorders for centuries in Asia [18]. In Japan, SSHT is well known as Sho-saiko-to or TJ-9, a chronic hepatitis medication [19]. SSHT is a mixture of different amounts of Radix bupleuri (Chaihu), Radix scutellariae (Huangqin), Rhizoma pinelliae (Banxia), Rhizoma zingiberis recens (Shengjiang), Fructus jujubae (Dazao), licorice (Gancao), and ginseng radix (Renshen) [20,21]. SSHT was evaluated as safe at doses of up to 2000 mg/kg in rat models [22,23] and 9000 mg/day in human participants aged 14–18 years [18]. According to a review by Kim et al., SSHT significantly lowered the elevated liver fibrosis markers and collagen types in fibrosis/cirrhosis-induced animal's serum [24]. Aqueous STT has been reported to prevent and attenuate several chronic diseases, including chronic inflammatory skin diseases and gastrointestinal disorders [18,21,25]. The variation in the phytochemical features of SSHT limits the identification of the specific effects of each element, leading to challenging and incompatible approval processes in Western countries. Despite these concerns, SSHT has been successfully applied in numerous therapeutic prescriptions, including clinical trials in Asia [26,27]. The traditional East Asian medicine (TEAM) system has developed a basic mechanism by which TCM and SSHT work synergistically to boost medicinal efficacy and alleviate the reverse effects [28,29]. Although a recent bibliometric analysis summarized the application of randomized control trials of SSHT and Western medicine in examination designs [30], an outline of how SSHT alone is potentially participating in modern medicine has not been presented.

As long as TCM, particularly SSHT, is composed of many components, systems pharmacology will allow researchers to access multiple mechanisms of action without isolating a single compound [31,32]. Understanding the mechanisms of how drugs and the body interact at system levels is a key aspect of medications in general. In this study, we aimed to classify the medicinal applications of SSHT in cellular, preclinical, and clinical studies. Herein, we address two points: (1) indications of multitargeted biomarkers and significant dosages, and (2) suggestions for effective preclinical studies and mechanisms for subsequent clinical examinations of SSHT. Through this methodical approach, researchers can comprehend the mode of action of SSHT on various multitargeted biomarkers and signaling pathways in certain disease models as well as patients. Because valuable in vitro and in vivo records guarantee successful clinical outcomes, the novelty and limitations of these studies can be collected, analyzed, and applied to further examinations using systemic pharmacology analysis. This scoping review provides general knowledge on the use of SSHT and an interdisciplinary perspective to therapy.

2. Literature Research Strategy

This review introduces the current status of cell-based, animal-based, and clinical studies on target diseases and the efficacy of SSHT. We used a search strategy to collect, identify, and classify literature on the applied diseases and the effects of SSHT on each disease. Considering that SSHT prescription is known by various scientific names, the following search terms were set through related reviews and databases: "soshiho-tang", "so-shi-ho-tang", "soshiho", "sosiho-tang", "so-si-ho-tang", "sosiho", "xiaochaihu", "xiao-chai-hu-tang", "xiaochaihu-tang", "Xiao-chai-hu-decoction", "Xiaochaihu-decoction", "Xiaochaihudecoction", "shosaikoto", "shosaiko-to", "sho-saiko-to" and "sho-sai-ko-to". A literature search was conducted for articles published until 20 December 2022 on the PubMed database only. The literature was identified and classified according to the following inclusion criteria: (1) Oriental medicine articles, (2) written in English, (3) on the efficacy of SSHT alone or/with treatment, and (4) original articles (e.g., survey, protocol). The exclusion criterion was studies that performed only chemical analysis. In addition, data were extracted from predetermined items in the literature (e.g., types of and several herbs included in prescription, clinical, or basic studies; cell type or animal type in basic studies; disease-inducing method; details of intervention; extraction method; concentration (dose); and outcome measures) and reviewed with others (Figure 1). Three researchers independently reviewed and evaluated the eligibility of the titles, abstracts, and full texts of the articles. In cases of disagreement during the literature selection and data extraction processes, they discussed the implications. The data extracted after the war are summarized and presented in the table, along with narrative descriptions.

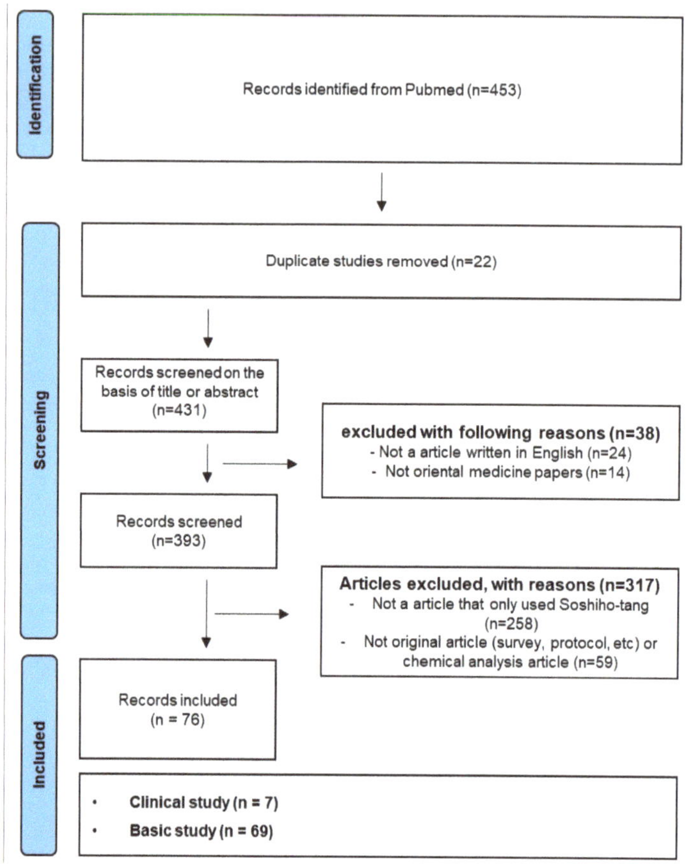

Figure 1. Flow chart of study selection indicates the retrieval process.

A total of 453 articles were retrieved using this search strategy. Literature that fulfilled the exclusion criteria was classified into cell, animal, and clinical studies by assessing the abstract and full text of the thesis according to the conditions stated. As a result of this process, 76 papers were included in the systematic review (Figure 1). The 76 results were divided into seven clinical studies and 69 basic studies. Regarding the efficacy of SSHT in basic research, 33 cell-based studies, 33 animal-based studies, and three in vitro and in vivo studies have been reported.

3. Results

3.1. In Vitro Studies on SSHT

Our analysis showed that one third (33.3%) of in vitro articles were published in Japan, followed by 22.2% in Korea, 11.1% in China, and 2.7% in Taiwan and the United States (Table 1). As shown in Table 1, SSHT is water-extracted and named Sho-saiko-to, So Shiho

Tang, or Xiao Chai Hu, depending on the country. Among these publications, seven demonstrated anticancer effects, mainly in hepatocellular carcinoma [33]. Additionally, SSHT was reported to cure various cancer types, such as ovarian cancer [34], melanoma, colon cancer, and adenocarcinoma. Growth inhibition and cytotoxicity against cancer cells were examined using SSHT treatment. Zhao et al. evaluated not only the antiproliferative effect but also the apoptotic effect [35]. This study found that SSHT induced apoptosis through the expression of Bax, Bcl-2, CDK4, and cyclin-D1. Liu et al. examined the apoptotic effects of SSHT in a murine malignant melanoma cell line (Mel-ret) [36]. SSHT downregulates the expression of Fas-L, cdk4, cdk6, and pRB. Yamashiki et al. used peripheral blood mononuclear cells from patients with hepatocellular carcinoma and type C liver cirrhosis, and demonstrated that SSHT induced the dose-dependent production of tumor necrosis factor-α (TNF-α) and granulocyte colony-stimulating factor (G-CSF) [37]. Mizushima et al. examined the cytotoxic effects of different concentrations of SSHT (0.5, 1, 1.5, 2, and 2.5 mg/mL) [38]. Except for SBC-5 cells, all tested cell lines were cytotoxic to SSHT in a dose-dependent manner. Shao et al. reported no effect of SSHT on the viability of HCT116 and LOVO cells [39].

Seven studies have investigated the immunomodulatory activity of SSHT. Kawakita et al. demonstrated that SSHT is an IFN inducer for the peroral treatment of spleen cells [40]. The immunological status induced by the inflammatory factors reflects an imbalance between CD4+ and CD8+ T cells. Modulation of the CD4/CD8 ratio by SSHT has been observed in hepatic mononuclear cells but not in splenocytes [41,42]. The induction of cytokines, such as interleukin-1β (IL-1β), TNF-α, and granulocyte colony-stimulating factor (G-CSF), are peculiar effects of SSHT [43]. Another study investigated the levels of cytokine mRNA of IL-12, IL-1β, IL-10, TNF-α, G-CSF, and IFN-γ; they were upregulated by SSHT using the Gel doc system [44]. Matsumoto et al. investigated the histamine release and intracellular Ca^{2+} reactions in mast cells after SSHT [45]. Because mast cells play a key role in IgE-mediated allergic reactions, these findings indicate that they have an active allergic effect. SSHT has been studied for the production of prostaglandin E2 (PGE2), leukotriene B4 (LTB4), and superoxide in polymorphonuclear cells of individuals infected with the human immunodeficiency virus [46]. Data showed that PGE2 and superoxide decreased and LTB4 increased after SSHT treatment, suggesting that SSHT suppressed human immunodeficiency virus activity and, more precisely, modulated the immune reaction.

The in vitro protection effects of SSHT on other diseases have also been reported lately. Sakaguchi et al. reported the effects of SSHT on the treatment of chronic hepatitis [47]. They verified the cytotoxic protection of the treated macrophage cell line J774A.1 by using SSHT. TNF-α production also showed significant inhibitory effects in cells treated with SSHT. Understanding that periodontal disease leads to inflammation of the gingiva, Ara et al. found the anti-inflammatory potential of SSHT in human gingival fibroblasts (HGFs) with LPS as an inducer [48]. The results suggest that SSHT inhibited PGE2 and cyclooxygenase2 (COX2). Two other studies have reported the anti-inflammatory effects of SSHT by using RAW264.7 cells, an LPS inducer and immunomodulator, and dexamethasone as a positive control. Oh et al. elicited the effect of SSHT on LPS-induced macrophages through the NF-κB and MAPK pathways [49]. They concluded that SSHT inhibited nitric oxide, immune response cytokines, and NF-κB through the dephosphorylation of the MAPK pathway in LPS-induced RAW264.7 cells. Choi et al. also employed RAW 264.7 cells in LPS-induced model, and found a similar inhibition of pro-inflammatory cytokines, such as IL-6 and TNF-α, via pretreatment or co-treatment with SSHT [50]. In a study of acute pancreatitis, Zhan et al. used LPS-stimulated rat pancreatic AR42J cells, and SSHT played an important role in the treatment of acute pancreatitis by acting on the key genes of MAPK3, IL-6, and TP53, which were associated with inflammation [51].

Table 1. Summary of designs and biomarkers of in vitro studies on SSHT.

Study Design	Cell Type	Inducer	Extract Type	Treatment (* Effective Concentrations)	Positive Control	Biomarker & Outcome	Authors	Country
Antitumor effect	Mel-ret cell		Aq	400 *, 2000 µg/mL		Fas-L, cdk4, cdk6, pRb	Liu et al. (1998) [36]	Japan
Antitumor effect (Proliferation)	HCC cell line (KIM-1), cholangio-carcinoma cell line (KMC-1)		Aq	400, 1000 *, 2000 *, 10,000 µg/mL		Morphological change, DNA synthesis	Yano et al. (1994) [33]	Japan
Antitumor effect (Cytotoxic effect)	PLC, JH, HuH-7, HepG2, HepG3, H69, H69/CDDP, SBC-4, SBC-5, PC-10, ABC-1, LCD, LCT-8		Aq	0.5, 1, 1.5, 2.0, 2.5 mg/mL		Cell viability	Mizushima et al. (1995) [38]	Japan
Immune response (Induction of cytokines)	Peripheral blood mononu-clear cell (PBMC)		Aq	3.1 *, 12.5 *, 50 *, 200 * µg/mL		TNF-α, G-CSF	Yamashiki et al. (1996) [37]	Japan
Anticancer effect (Proliferation)	Ovarian cancer cell (KF-1, MN-1, A2780, KF-r, MN-r, A2780cp)		Aq	25, 50, 100, 200, 500, 1000 *, 5000 * µg/mL		Annexin V-FITC	Zhu et al. (2005) [34]	Japan
Antitumor effect (Apoptosis)	Human hepatoma cell line (Huh7)		Aq	0.5 *, 1.0 *, 1.5 * mg/mL		Bcl-2, Bax, cyclin-D1, CDK4	Zhao et al. (2017) [35]	China
Anticancer effect (cancer comorbid with depression)	HCT116 & Lovo		Aq	10, 20, 40, 80, 180, 320 µg/mL		Cell viability	Shao et al. (2021) [39]	China

Table 1. *Cont.*

Study Design	Cell Type	Inducer	Extract Type	Treatment (* Effective Concentrations)	Positive Control	Biomarker & Outcome	Authors	Country
Immune response (Induction of interferon)	Spleen cell	IFN-a/β	Aq	7.5, 15, 30, 60, 120, 250, 500 μg/mL		IFN	Kawakita et al. (1990) [40]	Japan
Immune response (Inductions of cytokines)	Peripheral blood mononu-clear cells (PBMNC)		Aq	200 μg/mL		IL-1β, TNF-α, G-CSF	Yamashiki et al. (1996) [43]	Japan
Immune response	Peripheral blood mononu-clear cells & polymor-phonuclear cells (PMNC)		Aq	25, 50 *, 100 * μg/mL		PGE2, LTB4, superoxide	Miyamoto et al. (1996) [46]	USA
Immune response	Mast cell	DNP-As	Aq	0.01, 0.1, 1 *, 10 * mg/mL		Histamine release, Ca^{2+} response	Matsumoto et al. (1998) [45]	Japan
Immune response (Cytokine mRNA expression)	Human peripheral lymphocyte	LPS	Aq	200 μg/mL		IL-12, IL-1β, IL-10, TNF-α, G-CSF, IFN-γ	Huang et al. (2001) [44]	Japan
Immune response (Proliferation of T cell subsets)	Hepatic mononu-clear cells, splenocyte	Anti-CD3 mAb	Aq	62.5 *, 125 *, 250 * μg/mL		CD4/CD8	Ohtake et al. (2005) [41]	Japan
Immune response	Splenocyte, CD4 T cell		Aq	10 *, 25 *, 50 *, 100 * μg/mL		IL-4, IFN-γ	Kang et al. (2009) [42]	Korea
Immune response	J774A.1 cell	LPS	Aq	10 *, 20 *, 50 * μg/mL		Endotoxin-induced cytotoxicity (TNF-α)	Sakaguchi et al. (2004) [47]	Japan
Anti-inflammatory effects	HGFs		Aq	0.1, 0.3 *, 1 * mg/mL		PGE2, COX-2	Ara et al. (2008) [48]	Japan

Table 1. *Cont.*

Study Design	Cell Type	Inducer	Extract Type	Treatment (* Effective Concentrations)	Positive Control	Biomarker & Outcome	Authors	Country
Anti-inflammatory effects	RAW 264.7	LPS	Aq	10 *, 50 *, 100 * μg/mL	Dexamethasone	TNF-α, IL-6, Nitric Oxide, NF-κB, IκBα, ERK, p38, JNK	Oh et al. (2013) [49]	Korea
Anti-inflammatory effects	RAW 264.7	LPS	Aq	1, 10, 100, 250 *, 500 *, 1000 * μg/mL	Dexamethasone	IL-6, TNF-α, IFN-γ	Choi et al. (2021) [50]	Korea
Anti-inflammatory effects (Acute pancreatitis)	AR42J cell	LPS	Aq	12.5, 25 *, 50 *, 100 * μM		IL-6, IL-1β, TNF-α, MAPK3, TP53	Zhan et al. (2021) [51]	China
Immune response (Chronic HBV infection)	PBMC		Aq	50 *, 100 *, 300 * μg/mL		IFN-γ, anti-HBe & anti-HBc production	Kakumu et al. (1990) [52]	Japan
Liver diseases (Chronic active hepatitis B and C)	Peripheral blood mononuclear cells, polymorphonuclear cells (PMNC)		Aq	100 μg/mL		IL-10	Yamashiki et al. (1997) [53]	Japan
Liver diseases (Chronic hepatitis B)	HepG2.2.15 cell		Aq	10 *, 20 *%(vol/vol)		JAK2, STAT3, HBsAg	Chen et al. (2017) [54]	China
Liver diseases	Hepatocyte		Aq	3 *, 30 *, 300 * μg/mL		iNOS, nitric oxide	Hattori et al. (1995) [55]	Japan
Lipid metabolism	Hepatocyte	20% lipid emulsion	Aq	50, 100 *, 200 *, 400 *, 800 μg/mL		G6PD, ME, FAS, ATGL, LPL, PPARα	Zou et al. (2019) [56]	China
Liver fibrosis	Hepatic stellate cell (HSCs)		Aq	10, 100, 250, 500 *, 1000 * μg/mL		Type I and type III procollagen	Kayano et al. (1998) [57]	Japan

Table 1. *Cont.*

Study Design	Cell Type	Inducer	Extract Type	Treatment (* Effective Concentrations)	Positive Control	Biomarker & Outcome	Authors	Country
Liver fibrosis	Rat hepatic stellate cells (HSCs)		Aq	10, 100 *, 500 *, 1000 * μg/mL		MMP-13, MMP-2, TIMP-1, TIMP-2	Sakaida et al. (2004) [58]	Japan
Aging (Autocrine growth of human keratinocyte)	Normal human keratinocyte		Aq	100 *, 500 * μg/mL		IL-1α	Matsumoto et al. (1997) [59]	Japan
Atopic dermatitis (AD) symptoms	HaCaT cell	TNF-α/IFN-γ	Aq	10 *, 20, 50 *, 100 *, 500 μg/mL		ICAM-1, HO-1, NF-κB, Nrf2	Lee et al. (2019) [21]	Korea
Aging (UVB-induced skin damage and photoaging)	HaCaT cell	UVB irradiation	Aq	10 *, 50 *, 100 * μg/mL		MMP-1, MMP-9	Im et al. (2020) [60]	Korea
Mitogenic activity	Spleen cell	LPS		0.1, 1 *, 10 *, 100 * μg/mL		Mitogenic response ([^{3}H] thymidine uptake)	Hiroko et al. (1987) [61]	Japan
Antiviral activity	Human neonatal foreskin fibroblast cell line (CCFS-1/KMC)		Aq	25 *, 50 *, 100 *, 200 * μg/mL	Ribavirin	IFN-α, IFN-β, CVB1	Cheng et al. (2006) [62]	Taiwan
Anti-inflammatory effects (Calprotectin expression)	Human oral epithelial cell (TR146)		Aq	10, 25 *, 50 *, 100, 250 μg/mL		S100A8, S100A9, Calprotectin, ADM, AZU1, CAMP, CST3, DEFB1, DEFB4, DEFB103A, LCN2, IL-1α, IL-6, TNF-α G-CSF, MUC5B, IL-1R1	Hiroshima et al. (2010) [63]	Japan

Table 1. *Cont.*

Study Design	Cell Type	Inducer	Extract Type	Treatment (* Effective Concentrations)	Positive Control	Biomarker & Outcome	Authors	Country
Antithrombotic effect	Platelet	Collagen, thrombin, AA, ADP	Aq	200 *, 400 *, 800 * μg/mL	ASA	Serotonin, TXB2	Lee et al. (2013) [64]	Korea
Antiobesity effect	3T3-L1		Aq	50 *, 100 *, 200 * μg/mL	GW9662	PPAR-γ and C/EBP-α, FAS, perilipin, FABP4, triglyceride, leptin	Yoo et al. (2016) [65]	Korea
Immune response (mRNA & microRNA expression)	Mouse primary hepatocyte		Aq	500 μg/mL		P450 metabolism, cell cycle pathway, PPAR pathway, MAPK pathway	Song et al. (2014) [66]	Korea

Aq, Aqueous; eNOS, endothelial nitric oxide synthase; iNOS, inducible nitric oxide synthase; COX2, cyclooxygenase 2; MMPs, matrix metalloproteinase. adrenomedullin; ADM, azurocidin 1; AZU1, cathelicidin; CAMP, cystatin C; CST3, β-defensin 1; DEFB1, b-defensin 2; DEFB4, b-defensin 3; DEFB103A, lipocalin 2; LCN2, interleukin-1α; IL-1α, interleukin-6; IL-6, tumor necrosis factor α; TNF-α, granulocyte colony-stimulating factor; G-CSF, mucin 5; MUC5B, interleukin-1a receptor; IL-1R1, thymus-independent; TI, arachidonic acid; AA, acetylsalicylic acid; ASA, Thromboxane B2; TXB2. (*) concentration with significant effect. Accordingly, SSHT and quercetin were associated with anti-inflammation and blocked not only IL-6, TNF-α, and IL-1β but also MAPK3 and TP53.

Liver-related studies on SSHT have been divided into two categories: hepatitis virus [19,52–54] and liver disease (non-virus) [55–58]. The efficacy of SSHT was investigated in peripheral blood mononuclear cells from patients with chronic hepatitis. SSHT was found to enhance IFN-γ and alleviate HBe and HBc production dose-dependently. Moreover, SSHT induced IL-10, CSF, and TNF-α. Chen et al. treated HepG2 cells with 10% or 20% mXCHD-containing serum and found that the expression of hepatitis B surface antigen (HBsAg) decreased with 10% and 20% mXCHD [54]. The mRNA and protein expression of STAT3 increased in the group treated with 20% mXCHD serum, and no difference was observed in the expression level of JAK2. Zou et al. [56] tested the mRNA expression of adipogenesis markers (G6PD, DGAT2, and ME1) and lipolysis-related genes (ATGL, PPARα, and LPL) in 20% lipid emulsion (LE)-induced hepatocytes. SSHT treatment reverses LE-induced lipid accumulation and improves cell viability. Hatorri et al. studied the effect of SSHT on NO biosynthesis and found that SSHT dose-dependently induced NO production and iNOS mRNA expression in the presence of IFN [55]. Kayano et al. and Sakaida et al. clarified the inhibitory effect of SSHT on the formation of stellate cells isolated from male Wistar rats [57,58]. However, Kayano et al. reported that SSHT in 500 and 1000 μg/mL doses inhibited the transcription level of type I and III procollagen in scar tissue. Sakaida et al. demonstrated the upregulation of MMP2 and MMP13 and the downregulation of TIMP1, TIMP2, and IL-1α, which have an important function in immune regulatory and inflammatory responses were produced in keratinocytes treated with SSHT [59]. These extracts also regulate the proliferation of cultured human epidermal keratinocytes. Atopic dermatitis (AD) is a commonly observed skin condition. Lee et al. investigated the effect of SSHT on AD-like symptoms in TNF-κ/IFN-κ-activated human keratinocytes (HaCaT) and found that SSHT treatment increased the expression of heme oxygenase -1 (HO-1) and Nrf2 but decreased the expression of intercellular adhesion molecule-1 (I-CAM) and NF-κB [21]. Another dermatological study demonstrated protection against UVB-induced skin damage and photoaging after SSHT treatment [60]. SSHT, MMP1, and MMP9 were downregulated in UVB-irradiated HaCaT cells.

In addition, one study showed the mitogenic activity of SSHT by using murine splenic cells [61], and another study mentioned that SSHT neutralized Coxsackie B virus type 1 (CVB1)-induced cytopathic effects in foreskin fibroblast cells [62]. Another study reported the role of SSHT in calprotectin and AMP expression in oral epithelial cells [63]. Lee et al. examined the antithrombotic activity of SSHT [64], and Yoo et al. examined the antiobesity effects of SSHT [65]. In addition, Song et al. used microarray to analyze the correlation between temporally upregulated and downregulated patterns in primary mouse hepatocytes treated with SSHT [66]. A conclusion was drawn that the P450 metabolism, cell cycle, PPAR, and MAPK pathways are associated with the liver regenerative activity of SSHT. In Korea, Taiwan, and Japan, but not in China, antitumor examinations of SSHT have used methods associated with apoptosis detection, such as flow cytometry for annexin V and Western blot detection of Bcl-2 and Bax protein levels. Several immunity-related studies have been conducted on SSHT. Specifically, in most studies conducted in Korea, RAW 264.7 cells are employed as the target model, and LPS is used as an inflammatory inducer to show anti-inflammatory effects. Different concentrations of SSHT have been applied to various cell types to develop relevant methods and targets.

3.2. *In Vivo Studies on SSHT*

Cancer will be a leading cause of death in the 2020s, according to the WHO [67]. Aqueous extracts of SSHT cured cancer in ddY and BALB mouse models (Table 2). Drinking 2.5 g/kg/day of SSHT per month blocked cancer reproduction and metastasis, similar to that of IL-2 monotherapy. In addition, after tumor-transplanted mice drank 1600–2500 mg/kg SSHT for 2–4 weeks, their survival rate increased and their tumor size decreased [68,69]. At the lower dose of 500 mg/kg, oral administration showed antitumor activity by alleviating fibrinogen and glycogen levels in ddY mice after 5 d [70]. In addition to its action in cancers, SSHT has been demonstrated to have anti-fibrotic ability in rats fed up to 1% chow for a minimum of 8 weeks [71,72]. Sakaida et al. reported that 1% chow remarkably altered hydroxyproline and hyaluronic acid and reduced fibrotic markers, for example, COL3A1, myofibroblast-like cells, and glutathione S-transferase placental form (GST-P) positive foci, in induced rats compared with that of a choline-supplemented-amino acid-defined diet group [72]. Another study performed on BALB/c mice for 16 weeks confirmed that a very low dosage of SSHT (5 mL/kg/day) per os inhibits liver injury by decreasing scaring factor levels such as TGF-β1, Hsp47, α-SMA, Col1A1, and Col3A1 [73]. Moreover, the survival rate of ddY male mice with recombinant human tumor necrosis factor (rhTNF)-induced lethality recovered with 500 mg/kg/day feeding with SSHT [74].

In addition to fibrosis, other pathological features of chronic inflammatory diseases are downregulated when hosts are exposed to SSHT. Notably, studies have been conducted on the immune response in female mice because females have more efficient immune responses than males do [75,76]. In 1987, Kawakita et al. used C3H/He female mice as models for B-cell maturation and bacterial infection. SSHT was pre-injected intraperitoneally (I.P.) at different doses (100 and 250 mg/kg) before inflammatory induction. With 100 mg/kg I.P. of the SSHT extract, immune leukocyte levels were notably reduced after 6 h and 4 d of exposure [77]. With 250 mg/kg of the extract, the plaque-forming process was inhibited, and mature IgM+ IgD+ B cells were elevated on days 10 and 14 of treatment in response to exogenous stimulation [78]. I.P. injection of SSHT also rescued the renal failure of C3H/He and (BALB/c $\times$ DBA/2) F~(CDF) female mice [79] and showed significant anti-inflammatory activity at a low dose of 100 mg/mouse by increasing granulocyte macrophage colony-stimulating factor (GM-CSF) secretion [80]. In Nagatsu et al., prostaglandin E2 (PGE2) production decreased, and the membrane fluidity of murine host macrophages was successfully improved by SSHT in a dose- and time-dependent manner [81]. According to many reports, the oral administration of SSHT has been frequently used and has exhibited positive outcomes. In studies from 1994 and 1995 in Japan, SSHT aqueous extract was orally administered to C3H/He mice with chronic hepatitis at a high dose for 12–24 h and notably augmented natural killer (NK) cell activities [82,83]. At 500 mg/kg/day for 5 d, SSHT improved endotoxemia by altering lipid peroxide, xanthine oxidase, SOD, GPx, -tocopherol, and respiratory control index in male mice [84,85].

Recently, in ovalbumin-induced inflammation in BALB/c female mice, 3 weeks of feeding with 100–200 mg/kg/day SSHT decreased Th2-type cytokine levels while activating heme oxygenase-1 (HO-1) protein expression [86]. This data is consistent with the data from the positive control group treated with montelukast sodium, which effectively suppressed immunologic response stages in the muscles, lungs, and entire airway. In addition, an oral dosage of 50 and 100 mg/kg/day diminished IL 6, TNF-α, IL-1, and IFN-γ levels after 17 d [87]. Research in rats has also revealed the anti-inflammatory effects of SSHT. After treatment with 450 mg/kg/day, the aggregation of macrophages (granuloma) and certain lipids was alleviated compared with that of indomethacin, a granuloma inhibitor, and the control group in Wistar male rats [88,89]. The Cytochrome P450 (CYP P450) family of heme isozymes are responsible for drug biotransformation via oxidation. Hence, the CYP inducer rifampicin was used in a positive drug–drug interaction study. Another study by Li et al. performed in Sprague Dawley rats demonstrated the P450s-related drug–drug interaction effect of SSHT in dose-dependent trials in comparison with that of the rifampicin group [90].

Table 2. Summary of designs and biomarkers of in vivo studies (and 1 ex vivo study) on SSHT.

Target Study		Animal (Sex, Age, Body Weight)	Inducer	Type of Extracts	Administration (Frequency/Period)	Experimental Group	Positive Control	Biomarker & Outcome	Authors	Country
Lethality	Anti-lethality	ddY mice (male, 18–20 g)	rhTNF	Aq	500 * mg/kg/day (Oral, 1/day, day 2 & 6 of induced, 72 * h)	4 groups		Survival rate *	Sakaguchi S. et al. (1991) [74]	Japan
Cancer	Antitumor	ddY mice	Ehrlich tumors	Aq	1600 * mg/kg (Oral-drinking, 2 weeks)	10 groups		Survival rate *, TNF *, tumor weight	Haranaka K. et.al. (1985) [68]	Japan
Cancer	Antitumor activity, shock symptoms	ddY mice (male, 18–20 g)	LPS	Aq	500 * mg/kg/day (Oral, 1/day, 5 day)	4 groups		NO_2, Fibrinogen *, Glycogen *	Sakaguchi S. et al. (1996) [70]	Japan
Cancer	Carcinoma	BALB/c mice (female)		Aq	2.5 * g/kg/day (Drink, 30 day)	5 groups	IL-2	IL-6 *, tumor weight *	Huang et al. (1997) [69]	Japan
Fibrosis	Hepatic foci	Sprague Dawley rats (male)	N-nitroso morpholine	Aq	0.5% *, 1% chow (Oral, 8 weeks)	3 groups		GGT *, GST-P * lesion staining, T lymphocyte*	Tatsuta et al. (1991) [71]	Japan
Fibrosis	Liver fibrosis	Wistar rats (male, 140–150 g)	Choline-deficient-amino acid-defined diet	Aq	1% * Chow (Oral, 16 weeks)	5 groups	Choline-supplemented-amino acid-defined diet	Hydroxyproline *, hyaluronic acid *, ALT, AST, COL3A1 *, myofibroblast-like cells *, GST-P lesion *	Isao et al. (1998) [72]	Japan
Fibrosis	Liver fibrosis	BALB/c mice (female, ~20 g)	*S. japonicum*	Aq	XCH-L: 5 * mL/kg/day, XCH-M: 15 * mL/kg/day, XCH-H: 30 * mL/kg/day (Oral, 16 weeks)	6 groups		Serum ALT *, AST *, ALP *, HA * & PIIINP *, ALB * & GLOB *, TGF-β1 *, Hsp47 *, α-SMA *, Col1A1 *, Col3A1 *	Huang et al. (2020) [73]	China
Inflammation	*P. aeruginosa* infection	ICR and C3H/He mice (female)	*P. aeruginosa*	Aq	100 mg/kg (I.P., pretreat 6 h * or 4 days *)	3 groups		Leukocytes *	Kawakita et al. (1987) [77]	Japan

Table 2. *Cont.*

Target Study		Animal (Sex, Age, Body Weight)	Inducer	Type of Extracts	Administration (Frequency/Period)	Experimental Group	Positive Control	Biomarker & Outcome	Authors	Country
Inflammation	Peritoneal macrophage	C3H/HeJ & (BALB/c × DBA/2)F~(CDF) mice (female)		Aq	3 * mg, 5 mg/mouse/day (I.P., 1 time, 4 days)	3 groups		Acid phosphatase & N-acetyl-/3-D-glucosaminidase	Kumazawa. et al. (1988) [79]	Japan
Inflammation	Immune response	ICR mice (male), CBA mice (female)		Aq	1.2 g/kg/day (Oral, 1, 2, 3 *, 5 * day)—0.24, 0.6 *, 1.2 * g/kg/day (Oral, 3 days)	4 groups		PGE2 *, antigens, ARA, membrane fluidity *	Nagatsu et al. (1989) [81]	Japan
Inflammation	Colony-stimulating factors	C3H/He mice, (female)	Carrageenan	Aq	100 * mg/kg (I.P., serum I.V.)	3 groups		GM-CSF	Yonekura et al. (1990) [80]	Japan
Inflammation	Ovalbumin-induced inflammation	BALB/c (OVA)-induced mice (female)		Aq	100 *, 200 * mg/kg/day (Oral, 1/day, 18–23 days)	5 groups	Montelukast	Th2-type cytokines *, eotaxin, (HO)-1 *	Jeon et al. (2015) [85]	Korea
Inflammation	Cachexia-related symptoms	BALB/c CT-26-bearing mice		Aq	50 * and 100 * mg/kg/day (Oral, 1/day, 17 days)	4 groups		IL-6, TNF-α, IL-1, IFN-γ	Kim et.al. (2016) [86]	Korea
Inflammation	Peyer's patches (IgA production)	C3H/He mice (female)	LPS	Aq	200, 500, 1000 *, 2000 * mg/kg/day (Oral, 1/day, 2 day)	5 groups		SRBC-IgA & -HRBC IgA	Tauchi et al. (1993) [91]	Japan
Inflammation	Drug-drug interaction (CYPs)	Sprague Dawley Rats (male, 200–240 g)		Aq	Low dose, 1.7 * g/kg/day Medium dose, 3.4 * g/kg/day High dose, 6.8 * g/kg/day (Oral, 1/day, 3 & 6 days)	Control groups Treatment groups	CYP inducer (Rifampicin)	P450s (Cyp1a2, Cyp3a1, Cyp2d6, Cyp1b1)	Li et al. (2021) [89]	China

Table 2. *Cont.*

Target Study		Animal (Sex, Age, Body Weight)	Inducer	Type of Extracts	Administration (Frequency/Period)	Experimental Group	Positive Control	Biomarker & Outcome	Authors	Country
Inflammation	Endotoxemia	ddY mice (male, 18–20 g)	Endotoxin	Aq	500 * mg/kg/day (Oral, 1/day, 5 days)	4 groups		Lipid peroxide *, Xanthine oxidase *, SOD *, GPx *, α-Tocophero *, nonprotein SH *, acid phosphatase *, LDH *	Sakaguchi. et al. (1993) [84]	Japan
Inflammation	Granuloma	Wistar rats (male, ~200 g)	Carrageenin cotton pellet	Aq	450 * mg/kg/day (Oral, 1/day/8 days)	4 groups	Indomethacin	Granuloma weight *, acid-soluble glycoprotein *, sialic acid	Yoshida et al. (1993) [87]	Japan
Inflammation	NK activities	C3H/He mice (female)		Aq	500, 1000 * mg/kg (Oral 12 h * & 24 h)	3 groups		GM1, CD3, CD4, CD8, NK cell *	Kaneko et al. (1994) [82]	Japan
Inflammation	Granuloma	Wistar rats (male)	Carrageenin cotton pellet	Aq	450 * mg/kg/day (Oral, 1/day/8 days)	4 groups	Indomethacin	Vit E *, cholesterol, phospholipid, lipid peroxide *, granuloma weight *	Yoshida et al. (1994) [88]	Japan
Inflammation	Endotoxemia	ddY mice (male, 18–20 g)	Endotoxin	Aq	500 * mg/kg/day (Oral, 1/day, 5 days)	4 groups		$[Ca^{2+}]$ *, Mg^{2+}, Ca^{2+}-ATPase *, respiratory control index *	Sakaguchi et al. (1994) [84]	Japan
Inflammation	Macrophage function	Sprague Dawley rats (male, 150–155 g)	Gum arabic	Aq	1 g/kg/day (Oral, 3 weeks, 22 *–28 days)	4 groups		Superoxide anions	Fujiwara et al. (1995) [92]	Japan
Inflammation	NK activities	C3H/He mice (female)		Aq	1000 mg/kg, 1–12 * fraction (Oral, 1 time, 12 h)	12 groups		NK activities *	Yamaoka et al. (1995) [83]	Japan

Table 2. *Cont.*

Target Study		Animal (Sex, Age, Body Weight)	Inducer	Type of Extracts	Administration (Frequency/Period)	Experimental Group	Positive Control	Biomarker & Outcome	Authors	Country
Inflammation	B-cell maturation	C3H/He mice (female)	TNP-LPS (TI-1), TNP-Ficol (TI-2), SRCB (TD)	Aq	250 mg/kg (I.P., 4, 7, 10 *, 14 * days)	Control group Treatment group		Plaque-forming cells (PFC), IgM+ IgD+ * B cell, Thy1 antibody	Kawakita et al. (1987) [78]	Japan
Metabolic disorder	D-galactosamine -induced liver injury	ICR mice (male, 18–22 g)		Aq	Low dose 0.02 * g/kg/day Medium dose 1 * g/kg/day High dose 5 * g/kg/day (Oral, 1/day, 14 days)	6 groups	Biphenyl dicarboxylate	IL-6 *, TNF-α *, Fas*, Fas-L *, Bcl-2 *, Bax *	Zhou et al. (2012) [93]	China
Metabolic disorder	Perimenopausal disorder	Kunming Mice (female, 18–22 g)		Aq	2.3, 7 *, 21 * g/kg/day (Oral, 1/day, 8 weeks)	8 Groups	E2 & fluoxetine	HPA/HPO axis, Erβ, TPH2	Zhang et al. (2020) [94]	China
Metabolic disorder	Age-induced amnesia	Fischer F254 rats (male)		Aq	120 * mg/kg/day (Oral, 1/day, 72–110 * week-old)	4 groups	α-Tocopherol nicotinate	PAR failure *	Amagaya et al. (1990) [95]	Japan
Metabolic disorder	Liver injury	Wistar rats (male, 150–160 g)	D-galactosamine	Aq	1 * g/kg (Oral/I.P., 1 time, 24 h *)	8 groups		Albumin *, total protein *, 5′-nucleosidase *, glucose 6-phosphatase *, serum TG	Ohta et al. (1997) [96]	Japan
Metabolic disorder	Chronic pancreatitis	Wistar rats (male, 170–190 g)	Dibutyltin dichloride	Aq	10 * g/kg/day (Oral, 1/day, 28 days)	3 groups		Exocrine pancreatic function (PABA *), TGF-β1 *, TGFβRII *, Smad3 *, Smad7	Zhang et al. (2013) [97]	China
Metabolic disorder	Anti-hyperlipidemia & antiatherosclerosis	Hypercholesterolemic C57BL/6J mice (male, 20–24 g)		Aq	1.2 * g/kg/day (Oral, 1/day, 2–4 * weeks)	4 groups		Cholesterol *, T cell *, cholesterol oleate *, HDL, LDL, Acyl-CoA *, ACAT, NCEase *	Shen et al. (1996) [98]	Japan
Metabolic disorder	Hypercholesterolemia	ICR mice (male)		Aq	1.2 g/kg/day (Oral, 1/day, 2 weeks)	4 groups		PGE2 *, IL-1, NO *, LPC	Inoue et al. (1996) [90]	Japan

Table 2. *Cont.*

Target Study		Animal (Sex, Age, Body Weight)	Inducer	Type of Extracts	Administration (Frequency/Period)	Experimental Group	Positive Control	Biomarker & Outcome	Authors	Country
Metabolic disorder	Hypercholesterolemia	New Zealand White rabbits (male, 1.5–2 g)	LPS	Aq	3% chow (Oral, 20 * weeks)	3 groups		Monocyte *, cholesterol, LDL	Shen et al. (1996) [99]	Japan
Metabolic disorder	Tolbutamide bioavailability	Sprague Dawley rats (male, 302–376)		Aq	500 * mg/kg/day (Oral, 1/day, 6 days)	Single (2 groups) Multiple (2 groups)		Absorption rate & bioavailability of Tolbutamide	Nishimura et al. (1999) [100]	Japan
Metabolic disorder	Radical scavenging	Wistar rats (male)		Aq	500 * mg/kg (Oral, 1 time, plasma collection at 1, 2, 4, 6, 10, 12 *, 24 *h)	3 groups	α-Tocopherol & ascorbic acid	O_2- *, -OH *, DPPH *,	Egashira et al. (1999) [101]	Japan
Metabolic disorder	Gastric function	Sprague Dawley rat (male, 215–347 g)		Aq	250 *, 750 * mg/kg (Oral, 1 time, 20 & 40 min)	Control group Treatment group		Gastric emptying rate (GER)	Nishimura et al. (2001) [102]	Japan
Metabolic disorder	Hepatic microvascular dysfunction	Wistar rats (male, 200–250 g)	Gut ischemia/reperfusion	Aq	1 * g/kg/day (I.G., 1/day, 7 days)	5 groups		Leukocytes * (pericentral * & midzonal region), NPS *, TNF-α *, ALT	Horie et al. (2001) [103]	Japan
Metabolic disorder	Tolbutamide permeability	Ex vivo, Sprague Dawley rats (male)		Aq	50 * mg/kg (I.P., 10–60 min)	Control group Treatment group		Epithelial membrane permeability of Tolbutamide	Nishimura et al. (2010 [104])	Japan

Aq, aqueous; I.P., intraperitoneal injection; TNF, tumor necrosis factor; PGE2, Prostaglandin E2; ARA, Arachidonic acid; I.V., intravenous; GM-CSF, Granulocyte macrophage colony-stimulating factor; PAR, passive avoidance responses; GGT, γ-glutamyl transpeptidase; GST-P, Placental glutathione S-transferase; HRBC-IgA, horse erythrocyte-IgA; SRBC-IgA, Sheep red blood cells-IgA; SOD, Superoxide dismutase; GPx, Glutathione peroxidase; nonprotein SH, nonprotein sulfhydryl; LDH, Lactate Dehydrogenase; NK, Natural Killer Cell; GM1, Ganglioside; CD, cluster of differentiation; Vit E, Vitamin E; ATPase, adenosine triphosphate catalyst; NO_2, Nitrogen Dioxide; HDL, High Density Lipoprotein; LDL, low-density lipoprotein; ACAT, Acyl-CoA: cholesterol Acyltransferase; NCEase, neutral cholesterol ester hydrolase; IL-1, Interleukin-1; NO, Nitric oxide; LPC, Lysophosphatidylcholines; IL-2, Interleukin-2; DPPH, 2, 2-diphenyl-1-picrylhydrazyl; I.G., Intragastric; NPS, nonperfused sinusoids ; ALT, alanine aminotransferase; (HO)-1, enzyme heme oxygenase-1; IFN-γ, interferon gamma; Fas, Fas Cell Surface Death Receptor; FasL: Fas ligand; Bcl-2, B-cell lymphoma 2; Bax, bcl-2-like protein 4; HPA/HPO, hypothalamic-pituitary-adrenal/hypothalamic-pituitary-ovarian;, Erβ, Estrogen receptor beta; TPH2, Tryptophan hydroxylase 2; E2, estradiol; P450s, CYP, cytochrome p450; TGF-β1, transforming growth factor beta 1. (*) concentration with significant effect.

Furthermore, SSHT has been used to treat many metabolic disorders, including hepatic and pancreatic injuries, hyperlipidemia, and atherosclerosis. Experiments performed on male ICR mice and rabbits showed positive results for hypercholesterolemia reduction with low-dose absorption of SSHT (1.2 g/kg/day for 2 weeks) and 3% chow for 20 weeks [98,99]. Significance was analyzed in comparison with that of the biphenyl dicarboxylate-treated group, which was proven to abolish ALT in chronic liver disease models. Similarly, 1.2 g/kg/day of SSHT administered orally for 4 weeks initiated anti-hypercholesterolemia and antiatherosclerosis activity by attenuating cholesterol, T cells, cholesterol oleate, and acyl-CoA levels in hypercholesterolemic C57BL/6J mice [96]. In addition, hepatic injury in Wistar rats was rescued with 1 g/kg/day oral, I.P., and intragastric (I.G.) administration, which altered albumin, glucose 6-phosphatase, and leukocytes (pericentral and midzonal regions) [97,103]. By recovering exocrine pancreatic function (PABA) and dropping TGF-β1, TGFβRII, and the Smad3 protein level, SSHT was also verified as a chronic pancreatitis therapy in rats [97]. Different doses of SSHT were applied to mice with liver damage and perimenopausal disorder and had better results than the positive control groups did [93,94]. Studies by Nishimura et al. in Sprague Dawley rats have demonstrated the increased insulin sensitivity potential of oral and I.P.-administered SSHT by extending tolbutamide absorption [100,104]. Other reports in rats have shown that oral treatment with SSHT suppressed age-induced amnesia, scavenged radicals, and boosted the gastric emptying rate at modest doses [95,101,102]. These findings correlated with the positive treatment results of α-tocopherol, an antioxidant that scavenges lipid peroxyl radicals.

In summary, the aqueous extract of SSHT exhibits a wide range of therapeutic effects owing to its multicomponent characteristics. Among the 36 in vivo examinations of SSHT therapeutic ability, five were from China, two were from Korea, and the remainder were from Japan. Studies conducted in Japan were primarily performed in the 1990s and 2000s by using single- or double-dose treatments over multiple timeframes. By contrast, reports from China and Korea have been conducted in a dose-dependent manner over a single timeframe. Because fibrosis and inflammatory conditions have a wide range of effects on the body, various biomarkers have been enrolled, for example, lymphocyte accumulation, TNF-α, IL-6, and IL-1. By contrast, studies on cancer or metabolic disorders have focused on disease-specific markers such as tumor weight and tumor necrosis factor (TNF) expression in cancer research.

3.3. Clinical Studies on SSHT

Seven studies on SSHT were analyzed: four randomized controlled trials (RCTs) and three case reports (Table 3). For the efficacy evaluation of SSHT, four reports—one case of gastrointestinal disease in atopic patients, one case of depression in a patient with malignant cancer, and one case each of liver cirrhosis and hepatitis—were employed. In addition, two clinical cases reported that hepatotoxicity in middle-aged individuals could result from SSHT ingestion; one case successfully rescued liver function in a patient with chronic hepatitis C.

Four RCTs have evaluated the efficacy of SSHT on gastrointestinal diseases in patients with AD, depressive symptoms in patients with cancer, cirrhosis, and chronic active hepatitis. Sixty AD patients with gastrointestinal disorders [25] were enrolled and diagnosed using the Hanifin and Rajka criteria, with an AD (SCORAD) index score between 15 and 49. The participants were randomly assigned to the SSHT and placebo (PLA) groups at a 1:1 ratio, and efficacy was evaluated after 4 and 8 weeks. The participants were orally administered SSHT or PLA thrice daily for 4 weeks. This clinical study showed no statistically significant changes in AD severity or digestive symptoms in patients with AD treated with SSHT. However, as a complementary alternative treatment for AD, SSHT has been reported to alter steroid ointment dependence and improve the quality of life in patients with AD. A study on depressive symptoms in patients with cancer [39] was conducted to investigate the effects of SSHT on depression-associated tumors and its potential mechanisms. Specifically, a PLA-controlled trial was conducted in cancer patients with comorbid depressive symptoms to evaluate the effects of SSHT on depression scales, tumor-related immune indicators, and gut microbial composition. Seventy-two participants with lung, breast, colorectal, thyroid, and other cancers were randomly assigned to either the SSHT or PLA groups at a 1:1 ratio. The participants received 19 g of SSHT or PLA twice daily via oral administration for 6 weeks. Sixty-one participants completed the study. After 6 weeks of intervention, a significant decrease in the SDS score was observed in both groups. Antidepressant effects were more pronounced in the SSHT group than in the PLA group, as revealed by the differential SDS values (ΔSDS). The circulating cytokines assay further indicated that SSHT treatment downregulated TNF-α and IL-6 levels relative to the baseline and/or the PLA groups. The results of fecal 16S rRNA sequencing showed no significant differences between the Chao and Shannon indices on an operational taxonomic unit (OUT)-based principal component analysis (PCA).

A study on patients with cirrhosis [105] was conducted to evaluate the preventive effect of SSHT on hepatocellular carcinoma (HCC) development. Two hundred and sixty patients with cirrhosis were randomly assigned to two groups at a 1:1 ratio and matched for age, sex, presence of hepatitis B surface antigen, and severity of liver damage. Patients in the trial group were administered SSHT at a daily oral dose of 7.5 g in addition to the conventional drugs administered to the controls. The patients were prospectively monitored for 60 months, and the cumulative incidence of HCC and survival rates in the two groups were calculated. As a result, the 5-year survival curve of the trial group was higher than that of the control group, and for patients without HBs antigen, the difference was significant. Clinical research on chronic active hepatitis [106] enrolled 222 patients with the disease and conducted a double-blind, multicenter clinical study. One hundred and sixteen patients received SSHT at a daily oral dose of 5.4 g for 12 weeks, followed by the same dose for another 12 weeks. One hundred and six patients received PLA containing SSHT (0.5 g) for 12 weeks, followed by a crossover to SSHT for another 12 weeks. The medications assigned to the patients were coded by a controller and randomly assigned to the patients. This study showed that serum AST and ALT levels decreased significantly with the administration of SSHT. In addition, in patients with chronic active type B hepatitis, a tendency toward a decrease in HBeAg and an increase in anti-HBe antibodies was also observed.

Three case reports on the efficacy and adverse effects of SSHT have been published. In one case report on the efficacy of SSHT, 24 patients with chronic hepatitis C [107] were enrolled in a case study. The participants were orally administered medication thrice a day for 12 months. Liver function, hepatitis C virus (HCV) load, and liver biopsy histology were assessed before and after the intervention. Improvement in AST and ALT was observed in 16 (67%) and 18 (75%) participants, respectively. In nine subjects who showed improvement in their Knodell's histology activity index (HAI) score, paired liver biopsies before and after treatment showed improvement. Case reports on the adverse effects and toxicity of SSHT were published in 1995 and 2006, respectively. The study in 1995 [108] reported the side effects of SSHT in four patients: a 51-, 52-, 58-, and 42-year-old woman; SSHT (7.5 g) was orally administered one or more times per day for 2 d up to 1.5 months. All patients who visited the hospital showed elevated levels of ALT and AST in their blood, and liver biopsies showed signs of hepatitis. Symptoms improved after the discontinuation of the drug. In a 2006 case report [109], a 52-year-old woman exhibited weakness, fatigue, and tea-colored urine after continuous consumption of SSHT twice daily for 1.5 months. Laboratory examination upon admission revealed elevated serum levels of aspartate aminotransferase (AST), alanine aminotransferase (ALT), γ-glutamyl transpeptidase, alkaline phosphatase, total bilirubin, and direct bilirubin. Liver biopsy revealed acute hepatocellular hepatitis symptoms. The symptoms improved after the discontinuation of the drug, and the liver biochemical tests normalized two months later.

Table 3. Summary of designs and biomarkers of clinical studies on SSHT.

Target Disease	Study Design (Sample Size, n)	Type of Preparation Form	Extraction Method	Dose	Duration (Frequency)	Control	Outcomes	Results	Authors	Country
Gastrointestinal disorders of AD patients	RCT (60: I 30, C 30)	NA	NA	NA	6 weeks (3/days)	PLA	(1) SCORAD index (2) Amount and frequency of ointment application for AD (3) Dermatology quality of life index (4) Safety evaluation	(1) (2) not statistically significant (3) reduced (4) normal range	Lee et al. (2021) [25]	Korea
Depressive symptoms of cancer patients	RCT (72: I 36, C 36)	Granule	Aq	9.5 g/pack	6 weeks (2/days)	PLA	(1) Depressive scales (SDS) (2) Circulating cytokines assay (3) Gut microbial composition	(1) $p < 0.05$ (2) $p < 0.05$ (TNF-α, IL-6) (3) not significant	Shao et al. (2021) [39]	China
Cirrhosis	RCT (260: I 130, C 130)	NA	NA	7.5 g/day	60 months (1/days)	PLA	(1) Cumulative incidence of HCC (2) Survival rate	(1) inhibitory effect (2) high survival rate	Oka et al. (1995) [105]	Japan
Chronic active hepatitis	RCT (222: I, C)	Granule	NA	5.4 g/day	24 weeks (3/days)	PLA	(1) ALT (2) AST (3) HBeAg	(1) (2) decreased blood levels (3) decreased HBeAg (increased anti-HBe antibody)	Hirayama et al. (1989) [106]	Japan
Hepatitis C	Case report (24)	Granule	Aq	2.5 g/pack	12 months (3/days)	-	(1) Liver function (2) HCV viral load (3) Liver biopsy histology	(1) improved (2) mixed (3) improved	Deng et al. (2011) [107]	USA
Adverse effect	Case report (1)	NA	Aq	NA	1.5 month (2/days)	-	(1) ALT, AST (2) Liver biopsy	(1) increased (2) revealed lesion	Hsu et al. (2006) [109]	Taiwan
Adverse effect	Case report (4)	Granule	NA	7.5 g/day	6–7 weeks (1/days)	-	(1) ALT, AST, ALP, γGT, bilirubin (2) Liver histology	(1) increased (2) revealed lesion	Itoh et al. (1995) [108]	Japan

AD, atopic dermatitis; ALT, alanine aminotransferase; AST, aspartate aminotransferase; HBeAg, hepatitis B e antigen; HCA, hepatitis C virus; HCC, hepatocellular carcinoma; SCORAD, atopic dermatitis score; APL, alkaline phosphatase; γGT, γ-glutamyl transpeptidase, PLA, placebo group; VAS, visual analog scale. NA, not applicable.

4. Discussion

SSHT is a traditional herbal prescription used in East Asian medicine, particularly in Korea. In present study, we first provide an overall summary of previous in vitro, in vivo (Figure 2), and clinical research of SSHT effects on certain diseases and metabolic disorders. Subsequently, this will give the readers an insight into how multi-targeted biomarkers can be successfully engaged in TCM therapeutic studies.

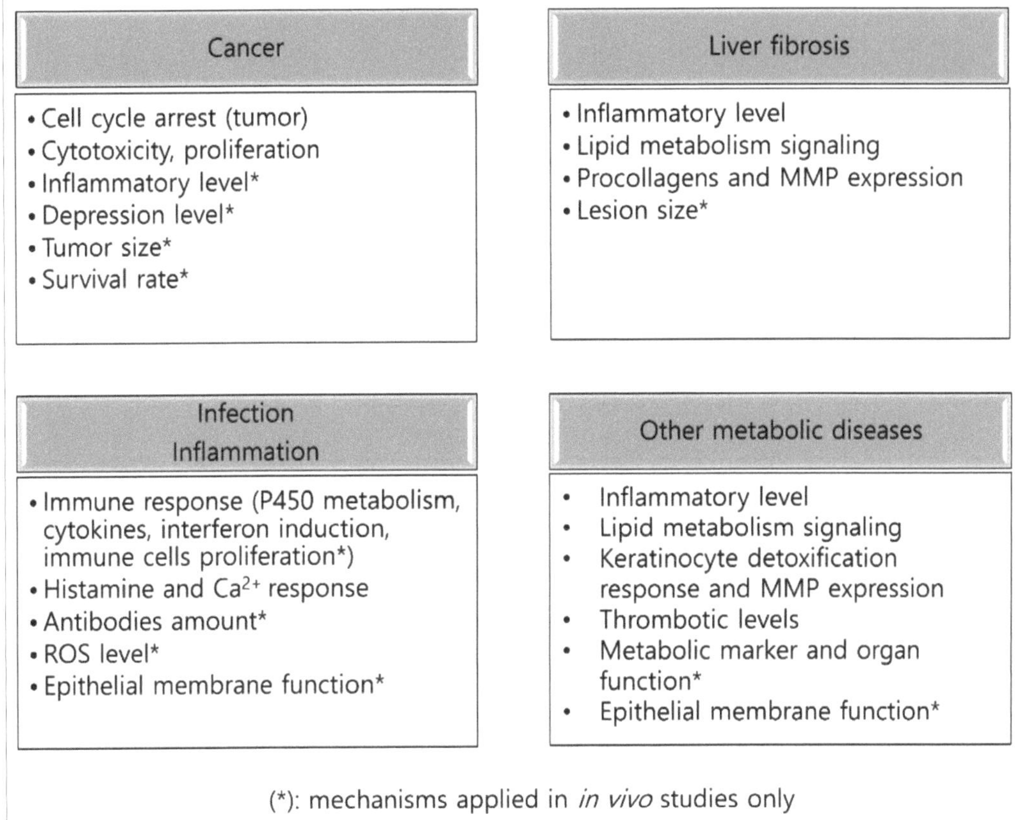

Figure 2. Target diseases and related mechanisms of SSHT in in vitro and in vivo experiments.

In many cell-based studies (Table 1), hepatocytes and hepatocarcinoma cells have been treated with aqueous SSHT. SSHT is usually extracted using distilled water and freeze-dried before applying it to the experiments. Based on research data, SSHT was earlier assigned for various hepatic diseases medication including hepatitis virus infection and cancer alleviation. Therefore, various biomarkers were assessed in the SSHT-treated hepatic cells. As shown in the large category of immune reactions in blood cells, there is antithrombotic activity in platelets, endotoxin-induced cytotoxicity in J774A.1 cells, and histamine release in mast cells. Anti-inflammatory effects of SSHT were evaluated in HGFs, AR42J cells, and RAW264.7 cells. In addition, IL-6 is the only common biomarker of the anti-inflammatory effect of SSHT in the summarized articles. In addition, SSHT has been proven to protect keratinocytes and has anti-tumor activity in various cancer cells. In spleen cells, one study tested mitogenic activity, and another study tested the induction effect of interferon. Regarding the in vitro system, a wide range of cells have been utilized to determine the therapeutic potential of SSHT by examining many biomarkers using various methods.

Among the 36 studies performed on animal models (Table 2), 2.8% investigated the efficacy of SSHT on anti-lethality, 8.3% reported anticancer and antifibrosis effects, and 36% studied metabolic-related diseases. The largest proportion of in vivo examinations were anti-inflammatory studies, accounting for 44% of the total. Broad preclinical applications of the traditional SSHT remedy have been reported for decades. Owing to its multicomponent features, this herbal medicine exhibits a wide range of therapeutic effects, including antitumor, anti-lethal, antifibrosis, anti-inflammation, and antimetabolic activities. In general, oral administration has been employed for most case studies of SSHT and other folk remedies because many components can be distributed safely by the gastrointestinal system. Feeding a modest dosage of 100 mg/kg/day protected rodent models from certain infections after 2 weeks. At 500 mg/kg/day per os, SSHT recovered murine cancers and inflammatory endotoxemia after 5 d of treatment. For the long-term treatment of cancer and hepatic fibrosis, a low dosage of SSHT (5 mL/kg/day) can be applied for 8–16 weeks. In metabolic disease therapies, a high dosage of 1.2 g/kg/day has been used for anti-hypercholesterolemia and anti-atherosclerotic activities in mouse and rabbit models for 2–4 weeks. Additionally, I.P. injection induced significant curing effects of SSHT on inflammation and metabolic disorders in rodent models because large amounts of herbal extracts can be promptly absorbed through the peritoneum into the body. SSHT can be injected at 100–1000 mg for the recovery of anti-inflammatory and insulin resistance in mice and rats. On the other hand, animal studies have been controversial owing to ethical concerns, and conducting experiments on animals requires comprehensive knowledge and caution.

Seven clinical studies on SSHT have been reported: four RCTs and three case reports (Table 3). The four RCTs evaluated the efficacy of SSHT on gastrointestinal illness in patients with AD, depressive symptoms in patients with cancer, cirrhosis, and chronic active hepatitis. The efficacy of SSHT in patients with AD showed improvements in the SCORAD index, gastrointestinal symptoms, and atopic dermatitis symptoms. Based on these results, our expectation is that SSHT will reduce the dependence on steroid ointments and improve the quality of life of patients with AD. A study on depressive symptoms in patients with cancer showed progress in depression, tumor-related immune indicators, and gut microbial composition [39]. Another study on liver cirrhosis showed that SSHT initiated an improvement in the cumulative incidence of HCC and the survival rate in patients with liver cirrhosis [105]. This gives rise to the utilization of SSHT in chronic liver illnesses treatments. In addition, the publication of SSHT medicinal application on chronic active hepatitis showed a decrease in serum AST and ALT values and HBeAg, but an increase in anti-HBe antibodies in patients with chronic active type B hepatitis [106]. In three case reports, SSHT was effective in alleviating hepatitis C symptoms by improving liver lesion and function [107]. However, two clinical cases in elderly groups reported hepatotoxicity resulting in elevated blood ALT and AST levels and liver tissue damage after SSHT ingestion [108,109]. Of the clinical research on SSHT, efficacy as well as toxicity in the liver accounted for the largest portion (5 cases), followed by gastrointestinal diseases and depression. These results show that SSHT administration at appropriate doses should be taken into consideration, which can help recover not only the liver but also gastrointestinal diseases, AD, and depression.

SSHT is a multitargeted herbal formula comprising various medicinal herbs with potential therapeutic effects. The evaluation of its effects involves identifying specific biomarkers, which are measurable indicators that can reflect changes or responses to the treatment (Figure 3). Since inflammation is a symbol of a wide range from acute to chronic diseases, inflammatory mediators were targeted for many medical studies. Herein, we have summarized the effective biomarkers which were enrolled in this review as follows.

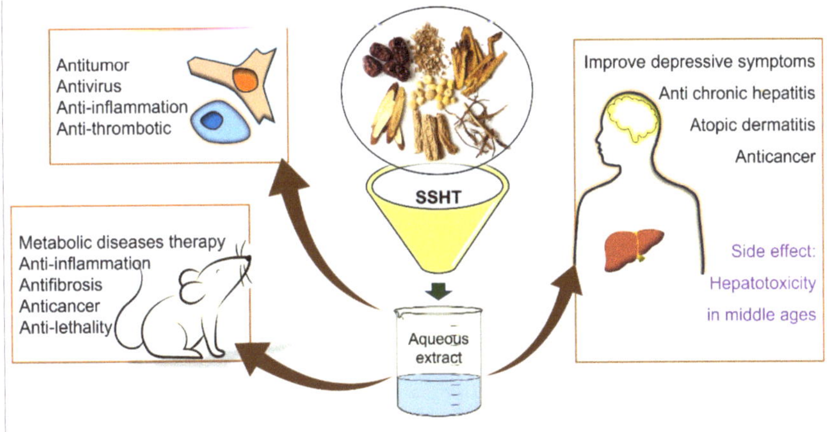

Figure 3. Schematic description of SSHT therapeutic application.

(I) Inflammatory markers: SSHT modulated the inflammatory response by altering cytokines like interleukins (IL-1β, IL-4, IL-6, IL-10, IL-12), Th2, TNF-α, TGF-β, IFN-γ, and G-CSF. In addition, P450s and COX-2/PGE2 system also take part in drug metabolism and tumor genesis mediation, respectively. The modulation of these factors presented the therapeutic capacity of SSHT on inflammatory responses, acute and chronic disease, apoptosis, and cancers.

(II) Immune function markers: SSHT might influence immune function by evaluating markers such as leukocytes (CD3, CD4+, and CD8+ T-cell), granulocytes, and natural killer (NK) cell activity, as well as histamine, which could shed light on its immunomodulatory anti-allergy, anti-chronic disease (liver fibrosis), and anticancer effects.

(III) Oxidative markers: The herbal prescription's antioxidative properties can be assessed by measuring biomarkers such as ROS, NO, iNOS, and endogenous antioxidant SOD and GPx levels. These markers can also be employed for inflammation state and apoptosis research.

(IV) Cell cycle progression and apoptosis markers: The inhibition of SSHT on certain cell cycle regulative biomarkers including Cyclin D, CDK (4 and 6), mitosis, and DNA synthesis levels could be targeted for cancers' research. Additionally, apoptosis markers like TNF family (Fas-L) and Bcl2 are aims of cytotoxicity and apoptosis studies of SSHT.

(V) Cellular signaling markers: The herbal prescription's multi-targeted effects may involve modulation of various cellular signaling pathways, such as MAPK (ERK, p38), NF-κB, IκBα, JAK-STAT, Nrf2/HO-1, and PI3K/AKT. Measuring the activity or expression levels of signaling molecules (FAS, ATGL, LPL, PPARs, MMPs, α-SMA, and certain indicative proteins) and transcription factors can provide insights into their mechanisms of action in fibrosis, metabolic disorders, and chronic diseases.

(VI) Metabolic markers: SSHT might have implications for metabolic health. Biomarkers such as blood glucose, insulin, vitamins, enzymes (AST/ALT, TPH2, ACAT, NCEase), hormones (HPA/HPO, Erβ), antigens and antibodies (SRBC-IgA and -HRBC IgA), collagen types, and lipid profiles (LDL, HDL, TG, and cholesterol) can be monitored. These metabolic markers were applied in fibrosis, inflammation state, cancer, acute and chronic disease, and infection research work.

(VII) Other biological indicators: The therapeutic effects of SSHT can be investigated by measuring granuloma weight (inflammations), tumor weight (cancers), fibrosis lesion level (fibrosis), respiratory index (endotoxemia), membrane fluidity (immune response), absorption rate (diabetes), SCORAD index (gastrointestinal disorders), gastric emptying rate (gut gastric function), depressive scale and gut microbial composition (mental diseases), and liver biopsy (liver diseases) as well.

SSHT represents the integration of traditional herbal knowledge with modern research, making it a potential candidate for complementary and alternative medicine. The multitargeted nature of the herbal prescription may offer a broad spectrum of effects, potentially addressing multiple aspects of a health condition simultaneously. As biomarker research advances, it might enable personalized treatment approaches with SSHT, tailoring the prescription based on individual patient profiles. Further research is necessary to establish the safety profile of SSHT and standardize its preparation to ensure consistent quality and efficacy. Rigorous clinical trials are essential to establish the therapeutic benefits of SSHT, providing evidence for its use in various health conditions.

It is important to note that scientific research in the field of herbal medicine is continually evolving, and more recent studies might have expanded our understanding of SSHT and its effects. For the most up-to-date and comprehensive information, it would be better to consult the latest scientific literature and consult with qualified healthcare professionals. Recently, efforts to understand the disease by integrating conventional molecular biological experiments, bio-big data analysis, and AI technologies have increased rapidly. In order to know the polypharmacological effects of multicomponents, a lot of time and effort is only required through conventional experiments [108,109]. Therefore, it is possible to develop a deeper understanding of the disease and better treatments through a more integrated approach.

Our work analyzed the literature on the protection of the traditional remedy SSHT in not only cell and animal-based tests but also in clinical models. We have summarized the mechanisms of certain multitargeted biomarkers involved in the conducted experiments and made a brief outline. Therefore, this review paper can give readers a comprehensive view of the SSHT therapeutic potential.

Author Contributions: Conceptualization, K.S.K.; methodology, N.K.S.T. and J.Y.P.; formal analysis, J.H.L.; investigation, N.K.S.T., M.J.L. and J.H.L.; writing—original draft preparation, N.K.S.T., M.J.L. and J.H.L.; writing—review and editing, J.Y.P. and K.S.K.; project administration, K.S.K.; funding acquisition, K.S.K. All authors have read and agreed to the published version of the manuscript.

Funding: This research was supported by a grant (21173MFDS561) from Ministry of Food and Drug Safety in 2023.

Institutional Review Board Statement: Not applicable.

Informed Consent Statement: Not applicable.

Data Availability Statement: The data presented in this study are available on request from the corresponding author.

Conflicts of Interest: The authors declare no conflict of interest.

References

1. Atanasov, A.G.; Zotchev, S.B.; Dirsch, V.M.; Supuran, C.T. Natural products in drug discovery: Advances and opportunities. *Nat. Rev. Drug Discov.* **2021**, *20*, 200–216. [CrossRef] [PubMed]
2. Kominsky, D.J.; Campbell, E.L.; Colgan, S.P. Metabolic shifts in immunity and inflammation. *J. Immunol.* **2010**, *184*, 4062–4068. [CrossRef] [PubMed]
3. Pålsson-McDermott, E.M.; O'Neill, L.A. Targeting immunometabolism as an anti-inflammatory strategy. *Cell Res.* **2020**, *30*, 300–314. [CrossRef]
4. Bashir Dar, K.; Hussain Bhat, A.; Amin, S.; Masood, A.; Afzal Zargar, M.; Ahmad Ganie, S. Inflammation: A multidimensional insight on natural anti-inflammatory therapeutic compounds. *Curr. Med. Chem.* **2016**, *23*, 3775–3800. [CrossRef] [PubMed]
5. Hotamisligil, G.S. Inflammation and metabolic disorders. *Nature* **2006**, *444*, 860–867. [CrossRef] [PubMed]
6. Wu, H.; Ballantyne, C.M. Metabolic inflammation and insulin resistance in obesity. *Circ. Res.* **2020**, *126*, 1549–1564. [CrossRef] [PubMed]
7. Ghasemian, M.; Owlia, S.; Owlia, M.B. Review of anti-inflammatory herbal medicines. *Adv. Pharmacol. Pharm. Sci.* **2016**, *2016*, 9130979. [CrossRef]
8. Yatoo, M.; Gopalakrishnan, A.; Saxena, A.; Parray, O.R.; Tufani, N.A.; Chakraborty, S.; Tiwari, R.; Dhama, K.; Iqbal, H. Anti-inflammatory drugs and herbs with special emphasis on herbal medicines for countering inflammatory diseases and disorders-a review. *Recent Pat. Inflamm. Allergy Drug Discov.* **2018**, *12*, 39–58. [CrossRef]

9. Food and Drug Administration. Finding and Learning about Side Effects (Adverse Reactions). 2021. Available online: https://www.fda.gov/drugs/information-consumers-and-patients-drugs/finding-and-learning-about-side-effects-adverse-reactions (accessed on 25 September 2023).
10. Goldman, J.L.; Jackson, M.A. Tip of the iceberg: Understanding the unintended consequences of antibiotics. *Pediatrics* **2015**, *136*, e492–e493. [CrossRef]
11. Poluzzi, E.; Raschi, E.; Godman, B.; Koci, A.; Moretti, U.; Kalaba, M.; Wettermark, B.; Sturkenboom, M.; de Ponti, F. Pro-arrhythmic potential of oral antihistamines (H1). *PLoS ONE* **2015**, *10*, e0119551. [CrossRef]
12. Zeynettin, K.; Tuncez, A. Adverse Cardiac Effects of Decongestants Agents. *Eur. J. Gen. Med.* **2013**, *10*, 32–35. [CrossRef]
13. Shao, I.-H.; Wu, C.-C.; Tseng, H.-J.; Lee, T.-J.; Lin, Y.-H.; Tam, Y.-Y. Voiding dysfunction in patients with nasal congestion treated with pseudoephedrine: A prospective study. *Drug Des. Dev. Ther.* **2016**, *10*, 2333–2339. [CrossRef]
14. Lu, C.Y.; Zhang, F.; Lakoma, M.D.; Butler, M.G.; Fung, V.; Larkin, E.K.; Kharbanda, E.O.; Vollmer, W.M.; Lieu, T.; Soumerai, S.B. Asthma treatments and mental health visits after a Food and Drug Administration label change for leukotriene inhibitors. *Clin. Ther.* **2015**, *37*, 1280–1291. [CrossRef] [PubMed]
15. Kochetkov, P.; Svistushkin, V.; Shchennikova, E. Intranasal glucocorticosteroids for the complex treatment of patients with chronic diseases of the nose and paranasal sinuses. *Meditsinskiy Sovet.* **2020**, *6*, 66–70. [CrossRef]
16. Benzie, I.F.; Wachtel-Galor, S. *Herbal Medicine: Biomolecular and Clinical Aspects*; CRC Press: Boca Raton, FL, USA, 2011.
17. El Mostafa, S.B.; Maamri, A. Herbal Medicine in Chronic Diseases Treatment: Determinants, Benefits and Risks. In *Disease Prevention and Health Promotion in Developing Countries*; Springer Nature: Berlin/Heidelberg, Germany, 2020; Volume 85. [CrossRef]
18. Kang, S.-J.; Jo, E.-H.; Yang, G.-J.; Shim, Y.-H.; Hong, J.-E.; Park, M.-C. Efficacy and safety of Soshiho-tang in patients with atopic dermatitis and gastrointestinal disorders: Study protocol for a double-blind, randomized, and placebo-controlled clinical trial. *Medicine* **2019**, *98*, e15479. [CrossRef] [PubMed]
19. Yamashiki, M.; Nishimura, A.; Suzuki, H.; Sakaguchi, S.; Kosaka, Y. Effects of the Japanese herbal medicine "Sho-Saiko-To" (TJ-9) on in vitro interleukin-10 production by peripheral blood mononuclear cells of patients with chronic hepatitis C. *Hepatology* **1997**, *25*, 1390–1397. [CrossRef] [PubMed]
20. Li, B.; Tao, W.; Zheng, C.; Shar, P.A.; Huang, C.; Fu, Y.; Wang, Y. Systems pharmacology-based approach for dissecting the addition and subtraction theory of traditional Chinese medicine: An example using Xiao-Chaihu-Decoction and Da-Chaihu-Decoction. *Comput. Biol. Med.* **2014**, *53*, 19–29. [CrossRef]
21. Lee, J.-H.; Jo, E.H.; Lee, B.; Noh, H.M.; Park, S.; Lee, Y.-M.; Kim, D.-K.; Park, M.C. Soshiho-Tang, a traditional herbal medicine, alleviates atopic dermatitis symptoms via regulation of inflammatory mediators. *Front. Pharmacol.* **2019**, *10*, 742. [CrossRef]
22. Shin, I.S.; Lee, M.Y.; Kim, Y.; Seo, C.S.; Kim, J.H.; Shin, H.K. Subacute toxicity and stability of Soshiho-tang, a traditional herbal formula, in Sprague–Dawley rats. *BMC Complement. Altern. Med.* **2012**, *12*, 266. [CrossRef]
23. Lee, M.-Y.; Seo, C.-S.; Shin, I.-S.; Kim, Y.-B.; Kim, J.-H.; Shin, H.-K. Evaluation of oral subchronic toxicity of soshiho-tang water extract: The traditional herbal formula in rats. *Evid. Based Complement. Altern. Med.* **2013**, *2013*, 590181. [CrossRef]
24. Kim, J.-H.; Lee, S.; Lee, M.-Y.; Shin, H.-K. Therapeutic effect of Soshiho-tang, a traditional herbal formula, on liver fibrosis or cirrhosis in animal models: A systematic review and meta-analysis. *J. Ethnopharmacol.* **2014**, *154*, 1–16. [CrossRef] [PubMed]
25. Lee, J.H.; Jo, E.H.; youn Jung, J.; Kang, S.J.; Yang, G.J.; Shim, Y.H.; Park, M.C. Efficacy and safety of Soshiho-tang in atopic dermatitis patients with gastrointestinal disorders: A double-blinded, randomized, and placebo-controlled clinical trial. *J. Ethnopharmacol.* **2021**, *274*, 114006. [CrossRef] [PubMed]
26. Tang, X.C.H. Herbal Monograph for Xiao Chai Hu Tang. July 2007. Available online: https://acupuncturetoday.com/article/31544-herbal-monograph-for-xiao-chai-hu-tang (accessed on 25 September 2023).
27. Jung, J.; Park, J.; Choi, J.-Y.; Lee, J.A. Soshiho-tang for treating common cold in children younger than 12 years: A systematic review and meta-analysis of randomized controlled trials. *Medicine* **2018**, *97*, e13045. [CrossRef] [PubMed]
28. Kim, H.U.; Ryu, J.Y.; Lee, J.O.; Lee, S.Y. A systems approach to traditional oriental medicine. *Nat. Biotechnol.* **2015**, *33*, 264–268. [CrossRef]
29. Song, B.-K.; Won, J.-H.; Kim, S. Historical medical value of Donguibogam. *J. Pharmacopunct.* **2016**, *19*, 16–20. [CrossRef]
30. Pan, Z.; Han, M.; Zhang, Y.; Liu, T.; Zhou, L.; Tan, D.; Wang, Q.; Liu, Z.; Fu, Y. Characteristics of Xiao Chai Hu decoction based on randomized controlled trials: A bibliometric analysis. *J. Tradit. Chin. Med. Sci.* **2023**, *10*, 100–105. [CrossRef]
31. Yu, H.; Chen, J.; Xu, X.; Li, Y.; Zhao, H.; Fang, Y.; Li, X.; Zhou, W.; Wang, W.; Wang, Y. A systematic prediction of multiple drug-target interactions from chemical, genomic, and pharmacological data. *PLoS ONE* **2012**, *7*, e37608. [CrossRef]
32. Wang, X.; Xu, X.; Li, Y.; Li, X.; Tao, W.; Li, B.; Wang, Y.; Yang, L. Systems pharmacology uncovers Janus functions of botanical drugs: Activation of host defense system and inhibition of influenza virus replication. *Integr. Biol.* **2013**, *5*, 351–371. [CrossRef]
33. Yano, H.; Mizoguchi, A.; Fukuda, K.; Haramaki, M.; Ogasawara, S.; Momosaki, S.; Kojiro, M. The herbal medicine sho-saiko-to inhibits proliferation of cancer cell lines by inducing apoptosis and arrest at the G0/G1 phase. *Cancer Res.* **1994**, *54*, 448–454.
34. Zhu, K.; Fukasawa, I.; Furuno, M.; Inaba, F.; Yamazaki, T.; Kamemori, T.; Kousaka, N.; Ota, Y.; Hayashi, M.; Maehama, T. Inhibitory effects of herbal drugs on the growth of human ovarian cancer cell lines through the induction of apoptosis. *Gynecol. Oncol.* **2005**, *97*, 405–409. [CrossRef]
35. Zhao, J.; Liu, L.; Zhang, Y.; Wan, Y.; Hong, Z. The herbal mixture Xiao-Chai-Hu Tang (XCHT) induces apoptosis of human hepatocellular carcinoma Huh7 cells in vitro and in vivo. *Afr. J. Tradit. Complement. Altern. Med.* **2017**, *14*, 231–241. [CrossRef] [PubMed]

36. Liu, W.; Kato, M.; Akhand, A.A.; Hayakawa, A.; Takemura, M.; Yoshida, S.; Suzuki, H.; Nakashima, I. The herbal medicine sho-saiko-to inhibits the growth of malignant melanoma cells by upregulating Fas-mediated apoptosis and arresting cell cycle through downregulation of cyclin dependent kinases. *Int. J. Oncol.* **1998**, *12*, 1321–1327. [CrossRef]
37. Yamashiki, M.; Nishimura, A.; Nomoto, M.; Suzuki, H.; Kosaka, Y. Herbal medicine 'Sho-saiko-to'induces tumour necrosis factor-α and granulocyte colony-stimulating factor in vitro in peripheral blood mononuclear cells of patients with hepatocellular carcinoma. *J. Gastroenterol. Hepatol.* **1996**, *11*, 137–142. [CrossRef] [PubMed]
38. Mizushima, Y.; Kashii, T.; Tokimitsu, Y.; Kobayashi, M. Cytotoxic effect of herbal medicine sho-saiko-to on human lung-cancer cell-lines in-vitro. *Oncol. Rep.* **1995**, *2*, 91–94. [CrossRef] [PubMed]
39. Shao, S.; Jia, R.; Zhao, L.; Zhang, Y.; Guan, Y.; Wen, H.; Liu, J.; Zhao, Y.; Feng, Y.; Zhang, Z. Xiao-Chai-Hu-Tang ameliorates tumor growth in cancer comorbid depressive symptoms via modulating gut microbiota-mediated TLR4/MyD88/NF-κB signaling pathway. *Phytomedicine* **2021**, *88*, 153606. [CrossRef] [PubMed]
40. Kawakita, T.; Nakai, S.; Kumazawa, Y.; Miura, O.; Yumioka, E.; Nomoto, K. Induction of interferon after administration of a traditional Chinese medicine, xiao-chai-hu-tang (shosaiko-to). *Int. J. Immunopharmacol.* **1990**, *12*, 515–521. [CrossRef] [PubMed]
41. Ohtake, N.; Yamamoto, M.; Takeda, S.; Aburada, M.; Ishige, A.; Watanabe, K.; Inoue, M. The herbal medicine Sho-saiko-to selectively inhibits CD8+ T-cell proliferation. *Eur. J. Pharmacol.* **2005**, *507*, 301–310. [CrossRef]
42. Kang, H.; Choi, T.-W.; Ahn, K.-S.; Lee, J.-Y.; Ham, I.-H.; Choi, H.-Y.; Shim, E.-S.; Sohn, N.-W. Upregulation of interferon-γ and interleukin-4, Th cell-derived cytokines by So-Shi-Ho-Tang (Sho-Saiko-To) occurs at the level of antigen presenting cells, but not CD4 T cells. *J. Ethnopharmacol.* **2009**, *123*, 6–14. [CrossRef]
43. Yamashiki, M.; Nishimura, A.; Sakaguchi, S.; Suzuki, H.; Kosaka, Y. Effects of the Japanese herbal medicine 'Sho-saiko-to'as a cytokine inducer. *Environ. Toxicol. Pharmacol.* **1996**, *2*, 301–306. [CrossRef]
44. Huang, X.X.; Yamashiki, M.; Nakatani, K.; Nobori, T.; Mase, A. Semi-quantitative analysis of cytokine mRNA expression induced by the herbal medicine Sho-saiko-to (TJ-9) using a gel doc system. *J. Clin. Lab. Anal.* **2001**, *15*, 199–209. [CrossRef]
45. Matsumoto, T.; Shibata, T. The ex vivo effect of the herbal medicine Sho-saiko-to on histamine release from rat mast cells. *Eur. Arch. Oto-Rhino-Laryngol.* **1998**, *255*, 359–364. [CrossRef] [PubMed]
46. Miyamoto, K.; Lange, M.; McKinley, G.; Stavropoulos, C.; Moriya, S.-i.; Matsumoto, H.; Inada, Y. Effects of sho-saiko-to on production of prostaglandin E2 (PGE2), leukotriene B4 (LTB4) and superoxide from peripheral monocytes and polymorphonuclear cells isolated from HIV infected individuals. *Am. J. Chin. Med.* **1996**, *24*, 1–10. [CrossRef] [PubMed]
47. Sakaguchi, S.; Furusawa, S.; Iizuka, Y. Preventive effects of a traditional Chinese medicine (Sho-saiko-to) on septic shock symptoms; approached from heme metabolic disorders in endotoxemia. *Biol. Pharm. Bull.* **2005**, *28*, 165–168. [CrossRef]
48. Ara, T.; Maeda, Y.; Fujinami, Y.; Imamura, Y.; Hattori, T.; Wang, P.L. Preventive effects of a Kampo medicine, Shosaikoto, on inflammatory responses in LPS-treated human gingival fibroblasts. *Biol. Pharm. Bull.* **2008**, *31*, 1141–1144. [CrossRef] [PubMed]
49. Oh, Y.C.; Cho, W.K.; Jeong, Y.H.; Im, G.Y.; Lee, K.J.; Yang, H.J.; Ma, J.Y. Anti-inflammatory effect of Sosihotang via inhibition of nuclear factor-kappaB and mitogen-activated protein kinases signaling pathways in lipopolysaccharide-stimulated RAW 264.7 macrophage cells. *Food Chem. Toxicol.* **2013**, *53*, 343–351. [CrossRef] [PubMed]
50. Choi, L.Y.; Kim, M.H.; Jung, D.-H.; Yang, W.M. Anti-Inflammatory Effects of Sosiho-Tang, a Traditional Herbal Formula, on Acute Lung Injury in LPS-Sensitized Mice and-Raw 264.7 Cells. *Evid. Based Complement. Altern. Med.* **2021**, *2021*, 6641689. [CrossRef] [PubMed]
51. Zhan, L.; Pu, J.; Hu, Y.; Xu, P.; Liang, W.; Ji, C. Uncovering the pharmacology of Xiaochaihu decoction in the treatment of acute pancreatitis based on the network pharmacology. *BioMed Res. Int.* **2021**, *2021*, 6621682. [CrossRef]
52. Kakumu, S.; Yoshioka, K.; Wakita, T.; Ishikawa, T. Effects of TJ-9 Sho-saiko-to (kampo medicine) on interferon gamma and antibody production specific for hepatitis B virus antigen in patients with type B chronic hepatitis. *Int. J. Immunopharmacol.* **1991**, *13*, 141–146. [CrossRef]
53. Yamashiki, M.; Nishimura, A.; Nobori, T.; Nakabayashi, S.; Takagi, T.; Inoue, K.; Ito, M.; Matsushita, K.; Ohtaki, H.; Kosaka, Y. In vitro effects of Sho-saiko-to on production of granulocyte colony-stimulating factor by mononuclear cells from patients with chronic hepatitis C. *Int. J. Immunopharmacol.* **1997**, *19*, 381–385. [CrossRef]
54. Chen, S.; Wang, Z.; Wan, S.; Huang, H.; Liang, H. Effect of modified Xiaochaihu decoction-containing serum on HepG2. 2.15 cells via the JAK2/STAT3 signaling pathway. *Mol. Med. Rep.* **2017**, *16*, 7416–7422. [CrossRef]
55. Hattori, Y.; Kasai, K.; Sekiguchi, Y.; Hattori, S.; Banba, N.; Shimoda, S.-I. The herbal medicine sho-saiko-to induces nitric oxide synthase in rat hepatocytes. *Life Sci.* **1995**, *56*, PL143–PL148. [CrossRef] [PubMed]
56. Zou, C.; Xu, M.; Chen, L.; Liu, Q.; Zhou, Y.; Sun, Z.; Ye, H.; Su, N.; Ye, C.; Wang, A. Xiaochaihu Decoction reduces hepatic steatosis and improves D-GalN/LPS-induced liver injury in hybrid grouper (*Epinephelus lanceolatus*♂ × *Epinephelus fuscoguttatus*♀). *Fish Shellfish Immunol.* **2019**, *91*, 293–305. [CrossRef] [PubMed]
57. Kayano, K.; Sakaida, I.; Uchida, K.; Okita, K. Inhibitory effects of the herbal medicine Sho-saiko-to (TJ-9) on cell proliferation and procollagen gene expressions in cultured rat hepatic stellate cells. *J. Hepatol.* **1998**, *29*, 642–649. [CrossRef] [PubMed]
58. Sakaida, I.; Hironaka, K.; Kimura, T.; Terai, S.; Yamasaki, T.; Okita, K. Herbal medicine Sho-saiko-to (TJ-9) increases expression matrix metalloproteinases (MMPs) with reduced expression of tissue inhibitor of metalloproteinases (TIMPs) in rat stellate cell. *Life Sci.* **2004**, *74*, 2251–2263. [CrossRef] [PubMed]

59. Matsumoto, Y.; Kato, M.; Tamada, Y.; Mori, H.; Ohashi, M. Enhancement of Interleukin-1α Mediated Autocrine Growth of Cultured Human Keratinocytes by Sho-saiko-to. *Jpn. J. Pharmacol.* **1997**, *73*, 333–336. [CrossRef] [PubMed]
60. Im, A.-R.; Ji, K.-Y.; Nam, K.-W.; Chae, S. Protective effects of Sosihotang extract against ultraviolet B-induced skin photoageing in hairless mice. *J. Pharm. Pharmacol.* **2020**, *72*, 1278–1286. [CrossRef]
61. Iwama, H.; Amagaya, S.; Ogihara, Y. Effect of shosaikoto, a Japanese and Chinese traditional herbal medicinal mixture, on the mitogenic activity of lipopolysaccharide: A new pharmacological testing method. *J. Ethnopharmacol.* **1987**, *21*, 45–53. [CrossRef]
62. Cheng, P.-W.; Ng, L.-T.; Lin, C.-C. Xiao chai hu tang inhibits CVB1 virus infection of CCFS-1 cells through the induction of Type I interferon expression. *Int. Immunopharmacol.* **2006**, *6*, 1003–1012. [CrossRef]
63. Hiroshima, Y.; Bando, M.; Kataoka, M.; Shinohara, Y.; Herzberg, M.; Ross, K.; Inagaki, Y.; Nagata, T.; Kido, J. Shosaikoto increases calprotectin expression in human oral epithelial cells. *J. Periodontal Res.* **2010**, *45*, 79–86. [CrossRef]
64. Lee, J.-J.; Kim, T.; Cho, W.-K.; Ma, J.Y. Antithrombotic and antiplatelet activities of Soshiho-tang extract. *BMC Complement. Altern. Med.* **2013**, *13*, 137. [CrossRef]
65. Yoo, S.-R.; Lee, M.-y.; Kang, B.-K.; Shin, H.-K.; Jeong, S.-J. Soshiho-tang aqueous extract exerts antiobesity effects in high fat diet-fed mice and inhibits adipogenesis in 3T3-L1 adipocytes. *Evid.-Based Complement. Altern. Med.* **2016**, *2016*, 2628901. [CrossRef] [PubMed]
66. Song, K.H.; Kim, Y.H.; Kim, B.-Y. Sho-saiko-to, a traditional herbal medicine, regulates gene expression and biological function by way of microRNAs in primary mouse hepatocytes. *BMC Complement. Altern. Med.* **2014**, *14*, 14. [CrossRef] [PubMed]
67. World Health Organization. Fact Sheet: Cancer. Available online: http://www.who.int/news-room/fact-sheets/detail/cancer (accessed on 3 February 2022).
68. Haranaka, K.; Satomi, N.; Sakurai, A.; Haranaka, R.; Okada, N.; Kobayashi, M. Antitumor activities and tumor necrosis factor producibility of traditional Chinese medicines and crude drugs. *Cancer Immunol. Immunother.* **1985**, *20*, 1–5. [CrossRef] [PubMed]
69. Huang, Y.; Marumo, K.; Murai, M. Antitumor effects and pharmacological interaction of xiao-chai-hu-tang (sho-saiko-to) and interleukin 2 in murine renal cell carcinoma. *Keio J. Med.* **1997**, *46*, 132–137. [CrossRef] [PubMed]
70. Sakaguchi, S.; Furusawa, S.; Yokota, K.; Sasaki, K.-I.; Takayanagi, M.; Takayanagi, Y. Effects of antitumor activity and protection of shock symptoms by a traditional Chinese medicine (sho-saiko-to) in recombinant human tumor necrosis factor administered mice. *Biol. Pharm. Bull.* **1996**, *19*, 1474–1478. [CrossRef]
71. Tatsuta, M.; Iishi, H.; Baba, M.; Nakaizumi, A.; Uehara, H. Inhibition by xiao-chai-hu-tang (TJ-9) of development of hepatic foci induced by N-nitrosomorpholine in Sprague-Dawley rats. *Jpn. J. Cancer Res.* **1991**, *82*, 987–992. [CrossRef] [PubMed]
72. Isao, S.; Yasuhiro, M.; Shinta, A.; Koji, H.; Atsushi, I.; Kiwamu, O. Herbal medicine Sho-saiko-to (TJ-9) prevent liver fibrosis and enzyme-altered lesions in rat liver cirrhosis induced by a choline-deficient l-amino acid-defined diet. *J. Hepatol.* **1998**, *28*, 298–306. [CrossRef]
73. Huang, Y.; Lu, J.; Xu, Y.; Xiong, C.; Tong, D.; Hu, N.; Yang, H. Xiaochaihu decorction relieves liver fibrosis caused by Schistosoma japonicum infection via the HSP47/TGF-β pathway. *Parasites Vectors* **2020**, *13*, 254. [CrossRef] [PubMed]
74. Sakaguchi, S.; Tutumi, E.; Yokota, K.; Furusawa, S.; Sasaki, K.i.; Takayanagi, Y. Preventive Effects of a Chinese Herb Medicine (Sho-saiko-to) against Lethality after Recombinant Human Tumor Necrosis Factor Administration in Mice. *Microbiol. Immunol.* **1991**, *35*, 389–394. [CrossRef]
75. Fehervari, Z. Vaccine sex differences. *Nat. Immunol.* **2019**, *20*, 111. [CrossRef]
76. Scotland, R.S.; Stables, M.J.; Madalli, S.; Watson, P.; Gilroy, D.W. Sex differences in resident immune cell phenotype underlie more efficient acute inflammatory responses in female mice. *Blood J. Am. Soc. Hematol.* **2011**, *118*, 5918–5927. [CrossRef] [PubMed]
77. Kawakita, T.; Yamada, A.; Mitsuyama, M.; Kumazawa, Y.; Nomoto, K. Protective effect of a traditional Chinese medicine, xiao-chai-hu-tang (Japanese name: Shosaiko-to), on Pseudomonas aeruginosa infection in mice. *Immunopharmacol. Immunotoxicol.* **1987**, *9*, 523–540. [CrossRef] [PubMed]
78. Kawakita, T.; Yamada, A.; Kumazawa, Y.; Nomoto, K. Functional maturation of immature B cells accumulated in the periphery by an intraperitoneal administration of a traditional Chinese medicine, xiao-chai-hu-tang (Japanese name: Shosaiko-to). *Immunopharmacol. Immunotoxicol.* **1987**, *9*, 299–317. [CrossRef] [PubMed]
79. Kumazawa, Y.; Takimoto, H.; Miura, S.-I.; Nishimura, C.; Yamada, A.; Kawakita, T.; Nomoto, K. Activation of murine peritoneal macrophages by intraperitoneal administration of a traditional Chinese herbal medicine, xiao-chai-hu-tang (Japanese name: Shosaiko-to). *Int. J. Immunopharmacol.* **1988**, *10*, 395–403. [CrossRef] [PubMed]
80. Yonekura, K.; Kawakita, T.; Mitsuyama, M.; Miura, O.; Yumioka, E.; Suzuki, A.; Nomoto, K. Induction of colony-stimulating factor (s) after administration of a traditional Chinese medicine, xiao-chai-hu-tang (Japanese name: Shosaiko-to). *Immunopharmacol. Immunotoxicol.* **1990**, *12*, 647–667. [CrossRef] [PubMed]
81. Nagatsu, Y.; Inoue, M.; Ogihara, Y. Modification of macrophage functions by Shosaikoto (kampo medicine) leads to enhancement of immune response. *Chem. Pharm. Bull.* **1989**, *37*, 1540–1542. [CrossRef] [PubMed]
82. Kaneko, M.; Kawakita, T.; Tauchi, Y.; Saito, Y.; Suzuki, A.; Nomoto, K. Augmentation of NK activity after oral administration of a traditional Chinese medicine, xiao-chai-hu-tang (shosaiko-to). *Immunopharmacol. Immunotoxicol.* **1994**, *16*, 41–53. [CrossRef]

83. Yamaoka, Y.; Kawakita, T.; Kaneko, M.; Nomoto, K. A polysaccharide fraction of shosaiko-to active in augmentation of natural killer activity by oral administration. *Biol. Pharm. Bull.* **1995**, *18*, 846–849. [CrossRef]
84. Sakaguchi, S.; Tsutsumi, E.; Yokota, K. Preventive effects of a traditional Chinese medicine (sho-saiko-to) against oxygen toxicity and membrane damage during endotoxemia. *Biol. Pharm. Bull.* **1993**, *16*, 782–786. [CrossRef]
85. Jeon, W.-Y.; Shin, H.-K.; Shin, I.-S.; Kim, S.K.; Lee, M.-Y. Soshiho-tang water extract inhibits ovalbumin-induced airway inflammation via the regulation of heme oxygenase-1. *BMC Complement. Altern. Med.* **2015**, *15*, 329. [CrossRef]
86. Kim, A.; Im, M.; Ma, J.Y. Sosiho-tang ameliorates cachexia-related symptoms in mice bearing colon 26 adenocarcinoma by reducing systemic inflammation and muscle loss. *Oncol. Rep.* **2016**, *35*, 1841–1850. [CrossRef] [PubMed]
87. Yoshida, K.; Mizukawa, H.; Honmura, A.; Uchiyama, Y.; Kaku, H.; Nakajima, S.; Haruki, E. The effect of sho-saiko-to on the concentration of acid soluble glycoprotein in serum and on granuloma formation in carrageenin cotton pellet-induced granuloma rats. *Am. J. Chin. Med.* **1993**, *21*, 171–177. [CrossRef] [PubMed]
88. Yoshida, K.; Mizukawa, H.; Honmura, A.; Uchiyama, Y.; Nakajima, S.; Haruki, E. The effect of sho-saiko-to on concentration of vitamin E in serum and on granuloma formation in carrageenin cotton pellet-induced granuloma rats. *Am. J. Chin. Med.* **1994**, *22*, 183–189. [CrossRef] [PubMed]
89. Li, H.; Tang, Y.; Wei, W.; Yin, C.; Tang, F. Effects of Xiaochaihu decoction on the expression of cytochrome P450s in rats. *Exp. Ther. Med.* **2021**, *21*, 588. [CrossRef] [PubMed]
90. Inoue, M.; Shen, Y.R.; Ogihara, Y. Restorative Effect of Shosaikoto (Kampo Medicine) on Diminution of Nitric Oxide Synthesis in Murine Peritoneal Macrophages induced by Hyperocholesterolemia. *Biol. Pharm. Bull.* **1996**, *19*, 1468–1473. [CrossRef] [PubMed]
91. Tauchi, Y.; Kawakita, T.; Saito, Y.; Suzuki, A.; Yamada, A.; Yoshikai, Y.; Nomoto, K. Enhancement of immunoglobulin A production in Peyer's patches by oral administration of a traditional Chinese medicine, xiao-chai-hu-tang (Shosaiko-to). *Immunopharmacol. Immunotoxicol.* **1993**, *15*, 251–272. [CrossRef] [PubMed]
92. Fujiwara, K.; Mochida, S.; Nagoshi, S.; Iijima, O.; Matsuzaki, Y.; Takeda, S.; Aburada, M. Regulation of hepatic macrophage function by oral administration of xiao-chai-hu-tang (sho-saiko-to, TJ-9) in rats. *J. Ethnopharmacol.* **1995**, *46*, 107–114. [CrossRef]
93. Zhou, Y.-X.; Qiu, Y.-Q.; Xu, L.-Q.; Guo, J.; Li, L.-J. Xiao-Chai-Hu Tang in treating model mice with D-galactosamine-induced liver injury. *Afr. J. Tradit. Complement. Altern. Med.* **2012**, *9*, 405–411. [CrossRef]
94. Zhang, K.; Wang, Z.; Pan, X.; Yang, J.; Wu, C. Antidepressant-like effects of Xiaochaihutang in perimenopausal mice. *J. Ethnopharmacol.* **2020**, *248*, 112318. [CrossRef]
95. Amagaya, S.; Umeda, S.H.M.; Ogihara, Y. Effects of Shosaikoto, an oriental herbal medicinal mixture, on age-induced amnesia in rats. *J. Ethnopharmacol.* **1990**, *28*, 349–356. [CrossRef]
96. Ohta, Y.; Nishida, K.; Sasaki, E.; Kongo, M.; Hayashi, T.; Nagata, M.; Ishiguro, I. Comparative study of oral and parenteral administration of sho-saiko-to (xiao-chaihu-tang) extract on D-galactosamine-induced liver injury in rats. *Am. J. Chin. Med.* **1997**, *25*, 333–342. [CrossRef] [PubMed]
97. Zhang, S.-k.; Cui, N.-q.; Zhuo, Y.-z.; Li, D.-h.; Liu, J.-h. Modified Xiaochaihu decoction (小柴胡汤) prevents the progression of chronic pancreatitis in rats possibly by inhibiting transforming growth factor-β1/Sma-and mad-related proteins signaling pathway. *Chin. J. Integr. Med.* **2013**, *19*, 935–939. [CrossRef]
98. Shen, Y.R.; Inoue, M.; Nagatsu, Y.; Ogihara, Y.; Aburada, M. Anti-hyperlipidemic and anti-atherosclerotic actions of shosaikoto (kampo medicine). *Biol. Pharm. Bull.* **1996**, *19*, 1160–1165. [CrossRef] [PubMed]
99. Shen, Y.R.; Inoue, M.; Ogihara, Y. Effect of Shosaikoto (Kampo Medicine) on the Adherence of Monocytes in Hypercholesterolemic Rabbit. *Biol. Pharm. Bull.* **1996**, *19*, 149–152. [CrossRef] [PubMed]
100. Nishimura, N.; Naora, K.; Hirano, H.; Iwamoto, K. A Chinese traditional medicine, sho-saiko-to (xiao-chaihu-tang), reduces the bioavailability of tolbutamide after oral administration in rats. *Am. J. Chin. Med.* **1999**, *27*, 355–363. [CrossRef] [PubMed]
101. Egashira, T.; Takayama, F.; Yamanaka, Y.; Komatsu, Y. Monitoring of radical scavenging activity of peroral administration of the Kampo medicine Sho-saiko-to in rats. *Jpn. J. Pharmacol.* **1999**, *80*, 379–382. [CrossRef] [PubMed]
102. Nishimura, N.; Naora, K.; Hirano, H.; IWAMOTO, K. Effects of sho-saiko-to (xiao chai hu tang), a Chinese traditional medicine, on the gastric function and absorption of tolbutamide in rats. *Yakugaku Zasshi* **2001**, *121*, 153–159. [CrossRef]
103. Horie, Y.; Kajihara, M.; Yamagishi, Y.; Kimura, H.; Tamai, H.; Kato, S.; Ishii, H. A Japanese herbal medicine, Sho-saiko-to, prevents gut ischemia/reperfusion-induced hepatic microvascular dysfunction in rats. *J. Gastroenterol. Hepatol.* **2001**, *16*, 1260–1266. [CrossRef]
104. Nishimura, N.; Uemura, T.; Iwamoto, K.; Naora, K. Change in tolbutamide permeability in rat jejunum and Caco-2 cells by Sho-saiko-to (Xiao Chai Hu Tang), a Chinese traditional medicine. *J. Pharm. Pharmacol.* **2010**, *62*, 651–657. [CrossRef]
105. Oka, H.; Yamamoto, S.; Kuroki, T.; Harihara, S.; Marumo, T.; Kim, S.R.; Monna, T.; Kobayashi, K.; Tango, T. Prospective study of chemoprevention of hepatocellular carcinoma with Sho-saiko-to (TJ-9). *Cancer* **1995**, *76*, 743–749. [CrossRef]
106. Hirayama, C.; Okumura, M.; Tanikawa, K.; Yano, M.; Mizuta, M.; Ogawa, N. A multicenter randomized controlled clinical trial of Shosaiko-to in chronic active hepatitis. *Gastroenterol. Jpn.* **1989**, *24*, 715–719. [CrossRef]
107. Deng, G.; Kurtz, R.C.; Vickers, A.; Lau, N.; Yeung, K.S.; Shia, J.; Cassileth, B. A single arm phase II study of a Far-Eastern traditional herbal formulation (sho-sai-ko-to or xiao-chai-hu-tang) in chronic hepatitis C patients. *J. Ethnopharmacol.* **2011**, *136*, 83–87. [CrossRef]

108. Itoh, S.; Marutani, K.; Nishijima, T.; Matsuo, S.; Itabashi, M. Liver injuries induced by herbal medicine, syo saiko to (xiao-chai-hu-tang). *Dig. Dis. Sci.* **1995**, *40*, 1845–1848. [CrossRef]
109. Hsu, L.-M.; Huang, Y.-S.; Tsay, S.-H.; Chang, F.-Y.; Lee, S.-D. Acute hepatitis induced by Chinese hepatoprotective herb, xiao-chai-hu-tang. *J. Chin. Med. Assoc.* **2006**, *69*, 86–88. [CrossRef]

pharmaceuticals

Systematic Review

Mechanistic Evidence of *Andrographis paniculata* (Burm. f.) Wall. ex Nees, *Pelargonium sidoides* DC., *Echinacea* Species and a Combination of *Hedera helix* L., *Primula veris* L./*Primula elatior* L. and *Thymus vulgaris* L./*Thymus zygis* L. in the Treatment of Acute, Uncomplicated Respiratory Tract Infections: A Systematic Literature Review and Expert Interviews

Liesbeth B. M. Veldman [1,*], Eefje Belt-Van Zoen [1] and Erik W. Baars [1,2]

1 Faculty of Healthcare, University of Applied Sciences Leiden, 2333 Leiden, The Netherlands
2 Louis Bolk Institute, 3981 Bunnik, The Netherlands
* Correspondence: veldman.l@hsleiden.nl

Abstract: Reducing inappropriate antibiotic (AB) use by using effective non-antibiotic treatments is one strategy to prevent and reduce antimicrobial resistance (AMR). *Andrographis paniculata* (Burm. f.) Wall. ex Nees, *Pelargonium sidoides* DC., *Echinacea* species and a combination of ivy (*Hedera helix* L.), primrose (*Primula veris* L./*Primula elatior* L.) and thyme (*Thymus vulgaris* L./*Thymus zygis* L.) have promising clinical effects in uncomplicated, acute upper respiratory tract infections (URTI) treatment. However, mechanistic evidence of these herbal treatments is lacking. The objective of this Pstudy is to provide an overview of mechanistic evidence for these effects. Thirty-eight databases were searched. Included studies were mechanistic studies (in vitro, animal, and human studies and reviews) on these herbs; published before June 2021. Non-mechanistic studies or studies on combinations of herbs other than ivy/primrose/thyme were excluded. Furthermore, three experts in traditional, complementary and integrative healthcare (TCIH) research and pharmacognosy were interviewed to collect additional expert knowledge. The results show that *A. paniculata* acts through immunomodulation and antiviral activity, possibly supplemented by antibacterial and antipyretic effects. *P. sidoides* acts through antiviral, indirect antibacterial, immunomodulatory and expectorant effects. *Echinacea* species likely act through immunomodulation. The combination of ivy/primrose/thyme combines secretolytic and spasmolytic effects from ivy with antibacterial effects from thyme. Studies on primrose were lacking. This mechanistic evidence supports the difference-making evidence from clinical studies, contributes to evidence-based recommendations for their use in URTI treatment, and guides future mechanistic studies on URTI treatments.

Keywords: antimicrobial resistance; mechanistic evidence; respiratory tract infections; multi-targeted

Citation: Veldman, L.B.M.; Belt-Van Zoen, E.; Baars, E.W. Mechanistic Evidence of *Andrographis paniculata* (Burm. f.) Wall. ex Nees, *Pelargonium sidoides* DC., *Echinacea* Species and a Combination of *Hedera helix* L., *Primula veris* L./*Primula elatior* L. and *Thymus vulgaris* L./*Thymus zygis* L. in the Treatment of Acute, Uncomplicated Respiratory Tract Infections: A Systematic Literature Review and Expert Interviews. *Pharmaceuticals* **2023**, *16*, 1206. https://doi.org/10.3390/ph16091206

Academic Editors: Elena Y. Enioutina, Kathleen M. Job and Catherine Sherwin

Received: 31 May 2023
Revised: 17 August 2023
Accepted: 18 August 2023
Published: 24 August 2023

1. Introduction

Antimicrobial resistance (AMR) is a worldwide leading public health problem affecting the lives of millions of people. In 2019, an estimated 4.95 million deaths were associated with bacterial AMR [1]. Policies at global, regional, and national levels focus on six main strategies to reduce antibiotic use. These strategies are (1) preventing infection and controlling resistant bacteria, (2) monitoring both infection prevention and control of resistant bacteria, (3) researching antibiotic resistance and antibiotic use, (4) only using antibiotics when appropriate, (5) reducing the use of antibiotics, and (6) developing new antibiotics [2]. However, in the European Union and European Economic Area over the period of 2010–2019 the average total AB consumption reduced only by 0.4% in the community and hospital sector combined. In each of these sectors alone the decrease was not statistically significant [3]. Finding ways to further, and more effectively, lower antibiotic prescription and consumption, is, therefore, of great importance.

URTIs are a leading cause of inappropriate use of antibiotics, especially in children [4]. In case of a bacterial pathogen, this often involves *Streptococcus pyogenes*, *Streptococcus pneumoniae*, or *Haemophilus influenzae* [5]. However, the vast majority of URTIs (an estimated 70%) are caused by viruses such as rhinoviruses, coronaviruses, influenzaviruses A or B, or respiratory syncytial viruses [6–8]. It is not surprising that antibiotics often only have small or negligible symptomatic benefit for URTI patients and are not included in most treatment guidelines [9]. Even though many URTIs are self-limiting, the patients' need for symptom relief remains. Therefore, non-antibiotic treatment strategies that help treat symptoms are required, especially in non-bacterial and non-severe cases.

Currently, traditional, complementary and integrative healthcare (TCIH) is not yet included as a strategy to counter AMR. However, it could prove to be of great value as a strategy for both reducing antibiotic consumption and promoting the appropriate use of antibiotics, as was observed in several observational studies. For example, a retrospective cross-sectional analysis of national primary care in England found that health centres that employed general practitioners (GPs) trained in TCIH or integrative medicine (IM) prescribed fewer antibiotics (relative risk = 0.78, 95% confidence interval (CI): 0.64 to 0.97) [10]. Furthermore, French patients who consulted a GP additionally trained in homeopathy used significantly fewer antibiotics for uncomplicated acute respiratory tract infections (URTIs) (OR = 0.43, 95% CI: 0.27–0.68) [11]. In children treated by anthroposophic GPs for URTIs and ear infections, significantly fewer antibiotics were prescribed as well (OR for non-prescription = 6.58, 95% CI: 3.45–12.56). In addition, there was a trend to quicker symptom relief and a higher caregiver satisfaction with anthroposophic GP treatment compared to conventional GP treatment [12]. In addition to reducing the use of antibiotics, TCIH treatments can contribute to reducing AMR development by offering new approaches to treat and prevent microbial infections such as URTIs.

TCIH treatments hold a unique potential to aid in the reduction in antibiotic use as these treatments approach the problem of URTI in a different way. Most conventional treatment strategies focus on creating specific immunity and fighting the microorganisms. In TCIH strategies, on the other hand, the main focus of treatment is on enhancing the individual's resilience; improving the general physiological ability to self-manage and adapt to infections by strengthening the individual's self-regulating abilities [13]. Resilience is a holistic concept that refers to an individual's ability to recover from or optimise the functioning in disease or disability [14]. Many resilience-enhancing TCIH treatment strategies are promising, but lack high-quality scientific evidence [13]. Therefore, more research is needed into their (cost)effectiveness.

1.1. Clinical Evidence for TCIH Treatments in URTI

The efficacy of some natural medicinal products for treating acute, uncomplicated URTIs has been shown in moderate- to high-quality clinical studies. Systematic reviews on their efficacy show promising effects. A recent meta-analysis of meta-analyses identified the four most promising TCIH treatments for RTIs [15]. These are *Andrographis paniculata* (Burm. f.) Wall. ex Nees and *Pelargonium sidiodes* DC. for both general and specific URTI symptoms (e.g., cough and sore throat) [16–21], *Echinacea* spp. for common cold [20], and a combination of ivy (*Hedera helix* L.), primrose (*Primula veris* L./*Primula elatior* L.), and thyme (*Thymus vulgaris* L./*Thymus zygis* L.) for cough only [22,23].

Andrographis paniculata is an extremely bitter herb, of which the aerial parts—and sometimes the roots—are used in Ayurveda, Siddha, homeopathy, naturopathy, and traditional Chinese and Thai medicine for various indications [24,25]. A systematic review and meta-analysis of clinical trials showed that *A. paniculata* significantly improved overall symptoms of acute URTI. Specifically, it improved cough (n = 596, standardised mean difference (SMD): −0.39, 95% CI: −0.67, −0.10; p = 0.008) and sore throat (n = 314, SMD: −1.13, 95% CI: −1.37, −0.89; $p < 0.00001$) and significantly shortened the duration of these symptoms when compared to standard treatment. In addition, no major adverse effects were found [17]. These findings were confirmed in another systematic review and meta-analysis which found *A. paniculata* significantly improved cough in URTI and common cold (SMD = −1.00, 95% CI: −1.85, −0.15; $p < 0.001$) [20].

Pelargonium sidoides is a medicinal plant from South Africa which belongs to the same family as the ornamental geraniums (*Geraniaceae*) [26]. In the 19th century, it was brought to Europe, where a standardised ethanolic extract of it was made, called EPs 7630 or Umckaloabo, which has been researched extensively. In a meta-analysis of clinical trials, treatment with EPs 7630 in adult acute bronchitis patients significantly reduced the bronchitis severity score (WMD 2.80 points, 95% CI: 2.44–3.15) [18]. Furthermore, in children under 18, EPs 7630 has been found to be effective in treating URTI (responder rates: RR = 2.56; 95% CI: 1.54–4.26; $p < 0.01$) and to be safe (patients with adverse events: RR, 1.06; 95% CI: 0.42–2.66; $p = 0.9$) [16]. Even in young children, under 6 years old, similar findings were reported [19].

Echinacea is a genus that includes nine different plants, of which three species, *E. purpurea* L. Moench, *E. angustifolia* (DC.) Hell., and *E. pallida* (Nutt.) Nutt., are most often used for medicinal purposes. The most used species is *Echinacea purpurea*. This species occurs in about 80% of all commercially available products containing some Echinacea species [27]. The evidence from clinical trials on *Echinacea*'s effectiveness in treating URTIs is contradictory. A systematic review of clinical trials found limited evidence for *Echinacea* reducing cough as a symptom of URTI and the common cold in adult patients (SMD = −0.68; 95% CI: −1.32, −0.04; $p = 0.04$) [20]. However, another systematic review found no effect of *Echinacea* preparations in the treatment and prevention of the common cold when compared to a placebo [28].

Ivy, primrose, and thyme are three plants that are medicinally used in European phytotherapy [29–31]. Primrose and thyme are also used in anthroposophic medicine. There are different products on the European market that contain different combinations of these herbs such as Bronchipret, Hedelix, Prospan, and Mintetten. A meta-analysis of clinical trials on the treatment with ivy, primrose, and thyme combinations found strong evidence for these to be effective in the treatment of cough in URTI and the common cold (RR = 1.40, 95% CI: 1.23–1.60; $p < 0.001$) [20].

1.2. Study Aims

In short, for each of these treatments there are clinical data that provide evidence of their effects in URTI treatment. Exploring the underlying mechanisms of these clinically observed effects could help when working towards evidence-based recommendations on the practical applications of these treatments. The underlying mechanisms might explain the unique potential of TCIH treatments to enhance a person's resilience [13]. Hence, the main aim of this study was to further investigate the working mechanisms that underlie the effects of these four treatment strategies.

1.3. Research Questions

The main research question was: what are the underlying mechanisms by which *Andrographis paniculata*, *Pelargonium sidoides*, *Echinacea* spp., and ivy/primrose/thyme positively influence acute and uncomplicated URTI symptoms?

The research hypothesis was that all of these plants decrease URTI symptoms through a combination of direct antibacterial and antiviral effects, as well as through an enhancement in the host's resilience [13]. In line with this hypothesis, sub-research questions were:

1. What are the direct antibacterial and antiviral effects of each treatment?
2. What are the effects on the immune system of each of these treatments?
3. What are the effects on expectoration and disease management of each of these herbs?
4. Are there effects resulting only from the combination of at least two of ivy, primrose, and thyme?

2. Materials and Methods

The PRISMA guidelines were followed. The study protocol was not registered in an online database.

2.1. Search Strategy

In total, three searches were executed in 38 databases. The first search was aimed at obtaining a broad picture of the available mechanistic evidence for the selected herbs in URTI treatment. To limit the number of results, only review articles were searched for. The concept of the working mechanism was further specified to effects on (1) bacterial growth, (2) viral replication, (3) immune (cell) function, or (4) URTI disease management.

If for a specific herb no review or only one review was found, a second literature search was performed. This second search was performed to ensure that for each herb a sufficient number of studies were included to obtain a good picture of the available evidence and to allow for the potential discovery of new insights. In this second search, all types of mechanistic studies, not only review articles but also mechanistic clinical trials, animal studies, and in vitro studies, were included.

Furthermore, if the most recent review that was retrieved in the first search was more than 5 years old at the time at which the initial search was performed (<2016), an additional search was performed. This search was performed to ensure that the present study contains recent developments and included all types of mechanistic studies that were published after the most recent review retrieved.

2.1.1. Search Terms

A qualified information specialist (University of Applied Sciences Leiden) developed a list of appropriate search terms for the electronic databases (search terms provided in Appendix B Search Terms). These search terms consisted of (1) various types of URTIs, (2) various alternative names for the different plants and main active compounds, and (3) different terms describing working mechanisms and the three main proposed working mechanisms (direct antibacterial/antiviral effects, immunomodulatory effects, and expectorant effects). An additional search term '"systematic review" OR "meta-analysis" OR "review" was included to narrow down the results to review articles for the first search. The exact search terms that were used can be found in Appendix B Search Terms.

2.1.2. Sources

The following databases were searched: Academic Search Ultimate, Beeld en Geluid op school, Business Source Premier, Chemische Feitelijkheden, CINAHL with full text, Chromedia, Cochrane Library, DART-Europe, Databank Vaktherapie, Delpher, Education Research Complete, ERIC, GreenFILE, HBO Kennisbank, JAR (OpMaat), Kennisbank Diversiteit en Emancipatie, Kluwer Navigator, Legal Intelligence, Library, Information Science & Technology Abstracts, MEDLINE with full text, NARCIS, National Guideline Clearinghouse, Nexis Uni, PEDro, Picarta, Psychology and Behavioral Sciences Collection, PsycINFO, PubMed, Regional Business News, SAGE journals, Schooltv, ScienceDirect, Sociaal Digitaal, SpringerLink, Teacher Reference Center, Tijdschrift voor HRM, TRIP database, and Wiley Online Library.

Additionally, the bibliographies of selected studies were searched for relevant references, ESCOP monographs were consulted, and pharmaceutical companies that produce products with the selected herbs were asked for studies on their mechanism of action.

2.2. Eligibility

2.2.1. Inclusion Criteria

Inclusion criteria required that the studies evaluated the working mechanism in the treatment of URTI of the herbs *A. paniculata*, *P. sidoides*, *Echinacea* species, ivy, primrose, or thyme or of active compounds present in these herbs. Only combinations with standard antibiotics and combinations of ivy, primrose, and thyme were included, as the effects of these combinations are relevant to treatment of URTI and for integrating the TCIH treatments in clinical practice. Studies on effects in the lungs were included as these effects could plausibly be translated to infections of the upper respiratory tract.

2.2.2. Exclusion Criteria

Studies reporting only on a combination of one of the six studied herbs with other herbs were excluded as effects could not with certainty be attributed to the studied herb. Other exclusion criteria concerned studies reporting only on mechanisms that are unrelated to URTI treatment, as they were not relevant to the research question that is focussed on the treatment of URTIs. Clinical trials that did not investigate the mechanism of antiviral, antibacterial, or immunomodulatory effects were excluded. Articles that were not scientific, e.g., popular magazine articles were excluded, as these did not offer reliable information on working mechanisms and would, therefore, not contribute to the methodological quality of this study. Articles written in languages other than English, German, or Dutch were excluded as the authors were not able to read and understand these. In the third search, articles that were published before the most recent review retrieved were excluded. A list of excluded studies with the reason for exclusion is provided as a Supplementary File (Table S1: Study selection).

2.3. *Data Selection and Extraction*

All identified studies were collected in an Endnote file. First, duplicates were removed, and then, a selection was performed on title, abstract, and full text. The results of the selection were recorded in an Excel file. Finally, the full texts of the selected studies were read and relevant data were recorded in a standard extraction file. The selection was performed by two authors independently (LV and EBZ). The results of this were compared and differences were discussed until an agreement was reached. If needed, a third author was consulted to resolve differences. Data extraction was performed by two authors independently (LV and EBA). The results of this were compared and differences were discussed until an agreement was reached. If needed, a third author was consulted to resolve differences.

2.4. *Interviews*

In order to integrate experiential knowledge and compare this to the findings from the literature, interviews with experts in the field were also conducted. For this purpose, several academic researchers connected to the EUROCAM or AZKIM network were approached and asked to participate in an online interview. From these, a medical doctor and professor of medicine with broad clinical experience in internal medicine, gastroenterology, and complementary medicine (Prof. Dr. Med. Roman Huber, Universitätklinikum Freiburg), as well as an Emeritus Professor of pharmacognosy (Emeritus Prof. Dr. Liselotte Krenn, University of Vienna) and a pharmacist specialising in herbal products (Dr. Mathias Schmidt, Herbresearch Germany) shared their experience. The topics discussed included the working mechanisms of the investigated herbs and more general methodological questions on mechanistic research. The interviews were semi-structured and were performed in an online (Microsoft Teams) or telephone meeting. When they were performed through an online meeting they were recorded. Notes were taken and the main messages are presented in the report.

2.5. *Analysis*

For each herb, findings from the literature and interviews were grouped together into relevant themes (antibacterial, antiviral, immunomodulatory, and other effects). No risk of bias assessment was performed. Specific information on the mechanism of action of individual active compounds was described when retrieved. If such detail in description is lacking, such information was not available in the included studies.

3. Results

3.1. Search Results

Three systematic searches were performed and yielded a total of 1405 reports. This included 996 articles from the first search, that included only review articles for all herbs; 319 articles from the second, that included all types of mechanistic studies on herbs for which only one or no reviews were retrieved during the first search; and another 120 articles from the third search, that included all types of mechanistic studies and that was performed if the most recent review article retrieved was more than 5 years old. After the screening of title, abstract, and full-text, 46 reports were chosen for data extraction. From the first search, 17 reviews were included. As this yielded only one review on thyme [32] and none on ivy or primrose, a second search for these herbs was performed, which yielded 21 additional studies. Only for *P. sidoides* was the most recent review more than five years old [26], hence, an additional search for more recent studies was performed for this herb. This yielded an additional eight studies. A PRISMA flow diagram of the selection and inclusion process is given in Figure 1. Another 45 studies were added after searching the bibliographies of the selected studies. Two more studies were included after consulting pharmaceutical companies, yielding a total of 93 studies for full review. A total of 17 of these 93 studies were reviews, 6 were mechanistic clinical trials, 10 were animal studies, and 60 were in vitro studies. A table describing the study characteristics can be found in Appendix A Study Characteristics.

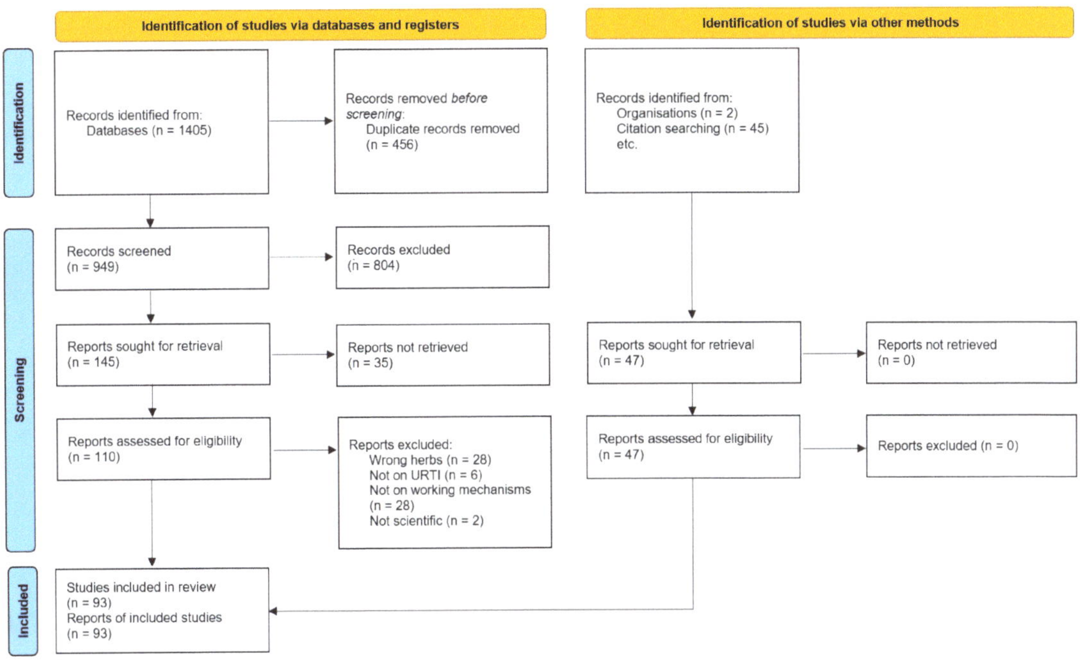

Figure 1. PRISMA flow diagram showing the identification and screening of studies retrieved.

3.2. *Andrographis paniculata (Burm. F) Nees*

Of *A. paniculata* different effects are known, including antibacterial, antiviral, immunomodulatory and antipyretic effects. An overview of these is given in Table 1. Below they are discussed in further detail.

Table 1. Overview of working mechanisms of *Andrographis paniculate (Burm. F) Nees.*

Antibacterial	Antiviral	Immunomodulatory	Other
Direct effects against *S. aureus, E. coli, S. typhimurium, B. subtilis, E. faecalis, K. pneumoniae, S. pneumoniae, P. vulgaris* [24,33–37]	Against avian influenza A virus (H9N2, H5N1 and H1N1) [38,39]	Increased proliferation of white blood cells [40]	Antipyretic [24]
Increased antibiotic sensitivity and reduced biofilm formation [35]		Reduced inflammatory response macrophages [41–44]	
Reduced bacterial adhesion to epithelium [35]		Anti-inflammatory [45,46]	

3.2.1. Antibacterial Effects

Several studies have found a direct antibacterial effect of *A. paniculata* and some of its compounds. For example, a methanolic extract of the leaves of *A. paniculata* showed a significant inhibition of *S. aureus, E. coli, S. typhimurium,* and *B. subtilis* in an agar well diffusion assay [24,33]. Furthermore, antibacterial effects against methicillin-resistant *S. aureus* (MRSA) and *E. faecalis* were found. When different solvents were tested, a methanol extract was more potent compared to water and hexane extracts [34]. More specifically, these effects were thought to be caused by the terpenoids, flavonoids, or phenolic acids present in *A. paniculata* [24].

The individual compound andrographolide inhibited *Staphylococcus aureus* with a very high MIC of 100 μg/mL. Reductions in DNA synthesis (31%), RNA synthesis (26%), and protein synthesis (36%) were found which were comparable to the antibiotic ciprofloxacin (with 25% incorporation). Furthermore, andrographolide affected the quorum sensing system (QSS), which resulted in a reduced production of extracellular polymeric substance and inhibited virulence factors [35].

However, when comparing the ethanolic extract of *A. paniculata* to andrographolide alone, the ethanolic extract showed a stronger inhibitory effect with *E. coli, K. pneumoniae,* and *P. vulgaris*. Only the inhibition of *S. pneumoniae* was stronger with andrographolide alone [36]. Looking at other compounds that could be involved in the antibacterial effect, the noriridoides andrographidoides A–E were investigated as well. These are mostly present in the roots of *A. paniculata*. However, they did not show any antibacterial effect on *E. coli, S. aureus, S. epidermidis, P. aeruginosa,* and *B. subtilis* (MICs > 100 μg/mL) [37].

Restoring Antibiotic Sensitivity and Reducing Biofilm

When looking closer at the inhibitory effects on bacteria, it was found that andrographolide could also help to restore the sensitivity of bacteria to antibiotics. Against *P. aeruginosa*, a direct inhibition of this kind was shown. The mechanism involved here was a reduced expression of the mexAB-oprM efflux pump, which is responsible for resistance to several antibiotics [35].

There could also be a more indirect mechanism involved. Some bacteria can form a multilayer structure called a biofilm. When pathogenic bacteria form such a structure it can form a barrier that protects them from the host's immune system and antibiotic drugs. The formation of a biofilm is, therefore, another mechanism of reducing sensitivity to antibiotics. Some compounds present in *A. paniculata* have been shown to reduce the biofilm of certain bacteria. The compounds andrographolide, 14-deoxyandrographolide, and andrograpanin reduced the biofilms of *P. auruginosa* and *S. aureus*. With 14-deoxyandrographolide and andrograpanin, the inhibition was dose-dependent and reached 54% and 56%, respectively, at 0.15 mM concentration. Their combination with gentamicin or azithromycin enhanced the effect up to 90% and 92% inhibition, respectively. Andrographolide was less potent and inhibited biofilm production of *P. auruginosa* up to 40% alone and up to 60% in combination with another antibiotic [35].

Reducing Bacterial Adhesion

Finally, *A. paniculata* can reduce URTIs caused by bacteria by reducing the adhesion of pathogenic bacteria to the epithelium of the lungs and thereby reducing respiratory colonization. This has been shown for example with andrographolide. This compound has been shown to inhibit bacterial adhesion of *E. coli* and *S. epidermidis* to epithelial cells of the lungs [35].

3.2.2. Antiviral Effects

Antiviral effects have also been reported. Both the water and ethanol extracts of the leaves, for example, inhibited the replication of avian influenza A virus (H5N1) in MDCK cells at non-toxic concentrations (IC50 = 38 ± 1 μg/mL). The compound 14-deoxy-11,12-dehydroandrographolide decreased the mRNA and protein expression of nucleoprotein and blocked viral ribonucleoprotein complexes from nuclei. Furthermore, this compound was shown to increase survival in mice after an infection with H5N1 to 33% at day 9, instead of 0% with no treatment [39].

A synthetic derivative of andrographolide, 14-α-lipolyl andrographolide, was tested both in vitro and in vivo. In a hemagglutinin inhibition assay an inhibition of viral absorption of both avian and human influenza A virus (H9N2, H5N1 and H1N1) into red blood cells was observed, with MICs ranging from 5.3 to 16.8 mM. The antiviral effect of *A. paniculata* was further shown in vivo. The oral administration of 14-α-lipolyl andrographolide to mice infected with either avian (H9N2 or H5N1) or human (H1N1) influenza A virus reduced death rate and prolonged life. Supplementation started 24 h before infection and was continued for seven days. 14-α-lipolyl andrographolide was the most potent and at a very high dose of 200 mg/kg bodyweight/day it increased survival to 100% in H1N1-infected and to 80% in both H9N2- and H5N1-infected mice. Andrographolide and 14-deoxy-11,12-dehydroandrographolide were also active though less potent compared to 14-α-lipolyl andrographolide. All were less potent than the control drug ribavirin, that resulted in 100% survival with each virus at a 150 mg/kg bodyweight/day dose [38].

3.2.3. Immunomodulatory Effects

Several studies show that *A. paniculata* can affect the functioning and proliferation of white blood cells. For example, an ethanolic extract of *A. paniculata* was found to stimulate both specific and non-specific immunity in mice injected with sheep red blood cells. Both antibody and delayed hypersensitivity were stimulated ($p < 0.001$) as well as macrophage migration index, phagocytosis of 14C-leucine labelled *E. coli*, and proliferation of splenic lymphocytes. Moreover, andrographolide and neoandrographolide were tested and showed similar effects, though less strong when compared to the ethanol extract [47]. Furthermore, in human peripheral blood lymphocytes the dichloromethane fraction of a methanol extract of *A. paniculata* increased proliferation. This effect was observed at low concentrations, with a 52% increase in proliferation at a concentration of 2.5 μg/mL. Further fractioning identified the three diterpenes andrographolide, 14-deoxyandrographolide, and 14-deoxy-11,12-didehydroandrographolide. All three compounds alone were also found to increase the proliferation of lymphocytes [40].

Furthermore, general anti-inflammatory effects have been observed. For example, both andrographolide and dehydroandrographolide inhibited COX-1 while andrographolide and neoandrographolide inhibited the COX-2 enzyme in ionophore A23187-induced human platelets [45]. Furthermore, the ethanol extract was shown to completely prevent the formation of carrageenan-induced paw oedema in BALB-c mice, when 5 mg was given intraperitoneally for five days before the induction of the oedema [46].

Regulation of Macrophage Functioning

More specifically focusing on macrophage functioning, *A. paniculata* can reduce the inflammatory response in macrophages. For example, the levels of NO, IL-1β, IL-6, and PGE2 produced by J774A.1 murine macrophages in response to LPS stimulation were reduced by a methanol extract of *A. paniculata* at concentrations that were not cytotoxic (<50 μg/mL) [44]. Further investigations into the compounds involved in these effects revealed that andrographolide and isoandrographolide both reduced NO, IL-1β, IL-6, and PGE2 after LPS stimulation. Furthermore, the *A. paniculate* constituent 7-O-methylwogonin reduced NO, IL-1β, and PGE2, whilst skullcapflavone-I reduced NO, IL-6, and PGE2 [43].

Looking closer at the compound andrographolide, in in vivo experiments, this compound reduced the increase in TNF-α and IL-6 that followed infection of the lungs with *S. aureus*, while keeping them high enough to adequately manage the infection [35]. Moreover, in mice infected with H1N1, treatment with 10 mg/kg bodyweight andrographolide decreased the expression of TNF-α, IL-6, and IL-10; NFκB signalling was also decreased [39]. In in vitro experiments, andrographolide inhibited IL-1β and IL-6 as well as TNF-α and IL-10 at 10 μg/mL in human ionophore A23187-induced human platelets. Furthermore, gene expression of cytokine receptors (TNFSF14, TNF, TNFRSF6, and IL1A) and chemokines (CCL8 and CXCL11) were downregulated as well as genes of the TLR family and the JAK/STAT and NFκB signalling pathways [45].

Furthermore, andrographolide was found to inhibit macrophage responses to IL-4 or LPS and regulated the polarization of macrophage phenotype, favouring the less inflammatory type 2 macrophages. Furthermore, it downregulated the mannose receptor in response to IL-4 and major histocompatibility complexes MHC-1, CD40, CD80, and CD85 in response to LPS. In accordance with these results, specific antibody presentation was downregulated in mice receiving 1 mg/kg bodyweight andrographolide via peritoneal injection for seven days. This effect was paired with downregulation of AKT and ERK1/2 phosphorylation in the in vivo experiment, indicating that the MAPK and PI3K pathways could be involved [42].

In addition, the compound andrograpanin reduced NO, TNF-α, IL-6, and IL-12(p70) in LPS-activated macrophages dose-dependently, at doses ranging from 15 to 90 μM, by downregulating iNOS and gene expression levels of TNF-α, IL-6, and IL-12(p70). Furthermore, it was suggested that MAPK pathways are involved, as the phosphorylation of p38 MAPKs was also downregulated in a dose-dependent way. The ERK1/2 and SAPK/JNK pathways were unaffected [41].

3.2.4. Antipyretic Effects

An antipyretic effect has been observed in rats with both the aqueous and chloroform extracts, when compared to petroleum ether and methanolic extracts. This was thought to be caused by the diterpenoid lactones. At doses of 400 or 800 mg/kg, the observed effect was significant [24].

3.3. *Pelargonium sidoides (Thunb.) R. Knuth*

Of *P. sidoides* different effects are known, including antibacterial, antiviral, immunomodulatory, expectorant and antitussive effects. An overview of these is given in Table 2. Below they are discussed in further detail.

Table 2. Overview of working mechanisms of *Pelargonium Sidoides* (*Thunb.*) *R. Knuth*.

Antibacterial	Antiviral	Immunomodulatory	Other
Reduced bacterial adhesion to epithelial cells [48,49]	Against influenza A virus (H1N1 and H3N2), respiratory syncytial virus (HCo-229E), parainfluenza virus type 3 and coxsackievirus A9 [50–53]	Reduced inflammatory damage [50,53–56]	Expectorant [54,57]
Increased bacterial adhesion to buccal cells [48]	Downregulation of docking proteins infected bronchial epithelial cells [51,52]	Increased macrophage functioning [58–60]	Antitussive [54]
Increased production of antimicrobial peptides [53,61,62]	Prevention of hemagglutination in human erythrocytes [50]	Increased inflammatory cytokines [60,61,63–66]	
	Upregulation of vitamin D receptor on human epithelial cells [53]	Increased production of antimicrobial peptides [53,61,62]	

3.3.1. Antibacterial Effects

Different studies have investigated a possible direct antibacterial effect of *P. sidoides*. However, most of these only found a weak antibacterial effect with MICs generally starting at 97 μg/mL [26,67–69]. However, an indirect antibacterial effect could be caused by *P. sidoides* affecting the adherence of certain bacteria to specific tissues.

For example, changes in adhesive behaviour after exposure to EPs 7630 were observed with *S. pyogenes*. In the control group, adhesion of *S. pyogenes* to human epithelial (Hep-2) was 80%. After 120 min incubation with 30 μg/mL EPs 7630 this adhesion was reduced on average by 46%. This effect was time- and dose-dependent and occurred after pretreatment of bacteria, but not after pretreatment of HEp-2 cells. This suggested that EPs 7630 influence bacterial adhesion factors rather than host adhesion factors [48]. A further study confirmed these findings with 30 μg/mL EPs 7630 in Hep-2 cells [49].

Furthermore, when looking into the compounds that could be responsible for this effect, it was found that both the methanol insoluble and methanol soluble fraction exhibited this effect. At concentrations of 30 μg/mL, inhibition of adhesion to Hep-2 cells of 35% and 30%, respectively, was observed. Furthermore, tannin-free fractions showed no effect on adhesion, which suggested that proanthocyanidins are responsible for the anti-adhesive effect. Especially, the (epi)gallocatechin constituent flavanyl units appeared to be crucial for this effect [49].

In addition to the decreased adhesion to human Hep-2 epithelial cells, the adhesion to buccal epithelial cells was increased. This increase was about sevenfold after pre-incubation for 120 min with 30 μg/mL EPs 7630. This effect was observed both with pre-incubation of the bacteria and the buccal cells. As buccal cells are replaced rapidly, increased adhesion to these cells could prevent infectious organisms from reaching the airways. Instead they are hypothesized to be swallowed with shedding buccal cells [48].

3.3.2. Antiviral Effects

Extract of *P. sidoides* (extraction method unknown) inhibited influenza A virus (H1N1 and H3N2) in MDCK cells with a mean IC50 between 7.80–11.67 μg/mL [50]. EPs 7630 also reduced virus replication of influenza virus (H1N1 and H3N2), as well as respiratory syncytial virus (HCo-229E), parainfluenza virus type 3, and coxsackievirus A9. It did not affect the virus replication of non-enveloped adenoviruses or rhinoviruses. However, *P. sidoides* did increase the survival of bronchial epithelial cells infected with rhinoviruses [51].

Underlying to this, *P. sidoides* appeared to interact with both the membrane of the cells and the virus envelope in order to prevent viral plaque build-up [50]. In rhinovirus-infected bronchial epithelial cells, EPs 7630 has been shown to downregulate docking proteins, such as cell surface calreticulin and inducible co-stimulator and its ligand, while simultaneously upregulating antibacterial proteins (see Section 3.3.3 Immunomodulatory Effects) [51,52]. Other membrane proteins that could interact with the virus, such as myeloid differentiation factor 88, TLR2/4, or intercellular adhesion molecule 1, remained unchanged [52]. Interaction with the cell membrane that prevented hemagglutination was also confirmed in human erythrocytes [50].

Another remarkable effect of EPs 7630 that could contribute to the antiviral effect was the upregulation of vitamin D receptors in human bronchial epithelial cells through Erk1/2 MAPK signaling. This has been observed with concentrations of EPs 7630 of 5 μg/mL or higher. Furthermore, the response of the vitamin D receptor to vitamin D was enhanced, which caused a 2.1 times stronger antiviral response against rhinovirus 16 in human bronchial epithelial cells treated with 5 μg/mL EPs 7630 [53].

3.3.3. Immunomodulatory Effects

In general, there are two ways in which *P. sidoides* influences the immune functioning. First, it can reduce harmful inflammation. For example, in a rat model for acute bacterial bronchitis, EPs 7630 at doses of 30 and 60 mg/kg bodyweight reduced the degree of tracheal lesions. This effect was paired with decreased serum levels of malondialdehyde, which could indicate that this effect was at least partially mediated by an upregulation of superoxide dismutase and, consequently, a reduced level of oxidative stress [54]. Furthermore, a reduction in E-cadherin was observed in human bronchial epithelial cells exposed to 5 μg/mL EPs 7630. This could indicate a decreased thickening of the airway wall during infection or inflammation [53]. Furthermore, EPs 7630 prevented asthma attacks in children triggered by rhinovirus by decreasing the inflammation caused by increases in IL-6, IL-8, and IL-16. Similarly, EPs 7630 has been show to decrease levels of IL-6 and IL-15 in serum, while increasing levels of immunoglobulin in athletes during strenuous exercise [51].

Further proof of an anti-inflammatory effect of *P. sidoides* in infection was found with studies on sickness behaviour. In response to infection, proinflammatory cytokines are produced which induce sickness behaviour. This includes anorexia, depressed activity, listlessness, and malaise. In male NMRI mice, sickness behaviour was induced by intraperitoneal injection with 400 μg/kg bodyweight LPS. Oral administration of a standardised *P. sidoides* extract (Umckaloabo) at doses ranging from 100 to 400 mg/kg bodyweight one hour before LPS administration dose-dependently antagonised reduced activity and listlessness [55]. Furthermore, administration of 100–400 mg/kg bodyweight EPs 7630 one hour before LPS injection caused this effect in mice. Further investigation into different molecular weight fractions showed that the high molecular weight fraction (>30 kDa) was responsible for this effect [56].

Second, *P. sidoides* can increase the immune response by enhancing phagocytic activity, oxidative burst, intracellular killing of pathogens, and the release of NO in macrophages, as well as inducing the release of TNF-α, IL-1, and IL-12 [67]. EPs 7630 has also been shown to increase levels of antimicrobial proteins in host cells. Below, these immune-stimulating effects will be discussed one by one in greater detail.

Effects on Macrophages

First, the enhancement in phagocytotic activity and oxidative burst was shown with EPs 7630. This extract increased the number of phagocytosing human peripheral blood phagocytes in a dose-dependent manner with concentrations between 1 and 30 μg/mL after 2–10 min exposure. The maximal increase was 56% after 2 min exposure to 30 μg/mL EPs 7630 (p = 0.002). Furthermore, the number of burst-active phagocytes increased dose-dependently at all timepoints between 2 and 30 min. The maximal increase in this was 120% after 4 min of exposure to 30 μg/mL [58].

In addition, the enhanced intracellular killing of pathogens was shown in the same experiment. *C. albicans* was used as the pathogen and the number of surviving *C. albicans* cells decreased significantly with 30 μg/mL EPs 7630, though not with lower concentrations. The highest reduction in viable yeast cells was 31% and was observed after 120 min incubation with 30 μg/mL [58]. In another experiment, it was shown that the methanol, petrol ether, ethyl acetate, and n-Butanol extracts of *P. sidoides* reduced the intracellular survival of *L. donovania* in murine macrophages. The EC50 concentration ranged from 0.1 to 3.3 μg/mL. Furthermore, gallic acid and methyl esters found in *P. sidoides* reduced the survival of L. donocania, with EC50's of 4.4 μg/mL and 12.5 μg/mL, respectively [59]. Moreover, when murine macrophages were infected with L. monocytogenes, EPs 7630 increased the intracellular killing dose-dependently at concentrations between 1 and 30 μg/mL. This effect was enhanced by IFN-γ, and when 10 μg/mL EPs 7630 was combined with 100 U/mL IFN-γ the effect was almost equal to 10 μg/mL LPS with 100 U/mL IFN-γ [60].

Finally, the production of NO by murine macrophages infected with *L. monocytogenes* was increased when exposed to 30 μg/mL EPs 7630 [60]. Similarly, iNOS expression increased in murine macrophages infected with *L. donovania* and exposed to EPs 7630. However, blocking iNOS did not affect the increased intracellular killing of *L. donovania* [59].

Cytokine Production and Effects on Other Immune Cells

In human blood immune cells, EPs 7630 increased TNF-α, IL-6, and IL-10 dose-dependently [63], and in macrophages, pro-inflammatory cytokines such as TNF-α, IL-1α,

IL-1β, and IL-12 increased [60]. In RAW 264.7 cells, treatment with 50 μg/mL EPs 7630 increased the mRNA levels of IL-1, IL-12, IL-18, TNF-α, IFN-α, and IFN-γ. This was observed in uninfected cells, but the increase was stronger in cells infected with L. major. Further investigation found that this effect occurred with the methanol-soluble fraction, but not with the methanol-insoluble fraction [64]. Further explanation might involve MAPK activation, which was found with EPs 7630 treatment in human monocytes, while p38 was strongly inhibited [63].

Furthermore, the interleukins 17 and 22 increased with EPs 7630 treatment of human memory T-cells. Especially, IL-22 increased strongly. Direct contact of the T-cell with EPs 7630 was necessary, as well as soluble mediators produced by monocytes upon EPs 7630 treatment [61]. Stimulation of T-cells with EPs 7630 alone did not produce such an effect [61,63]. Interestingly, this IL-22 was then found to increase the release of antimicrobial protein S100A9 in lung epithelial cells and pulmonary tissues [61].

In mechanistic clinical trials, there have also been changes in cytokine and chemokine levels observed. Acute bacterial rhinosinusitis patients receiving 20 mg EPs 7630 three times a day for ten days showed increased concentrations of MCP-1 and interferon gamma-induced protein 10 (IP-10) ($p < 0.01$) [65]. Furthermore, in post-viral rhinosinusitis patients receiving the same treatment, MCP-1, IP-10, and macrophage inflammatory protein (MIP)-1β were increased in nasal secretions [66]. The chemo- and cytokines MIP-1α, epithelial neutrophil activating peptide were increased both in acute and post-viral rhinosinusitis. This could indicate that EPs 7630 can regulate monocytes and neutrophils in the nasal mucosa and, hence, influence the infection [65,66].

Antimicrobial Proteins

Furthermore, EPs 7630 has been shown to increase the release of different antimicrobial proteins by different cells. In human epithelial cells, both infected with rhinovirus and uninfected, EPs 7630 has been shown to upregulate the expression of antimicrobial proteins such as β-defensin-1 and suppressor of cytokine signalling 1 [53]. EPs 7630 increased the release of the antibacterial proteins neutrophil peptides 1–3 (HNP 1–3) and bactericidal/permeability-increasing protein (BPI) from human neutrophils and granulocytes. After a five-hour incubation with EPs 7630 at a concentration of 30 μg/mL, HNP 1–3 was increased by 150% while BPI increased 127%. While 10 ng/mL LPS increased the release of HNPs 82% and BPI 356%, the combination of 30 μg/mL EPs 7630 and 10 ng/mL LPS stimulated the release even more and caused HNPs to increase by 294% and BPI by 531%. This could indicate that EPs 7630 can cause a stronger reaction against pathogens [62]. Furthermore, indirectly, by stimulating the release of IL-22, EPs 7630 can increase the production of antimicrobial protein S100A9 in lung tissue as explained before (see Section Cytokine Production and Effects on Other Immune Cells) [61].

3.3.4. Expectorant Activity

Other effects of *P. sidoides* include effects on mucocilliary clearing. In mice that were intraperitoneally injected with phenol red, the elimination of the dye through the respiratory tract was dose-dependently increased with the administration of 20, 40, or 120 mg/kg bodyweight EPs 7630 for three days. This increase was statistically significant at doses of 40 and 120 mg/kg bodyweight when compared to mice receiving no treatment ($p < 0.01$) [54]. An underlying mechanism could be an increase in ciliary beat frequency of nasal epithelium cells. In an adherent monolayer cell culture of human nasal epithelium, EPs 7630 increased the frequency of ciliary beats by up to 123% at a concentration of 30 μg/mL and to 133% at a concentration of 100 μg/mL [57].

Antitussive effects were found in guinea pigs in a citric acid-induced cough model. A significant and dose-dependent reduction in the frequency of cough was observed in guinea pigs receiving 10, 20, or 45 mg/kg bodyweight EPs 7630 ($p < 0.01$). Moreover, in mice with ammonia-induced cough, a reduction in cough frequency as well as a prolongation of cough latency time was observed with doses of EPs 7630 of 20, 40, or 120 mg/kg bodyweight [54].

3.3.5. Expert Opinion

P. sidoides is only used in preparations, the most well-known and well-researched being Kaloba®, and not on a more uncontrollable basis such as in a tea. This is an advantage, as these preparations are standardised and well researched. Clinical records are very good, and the mechanism is thought to be a combination of immune enhancement, antibacterial, antiviral, and expectorant effects. As most research is performed with the full extract, it is not possible to attribute the observed effects to one specific compound. There is an important role for coumarins, especially umckalin, but groups of compounds such as tannins and phenolics are also expected to contribute to the spasmolytic, antiphlogistic and antibacterial effects (Emeritus Prof. Dr. Liselotte Krenn, personal communication 2021).

A major issue with *P. sidoides* is, however, the lack of quality control. The European monographs use too broad a definition to ensure that actual *P. sidoides* is used. Related species such as *P. reniforme* and others can also be included in products sold as *P. sidoides*. The use of certain marker compounds, which is performed for example with standardised extracts such as EPs 7630, does not ensure that the same species is used either, as these marker compounds can still be present in other species. Overall, the chemical composition is likely different between different species, which is reflected by the fact that local people will not use any other species. Since almost all research is performed with EPs 7630, it is plausible, but not confirmed, that these effects would translate to other *P. sidoides* preparations (Mathias Schmidt, personal communication 2021).

3.4. Echinacea Species

Of Echinacea species different effects are known, including antibacterial, antiviral, immunomodulatory and expectorant effects. An overview of these is given in Table 3. Below they are discussed in further detail.

Table 3. Overview of mechanisms of *Echinacea* species.

Antibacterial	Antiviral	Immunomodulatory	Other
Reduced adhesion of *S. aureus* and *H. influenzae* to epithelial cells [70]	Against influenza virus A (both human and avian), influenza virus B, herpes simplex virus 1 and 2, respiratory syncytial virus and rhinoviruses [71]	Immunostimulatory effects: ○ Increased total white blood cell count [72,73] ○ Increased activity of T-lymphocytes, NK-cells, dendritic cells and macrophages [72,74–77] ○ Increased secretion of pro-inflammatory cytokines [72–77]	Expectorant [71]
	Increased presentation of viral antigens by infected cells [73]	Anti-inflammatory effects:Inhibition of COX-1, COX-2 and 5-LOX [72,73,76]	
	Decreased viral binding [71,78]		
	Increased antibody-dependent and innate NK-mediated activity [73]		

3.4.1. Antibacterial Effects

Only one study has reported on the direct antibacterial effects of Echinacea. Here, it was found that a standardised alcoholic extract of *E. purpurea* (Echinaforce, A. Vogel Bioforce AG) reduced the expression of intracellular adhesion molecule 1 (ICAM-1) in human lung epithelial (BEAS-2B) cells. Subsequently, the adhesion of both *Staphylococcus aureus* and *Haemophilus influenzae* was reduced [70].

3.4.2. Antiviral Effects

Some studies point to a direct antiviral effect of Echinacea [74]. For example, it was found that *E. purpurea* can directly inhibit influenza virus A (both human and avian), influenza virus B, herpes simplex virus 1 and 2, respiratory syncytial virus, and rhinoviruses [71]. Furthermore, in vitro pre-incubation of mouse fibroblasts with *E. purpurea* juice, methanolic extract, or aqueous extract for 24 h resulted in resistance to influenza A2, herpes, and vesicular stomatitis virus [72]. Another study found that the presentation of viral antigens by infected cells increased after exposure to *E. purpurea* juice in vitro. However, in this study, viral replication or viral load did not change [73]. When assessing light-activated antiviral activity, an n-hexane extract of *E. purpurea* had an MIC of 0.12 mg/mL, an ethanolic extract of E. pallida had an MIC of 26 μg/mL, and the isolated compound cichoric acid had an MIC of 45 μg/mL against HSV-1. E. angustifolia inhibits influenza A, herpes simplex virus 1, and rhinovirus, whilst *E. pallida* inhibits herpes simplex virus 1 and 2 [71].

The underlying mechanisms could involve inhibiting the influenza-virus-specific hemagglutinatinin and neuramidase [71]. At concentrations between 1.6 μg/mL and 1.6 mg/mL, a standardised ethanolic extract of *E. purpurea* (Echinaforce) inactivated human H1N1 type IV virus, highly pathogenic avian influenza virus (H5 and H7 types), and swine-origin influenza virus (S-OIV and H1N1) in cell culture assays. Direct contact between the virus and the extract was needed for this effect. Possibly this is because the extract inhibits the receptor binding activity of the virus, as was shown in hemagglutination assays. Interestingly, in sequential passage studies it was shown that in cell culture with H5N1 virus, no resistance of the virus to the *E. purpurea* extract developed, whilst this was the case with the control drug Tamiflu. Furthermore, the Tamiflu-resistant virus was still equally susceptible to the *E. purpurea* extract compared to the wild type virus [78]. Another underlying mechanism of the antiviral effect might be an increase in both the antibody-dependent and the innate NK-mediated activity, which has been found with *E. purpurea* extract and juice against herpes virus [73].

3.4.3. Immunomodulatory Effects

The effects of Echinacea on the immune system are diverse. Depending on the circumstances, both immunostimulatory and anti-inflammatory effects have been observed.

Immunostimulatory Effects

Immunostimulatory effects have been reported on both non-specific and specific immunity. A stimulating effect was found in several immune cells. Firstly, *E. purpurea* can increase the total white blood cell count and specifically increase the proportions of lymphocytes and monocytes, whilst reducing neutrophil and eosinophil counts [72]. However, changes in T and B cell count are inconsistent [6,73]. Furthermore, *E. purpurea* can stimulate immune function by enhancing T-lymphocytes' activity and neutrophils and macrophage-induced phagocytosis. It also possesses short-term, non-specific immune system stimulating properties such as increasing the activity of components of the alternate complement system [74,75,79]. These effects have also been confirmed in mechanistic clinical trials (see Section Evidence from Mechanistic Clinical Trials).

There are also reports of increased NK cell activity [72,74,76]. After 14 days of supplementation in mice, enhanced resistance of splenic lymphocytes to apoptosis was found [72]. Furthermore, a reduction in splenic NK cell activity as part of a stress response was prevented by Echinacea extract [76]. Moreover, in healthy people, patients with chronic fatigue syndrome, and AIDS patients an increase in NK cell activity was found after *E. purpurea* supplementation [77], although other studies did not find an increase in NK cells [72].

Other immunostimulant effects include, for example, both phenotypic and functional maturation of murine and human dendritic cells. It has also been found to reduce stress-induced reduction in splenocyte proliferation [76]. In addition, there is evidence that Echinacea can enhance macrophage functioning (in vitro, in vivo, and from human studies) as *E. purpurea*, E. pallida, and E. angustifolia all increased phagocytosis in vitro [77]. Furthermore, an increase in the levels of IL-1, IL-10, and TNF-α was reported (both in rat in vivo studies and in vitro macrophage studies) with the fresh juice of *E. purpurea* [72–74] which could be comparable to LPS simulation [77]. IL-6 and IFN-γ also increased [72–74,77]. This effect was especially observed with the polysaccharide fraction of *E. purpurea*. More specifically, an increase in the LPS-induced NO release by rat splenic macrophages was observed. Moreover, a dose-dependent increase in phagocytic activity of these macrophages was observed with an aqueous extract of an (unspecified) Echinacea extract [72]. In addition, stimulation of polymorphonuclear granulocytes was found with *E. purpurea* [73].

Furthermore, an immunostimulant effect is reflected in the increased levels of pro-inflammatory cytokines that has been reported in several studies. Echinacea species can, for example, increase IL-2 levels [72] as well as increase levels of TNF-α, IL-1α, IL-1β, IL-6, IFN-γ, and NO (in both rat in vivo studies and in vitro macrophage studies) [73,75]. It also can restore serum protein and splenic mRNA levels of cytokines in rats (IL-6, IL-10, and IL-17) and humans (IL-2, IL-16, IFN-γ, and TNF-a) [76]. With regard to different species, *E. purpurea* enhances IL-1, IL-6, TNF-α, and IFN-γ more than E. angustifolia or E. pallida [73].

However, the changes in cytokine levels also reflect the different effects Echinacea can have on the immune system. For example, an aqueous extract of *E. purpurea* (80% polysaccharides) enhanced dose-dependently the production of IL-2 and IFN-γ by human T-cells (Jurkat E6) when stimulated by phorbol 12-myristate 13-acetate plus ionomycin (PMA-I) in vitro. This stimulation was, however, absent when the cells were not stimulated by PMA-I. In conditions where the T-cells were seeded with a low density (0.5 × 106 cells/mL), *E. purpurea* also reduced the IFN-γ response and the percentage of CD25+ T-cells. This effect was, however, not seen when T-cells were seeded with a high density (5.0 × 106 cells/mL) [80]. Furthermore, in human lung epithelial cells (BEAS-2B), a standardised *E. purpurea* extract (Echinaforce) effectively prevented super-expression of inflammatory cytokines, otherwise known as a cytokine storm, in response to infection with influenza A virus. It achieved this by suppressing the expression of the NFκB pathway and possibly also TLR-4 [70].

Anti-Inflammatory Effects

More anti-inflammatory effects in epithelial tissues have been reported. For example, the expression of inflammatory cytokine genes and some of their properties in bronchial epithelial cells can be reversed by *E. purpurea*. Furthermore, undefined Echinacea extracts can inhibit the activity of COX-1 and COX-2 [72,73]. Cyclo-oxygenase (COX)-1, COX-2, and lipoxygenase enzymes are important enzymes involved in the production of pro-inflammatory prostaglandins. Inhibition of COX-1 and COX-2 was found with *E. purpurea*, whilst inhibition of 5-LOX was found with *E. purpurea*, E. pallida, and E. angustifolia. This inhibition of 5-LOX appears to be related to the concentration of alkamides [72]. Furthermore, lipoxygenase-inhibiting anti-inflammatory activity was attributable to isobutyl amide and decatetraene acid in *E. purpurea* [76]. In addition, inhibition of hyaluronidase is reported as an anti-inflammatory effect of Echinacea species, caused by cichoric acid as the most potent inhibitor [73].

Evidence from Mechanistic Clinical Trials

The effect of Echinacea species on the immune system is also observed in mechanistic clinical trials that found changes in white blood cell count, cytokine levels, and the complement system. For example, a seven day treatment with 5 mL of a standardized *E. purpurea* extract (Echinilin) increased the total white blood cell, monocyte, neutrophil, and NK cell counts significantly in healthy volunteers [81].

Changes in cytokine levels were also observed with daily supplementation with an *E. angustifolia* syrup (corresponding to 4.7 mg Echinacoside and 8.0 mg of a high-molecular-weight (20 kDa) polysaccharide). This caused an increase in IL-2 and IL-8 mRNA levels and a decrease in TNF-α and IL-6 mRNA levels in healthy volunteers (n = 10). The changes in IL-2 and IL-6 were confirmed by protein levels of these cytokines in the blood. Supplementation went on for a month, but these effects were maximal after 14 days [82].

In another study, healthy volunteers ($n = 30$) received supplementation with a standardised ethanolic *E. purpurea* extract (Echinaforce) for eight days. Afterwards, blood samples were taken and stimulated in vitro with LPS, SEB, or zymosan. The pro-inflammatory mediators TNF-α and IL-1β decreased by up to 24% ($p < 0.05$) while anti-inflammatory IL-10 levels increased by 13% ($p < 0.05$), and IL-8 and MCP-1 increased by 15% ($p < 0.05$) when compared to baseline measurements. In a subgroup of volunteers who showed low levels of MCP-1, IL-8, IL-10, and IFN-γ, treatment with Echinaforce significantly increased these levels (30–49%, $p < 0.05$), whereas volunteers with higher levels of these cytokines before treatment did not show any significant change in their levels after treatment. Furthermore, in volunteers with reported high stress levels and who experienced more than two colds per year, treatment increased IFN-γ levels (>50%). A relationship with stress was also found in volunteers with a low level of cortisol, in whom levels of IL-1β, IL-6, IL-12, and TNF-α decreased with treatment, while in volunteers with higher cortisol levels such changes were not found [83].

Furthermore, after four weeks of taking daily a combination of *E. purpurea* and *E. angustifolia* (*E. purpurea* whole herb extract 4% (908 mg/day), *E. purpurea* whole herb (464 mg/day) and *E. angustifolia* root (36 mg/day)), complement properdin increased by 21% ($p < 0.05$) in healthy volunteers ($n = 8$) compared to a placebo treatment [84].

Compounds Involved and Differences between Species

Some studies have also looked specifically at compounds that could be involved in the immune modulating effects. Many point to the polysaccharides as important for this. Intravenous injection with the polysaccharide fraction was, for example, twice as effective compared to the whole aqueous extract in reducing carrageenan-induced rat paw oedema. It was half as effective as indomectin in the croton oil test when applied topically [72]. Polysaccharides have further been shown to enhance phagocyte function in in vitro and in vivo studies by increasing phagocytosis, increasing TNF-α, IL-1, and IL-6 secretion. Furthermore, they increased the motility of polymorphonuclear cells and their cytotoxic activity [77]. Finally, the enhanced immune response of human T-cells to PMA-I was also found with the polysaccharides and not with phenolic compounds in *E. purpurea* [80].

Moreover, alkamides derived from Echinacea have immunomodulatory and anti-inflammatory activity. This is reflected in the inhibiting effect of alcohol extracts of Echinacea on the production of inflammatory mediators such as TNF-α and NO [75]. The alkylamides dodeca-2E,4E,8Z,10E/Z-tetraenoic acid isobutylamides, trienoic, and dienoic acid derivatives in *E. purpurea* increased TNF-α mRNA synthesis in primary human monocytes and macrophages through activation of the endocannabinoid receptor 2, though no increase in TNF-α protein levels was found [85].

With regards to the different species of Echinacea, the evidence differs. For example, arabinogalactan-proteins from *E. pallida* strongly stimulated proliferation of mouse lymphocytes in vitro, while the arabinogalactans from *E. purpurea* did not show this effect [86]. Furthermore, cichoric acid, which is involved in immunomodulation, enhancing phagocytosis, and inhibiting hyaluronidase, is the main phenolic compound in *E. purpurea*. Echinacoside is the main phenolic compound in *E. pallida* and *E. angustifolia* and does not have immunostimulatory effects, though anti-inflammatory and antioxidant properties have been reported [87].

3.4.4. Expectorant Effects

Aside from a direct virucidal effect and an immunomodulatory effect, *E. purpurea* reduced excessive mucin production by airway cells and tissues [71].

3.4.5. Expert Opinion

Regarding Echinacea, the main effect in mechanistic studies appears to be immunomodulation. There are some conflicting results, but this could be due to a U-shaped response curve, where in low concentrations the effects are more immunomodulatory, whilst in higher concentrations the effect is more immunosuppressive. The reported changes in white blood cell count are inconsistent. More so, animal studies are susceptible for finding such changes, often inconsistent, and the translation to clinically relevant effects is not clear. Increased functioning of macrophages is a mechanism that can enhance immune function but is difficult to prove in clinical studies (Emeritus Prof. Dr. Liselotte Krenn, personal communication 2021) and in vitro and in vivo models do not represent the situation of infection very well (Dr. Mathias Schmidt, personal communication 2021). Furthermore, contaminations with endotoxins can easily occur with testing Echinacea in vitro. These can have an LPS-like activity and can contaminate the results, leading to an unjustified conclusion of immunostimulation (Prof. Dr. Roman Huber, personal communication 2021).

3.5. *Hedera helix* L.

Of *H. helix* different effects are known, including antibacterial, antiviral, immunomodulatory, bronchospasmolytic and secretolytic effects. An overview of these is given in Table 4. Below they are discussed in further detail.

Table 4. Overview of mechanisms of *Hedera helix* L.

Antibacterial	Antiviral	Immunomodulatory	Other
Direct effects against *S. pneumonia*, *S. pyogenes*, *S. aureus*, *S. epidermidis*, *M. tuberculosis*, *M. avium*, *H. influenzae*, and *A. baumannii* [88,89]	No antiviral effects reported.	Anti-inflammatory effects [90–93] Reduced pathological changes to lung tissue [93,94]	Bronchospasmolytic and secretolytic [95–98]

3.5.1. Antibacterial and Antiviral Effects

A direct antibacterial effect of an aqueous extract of *H. helix* leaves was assessed for *S. pneumonia*, *S. pyogenes*, *S. aureus*, *S. epidermidis*, *M. tuberculosis*, *M. avium*, *H. influenza*, and *A. baumannii*. The MICs ranged from 16 to 64 μg/mL, with the lowest MICs (16 μg/mL) found with *M. avium* and *H. influenzae* [88]. The petroleum and ethanolic extracts were found to be less effective against *S. aureus*, *S. epidermidis*, *E. coli*, *K. pneumoniae*, *P. auruginosa*, and *P. mirabilis*, with MICs of 156.2 μg/mL or higher [89]. No reports on direct antiviral effects were found.

3.5.2. Anti-Inflammatory Effects

Treatment with *H. helix* extracts has been shown to reduce the level of pro-inflammatory cytokines. In murine macrophages (J774.2 cells), significant decreases in IL-6 were observed of 25 ± 4%, 32 ± 4%, and 40 ± 7% with concentrations of 80, 160, and 400 μg/mL EA575, respectively [90]. In both J774.2 and HEK293 cells, the anti-inflammatory effects have been shown to be a result of a dose-dependent inhibition of the NFkB pathway, probably due to a specificity switch of IKKβ [91]. In in vivo studies, an anti-inflammatory effect was also observed for saponins present in *H. helix*. In ovalbumin-sensitized guinea pigs, for example, a peritoneal injection of either a high (3 mg/kg bodyweight) or a low dose (0.3 mg/kg bodyweight) of α-hederin reduced total white blood cell and eosinophil counts compared to sensitized animals without treatment ($p < 0.01$ and $p < 0.001$, respectively). There was an increase in the percentage of neutrophils, lymphocytes, and monocytes, whilst the eosinophil and basophil counts decreased ($p < 0.01$–0.05) [92]. Moreover, blood levels of IL-4 and IL-17 were decreased with the high dose ($p < 0.05$), while INF-γ levels increased with both low and high doses compared to the control ($p < 0.05$) [93].

Furthermore, treatment with α-hederin reduced pathological changes in lung tissue due to asthma induction, such as reduced thickness of vessels and airway wall, mucus plaque, and respiratory epithelium denudation [93]. Similarly, in ovalbumin-sensitized

BALB/c mice, treatment with *H. helix* (100 mg/kg) reduced the increased number of goblet cells and reduced the increased thickness of basement membrane. However, compared to dexamethasone only the reduction in thickness of the basement membrane was greater with *H. helix* while other histopathological parameters improved more with dexamethasone [94].

Looking at different compounds that could be involved in an anti-inflammatory effect, oral administration of 0.02 mg/kg α-hederin was found to be ineffective for reducing carrageenan-induced rat paw oedema after one hour. The same was found for hederasaponin-C, while hederacolchisides-E and -F showed slight anti-inflammatory effects after one hour ($p < 0.05$). After four hours, hederacolchiside-F was found as effective as the control drug indomethacin (20 mg/kg), while hederacolchisides-C and -E were both effective, though less effective compared to indomethacin [99].

3.5.3. Bronchospasmolytic and Secretolytic Effects

Some studies have found that *H. helix* can relax the smooth muscle in the lungs, leading to bronchodilation. In vitro, the three saponins α-hederin, hederagenin, and hederacoside C did not influence histamine- or methacholine-induced contraction in muscle strips. Pretreatment with 1 μM α-hederin for 18 h, however, enhanced isoprenaline-induced relaxation. Hederagenin and hederacoside C did not show this effect [95]. In vivo, these findings were confirmed. In ovalbumin-sensitized guinea pigs, intraperitoneal injection with either a high (3 mg/kg bodyweight) or low dose (0.3 mg/kg bodyweight) of α-hederin decreased the responsiveness of tracheal smooth muscle to methacholine, histamine, and ovalbumine. The change in responsiveness to ovalbumin was even stronger than with the control treatment thymoquinone [92].

An underlying mechanism causing these effects appears to be that *H. helix* extract can reduce the internalization of β2 adrenergic receptors. This was shown with pre-incubation of human embryonic kidney (HEK293) cells with 1 μM α-hederin or 1 μM β-hederin for 24 h. In addition, in type 2 alveolar cells (A549 cells) pre-treated with 1 μM α-hederin or 1 μM β-hederin, binding of a dye (Alexa532-NA) to the β2 adrenergic receptor increased. Interestingly, in saturation experiments, α-hederin did not change the density of β2 adrenergic receptors. Furthermore, in human airway smooth muscle (HASM) cells, pretreatment with 1 μM α-hederin or 1 μM β-hederin for 24 h increased cAMP levels when the cells were stimulated compared to no pretreatment [96,97]. An increase in cAMP can indicate (increased) activation of the β2 adrenergic receptor [98].

These results indicate that pretreatment with α-hederin prevents the number of β2 adrenergic receptors from declining under stimulating conditions. This increased responsiveness could lead to a bronchospasmolytic effect in the smooth muscle cells. In alveolar cells, this increased stimulation of the β2 adrenergic receptor can lead to increased secretion of surfactant. This can cause the bronchial mucus to be diluted and more easily expelled [98].

The effect on β2 adrenergic receptors is only found with α-hederin and β-hederin. Hederacosid-C and hederagenin did not show these effects on β2 adrenergic receptor internalization [97]. Protocatechuic acid, neochlorogenic acid, chlorogenic acid, cryptochlorogenic acid, rutin, kaempferol-3-O-rutinoside, 3,4-, 3,5-, and 4,5-dicaffeoylquinic acid, and hederacoside B did not affect β2 adrenergic receptors [96]. However, resorption studies have shown that hederacoside C does not reach significant levels in the blood but is readily transformed into α-hederin instead. It can, therefore, be seen as a prodrug. Furthermore, human resorption studies have shown that α-hederin reaches blood plasma concentrations of 0.66 μM, whilst concentrations of 0.5 μM have been shown to induce an inhibition of approximately 60% of the β2 adrenergic receptor internalization [98].

3.6. Primula veris L. and Primula elatior L.

No reports on the effects of isolated *P. veris* or *P. elatior* were found.

3.7. *Thymus vulgaris* L. and *Thymus zygis* L.

3.7.1. Antibacterial Effects

In vitro studies assessing the antibacterial effects have focused on different extracts and some on individual compounds. Antibacterial effects have been shown against a broad spectrum of bacteria, including those relevant to URTI. In the following paragraphs, ethanolic extracts, essential oil, and individual compounds, will be discussed.

Ethanolic Extracts

First, there are studies into the ethanolic extract of *T. vulgaris*. Using disk diffusion, MICs against *S. aureus* of 5 mg/mL, against *E. coli* and *K. pneumoniae* of 10 mg/mL, and against *P. vulgaris* and *P. auruginosa* of 20 mg/mL were established [100]. Furthermore, a 25 mg/mL ethanolic extract showed a zone of inhibition ranging from 4.00 to 21.00 mm against ten multidrug-resistant clinical isolates of *S. aureus*, *E. coli*, *P. mirabellis*, and *K. pneumoniae* and two standard strains: *S. aureus* ATCC 25923 and *E. coli* ATCC 25922 [101].

Essential Oils

Most research on the direct antibacterial effects of *T. vulgaris* and *T. zygis* has, however, focused on the essential oils. The antibacterial effects of the essential oil has, for example, been shown against *P. fluorescens*, *L. monocytogenes*, *B. thermosphacta*, *E. coli*, *Salmonella*, *P. auruginosa*, and *S. aureus* [102–105]. Overall, Gram-positive bacteria appear to be more vulnerable compared to Gram-negative [106]. An overview of the different MICs that have been established with different methods is given in Table 5. Toxicity against non-bacterial cells was tested and a minimum non-toxic concentration to Vero cells was found of 0.0002 mL/mL [107].

Some studies also investigated the antibacterial effect of the essential oil of *T. vulgaris* against some standard-drug-resistant bacteria. Though it showed activity against some multidrug-resistant bacteria such as MRSA, to others, such as resistant *P. aeruginosa*, it did not [108]. Interaction with standard antibiotics was also investigated against extended-spectrum β-lactamase (ESBL)-producing and New Delhi metallo-β-lactamase (MBL)-1-producing *K. pneumoniae* isolates. Here, the combination of the essential oil of *T. vulgaris* with gentamicin had an additive effect rather than a synergistic effect [109].

Furthermore, the essential oil of *T. zygis* was tested against several bacterial strains as well. MIC values against a collection of colistin-sensitive *A. baumanii* and *K. pneumoniae* ranged between 256 and 1024 µg/mL. Synergy was observed against these organisms when the essential oil was given in combination with colistin, but not with other antibiotics [110].

Table 5. Overview of the minimum inhibitory concentration (MIC) values that have been established with direct contact for essential oil of *T. vulgaris*.

Bacterial Species	Method	MIC	
Acinetobacter baumanii	Agar dilution	0.12% (*v*/*v*)	[111]
Enterococcus faecalis	Agar dilution	0.5% (*v*/*v*)	[111]
Aeromonas sobria	Agar dilution	0.12% (*v*/*v*)	[111]
Escherichia coli	Agar dilution Broth microdilution Microwell dilution	0.12% (*v*/*v*) 0.03% (*v*/*v*) 62.5 µg/mL	[111] [111] [112]
Klebsiella pneumoniae	Agar dilution Microwell dilution	0.25% (*v*/*v*) 500 µg/mL 0.025 mL/mL	[111] [112] [107]
Pseudomonas aeruginosa	Agar dilution Microwell dilution	>2.0% (*v*/*v*) >500 µg/mL	[111] [112]
Salmonella typhimurium	Agar dilution Microwell dilution	>2.0% (*v*/*v*) 125 µg/mL	[111] [112]

Table 5. *Cont.*

Bacterial Species	Method	MIC	
Serratia marcescens	Agar dilution	0.25% (*v*/*v*)	[111]
Staphylococcus aureus	Agar dilution Broth microdilution Microwell dilution	0.25% (*v*/*v*) 0.03% (*v*/*v*) 0.0125 mL/mL 31.2 µg/mL	[111] [111] [107] [112]
Streptococcus pyogenes	Broth microdilution	0.43 mg/mL 0.0125 mL/mL	[113] [107]
Streptococcus pneumoniae	Broth microdilution	0.11 mg/mL 0.00625 mL/mL	[113] [107]
Streptococcus mutans	Broth microdilution	0.04 mg/mL	[113]
Haemophilius influenzae	Broth microdilution	0.11 mg/mL 0.00625 mL/mL	[113] [107]
Haemophilius parainfluenzae	Broth microdilution	0.11 mg/mL	[113]
Moraxella catarrhalis	Broth microdilution	0.09 mg/mL	[113]
Meticillin-resistant Staphylococcus aureus (MRSA)	Tube dilution	0.4 mg/mL	[108]
Pseudomonas aeruginosa	Tube dilution	1.4 mg/mL	[108]
Bacillus cereus	Microwell dilution	15.6 µg/mL	[112]
Proteus vulgaris	Microwell dilution	31.2 µg/mL	[112]
Salmonella typhi	Microwell dilution	250 µg/mL	[112]
Streptococcus agalactiae	Broth microdilution	0.00625 mL/mL	[107]
Stenotrophomonas maltophilia	Broth microdilution	0.003125 mL/mL	[107]
Extended-spectrum beta-lactamase (ESBL)-producing *K. pneumoniae*	Broth microdilution	3.6 mg/mL	[109]
New Delhi metallo-beta-lactamase (MBL)-1-producing *K. pneumoniae*	Broth microdilution	5.4 mg/mL	[109]

Compounds

The essential oil of *T. vulgaris* consists of several compounds that could have antibiotic effects. An analysis showed that the essential oil contained about 43.3% thymol, 25.5% p-cymene, and 4.1% carvacrol [114]. Thymol in particular has been researched extensively, and possesses antibacterial activity against a large range of species, including biofilm-embedded ones [32,115]. P-cymene did not show much antibacterial activity against Gram-negative bacteria, whereas carvacrol appeared to be effective against *S. aureus*, *E. faecalis*, *E. coli*, *P. aerigunosa*, *P. vulgaris*, *K. pneumoniae*, and *Salmonella* sp. [114]. Thymol, eugenol, and cavacrol have also been shown to inhibit food borne pathogens [102].

3.7.2. Antiviral Effects

Only a few studies have reported the antiviral effects of *T. vulgaris* or *T. zygis*. Ethanolic extract of thyme (species not specified) was found to reduce the cytopathic effect caused by influenza A virus dose-dependently at non-toxic concentrations (0.03–0.33% *v*/*v*) in MDCK cells. Against rhinoviruses, no effect was observed [50]. Furthermore, a *T. vulgaris* aqueous extract was effective at inhibiting avian infectious bronchitis virus infection in Vero cells, with an EC50 value of 63.1 µg [116]. Furthermore, the essential oil of *T. vulgaris* has shown intercellular antiviral effects against influenza type A virus (H1N1) [102].

3.7.3. Immunomodulatory Effects

Only a few articles have reported the effects on the immune system. In an acute pneumonitis mouse model, inhalation of the essential oil of *T. vulgaris* (maximum concentration 6.55 μL/L) reduced inflammatory airway hyperresponsiveness and myeloperoxidase activity. This was also reflected in a reduction in histopathological changes in the lungs [117]. Furthermore, thymol has also been shown to have anti-inflammatory effects in carrageenan-induced paw oedema in rats. A dose of 200 mg/kg bodyweight of thymol reduced the oedema equally to 300 mg/kg bodyweight acetylsalicylic acid. Leukocyte migration into the peritoneal cavity was also reduced with doses of 50 mg/kg bodyweight and higher [32].

3.8. *Combinations of Ivy, Primrose, and Thyme*

Looking at studies that investigated combinations of ivy, primrose, and thyme, one study looked into the effects of film-coated tablets with a combination of thyme and primrose in a ratio of 2.67:1 (Bronchipret). It involved rats in which pulmonary inflammation was induced by LPS. When they received either 14, 68, or 339 mg/kg bodyweight per day (corresponding to 0.2, 1, and 5 times the human daily dose) orally of this combination, the infiltration of the lungs by inflammatory cells, myeloperoxidase (MPO) activity, and mucin 5A (MUC5AC) protein secretion in the lungs was significantly reduced after 48 h ($p < 0.05$). When using higher doses (68, 203, and 678 mg/kg bodyweight per day), not only MPO activity and MUC5AC secretion was reduced, but also goblet cell hyperplasia was partially prevented after 72 h. The reduction in MUC5AC secretion was confirmed in an in vitro model using human respiratory epithelium and Calu-3 cells, which were exposed to either 1 or 10 μg/mL for 14 days of this combination of thyme and primrose. Here, also mRNA levels of MUC5AC were reduced [118].

The same combination of thyme and primrose (Bronchipret, Bionorica SE, Neumarkt, Germany) was shown to inhibit arachidonate 5-lipoxygenase (LO-5) in an enzymatic assay. This inhibits the biosynthesis of leukotriene, which was confirmed in an in vivo study with rats receiving the same doses as described above. This animal study also confirmed the reduction in leukocyte infiltration of the lungs, as was found similarly in the previously discussed study [119].

Furthermore, a syrup consisting of thyme and *H. helix* in a ratio of 10:1 (Bronchipret) reversed the increase in leukocyte and goblet cell numbers in lung tissue in rats with LPS-induced broncho alveolitis. The syrup was given 1, 25, and 49 h after induction and the effects were observed with all three doses: 1.7, 5.0, and 16.7 mL/kg bodyweight. The syrup also prevented an increase in bronchoalveolar lavage fluid and blood. Furthermore, in vitro this syrup reduced the levels of leukotriene B4, cysteine leukotriene receptor, and 5-lipoxygenase with IC50 values of 36 μg/mL, 10 μg/mL, and 19 μg/mL, respectively [120].

Expert Opinion

Thyme contains essential oils that are antibacterial and could thus aid in respiratory tract infections. Other compounds in thyme, such as flavonoids and tannins, could also contribute to an antibacterial effect. Especially tannins of the rosmarinic acid type could act as spasmolytics. Primrose is very little researched, and its use is mostly based on traditional use. However, the saponins in primrose are very similar in structure to those in ivy and, therefore, it can be expected that they too can have a secretolytic effect. Both can slightly irritate the mucosa and, hence, stimulate it to dilute the mucus (Emeritus Prof. Dr. Liselotte Krenn, personal communication 2021). Saponins in primrose, furthermore, irritate the vagus nerve in the stomach. This results in a response in the entire body, including the respiratory tract, where it acts as a secretolytic. Hence, it dilutes the mucus and eases expectoration. Thyme acts as an antimicrobial in in vitro studies. However, it is not yet clear how thyme constituents end up in the respiratory tract when it is taken orally (Dr. Mathias Schmidt, personal communication 2021). Combinations with ivy, primrose, and thyme create a useful mixture that has antimicrobial and secretolytic effects (Prof. Dr. Roman Huber and Dr. Mathias Schmidt, personal communication 2021).

4. Discussion

TCIH treatments offer a unique perspective and potential opportunities for reducing the inappropriate use of antibiotics, and so to address antimicrobial resistance. This systematic literature review focusses on the underlying mechanisms of four TCIH treatments that have shown moderate- to high-quality evidence of clinical effectiveness in the treatment of URTIs: *Andrographis paniculata, Pelargonium sidoides, Echinacea* species, and the combination of ivy, primrose, and thyme [16–23]. The mechanisms were hypothesized to include not only direct antibacterial and antiviral effects, but also the immune response of the patient and the modulation of URTI symptoms such as cough and fever [13].

4.1. *Andrographis paniculata*

For *Andrographis paniculata*, the beneficial effects appear to result from a combination of antibacterial, antiviral, anti-inflammatory, and possibly antipyretic activity. Antiviral effects have been shown both in vitro and in vivo with clinically realistic doses [38,39] and are hence a likely underlying mechanism. Furthermore, there is an interesting indication from animal studies that andrographolide can reduce inflammation (measured by IL-6 and TNF-α), whilst keeping sufficient inflammatory activity to fight off an infection [35]. The clinical relevance of direct antimicrobial effects is as yet hard to assess. It was mostly investigated by agar well diffusion assays and these give only limited insight into the size of the effect [24,33]. The MICs that have been reported are all above 100 µg/mL [35] which, according to expert opinion, suggests that these effects are not clinically relevant. On the other hand, indirect antibacterial effects such as sensitisation to antibiotics and reduction in adherence to host epithelium could indicate an overall antibacterial effect [35]. Finally, antipyretic effects are shown in only one study and this study used high doses. As it is still unknown by what molecular mechanism this inhibition is caused, it is not yet possible to assess if and in which cases of URTI this effect is beneficial [13]. More research into this mechanism is, therefore, recommended [24].

4.2. *Pelargonium sidoides*

There is interesting evidence that the standardised ethanolic extract from *P. sidoides*, EPs 7630, increases the adherence of bacteria to immune cells and simultaneously decreases the adherence to host epithelial cells [48,49]. In terms of immunomodulation *P. sidoides* reduces infection-related tissue damage during infection (e.g., inflammatory damage to the lungs), hence can reduce sickness behaviour [51,52,54–56]. On the other hand, it increases antimicrobial functioning of macrophages in vitro [48,59–61,63,64,66,69]. Furthermore, *P. sidoides* also has a direct antiviral effect, possibly involving upregulation of the vitamin D receptor [50–52], and expectorant effects [54,57], and thus contributes to URTI treatment. Based on expert opinion, direct antibacterial effects are not considered as clinically relevant as MICs are above 100 µg/mL. However, the stimulation of the immune system to produce antimicrobial proteins could be an indirect antibacterial effect in practice [52,61,62]. This and the antiviral effects could reduce the duration of URTI symptoms, while the reduction in inflammatory damage and expectorant effects could help to resolve URTI symptoms such as sore throat and cough.

4.3. *Echinacea* Species

Both the literature and the experts agree that the effect of *E. purpurea* is mostly immunomodulatory. However, none of the experts was fully convinced of its efficacy, and interpreting the different findings remains difficult since both anti-inflammatory and immunostimulatory effects have been reported in the literature. Immunostimulatory measurements are hard to model in vivo. In vitro assays are vulnerable to endotoxin contamination, and are not necessarily directly translatable to a live situation. From mechanistic clinical trials, the effect in healthy volunteers appears to be mostly anti-inflammatory, though differences in immune response between healthy and immunosuppressed people indicate that the effect can change in a different immunological situation [81–84]. Different effects in people with different immunological states might explain the inconclusive and sometimes contradictory findings in clinical trials. Moreover, antiviral effects are plausible as extracellular antiviral effects against inactivated human H1N1 type IV virus start at concentrations of 1.6 μg/mL ethanolic *E. purpurea* extract [71–75]. This is especially interesting as in cell culture assays resistance did not occur, whilst it did occur with the standard drug Tamiflu [78]. There is no good evidence to suggest a clinically relevant antibacterial effect. For the other species, *E. pallida* and *E. angustifolia*, similar effects are expected, though not enough studies were retrieved to confirm this. Furthermore, the variety in species and preparation methods used means it is not possible to draw strong conclusions as it is possible that the variability in the results is caused by differences between preparations.

4.4. Ivy, Primrose, and Thyme

The effect of ivy, primrose, and thyme in the treatment of cough is explained by an additive effect of their individual effects. First, ivy can prevent internalization of β-adrenergic receptors, and thus causes a secretolytic effect [92,95–98]. The resulting bronchodilation can decrease the airway resistance and, hence, improve airflow in the lungs and reduce shortness of breath. The increased amount of surfactant dilutes the mucus and eases its expulsion. According to expert opinion, saponins in primrose might act in a similar way or might stimulate the vagus nerve to bring about a secretolytic effect, but we found no evidence in the literature for this. The added value of primrose in this mixture, and whether potential side effects would outweigh the positive effects or not, therefore, remains unsure. Finally, *T. vulgaris* acts mainly via direct antibacterial effects of the essential oil [102,106–110,121]. According to expert opinion, these effects are promising as many reported MIC values are under 100 μg/mL. There are no reported interactions between ivy, primrose, and thyme. Hence, there is no evidence that using them in a mixture should be preferred over using the three herbs separately. However, when combined each of them may contribute to a multi-targeted treatment that has bronchospasmolytic, secretolytic, and antibacterial effects.

4.5. Practical Implications

These findings give an overview of the mechanistic evidence and (possible) modes of action of effects that have been observed in clinical trials [13]. This creates a basis for clinical advice on the use of the investigated herbs in URTIs. However, before strong recommendations can be made, better defined descriptions of the treatments and their quality control are needed. Especially with *Echinacea*, there is a wide variety of products using different species of *Echinacea*, different plant parts, different extraction mediums and different extraction methods. As this results in many different products with different compositions, findings about one of these products cannot automatically be generalised to all. On the other hand, in the case of *P. sidoides* and *H. helix*, most research is performed using the standardised extracts EPs 7630 and EA 575. Consecutive studies with these extracts can be compared, which allows for a recommendation on their clinical use.

All four herbs hold great potential to aid in the reduction in the use of antibiotics. In the first place, they offer an alternative treatment option for URTI treatment [2]. Ways to ensure that new antibiotic treatments are less susceptible for developing AMR include using multi-target treatments, treatments that decrease virulence, or treatments that improve innate immunity [122]. Both *A. paniculata* and *P. sidoides* by themselves target different mechanisms, and the combination of thyme with either ivy or primrose is expected to be a multi-target treatment as well, targeting both the β-adrenergic receptor and directly targeting the bacteria. Secondly, compounds in *A. paniculata* and *T. vulgaris* may improve the effectiveness of standard antibiotics and, thus, might reduce the use of antibiotics [2]. Thirdly, *A. paniculata*, *P. sidoides* and *Echinacea* species may all reduce infection-related tissue damage, while both *P. sidoides* and *Echinacea* species are also suggested to increase the innate immune response. Therefore, all of these are promising new treatments for URTIs, especially *P. sidoides*, as it appears to be multi-targeted, decreasing infection-related tissue damage and modulating innate immunity.

4.6. Strengths and Limitations

While many studies on AMR only focus on targeting pathogens, this study also considered other possible mechanisms by which URTIs could be tackled, such as immunomodulation. Another strength of this study is that it was conducted systematically, with a transparent methodology and used many databases. Furthermore, study selection was performed independently by two authors, after which the findings were compared. Finally, findings from the literature were compared with and supplemented by interviews with different experts in this field.

However, some limitations of this study should be taken into consideration as well. The first is that, due to the varied methodology of studies of interest for the research question, setting uniform quality criteria was challenging. Due to time limitations and to avoid excessive exclusion general criteria were not established and applied in this study. Stronger conclusions might be drawn if quality standards of the tested products were introduced as inclusion criteria. Secondly, the search terms were based on several proposed mechanisms. It could be, however, that additional mechanistic pathways are involved, but were not retrieved as they were not included in the initial search terms. Furthermore, studies that were not written in English, German, or Dutch were excluded which might have left out relevant information published in articles in other languages. Finally, none of the interviewed experts had experience with *A. paniculata*. A larger panel of experts, with a broader experience, might have improved this aspect of the project.

5. Conclusions

A. paniculata probably acts mainly through immunomodulation and antiviral activity, and possibly also through antibacterial and antipyretic effects. *P. sidoides* most likely acts through antiviral, indirect antibacterial, anti-virulence, and expectorant effects, and *Echinacea* species most likely act through immunomodulation. The combination of ivy, primrose, and thyme combines secretolytic, spasmolytic, and antibacterial effects. This mechanistic evidence supports the promising data from clinical trials and opens the door to evidence-based recommendations for the use of these herbs in clinical URTI treatment. Furthermore, it offers suggestions for future research on the working mechanisms of other potential URTI TCIH treatments.

6. Future Directions

For the clinical use of the researched herbs, strong(er) quality standards should be developed to streamline research and allow for evidence-based recommendations. Published data on the effects of extracts need to be carefully checked for an authentic botanical source, the plant parts processed, and the specific production procedure.

Furthermore, since this study focussed on only two of the three pillars for evidence based medicine, (1) research evidence, (2) expert opinion, and (3) patient values [123], future research should pay more attention to the third pillar, 'patient values'. Clinical trials seem to show that the treatments are effective [13]. However, the experience of patients with the treatments, the side effects, and the costs should also be taken into account.

Since there are indications that certain effects only occur at higher doses, more research into the dose–response relationship with all treatments is needed. Furthermore, toxicity, pharmacodynamics, and potential interactions with medications or other herbs should be monitored to prevent harmful side effects, and be taken into account when making recommendations for clinical practice. Further details on the mechanisms should also be researched, such as specific working mechanisms of individual active compounds. Pharmacodynamics is especially relevant as this type of research could determine if in the in vitro studies compounds are used that actually are absorbed and end up at the researched site.

Finally, the fact that the identified mechanisms occur in the studied treatments, suggests that these mechanisms should also be researched in other TCIH URTI treatments. These include treatments involving alternative antibacterial mechanisms that target the bacteria–host interaction, such as changes in adherence or the production of antimicrobial proteins. Given the lack of evidence retrieved on the working mechanisms of *P. veris* and *P. elatior*, this kind of research is recommended for these herbs in the future.

Supplementary Materials: The following supporting information can be downloaded at: https://www.mdpi.com/article/10.3390/ph16091206/s1, Table S1: Study selection.

Author Contributions: Conceptualisation, E.W.B.; methodology, E.W.B. and L.B.M.V.; investigation, L.B.M.V., E.B.-V.Z. and E.W.B.; writing—original draft preparation, L.B.M.V.; writing—review and editing, L.B.M.V., E.B.-V.Z. and E.W.B.; supervision, E.W.B. All authors have read and agreed to the published version of the manuscript.

Funding: This research received no external funding.

Institutional Review Board Statement: Not applicable.

Informed Consent Statement: Not applicable.

Data Availability Statement: The data presented in this study are available in the Supplementary Files Table S1: Study selection.

Acknowledgments: We would like to thank Roman Huber (University Medical Center Freiburg, Germany), Mathias Schmidt (HerbResearch, Germany), and Liselotte Krenn (Emeritus) (University of Vienna, Austria) for sharing their expertise with the authors; Merlin Wilcox (University of Southampton, United Kingdom) and Florian Stintzing (University Hohenheim, Germany) for proofreading the manuscript; Toine Groen (University of Applied Sciences Leiden, The Netherlands) for his work on setting up the search terms; and Jocelijn Meijerink (Wageningen University and Research, the Netherlands) and Renger Witkamp (Wageningen University and Research, The Netherlands) for feedback and supervision during the internship project.

Conflicts of Interest: The authors declare that they have the following possible conflicts of interest. However, these conflicts of interest did not influence the design, analyses, and the reporting of this study in the current article. Liesbeth Veldman and Eefje Belt-van Zoen have no conflict of interest to declare. Erik W. Baars is a member of the European Scientific Cooperative on Anthroposophic Medicinal Products (ESCAMP), Freiburg, Germany, and a professor of anthroposophic medicine at the University of Applied Sciences Leiden, The Netherlands. In the past, he received research funding from TCIH pharmaceutical industries.

Appendix A Study Characteristics

Study	Methods	Population	Intervention	Outcomes
Perić et al. (2020) [66]	Prospective case–control study	26 patients with acute post-viral rhinosinusitis	3×/day 20 mg oral EPs 7630 tablets for 10 days	Chemokine levels in nasal secretions, nasal symptoms and endoscopic findings
Perić et al. (2021) [65]	Randomized prospective study	78 patients with uncomplicated acute bacterial rhinosinusitis	During 10 days: 26 patients received 3 × 20 mg/day EPs 7630 tablets; 26 patients received 2 × 150 mg/day roxithromysin tablets	Chemokine levels in nasal secretion and clinical parameters were compared on day 0 and day 10
Goel et al. (2005) [81]	Randomized, double-blind, placebo controlled trial	150 volunteers, aged 18–65 years, with a history of two or more infections of the common cold in the previous year	At the onset of a cold, on day 1 eight doses of 5 mL Echinilin^{TM} ('Factors R&D Technologies', Burnaby, BC, Canada) were taken, and on the 6 consecutive days three doses/day	Self-assessed severity of cold symptoms during the 7 days

Table A1. *Cont.*

Study	Methods	Population	Intervention	Outcomes
Dapas et al. (2014) [82]	Pilot study	10 healthy volunteers	10 mL Polinacea® (Indena, Milano, Italy) syrup/day during 1 month	Expression levels of IL-2, IL-8, IL-6, and TNF-α in lympho-monocytes and plasma samples
Ritchie et al. (2011) [83]	Intervention study	30 healthy volunteers	Five days of 4 × 1 mL, followed by 3 days of 10 × 1 mL Echinaforce®	Elastase, IL-1β, IL-6, IL-8, IL-10, IL-12 MCP-1, TNF-α, and IFN-γ in daily taken blood samples
Kim et al. (2002) [84]	Preliminary, randomized, double-blind, placebo-controlled trial	48 healthy female volunteers, aged 22–51 years	Daily, a combination of *E. purpurea* and *E. angustifolia* (E. purpurea whole herb extract 4% (908 mg/day), *E. purpurea* whole herb (464 mg/day) or *E. angustifolia* root (36 mg/day) during 4 weeks	Complement properdin, white blood cell count, neutrophils, lymphocytes, monocytes, quality of life assessment
Sheeja et al. (2006) [46]	Animal study	12 BALB/c mice	5 doses of 10 mg methanolic extract of *A. paniculata* for 5 days	PMA-induced superoxide and nitric oxide formation
Wang et al. (2010) [42]	Animal study	12 BALB/c mice	Intraperitoneal administration of 1 mg/kg/day andrographolide, during 7 days	Antibodies and IL-4-producing splenocytes
Mishra et al. (2013) [34]	In vitro	*E. coli, P. aeruginosa, M. tuberculosis, S. Aureus,* MRSA, and methicillin-resistant *E. faecalis*	Agar well diffusion with *A. paniculata*	MIC
Abubacker and Vasantha (2010) [36]	In vitro	*E. coli, K. pneumoniae, P. vulgaris,* and *S. pneumoniae*	Disc diffusion assay with *A. paniculata*	Inhibition zone
Rajalakshmi and Cathrine (2016) [33]	In vitro	*E. coli, S. aureus, B. subtilis*	Screening for phytochemical components of *A. paniculata* and disc diffusion assay	Inhibition zone
Xu et al. (2012) [37]	In vitro	*S. epidermidis, P. aeruginosa, B. subtilis*	Microtitre plate broth dilution with noriridoids from the roots of *A. paniculata*	MIC
Chandrasekaran et al. (2010) [44]	In vitro	J774A.1 murine macrophages	Effect of an extract of *A. paniculata* leaves on inflammatory response to LPS	Inhibition of NO, PGE_2, IL-1β, and IL-6
Chandrasekaran et al. (2011) [43]	In vitro	J774A.1 macrophages	Effect of 7 phytoconstituents (andrographolide, neoandrographolide, isoandrographolide, andrograpanin, 14-deoxy-11,12-didehydroandrographolide, 7-O-methylwogonin, and skullcapflavone-I) isolated from *A. paniculata* on inflammatory mediators	NO, PGE2, IL-1β, IL-6, LTB_4, TXB_2, and histamine
Parichatikanond et al. (2010) [45]	In vitro	Ionophore A23 187-induced human platelets	The effect of diterpenoids from *A. paniculata* on the production of inflammatory cytokines and COX activities	COX-2 activity, TNF-α, IL-6, IL-1β, and IL-10, gene expression of cytokines and cytokine receptors
Liu et al. (2007) [41]	In vitro	L-929 cells and bone-marrow-derived macrophages from BALB-c mice	The effect of andrograpanin from *A. paniculata* on overproduction of NO, pro-inflammatory cytokines, and involved pathways	NO, TNF-, IL-6, and IL-12p70

Table A1. *Cont.*

Study	Methods	Population	Intervention	Outcomes
Kumar et al. (2004) [40]	In vitro	Peripheral blood lymphocytes of healthy volunteers	Different fractions of methanolic extract of *A. paniculata* were screened for immunostimulatory effects	IL-2
Chen et al. (2009) [38]	Animal and in vitro study	BALB/c mice	Mice were infected with avian influenza A/chicken/Guang-dong/96 (H9N2) virus and A/duck/Guangdong/99 (H5N1) virus and different doses of *A. paniculata* were administered	LD50 of influenza virus in mice, lung virus titer, in vivo and in vitro antiviral evaluation, toxicity of *A. paniculata*
Conrad et al. (2007) [49]	In vitro	Human peripheral blood	The effect of EPs 7630 on the activity of human peripheral blood cells	Phagocytosis and oxidative burst
Janecki et al. (2011) [49]	In vitro	Human HEp-2 epithelial cells and group A-streptococci (GAS)	The effect of EPs 7630, the methanol and non-methanol fraction, on GAS adhesion to Hep-2 cells	Percentage of change in adhesion
Neugebauer et al. (2005) [57]	In vitro	Ciliated cell cultures of human epithelium	The effect of EPs 7630 on ciliary beat frequency	Percentage of change in ciliary beat frequency
Koch and Wohn (2007) [62]	In vitro	Human neutrophils and granulocytes	The effects of EPs 7630 in concentrations between 0.3 and 30 μg/mL after 5 h incubation on antibacterial peptide production	Antibacterial protein's neutrophil peptides 1–3 and bactericidal/permeablity-increasing protein
Kayser et al. (2001) [59]	In vitro	*Leishmania donovani*, murine macrophages	Effects of EPs 7630 in in vitro models for intracellular infection with *Leishmania* parasites, an extracellular *Leishmania* growth assay, a fibroblast-virus protection assay (IFN activity), a fibroblast-lysis assay (TNF activity) and a biochemical assay for inorganic nitric oxides (iNO) were employed	TNF release, IFN induction, NO
Thäle et al. (2008) [60]	In vitro	Bone-marrow-derived mouse macrophages, *Listeria monocytogenes*	Effects of EPs 7630 on immunomodulators	NO, IL-1, IL-12, TNF-α, CD40, CD119
Trun et al. (2006) [64]	In vitro	Non-infected and *Leishmania*-infected RAW 264.7 cells	Effect of EPs 7630 on cytokine production	Gene expression of NO synthase and IL-1, IL-12, IL-18, TNF-α, IFN-α, and IFN-γ
Kolodziej and Kinderlen (2007) [69]	In vitro	Non-infected and *Leishmania*-infected murine macrophages	Antibacterial effects of EPs 7630 and their effects on non-specific immune functions	iNOS, IFN-α, IFN-γ, TNF-α, IL-1, IL-10, IL-12, and IL-18
Nöldner and Koch (2004) [55]	Animal study	NMRI mice	Effect of oral administration of a *P. sidoides* extract (100–400 mg/kg); 1 h later sickness behaviour was induced by intraperitoneal injection of LPS (400 μg/kg)	One hour later, behavioural effects were examined in the 'light/dark box model' by monitoring exploratory activity for 3 min
Nöldner and Schötz (2007) [56]	Animal study	NMRI mice	Effect of oral administration of a EPs 7630 extract (100–400 mg/kg) and subfractions; 1 h later sickness behaviour was induced by intraperitoneal injection of LPS (400 μg/kg)	Time spent in light compartment, number of changes

Table A1. *Cont.*

Study	Methods	Population	Intervention	Outcomes
Walther et al. (2020) [50]	In vitro	MDCK and HeLa cells	Antiviral effects of *P. sidoides* against different types of rhinovirus and influenza virus	Cytotoxicity, viral plaque production, viral neuraminidase activity
Bao et al. (2015) [54]	Animal study	ICR mice SPF-class and guinea pigs	Antitussive, secretolytic, and anti-inflammatory effects of EPs 7630 were assessed in animal experiments following oral administration at human equivalent doses	Degree of tracheal and bronchial lesions, bronchosecretolytic (phenol red), concentrations of SOD and MDA in serum
Roth et al. (2019) [52]	In vitro	Human bronchial cells from patients with severe asthma (*n* = 6), moderate COPD (*n* = 6) and non-diseased controls (*n* = 6)	The effect of EPs 7630 on human bronchial cells was assessed with western blot, immunofluorescence, and polymerase chain reaction	Protein expression, cell survival
Roth et al. (2021) [53]	In vitro	Human bronchial epithelial cells	The effect of EPs 7630 on human bronchial cells was assessed with western blot and immunofluorescence	Protein expression, intracellular signalling, antiviral effect
Witte et al. (2015) [63]	In vitro	Human monocytes (PBMCs), isolated from healthy donors	The effects of EPs 7630 on human monocytes was assessed by ELISA, western blot, and flow cytometry analyses	TNF-α, IL-6, and IL-10
Witte et al. (2020) [61]	In vitro	PBMCs	The effects of EPs 7630 on antimicrobial airway defense through monocytes	IL-22, IL-17, IFN-γ, IL-1, IL-23
Vimalanathan et al. (2017) [70]	In vitro	MDCK and BEAS-2B (human) cells. Influenza virus A and *H. influenzae* and *S. aureus*	Effect of an *E. purpurea* extract (Echinaforce™) on H3N2-induced adhesion of live *H. influenzae* and *S. aureus*	Cytotoxicity, bacterial adhesion, expression of ICAM-1, fibronectin, PAFr, TLR4 and NFkB p65, IL-6 and IL-8
Fonseca et al. (2014) [80]	In vitro	Human Jurkat T-cells	Effect of different concentrations of *E. purpurea* extract (0, 10, 25, 100 and 250 μg/mL) on human T-cells was assessed	IL-2, IFN-γ, CD25 expression
Gertsch et al. (2004) [85]	In vitro	Human monocytes/macrophages	*Echinacea* alkylamides from Echinaforce™	TNF-α protein and mRNA, cAMP, p38/MAPK, and JNK signaling, as well as NF-jB and ATF-2/CREB-1
Classen et al. (2006) [86]	In vitro	Mouse spleen cell cultures and mouse macrophages	Effects of different arabinogalactan-proteins from *E. paalida* were assessed	Proliferation, IgM production, induction of IL-6 and nitrite production
Keyhanmanesch et al. (2015) [93]	Animal study	Dunkin–Hartley guinea pigs	Intraperitoneal injection of different doses of α-hederin	IL-4, IFN-γ, and IL-17 levels in blood and histopathological evaluation of lungs and trachea
Sieben et al. (2009) [97]	In vitro	Human airway smooth muscle cells (HASM)	Cells were pre-treated with α-hederin, hederacoside, and hederagenin	β2 adrenergic receptor density, intracellular cAMP
Gepdiremen et al. (2005) [99]	Animal study	Wistar albino rats	Anti-inflammatory potential of a-hederin (monodesmoside) and hederasaponin-C from *H. helix* was assessed in carrageenan-induced acute paw edema in rats	Edema rate percentage
Wolf et al. (2011) [95]	In vitro	Bovine tracheal smooth muscle strips	Effects of the three main saponins of ivy, α-hederin, hederacoside C, and hederagenin, on the contraction and relaxation behaviour of isolated bovine tracheal smooth muscle strips by isometric tension measurements	Histamine-, methacholine-, and isoprenaline-induced relaxation of precontracted muscle strips

Table A1. *Cont.*

Study	Methods	Population	Intervention	Outcomes
Hocauglu et al. (2012) [94]	Animal study	BALB/c mice	Mice were challenged with ovalbumin after which they received either a placebo, *H. helix* extract, or dexamethasone.	Goblet cell numbers, thickness of basement membrane, epithelium, and subepithelial smooth muscle layers
Saadat et al. (2015) [92]	Animal study	Dunkin–Hartley guinea pigs	Guinea pigs were sensitized with ovalbumin, after which a low (0.3 mg/kg) or high (3.0 mk/kg) dose of α-hederin was given	Tracheal response to methacholine, histamine and ovalbumin, white blood cell count
Shulte-Michels et al. (2016) [90]	In vitro	HEK293 cells	To assess the effect of *H. helix* extract on protein kinase A and G protein-coupled receptor kinases phosphorylation of β2 adrenergic receptors, an in-cell western was performed	Protein kinase A-mediated phosphorylation, G coupled receptor kinases phosphorylation
Greunke et al. (2015) [96]	In vitro	Human airway smooth muscle cells	The effect of an ivy leaf extract (EA 575) on human airway smooth muscle cells was assessed using live cell imaging, fluorescence correlation spectroscopy, and a cAMP assay	cAMP, internalization and binding of β-adrenergic receptors
Orhan et al. (2012) [88]	In vitro	*S. pneumonia, S. pyogenes, S. aureus, S. epidermidis, M. tuberculosis, K. pneumoniae, H. influenzae, P. auruginosa, A. baumannii*	Antibacterial effects of *H. helix* were assessed	DPPH inhibition, MIC
Schulte-Michels et al. (2019) [91]	In vitro	Mouse macrophages (J774.2), human embryonic kidney cells (HEK 293), acute monocytic leukemia cells (THP-1), and human lung epithelium-derived cells (A549)	Effect of EA 575 on transcriptional activity of NFkB was assessed	NFkB, IkBa and RelA, TNF-α
Schulte-Michels et al. (2016) [90]	In vitro	Murine macrophages (J774.2)	Different concentrations of EA 575 were tested for their effect on IL-6 release in macrophages	IL-6
Ünsal et al. (2010) [89]	Field study and in vitro study	*S. aureus, S. epidermidis, E. coli, K. pneumoniae*	During a three-month field study, 64 plant samples of plants that are traditionally used in common infections were collected and tested for antimicrobial activity	MIC
Acs et al. (2016) [108]	In vitro	Methicillin-resistant *Staphylococcus aureus* and the antibiotic-resistant *Pseudomonas aeruginosa*	With a tube dilution test, antimicrobial activity of thyme was assessed	MIC
Acs et al. (2018) [113]	In vitro	*S. pneumoniae, S. mutans, S. pyogenes, H. influenzae, H. parainfluenzae,* and *M. catarrhalis*	With broth microdilution test and vapor phase test, antimicrobial activity of thyme was assessed	MIC and MBC
Al-Bayati et al. (2008) [112]	In vitro	*S. aureus, B. cereus, E. coli, P. vulgaris, P. mirabilis, S. typhi, S. typhimurium, K. pneumoniae,* and *P. aeruginosa*	With microwell dilution method, the antimicrobial activity of *T. vulgaris* was assessed	MIC
Csikos et al. (2020) [117]	Animal study	C57BL/6J mice	Acute airway inflammation was induced in mice, essential oil of thyme was inhaled by one group of the animals	Airway function, hyperresponsiveness, and myeloperoxidase activity

Table A1. *Cont.*

Study	Methods	Population	Intervention	Outcomes
Dahiya and Purkayastha (2012) [101]	In vitro	MDR clinical isolates of *S. aureus* (3 isolates), *S. aureus* (MRSA), *Escherichia coli* (3 isolates), *K. pneumoniae* (2 isolates), and *P. mirabilis*	With the agar well diffusion method, the antimicrobial activity of thyme was assessed	MIC
Fabio et al. (2007) [107]	In vitro	*S. pyogenes*, *S. agalactiae*, *S. Pneumoniae*, *K. pneumoniae*, *H. influenzae*, *S. aureus*, *S. maltophilia*	With the Kirby–Bauer paper method	Cytotoxicity, MIC, and MBC
Hammer et al. (1999) [111]	In vitro	*Aer. Sobria*, *Candida albica*, *E. faecalis*, *E. coli*, *K. pneumoniae*, *P. aeruginosa*, *S. enterica*, *S. marcescens*, and *S. aureu*	With the agar dilution method and the broth dilution method, the antimicrobial activity of essential oil of *T. vulgaris* was assessed	MIC and MCC
Hoferl et al. (2009) [114]	In vitro	*S. aureus*, *E. coli*, *P. aeruginosa*, *P. vulgaris*, *K. pneumoniae*, and *S. sp.*	With agar diffusion disc method and agar dilution method, the antimicrobial activity of thyme was assessed	MIC and inhibition zone (IZ)
Inouye et al. (2001) [103]	In vitro	*H. influenzae*, *S. aureus*, *S. pneumoniae*, *E. coli*, and *S. pyogenes*	A minimum inhibitory dose was established to assess the antimicrobial activity of thyme	Minimum inhibitory dose (MID)
Iseppe et al. (2020) [104]	In vitro	*E. coli*, *K. pneumoniae*, *P. aeruginosa*	With agar diffusion disc method, the antimicrobial activity of essential oil of thyme was assessed	MIC
Javed et al. (2018) [100]	In vitro	*S. aureus*, *P. aeruginosa*, *E. coli*, *P. vulgaris*, *K. pneumoniae*	With the disk diffusion method, the antibacterial activity of *T. vulgaris* was assessed	MIC
Kwiatkowski et al. (2018) [109]	In vitro	*K. pneumoniae*	With broth microdilution method, the antimicrobial activity of essential oil of *T. vulgaris* was assessed	MIC, MBC
Lelesius et al. (2019) [116]	In vitro	Avian infectious bronchitis virus (IBV)/Vero Cells	Antiviral effects of *T. vulgaris* were assessed	Cytotoxicity, antiviral effect against IBV, and prior to infection in Vero cells
Man et al. (2016) [106]	In vitro	*S. aureus*, *E. faecalis*, *E. coli*, *K. pneumoniae*, *P. aeruginosa*	Antibacterial effects of *T. vulgaris* were assessed	MIC, MBC
Marchese et al. (2016) [32]	Review	n.a.	Antibacterial and antifungal activities of thymol are researched in the literature	Chemistry, bioavailability, safety assessment, biological activity, antibacterial, and antifungal activity
Mohamed et al. (2019) [115]	In vitro	*K. pneumoniae*	Assessment of antibacterial effects of thymol, also in combination with ampicillin with disc diffusion assay and checkerboard assay	MIC, IZ
Mohammed et al. (2018) [105]	In vitro	*K. pneumoniae*	Assessment of antibacterial effects of essential oil of thyme, also in combination with ciprofloxacin with disc diffusion assay and checkerboard assay	MIC, MBC
Seibel et al. (2015) [120]	Animal study	Wistar rats	Bronchoalveolitis was induced in rats, which were then given different doses of Bronchipret (combination of ivy/primrose/thyme)	Granulocyte infiltration, effects on leukocytes, goblet cells in bronchial tissue, and leukotriene production and 5-LO enzyme activity

Table A1. *Cont.*

Study	Methods	Population	Intervention	Outcomes
Van Vuuren et al. (2008) [121]	In vitro	*S. aureus*, *K. pnuemoniae*, *C. albicans*	Essential oil of *T. vulgaris* was assessed for antimicrobial activity, also in combination with conventional antimicrobials	MIC
Vazquez-Ucha et al. (2020) [110]	In vitro	*A. baumannii* and *K. pneumoniae*	Combined disk diffusion test and checkerboard assays were performed with the essential oil of *T. zygis* in combination with colistin	MIC
Wani et al. (2021) [102]	Review	n.a.	Literature review of antiviral potential of essential oils (including thyme)	Chemical composition, antiviral effects
Samuel and Priyadarshoni (2019) [75]	Review	n.a.	Literature review on biologic effects of *Echinacea* species	Active components, pharmacological actions, medicinal effects
Rondanelli et al. (2018) [76]	Review	n.a.	Literature review on the use of *Echinacea* in self-care for common colds	Effects on cellular immunity and adaptive immunity
Roxas and Jurenka (2007) [79]	Review	n.a.	Literature review on the use of *Echinacea* in treatment of the common cold	Incidence, signs and symptoms, potential complications, conventional treatment, alternative treatments
Barnes et al. (2005) [72]	Review	n.a.	Literature review on *E. angustifolia*, *E. pallida*, and *E. purpurea*	Chemistry, pharmacology, and clinical properties
Islam and Carter (2005) [87]	Review	n.a.	Literature review on the use of *Echinacea* in upper respiratory tract infections	Qualitative and quantitative properties, mechanism of action, clinical trials, and its effect on the immune system
Barret (2003) [73]	Review	n.a.	Literature review on the medicinal properties of *Echinacea*	Pharmacology, safety, contraindications, risk of adverse events, phytochemistry
Bash et al. (2005) [74]	Review	n.a.	Natural standard review on *E. angustifolia*, *E. pallida*, and *E. purpurea*	Toxicology, dosing, interactions, mechanism of action
Borchers et al. (2000) [77]	Review	n.a.	Literature review on *Echinacea* species	Anti-inflammatory activities, *Echinacea* species
Moyo and Van Staden (2014) [26]	Review	n.a.	Literature review on the uses and mechanism of action of *P. sidoides*	Phytochemistry, pharmacological properties, commercial potential, biotechnology application
Kolodziej et al. (2011) [67]	Review	n.a.	Literature review on the antimicrobial, antiviral, and immunomodulatory activities of *P. sidoides*	Respiratory tract related antibacterial activity, effect on mucociliary system, antiviral effects, immunomodulatory effects
Brendler et al. (2008) [68]	Review	n.a.	Literature review on pre-clinical and clinical studies of *P. sidoides*	Historical and commercial perspectives, scientific perspectives
Hossain et al. (2021) [35]	Review	n.a.	Literature review on *A. paniculata*	Phytochemistry, antimicrobial pharmacology, and clinical safety and efficacy
Jiang et al. (2021) [39]	Review	n.a.	Literature review on *A. paniculata* and andrographolide	Ethnopharmacology, phytochemicals, antiviral properties, toxicology
Kumar et al. (2021) [24]	Review	n.a.	Literature review on *A. paniculata*	Traditional uses, phytochemistry, pharmacology, and quality control

Table A1. *Cont.*

Study	Methods	Population	Intervention	Outcomes
Okhuarobo et al. (2014) [47]	Review	n.a.	Literature review on *A. paniculata*	Phytochemistry and pharmacology

Appendix B Search Terms

Appendix B.1 Search 1: Reviews on All Herbs

(Bronchiolit* OR bronchit* OR bronchopneumon* OR "Common Cold" OR Cough OR Croup OR laryngit* OR "Parainfluenza Virus" OR laryngotracheobronchit* OR nasopharyngit* OR nasosinusit* OR pharyngit* OR Pleurisy OR pneumon* OR pleuropneumon* OR Pseudocroup OR "respiratory infection*" OR "Respiratory Tract Infections" OR "Respiratory Tract Infection*" OR Rhinit* OR rhinopharyngit* OR rhinosinusit* OR rhinorrh* OR sinusit* OR Sneez* OR "blocked nose" OR "pain* throat*" OR "sore throat*" OR "strep throat" OR "Tonsillitis" OR tonsillit* OR "Scarlet Fever" OR "scarlet fever" OR tracheobronchit* OR URTI) AND ("Andrographis paniculat*" OR Chuan Xin Lian OR Creat* OR "green chiretta" OR nilavembu OR kariya* OR sanshin* OR "ch'onsimyon" OR Andrographol* OR "Pelargonium sidoides" OR "African geranium*" OR "black geranium*" OR "calvary bossia" OR "cape perlargonium" OR Umckaloab* OR Rabassamin OR zucol OR "Echinacea" OR Echinacea OR echinacoside OR "Primula" OR Primula OR "P. veris" OR "P. elatior" OR "Thymus Plant" OR Thyme OR "T. vulgaris" OR "T. zygis" OR Umckaloabo OR Ivy OR "Hedera" OR "Hedera helix" OR Primrose OR Thymus OR "cow slip") AND ("Anti-Bacterial Agent*" OR "Antibacterial agent*" OR "Anti-Infective Agent*" OR "Anti-Infective Agent*" OR "Antimicrobial agent*" OR "Anti-microbial agent*" OR "Antiviral Agent*" OR "Anti-viral Agent*" OR Resilien* OR immun* OR " antipyretic* OR febrifug* OR Bioactivity OR "mechanism of action" OR Mechanistic OR "working mechanism*") AND ("systematic review" OR meta-analysis OR review)

Appendix B.2 Search 2: Mechanistic studies on Ivy, Primrose, and Thyme

(Bronchiolit* OR bronchit* OR bronchopneumon* OR "Common Cold" OR Cough OR Croup OR laryngit* OR "Parainfluenza Virus" OR laryngotracheobronchit* OR nasopharyngit* OR nasosinusit* OR pharyngit* OR Pleurisy OR pneumon* OR pleuropneumon* OR Pseudocroup OR "respiratory infection*" OR "Respiratory Tract Infections" OR "Respiratory Tract Infection*" OR Rhinit* OR rhinopharyngit* OR rhinosinusit* OR rhinorrh* OR sinusit* OR Sneez* OR "blocked nose" OR "pain* throat*" OR "sore throat*" OR "strep throat" OR "Tonsillitis" OR tonsillit* OR "Scarlet Fever" OR "scarlet fever" OR tracheobronchit* OR URTI) AND ("Primula" OR Primula OR "P. veris" OR "P. elatior" OR "Thymus Plant" OR Thyme OR "T. vulgaris" OR "T. zygis" OR Umckaloabo OR Ivy OR "Hedera" OR "Hedera helix" OR Primrose OR Thymus OR "cow slip") AND ("Anti-Bacterial Agent*" OR "Antibacterial agent*" OR "Anti-Infective Agent*" OR "AntiInfective Agent*" OR "Antimicrobial agent*" OR "Anti-microbial agent*" OR "Antiviral Agent*" OR "Anti-viral Agent*" OR Resilien* OR immun* OR " antipyretic* OR febrifug* OR Bioactivity OR "mechanism of action" OR Mechanistic OR "working mechanism*")

Appendix B.3 Search 3: Recent Studies on Pelargonium

("Pelargonium sidoides" OR "African geranium*" OR "black geranium*" OR "calvary bossia" OR "cape perlargonium" OR Umckaloab* OR Rabassamin OR zucol OR Umckaloabo) AND ("Anti-Bacterial Agent*" OR "Antibacterial agent*" OR "Anti-Infective Agent*" OR "AntiInfective Agent*" OR "Antimicrobial agent*" OR "Anti-microbial agent*" OR "Antiviral Agent*" OR "Anti-viral Agent*" OR Resilien* OR immun* OR " antipyretic* OR febrifug* OR Bioactivity OR "mechanism of action" OR Mechanistic OR "working mechanism*") AND("pharmacological effect*" OR "therapeutic effect*" "molecular mechanism*" OR "treatment efficacy" OR "treatment outcome*" OR "outcome* assessment*" OR "therapeutic equivalen*")

References

1. Ikuta, K.S.; Swetschinski, L.; Gray, A.; Han, C.; Bisignano, C.; Rao, P.; Wool, E.; Johnson, S.C.; Fell, F.; Hackett, S.; et al. Global Burden of Bacterial Antimicrobial Resistance in 2019: A Systematic Analysis. *Lancet* **2022**, *399*, 629–655.
2. WHO. *Global Action Plan on Antimicrobial Resistance*, 1st ed.; WHO Document Production Services: Geneva, Switzerland, 2015; pp. 1–19.
3. European Centre for Disease Prevention and Control. *Antimicrobial Consumption in the EU and EEA: Annual Epidemiological Report 2019*; ECDC: Solna, Sweden, 2019; pp. 1–25.
4. Pouwels, K.B.; Dolk, F.C.K.; Smith, D.R.M.; Robotham, J.V.; Smieszek, T. Actual versus 'Ideal' Antibiotic Prescribing for Common Conditions in English Primary Care. *J. Antimicrob. Chemother.* **2018**, *73*, 19–26. [CrossRef]
5. Jain, N.; Lodha, R.; Kabra, S.K. Upper Respiratory Tract Infections. *Indian J. Pediatr.* **2001**, *68*, 1135–1138. [CrossRef]
6. Nicholson, K.G.; Kent, J.; Hammersley, V.; Cancio, E. Acute Viral Infections of Upper Respiratory Tract in Elderly People Living in the Community: Comparative, Prospective, Population Based Study of Disease Burden. *BMJ* **1997**, *315*, 1060–1064. [CrossRef]
7. Kardos, P.; Malek, F. Common Cold—An Umbrella Term for Acute Infections of Nose, Throat, Larynx and Bronchi. *Pneumologie* **2016**, *71*, 221–226. [CrossRef]
8. McDonagh, M.S.; Peterson, K.; Winthrop, K.; Cantor, A.; Lazur, B.H.; Buckley, D.I. Interventions to Reduce Inappropriate Prescribing of Antibiotics for Acute Respiratory Tract Infections: Summary and Update of a Systematic Review. *J. Int. Med. Res.* **2018**, *46*, 3337–3357. [CrossRef]
9. Baars, E.W.; Belt-Van Zoen, E.; Willcox, M.; Huber, R.; Hu, X.; van der Werf, E.T. CAM Treatments for Cough and Sore Throat as Part of an Uncomplicated Acute Respiratory Tract Infection: A Systematic Review of Prescription Rates and a Survey among European Integrative Medical Practitioners. *Eur. J. Integr. Med.* **2020**, *39*, 101194. [CrossRef]
10. van der Werf, E.T.; Duncan, L.J.; Flotow, P.; Baars, E.W. Do NHS GP Surgeries Employing GPs Additionally Trained in Integrative or Complementary Medicine have Lower Antibiotic Prescribing Rates? Retrospective Cross-Sectional Analysis of National Primary Care Prescribing Data in England in 2016. *BMJ Open* **2018**, *8*, e020488. [CrossRef]
11. Grimaldi-Bensouda, L.; Bégaud, B.; Rossignol, M.; Avouac, B.; Lert, F.; Rouillon, F.; Bénichou, J.; Massol, J.; Duru, G.; Magnier, A.; et al. Management of Upper Respiratory Tract Infections by Different Medical Practices, Including Homeopathy, and Consumption of Antibiotics in Primary Care: The EPI3 Cohort Study in France 2007–2008. *PLoS ONE* **2014**, *9*, e89990. [CrossRef]
12. Hamre, H.J.; Glockmann, A.; Schwarz, R.; Riley, D.S.; Baars, E.W.; Kiene, H.; Kienle, G.S. Antibiotic use in Children with Acute Respiratory or Ear Infections: Prospective Observational Comparison of Anthroposophic and Conventional Treatment Under Routine Primary Care Conditions. *Evid. Based Complement. Altern. Med.* **2014**, *2014*, 243801. [CrossRef]
13. Baars, E.W.; Zoen, E.B.; Breitkreuz, T.; Martin, D.; Matthes, H.; Schoen-Angerer, T.v.; Soldner, G.; Vagedes, J.; Wietmarschen, H.v.; Patijn, O.; et al. The Contribution of Complementary and Alternative Medicine to Reduce Antibiotic use: A Narrative Review of Health Concepts, Prevention, and Treatment Strategies. *Evid. Based Complement. Altern. Med.* **2019**, *2019*, 5365608. [CrossRef]
14. Dantzer, R.; Cohen, S.; Russo, S.J.; Dinan, T.G. Resilience and Immunity. *Brain Behav. Immun.* **2018**, *74*, 28–42. [CrossRef]
15. Baars, E.W.; Belt-Van Zoen, E.; Hu, X.Y.; Lai, L.; Willcox, M.; Huber, R.; Roberts, N.; Huntley, A.; van Wietmarschen, H.; van der Werf, E.T. Can Complementary and Alternative Medicine Treatment Strategies Control Symptoms of Uncomplicated Acute RTIs and Reduce Antibiotic use? A Systematic Review of Systematic Reviews Examining Observational Studies and Clinical Trials. Louis Bolk Institute, Bunnik, The Netherlands. 2023, *in preparation*.
16. Anheyer, D.; Cramer, H.; Lauche, R.; Saha, F.J.; Dobos, G. Children with Respiratory Tract Infection: Systematic Review and Meta-Analysis. *Acad. Pediatr.* **2018**, *18*, 8–19. [CrossRef]
17. Hu, X.; Wu, R.; Logue, M.; Blondel, C.; Lai, L.Y.W.; Stuart, B.; Flower, A.; Fei, Y.; Moore, M.; Shepherd, J.; et al. *Andrographis Paniculata* (Chuān Xīn Lián) for Symptomatic Relief of Acute Respiratory Tract Infections in Adults and Children: A Systematic Review and Meta-Analysis. *PLoS ONE* **2017**, *12*, e0181780. [CrossRef]
18. Agbabiaka, T.B.; Guo, R.; Ernst, E. *Pelargonium Sidoides* for Acute Bronchitis: A Systematic Review and Meta-Analysis. *Phytomedicine* **2008**, *15*, 378–385. [CrossRef]
19. Kamin, W.; Funk, P.; Seifert, G.; Zimmermann, A.; Lehmacher, W. EPs 7630 is Effective and Safe in Children under 6 Years with Acute Respiratory Tract Infections: Clinical Studies Revisited. *Curr. Med. Res. Opin.* **2018**, *34*, 475–485. [CrossRef]
20. Wagner, L.; Cramer, H.; Klose, P.; Lauche, R.; Gass, F.; Dobos, G.; Langhorst, J. Herbal Medicine for Cough: A Systematic Review and Meta-Analysis. *Complement. Med. Res.* **2015**, *22*, 359–368. [CrossRef]
21. Timmer, A.; Günther, J.; Motschall, E.; Rücker, G.; Antes, G.; Kern, W.V.; Timmer, A. *Pelargonium Sidoides* Extract for Treating Acute Respiratory Tract Infections. *Cochrane Database Syst. Rev.* **2013**, *2013*, CD006323. [CrossRef]
22. Holzinger, F.; Chenot, J. Systematic Review of Clinical Trials Assessing the Effectiveness of Ivy Leaf (*Hedera Helix*) for Acute Upper Respiratory Tract Infections. *Evid. Based Complement. Altern. Med.* **2011**, *2011*, 382789. [CrossRef]
23. Schaefer, A.; Kehr, M.S.; Giannetti, B.M.; Bulitta, M.; Staiger, C. A Randomized, Controlled, Double-Blind, Multi-Center Trial to Evaluate the Efficacy and Safety of a Liquid Containing Ivy Leaves Dry Extract (EA 575®) vs. Placebo in the Treatment of Adults with Acute Cough. *Pharmazie* **2016**, *71*, 504–509.
24. Kumar, S.; Singh, B.; Bajpai, V. *Andrographis Paniculata* (Burm.F.) Nees: Traditional Uses, Phytochemistry, Pharmacological Properties and Quality Control/Quality Assurance. *J. Ethnopharmacol.* **2021**, *275*, 114054. [CrossRef] [PubMed]
25. Subramanian, R.; Zaini Asmawi, M.; Sadikun, A. Bitter Plant with a Sweet Future? *A Comprehensive Review of an Oriental Medicinal Plant: Paniculata. Phytochem. Rev.* **2012**, *11*, 39–75.

26. Moyo, M.; Van Staden, J. Medicinal Properties and Conservation of *Pelargonium Sidoides* DC. *J. Ethnopharmacol.* **2014**, *152*, 243–255. [CrossRef] [PubMed]
27. Parsons, J.L.; Cameron, S.I.; Harris, C.S.; Smith, M.L. Echinacea Biotechnology: Advances, Commercialization and Future Considerations. *Pharm. Biol.* **2018**, *56*, 485–494. [CrossRef] [PubMed]
28. Karsch-Völk, M.; Barrett, B.; Kiefer, D.; Bauer, R.; Ardjomand-Woelkart, K.; Linde, K.; Karsch-Völk, M. Echinacea for Preventing and Treating the Common Cold. *Cochrane Database Syst. Rev.* **2014**, *2014*, CD000530. [CrossRef]
29. Lang, C.; Röttger-Lüer, P.; Staiger, C. A Valuable Option for the Treatment of Respiratory Diseases: Review on the Clinical Evidence of the Ivy Leaves Dry Extract EA 575. *Planta Med.* **2015**, *81*, 968–974. [CrossRef]
30. Colombo, P.S.; Flamini, G.; Rodondi, G.; Giuliani, C.; Santagostini, L.; Fico, G. Phytochemistry of European Primula Species. *Phytochemistry* **2017**, *143*, 132–144. [CrossRef]
31. Jaric, S.; Pavlovic, P.; Mitrovic, M. Review of Ethnobotanical, Phytochemical, and Pharmacological Study of *Thymus serpyllum* L. *Evid. Based Complement. Altern. Med.* **2015**, *2015*, 101978. [CrossRef]
32. Marchese, A.; Orhan, I.E.; Daglia, M.; Barbieri, R.; Di Lorenzo, A.; Nabavi, S.F.; Gortzi, O.; Izadi, M.; Nabavi, S.M. Antibacterial and Antifungal Activities of Thymol: A Brief Review of the Literature. *Food Chem.* **2016**, *210*, 402–414. [CrossRef]
33. Rajalakshmi, V.; Cathrine, L. Phytochemical Screening and Antimicrobial Activity of Ethanolic Extract of *Andrographis paniculata*. *J. Pharmacogn. Phytochem.* **2016**, *5*, 175–177.
34. Mishra, P.K.; Singh, R.K.; Gupta, A.; Chaturvedi, A.; Pandey, R.; Tiwari, S.P.; Mohapatra, T.M. Antibacterial Activity of *Andrographis Paniculata* (Burm. F.) Wall Ex Nees Leaves Against Clinical Pathogens. *J. Pharm. Res.* **2013**, *7*, 459–462. [CrossRef]
35. Hossain, S.; Urbi, Z.; Karuniawati, H.; Mohiuddin, R.B.; Moh Qrimida, A.; Allzrag, A.M.M.; Ming, L.C.; Pagano, E.; Capasso, R. *Andrographis Paniculata* (Burm. F.) Wall. Ex Nees: An Updated Review of Phytochemistry, Antimicrobial Pharmacology, and Clinical Safety and Efficacy. *Life* **2021**, *11*, 348. [CrossRef]
36. Abubacker, M.N.; Vasantha, S. Antibacterial Activity of Ethanolic Leaf Extract of *Andrographis Paniculata* Nees (Acanthaceae) and its Bioactive Compound Andrographolide. *Drug Invent. Today* **2010**, *2*, 440–442.
37. Xu, C.; Chou, G.; Wang, C.; Wang, Z. Rare Noriridoids from the Roots of *Andrographis paniculata*. *Phytochemistry* **2012**, *77*, 275–279. [CrossRef]
38. Chen, J.; Xue, H.; Ye, W.; Fang, B.; Liu, Y.; Yuan, S.; Yu, P.; Wang, Y. Activity of Andrographolide and its Derivatives against Influenza Virus in Vivo and in Vitro. *Biol. Pharm. Bull.* **2009**, *32*, 1385–1391. [CrossRef]
39. Jiang, M.; Sheng, F.; Zhang, Z.; Ma, X.; Gao, T.; Fu, C.; Li, P. *Andrographis Paniculata* (Burm.F.) Nees and its Major Constituent Andrographolide as Potential Antiviral Agents. *J. Ethnopharmacol.* **2021**, *272*, 113954. [CrossRef]
40. Ajaya Kumar, R.; Sridevi, K.; Vijaya Kumar, N.; Nanduri, S.; Rajagopal, S. Anticancer and Immunostimulatory Compounds from *Andrographis paniculata*. *J. Ethnopharmacol.* **2004**, *92*, 291–295. [CrossRef]
41. Liu, J.; Wang, Z.; Ge, B. Andrograpanin, Isolated from *Andrographis Paniculata*, Exhibits Anti-Inflammatory Property in Lipopolysaccharide-Induced Macrophage Cells through Down-Regulating the p38 MAPKs Signaling Pathways. *Int. Immunopharmacol.* **2008**, *8*, 951–958. [CrossRef]
42. Wang, W.; Wang, J.; Dong, S.; Liu, C.; Italiani, P.; Sun, S.; Xu, J.; Boraschi, D.; Ma, S.; Qu, D. Immunomodulatory Activity of Andrographolide on Macrophage Activation and Specific Antibody Response. *Acta Pharmacol. Sin.* **2010**, *31*, 191–201. [CrossRef]
43. Chandrasekaran, C.V.; Thiyagarajan, P.; Deepak, H.B.; Agarwal, A. In Vitro Modulation of LPS/Calcimycin Induced Inflammatory and Allergic Mediators by Pure Compounds of *Andrographis Paniculata* (King of Bitters) Extract. *Int. Immunopharmacol.* **2011**, *11*, 79–84. [CrossRef]
44. Chandrasekaran, C.V.; Gupta, A.; Agarwal, A. Effect of an Extract of *Andrographis Paniculata* Leaves on Inflammatory and Allergic Mediators in Vitro. *J. Ethnopharmacol.* **2010**, *129*, 203–207. [CrossRef]
45. Parichatikanond, W.; Suthisisang, C.; Dhepakson, P.; Herunsalee, A. Study of Anti-Inflammatory Activities of the Pure Compounds from *Andrographis Paniculata* (Burm.F.) Nees and their Effects on Gene Expression. *Int. Immunopharmacol.* **2010**, *10*, 1361–1373.
46. Sheeja, K.; Shihab, P.K.; Kuttan, G. Antioxidant and Anti-Inflammatory Activities of the Plant *Andrographis Paniculata* Nees. *Immunopharmacol. Immunotoxicol.* **2006**, *28*, 129–140. [CrossRef]
47. Okhuarobo, A.; Ehizogie Falodun, J.; Erharuyi, O.; Imieje, V.; Falodun, A.; Langer, P. Harnessing the Medicinal Properties of *Andrographis Paniculata* for Diseases and Beyond: A Review of its Phytochemistry and Pharmacology. *Asian Pac. J. Trop. Dis.* **2014**, *4*, 213–222. [CrossRef]
48. Conrad, A.; Jung, I.; Tioua, D.; Lallemand, C.; Carrapatoso, F.; Engels, I.; Daschner, F.D.; Frank, U. Extract of *Pelargonium Sidoides* (EPs ®7630) Inhibits the Interactions of Group A-Streptococci and Host Epithelia in Vitro. *Phytomedicine* **2007**, *14*, 52–59. [CrossRef]
49. Janecki, A.; Conrad, A.; Engels, I.; Frank, U.; Kolodziej, H. Evaluation of an Aqueous-Ethanolic Extract from *Pelargonium Sidoides* (EPs ®7630) for its Activity against Group A-Streptococci Adhesion to Human HEp-2 Epithelial Cells. *J. Ethnopharmacol.* **2011**, *133*, 147–152. [CrossRef]
50. Walther, C.; Döring, K.; Schmidtke, M. Comparative in Vitro Analysis of Inhibition of Rhinovirus and Influenza Virus Replication by Mucoactive Secretolytic Agents and Plant Extracts. *BMC Complement. Altern. Med.* **2020**, *20*, 380. [CrossRef]
51. Brendler, T.; Al-Harrasi, A.; Bauer, R.; Gafner, S.; Hardy, M.L.; Heinrich, M.; Hosseinzadeh, H.; Izzo, A.A.; Michaelis, M.; Nassiri-Asl, M.; et al. Botanical Drugs and Supplements Affecting the Immune Response in the Time of COVID-19: Implications for Research and Clinical Practice. *Phytother. Res.* **2021**, *35*, 3013–3031. [CrossRef]

52. Roth, M.; Fang, L.; Stolz, D.; Tamm, M. *Pelargonium Sidoides* Radix Extract EPs 7630 Reduces Rhinovirus Infection through Modulation of Viral Binding Proteins on Human Bronchial Epithelial Cells. *PLoS ONE* **2019**, *14*, e0210702. [CrossRef]
53. Roth, M.; Sun, Q.; Tamm, M. Up-Regulated Vitamin D Receptor by *Pelargonium Sidoides* Extract EPs®7630 Contributes to Rhinovirus Defense in Bronchial Epithelial Cells. *Pharmaceuticals* **2021**, *14*, 172. [CrossRef]
54. Bao, Y.; Gao, Y.; Koch, E.; Pan, X.; Jin, Y.; Cui, X. Evaluation of Pharmacodynamic Activities of EPs®7630, a Special Extract from Roots of Pelargonium Sidoides, in Animals Models of Cough, Secretolytic Activity and Acute Bronchitis. *Phytomedicine* **2015**, *22*, 504–509. [CrossRef] [PubMed]
55. Nöldner, M.; Koch, E. Inhibition of Endotoxin-induced Sickness Behaviour in Mice by an Extract from Roots of *Pelargonium Sidoides* (Umckaloabo). *Focus Altern. Complement. Ther.* **2004**, *9*, 20. [CrossRef]
56. Noldner, M.; Schotz, K. Inhibition of Lipopolysaccharid-Induced Sickness Behavior by a Dry Extract from the Roots of *Pelargonium Sidoides* (EPs ®7630) in Mice. *Phytomedicine* **2007**, *14*, 27–31. [CrossRef]
57. Neugebauer, P.; Mickenhagen, A.; Siefer, O.; Walger, M. A New Approach to Pharmacological Effects on Ciliary Beat Frequency in Cell Cultures—Exemplary Measurements under *Pelargonium Sidoides* Extract (EPs 7630). *Phytomedicine* **2005**, *12*, 46–51. [CrossRef] [PubMed]
58. Conrad, A.; Hansmann, C.; Engels, I.; Daschner, F.D.; Frank, U. Extract of *Pelargonium Sidoides* (EPs ®7630) Improves Phagocytosis, Oxidative Burst, and Intracellular Killing of Human Peripheral Blood Phagocytes in Vitro. *Phytomedicine* **2007**, *14*, 46–51. [CrossRef] [PubMed]
59. Kayser, O.; Kolodziej, H.; Kiderlen, A.F. Immunomodulatory Principles of Pelargonium Sidoides. *Phytother. Res.* **2001**, *15*, 122–126. [CrossRef] [PubMed]
60. Thale, C.; Kiderlen, A.; Kolodziej, H. Anti-Infective Mode of Action of EPs 7630 at the Molecular Level. *Planta Med.* **2008**, *74*, 675–681. [CrossRef]
61. Witte, K.; Koch, E.; Volk, H.; Wolk, K.; Sabat, R. The Herbal Extract EPs®7630 Increases the Antimicrobial Airway Defense through Monocyte-Dependent Induction of IL-22 in T Cells. *J. Mol. Med.* **2020**, *98*, 1493–1503. [CrossRef]
62. Koch, E.; Wohn, C. *Pelargonium Sidoides* Root Extract EPs®7630 Stimulates Release of Antimicrobial Peptides from Neutrophil Granulocytes in Human Whole Blood. *Planta Med.* **2007**, *73*, P_072. [CrossRef]
63. Witte, K.; Koch, E.; Volk, H.; Wolk, K.; Sabat, R. The *Pelargonium Sidoides* Extract EPs 7630 Drives the Innate Immune Defense by Activating Selected MAP Kinase Pathways in Human Monocytes. *PLoS ONE* **2015**, *10*, e0138075. [CrossRef]
64. Trun, W.; Kiderlen, A.F.; Kolodziej, H. Nitric Oxide Synthase and Cytokines Gene Expression Analyses in Leishmania-Infected RAW 264.7 Cells Treated with an Extract of *Pelargonium Sidoides* (Eps ®7630). *Phytomedicine* **2006**, *13*, 570–575. [CrossRef] [PubMed]
65. Perić, A.; Vezmar Kovačević, S.; Barać, A.; Perić, A.V.; Vojvodić, D. Effects of *Pelargonium Sidoides* Extract vs. Roxithromycin on Chemokine Levels in Nasal Secretions of Patients with Uncomplicated Acute Rhinosinusitis. *Laryngoscope Investig. Otolaryngol.* **2021**, *6*, 25–33. [CrossRef] [PubMed]
66. Perić, A.; Vezmar Kovačević, S.; Barać, A.; Gaćeša, D.; Perić, A.V.; Vojvodić, D. Effects of *Pelargonium Sidoides* Extract on Chemokine Levels in Nasal Secretions of Patients with Non-Purulent Acute Rhinosinusitis. *J. Drug Assess.* **2020**, *9*, 145–150. [CrossRef] [PubMed]
67. Kolodziej, H. Antimicrobial, Antiviral and Immunomodulatory Activity Studies of *Pelargonium Sidoides* (EPs®7630) in the Context of Health Promotion. *Pharmaceuticals* **2011**, *4*, 1295–1314. [CrossRef]
68. Brendler, T.; van Wyk, B.E. A Historical, Scientific and Commercial Perspective on the Medicinal use of *Pelargonium Sidoides* (Geraniaceae). *J. Ethnopharmacol.* **2008**, *119*, 420–433. [CrossRef]
69. Kolodziej, H.; Kiderlen, A.F. In Vitro Evaluation of Antibacterial and Immunomodulatory Activities of Pelargonium Reniforme, *Pelargonium Sidoides* and the Related Herbal Drug Preparation EPs ®7630. *Phytomedicine* **2007**, *14*, 18–26. [CrossRef]
70. Vimalanathan, S.; Schoop, R.; Suter, A.; Hudson, J. Prevention of Influenza Virus Induced Bacterial Superinfection by Standardized *Echinacea Purpurea*, via Regulation of Surface Receptor Expression in Human Bronchial Epithelial Cells. *Virus Res.* **2017**, *233*, 51–59. [CrossRef]
71. Hudson, J.; Vimalanathan, S. Echinacea—A Source of Potent Antivirals for Respiratory Virus Infections. *Pharmaceuticals* **2011**, *4*, 1019–1031. [CrossRef]
72. Barnes, J.; Anderson, L.A.; Gibbons, S.; Phillipson, J.D. Echinacea Species (*Echinacea Angustifolia* (DC.) Hell., *Echinacea Pallida* (Nutt.) Nutt., *Echinacea Purpurea* (L.) Moench): A Review of their Chemistry, Pharmacology and Clinical Properties. *J. Pharm. Pharmacol.* **2005**, *57*, 929–954. [CrossRef]
73. Barrett, B. Medicinal Properties of Echinacea: A Critical Review. *Phytomedicine* **2003**, *10*, 66–86. [CrossRef]
74. Basch, E.; Ulbricht, C.; Basch, S.; Dalton, S.; Ernst, E.; Foppa, I.; Szapary, P.; Tiffany, N.; Orlando, C.W.; Vora, M. An Evidence-Based Systematic Review of Echinacea (*E. Angustifolia* DC, *E. Pallida*, *E. Purpurea*) by the Natural Standard Research Collaboration. *J. Herb. Pharmacother.* **2005**, *5*, 57–88. [CrossRef] [PubMed]
75. Samuel, D.S.; Priyadarshoni, S.P. *Echinacea Purpurea*—A Potent Medicinal Herb. *Drug Invent. Today* **2019**, *11*, 448–452.
76. Rondanelli, M.; Miccono, A.; Lamburghini, S.; Avanzato, I.; Riva, A.; Allegrini, P.; Faliva, M.A.; Peroni, G.; Nichetti, M.; Perna, S. Self-Care for Common Colds: The Pivotal Role of Vitamin D, Vitamin C, Zinc, and Echinacea in Three Main Immune Interactive Clusters (Physical Barriers, Innate and Adaptive Immunity) Involved during an Episode of Common Colds—Practical Advice on

Dosages and on the Time to Take these Nutrients/Botanicals in Order to Prevent or Treat Common Colds. *Evid. Based Complement. Altern. Med.* **2018**, *2018*, 5813095.
77. Borchers, A.T.; Keen, C.L.; Stern, J.S.; Gershwin, M.E. Inflammation and Native American Medicine: The Role of Botanicals1,2,3. *Am. J. Clin. Nutr.* **2000**, *72*, 339–347. [CrossRef]
78. Pleschka, S.; Stein, M.; Schoop, R.; Hudson, J.B. Anti-Viral Properties and Mode of Action of Standardized *Echinacea Purpurea* Extract against Highly Pathogenic Avian Influenza Virus (H5N1, H7N7) and Swine-Origin H1N1 (S-OIV). *Virol. J.* **2009**, *6*, 197. [CrossRef]
79. Roxas, M.; Jurenka, J. Colds and influenza: A review of diagnosis and conventional, botanical, and nutritional considerations. *Altern. Med. Rev. J. Clin. Ther.* **2007**, *12*, 25–48.
80. Fonseca, F.N.; Papanicolaou, G.; Lin, H.; Lau, C.B.S.; Kennelly, E.J.; Cassileth, B.R.; Cunningham-Rundles, S. *Echinacea Purpurea* (L.) Moench Modulates Human T-Cell Cytokine Response. *Int. Immunopharmacol.* **2014**, *19*, 94–102. [CrossRef]
81. Goel, V.; Lovlin, R.; Chang, C.; Slama, J.V.; Barton, R.; Gahler, R.; Bauer, R.; Goonewardene, L.; Basu, T.K. Proprietary Extract from the Echinacea Plant (*Echinacea Purpurea*) Enhances Systemic Immune Response during a Common Cold. *Phytother. Res.* **2005**, *19*, 689–694. [CrossRef]
82. Dapas, B.; Dall'Acqua, S.; Bulla, R.; Agostinis, C.; Perissutti, B.; Invernizzi, S.; Grassi, G.; Voinovich, D. Immunomodulation Mediated by a Herbal Syrup Containing a Standardized Echinacea Root Extract: A Pilot Study in Healthy Human Subjects on Cytokine Gene Expression. *Phytomedicine* **2014**, *21*, 1406–1410. [CrossRef]
83. Ritchie, M.R.; Gertsch, J.; Klein, P.; Schoop, R. Effects of Echinaforce®Treatment on Ex Vivo-Stimulated Blood Cells. *Phytomedicine* **2011**, *18*, 826–831. [CrossRef]
84. Kim, L.S.; Waters, R.F.; Burkholder, P.M. Immunological Activity of Larch Arabinogalactan and Echinacea: A Preliminary, Randomized, Double-Blind, Placebo-Controlled Trial. *Altern. Med. Rev.* **2002**, *7*, 138–149.
85. Gertsch, J.; Schoop, R.; Kuenzle, U.; Suter, A. Echinacea Alkylamides Modulate TNF-A Gene Expression via Cannabinoid Receptor CB2 and Multiple Signal Transduction Pathways. *FEBS Lett.* **2004**, *577*, 563–569. [CrossRef] [PubMed]
86. Classen, B.; Thude, S.; Blaschek, W.; Wack, M.; Bodinet, C. Immunomodulatory Effects of Arabinogalactan-Proteins from Baptisia and Echinacea. *Phytomedicine* **2006**, *13*, 688–694. [CrossRef] [PubMed]
87. Islam, J.; Carter, R. Use of Echinacea in Upper Respiratory Tract Infection. *South. Med. J.* **2005**, *98*, 311–318. [CrossRef] [PubMed]
88. Orhan, D.D.; Özçelik, B.; Hoşbaş, S.; Vural, M. Assessment of Antioxidant, Antibacterial, Antimycobacterial, and Antifungal Activities of some Plants used as Folk Remedies in Turkey against Dermatophytes and Yeast-Like Fungi. *Turk. J. Biol.* **2012**, *36*, 672–686. [CrossRef]
89. Ünsal, C.; Vural, H.; Sariyar, G.; Özbek, B.; Ötük, G. Traditional Medicine in Bilecik Province (Turkey) and Antimicrobial Activities of Selected Species. *Turk. J. Pharm. Sci.* **2010**, *7*, 139–150.
90. Schulte-Michels, J.; Runkel, F.; Gokorsch, S.; Häberlein, H. Ivy Leaves Dry Extract EA 575®Decreases LPS-Induced IL-6 Release from Murine Macrophages. *Pharmazie* **2016**, *71*, 158–161.
91. Schulte-Michels, J.; Keksel, C.; Häberlein, H.; Franken, S. Anti-Inflammatory Effects of Ivy Leaves Dry Extract: Influence on Transcriptional Activity of NFκB. *Inflammopharmacology* **2019**, *27*, 339–347. [CrossRef]
92. Saadat, S.; Mohammadi, M.; Fallahi, M.; Keyhanmanesh, R.; Aslani, M.R. The Protective Effect of A-Hederin, the Active Constituent of *Nigella Sativa*, on Tracheal Responsiveness and Lung Inflammation in Ovalbumin-Sensitized Guinea Pigs. *J. Physiol. Sci.* **2015**, *65*, 285–292. [CrossRef]
93. Keyhanmanesh, R.; Saadat, S.; Mohammadi, M.; Shahbazfar, A.; Fallahi, M. Protective Effect of α-Hederin, the Active Constituent of *Nigella Sativa*, on Lung Inflammation and Blood Cytokines in Ovalbumin Sensitized Guinea Pigs. *Phytother. Res.* **2015**, *29*, 1761–1767. [CrossRef]
94. Hocaoglu, A.B.; Karaman, O.; Erge, D.O.; Erbil, G.; Yilmaz, O.; Kivcak, B.; Bagriyanik, H.A.; Uzuner, N. Effect of *Hedera Helix* on Lung Histopathology in Chronic Asthma. *Iran. J. Allergy Asthma Immunol.* **2012**, *11*, 316–323. [PubMed]
95. Wolf, A.; Gosens, R.; Meurs, H.; Häberlein, H. Pre-Treatment with A-Hederin Increases B-Adrenoceptor Mediated Relaxation of Airway Smooth Muscle. *Phytomedicine* **2011**, *18*, 214–218. [CrossRef] [PubMed]
96. Greunke, C.; Hage-Hülsmann, A.; Sorkalla, T.; Keksel, N.; Häberlein, F.; Häberlein, H. A Systematic Study on the Influence of the Main Ingredients of an Ivy Leaves Dry Extract on the B2 -Adrenergic Responsiveness of Human Airway Smooth Muscle Cells. *Pulm. Pharmacol. Ther.* **2015**, *31*, 92–98. [CrossRef]
97. Sieben, A.; Prenner, L.; Sorkalla, T.; Wolf, A.; Jakobs, D.; Runkel, F.; Häberlein, H. A-Hederin, but Not Hederacoside C and Hederagenin from *Hedera Helix*, Affects the Binding Behavior, Dynamics, and Regulation of B 2-Adrenergic Receptors. *Biochemistry* **2009**, *48*, 3477–3482. [CrossRef]
98. Runkel, F.; Prenner, L.; Häberlein, H. Ein Beitrag Zum Wirkmechanismus Von Efeu. *Pharm. Ztg.* **2005**, *150*, 19–25.
99. Gepdiremen, A.; Mshvildadze, V.; Süleyman, H.; Elias, R. Acute Anti-Inflammatory Activity of Four Saponins Isolated from Ivy: Alpha-Hederin, Hederasaponin-C, Hederacolchiside-E and Hederacolchiside-F in Carrageenan-Induced Rat Paw Edema. *Phytomedicine* **2005**, *12*, 440–444. [CrossRef]
100. Javed, H.; Tabassum, S.; Erum, S.; Murtaza, I.; Muhammad, A.; Amin, F.; Nisar, M.F. Screening and Characterization of Selected Drugs having Antibacterial Potential. *Pak. J. Pharm. Sci.* **2018**, *31*, 933–939.
101. Dahiya, P.; Purkayastha, S. Phytochemical Screening and Antimicrobial Activity of some Medicinal Plants against Multi-Drug Resistant Bacteria from Clinical Isolates. *Indian J. Pharm. Sci.* **2012**, *74*, 443–450.

102. Wani, A.R.; Yadav, K.; Khursheed, A.; Rather, M.A. An Updated and Comprehensive Review of the Antiviral Potential of Essential Oils and their Chemical Constituents with Special Focus on their Mechanism of Action against various Influenza and Coronaviruses. *Microb. Pathog.* **2021**, *152*, 104620. [CrossRef]
103. Inouye, S.; Yamaguchi, H.; Takizawa, T. Screening of the antibacterial effects of a variety of essential oils on respiratory tract pathogens, using a modified dilution assay method. *J Infect Chemother* **2001**, *7*, 251–254. [CrossRef]
104. Iseppi, R.; Di Cerbo, A.; Aloisi, P.; Manelli, M.; Pellesi, V.; Provenzano, C.; Camellini, S.; Messi, P.; Sabia, C. In Vitro Activity of Essential Oils Against Planktonic and Biofilm Cells of Extended-Spectrum β-Lactamase (ESBL)/Carbapenamase-Producing Gram-Negative Bacteria Involved in Human Nosocomial Infections. *Antibiotics* **2020**, *9*, 272. [CrossRef] [PubMed]
105. Mohamed, S.H.; Mohamed, M.S.M.; Khalil, M.S.; Azmy, M.; Mabrouk, M.I. Combination of essential oil and ciprofloxacin to inhibit/eradicate biofilms in multidrug-resistant Klebsiella pneumoniae. *J. Appl. Microbiol.* **2018**, *125*, 84–95. [CrossRef] [PubMed]
106. Man, A.; Santacroce, L.; Jacob, R.; Mare, A.; Man, L. Antimicrobial Activity of Six Essential Oils against a Group of Human Pathogens: A Comparative Study. *Pathogens* **2019**, *8*, 15. [CrossRef] [PubMed]
107. Fabio, A.; Cermelli, C.; Fabio, G.; Nicoletti, P.; Quaglio, P. Screening of the Antibacterial Effects of a Variety of Essential Oils on Microorganisms Responsible for Respiratory Infections. *Phytother. Res.* **2007**, *21*, 374–377. [CrossRef]
108. Ács, K.; Bencsik, T.; Böszörményi, A.; Kocsis, B.; Horváth, G. Essential Oils and their Vapors as Potential Antibacterial Agents Against Respiratory Tract Pathogens. *Nat. Prod. Commun.* **2016**, *11*, 1709–1712. [CrossRef]
109. Kwiatkowski, P.; Pruss, A.; Grygorcewicz, B.; Wojciuk, B.; Dołęgowska, B.; Giedrys-Kalemba, S.; Kochan, E.; Sienkiewicz, M. Preliminary Study on the Antibacterial Activity of Essential Oils Alone and in Combination with Gentamicin Against Extended-Spectrum Β-Lactamase-Producing and New Delhi Metallo-Β-Lactamase-1-Producing Klebsiella Pneumoniae Isolates. *Microb. Drug Resist.* **2018**, *24*, 1368–1375. [CrossRef]
110. Vázquez-Ucha, J.C.; Martínez-Guitián, M.; Lasarte-Monterrubio, C.; Conde-Pérez, K.; Arca-Suárez, J.; Álvarez-Fraga, L.; Pérez, A.; Crecente-Campo, J.; Alonso, M.J.; Bou, G.; et al. *Syzygium Aromaticum* (Clove) and *Thymus Zygis* (Thyme) Essential Oils Increase Susceptibility to Colistin in the Nosocomial Pathogens *Acinetobacter Baumannii* and *Klebsiella pneumoniae*. *Biomed. Pharmacother.* **2020**, *130*, 110606. [CrossRef]
111. Hammer, K.A.; Carson, C.F.; Riley, T.V. Antimicrobial Activity of Essential Oils and Other Plant Extracts. *J. Appl. Microbiol.* **1999**, *86*, 985–990. [CrossRef]
112. Al-Bayati, F.A. Synergistic Antibacterial Activity between *Thymus Vulgaris* and *Pimpinella Anisum* Essential Oils and Methanol Extracts. *J. Ethnopharmacol.* **2008**, *116*, 403–406. [CrossRef]
113. Ács, K.; Balázs, V.L.; Kocsis, B.; Bencsik, T.; Böszörményi, A.; Horváth, G. Antibacterial Activity Evaluation of Selected Essential Oils in Liquid and Vapor Phase on Respiratory Tract Pathogens. *BMC Complement. Altern. Med.* **2018**, *18*, 227. [CrossRef]
114. Hoferl, M.; Buchbauer, G.; Jirovetz, L.; Schmidt, E.; Stoyanova, A.; Denkova, Z.; Slavchev, A.; Geissler, M. Correlation of Antimicrobial Activities of various Essential Oils and their Main Aromatic Volatile Constituents. *J. Essent. Oil Res.* **2009**, *21*, 459–463. [CrossRef]
115. Mohamed, S.H.; Khalil, M.S.; Azmy, M. In vitro Efficiency of Ampicillin, Thymol and Their Combinations against Virulence Strains of Klebsiella pneumoniae August 2019. *Int. J. Pharm. Sci.* **2019**, *11*, 315–321. [CrossRef]
116. Lelešius, R.; Karpovaitė, A.; Mickienė, R.; Drevinskas, T.; Tiso, N.; Ragažinskienė, O.; Kubilienė, L.; Maruška, A.; Šalomskas, A. In Vitro Antiviral Activity of Fifteen Plant Extracts against Avian Infectious Bronchitis Virus. *BMC Vet. Res.* **2019**, *15*, 178. [CrossRef] [PubMed]
117. Csikós, E.; Csekő, K.; Ashraf, A.R.; Kemény, Á.; Kereskai, L.; Kocsis, B.; Böszörményi, A.; Helyes, Z.; Horváth, G. Effects of *Thymus Vulgaris*, L., *Cinnamomum Verum*, J.Presl and *Cymbopogon Nardus* (L.) Rendle Essential Oils in the Endotoxin-Induced Acute Airway Inflammation Mouse Model. *Molecules* **2020**, *25*, 3553. [CrossRef]
118. Seibel, J.; Kryshen, K.; Pongrácz, J.E.; Lehner, M.D. In Vivo and in Vitro Investigation of Anti-Inflammatory and Mucus-Regulatory Activities of a Fixed Combination of Thyme and Primula Extracts. *Pulm. Pharmacol. Ther.* **2018**, *51*, 10–17. [CrossRef]
119. Seibel, J.; Wonnemann, M.; Werz, O.; Lehner, M.D. A Tiered Approach to Investigate the Mechanism of Anti-Inflammatory Activity of an Herbal Medicinal Product Containing a Fixed Combination of Thyme Herb and Primula Root Extracts. *Clin. Phytosci.* **2018**, *4*, 4. [CrossRef]
120. Seibel, J.; Pergola, C.; Werz, O.; Kryshen, K.; Wosikowski, K.; Lehner, M.D.; Haunschild, J. Bronchipret®Syrup Containing Thyme and Ivy Extracts Suppresses Bronchoalveolar Inflammation and Goblet Cell Hyperplasia in Experimental Bronchoalveolitis. *Phytomedicine* **2015**, *22*, 1172–1177. [CrossRef]
121. van Vuuren, S.F.; Suliman, S.; Viljoen, A.M. Antimicrobial Activity of Four Commercial Essential Oils in Combination with Conventional Antimicrobials. *Lett. Appl. Microbiol.* **2009**, *48*, 440–446. [CrossRef]
122. Oldfield, E.; Feng, X. Resistance-Resistant Antibiotics. *Trends Pharmacol. Sci.* **2014**, *35*, 664–674. [CrossRef]
123. Sackett, D.L. *Evidence Based Medicine*, 2nd ed.; Churchill Livingstone: Edinburgh, UK, 2000.

pharmaceuticals

MDPI

Review

Mitigation of Insulin Resistance by Natural Products from a New Class of Molecules, Membrane-Active Immunomodulators

Elzbieta Izbicka * and Robert T. Streeper

New Frontier Labs LLC, San Antonio, TX 78240, USA
* Correspondence: eizbicka.g4@gmail.com

Abstract: Insulin resistance (IR), accompanied by an impaired cellular glucose uptake, characterizes diverse pathologies that include, but are not limited to, metabolic disease, prediabetes and type 2 diabetes. Chronic inflammation associated with deranged cellular signaling is thought to contribute to IR. The key molecular players in IR are plasma membrane proteins, including the insulin receptor and glucose transporter 4. Certain natural products, such as lipids, phenols, terpenes, antibiotics and alkaloids have beneficial effects on IR, yet their mode of action remains obscured. We hypothesized that these products belong to a novel class of bioactive molecules that we have named membrane-active immunomodulators (MAIMs). A representative MAIM, the naturally occurring medium chain fatty acid ester diethyl azelate (DEA), has been shown to increase the fluidity of cell plasma membranes with subsequent downstream effects on cellular signaling. DEA has also been shown to improve markers of IR, including blood glucose, insulin and lipid levels, in humans. The literature supports the notion that DEA and other natural MAIMs share similar mechanisms of action in improving IR. These findings shed a new light on the mechanism of IR mitigation using natural products, and may facilitate the discovery of other compounds with similar activities.

Keywords: insulin resistance; type 2 diabetes; natural product; membrane-active immunomodulator; diethyl azelate; drug discovery; drug development

Citation: Izbicka, E.; Streeper, R.T. Mitigation of Insulin Resistance by Natural Products from a New Class of Molecules, Membrane-Active Immunomodulators. *Pharmaceuticals* **2023**, *16*, 913. https://doi.org/10.3390/ph16070913

Academic Editors: Elena Y. Enioutina, Kathleen M. Job and Catherine Sherwin

Received: 10 April 2023
Revised: 14 June 2023
Accepted: 15 June 2023
Published: 21 June 2023

1. Introduction

Insulin resistance (IR) is clinically defined as the inability of a known quantity of exogenous or endogenous insulin to increase glucose uptake and its utilization in an individual as much as it does in a normal population [1]. IR is associated with conditions beyond prediabetes and type 2 diabetes (T2D), including cardiovascular and metabolic pathologies, collectively referred to as a metabolic syndrome, nonalcoholic fatty liver disease, as well as atherosclerosis, hypertension, polycystic ovarian syndrome and infectious diseases with sepsis sequelae [2–8]. The cause of IR is poorly understood, but the major contributors are thought to comprise systemic chronic inflammation [9] associated with abnormal lipid levels, oxidative and endoplasmic reticulum stress, insulin receptor mutations and mitochondrial dysfunctions [10].

The plasma membrane plays an essential role in cellular communication, as its structure and composition affect cellular signal transduction in health and disease [11]. We hypothesized that certain small lipophilic or amphiphilic molecules, which we have named membrane-active immunomodulators (MAIMs), affect cellular communications by modulating plasma membrane fluidity in a feedback-regulated mechanism that we refer to as adaptive membrane fluidity modulation (AMFM) [12,13].

Thanks to their membrane-fluidizing properties, MAIMs can indirectly impact the structures and functions of membrane proteins, such as receptors and ion channels. MAIMs can also directly interact with plasma membrane proteins [12,13]. In some cases, MAIMs display a nonlinear or inversed U-shaped dose response effect, which suggests their role in the maintenance of an optimal plasma membrane fluidity [13,14].

A natural product can be defined as a small molecule produced by a biological source [15]. In adherence to this definition, we have focused on single-chemical entities that were examined in pure forms or identified as active moieties in various extracts, mixtures or decoctions.

Natural products have been extensively exploited in drug development [16,17]. Some natural products comprising lipids, phenols, terpenes, antibiotics, alkaloids and gut microbiome metabolites were reported to mitigate IR, but their mode of action remains obscured. We have sought to understand how such diverse compounds can elicit comparable IR benefits. Upon the examination of the physicochemical properties of individual molecules, we realized that the mitigation of IR could be due to the "MAIM-ness" of superficially unrelated compounds.

The aim of this review is to highlight how natural products in the MAIMs family might alleviate IR through direct or indirect interactions with plasma membrane proteins. Two key players in the pathology of IR are of special interest, because their functions are affected by fluctuations in membrane fluidity [18–21]: the insulin receptor, an integral plasma membrane protein, and glucose transporter type 4 (GLUT4), which resides in insulin-responsive vesicles inside cells and shuttles between the membrane and cytoplasm [22]. Other membrane proteins, including potassium and calcium channels [23,24], ectopically expressed olfactory receptors and other G-protein-coupled receptors, implicated as players in IR [25–27] are also susceptible to the effects of naturally derived MAIMs.

2. Methods

A PUBMED search was conducted to identify peer-reviewed research articles, re-views and meta-analyses published through February 2023. The search terms included "plasma membrane" and "fluidity" or "plasticity" or "rigidity". Secondary searches combined keywords consisting of individual chemical entities listed below and "insulin resistance" or "insulin sensitivity", and specific pathologies, including metabolic syndrome or metabolic diseases, atherosclerosis, hypertension, polycystic ovarian syndrome, prediabetes and T2D. The collected abstracts and full papers were surveyed by the authors to confirm the relevance of the article to the topic of this review. The chemical structures were obtained from PubChem's database (https://pubchem.ncbi.nlm.nih.gov); URL accessed on 5 June 2023.

3. Results

The literature reports discussed below describe the IR-modulating effects of natural products that were selected based on their MAIM features, such as being typically lipophilic or amphiphilic small molecules, combined with reported effects of these natural products on plasma membrane fluidity, interactions with plasma membrane proteins and the modulation of biomarkers relevant for IR, as demonstrated preclinically and also preferably in the clinic. Given that MAIMs lack a single target, the structure–function relationship (SAR) used as a standard in the development of targeted drugs was not applicable here.

The representative compounds were grouped into classes of lipids, phenols, terpenes, antibiotics and alkaloids. We also added a section on gut metabolites comprising some lipids produced by gut microbiota as secondary metabolites, which, nevertheless, stood out as a separate group because of their local and systemic role within the human body.

The compounds that met the criteria of reported effects on IR mitigation and MAIM features are referenced in the text as links to the PubChem database. We presented examples of functional similarities in the regulation of IR between the lead MAIM, diethyl azelate (DEA), and other natural MAIMs.

3.1. Lipids

Lipids are hydrophobic or amphiphilic small molecules, including fatty acids and their derivatives, in particular esters, sterols, steroids and phospholipids.

Azelaic acid (AZA) [28] and the best characterized azelate, diethyl azelate DEA [29], (Figure 1A) are both MAIMs. Yet, as can be expected from the large differences in respective water–octanol partitioning coefficients, the respective interactions of AZA and DEA with plasma membrane are quite different [30]. DEA is a membrane fluidizer that interacts with the plasma membrane and membrane proteins, while AZA, due to its lower lipophilicity, has limited membrane interactions [12,30].

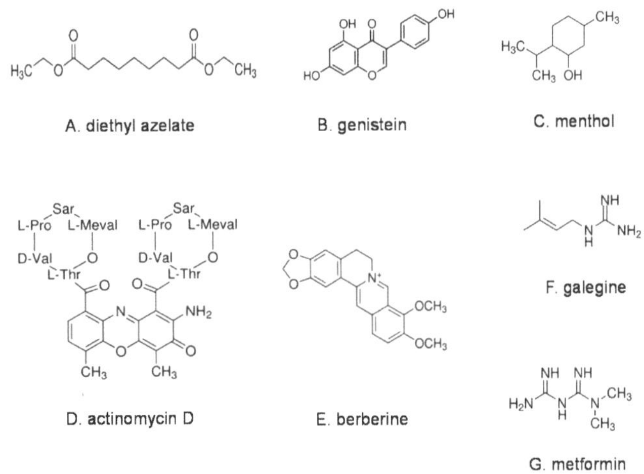

Figure 1. Representative natural products in the families of lipids (**A**), phenols (**B**), terpenes (**C**), antibiotics (**D**) and alkaloids (**E–G**).

AZA and azelates occur naturally in plants, animals and humans. Archaeological records provide evidence that even ancient humans consumed AZA and its esters in the form of grains, olives, soybeans, fermented foods and alcoholic beverages [12,13,30]. Endogenous AZA produced from longer chain carboxylic acids, mainly oleic acid, is present at micromolar levels in human cerebrospinal fluid, saliva and also in breast milk [30]. The levels of AZA and azelates in the body appear to increase in response to environmental insults [31] and fasting [32].

AZA and its esters act as immunomodulators in multicellular organisms. AZA primes plant systemic immunity after infection [33]. AZA modulates the innate immune responses in human skin and induces the expression of peroxisome proliferator-activated receptor gamma (PPARγ), a key regulator of inflammation, activated by fatty acids and products of lipid peroxidation [34]. DEA and related azelates exert immunomodulatory actions in vitro and in vivo [12]. DEA is a metabolic precursor of AZA, and is rapidly converted into AZA under physiological conditions [30].

Although DEA and AZA are pharmacologically distinct entities, they share some common effects in the mitigation of IR, albeit at quite different doses. Oral AZA administered to diabetic mice at 80 mg/kg over 11–15 weeks improved glucose tolerance and decreased plasma triglycerides, glucose and cholesterol plaque formation in the arteries [35]. In a human study in overweight adult males, daily oral DEA at 1 mg/kg over 3 weeks significantly reduced fasting glucose and insulin in subjects with IR and/or hemoglobin A1c (A1c) $\geq$ 5.6%, and improved diagnostic lipid ratios in all cases. The impact of DEA on biomarkers of disease correlated with the degree of IR [36]. These findings are in line with the physicochemical differences between AZA and DEA. Notably, sebacic acid [37], a C10 dicarboxylic acid, purportedly has some hypoglycemic effects [38], albeit at doses nearly 100 times higher than those achieved with DEA in humans [36].

Some effects of DEA and AZA on IR may be mediated by mitochondria. Mitochondrial dysfunction has been found to be associated with obesity-induced IR and T2D [39], while the enrichment of mitochondria in skeletal muscle was reported to lower the risk of T2D [40].

AZA was reported to bind to a murine olfactory receptor Olfr544 [41]. Olfactory receptors are G-protein-coupled plasma membrane receptors that constitute over 5% of the mammalian genome. Olfr544 is widely expressed in nonolfactory murine tissues, such as the small intestine, colon, adipose tissue, liver and skeletal muscle [32]. The activation of Olfr544 with AZA stimulated mitochondrial biogenesis in mouse skeletal muscle [25,42]. In vivo treatment with AZA increased insulin sensitivity and ketone body levels [32] and upregulated genes involved in insulin signal transduction [43]. It was proposed that AZA is a fasting signaling molecule that can activate Olfr544 in various tissues [32]. In the pancreas, AZA upregulated glucagon secretion through pancreatic islets [41]. In the gut, AZA's activation of Olfr544 increased the secretion of an insulinotropic hormone glucagon-like peptide-1 (GLP-1) [26]. Since IR and T2D are associated with the impaired postprandial secretion of GLP-1 [44,45], the endogenous activity of AZA might be beneficial in these conditions. The putative human analogue of murine Olfr544 is encoded by the OR52K1 gene, but its function, like that of many other ectopically expressed olfactory receptors, is presently unknown.

Phospholipids are the main components of cell plasma membranes, and are also canonical MAIMs. Human studies have demonstrated the association between IR and the levels of the two most abundant phospholipids, phosphatidylcholine (PC) [46] and phosphatidylethanolamine (PE) [47,48]. Interestingly, the PC/PE ratio in skeletal muscle has been found to be elevated in T2D [49]. Abnormally high or low PC/PE ratios (and even small alterations thereof) influence the mitochondrial energy metabolism and have been linked to IR and metabolic syndrome [50,51]. A U-shaped dose response of phospholipids in the control of IR was reminiscent of the dose responsiveness of some MAIMs [13].

Other lipid MAIMs, such as n-3 and n-6 polyunsaturated fatty acids (PUFAs), represented by α-linoleic acid [52] and linoleic acid [53], respectively, affect membrane fluidity upon incorporation into phospholipids [54] or as free fatty acids. The dietary n-3 PUFA counteracted IR by modulating mitochondrial bioenergetics and decreasing endoplasmic reticulum stress [55]. Higher adipose tissue levels of α-linoleic acid have been inversely associated with IR in healthy adults [56]. Rats fed a high-fat diet enriched in n-3 and n-6 PUFAs developed hyperglycemia and hyperinsulinemia, consistent with IR. The expression of insulin receptors was significantly reduced in the liver, but not in the muscle, and the n-3 PUFA diet maintained normal GLUT-4 levels in the muscle [57]. Isomers of linoleic acids activated nuclear factor kappa-B (NFκB), elevated interleukin-6 (IL-6) and induced IR in human adipocytes [58].

Cholesterol [59] is the most common steroid in human physiology and a classical lipid MAIM. Cholesterol organizes and rigidifies plasma membranes [60] where cholesterol-enriched lipid rafts regulate protein diffusion and distribution [61]. An association between IR, increased cholesterol synthesis and decreased cholesterol absorption was reported in normoglycemic men [62] and subjects with metabolic syndrome [63]. Insulin sensitivity affected the cholesterol metabolism to a greater extent than obesity [64].

Cholesterol is a precursor of primary bile salts produced by the liver. The regulation of bile acid levels is linked to the lipid and glucose metabolism. Increased plasma levels of α-hydroxylated bile acids were found to be associated with IR [65], while bile acid sequestrants reduced glucose and cholesterol levels in T2D [66,67].

As a footnote, we wanted to mention natural statins, which are not classical lipids, but inhibitors of 3-hydroxy-3-methylglutaryl coenzyme A (HMG-CoA) reductase, a key enzyme in cholesterol biosynthesis. Statins reduce systemic cholesterol with a subsequent increase in membrane fluidity. Statins are "secondary MAIMs", which we defined as compounds that do not directly interact with the plasma membrane, but that affect the membrane composition. A natural statin, lovastatin [68], a secondary metabolite produced by fungi, was shown to modulate IR [69], presumably due to the increased signaling through the insulin receptor pathway [70].

3.2. Phenols

Natural phenolic compounds produced in plants are present in many foods consumed by humans [71]. Natural phenols can be viewed as MAIMs [13]. Due to their lipophilicity and usually low molecular masses, phenols can rapidly diffuse in and out of membranes and exert physiological effects promptly after absorption.

The large family of over 8000 phenolic compounds includes flavonoids and nonflavonoids. The simple nonflavonoid phenol salicylic acid [72] was recognized for the control of hyperglycemia for over a century. This activity was linked to mitochondrial uncoupling, anti-inflammatory effects mediated via NF-κB signaling and the regulation of AMP-activated protein kinase (AMPK) [73], which was reported to enhance insulin effects on GLUT4 by lowering cholesterol in plasma membranes [20]. Since salicylate is soluble in the plasma membrane [74], its aspirin-like effect [13] may explain the activity of salicylate in the control of IR. Another simple nonflavonoid, caffeic acid [75], also appears to have antihyperglycemic, hypolipidemic and hypotensive activity in vitro and in vivo [76].

Flavonoids are the most abundant polyphenols. Some flavonoids were reported to mitigate IR by affecting glucose transport and blood levels, improving insulin signaling and the function of pancreatic β-cells [77,78].

A simple flavonoid trans-chalcone [79] was shown to reduce body weight, blood glucose and insulin in healthy rats, suggesting its insulin-sensitizing activity in vivo, but the effects under IR conditions are still unknown [78].

Quercetin [80], the most abundant flavonoid in the human diet, is especially high in red onions, apples, grapes, tomatoes and dark berries. Quercetin has been shown to stimulate AMPK, increase GLUT4 translocation and protein content in skeletal muscle [81] and decrease the stiffness of plasma membranes in vitro [82].

Epigallocatechin gallate (EGCG) [83] is the most abundant catechin in green tea. EGCG decreases IR as it activates the PI3K/Akt pathway, increases GLUT4 translocation through the enhanced phosphorylation of AMPK [84] and decreases oxidative stress in vivo [85]. EGCG has showed a U-shaped dose dependence in human hepatocytes; sub-micromolar levels decreased glucose production and 5 μM of EGCG significantly increased glucose uptake, while 10 μM EGCG was toxic [86].

Luteolin [87] was reported to intercalate and disrupt bacterial cytosolic membranes [88] and significantly increase the expression of adiponectin, leptin and PPARγ in murine adipocytes in vitro [89]. Luteolin reduced obesity-associated IR in mice by activating AMPKα1 signaling in adipose tissue macrophages [90], and was suggested to modulate IR in humans [91].

Resveratrol [92] apparently targets the entire cell plasma membrane in vitro [93]. In animal and human studies, resveratrol improved markers of IR by normalizing blood glucose, reducing insulin secretion and improving insulin sensitivity. Resveratrol was also effective in managing IR-related dyslipidemia and obesity [94].

Curcumin [95] was shown to fluidize plasma membranes and decrease membrane rigidity, but also stiffened model membranes with a high cholesterol content [96,97]. Curcumin modulated the function and expression of unrelated membrane proteins in vitro [98]. In a randomized double-blind, placebo-controlled trial, daily doses of 1500 mg curcumin significantly reduced fasting blood glucose and body weight in patients with T2D [99].

Myricetin [100] present in fruits and vegetables increased membrane fluidity and reduced mitochondria dysfunction by raising mitochondrial membrane potential in vitro [101]. Myricetin also improved insulin sensitivity by restoring insulin receptors, GLUT4 expression and translocation in the muscle of rats fed a high-fructose diet [102].

Isoflavonoid fisetin [103] activated AMPK in vitro [104] and mitigated IR in vivo by blocking the inflammatory response to a high-fat diet [105].

Genistein [106] (Figure 1B), the isoflavone present at high levels in soybeans, has been recognized for its estrogenic activity. Genistein potentiated hepatic insulin signaling in rodents [107] and showed opposite effects in normal and IR mice, decreasing insulin sensitivity in the former but improving the insulin sensitivity and elevated GLUT4 translocation in the group of IR mice [108].

Human studies have yielded somewhat conflicting data on genistein. A meta-analysis of 10 randomized clinical trials involving 794 non-Asian perimenopausal or postmenopausal women showed that daily supplementation with 40 mg to 120 mg of soy isoflavones was ineffective, but comparable doses of genistein alone lowered fasting blood glucose by increasing glucose uptake in skeletal muscle [109]. Another meta-analysis of 24 clinical trials conducted in 1518 men and women who were overweight, obese or diagnosed with T2D found no significant effect of soy intake on fasting glucose and insulin levels [110].

Kaempferol [111] increased lipid organization in model membranes and facilitated the penetration of water molecules, an effect inhibited by cholesterol [112]. In vivo, kaempferol improved blood lipids and insulin levels in a dose-dependent manner, inhibited the phosphorylation of insulin receptor substrate-1 (IRS-1) and reduced the nucleic and cytosolic levels of NF-κB, tumor necrosis factor-α (TNF-α) and IL-6 levels in diabetic rats [113].

Overall, preclinical and clinical data suggest that dietary flavonoids may be beneficial for the management of IR, as they induce glucose uptake in skeletal muscle. They were also shown to decrease the production of hepatic glucose through the activation of the PI3K/Akt pathway, leading to GLUT4 translocation, the suppression of gluconeogenesis and the stimulation of glycogen production [78]. These examples underscore the MAIM effects of flavonoids.

3.3. *Terpenes*

Terpenes are a large class of over 30,000 natural compounds containing variable numbers of the isoprene unit $(C5H8)_n$. Terpenes are mostly produced by plants, especially conifers and citrus trees. A distilled pine resin product, commonly used as a solvent under the name of terpentine/turpentine oil, containing a mixture of terpenes, has been recognized for its medicinal benefits for over two millennia [114].

The monoterpenes 1,8-cineole, also known as eucalyptol [115] and L-menthol [116] (Figure 1C) reportedly increased the fluidity of the outermost skin layer [117,118], acted as structural spacers in model membranes and promoted reorganization in cell membranes [119]. The chronic administration of menthol (50 and 100 mg/kg/day for 12 weeks) to mice on a high-fat diet prevented weight gain, IR, the hypertrophy of adipose tissue and the deposition of triacylglycerol in the liver. The metabolic effects of menthol in the liver and adipose tissue mirrored those of glucagon [120].

Terpenes, including limonene [121], a-terpineol [122] and 1,8-cineole, were shown to rapidly incorporate into the plasma membrane of a protozoan parasite *Leishmania amazonensis* [123]. The antidiabetic potential of multiple monoterpenes was linked to an increase in insulin sensitivity and the lowering of blood glucose and insulin levels [124].

Some triterpenes, including ursolic acid [125] and pachymic acid [126] exhibited antidiabetic and antihyperglycemic activities in preclinical studies [127]. Pachymic acid inducted the gene expression and translocation of GLUT4, the stimulation of glucose uptake and the accumulation of triglycerides in vitro [128].

A triterpene glycoside saponin [129] increased GLUT4 translocation, insulin secretion and glucose uptake in murine and human cell lines [130]. In vivo, various triterpenes increased insulin biosynthesis, secretion and signaling, decreased the levels of total cholesterol and triglycerides and lowered the body weight [127]. Terpenes from a marine algae upregulated the PPARγ gene and protein expression in the livers of diabetic rats with improved insulin sensitivity and carbohydrate metabolism [131].

D-limonene reportedly decreased blood glucose levels [132] and displayed antiatherogenic and hypolipidemic activities in rats [133]. A sesquiterpene α-cedrene [134] from cedarwood oil significantly increased the translocation of GLUT4 and increased glucose uptake in human hepatocytes in vitro, and improved glucose intolerance induced by a high-fat diet in vivo through the activation of the murine olfactory receptor Olfr16 [135]. A similar effect of α-cedrene in mice with IR was ascribed to the interaction of α-cedrene with the murine olfactory receptor 23 (Mor23) [136]. These reports suggest the possible involvement of odorant receptors in the control of IR.

Tetraterpene carotenoids exemplified by α-and β-carotene [137] are ubiquitous pigments present in photosynthetic bacteria, fungi, plants and animals. Carotenoids could modify membrane fluidity and membrane order in bacterial cells, in which carotenoid biosynthesis is integral to adaptation to cold [138]. Dietary carotenoids apparently reduce the risk of several chronic diseases, including IR, but do not prevent cardiovascular disease or cancer [139]. However, obesity and IR were shown to be inversely associated with the levels of carotenoids in serum and adipose tissue in adults, suggesting possible health benefits of dietary carotenoids [140].

3.4. Antibiotics

Antibiotics are broadly defined as compounds that can treat and prevent bacterial infections [141]. The classification of two major groups of antibiotics, polyketides and nonribosomal peptides, was based on their mechanism of action related to bacterial functions or growth processes.

Some broad-spectrum polyketide antibiotics, such as streptomycin [142], ampicillin [143] and vancomycin [144] were shown to worsen IR and alter gut microbiota, increasing susceptibility to metabolic syndrome and T2D [145,146]. Likewise, a monotherapy with rapamycin (also known as sirolimus) [147] exacerbated hyperglycemia, hypertriglyceridemia and the degranulation of pancreatic islets in a mouse model of T2D. Surprisingly, rapamycin combined with metformin (further discussed in Section 3.5) reversed the negative effects of rapamycin on systemic insulin sensitivity [148].

Polyketide tetracyclines from *Streptomyces* bacteria [149] can cross the plasma membrane, and their activity has been shown to be related to the transmembrane flux in human cells [150]. Tetracycline doxycycline [151] showed an unusual dose response activity in mice on a high-fat diet. Doxycycline increased their body weight at 200 μg/mL, decreased the fasting blood glucose at 20 μg/mL and increased the neogenesis of pancreatic β-cells at 2 μg/mL [152]. In a clinical case study, doxycycline induced hypoglycemia with implications for the management of IR [153].

A nonribosomal peptide actinomycin D [154] has been recognized for its antibacterial and anticancer activities ascribed to its drug–DNA interactions [155], but its interactions with cell membranes and the consequences thereof are less known. The uptake of ^{3}H-actinomycin D by human cell lines in vitro was shown to vary with cell types, reflecting permeability differences in cell membranes [156]. In fungal cells, antibiotics damage the plasma membrane and induce membrane folding, cell swelling and the leakage of cellular contents [157]. In a rat feeding study, actinomycin D given before refeeding blocked the return of normal glucose-stimulated insulin secretion, despite an adequate food intake [158].

More importantly, actinomycin D (Figure 1D) has been shown to stimulate GLUT4 translocation and glucose uptake in murine adipocytes without the involvement of conventional signaling proteins and with no effect on GLUT4 endocytosis, suggesting that this antibiotic may increase the exocytosis of insulin-responsive vesicles in a process linked to the biosynthesis of RNA and protein [22].

3.5. Alkaloids

Alkaloids, broadly defined as natural products that contain at least one nitrogen atom, are produced by bacteria, fungi, plants and animals. The benefits of some alkaloids in the control of IR and diabetes have been attributed to the modulation of insulin signaling pathways, an improvement in the function of pancreatic β-cells and a reduction in oxidative stress and inflammation. Although most data came from preclinical studies, alkaloids are being pursued in the clinic as potential new drugs [159,160].

Emetine [161], an alkaloid present in the ipecac root, is commonly used as an expectorant, emetic and an antiparasitic treatment. Emetine inhibits ribosomal and mitochondrial protein synthesis and interferes with viral entry through host membranes [162,163].

Like actinomycin D, emetine stimulates GLUT4 translocation and glucose uptake in adipocytes [22]. The alkaloid catharanthine [164] and related alkaloids from Madagascar periwinkle (*Catharanthus roseus*) are used not only for cancer but also T2D treatments because of their antihyperlipidemic and antidiabetic effects in vivo [160].

Berberine [165] (Figure 1E), a quinoline alkaloid present in the root and bark of the berberis plant *Berberis vulgaris*, is one of the most promising alkaloids for the control of IR [166]. Berberine was shown to increase plasma membrane fluidity in rabbit erythrocytes in a dose-dependent manner. The effects of berberine on membrane proteins may explain its cardiovascular benefits [167,168].

Preclinical and clinical reports suggest the favorable activity of berberine in the treatment of T2D, obesity, hyperlipidemia, nonalcoholic fatty liver disease and gout. Berberine was shown to inhibit lipogenesis and improve insulin secretion, IR and gut microbiota disorders [169]. An insight on berberine's mechanism of action came from the identification of a key role of the voltage-dependent K+ channel KCNH6 in the control of insulin secretion [170]. The blockade of KCNH6 channels with berberine increased insulin secretion, but only under hyperglycemic conditions, suggesting that berberine is a glucose-dependent insulin secretagogue that does not cause hypoglycemia or affects basal insulin secretion [25].

Plant-derived biguanide alkaloids are represented by galegine [171] (Figure 1F), first isolated from French lilac (*Galega officinalis*) in the 1920s following centuries of use of lilac products in folk medicine. Galegine induced weight loss and lowered blood sugar in vivo [172], but further development was overshadowed by its synthetic derivative, metformin [173] (Figure 1G). Metformin is the first-line medication for treating T2D (especially in overweight individuals), polycystic ovary syndrome, gestational diabetes and other conditions including cancer and is on the World Health Organization's List of Essential Medicines [174–179].

Metformin's diverse mechanisms of action are rather puzzling [180,181]. Metformin was shown to reduce hepatic glucose production, but also to play an unspecified role in the gut, exerting different effects when administered in acute versus chronic treatments, working in an AMP-dependent or AMP-independent manner and affecting mitochondrial function [180–183].

Metformin increased the membrane fluidity of human erythrocytes taken from subjects with T1D treated with the drug. When the erythrocytes isolated from these subjects were later incubated with metformin in vitro, the metformin had no further membrane-fluidizing effect, suggesting that the optimum fluidity was already attained in the body [184]. Metformin mitigated IR in rat adipocytes in vivo by enhancing the insulin-induced translocation of glucose transporters to the plasma membrane [185]. Membrane physiology has been proposed to play an unspecified role in the effects of metformin in IR and T2D [186]. Despite structural differences, metformin and berberine share similarities in the control of metabolic syndrome and T2D that may be related to common targets in the mitochondrial respiratory chain [174].

3.6. Gut Microbiome Metabolites: The Second Lives of Some Natural Products

The human gut hosts the largest number and species of bacteria compared to other human organs [187]. The Human Microbiome project revealed astronomical numbers (over 10^{13}) of resident gut bacteria [188], which may not be commensal, but are otherwise engaged in mutually beneficial relationships. The gut microbiome and its interactions with the human body constitute a feedback loop with an impact on obesity, metabolic diseases, IR and a multitude of other conditions [189,190].

The bacterial fermentation of dietary fiber consisting of complex polysaccharides generates short-chain fatty acids (SCFAs), including acetate [191], propionate [192] and butyrate [193], which are absorbed by the host [194]. As small amphiphilic molecules, SCFAs can interact with cell plasma membranes through simple diffusion [195,196] or through active transport [197,198] due to the proton-linked monocarboxylate transporters present in the human intestinal epithelium [199].

Gut SCFAs are more than substrates for energy production, as they promote the proliferation and differentiation of the intestinal epithelium and improve the pancreatic secretion of insulin and glucagon [200]. A prospective study of 2166 participants revealed that a higher microbiome diversity was associated with fewer cases of IR, and the subjects with T2D had a lower microbiome diversity than the healthy controls, suggesting the link between the diversity and composition of the gut microbiome and the pathogenesis of T2D [201].

Secondary bile acids, including taurocholic [202], glycocholic [203], taurochenodeoxycholic [204] and glycochenodeoxycholic [205] acids, are derived from the bacterial metabolism of primary bile acids in the colon, and are viewed as potentially detrimental products [206].

4. Discussion

The above examples of natural products (Table 1) support the hypothesis that certain natural MAIMs can modulate IR and related pathologies. A few lipids, phenols, terpenes, antibiotics and alkaloids whose chemical structures were shown in this paper are either already used as drugs or are candidates for further development as drugs or medicinal foods/nutraceuticals for the control of IR. However, the conventional SAR analysis would likely not be capable of identifying a common denominator for such dissimilar compounds without accounting for their MAIM properties.

Table 1. Examples of natural membrane-active immunomodulators (MAIMs) implicated in the mitigation of insulin resistance (IR).

Class	Example	Effects Relevant to IR Mitigation	Comments	Reference
Lipids	azelaic acid diethyl azelate sebacic acid phosphatidylcholine phosphatidylethanolamine a-linolenic acid linoleic acid cholesterol lovastatin	regulation of genes in insulin signal transduction plasma membrane fluidizer, immunomodulator GLUT4 upregulation mitochondrial energy metabolism mitochondrial energy metabolism mitochondrial energy metabolism mitochondrial energy metabolism unknown direct association reduction in systemic cholesterol level	metabolite of diethyl azelate canonical MAIM, membrane fluidizer in vitro effect canonical MAIM canonical MAIM tissue-dependent effects promotion of IR in human adipocytes canonical MAIM, membrane rigidifier statin; secondary metabolite	[12,13,28,30–32] [12,13,29–36] [37,38] [47,49–51] [47–49,51] [50–52] [53,54,56–58] [59,67] [68–70]

Table 1. *Cont.*

Class	Example	Effects Relevant to IR Mitigation	Comments	Reference
Phenols	salicylic acid	mitochondrial uncoupling	aspirin-like membrane effect	[13,20,72–74]
	caffeic acid	AMPK stimulation	antiobesogenic effect via gut	[75,76]
	trans-chalcone	indirect via lowering blood glucose and insulin	effective in healthy rats	[78,79]
	quercetin	AMPK stimulation	unclear antidiabetic potential	[80–82]
	epigallocatechin gallate	AMPK stimulation	U-shaped dose effect in vitro	[83–86]
	luteolin	AMPK stimulation	potentially effective in humans	[87–91]
	resveratrol	indirect via lowering blood glucose and insulin	potentially effective in humans	[92–94]
	curcumin	improvement in b-cell function	potentially effective in humans	[95–99]
	myricetin	insulin receptor and GLUT4 expression control	in vivo data	[100–102]
	fisetin	AMPK stimulation	anti-inflammatory in vivo	[103–105]
	genistein	elevated GLUT4 translocation	human data	[106–110]
	kaempferol	regulation of insulin signaling	in vivo data	[111–113]
Terpenes	1,8-cineole	unknown direct association	preclinical data	[115,119,123]
	L-menthol	glucagon-like effects in liver	preclinical data	[116,119,120]
	D-limonene	protection against DNA damage glycation	preclinical data	[121,132,133]
	α-terpineol	inhibition of a-amylase	in vitro data	[122,123]
	ursolic acid	GLUT4 translocation	preclinical data	[125,127]
	pachymic acid	GLUT4 translocation	preclinical data	[126,128]
	saponin	GLUT4 translocation	in vitro data	[129,130]
	α-cedrene	GLUT4 translocation	preclinical data	[134,136]
	β-carotene	regulation of lipogenesis	preclinical and human data	[137–140]
Antibiotics	streptomycin	alteration of gut microbiota	worsened IR	[142,145,146]
	ampicillin	alteration of gut microbiota	worsened IR	[143,145,146]
	vancomycin	alteration of gut microbiota	worsened IR	[144–146]
	rapamycin	increased hyperglycemia	improved IR with metformin in vivo	[147,148]
	doxycycline	induced hypoglycemia	dose-dependent in vivo	[151–153]
	actinomycin D	GLUT4 translocation	in vitro data	[154–158]
Alkaloids	emetine	GLUT4 translocation in type 1 diabetes model	preclinical data	[160–163]
	catharanthine	suppression of hyperlipidemia	in vivo data	[160,164]
	berberine	glucose-dependent insulin secretagogue	preclinical and human data	[165–170]
	galegine	increased weight loss, decreased blood glucose	less potent than metformin	[171,172]
	metformin	suppressed hepatic glucose production	synthetic analog of galegine	[173–186]
Gut microbiome metabolites	acetic acid	better pancreatic secretion of insulin, glucagon	marker of microbiome diversity	[191,194–199]
	propionic acid	better pancreatic secretion of insulin, glucagon	marker of microbiome diversity	[192,194–199]
	butyric acid	better pancreatic secretion of insulin, glucagon	marker of microbiome diversity	[193–199]
	taurocholic acid	cholesterol catabolite	potentially detrimental	[202,206]
	glycocholic acid	cholesterol catabolite	potentially detrimental	[203,206]
	taurochenodeoxycholic acid	cholesterol catabolite	potentially detrimental	[204,206]
	glycochenodeoxycholic acid	cholesterol catabolite	potentially detrimental	[205,206]

Taken together, historical data on the effects of natural MAIMs from in vitro and in vivo studies, anecdotal reports on human efficacy and actual clinical findings are often provocative and introduce the possibility of developing some natural MAIMs as novel modalities for the control of IR. Nevertheless, these efforts may face challenges common in the development of natural products for therapeutic applications. For example, the levels of active principles (e.g., phenols) may vary depending on the geographical location of the plant, time of harvest, processing and even time of the day [207]. Crude extracts may contain other bioactive compounds that could affect the measured endpoints because of interactions with the intended test article. So called "impurities" may be pharmacologically active or have antagonistic effects in experiments, leading to false-positive or negative results.

Even if purified and better characterized natural MAIMs and normalized quantities were to be used in assay systems, head-to-head comparisons may be difficult because of nonlinear dose responses [208] or schedule-dependent effects [178].

Another problem arises from the assay systems used to generate the data on health benefits of natural MAIMs. For in vitro assays, primary cells are difficult to standardize, while cell lines can behave differently in various testing laboratories, especially if used past the optimum number of passages [209]. In consequence encouraging preclinical efficacy of some products could not be replicated in controlled human studies [79,210].

Limited SAR preclinical–clinical correlations can be illustrated using examples of monoterpenes and flavonoids. Antidiabetic effects of monoterpenes have been ascribed to multiple pharmacological and molecular mechanisms of action, but their SARs are largely unknown [124]. In cell-free tests of flavonoids for AMPK activation, genistein was >70% less active than fisetin [104]. However, unlike fisetin [211], genistein had shown promising activity in the clinic [109]. In general, flavonoids often demonstrate impressive preclinical activities, but their clinical efficacy is limited by poor bioavailability [212].

Last, but not least, the effects of natural MAIMs may differ in healthy subjects and those with IR. For example, berberine did not alter insulin secretion under low or normal glucose conditions, but was effective in subjects with hyperglycemia [24]. Metformin reduced the incidence of T2D with the greatest benefit in the subset of subjects with higher baseline fasting glucose or A1c [213]. DEA significantly reduced fasting glucose and insulin in subjects with IR and/or A1c $\geq$5.6%, suggesting the correlation in DEA efficacy with the degree of IR [36].

Many natural products are MAIMs, and most are "good MAIMs" that provide health benefits, as evidenced by human use for many centuries. Natural "good MAIMs" are consumed across the world in the form of traditional Chinese medicine, Mediterranean diet and fermented foods. In contrast, relatively fewer cases of natural "bad MAIMs" are represented by oils produced by microbes, plants, animals [214] and certain gut metabolites [206].

Most "bad MAIMs" are synthetic chemicals. Notorious halogenated compounds, such as perfluoroalkyl compounds (PFASs), can readily incorporate into membranes but cannot be rapidly eliminated by the body [12,30]. Another "bad MAIM", the endocrine disruptor 2,3,7,8-tetrachlorodibenzo-p-dioxin (TCDD) [215], alters plasma membrane function [216] and contributes to IR [217]. The induction of azelates through TCCD in humans [31] can be viewed as a chemoprotective response of the body taking advantage of the immunomodulatory role of azelates. Bisphenols are another family of " bad MAIMs" that are of toxicological concern [218], underscored by a link between exposure to bisphenol A [219] and the elevated risk of gestational diabetes [220].

5. Conclusions

Certain natural MAIMs share similar characteristics in improving IR. The membrane-fluidizing potential of a natural product may be a useful criterion to consider in the development of novel functional foods or drugs for the mitigation of IR.

6. Patents

Some of the data on DEA pertaining to the control of IR and T2D presented in this manuscript are covered by US and worldwide patents. Representative examples of 46 patents granted to date include:

- Robert T Streeper and Elzbieta Izbicka "Azelaic acid esters in the control of insulin resistance". US Patent No. 10251857. Application granted 4 September 2019.
- Robert T Streeper and Elzbieta Izbicka "Azelaic acid esters in the control of insulin resistance". US Patent No. 11026912. Application granted 6 August 2021.

Author Contributions: Both authors (E.I. and R.T.S.) contributed equally to the conceptualization, methodology, resources and writing. All authors have read and agreed to the published version of the manuscript.

Funding: This research was entirely funded by New Frontier Labs, LLC.

Institutional Review Board Statement: Not applicable.

Informed Consent Statement: Not applicable.

Data Availability Statement: Data sharing not applicable.

Conflicts of Interest: E.I. and R.T.S. are the owners and officers of New Frontier Labs, LLC.

References

1. Lebovitz, H.E. Insulin resistance: Definition and consequences. *Exp. Clin. Endocrinol. Diabetes* **2001**, *109* (Suppl. S2), S135–S148. [CrossRef]
2. Kouzi, S.A.; Yang, S.; Nuzum, D.S.; Dirks-Naylor, A.J. Natural supplements for improving insulin sensitivity and glucose uptake in skeletal muscle. *Front. Biosci.* **2015**, *7*, 94–106. [CrossRef]
3. Bugianesi, E.; Moscatiello, S.; Ciaravella, M.F.; Marchesini, G. Insulin resistance in nonalcoholic fatty liver disease. *Curr. Pharm. Des.* **2010**, *16*, 1941–1951. [CrossRef] [PubMed]
4. Affinati, A.H.; Wallia, A.; Gianchandani, R.Y. Severe hyperglycemia and insulin resistance in patients with SARS-CoV-2 infection: A report of two cases. *Clin. Diabetes Endocrinol.* **2021**, *7*, 8. [CrossRef]
5. Acquah, S.; Boampong, J.N.; Eghan Jnr, B.A.; Eriksson, M. Evidence of insulin resistance in adult uncomplicated malaria: Result of a two-year prospective study. *Malar. Res. Treat.* **2014**, *2014*, 136148. [CrossRef]
6. Van Cromphaut, S.J.; Vanhorebeek, I.; Van den Berghe, G. Glucose metabolism and insulin resistance in sepsis. *Curr. Pharm. Des.* **2008**, *14*, 1887–1899. [CrossRef] [PubMed]
7. Niang, F.; Sarfo, F.S.; Frimpong, M.; Guenin-Mace, L.; Wansbrough-Jones, M.; Stinear, T.; Phillips, R.O.; Demangel, C. Metabolomic profiles delineate mycolactone signature in Buruli ulcer disease. *Sci. Rep.* **2015**, *5*, 17693. [CrossRef] [PubMed]
8. Phillips, R.O.; Sarfo, F.S.; Landier, J.; Oldenburg, R.; Frimpong, M.; Wansbrough-Jones, M.; Abass, K.; Thompson, W.; Forson, M.; Fontanet, A.; et al. Combined inflammatory and metabolic defects reflected by reduced serum protein levels in patients with Buruli ulcer disease. *PLoS Negl. Trop. Dis.* **2014**, *8*, e2786. [CrossRef]
9. Hansson, E.; Skioldebrand, E. Coupled cell networks are target cells of inflammation, which can spread between different body organs and develop into systemic chronic inflammation. *J. Inflamm.* **2015**, *12*, 44. [CrossRef]
10. Yaribeygi, H.; Farrokhi, F.R.; Butler, A.E.; Sahebkar, A. Insulin resistance: Review of the underlying molecular mechanisms. *J. Cell Physiol.* **2019**, *234*, 8152–8161. [CrossRef]
11. Grecco, H.E.; Schmick, M.; Bastiaens, P.I. Signaling from the living plasma membrane. *Cell* **2011**, *144*, 897–909. [CrossRef] [PubMed]
12. Izbicka, E.; Streeper, R.T.; Louden, C. Adaptive Membrane Fluidity Modulation: A Feedback Regulated Homeostatic System and Target for Pharmacological Intervention. *In Vivo* **2021**, *35*, 3073–3095. [CrossRef] [PubMed]
13. Izbicka, E.; Streeper, R.T. Adaptive Membrane Fluidity Modulation: A Feedback Regulated Homeostatic System Hiding in Plain Sight. *In Vivo* **2021**, *35*, 2991–3000. [CrossRef] [PubMed]
14. Streeper, R.T.; Izbicka, E. Diethyl Azelate for the Treatment of Brown Recluse Spider Bite, a Neglected Orphan Indication. *In Vivo* **2022**, *36*, 86–93. [CrossRef]
15. All natural. *Nat. Chem. Biol.* **2007**, *3*, 351. [CrossRef]
16. Atanasov, A.G.; Zotchev, S.B.; Dirsch, V.M.; Supuran, C.T.; the International Natural Product Sciences Taskforce. Natural products in drug discovery: Advances and opportunities. *Nat. Rev. Drug Discov.* **2021**, *20*, 200–216. [CrossRef]
17. Newman, D.J. Natural products and drug discovery. *Natl. Sci. Rev.* **2022**, *9*, nwac206. [CrossRef]
18. Ginsberg, B.H.; Brown, T.J.; Simon, I.; Spector, A.A. Effect of the membrane lipid environment on the properties of insulin receptors. *Diabetes* **1981**, *30*, 773–780. [CrossRef]

19. Patel, J.M.; Edwards, D.A.; Block, E.R.; Raizada, M.K. Effect of nitrogen dioxide on surface membrane fluidity and insulin receptor binding of pulmonary endothelial cells. *Biochem. Pharmacol.* **1988**, *37*, 1497–1507. [CrossRef]
20. Habegger, K.M.; Hoffman, N.J.; Ridenour, C.M.; Brozinick, J.T.; Elmendorf, J.S. AMPK enhances insulin-stimulated GLUT4 regulation via lowering membrane cholesterol. *Endocrinology* **2012**, *153*, 2130–2141. [CrossRef]
21. Das, U.N. Syntaxin interacts with arachidonic acid to prevent diabetes mellitus. *Lipids Health Dis.* **2022**, *21*, 73. [CrossRef] [PubMed]
22. Mcriin, A.B.; Zaarur, N.; Bogan, J.S.; Kandror, K.V. Inhibitors of RNA and protein synthesis cause Glut4 translocation and increase glucose uptake in adipocytes. *Sci. Rep.* **2022**, *12*, 15640. [CrossRef] [PubMed]
23. Kimchi, O.; Veatch, S.L.; Machta, B.B. Ion channels can be allosterically regulated by membrane domains near a de-mixing critical point. *J. Gen. Physiol.* **2018**, *150*, 1769–1777. [CrossRef]
24. Zhao, M.M.; Lu, J.; Li, S.; Wang, H.; Cao, X.; Li, Q.; Shi, T.T.; Matsunaga, K.; Chen, C.; Huang, H.; et al. Berberine is an insulin secretagogue targeting the KCNH6 potassium channel. *Nat. Commun.* **2021**, *12*, 5616. [CrossRef] [PubMed]
25. Thach, T.T.; Wu, C.; Hwang, K.Y.; Lee, S.J. Azelaic Acid Induces Mitochondrial Biogenesis in Skeletal Muscle by Activation of Olfactory Receptor 544. *Front. Physiol.* **2020**, *11*, 329. [CrossRef] [PubMed]
26. Wu, C.; Jeong, M.Y.; Kim, J.Y.; Lee, G.; Kim, J.S.; Cheong, Y.E.; Kang, H.; Cho, C.H.; Kim, J.; Park, M.K.; et al. Activation of ectopic olfactory receptor 544 induces GLP-1 secretion and regulates gut inflammation. *Gut Microbes* **2021**, *13*, 1987782. [CrossRef] [PubMed]
27. Riddy, D.M.; Delerive, P.; Summers, R.J.; Sexton, P.M.; Langmead, C.J. G Protein-Coupled Receptors Targeting Insulin Resistance, Obesity, and Type 2 Diabetes Mellitus. *Pharmacol. Rev.* **2018**, *70*, 39–67. [CrossRef] [PubMed]
28. Azelaic Acid. Available online: https://pubchem.ncbi.nlm.nih.gov/#query=azelaic%20acid (accessed on 5 June 2023).
29. Diethyl Azelate. Available online: https://pubchem.ncbi.nlm.nih.gov/#query=diethyl%20azelate (accessed on 5 June 2023).
30. Izbicka, E.; Streeper, R. Azelaic Acid Esters as Pluripotent Immunomodulatory Molecules: Nutritional Supplements or Drugs? *Nutraceuticals* **2021**, *1*, 42–53. [CrossRef]
31. Matsubara, T.; Tanaka, N.; Krausz, K.W.; Manna, S.K.; Kang, D.W.; Anderson, E.R.; Luecke, H.; Patterson, A.D.; Shah, Y.M.; Gonzalez, F.J. Metabolomics identifies an inflammatory cascade involved in dioxin- and diet-induced steatohepatitis. *Cell Metab.* **2012**, *16*, 634–644. [CrossRef]
32. Wu, C.; Hwang, S.H.; Jia, Y.; Choi, J.; Kim, Y.J.; Choi, D.; Pathiraja, D.; Choi, I.G.; Koo, S.H.; Lee, S.J. Olfactory receptor 544 reduces adiposity by steering fuel preference toward fats. *J. Clin. Investig.* **2017**, *127*, 4118–4123. [CrossRef]
33. Jung, H.W.; Tschaplinski, T.J.; Wang, L.; Glazebrook, J.; Greenberg, J.T. Priming in systemic plant immunity. *Science* **2009**, *324*, 89–91. [CrossRef] [PubMed]
34. Mastrofrancesco, A.; Ottaviani, M.; Aspite, N.; Cardinali, G.; Izzo, E.; Graupe, K.; Zouboulis, C.C.; Camera, E.; Picardo, M. Azelaic acid modulates the inflammatory response in normal human keratinocytes through PPARgamma activation. *Exp. Dermatol.* **2010**, *19*, 813–820. [CrossRef] [PubMed]
35. Muthulakshmi, S.; Saravanan, R. Protective effects of azelaic acid against high-fat diet-induced oxidative stress in liver, kidney and heart of C57BL/6J mice. *Mol. Cell Biochem.* **2013**, *377*, 23–33. [CrossRef] [PubMed]
36. Streeper, R.T.; Louden, C.; Izbicka, E. Oral Azelaic Acid Ester Decreases Markers of Insulin Resistance in Overweight Human Male Subjects. *In Vivo* **2020**, *34*, 1173–1186. [CrossRef]
37. Sebacic Acid. Available online: https://pubchem.ncbi.nlm.nih.gov/#query=sebacic%20acid (accessed on 5 June 2023).
38. Iaconelli, A.; Gastaldelli, A.; Chiellini, C.; Gniuli, D.; Favuzzi, A.; Binnert, C.; Mace, K.; Mingrone, G. Effect of oral sebacic Acid on postprandial glycemia, insulinemia, and glucose rate of appearance in type 2 diabetes. *Diabetes Care* **2010**, *33*, 2327–2332. [CrossRef]
39. Montgomery, M.K.; Turner, N. Mitochondrial dysfunction and insulin resistance: An update. *Endocr. Connect.* **2015**, *4*, R1–R15. [CrossRef]
40. Russell, A.P.; Foletta, V.C.; Snow, R.J.; Wadley, G.D. Skeletal muscle mitochondria: A major player in exercise, health and disease. *Biochim. Biophys. Acta* **2014**, *1840*, 1276–1284. [CrossRef]
41. Kang, N.; Bahk, Y.Y.; Lee, N.; Jae, Y.; Cho, Y.H.; Ku, C.R.; Byun, Y.; Lee, E.J.; Kim, M.S.; Koo, J. Olfactory receptor Olfr544 responding to azelaic acid regulates glucagon secretion in alpha-cells of mouse pancreatic islets. *Biochem. Biophys. Res. Commun.* **2015**, *460*, 616–621. [CrossRef]
42. Thach, T.T.; Hong, Y.J.; Lee, S.; Lee, S.J. Molecular determinants of the olfactory receptor Olfr544 activation by azelaic acid. *Biochem. Biophys. Res. Commun.* **2017**, *485*, 241–248. [CrossRef]
43. Muthulakshmi, S.; Chakrabarti, A.K.; Mukherjee, S. Gene expression profile of high-fat diet-fed C57BL/6J mice: In search of potential role of azelaic acid. *J. Physiol. Biochem.* **2015**, *71*, 29–42. [CrossRef]
44. Nachawi, N.; Rao, P.P.; Makin, V. The role of GLP-1 receptor agonists in managing type 2 diabetes. *Cleve. Clin. J. Med.* **2022**, *89*, 457–464. [CrossRef]
45. Lim, G.E.; Huang, G.J.; Flora, N.; LeRoith, D.; Rhodes, C.J.; Brubaker, P.L. Insulin regulates glucagon-like peptide-1 secretion from the enteroendocrine L cell. *Endocrinology* **2009**, *150*, 580–591. [CrossRef]
46. Phosphatidylcholine. Available online: https://pubchem.ncbi.nlm.nih.gov/#query=phosphatidylcholine&sort=cid&page=1 (accessed on 5 June 2023).

47. Phosphatidylethanolamine. Available online: https://pubchem.ncbi.nlm.nih.gov/#query=%22Phosphatidylethanolamine%20%5BWHO-DD%5D%22 (accessed on 5 June 2023).
48. Zhao, J.; Zhu, Y.; Hyun, N.; Zeng, D.; Uppal, K.; Tran, V.T.; Yu, T.; Jones, D.; He, J.; Lee, E.T.; et al. Novel metabolic markers for the risk of diabetes development in American Indians. *Diabetes Care* **2015**, *38*, 220–227. [CrossRef] [PubMed]
49. Newsom, S.A.; Brozinick, J.T.; Kiseljak-Vassiliades, K.; Strauss, A.N.; Bacon, S.D.; Kerege, A.A.; Bui, H.H.; Sanders, P.; Siddall, P.; Wei, T.; et al. Skeletal muscle phosphatidylcholine and phosphatidylethanolamine are related to insulin sensitivity and respond to acute exercise in humans. *J. Appl. Physiol.* **2016**, *120*, 1355–1363. [CrossRef]
50. Van der Veen, J.N.; Kennelly, J.P.; Wan, S.; Vance, J.E.; Vance, D.E.; Jacobs, R.L. The critical role of phosphatidylcholine and phosphatidylethanolamine metabolism in health and disease. *Biochim. Biophys. Acta Biomembr.* **2017**, *1859*, 1558–1572. [CrossRef]
51. Chang, W.; Hatch, G.; Wang, Y.; Yu, F.; Wang, M. The relationship between phospholipids and insulin resistance: From clinical to experimental evidence. *J. Cell. Mol. Med.* **2019**, *23*, 702–710. [CrossRef]
52. Alpha Linolenic Acid. Available online: https://pubchem.ncbi.nlm.nih.gov/#query=%22alpha%20Linolenic%20Acid%22 (accessed on 5 June 2023).
53. Linoleic Acid. Available online: https://pubchem.ncbi.nlm.nih.gov/#query=linoleic%20acid (accessed on 5 June 2023).
54. Calder, P.C. Polyunsaturated fatty acids and inflammatory processes: New twists in an old tale. *Biochimie* **2009**, *91*, 791–795. [CrossRef]
55. Lepretti, M.; Martucciello, S.; Burgos Aceves, M.A.; Putti, R.; Lionetti, L. Omega-3 Fatty Acids and Insulin Resistance: Focus on the Regulation of Mitochondria and Endoplasmic Reticulum Stress. *Nutrients* **2018**, *10*, 350. [CrossRef] [PubMed]
56. Heskey, C.E.; Jaceldo-Siegl, K.; Sabate, J.; Fraser, G.; Rajaram, S. Adipose tissue alpha-linolenic acid is inversely associated with insulin resistance in adults. *Am. J. Clin. Nutr.* **2016**, *103*, 1105–1110. [CrossRef] [PubMed]
57. Taouis, M.; Dagou, C.; Ster, C.; Durand, G.; Pinault, M.; Delarue, J. N-3 polyunsaturated fatty acids prevent the defect of insulin receptor signaling in muscle. *Am. J. Physiol. Endocrinol. Metab.* **2002**, *282*, E664–E671. [CrossRef]
58. Chung, S.; Brown, J.M.; Provo, J.N.; Hopkins, R.; McIntosh, M.K. Conjugated linoleic acid promotes human adipocyte insulin resistance through NFkappaB-dependent cytokine production. *J. Biol. Chem.* **2005**, *280*, 38445–38456. [CrossRef] [PubMed]
59. Cholesterol. Available online: https://pubchem.ncbi.nlm.nih.gov/compound/5997 (accessed on 5 June 2023).
60. Yeagle, P.L. Cholesterol and the cell membrane. *Biochim. Biophys. Acta* **1985**, *822*, 267–287. [CrossRef] [PubMed]
61. Owen, D.M.; Williamson, D.J.; Magenau, A.; Gaus, K. Sub-resolution lipid domains exist in the plasma membrane and regulate protein diffusion and distribution. *Nat. Commun.* **2012**, *3*, 1256. [CrossRef] [PubMed]
62. Pihlajamaki, J.; Gylling, H.; Miettinen, T.A.; Laakso, M. Insulin resistance is associated with increased cholesterol synthesis and decreased cholesterol absorption in normoglycemic men. *J. Lipid Res.* **2004**, *45*, 507–512. [CrossRef] [PubMed]
63. Hoenig, M.R.; Sellke, F.W. Insulin resistance is associated with increased cholesterol synthesis, decreased cholesterol absorption and enhanced lipid response to statin therapy. *Atherosclerosis* **2010**, *211*, 260–265. [CrossRef]
64. Gylling, H.; Hallikainen, M.; Pihlajamaki, J.; Simonen, P.; Kuusisto, J.; Laakso, M.; Miettinen, T.A. Insulin sensitivity regulates cholesterol metabolism to a greater extent than obesity: Lessons from the METSIM Study. *J. Lipid Res.* **2010**, *51*, 2422–2427. [CrossRef]
65. Haeusler, R.A.; Astiarraga, B.; Camastra, S.; Accili, D.; Ferrannini, E. Human insulin resistance is associated with increased plasma levels of 12alpha-hydroxylated bile acids. *Diabetes* **2013**, *62*, 4184–4191. [CrossRef]
66. Staels, B.; Kuipers, F. Bile acid sequestrants and the treatment of type 2 diabetes mellitus. *Drugs* **2007**, *67*, 1383–1392. [CrossRef]
67. Tomkin, G.H.; Owens, D. Obesity diabetes and the role of bile acids in metabolism. *J. Transl. Int. Med.* **2016**, *4*, 73–80. [CrossRef]
68. Lovastatin. Available online: https://pubchem.ncbi.nlm.nih.gov/compound/53232 (accessed on 5 June 2023).
69. Bobek, P.; Galbavy, S.; Ozdin, L. Effect of oyster mushroom (*Pleurotus ostreatus*) on pathological changes in dimethylhydrazine-induced rat colon cancer. *Oncol. Rep.* **1998**, *5*, 727–730. [CrossRef]
70. Lalli, C.A.; Pauli, J.R.; Prada, P.O.; Cintra, D.E.; Ropelle, E.R.; Velloso, L.A.; Saad, M.J. Statin modulates insulin signaling and insulin resistance in liver and muscle of rats fed a high-fat diet. *Metabolism* **2008**, *57*, 57–65. [CrossRef] [PubMed]
71. Hussain, S.A.; Sulaiman, A.A.; Alhaddad, H.; Alhadidi, Q. Natural polyphenols: Influence on membrane transporters. *J. Intercult. Ethnopharmacol.* **2016**, *5*, 97–104. [CrossRef] [PubMed]
72. Salicylic Acid. Available online: https://pubchem.ncbi.nlm.nih.gov/compound/338 (accessed on 5 June 2023).
73. Rena, G.; Sakamoto, K. Salicylic acid: Old and new implications for the treatment of type 2 diabetes? *Diabetol. Int.* **2014**, *5*, 212–218. [CrossRef]
74. Li, A.; Seipelt, H.; Muller, C.; Shi, Y.; Artmann, M. Effects of salicylic acid derivatives on red blood cell membranes. *Pharmacol. Toxicol.* **1999**, *85*, 206–211. [CrossRef] [PubMed]
75. Caffeic Acid. Available online: https://pubchem.ncbi.nlm.nih.gov/compound/689043 (accessed on 5 June 2023).
76. Muhammad Abdul Kadar, N.N.; Ahmad, F.; Teoh, S.L.; Yahaya, M.F. Caffeic Acid on Metabolic Syndrome: A Review. *Molecules* **2021**, *26*, 5490. [CrossRef]
77. Williamson, G.; Sheedy, K. Effects of Polyphenols on Insulin Resistance. *Nutrients* **2020**, *12*, 3135. [CrossRef]
78. Russo, B.; Picconi, F.; Malandrucco, I.; Frontoni, S. Flavonoids and Insulin-Resistance: From Molecular Evidences to Clinical Trials. *Int. J. Mol. Sci.* **2019**, *20*, 61. [CrossRef]
79. Trans-Chalcone. Available online: https://pubchem.ncbi.nlm.nih.gov/compound/637760 (accessed on 5 June 2023).
80. Quercetin. Available online: https://pubchem.ncbi.nlm.nih.gov/compound/5280343 (accessed on 5 June 2023).

81. Eid, H.M.; Haddad, P.S. The Antidiabetic Potential of Quercetin: Underlying Mechanisms. *Curr. Med. Chem.* **2017**, *24*, 355–364. [CrossRef]
82. Kreczmer, B.; Dyba, B.; Barbasz, A.; Rudolphi-Szydlo, E. Advantageous/Unfavorable Effect of Quercetin on the Membranes of SK-N-SH Neuroblastoma Cells. *Molecules* **2021**, *26*, 4945. [CrossRef]
83. Epigallocatechin Gallate. Available online: https://pubchem.ncbi.nlm.nih.gov/compound/65064 (accessed on 5 June 2023).
84. Zhang, Z.F.; Li, Q.; Liang, J.; Dai, X.Q.; Ding, Y.; Wang, J.B.; Li, Y. Epigallocatechin-3-O-gallate (EGCG) protects the insulin sensitivity in rat L6 muscle cells exposed to dexamethasone condition. *Phytomedicine* **2010**, *17*, 14–18. [CrossRef] [PubMed]
85. Yan, J.; Zhao, Y.; Suo, S.; Liu, Y.; Zhao, B. Green tea catechins ameliorate adipose insulin resistance by improving oxidative stress. *Free Radic. Biol. Med.* **2012**, *52*, 1648–1657. [CrossRef]
86. Collins, Q.F.; Liu, H.Y.; Pi, J.; Liu, Z.; Quon, M.J.; Cao, W. Epigallocatechin-3-gallate (EGCG), a green tea polyphenol, suppresses hepatic gluconeogenesis through 5′-AMP-activated protein kinase. *J. Biol. Chem.* **2007**, *282*, 30143–30149. [CrossRef]
87. Luteolin. Available online: https://pubchem.ncbi.nlm.nih.gov/compound/5280445 (accessed on 5 June 2023).
88. Zhang, T.; Qui, Y.; Luo, Q.; Zhao, L.; Yan, X.; Ding, Q.; Jiang, H.; Yang, H. The mechanism by which luteolin disrupts the cytoplasmic membrane of methicilin resistant *Staphylococcus aureus*. *J. Phys. Chem. B* **2018**, *122*, 1427–1438. [CrossRef]
89. Ding, L.; Jin, D.; Chen, X. Luteolin enhances insulin sensitivity via activation of PPARgamma transcriptional activity in adipocytes. *J. Nutr. Biochem.* **2010**, *21*, 941–947. [CrossRef] [PubMed]
90. Zhang, L.; Han, Y.J.; Zhang, X.; Wang, X.; Bao, B.; Qu, W.; Liu, J. Luteolin reduces obesity-associated insulin resistance in mice by activating AMPKalpha1 signalling in adipose tissue macrophages. *Diabetologia* **2016**, *59*, 2219–2228. [CrossRef]
91. Wang, Z.; Zeng, M.; Wang, Z.; Qin, F.; Chen, J.; He, Z. Dietary Luteolin: A Narrative Review Focusing on Its Pharmacokinetic Properties and Effects on Glycolipid Metabolism. *J. Agric. Food Chem.* **2021**, *69*, 1441–1454. [CrossRef]
92. Resveratrol. Available online: https://pubchem.ncbi.nlm.nih.gov/compound/445154 (accessed on 5 June 2023).
93. Milardi, G.L.; Stringaro, A.; Colone, M.; Bonincontro, A.; Risuleo, G. The cell membrane is the main target of resveratrol as shown by interdisciplinary biomolecular/cellular and biophysical approaches. *J. Membr. Biol.* **2014**, *247*, 1–8. [CrossRef] [PubMed]
94. Abbasi Oshaghi, E.; Goodarzi, M.T.; Higgins, V.; Adeli, K. Role of resveratrol in the management of insulin resistance and related conditions: Mechanism of action. *Crit. Rev. Clin. Lab. Sci.* **2017**, *54*, 267–293. [CrossRef]
95. Curcumin. Available online: https://pubchem.ncbi.nlm.nih.gov/compound/969516 (accessed on 5 June 2023).
96. Hung, W.C.; Chen, F.Y.; Lee, C.C.; Sun, Y.; Lee, M.T.; Huang, H.W. Membrane-thinning effect of curcumin. *Biophys. J.* **2008**, *94*, 4331–4338. [CrossRef] [PubMed]
97. Leite, N.B.; Martins, D.B.; Fazani, V.E.; Vieira, M.R.; Dos Santos Cabrera, M.P. Cholesterol modulates curcumin partitioning and membrane effects. *Biochim. Biophys. Acta Biomembr.* **2018**, *1860*, 2320–2328. [CrossRef] [PubMed]
98. Ingolfsson, H.I.; Koeppe, R.E., 2nd; Andersen, O.S. Curcumin is a modulator of bilayer material properties. *Biochemistry* **2007**, *46*, 10384–10391. [CrossRef] [PubMed]
99. Hodaei, H.; Adibian, M.; Nikpayam, O.; Hedayati, M.; Sohrab, G. The effect of curcumin supplementation on anthropometric indices, insulin resistance and oxidative stress in patients with type 2 diabetes: A randomized, double-blind clinical trial. *Diabetol. Metab. Syndr.* **2019**, *11*, 41. [CrossRef]
100. Myricetin. Available online: https://pubchem.ncbi.nlm.nih.gov/compound/5281672 (accessed on 5 June 2023).
101. Kimura, A.M.; Tsuji, M.; Yasumoto, T.; Mori, Y.; Oguchi, T.; Tsuji, Y.; Umino, M.; Umino, A.; Nishikawa, T.; Nakamura, S.; et al. Myricetin prevents high molecular weight Abeta1-42 oligomer-induced neurotoxicity through antioxidant effects in cell membranes and mitochondria. *Free Radic. Biol. Med.* **2021**, *171*, 232–244. [CrossRef]
102. Liu, I.M.; Tzeng, T.F.; Liou, S.S.; Lan, T.W. Myricetin, a naturally occurring flavonol, ameliorates insulin resistance induced by a high-fructose diet in rats. *Life Sci.* **2007**, *81*, 1479–1488. [CrossRef] [PubMed]
103. Fisetin. Available online: https://pubchem.ncbi.nlm.nih.gov/compound/5281614 (accessed on 5 June 2023).
104. Yong, Y.; Shin, S.; Jung, Y.; Jung, H.; Ahn, S.; Chong, Y.; Lim, Y. Flavonoids activating adenosine monophosphate-activating protein kinase. *J. Korean Soc. Appl. Biol. Chem.* **2015**, *58*, 13–19. [CrossRef]
105. Ge, C.; Xu, M.; Qin, Y.; Gu, T.; Lou, D.; Li, Q.; Hu, L.; Nie, X.; Wang, M.; Tan, J. Fisetin supplementation prevents high fat diet-induced diabetic nephropathy by repressing insulin resistance and RIP3-regulated inflammation. *Food Funct.* **2019**, *10*, 2970–2985. [CrossRef]
106. Genistein. Available online: https://pubchem.ncbi.nlm.nih.gov/compound/5280961 (accessed on 5 June 2023).
107. Arunkumar, E.; Karthik, D.; Anuradha, C.V. Genistein sensitizes hepatic insulin signaling and modulates lipid regulatory genes through p70 ribosomal S6 kinase-1 inhibition in high-fat-high-fructose diet-fed mice. *Pharm. Biol.* **2013**, *51*, 815–824. [CrossRef]
108. Wang, M.; Gao, X.J.; Zhao, W.W.; Zhao, W.J.; Jiang, C.H.; Huang, F.; Kou, J.P.; Liu, B.L.; Liu, K. Opposite effects of genistein on the regulation of insulin-mediated glucose homeostasis in adipose tissue. *Br. J. Pharmacol.* **2013**, *170*, 328–340. [CrossRef]
109. Ricci, E.; Cipriani, S.; Chiaffarino, F.; Malvezzi, M.; Parazzini, F. Effects of soy isoflavones and genistein on glucose metabolism in perimenopausal and postmenopausal non-Asian women: A meta-analysis of randomized controlled trials. *Menopause* **2010**, *17*, 1080–1086. [CrossRef]
110. Liu, Z.M.; Chen, Y.M.; Ho, S.C. Effects of soy intake on glycemic control: A meta-analysis of randomized controlled trials. *Am. J. Clin. Nutr.* **2011**, *93*, 1092–1101. [CrossRef]
111. Kaempferol. Available online: https://pubchem.ncbi.nlm.nih.gov/compound/5280863 (accessed on 5 June 2023).

112. Ulrih, N.; Maricic, M.; Ota, A.; Sentjurc, M.; Abram, V. Kaempferol and quercetin interactions with model lipid membranes. *Food Res. Int.* **2015**, *71*, 146–154. [CrossRef]
113. Luo, C.; Yang, H.; Tang, C.; Yao, G.; Kong, L.; He, H.; Zhou, Y. Kaempferol alleviates insulin resistance via hepatic IKK/NF-kappaB signal in type 2 diabetic rats. *Int. Immunopharmacol.* **2015**, *28*, 744–750. [CrossRef]
114. Holst, X. On Spirit of Turpentine in the Yellow Fever. *Med. Phys. J.* **1806**, *15*, 16.
115. Eucalyptol. Available online: https://pubchem.ncbi.nlm.nih.gov/compound/2758 (accessed on 5 June 2023).
116. L-Menthol. Available online: https://pubchem.ncbi.nlm.nih.gov/compound/16666 (accessed on 5 June 2023).
117. Anjos, J.L.; Neto Dde, S.; Alonso, A. Effects of 1,8-cineole on the dynamics of lipids and proteins of stratum corneum. *Int. J. Pharm.* **2007**, *345*, 81–87. [CrossRef]
118. dos Anjos, J.L.; de Sousa Neto, D.; Alonso, A. Effects of ethanol/l-menthol on the dynamics and partitioning of spin-labeled lipids in the stratum corneum. *Eur. J. Pharm. Biopharm.* **2007**, *67*, 406–412. [CrossRef]
119. Mendanha, S.A.; Alonso, A. Effects of terpenes on fluidity and lipid extraction in phospholipid membranes. *Biophys. Chem.* **2015**, *198*, 45–54. [CrossRef]
120. Khare, P.; Mangal, P.; Baboota, R.K.; Jagtap, S.; Kumar, V.; Singh, D.P.; Boparai, R.K.; Sharma, S.S.; Khardori, R.; Bhadada, S.K.; et al. Involvement of Glucagon in Preventive Effect of Menthol Against High Fat Diet Induced Obesity in Mice. *Front. Pharmacol.* **2018**, *9*, 1244. [CrossRef] [PubMed]
121. Limonene. Available online: https://pubchem.ncbi.nlm.nih.gov/compound/22311 (accessed on 5 June 2023).
122. Alpha-Terpineol. Available online: https://pubchem.ncbi.nlm.nih.gov/compound/17100 (accessed on 5 June 2023).
123. Camargos, H.S.; Moreira, R.A.; Mendanha, S.A.; Fernandes, K.S.; Dorta, M.L.; Alonso, A. Terpenes increase the lipid dynamics in the *Leishmania plasma* membrane at concentrations similar to their IC50 values. *PLoS ONE* **2014**, *9*, e104429. [CrossRef]
124. Al Kury, L.T.; Abdoh, A.; Ikbariah, K.; Sadek, B.; Mahgoub, M. In Vitro and In Vivo Antidiabetic Potential of Monoterpenoids: An Update. *Molecules* **2021**, *27*, 182. [CrossRef] [PubMed]
125. Ursolic Acid. Available online: https://pubchem.ncbi.nlm.nih.gov/compound/64945 (accessed on 5 June 2023).
126. Pachymic Acid. Available online: https://pubchem.ncbi.nlm.nih.gov/compound/5484385 (accessed on 5 June 2023).
127. Nazaruk, J.; Borzym-Kluczyk, M. The role of triterpenes in the management of diabetes mellitus and its complications. *Phytochem. Rev.* **2015**, *14*, 675–690. [CrossRef] [PubMed]
128. Huang, Y.C.; Chang, W.L.; Huang, S.F.; Lin, C.Y.; Lin, H.C.; Chang, T.C. Pachymic acid stimulates glucose uptake through enhanced GLUT4 expression and translocation. *Eur. J. Pharmacol.* **2010**, *648*, 39–49. [CrossRef] [PubMed]
129. Saponin. Available online: https://pubchem.ncbi.nlm.nih.gov/compound/198016 (accessed on 5 June 2023).
130. Keller, A.C.; Ma, J.; Kavalier, A.; He, K.; Brillantes, A.M.; Kennelly, E.J. Saponins from the traditional medicinal plant *Momordica charantia* stimulate insulin secretion in vitro. *Phytomedicine* **2011**, *19*, 32–37. [CrossRef]
131. Germoush, M.O.; Elgebaly, H.A.; Hassan, S.; Kamel, E.M.; Bin-Jumah, M.; Mahmoud, A.M. Consumption of Terpenoids-Rich Padina pavonia Extract Attenuates Hyperglycemia, Insulin Resistance and Oxidative Stress, and Upregulates PPARgamma in a Rat Model of Type 2 Diabetes. *Antioxidants* **2019**, *9*, 22. [CrossRef] [PubMed]
132. Bacanli, M.; Anlar, H.G.; Aydin, S.; Cal, T.; Ari, N.; Undeger Bucurgat, U.; Basaran, A.A.; Basaran, N. d-limonene ameliorates diabetes and its complications in streptozotocin-induced diabetic rats. *Food Chem. Toxicol.* **2017**, *110*, 434–442. [CrossRef] [PubMed]
133. Ahmad, S.; Beg, Z.H. Hypolipidemic and antioxidant activities of thymoquinone and limonene in atherogenic suspension fed rats. *Food Chem.* **2013**, *138*, 1116–1124. [CrossRef]
134. Cedrene. Available online: https://pubchem.ncbi.nlm.nih.gov/compound/521207 (accessed on 5 June 2023).
135. Tong, T.; Wang, Y.; Kang, S.G.; Huang, K. Ectopic Odorant Receptor Responding to Flavor Compounds: Versatile Roles in Health and Disease. *Pharmaceutics* **2021**, *13*, 1314. [CrossRef]
136. Kang, W.; Zhang, K.; Tong, T.; Park, T. Improved Glucose Intolerance through a Distinct Mouse Olfactory Receptor 23-Induced Signaling Pathway Mediating Glucose Uptake in Myotubes and Adipocytes. *Mol. Nutr. Food Res.* **2020**, *64*, e1901329. [CrossRef]
137. Alpha-Carotene. Available online: https://pubchem.ncbi.nlm.nih.gov/compound/6419725 (accessed on 5 June 2023).
138. Seel, W.; Baust, D.; Sons, D.; Albers, M.; Etzbach, L.; Fuss, J.; Lipski, A. Carotenoids are used as regulators for membrane fluidity by *Staphylococcus xylosus*. *Sci. Rep.* **2020**, *10*, 330. [CrossRef]
139. Mayne, S.T. Beta-carotene, carotenoids, and disease prevention in humans. *FASEB J.* **1996**, *10*, 690–701. [CrossRef]
140. Harari, A.; Coster, A.C.F.; Jenkins, A.; Xu, A.; Greenfield, J.R.; Harats, D.; Shaish, A.; Samocha-Bonet, D. Obesity and Insulin Resistance Are Inversely Associated with Serum and Adipose Tissue Carotenoid Concentrations in Adults. *J. Nutr.* **2020**, *150*, 38–46. [CrossRef]
141. Hutchings, M.I.; Truman, A.W.; Wilkinson, B. Antibiotics: Past, present and future. *Curr. Opin. Microbiol.* **2019**, *51*, 72–80. [CrossRef]
142. Streptomycin. Available online: https://pubchem.ncbi.nlm.nih.gov/compound/19649 (accessed on 5 June 2023).
143. Ampicillin. Available online: https://pubchem.ncbi.nlm.nih.gov/compound/6249 (accessed on 5 June 2023).
144. Vancomycin. Available online: https://pubchem.ncbi.nlm.nih.gov/compound/14969 (accessed on 5 June 2023).
145. Fenneman, A.C.; Weidner, M.; Chen, L.A.; Nieuwdorp, M.; Blaser, J. Antibiotics in the pathogenesis of diabetes and inflammatory diseases of the gastrointestinal tract. *Nat. Rev. Gastroenterol. Hepatol.* **2022**, *20*, 81–100. [CrossRef]

146. Candon, S.; Perez-Arroyo, A.; Marquet, C.; Valette, F.; Foray, A.P.; Pelletier, B.; Milani, C.; Ventura, M.; Bach, J.F.; Chatenoud, L. Antibiotics in early life alter the gut microbiome and increase disease incidence in a spontaneous mouse model of autoimmune insulin-dependent diabetes. *PLoS ONE* **2015**, *10*, e0125448. [CrossRef]
147. Sirolimus. Available online: https://pubchem.ncbi.nlm.nih.gov/compound/5284616 (accessed on 5 June 2023).
148. Reifsnyder, P.C.; Flurkey, K.; Doty, R.; Calcutt, N.A.; Koza, R.A.; Harrison, D.E. Rapamycin/metformin co-treatment normalizes insulin sensitivity and reduces complications of metabolic syndrome in type 2 diabetic mice. *Aging Cell* **2022**, *21*, e13666. [CrossRef] [PubMed]
149. Wang, H.; Wang, L.; Fan, K.; Pan, G. Tetracycline natural products: Discovery, biosynthesis and engineering. *Chin. J. Nat. Med.* **2022**, *20*, 773–794. [CrossRef] [PubMed]
150. Gabler, W.L. Fluxes and accumulation of tetracyclines by human blood cells. *Res. Commun. Chem. Pathol. Pharmacol.* **1991**, *72*, 39–51. [PubMed]
151. Doxycycline. Available online: https://pubchem.ncbi.nlm.nih.gov/compound/54671203 (accessed on 5 June 2023).
152. Chen, Y.; Chen, Y.; Wang, N.; Gu, S.; Wang, M.; Fu, Y.; Wei, C.; Xu, W. Doxycycline in Extremely Low Dose Improves Glycemic Control and Islet Morphology in Mice Fed a High-Fat Diet. *Diabetes Metab. Syndr. Obes.* **2021**, *14*, 637–646. [CrossRef]
153. Tan, C.H.; Shelley, C.; Harman, K.E. Doxycycline-induced hypoglycaemia. *Clin. Exp. Dermatol.* **2016**, *41*, 43–44. [CrossRef]
154. Actinomycin D. Available online: https://pubchem.ncbi.nlm.nih.gov/compound/2019 (accessed on 5 June 2023).
155. Sobell, H.M. Actinomycin and DNA transcription. *Proc. Natl. Acad. Sci. USA* **1985**, *82*, 5328–5331. [CrossRef] [PubMed]
156. Polet, H. Role of the cell membrane in the uptake of 3H-actinomycin D by mammalian cells in vitro. *J. Pharmacol. Exp. Ther.* **1975**, *192*, 270–279.
157. Zeng, H.; Feng, P.X.; Wan, C.X. Antifungal effects of actinomycin D on *Verticillium dahliae* via a membrane-splitting mechanism. *Nat. Prod. Res.* **2019**, *33*, 1751–1755. [CrossRef]
158. Grey, N.J.; Goldring, S.; Kipnis, D.M. The effect of fasting, diet, and actinomycin D on insulin secretion in the rat. *J. Clin. Investig.* **1970**, *49*, 881–889. [CrossRef]
159. Christodoulou, M.I.; Tchoumtchoua, J.; Skaltsounis, A.L.; Scorilas, A.; Halabalaki, M. Natural Alkaloids Intervening the Insulin Pathway: New Hopes for Anti-Diabetic Agents? *Curr. Med. Chem.* **2019**, *26*, 5982–6015. [CrossRef] [PubMed]
160. Behl, T.; Gupta, A.; Albratty, M.; Najmi, A.; Meraya, A.M.; Alhazmi, H.A.; Anwer, M.K.; Bhatia, S.; Bungau, S.G. Alkaloidal Phytoconstituents for Diabetes Management: Exploring the Unrevealed Potential. *Molecules* **2022**, *27*, 5851. [CrossRef] [PubMed]
161. Emetine. Available online: https://pubchem.ncbi.nlm.nih.gov/compound/10219 (accessed on 5 June 2023).
162. Yang, S.; Xu, M.; Lee, E.M.; Gorshkov, K.; Shiryaev, S.A.; He, S.; Sun, W.; Cheng, Y.S.; Hu, X.; Tharappel, A.M.; et al. Emetine inhibits Zika and Ebola virus infections through two molecular mechanisms: Inhibiting viral replication and decreasing viral entry. *Cell Discov.* **2018**, *4*, 31. [CrossRef] [PubMed]
163. Valipour, M.; Irannejad, H.; Emami, S. Application of emetine in SARS-CoV-2 treatment: Regulation of p38 MAPK signaling pathway for preventing emetine-induced cardiac complications. *Cell Cycle* **2022**, *21*, 2379–2386. [CrossRef] [PubMed]
164. Catharanthine. Available online: https://pubchem.ncbi.nlm.nih.gov/compound/5458190 (accessed on 5 June 2023).
165. Berberine. Available online: https://pubchem.ncbi.nlm.nih.gov/compound/2353 (accessed on 5 June 2023).
166. Neag, M.A.; Mocan, A.; Echeverria, J.; Pop, R.M.; Bocsan, C.I.; Crisan, G.; Buzoianu, A.D. Berberine: Botanical Occurrence, Traditional Uses, Extraction Methods, and Relevance in Cardiovascular, Metabolic, Hepatic, and Renal Disorders. *Front. Pharmacol.* **2018**, *9*, 557. [CrossRef] [PubMed]
167. Marin-Neto, J.A.; Maciel, B.C.; Secches, A.L.; Gallo Junior, L. Cardiovascular effects of berberine in patients with severe congestive heart failure. *Clin. Cardiol.* **1988**, *11*, 253–260. [CrossRef]
168. Yang, Y.; Ye, X.; Li, X. Effect of berberine on membrane fluidity and membrane protein fluorescence of rabbit red-blood cells. *J. Fourth Mil. Med. Univ.* **2009**, *30*, 1627–1629.
169. Xu, X.; Yi, H.; Wu, J.; Kuang, T.; Zhang, J.; Li, Q.; Du, H.; Xu, T.; Jiang, G.; Fan, G. Therapeutic effect of berberine on metabolic diseases: Both pharmacological data and clinical evidence. *Biomed. Pharmacother.* **2021**, *133*, 110984. [CrossRef]
170. Yang, J.K.; Lu, J.; Yuan, S.S.; Asan; Cao, X.; Qiu, H.Y.; Shi, T.T.; Yang, F.Y.; Li, Q.; Liu, C.P.; et al. From Hyper- to Hypoinsulinemia and Diabetes: Effect of KCNH6 on Insulin Secretion. *Cell Rep.* **2018**, *25*, 3800–3810.e3806. [CrossRef] [PubMed]
171. Galegine. Available online: https://pubchem.ncbi.nlm.nih.gov/compound/10983 (accessed on 5 June 2023).
172. Mooney, M.H.; Fogarty, S.; Stevenson, C.; Gallagher, A.M.; Palit, P.; Hawley, S.A.; Hardie, D.G.; Coxon, G.D.; Waigh, R.D.; Tate, R.J.; et al. Mechanisms underlying the metabolic actions of galegine that contribute to weight loss in mice. *Br. J. Pharmacol.* **2008**, *153*, 1669–1677. [CrossRef] [PubMed]
173. Metformin. Available online: https://pubchem.ncbi.nlm.nih.gov/compound/4091 (accessed on 5 June 2023).
174. Wang, H.; Zhu, C.; Ying, Y.; Luo, L.; Huang, D.; Luo, Z. Metformin and berberine, two versatile drugs in treatment of common metabolic diseases. *Oncotarget* **2018**, *9*, 10135–10146. [CrossRef]
175. Scarpello, J.H.; Howlett, H.C. Metformin therapy and clinical uses. *Diabetes Vasc. Dis. Res.* **2008**, *5*, 157–167. [CrossRef]
176. Lord, J.M.; Flight, I.H.; Norman, R.J. Metformin in polycystic ovary syndrome: Systematic review and meta-analysis. *BMJ* **2003**, *327*, 951–953. [CrossRef]
177. Baker, C.; Retzik-Stahr, C.; Singh, V.; Plomondon, R.; Anderson, V.; Rasouli, N. Should metformin remain the first-line therapy for treatment of type 2 diabetes? *Ther. Adv. Endocrinol. Metab.* **2021**, *12*, 2042018820980225. [CrossRef] [PubMed]

178. Rena, G.; Hardie, D.G.; Pearson, E.R. The mechanisms of action of metformin. *Diabetologia* **2017**, *60*, 1577–1585. [CrossRef] [PubMed]
179. WHO. Model List of Essential Medicines—22nd List. 2021. Available online: https://www.who.int/publications/i/item/WHO-MHP-HPS-EML-2021.02h (accessed on 5 June 2023).
180. LaMoia, T.E.; Shulman, G.I. Cellular and Molecular Mechanisms of Metformin Action. *Endocr. Rev.* **2021**, *42*, 77–96. [CrossRef] [PubMed]
181. Giusti, L.; Tesi, M.; Ciregia, F.; Marselli, L.; Zallocco, L.; Suleiman, M.; De Luca, C.; Del Guerra, S.; Zuccarini, M.; Trerotola, M.; et al. The Protective Action of Metformin against Pro-Inflammatory Cytokine-Induced Human Islet Cell Damage and the Mechanisms Involved. *Cells* **2022**, *11*, 2465. [CrossRef] [PubMed]
182. Fujita, Y.; Inagaki, N. Metformin: Clinical topics and new mechanisms of action. *Diabetol. Int.* **2017**, *8*, 4–6. [CrossRef]
183. Hur, K.Y.; Lee, M.S. New mechanisms of metformin action: Focusing on mitochondria and the gut. *J. Diabetes Investig.* **2015**, *6*, 600–609. [CrossRef] [PubMed]
184. Muller, S.; Denet, S.; Candiloros, H.; Barrois, R.; Wiernsperger, N.; Donner, M.; Drouin, P. Action of metformin on erythrocyte membrane fluidity in vitro and in vivo. *Eur. J. Pharmacol.* **1997**, *337*, 103–110. [CrossRef] [PubMed]
185. Matthaei, S.; Greten, H. Evidence that metformin ameliorates cellular insulin-resistance by potentiating insulin-induced translocation of glucose transporters to the plasma membrane. *Diabète Metab.* **1991**, *17*, 150–158. [PubMed]
186. Wiernsperger, N.F. Membrane physiology as a basis for the cellular effects of metformin in insulin resistance and diabetes. *Diabetes Metab.* **1999**, *25*, 110–127.
187. Quigley, E.M. Gut bacteria in health and disease. *Gastroenterol. Hepatol.* **2013**, *9*, 560–569.
188. Turnbaugh, P.J.; Ley, R.E.; Hamady, M.; Fraser-Liggett, C.M.; Knight, R.; Gordon, J.I. The human microbiome project. *Nature* **2007**, *449*, 804–810. [CrossRef]
189. Caricilli, A.M.; Saad, M.J. The role of gut microbiota on insulin resistance. *Nutrients* **2013**, *5*, 829–851. [CrossRef]
190. Diamant, M.; Blaak, E.E.; de Vos, W.M. Do nutrient-gut-microbiota interactions play a role in human obesity, insulin resistance and type 2 diabetes? *Obes. Rev.* **2011**, *12*, 272–281. [CrossRef]
191. Acetic Acid. Available online: https://pubchem.ncbi.nlm.nih.gov/compound/176 (accessed on 5 June 2023).
192. Propionic Acid. Available online: https://pubchem.ncbi.nlm.nih.gov/compound/1032 (accessed on 5 June 2023).
193. Butyric Acid. Available online: https://pubchem.ncbi.nlm.nih.gov/compound/264 (accessed on 5 June 2023).
194. Bastos, R.M.C.; Rangel, E.B. Gut microbiota-derived metabolites are novel targets for improving insulin resistance. *World J. Diabetes* **2022**, *13*, 65–69. [CrossRef]
195. Ganapathy, V.; Thangaraju, M.; Prasad, P.D.; Martin, P.M.; Singh, N. Transporters and receptors for short-chain fatty acids as the molecular link between colonic bacteria and the host. *Curr. Opin. Pharmacol.* **2013**, *13*, 869–874. [CrossRef]
196. Rechkemmer, G.; von Engelhardt, W. Concentration- and pH-dependence of short-chain fatty acid absorption in the proximal and distal colon of guinea pig (*Cavia porcellus*). *Comp. Biochem. Physiol. A Comp. Physiol.* **1988**, *91*, 659–663. [CrossRef] [PubMed]
197. Charney, A.N.; Micic, L.; Egnor, R.W. Nonionic diffusion of short-chain fatty acids across rat colon. *Am. J. Physiol.* **1998**, *274*, G518–G524. [CrossRef] [PubMed]
198. Ritzhaupt, A.; Wood, I.S.; Ellis, A.; Hosie, K.B.; Shirazi-Beechey, S.P. Identification and characterization of a monocarboxylate transporter (MCT1) in pig and human colon: Its potential to transport L-lactate as well as butyrate. *J. Physiol.* **1998**, *513 Pt 3*, 719–732. [CrossRef]
199. Gill, R.K.; Saksena, S.; Alrefai, W.A.; Sarwar, Z.; Goldstein, J.L.; Carroll, R.E.; Ramaswamy, K.; Dudeja, P.K. Expression and membrane localization of MCT isoforms along the length of the human intestine. *Am. J. Physiol. Cell Physiol.* **2005**, *289*, C846–C852. [CrossRef]
200. Manns, J.G.; Boda, J.M.; Willes, R.F. Probable role of propionate and butyrate in control of insulin secretion in sheep. *Am. J. Physiol.* **1967**, *212*, 756–764. [CrossRef]
201. Chen, Z.; Radjabzadeh, D.; Chen, L.; Kurilshikov, A.; Kavousi, M.; Ahmadizar, F.; Ikram, M.A.; Uitterlinden, A.G.; Zhernakova, A.; Fu, J.; et al. Association of Insulin Resistance and Type 2 Diabetes with Gut Microbial Diversity: A Microbiome-Wide Analysis from Population Studies. *JAMA Netw. Open* **2021**, *4*, e2118811. [CrossRef]
202. Taurocholic Acid. Available online: https://pubchem.ncbi.nlm.nih.gov/compound/6675 (accessed on 5 June 2023).
203. Glycocholic Acid. Available online: https://pubchem.ncbi.nlm.nih.gov/compound/10140 (accessed on 5 June 2023).
204. Taurochenodeoxycholic Acid. Available online: https://pubchem.ncbi.nlm.nih.gov/compound/387316 (accessed on 5 June 2023).
205. Glycochenodeoxycholic Acid. Available online: https://pubchem.ncbi.nlm.nih.gov/compound/12544 (accessed on 5 June 2023).
206. Zou, J.; Chassaing, B.; Singh, V.; Pellizzon, M.; Ricci, M.; Fythe, M.D.; Kumar, M.V.; Gewirtz, A.T. Fiber-Mediated Nourishment of Gut Microbiota Protects against Diet-Induced Obesity by Restoring IL-22-Mediated Colonic Health. *Cell Host Microbe* **2018**, *23*, 41–53.e44. [CrossRef]
207. Yu, M.; Gouvinhas, I.; Rocha, J.; Barros, A. Phytochemical and antioxidant analysis of medicinal and food plants towards bioactive food and pharmaceutical resources. *Sci. Rep.* **2021**, *11*, 10041. [CrossRef]
208. Martucci, M.; Ostan, R.; Biondi, F.; Bellavista, E.; Fabbri, C.; Bertarelli, C.; Salvioli, S.; Capri, M.; Franceschi, C.; Santoro, A. Mediterranean diet and inflammaging within the hormesis paradigm. *Nutr. Rev.* **2017**, *75*, 442–455. [CrossRef]

209. Kwist, K.; Bridges, W.C.; Burg, K.J. The effect of cell passage number on osteogenic and adipogenic characteristics of D1 cells. *Cytotechnology* **2016**, *68*, 1661–1667. [CrossRef] [PubMed]
210. Emami, J. In vitro–In vivo correlation: From theory to applications. *J. Pharm. Pharm. Sci.* **2006**, *9*, 169–189.
211. Choi, M.S.; Choi, J.Y.; Kwon, E.Y. Fisetin Alleviates Hepatic and Adipocyte Fibrosis and Insulin Resistance in Diet-Induced Obese Mice. *J. Med. Food* **2020**, *23*, 1019–1032. [CrossRef]
212. Safe, S.; Jayaraman, A.; Chapkin, R.S.; Howard, M.; Mohankumar, K.; Shrestha, R. Flavonoids: Structure-function and mechanisms of action and opportunities for drug development. *Toxicol. Res.* **2021**, *37*, 147–162. [CrossRef]
213. Diabetes Prevention Program Research Group. Long-term Effects of Metformin on Diabetes Prevention: Identification of Subgroups That Benefited Most in the Diabetes Prevention Program and Diabetes Prevention Program Outcomes Study. *Diabetes Care* **2019**, *42*, 601–608. [CrossRef]
214. Klaschka, U. Naturally toxic: Natural substances used in personal care products. *Environ. Sci. Eur.* **2015**, *27*, 1. [CrossRef]
215. 2,3,7,8-Tetrachlorodibenzo-P-Dioxin. Available online: https://pubchem.ncbi.nlm.nih.gov/compound/15625 (accessed on 5 June 2023).
216. Matsumura, F.; Brewster, D.W.; Madhukar, B.V.; Bombick, D.W. Alteration of rat hepatic plasma membrane functions by 2,3,7,8-tetrachlorodibenzo-p-dioxin (TCDD). *Arch. Environ. Contam. Toxicol.* **1984**, *13*, 509–515. [CrossRef] [PubMed]
217. Lee, H.; Ha, T.Y.; Jung, C.H.; Nirmala, F.S.; Park, S.Y.; Huh, Y.H.; Ahn, J. Mitochondrial dysfunction in skeletal muscle contributes to the development of acute insulin resistance in mice. *J. Cachexia Sarcopenia Muscle* **2021**, *12*, 1925–1939. [CrossRef]
218. Welshons, W.V.; Nagel, S.C.; vom Saal, F.S. Large effects from small exposures. III. Endocrine mechanisms mediating effects of bisphenol A at levels of human exposure. *Endocrinology* **2006**, *147*, S56–S69. [CrossRef]
219. Bisphenol A. Available online: https://pubchem.ncbi.nlm.nih.gov/compound/6623 (accessed on 5 June 2023).
220. Yang, J.; Wang, H.; Du, H.; Xu, L.; Liu, S.; Yi, J.; Chen, Y.; Jiang, Q.; He, G. Serum Bisphenol A, glucose homeostasis, and gestational diabetes mellitus in Chinese pregnant women: A prospective study. *Environ. Sci. Pollut. Res. Int.* **2021**, *28*, 12546–12554. [CrossRef] [PubMed]

pharmaceuticals

MDPI

Article

Inhibition of TRPA1, Endoplasmic Reticulum Stress, Human Airway Epithelial Cell Damage, and Ectopic *MUC5AC* Expression by Vasaka (*Adhatoda vasica*; Malabar Nut) Tea

Tosifa A. Memon [1], Lili Sun [1], Marysol Almestica-Roberts [1], Cassandra E. Deering-Rice [1,2], Philip J. Moos [1] and Christopher A. Reilly [1,2,*]

[1] Department of Pharmacology and Toxicology, College of Pharmacy, University of Utah Health, Salt Lake City, UT 84112, USA; memon.tosifa@gmail.com (T.A.M.); lili.sun@pharm.utah.edu (L.S.); m.almestica@utah.edu (M.A.-R.); cassandra.rice@utah.edu (C.E.D.-R.); philip.moos@pharm.utah.edu (P.J.M.)

[2] Center for Human Toxicology, College of Pharmacy, University of Utah Health, Salt Lake City, UT 84112, USA

* Correspondence: chris.reilly@pharm.utah.edu; Tel.: +1-801-581-5236

Abstract: This study tested whether a medicinal plant, Vasaka, typically consumed as a tea to treat respiratory malaise, could protect airway epithelial cells (AECs) from wood smoke particle-induced damage and prevent pathological mucus production. Wood/biomass smoke is a pneumotoxic air pollutant. Mucus normally protects the airways, but excessive production can obstruct airflow and cause respiratory distress. Vasaka tea pre- and co-treatment dose-dependently inhibited mucin 5AC (*MUC5AC*) mRNA induction by AECs treated with wood smoke particles. This correlated with transient receptor potential ankyrin-1 (TRPA1) inhibition, an attenuation of endoplasmic reticulum (ER) stress, and AEC damage/death. Induction of mRNA for anterior gradient 2, an ER chaperone/disulfide isomerase required for *MUC5AC* production, and TRP vanilloid-3, a gene that suppresses ER stress and wood smoke particle-induced cell death, was also attenuated. Variable inhibition of TRPA1, ER stress, and *MUC5AC* mRNA induction was observed using selected chemicals identified in Vasaka tea including vasicine, vasicinone, apigenin, vitexin, isovitexin, isoorientin, 9-oxoODE, and 9,10-EpOME. Apigenin and 9,10-EpOME were the most cytoprotective and mucosuppressive. Cytochrome P450 1A1 (CYP1A1) mRNA was also induced by Vasaka tea and wood smoke particles. Inhibition of CYP1A1 enhanced ER stress and *MUC5AC* mRNA expression, suggesting a possible role in producing protective oxylipins in stressed cells. The results provide mechanistic insights and support for the purported benefits of Vasaka tea in treating lung inflammatory conditions, raising the possibility of further development as a preventative and/or restorative therapy.

Keywords: Vasaka; TRPA1; airway epithelium; mucus hypersecretion; *MUC5AC*; lung injury; wood smoke; biomass smoke

Citation: Memon, T.A.; Sun, L.; Almestica-Roberts, M.; Deering-Rice, C.E.; Moos, P.J.; Reilly, C.A. Inhibition of TRPA1, Endoplasmic Reticulum Stress, Human Airway Epithelial Cell Damage, and Ectopic *MUC5AC* Expression by Vasaka (*Adhatoda vasica*; Malabar Nut) Tea. *Pharmaceuticals* **2023**, *16*, 890. https://doi.org/10.3390/ph16060890

Academic Editor: Jong-Eun Kim

Received: 30 May 2023
Revised: 13 June 2023
Accepted: 14 June 2023
Published: 17 June 2023

1. Introduction

This study tested the hypothesis that tea prepared from the medicinal plant, Vasaka (*Adhatoda vasica*; Malabar Nut), could attenuate airway epithelial cell (AEC) damage and ectopic *MUC5AC* expression in an in vitro model of WSPM-induced AEC/lung injury. Furthermore, it was investigated whether specific chemicals in Vasaka could replicate the effects of the tea. Despite the purported benefits of Vasaka in treating respiratory conditions [1–3], the mechanisms via which Vasaka acts have not been elucidated. Additionally, potential synergistic and/or antagonistic effects among Vasaka components have not been reported. Thus, while Vasaka tea may be useful as a homeopathic therapy, it may be possible to further optimize the beneficial effects using Vasaka-derived compounds that target regulatory pathways controlling AEC injury and excessive *MUC5AC* expression.

Breathing polluted air increases risks of infection, asthma, and chronic obstructive pulmonary disease (COPD), among other effects [4–8]. AEC damage may contribute to air pollution-associated morbidities. Wood and biomass smoke particulate materials (WSPM) are pneumotoxic and have the ability to preferentially stimulate mucin 5AC (*MUC5AC*) expression by human AECs in vitro and in mice following oropharyngeal delivery of suspended WSPM through the activation of transient receptor potential ankyrin-1 (TRPA1) and endoplasmic reticulum (ER) stress [9,10], Additionally, AEC damage triggers activation of epidermal growth factor receptor (EGFR) to drive *MUC5AC* expression. Accordingly, EGFR ligands can promote *MUC5AC* expression [9].

The effect of WSPM on AECs and *MUC5AC* expression is of interest because of the frequency at which humans are exposed to WSPM, and both AEC damage and excessive mucus production are consequential to human respiratory health. Common sources of exposure to WSPM include wood/biomass-burning in stoves, fireplaces, campfires, and wildfires. Depending upon the exposure (dose and duration), WSPM can cause mild reversible to severe irreversible lung injury [11–13]. Short-term exposure has been linked to increased rates of hospital admissions for respiratory complications [12,14–16], while long-term exposure has been associated with chronic disease exacerbation and causation, including asthma, emphysema, COPD, and "hut lung" [17,18].

Airway mucus contains gel-forming glycoproteins known as mucins. *MUC5AC* and mucin 5B (MUC5B) are secreted mucins. Differential expression of *MUC5AC* and MUC5B has been shown to affect the viscoelasticity of airway mucus [19,20]. MUC5B has been shown to be preferentially expressed in the airways of healthy people and mice, and to play an essential role in trapping pathogens and pollutants entering the airway [21,22]. However, *MUC5AC* has been found to be overexpressed in COPD patients and mice primed with allergens, where it plays a role in obstruction and airway hyper-reactivity [23–25]. Accordingly, targeting pathways leading to WSPM-induced AEC/lung injury and *MUC5AC* production may be advantageous [26].

2. Results

2.1. Vasaka Tea Attenuated MUC5AC mRNA Induction by AECs

Inhibition of WSPM-induced *MUC5AC* mRNA induction by Vasaka tea in HBEC3-KT AECs was evaluated. Vasaka tea was prepared, diluted in cell culture medium, and applied to cells for 2 h. After 2 h, fresh medium with varying percentages of Vasaka tea with and without WSPM (20 μg/cm^2) was applied. The expression of *MUC5AC* mRNA was quantified 24 h later using qPCR (Figure 1). Note that we previously showed that *MUC5AC* mRNA induction is correlated with increased *MUC5AC* protein expression (periodic acid–Schiff staining and immunocytochemical analysis of cells) and secretion (enzyme-linked immunosorbent assay; ELISA) by AECs [9]. Here, Vasaka tea pre- and co-treatment at concentrations $\geq$ 0.625 mg/mL suppressed *MUC5AC* mRNA induction. The IC_{50} was approximately 0.7 mg/mL.

2.2. Vasaka Tea Attenuated TRPA1 Activation

Inhibition of TRPA1 by Vasaka tea was subsequently tested. Pretreatment (>30 min), but not co-treatment of HBEC3-KT cells with Vasaka tea (1.25 and 2.5 mg/mL) decreased allyl-isothiocyanate (AITC)- (i.e., TRPA1-dependent) and WSPM-induced calcium flux akin to the TRPA1 antagonist HC-030031 (Figure 2).

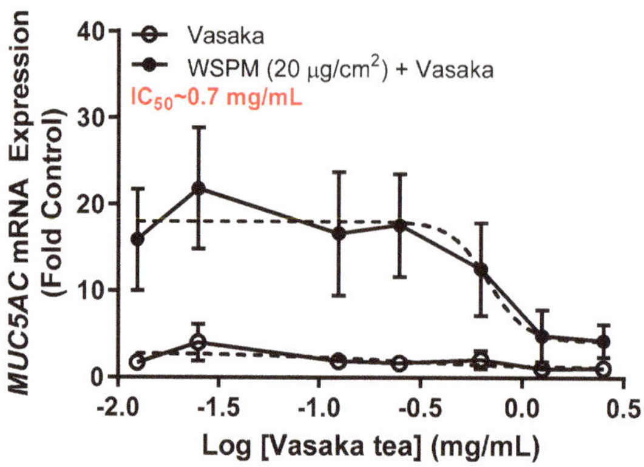

Figure 1. Concentration-dependent inhibition of *MUC5AC* mRNA expression by Vasaka tea. HBEC3-KT cells were pre- (2 h) and cotreated with Vasaka tea diluted in treatment medium with (solid circles) and without (open circles) WSPM (2.5 mg/mL) for 24 h ($n = 3$). *MUC5AC* mRNA expression was quantified using qPCR. Data were modeled using the log (antagonist) vs. response equation in GraphPad 9.5 software to predict the IC_{50} value.

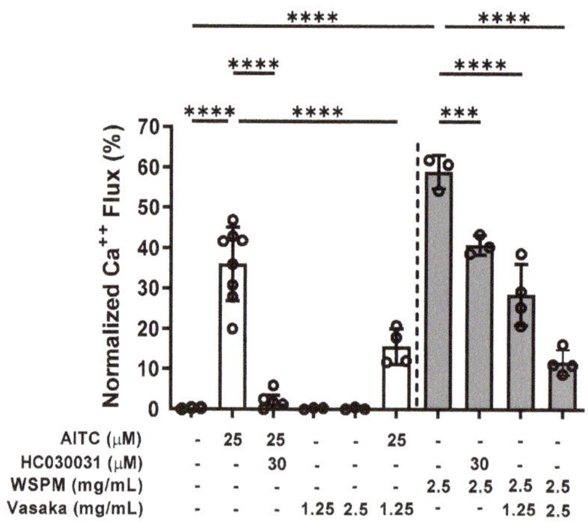

Figure 2. Inhibition of TRPA1-mediated calcium flux by Vasaka tea in HBEC3-KT cells treated with the TRPA1 agonist AITC (25 μM; white bars) or WSPM (2.5 mg/mL or 195 μg/cm^2; gray bars). Replicates within each group are shown as open circles. HC-030031 is a TRPA1 antagonist. Vasaka tea was diluted in medium, and cells were pretreated with HC-030031 and Vasaka tea for 30 min prior to agonist (AITC or WSPM) application. Data were analyzed by one-way ANOVA with post hoc testing for significance among preselected groups using the Bonferroni test ($n = 4$–8). *** $p < 0.001$, **** $p < 0.0001$.

2.3. *Vasaka Tea Attenuated WSPM-Induced ER Stress, Oxidative Stress, and Other Cellular Pathways*

HBEC-3KT cells were treated with a vehicle control (0.2% dimethyl sulfoxide; DMSO in cell culture medium), WSPMP (10 μg/cm^2), Vasaka tea (1.25 mg/mL), or a combination of both WSPM and Vasaka tea for 24 h. RNA sequencing was used to compare transcriptional changes associated with WSPM and Vasaka tea treatment. WSPM treatment induced robust changes to the AEC transcriptome, with many of the effects being attenuated by Vasaka tea cotreatment. Vasaka tea alone had few effects on the genes/pathways affected by WSPM. A comparison of the top 1000 genes exhibiting differential expression with WSPM treatment is shown in Figure 3A. The full dataset is publicly available.

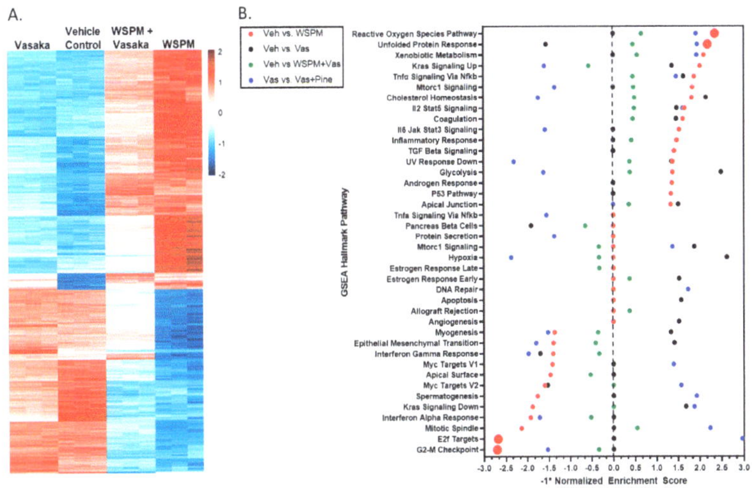

Figure 3. (**A**) Heatmap comparing the expression of the 1000 most changed transcripts in HBEC3-KT cells treated with WSPM compared to the vehicle control, as a function of treatment group. (**B**) Quantitative comparison of normalized enrichment score values multiplied by −1 (−1*NES) from pathway/GSEA of HBEC3-KT cells treated with vehicle (cell culture medium + 0.2% DMSO), WSPM (10 μg/cm^2), Vasaka tea (1.25 mg/mL), or WSPM and Vasaka tea. Differential gene expression was determined using hciR and DESeq2 (1.30.1). Pathway analysis was performed using fgsea (1.18.0) using the Hallmarks Molecular Signatures Database. A negative value indicates enrichment in the comparison control group.

Pathway analysis using Bioconductor Fast Geneset Enrichment Analysis (fgsea; or GSEA for short) was used to categorize cellular responses as pathways affected by WSPM and the Vasaka tea treatments. The hallmark *reactive oxygen species* (ROS) pathway (i.e., genes upregulated by ROS) was the most significant pathway associated with WSPM treatment (p-adjusted value = 0.0012; nominal enrichment score = 2.325; Figure 3B), according to the returned statistics using a default of 1000 permutations. Akin to prior observations [10], the hallmark *unfolded protein response* (UPR) pathway (i.e., genes upregulated during UPR/ER stress) was the second most activated pathway (p-adjusted value = 0.0012; nominal enrichment score = 2.173). WSPM treatment was also associated with a decrease in the hallmark *E2F target* pathway (i.e., genes encoding cell cycle-related targets of E2F transcription factors; p-adjusted value = 0.0012; nominal enrichment score = −2.694) and *G2M checkpoint* (genes involved in the G2/M checkpoint and progression through the cell cycle; p-adjusted value = 0.0012; nominal enrichment score = −2.716). These latter phenomena presumably developed from cell-cycle arrest driven by activation of the unfolded protein/ER stress response, as previously described for WSPM and the ER stress/the unfolded protein response pathway in general [10,27–29].

The relative expression of specific genes driving the pathway predictions (i.e., leading edge genes; $p < 0.05$) is compared in Figure 4A–D. For example, for the ROS/oxidative stress pathway, thioredoxin reductase, genes involved in glutathione metabolism (GCLC glutamate–cysteine ligase catalytic subunit; GCLC, GCLM glutamate-cysteine ligase modifier subunit; GCLM), and glutaredoxin (GLRX) were upregulated by WSPM and attenuated by Vasaka tea cotreatment. Similarly, X-box-binding protein 1 (XBP1), protein disulfide isomerase family A member 6 (PDIA6), heat-shock protein family A member 5 (HSPA5/BiP/GRP78), and stanniocalcin 2 (STC2), among other genes commonly associated with the unfolded protein/ER stress pathway, were upregulated by WSPM treatment, and attenuated with Vasaka tea cotreatment. Other pathways of interest included hallmark *hypoxia*, *xenobiotic metabolism*, *Kras signaling (up and down)*, *glycolysis*, *cholesterol metabolism*, and *mitotic spindle* (leading edge analyses data are shown in Figure S1A–E). Regarding glycolysis, a related metabolomics analysis of BEAS-2B AECs treated with WSPM identified a time-dependent shift in metabolism in treated cells, wherein glycolytic metabolism was affected (i.e., the Warburg effect was observed; Figure S2).

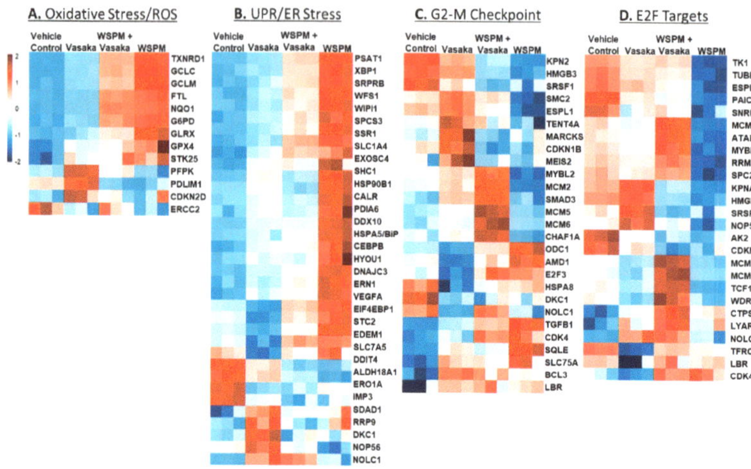

Figure 4. Heatmaps comparing the expression of significantly altered genes associated with the (**A**) hallmark *ROS/oxidative stress response* pathway, (**B**) the *unfolded protein response* pathway, (**C**) the hallmark *G2M checkpoint* pathway, and (**D**) the hallmark *E2F targets* pathway in HBEC3-KT cells treated with vehicle (cell culture medium + 0.2% DMSO), WSPM (10 μg/cm^2), Vasaka tea (1.25 mg/mL), or WSPM and Vasaka tea.

Additional significantly modified genes induced by WSPM that were not linked with any of the pathways identified by GSEA included anterior gradient protein 2 homolog (AGR2) and transient receptor potential vanilloid-3 (TRPV3). AGR2 is an ER-associated protein disulfide isomerase necessary for *MUC5AC* expression and secretion [30], while TRPV3 induction by WSPM and other causes of cell injury including prototypical ER stress-inducing agents has previously been found to be protective [10,31]; induction of both genes was inhibited by Vasaka tea cotreatment (Figure 5).

2.4. Vasaka Tea Attenuated WSPM-Induced AEC Damage In Vitro

Vasaka tea cotreatment of HBEC-3KT cells also protected AECs from WSPM damage (Figure 6). HBEC3-KT cells treated with WSPM (20 μg/cm^2) exhibited time-dependent disruption of cell morphology and monolayer integrity beginning within ~4 h of treatment, with evidence of mounting damage occurring over ~24 h (Figure S3 Movies). AEC damage was characterized by a decrease in mean area, perimeter, and internal density. While the AEC monolayer remained distinguishable from control cells when cotreated with WSPM and Vasaka tea, protection was observed as indicated by the partial attenuation of WSPM-induced changes in cell morphology and monolayer integrity.

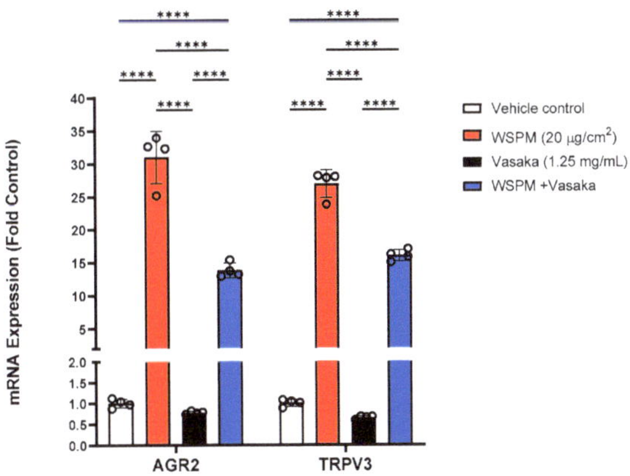

Figure 5. Comparison of *AGR2* and *TRPV3* mRNA expression in HBEC3-KT cells treated with vehicle (cell culture medium + 0.2% DMSO), WSPM (10 μg/cm^2), Vasaka tea (1.25 mg/mL), or WSPM and Vasaka tea using qPCR. Replicates within each group are shown as open circles. **** $p < 0.0001$ using 2-way ANOVA and Tukey post-test to compare the effects of treatment on mRNA expression for each gene ($n = 4$).

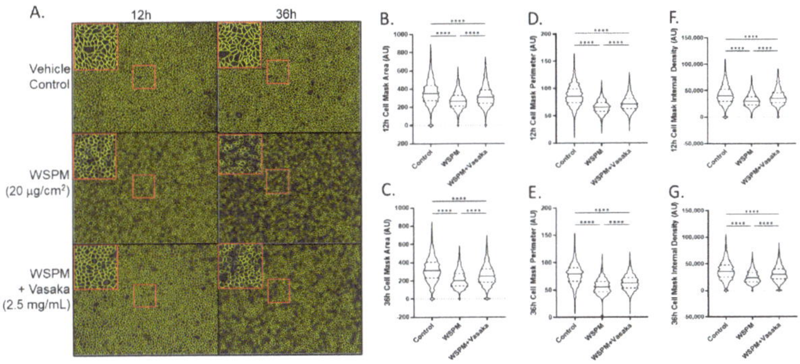

Figure 6. Comparison of HBEC3-KT morphological features and monolayer integrity as a function of WSPM and Vasaka tea treatments and time. Confluent monolayers of HBEC3-KT cells were treated with WSPM (20 μg/cm^2) or WSPM + Vasaka tea (2.5 mg/mL) and imaged using an Incucyte live cell imaging system. (**A**) Representative images 12 h and 36 h post treatment with a cell mask overlaid in yellow. Red boxes indicate expanded regions of the image. Quantification of (**B**,**C**) cell area, (**D**,**E**) cell perimeter, and (**F**,**G**) internal density of cells at 12 and 36 h. **** $p < 0.0001$ using ANOVA and Tukey post-test to compare the average feature values as a function of treatments. Movies showing changes associated with the treatments are shown in the Supplementary Materials.

2.5. Vasaka Components Exhibited Variable Inhibition of TRPA1, ER and Oxidative Stress, and *MUC5AC* Induction

Vasaka tea contains numerous chemicals that may or may not inhibit TRPA1, prevent ER and/or oxidative stress, or attenuate *MUC5AC* induction. Reported chemicals include vasicine, vasicinone, apigenin, and a variety of glycated flavonoids [32]. Vasicine, vasicinone, isoorientin, isovitexin, and apigenin were quantified in the Vasaka tea using liquid chromatography–tandem mass spectrometry (LC/MS/MS). The concentrations estimated for a 1 mg/mL solution of Vasaka tea were as follows (in μM): vasicinone (290 ± 52), vasicine (33 ± 4), isoorientin (0.27 ± 0.007), isovitexin (0.6 ± 0.2), and apigenin (<LLOQ; Figure 7A and Figure S4); vitexin is apigenin-8-C-glucoside, isovitexin is apigenin-6-C-glucoside, and isoorientin is luteolin-6-C-glucoside. The structures of these compounds

and mirror match spectra from the untargeted LC/MS/MS analyses described below are shown in Figure S4B. While free apigenin was not detected in the Vasaka tea, it may be liberated from C- and O-linked glucosides (e.g., schaftoside, isoschaftoside, vitexin, isovitexin, vicinin, and apiin) [33–37], and it has been reported to occur in Vasaka extracts by others [32]. Accordingly, apigenin was included in further studies.

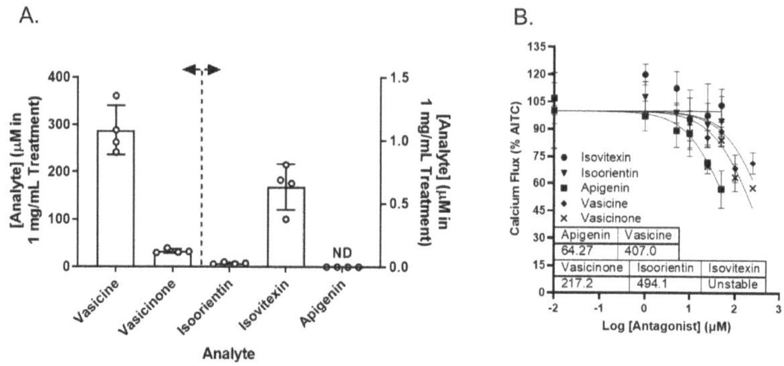

Figure 7. (**A**) Estimated concentrations of vasicine, vasicinone, isoorientin, isovitexin, and apigenin in a 1 mg/mL solution of Vasaka tea. Analytes were quantified by LC/MS/MS (n = 4 extracts). The dashed line and arrows indicate which y-axis the data are plotted on and replicates within each group are shown as open circles. A representative LC/MS/MS chromatogram is shown in Figure S4. (**B**) Inhibition of AITC-induced (TRPA1-dependent) calcium flux in HBEC3-KT cells treated with increasing concentrations of apigenin, vasicine, and vasicinone and stimulated with AITC (25 µM). Data were modeled using the log (antagonist) vs. response equation in GraphPad 9.5 software to estimate the IC_{50} value (n = 3–4).

Vasicine, vasicinone, isoorientin, isovitexin, and apigenin were evaluated as TRPA1 antagonists. Vasicine, vasicinone, and apigenin dose-dependently inhibited TRPA1, albeit with variable and relatively low potency. Isovitexin and isoorientin had minimal inhibitory effect up to 50 µM. The IC_{50} values for vasicine, vasicinone, isoorientin, and apigenin were estimated to be ~407, 217, 494, and 64 µM, respectively (Figure 7B).

Vasicine, vasicinone, isoorientin, isovitexin, and apigenin were also tested for the ability to attenuate ER stress (DNA damage-inducible transcript-3; *DDIT3*), oxidative stress (heme oxygenase-1; *HMOX1*), and *MUC5AC* mRNA induction using concentrations predicted to be in Vasaka tea when applied to cells at a concentration of ~1–2 mg/mL (Figure 8A–C). Vasicine (300 µM), vasicinone (50 µM), and vitexin (2.5 µM) failed to inhibit *DDIT3* induction, but isovitexin, isoorientin, and apigenin (all at 2.5 µM) reduced this response ~30%. All compounds also slightly reduced *HMOX1* induction, but only apigenin (2.5 µM) appeared to reduce *MUC5AC* mRNA induction. Lastly, apigenin and vitexin, but not isoorientin, vasicine, vasicinone, or isovitexin exhibited protective effects with respect to AEC monolayer damage (Figure 8D,E).

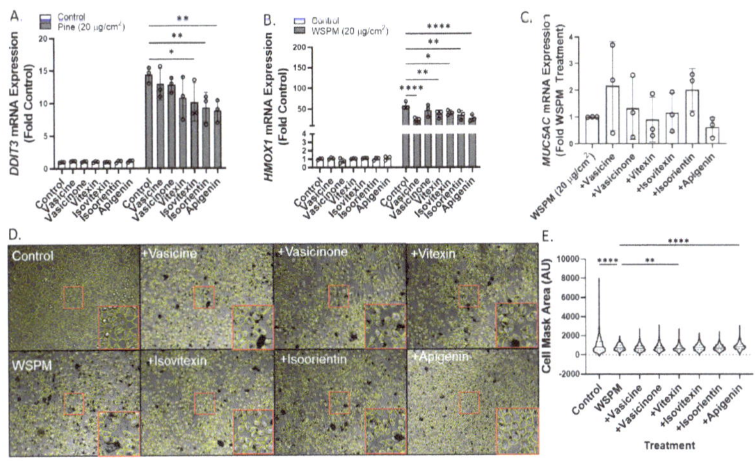

Figure 8. Comparison of (**A**) *DDIT3*, (**B**) *HMOX1*, and (**C**) *MUC5AC* mRNA expression in HBEC3-KT cells treated with vehicle (cell culture medium + 0.2% DMSO), WSPM (20 µg/cm^2), and various concentrations of Vasaka tea components using qPCR (vasicine = 300 µM; vasicinone = 50 µM; vitexin = 2.5 µM; isovitexin = 2.5 µM; isoorientin = 2.5 µM; apigenin = 2.5 µM, based on Figure 7A. replicates within each group are shown as open circles. * $p < 0.05$, ** $p < 0.01$ and **** $p < 0.0001$ using two-way ANOVA and Dunnett post-test to compare the effects of treatment on mRNA expression for each gene compared to the control ($n = 3$). (**D**) Representative images 24 h post treatment collected using a Molecular Devices Image Express PICO with cell masks overlaid in yellow. Red boxes indicate expanded regions of the image. (**E**) Cell area as a function of treatments. ** $p < 0.01$ and **** $p < 0.0001$ using ANOVA and Dunnett post-test to compare to the effects of WSPM treatment.

2.6. *Vasaka Tea Is a Complex Mixture*

Vasaka tea was also analyzed using untargeted LC/MS/MS and the Global Natural Products Social Molecular Networking (GNPS) Knowledge Base library search function [38] to identify additional Vasaka tea components (i.e., dereplication). Representative positive and negative electrospray ionization (+ and − ESI) LC/MS chromatograms are shown in Figure S5A,B. The GNPS results summary file is also included in the Supplementary Materials, and mzML raw data files are available upon request. To summarize, multiple previously reported chemicals were identified, including vasicine, vasicinone, isovitexin, vitexin, and numerous other flavonoids and glycated flavonoids.

Previously unreported linoleic acid-derived oxylipins were also identified in Vasaka tea, including 9,10- and 12,13-EpOME (epoxy-9Z-octadecenoic acids), 9,10- and 12,13-DiHOME (dihydroxyoctadec-9-enoic acids), 9- and 13-HODE (hydroxyoctadecadienoic acids), 9-oxoODE (9-oxo-10E,12Z-octadecadienoic acid), and 9- and 13-HpODE (hydroperoxy-9Z,11E-octadecadienoic acids). These results were verified using water to prepare Vasaka tea as opposed to cell culture medium which contained linoleic acid. Mirror match spectra of these compounds as determined by GNPS analysis are shown in Figure S6A–E, and a chromatogram from targeted oxylipin analysis is shown in Figure S6F. Quantification of linoleic acid-derived oxylipins in Vasaka tea prepared in water by LC/MS/MS estimated concentrations in a 1 mg/mL Vasaka tea solution to be as follows (in mM): 12,13-DiHOME (1.1 ± 0.2), 9,10-DiHOME (0.32 ± 0.07), 13(S)-HODE (86 ± 8), 9(S)-HODE (131 ± 9), 13-oxoODE (31 ± 4), 9-oxoODE (33 ± 3), 12,13-EpOME (0.25 ± 0.06), and 9,10-EpOME (0.55 ± 0.07) (Figure 9A).

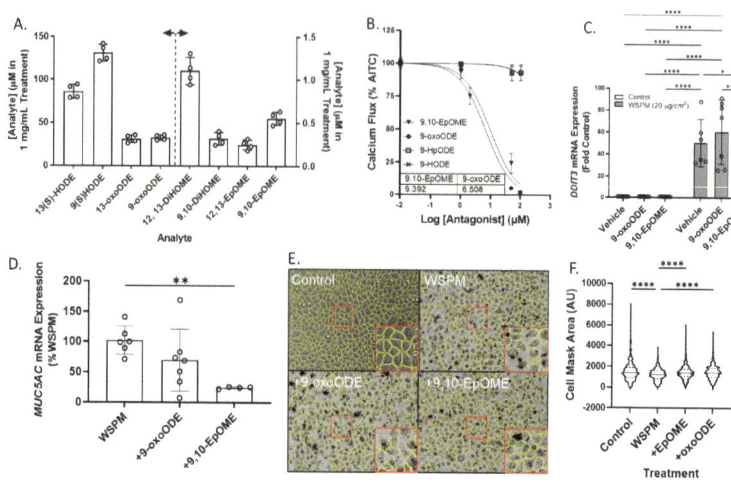

Figure 9. (**A**) Estimated concentrations of 13(S)- and 9(S)-HODE, 13-oxo and 9-oxoODE, 12,13-and 9,10-DiHOME, and 12,13- and 9,10-EpOME in a 1 mg/mL solution of Vasaka tea. Analytes were quantified by LC/MS/MS (n = 4 extracts). The dashed line and arrows indicate which y-axis the data are plotted on and replicates within each group are shown as open circles. A representative LC/MS/MS chromatogram is shown in Figure S6F. (**B**) Inhibition of AITC-induced (TRPA1-dependent) calcium flux in HBEC3-KT cells treated with various concentrations of oxylipins and stimulated with AITC (25 μM). Data were modeled with the log (antagonist) vs. response equation in GraphPad 9.5 software to estimate the IC_{50} value (n = 3–6). (**C**) *DDIT3* and (**D**) *MUC5AC* mRNA expression in HBEC3-KT cells treated with WSPM (20 μg/cm^2) with and without pre- (30 min) and cotreatment with 9-oxoODE or 9,10-EpOME (1 μM). * $p < 0.05$, ** $p < 0.01$, *** $p < 0.001$ and **** $p < 0.0001$ using two-way ANOVA and a Tukey post hoc test comparing all groups (panel **D**) and ANOVA with a Dunnett post-test comparing the effects of treatment relative to WSPM treatment (panel **C**). n = 4–7. (**E**) Representative images 24 h post treatment collected using a Molecular Devices Image Express PICO with cell masks overlaid in yellow. Red boxes indicate expanded regions of the image. (**F**) Cell area as a function of treatments. **** $p < 0.0001$ using ANOVA and Dunnett post-test to compare to the effects of WSPM treatment. Data showing TRPA1 agonist and antagonist effects of 9-oxoODE, 9-HpODE, 9,10-EpOME, and 9-HODE at 50 μM are shown in Figure S7.

Both 9,10-EpOME and 9-oxoODE were found to inhibit TRPA1 activation by AITC (Figure 9B; IC_{50} ~9.4 and 6.5 μM, respectively), but only 9,10-EpOME reduced *DDIT3* and *MUC5AC* mRNA induction by WSPM (Figure 9C,D). 9,10-EpOME and, to a lesser extent, 9-oxoODE were also cytoprotective (Figure 9E,F). Of note, 9-HpODE was a TRPA1 agonist according to the inhibition of elicited calcium flux by the TRPA1 antagonist A967079, while 9-HODE had minimal effect on TRPA1 activity (Figure S7).

2.7. CYP1A1 Limited WSPM Toxicity

Cytochrome P450 1A1 (CYP1A1) was among the top dysregulated genes in AECs treated with WSPM and Vasaka tea (Figure 10A and Figure S1B). Pre- and cotreatment of HBEC3-KT cells with the CYP1A1 inhibitor 7-ethoxyresorufin (7-ER) [39,40] enhanced *CYP1A1* mRNA induction by WSPM akin to Vasaka tea (Figure 10B), enhanced the induction of *DDIT3* and *TRPV3* (ER stress markers; Figure 10C,D), and promoted *MUC5AC* mRNA expression (Figure 10E), suggesting that inhibition of CYP1A1 by Vasaka tea (likely by flavonoids) [41,42] may underlie the superinduction phenomenon, and that oxylipins produced by CYP1A1 (e.g., 9,10-EpOME) [43] may normally restrict injury and *MUC5AC* induction by WSPM.

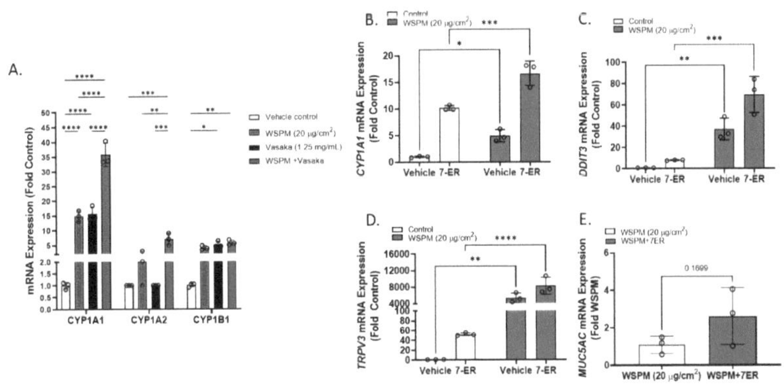

Figure 10. (**A**) Comparison of *CYP1A1*, *1A2*, and *1B1* mRNA expression by HBEC3-KT cells treated with vehicle (cell culture medium + 0.2% DMSO), WSPM (10 μg/cm^2), Vasaka tea (1.25 mg/mL), or WSPM and Vasaka tea. Replicates within each group are shown as open circles. Data were analyzed using two-way ANOVA with a Tukey post-test comparing the effects of treatments ($n = 3$). * $p < 0.05$, ** $p < 0.01$, *** $p < 0.001$, **** $p < 0.0001$. Expression of mRNA for (**B**) *CYP1A1*, (**C**) *DDIT3*, (**D**) *TRPV3*, and (**E**) *MUC5AC* as a function of WSPM treatment with and without pre- (2 h) and cotreatment with the CYP1A1 inhibitor 7-ethoxyresorufin (7-ER) ($n = 3$). Data were analyzed using two-way ANOVA and a Bonferroni post-test to compare the effects of each treatment. * $p < 0.05$, ** $p < 0.01$, *** $p < 0.001$, **** $p < 0.0001$.

3. Discussion

WSPM can be a prevalent household and ambient pollutant, and, in recent years, wildfires in North America have set records for the number of acres burned. While the type of biomass burned affects the characteristics and seemingly the relative potency of the resulting emissions as a pneumotoxin, we found that particle concentrates derived from burning pine, mesquite, sage, apple, range grass, sheep and cow dung, juniper, and other materials share the capacity to activate TRPA1, trigger ER stress, and induce *MUC5AC* expression [9,10]. While the selectivity for *MUC5AC* induction can also vary by WSPM and pollutant source/type, we and others have also found that TRPA1 can be activated and ER stress initiated by a variety of pneumotoxic ambient pollutants including diesel exhaust particles, cigarette smoke condensate, E-cigarette vaping products, and many other substances [9,10,44–48]. Thus, it is possible that the findings here could apply to a range of pneumotoxicants that humans can be exposed to on a frequent basis.

Currently, there are few if any therapeutics that prevent and/or directly treat lung injury, and available mucus-directed therapies are generally limited to expectorants and mucokinetics, although, in severe cases (e.g., ARDS), liquid ventilation can be used [49,50]. The most widely used mucus treatments include guaifenesin and anti-inflammatory oral and inhaled corticosteroids. Guaifenesin, derived from the Guaiac tree (FDA-approved and currently marketed as, e.g., Mucinex) acts as an expectorant by promoting discharge of mucus from the airways and facilitating mucociliary clearance. Guaifenesin is also weakly *MUC5AC*-suppressive [51] and can be paired with β_2-agonists to aid in mucus clearance. Glucocorticoids, β_2-agonists, and anticholinergic bronchodilators also relieve congestion and excess mucus production, and they are mainstay therapeutics for asthma [49]. While long-term therapy is possible with these agents, they are not known to prevent AEC injury as an origin for ectopic *MUC5AC* production. Furthermore, these agents are not guaranteed to work in all patients (e.g., people with glucocorticoid resistance), are costly, and have side-effects that may preclude their use in some circumstances and in some individuals. Chronic β_2-agonist therapy specifically may be counterproductive in terms of *MUC5AC* suppression [52–57]. Thus, a problem with current therapies is that, while they aid in inflammation and mucus clearance to provide relief, cell damage and excess mucus production can continue, adversely affecting lung functions because AEC injury is not addressed [49,58]. Regarding the management of environmentally induced pulmonary effects on the respiratory tract, addressing acute and recurrent AEC injury and ectopic *MUC5AC* expression and hypersecretion may be key.

Vasaka (generally as a tea) is used in traditional medicine to treat asthma and tuberculosis due to its purported antitussive and mucolytic properties [1,2,59]. Bromhexine and its metabolite ambroxol are over-the-counter medicines available in some locations around the world, used to treat respiratory ailments involving excess mucus [2,3,60–66]. These synthetic molecules were inspired by vasicine and vasicinone, two of the most abundant chemicals in Vasaka, and they act by disrupting the structure of mucopolysaccharide fibers in sputum and decreasing viscosity such that the mucus can be cleared. Ambroxol has also been shown to stimulate surfactant production by alveolar type II cells, as well as inhibit immunoglobulin E (IgE)-dependent histamine release and the production of interleukin (IL)-4 and -13 by mast cells and basophils, in part, by modulating kinase signaling. Bromhexine, ambroxol, and another vasicine-based synthetic agent R8 have also been shown to be mildly *MUC5AC*-suppressive [51,67,68], but how these agents affect *MUC5AC* and AECs in general is not completely understood. Additionally, they are not widely available.

This study shows that Vasaka tea itself may be a source of therapeutic mucosuppressing agents that can also protect AECs from the damaging effects of WSPM, and possibly other TRPA1 agonists. Use of Vasaka in traditional medicine typically involves consumption as tea. If reports on the benefits of Vasaka on respiratory illnesses are true, it may be possible that one or more of the compounds in the tea have the capacity to distribute to the lungs through systemic circulation where they may limit AEC damage and/or associated proinflammatory effects triggered by the inciting stimulus. According to the results herein, this may involve TRPA1 inhibition, which, in the case of environmental exposures to pollutants that activate TRPA1 (WSPM, diesel exhaust, cigarette smoke, vaping chemicals, etc.), could be beneficial. Additional benefits may arise from antioxidants in the tea, flavonoids that modulate CYP enzyme functions and other cellular processes, bioactive lipids, and EGFR modulators. For example, apigenin, identified as protective in this study via apparent interactions with TRPA1, has also been reported to inhibit EGFR activation [69], which would become active downstream of TRPA1 in the scenario tested here. It is also possible that Vasaka tea could act at the systemic level to impact respiratory symptomatology. While not directly tested, modulation of TRPA1 in immune or other cell types (e.g., vascular endothelial cells in the alveolar capillaries) could be part of this process. Regardless, the abundance of bioactive flavonoids and oxylipins in Vasaka tea may contribute to the overall pneumoprotective and mucosuppressive effects of Vasaka tea.

Regarding potential therapeutic opportunities based on Vasaka and use of Vasaka itself, several protective and mucosuppressing compounds were identified in the tea that could potentially be delivered systemically or directly to the lungs on an as-needed basis. These include selected flavonoids (e.g., apigenin) and 9,10-EpOME. The finding that some oxylipins were TRPA1 antagonists was surprising as others have reported that they activate rodent TRPA1 [70], and we previously found that arachidonic acid-derived oxylipins produced from *Cyp1b1* metabolism could sensitize TRPA1 and promote chronic pain in mice [48]. While not shown, both 9,10-EpOME and 9-oxoODE were also able to activate TRPA1 at concentrations ~100 μM. Accordingly, careful consideration of dose would be needed to use these substances as therapeutics. Regardless, the data suggest a novel interaction between CYP enzymes and TRPA1 involving lipid-derived epoxides, wherein pre-emptive induction of CYPs by Vasaka (perhaps due to the presence of CYP1A1-inhibiting flavonoids) [71,72] may promote a net anti-inflammatory environment wherein TRPA1, ER stress, and *MUC5AC* induction are suppressed. This is consistent with the broad anti-inflammatory effects of other CYP1A inducers such as the endogenous arylhydrocarbon receptor ligand 6-formylindolo[3,2-b]carbazole (FICZ) [73]. Accordingly, dietary supplementation using, for example, linoleic acid, flavonoids, or perhaps even standardized extracts of Vasaka may be advantageous. To conclude, these ideas will require further study to establish feasibility, efficacy, and safety. However, the cumulative results from this study support efforts to develop Vasaka for preventing and treating respiratory conditions arising from exposure to toxic air pollutants that target the TRPA1 receptor.

4. Materials and Methods

4.1. Chemicals and Reagents

Vasicine, vasicinone, isoorientin, isovitexin, vitexin, apigenin, 12,13-DiHOME, 9,10-DiHOME, 13(S)-HODE, 9(S)-HODE, 13-oxoODE, 9-oxoODE, 12,13-EpOME and 9,10-EpOME, 9-HpODE, and 7-ethoxyresorufin were purchased from Cayman Chemical (Ann Arbor, MI, USA). AITC, ionomycin calcium salt, HC-030039, and A967079 were from Sigma-Aldrich (St. Louis, MO, USA). DMSO was from Fisher Scientific (Waltham, MA, USA).

4.2. WSPM

Preparation of pine WSPM was described in [47]. Briefly, ~10 g of 1 inch toothpick-to pencil-sized pieces of Austrian pine (from a tree growing in the Salt Lake Valley) were burned in a pipe furnace at 750 °C with constant air flow. WSPM was collected using an Anderson cascade impactor operated at 1 L/min, and fractions 6 and 7 (0.65–1.1 µm and 0.43–0.65 µm) were used. For experiments, WSPM concentrate was suspended in DMSO at ~100× the target concentration and diluted in cell culture medium for treatments.

4.3. Preparation of Vasaka Tea

Vasaka tea was prepared by incubating a suspension of organic Vasaka powder (Banyan Botanicals; 20 mg/mL) in cell culture medium for 30 min at 37 °C. The tube was vortexed every 5 min, and after 30 min the suspension was centrifuged at 20,000× *g* for 2 min, followed by filtration of the supernatant using a 0.22 µm syringe filter. The Vasaka tea was used fresh by diluting into cell culture medium or stored frozen as a concentrate at −80 °C for up to 1 month. Blank medium processed in parallel was used as a negative control.

4.4. Cell Culture

BEAS-2B (used only in a metabolomics study) and HBEC3-KT cells were purchased from ATCC (Rockville, MD, USA). Cells were maintained in a humidified cell culture incubator at 37 °C with a 95% air:5% CO_2 atmosphere and sub-cultured every 2–3 days when cells reached ~80% confluence using trypsin. BEAS-2B cells were grown in LHC-9 medium (LHC-8 supplemented with 33 nM retinoic acid and 2.75 µM epinephrine), while HBEC3-KT cells were cultured in airway epithelial cell basal medium supplemented with a bronchial epithelial cell growth kit, 30 µg/mL geneticin, and 250 ng/mL puromycin.

4.5. Gene Expression Analysis/RNA qPCR

Cells were plated and treated at ~90% confluence. After treatment, total RNA was isolated using the Invitrogen PureLink RNA Mini Kit and quantified by UV absorbance on a Nanodrop One^{c}. cDNA (2 µg) was synthesized using the Applied Biosystems High-Capacity cDNA Synthesis Kit with RNase inhibitor. Transcript abundance was quantified using TaqMan gene expression master mix (ThermoFisher, Waltham, MA, USA) on a Life Technologies QuantStudio 6 Flex instrument. The following TaqMan probe-based assays were used: human *MUC5AC* (Hs_01365616_m1); human HMOX1 (Hs01110250_m1); human DDIT3 (Hs_00358796_g1); human TRPV3 (Hs00376854_m1). The PCR programs used were according to supplier recommendations. Expression values were normalized to human β2-microglobulin (β*2M*; Hs00984230_m1), and to the average of the control samples.

4.6. TRPA1 Activity Assays

Calcium flux was measured using the Fluo-4 Direct assay kit and imaging on an EVOS FL Auto microscope at 10× magnification using a green fluorescent protein (GFP) filter as described [10,45,46,74]. Cells were plated in a flat bottom 96-well plate at ~25,000 cells/cm^2 and assayed at 80–90%. Prior to assay, cells were loaded with Fluo-4 diluted 1:1 in calcium assay buffer (Hank's balanced salt solution, with $CaCl_2$ and $MgCl_2$, buffered to pH 7.3 with 20 mM HEPES; ThermoFisher) at ~23 °C for 1 h in the dark. After 1 h, the Fluo-4 was removed, and the cells were washed with calcium assay buffer containing 1 mM probenecid and 0.75 mM trypan red (ATT Bioquest; Sunnyvale, CA, USA). Cells were pretreated for 30 min or 2 h with various agents by diluting in the wash buffer and in the desired treatment solutions (i.e., AITC or WSPM). Assays were performed using an EVOS FL auto microscope with an on-stage environmental chamber maintained at 37 °C with a 95% air/5% CO_2 atmosphere. Agonist treatments (AITC or WSPM) were added to cells at 3× the desired final concentration in calcium assay buffer. Images were captured every 6 s for 72 s. Changes in fluorescence were quantified using a custom MATLAB program as previously described [46,74]. Reported values are from the 60 s timepoint and were corrected by subtracting the fluorescence response to a blank medium control (i.e., no agonist), then normalized to the response value at 72 s following ionomycin (20 μM) treatment applied after the 60 s image was taken.

4.7. Gene Expression Analysis/RNA Sequencing

RNA sequencing was performed at the High-Throughput Genomics Core Facility at the Huntsman Cancer Institute, University of Utah. Total RNA was extracted using the RNeasy Mini kit (Qiagen, Hilden, Germany) with on-column DNase digestion. RNA quality was assessed by Agilent TapeStation, and library construction was performed using the Illumina TruSeq Stranded *mRNA* Sample Preparation kit. RNAseq was performed on a NovaSeq6000 S4 instrument with a 150 × 150 paired-end format and 100 million read-pair depth. Results were processed with University of Utah Bioinformatics core support. Optical duplicates were removed, adaptors were trimmed, and STAR alignments were generated. Differential gene expression was determined using hciR and DESeq2 (1.30.1) and a 5% false-discovery rate. Pathway analysis was performed using fgsea (1.18.0) using the Hallmarks Molecular Signatures Database. The data presented in this publication were deposited in NCBI's Gene Expression Omnibus and are accessible through GEO Series accession number GSE232172.

4.8. Metabolomics Analysis

Confluent monolayers of BEAS-2B cells grown in T-25 flasks were treated for 0, 4 or 24 h with medium containing 0.2% DMSO or WSPM (20 μg/cm^2). Treatment medium was aspirated at 0, 4, and 24 h; the cells were rinsed 1× with 5 mL of cold phosphate-buffered saline, and immediately frozen at −80 °C. To each cell flask (n = 3; ~2.0 × 10^6 cells), 450 mL of cold 90% methanol containing the internal standard D_4-succinic acid (Sigma-Aldrich) was added. The samples were vortexed, incubated at −20 °C for 1 h, and centrifuged at 20,000× g for 10 min at 4 °C. Supernatant (400 mL) was then transferred and mixed with D_{27}-myristic acid (Sigma-Aldrich). Pooled quality control samples were prepared by removing a fraction of collected supernatant from each sample while process blanks were prepared using only extraction solvent, processed in parallel with the samples. All samples were then dried under vacuum prior to analysis. Samples were analyzed by gas chromatography/mass spectrometry (GC/MS) using an Agilent 7200 GC-QTOF fit with an Agilent 7693A autosampler. Dried samples were suspended in 40 μL of a 40 mg/mL methoxylamine hydrochloride (MOX) (MP Biomedicals, Irvine, CA) in dry pyridine and incubated for 1 h at 37 °C. This solution (25 μL) was added to auto sampler vials to which 60 μL of N-methyl-N-trimethylsilyltrifluoracetamide (MSTFA with 1% TMCS, ThermoFisher) was added via the autosampler and incubated for 30 min at 37 °C. After incubation, samples were vortexed, and 1 μL of the prepared sample was injected into the GC inlet in the split mode with the inlet temperature held at 250 °C. A 5:1 split ratio was used for analysis, and any metabolite that saturated the instrument response at the 5:1 split was re-analyzed at a 50:1 split ratio. The gas chromatograph had an initial temperature of 60 °C for 1 min followed by a 10 °C/min ramp to 325 °C and a hold time of 10 min. A 30 m Agilent Zorbax DB-5MS with 10 m Duraguard capillary column was employed for chromatographic separation. Helium was used as the carrier gas at a rate of 1 mL/min. Data were quantified relative to the internal standard and relative analyte/metabolite peak areas. Processed data were then analyzed for statistical differences and metabolic pathway perturbations using Metaboanalyst 5.0 [75]. Raw data are provided in the Supplementary Materials.

4.9. Image Analysis

Images were collected in real time using an Incucyte zoom (Essen Bio Science, Ann Arbor, MI, USA) and converted to movies using an Image Express PICO (Molecular Devices, San Jose, CA, USA). Image files (.jpg or .png) were analyzed using Cellpose 2.0 [76,77] with model training using images collected from multiple experiments. Image masks were created and saved, and then further processed using the Labels to ROIs plugin for Image J [78]. Following a 1 px erosion of the masks, cell area, perimeter, and integrated density were quantified.

4.10. Quantification of Known Vasaka Tea Chemicals by LC/MS/MS

Vasicine, vasicinone, isoorientin, isovitexin, and apigenin were quantified using a Thermo Vanquish Flex UPLC System interfaced with an LTQ Velos Pro Linear Ion Trap Mass Spectrometer (ThermoFisher, San Jose, CA, USA). Chromatographic separation of the analytes was achieved using a BEH C_{18} column (150 × 3 mm i.d.; 1.7 µm particle size; Waters, Milford, MA) at 50 °C with gradient elution. The mobile phases were (A) 0.1% formic acid in H_2O and (B) methanol and a flow rate of 300 mL/minute. The percentage of B varied as follows: 2% B at 0 min, 2%→95% (0 to 7.5 min), hold at 95% (7.5 to 8.5 min), 95%→2% (8.5 to 8.6 min), and hold at 2% from 8.6 to 10 min. A convex gradient (setting = 6 during the 0–7.5 min ramp) was used. The mass spectrometer was operated in positive electrospray ionization, selective reaction-monitoring mode. The MS/MS parameters were optimized by infusion of vasicine into the MS/MS system and the following precursor→product transitions were used: *m/z* 189.1→*m/z* 171.1 for vasicine, *m/z* 203.2→*m/z* 185.1 for vasicinone, *m/z* 449.1→*m/z* 431.1 for isoorientin, *m/z* 433.2→*m/z* 415.1 for isovitexin, and *m/z* 271.1→*m/z* 271.1 + 243.1 for apigenin. Data acquisition and processing were performed using Xcalibur software, and calibration curves were prepared in water using analyte peak area versus concentration.

4.11. Discovery Mass Spectrometry

The identification of additional components of Vasaka tea was achieved using positive and negative electrospray LC/MS/MS using a Thermo Vanquish Flex UPLC System interfaced with an LTQ Velos Pro Linear Ion Trap Mass Spectrometer, coupled with dataset interrogation/spectral matching using the Global Natural Products Social (GNPS) Molecular Networking Knowledge Base [38]. Chromatographic fractionation of Vasaka tea was achieved using a BEH C_{18} column (150 × 3 mm i.d.; 1.7 µm particle size; Waters, Milford, MA, USA) at 50 °C with gradient elution. The mobile phases were (A) 0.1% formic acid in H_2O and (B) methanol and a flow rate of 100 mL/min. The percentage of B varied as follows: 2% B at 0 min, 2%→100% (0 to 50 min), hold at 100% (50 to 55 min), 100%→2% (55.0 to 55.1 min), and hold at 2% (55.1 to 60 min). The mass spectrometer was programmed to assay both positive and negative ions *m/z* 100–750 (in separate acquisitions) using the "double play" data-dependent MS/MS mode. MS/MS scans were triggered by analytes having a signal intensity set at ~5× baseline using a collision energy of 30% or 45% (separate acquisitions). The top four peaks of each scan were analyzed, and dynamic exclusion was active. The parameters were as follows: repeat count = 3; repeat duration = 5 s; exclusion list size = 25; and exclusion duration = 5 s. Data were analyzed using GNPS. The .raw files were converted to mzML files using the GNPS quickstart feature. The files were then uploaded into GNPS and processed using the Library Search feature. Default criteria were used with the exception that the minimum matched peaks = 4 and top hits per spectrum = 5.

4.12. Quantification of Oxylipins in Vasaka Tea by LC/MS/MS

Quantification of 9(10)- and 12(13)-EpOME; 9(10)- and 12(13)-DiHOME, 9(S)- and 13(S)-HODE, and 9- and 13-oxoODE was achieved using a Thermo Vanquish Flex UPLC System interfaced with an LTQ Velos Pro Linear Ion Trap Mass Spectrometer. Chromatographic separation was achieved using a BEH C_{18} column (150 × 3 mm i.d.; 1.7 μm particle size; Waters, Milford, MA) at 35 °C with gradient elution. The mobile phases were (A) 0.1% acetic acid in H_2O and (B) 9:1 acetonitrile/isopropanol, and a flow rate of 250 mL/minute was used. The percentage of B varied as follows: 52.5% B at 0 min, 52.5%→57.5% (0 to 6 min), 62.5% at 6.1 min, 62.5%→77% (6.1 to 12.5 min), 77%→95% (12.5 to 16 min), 95% hold (16 to 19 min), 95%→5.25% (19 to 19.1 min), and 52.5% hold until 22 min. Negative electrospray ionization selective reaction monitoring was used. The MS/MS parameters were optimized by infusion of lipid standard (Cayman Chemical) solutions into the MS/MS system. The precursor→product transitions used were as follows: *m/z* 313.2→*m/z* 194.0 + 183.1 for 12(13)-DiHOME, *m/z* 313.2→*m/z* 201.1 + 171.1 for 9(10)-DiHOME, *m/z* 295.3→*m/z* 195.1 + 171.1 for 13(S) and 9(S)-HODE, as well as 12(13)- and 9(10)-EpOME, and *m/z* 293.2→*m/z* 185.1 + 113.1 for 13- and 9-oxoODE. The precursor-to-product ion transitions used for the internal standards were as follows: *m/z* 317.2→*m/z* 185.1 for 9(10)-EpOME-d_4, *m/z* 317.2→*m/z* 203.1 for 12(13)-EpOME-d_4, *m/z* 299.2→*m/z* 172.0 for 9(10)-DiHOME-d_4, and *m/z* 299.2→*m/z* 198.0 for 12(13)-DiHOME-d_4. Data acquisition and processing were performed using Xcalibur software with calibration curves prepared in water using the ratio of analyte to internal standard peak.

4.13. Statistical Analysis

Graphing and statistical analyses were performed using GraphPad Prism 9.5.0 software. Values are represented as the mean ± SD unless stated otherwise. For comparisons between two groups, the unpaired *t*-test was used. One- or two-way ANOVA with Tukey's or a Bonferroni post-test was used for multiple comparisons. A *p*-value <0.05 was considered significant.

5. Conclusions

A tea prepared from a Vasaka supplement was found to inhibit the TRPA1 receptor and attenuate WSPM-induced AEC damage and ectopic *MUC5AC* expression in vitro. These effects were attributable to an attenuation of TRPA1-induced ER stress and, to a lesser extent, oxidative stress by selected flavones (i.e., apigenin) and linoleic-derived oxylipins (i.e., 9,10-EpOME) present in the tea. It is possible that these mechanisms may underlie the purported beneficial effects of Vasaka and Vasaka tea in treating respiratory malaise, and that a standardized Vasaka tea/supplement or pure apigenin and/or 9,10-EpOME may provide therapeutic benefit.

Supplementary Materials: The following supporting information can be downloaded at https://www.mdpi.com/article/10.3390/ph16060890/s1: Figure S1A–E. comparison of the expression of leading-edge genes associated with the (A) hypoxia, (B) xenobiotic metabolism, (C) Kras up and down, (D) glycolysis and cholesterol homeostasis, and (E) mitotic spindle hallmark pathways obtained from RNA sequencing analysis of HBEC3-KT cells treated with WSPM and Vasaka tea; Figure S2. Comparison of metabolomic pathway signatures in control and WSPM-treated BEAS-2B cells, as generated by data analysis using Metaboanalyst 5.0; Figure S3. Movies of HBEC3-KT cells treated with vehicle, WSPM, or WSPM + Vasaka tea; Figure S4A,B. LC/MS/MS selective reaction monitoring chromatogram and mirror match spectra for vasicine, vasicinone, isoorientin, isovitexin, and apigenin analysis; Figure S5a,b. +ESI and −ESI LC/MS chromatograms from untargeted LC/MS/MS analysis of Vasaka tea; Figure S6A–F. Mirror match MS/MS spectra for the identification of oxylipins in Vasaka tea and LC/MS/MS selective reaction monitoring chromatogram from oxylipin quantification by

LC/MS/MS; Figure S7. Data showing the activation and inhibition of TRPA1 activity by selected oxylipins.

Author Contributions: Conceptualization, T.A.M., L.S., M.A.-R. and C.A.R.; methodology, T.A.M., L.S., M.A.-R., P.J.M., C.E.D.-R. and C.A.R.; software, not applicable; validation, not applicable; formal analysis, T.A.M., L.S., M.A.-R., P.J.M., C.E.D.-R. and C.A.R.; investigation, T.A.M., L.S., M.A.-R., P.J.M., C.E.D.-R. and C.A.R.; resources, C.A.R.; data curation, not applicable; writing—original draft preparation, T.A.M., L.S., M.A.-R., P.J.M., C.E.D.-R. and C.A.R.; writing—review and editing, T.A.M., L.S., M.A.-R., P.J.M., C.E.D.-R. and C.A.R.; visualization, not applicable; supervision, C.A.R.; project administration, C.A.R.; funding acquisition, C.E.D.-R. and C.A.R. All authors have read and agreed to the published version of the manuscript.

Funding: This research was funded by The National Institute of Environmental Health Sciences (NIEHS) through grants numbers ES017431 and ES027015.

Institutional Review Board Statement: Not applicable.

Informed Consent Statement: Not applicable.

Data Availability Statement: All data presented in the study are available in the main manuscript or Supplementary Materials. The RNA sequencing data presented in this publication were deposited in the National Center for Biotechnology Information (NCBI) Gene Expression Omnibus (GEO) and are accessible through GEO Series accession number GSE232172. Raw data will be made available upon request.

Acknowledgments: The authors would like to acknowledge the University of Utah Metabolomics and Huntsman Cancer Institute High-Throughput Genomics and Bioinformatics Cores and staff. The authors also thank Erin G. Romero for assistance with final editing.

Conflicts of Interest: The authors declare no conflict of interest. The funders had no role in the design of the study; in the collection, analyses, or interpretation of data; in the writing of the manuscript; or in the decision to publish the results.

References

1. Cambridge, G.W.; Jansen, A.B.; Jarman, D.A. Bronchodilating action of vasicinone and related compounds. *Nature* **1962**, *196*, 1217. [CrossRef] [PubMed]
2. Grange, J.M.; Snell, N.J. Activity of bromhexine and ambroxol, semi-synthetic derivatives of vasicine from the Indian shrub Adhatoda vasica, against Mycobacterium tuberculosis in vitro. *J. Ethnopharmacol.* **1996**, *50*, 49–53. [CrossRef] [PubMed]
3. Rachana, B.S.; Mamta, P.; Priyanka, K.M.; Sonam, S. Review & Future Perspectives of Using Vasicine, and Related Compounds. *Indo-Glob. J. Pharm. Sci.* **2011**, *1*, 85–98.
4. Tuazon, J.A.; Kilburg-Basnyat, B.; Oldfield, L.M.; Wiscovitch-Russo, R.; Dunigan-Russell, K.; Fedulov, A.V.; Oestreich, K.J.; Gowdy, K.M. Emerging Insights into the Impact of Air Pollution on Immune-Mediated Asthma Pathogenesis. *Curr. Allergy Asthma Rep.* **2022**, *22*, 77–92. [CrossRef] [PubMed]
5. Grant, T.L.; Wood, R.A. The influence of urban exposures and residence on childhood asthma. *Pediatr. Allergy Immunol.* **2022**, *33*, e13784. [CrossRef] [PubMed]
6. Thurston, G.D.; Balmes, J.R.; Garcia, E.; Gilliland, F.D.; Rice, M.B.; Schikowski, T.; Van Winkle, L.S.; Annesi-Maesano, I.; Burchard, E.G.; Carlsten, C.; et al. Outdoor Air Pollution and New-Onset Airway Disease. An Official American Thoracic Society Workshop Report. *Ann. Am. Thorac. Soc.* **2020**, *17*, 387–398. [CrossRef] [PubMed]
7. Duan, R.R.; Hao, K.; Yang, T. Air pollution and chronic obstructive pulmonary disease. *Chronic Dis. Transl. Med.* **2020**, *6*, 260–269. [CrossRef]
8. Manisalidis, I.; Stavropoulou, E.; Stavropoulos, A.; Bezirtzoglou, E. Environmental and Health Impacts of Air Pollution: A Review. *Front. Public Health* **2020**, *8*, 14. [CrossRef]
9. Memon, T.A.; Nguyen, N.D.; Burrell, K.L.; Scott, A.F.; Almestica-Roberts, M.; Rapp, E.; Deering-Rice, C.E.; Reilly, C.A. Wood Smoke Particles Stimulate *MUC5AC* Overproduction by Human Bronchial Epithelial Cells Through TRPA1 and EGFR Signaling. *Toxicol. Sci.* **2020**, *174*, 278–290. [CrossRef]
10. Nguyen, N.D.; Memon, T.A.; Burrell, K.L.; Almestica-Roberts, M.; Rapp, E.; Sun, L.; Scott, A.F.; Rower, J.E.; Deering-Rice, C.E.; Reilly, C.A. Transient Receptor Potential Ankyrin-1 and Vanilloid-3 Differentially Regulate Endoplasmic Reticulum Stress and Cytotoxicity in Human Lung Epithelial Cells after Pneumotoxic Wood Smoke Particle Exposure. *Mol. Pharmacol.* **2020**, *98*, 586–597. [CrossRef]
11. Orozco-Levi, M.; Garcia-Aymerich, J.; Villar, J.; Ramirez-Sarmiento, A.; Anto, J.M.; Gea, J. Wood smoke exposure and risk of chronic obstructive pulmonary disease. *Eur. Respir. J.* **2006**, *27*, 542–546. [CrossRef]

12. Swiston, J.R.; Davidson, W.; Attridge, S.; Li, G.T.; Brauer, M.; van Eeden, S.F. Wood smoke exposure induces a pulmonary and systemic inflammatory response in firefighters. *Eur. Respir. J.* **2008**, *32*, 129–138. [CrossRef]
13. Thorning, D.R.; Howard, M.L.; Hudson, L.D.; Schumacher, R.L. Pulmonary responses to smoke inhalation: Morphologic changes in rabbits exposed to pine wood smoke. *Hum. Pathol.* **1982**, *13*, 355–364. [CrossRef]
14. Ghio, A.J.; Soukup, J.M.; Case, M.; Dailey, L.A.; Richards, J.; Berntsen, J.; Devlin, R.B.; Stone, S.; Rappold, A. Exposure to wood smoke particles produces inflammation in healthy volunteers. *Occup. Environ. Med.* **2012**, *69*, 170–175. [CrossRef]
15. Liu, J.C.; Wilson, A.; Mickley, L.J.; Dominici, F.; Ebisu, K.; Wang, Y.; Sulprizio, M.P.; Peng, R.D.; Yue, X.; Son, J.Y.; et al. Wildfire-specific Fine Particulate Matter and Risk of Hospital Admissions in Urban and Rural Counties. *Epidemiology* **2017**, *28*, 77–85. [CrossRef]
16. Reid, C.E.; Jerrett, M.; Tager, I.B.; Petersen, M.L.; Mann, J.K.; Balmes, J.R. Differential respiratory health effects from the 2008 northern California wildfires: A spatiotemporal approach. *Environ. Res.* **2016**, *150*, 227–235. [CrossRef]
17. Laumbach, R.J.; Kipen, H.M. Respiratory health effects of air pollution: Update on biomass smoke and traffic pollution. *J. Allergy Clin. Immunol.* **2012**, *129*, 3–11, Quiz 12–13. [CrossRef] [PubMed]
18. Olloquequi, J.; Silva, O.R. Biomass smoke as a risk factor for chronic obstructive pulmonary disease: Effects on innate immunity. *Innate Immun.* **2016**, *22*, 373–381. [CrossRef]
19. Hauber, H.P.; Foley, S.C.; Hamid, Q. Mucin overproduction in chronic inflammatory lung disease. *Can. Respir. J.* **2006**, *13*, 327–335. [CrossRef] [PubMed]
20. Kesimer, M.; Ford, A.A.; Ceppe, A.; Radicioni, G.; Cao, R.; Davis, C.W.; Doerschuk, C.M.; Alexis, N.E.; Anderson, W.H.; Henderson, A.G.; et al. Airway Mucin Concentration as a Marker of Chronic Bronchitis. *N. Engl. J. Med.* **2017**, *377*, 911–922. [CrossRef] [PubMed]
21. Ermund, A.; Meiss, L.N.; Rodriguez-Pineiro, A.M.; Bahr, A.; Nilsson, H.E.; Trillo-Muyo, S.; Ridley, C.; Thornton, D.J.; Wine, J.J.; Hebert, H.; et al. The normal trachea is cleaned by MUC5B mucin bundles from the submucosal glands coated with the *MUC5AC* mucin. *Biochem. Biophys. Res. Commun.* **2017**, *492*, 331–337. [CrossRef] [PubMed]
22. Roy, M.G.; Livraghi-Butrico, A.; Fletcher, A.A.; McElwee, M.M.; Evans, S.E.; Boerner, R.M.; Alexander, S.N.; Bellinghausen, L.K.; Song, A.S.; Petrova, Y.M.; et al. Muc5b is required for airway defence. *Nature* **2014**, *505*, 412–416. [CrossRef] [PubMed]
23. Caramori, G.; Casolari, P.; Di Gregorio, C.; Saetta, M.; Baraldo, S.; Boschetto, P.; Ito, K.; Fabbri, L.M.; Barnes, P.J.; Adcock, I.M.; et al. *MUC5AC* expression is increased in bronchial submucosal glands of stable COPD patients. *Histopathology* **2009**, *55*, 321–331. [CrossRef]
24. Evans, C.M.; Raclawska, D.S.; Ttofali, F.; Liptzin, D.R.; Fletcher, A.A.; Harper, D.N.; McGing, M.A.; McElwee, M.M.; Williams, O.W.; Sanchez, E.; et al. The polymeric mucin *MUC5AC* is required for allergic airway hyperreactivity. *Nat. Commun.* **2015**, *6*, 6281. [CrossRef] [PubMed]
25. Welsh, K.G.; Rousseau, K.; Fisher, G.; Bonser, L.R.; Bradding, P.; Brightling, C.E.; Thornton, D.J.; Gaillard, E.A. *MUC5AC* and a Glycosylated Variant of MUC5B Alter Mucin Composition in Children with Acute Asthma. *Chest* **2017**, *152*, 771–779. [CrossRef]
26. Samsuzzaman, M.; Uddin, M.S.; Shah, M.A.; Mathew, B. Natural inhibitors on airway mucin: Molecular insight into the therapeutic potential targeting *MUC5AC* expression and production. *Life Sci.* **2019**, *231*, 116485. [CrossRef]
27. Almanza, A.; Carlesso, A.; Chintha, C.; Creedican, S.; Doultsinos, D.; Leuzzi, B.; Luis, A.; McCarthy, N.; Montibeller, L.; More, S.; et al. Endoplasmic reticulum stress signalling—From basic mechanisms to clinical applications. *FEBS J.* **2019**, *286*, 241–278. [CrossRef]
28. Marciniak, S.J.; Ron, D. Endoplasmic reticulum stress signaling in disease. *Physiol. Rev.* **2006**, *86*, 1133–1149. [CrossRef]
29. Oyadomari, S.; Mori, M. Roles of CHOP/GADD153 in endoplasmic reticulum stress. *Cell Death Differ.* **2004**, *11*, 381–389. [CrossRef]
30. Schroeder, B.W.; Verhaeghe, C.; Park, S.W.; Nguyenvu, L.T.; Huang, X.; Zhen, G.; Erle, D.J. AGR2 is induced in asthma and promotes allergen-induced mucin overproduction. *Am. J. Respir. Cell Mol. Biol.* **2012**, *47*, 178–185. [CrossRef] [PubMed]
31. Burrell, K.L.; Nguyen, N.D.; Deering-Rice, C.E.; Memon, T.A.; Almestica-Roberts, M.; Rapp, E.; Serna, S.N.; Lamb, J.G.; Reilly, C.A. Dynamic Expression of Transient Receptor Potential Vanilloid-3 and Integrated Signaling with Growth Factor Pathways during Lung Epithelial Wound Repair following Wood Smoke Particle and Other Forms of Lung Cell Injury. *Mol. Pharmacol.* **2021**, *100*, 295–307. [CrossRef] [PubMed]
32. Singh, A.; Kumar, S.; Bajpai, V.; Kumar, B. Simultaneous determination of pyrroquinazoline alkaloids and flavonoids in Adhatoda beddomei and Adhatoda vasica and their marketed herbal formulations using ultra-high-performance liquid chromatography coupled with triple quadrupole linear ion trap mass spectrometry. *Biomed. Chromatogr.* **2017**, *31*, e3827. [CrossRef]
33. Borges, G.; Fong, R.Y.; Ensunsa, J.L.; Kimball, J.; Medici, V.; Ottaviani, J.I.; Crozier, A. Absorption, distribution, metabolism and excretion of apigenin and its glycosides in healthy male adults. *Free. Radic. Biol. Med.* **2022**, *185*, 90–96. [CrossRef] [PubMed]
34. Braune, A.; Engst, W.; Blaut, M. Identification and functional expression of genes encoding flavonoid O- and C-glycosidases in intestinal bacteria. *Environ. Microbiol.* **2016**, *18*, 2117–2129. [CrossRef]
35. Day, A.J.; Canada, F.J.; Diaz, J.C.; Kroon, P.A.; McLauchlan, R.; Faulds, C.B.; Plumb, G.W.; Morgan, M.R.; Williamson, G. Dietary flavonoid and isoflavone glycosides are hydrolysed by the lactase site of lactase phlorizin hydrolase. *FEBS Lett.* **2000**, *468*, 166–170. [CrossRef] [PubMed]

36. Schroder, C.; Matthies, A.; Engst, W.; Blaut, M.; Braune, A. Identification and expression of genes involved in the conversion of daidzein and genistein by the equol-forming bacterium Slackia isoflavoniconvertens. *Appl. Environ. Microbiol.* **2013**, *79*, 3494–3502. [CrossRef]
37. DeRango-Adem, E.F.; Blay, J. Does Oral Apigenin Have Real Potential for a Therapeutic Effect in the Context of Human Gastrointestinal and Other Cancers? *Front Pharmacol* **2021**, *12*, 681477. [CrossRef]
38. Wang, M.; Carver, J.J.; Phelan, V.V.; Sanchez, L.M.; Garg, N.; Peng, Y.; Nguyen, D.D.; Watrous, J.; Kapono, C.A.; Luzzatto-Knaan, T.; et al. Sharing and Community Curation of Mass Spectrometry Data with Global Natural Products Social Molecular Networking. *Nat. Biotechnol.* **2016**, *34*, 828–837. [CrossRef]
39. Bourrie, M.; Meunier, V.; Berger, Y.; Fabre, G. Cytochrome P450 isoform inhibitors as a tool for the investigation of metabolic reactions catalyzed by human liver microsomes. *J. Pharmacol. Exp. Ther.* **1996**, *277*, 321–332.
40. Tassaneeyakul, W.; Birkett, D.J.; Veronese, M.E.; McManus, M.E.; Tukey, R.H.; Quattrochi, L.C.; Gelboin, H.V.; Miners, J.O. Specificity of substrate and inhibitor probes for human cytochromes P450 1A1 and 1A2. *J. Pharmacol. Exp. Ther.* **1993**, *265*, 401–407.
41. Androutsopoulos, V.P.; Papakyriakou, A.; Vourloumis, D.; Spandidos, D.A. Comparative CYP1A1 and CYP1B1 substrate and inhibitor profile of dietary flavonoids. *Bioorganic Med. Chem.* **2011**, *19*, 2842–2849. [CrossRef]
42. Wilsher, N.E.; Arroo, R.R.; Matsoukas, M.T.; Tsatsakis, A.M.; Spandidos, D.A.; Androutsopoulos, V.P. Cytochrome P450 CYP1 metabolism of hydroxylated flavones and flavonols: Selective bioactivation of luteolin in breast cancer cells. *Food Chem. Toxicol.* **2017**, *110*, 383–394. [CrossRef] [PubMed]
43. Hildreth, K.; Kodani, S.D.; Hammock, B.D.; Zhao, L. Cytochrome P450-derived linoleic acid metabolites EpOMEs and DiHOMEs: A review of recent studies. *J. Nutr. Biochem.* **2020**, *86*, 108484. [CrossRef] [PubMed]
44. Alavi, M.S.; Shamsizadeh, A.; Karimi, G.; Roohbakhsh, A. Transient receptor potential ankyrin 1 (TRPA1)-mediated toxicity: Friend or foe? *Toxicol. Mech. Method.* **2020**, *30*, 1–18. [CrossRef] [PubMed]
45. Deering-Rice, C.E.; Memon, T.; Lu, Z.; Romero, E.G.; Cox, J.; Taylor-Clark, T.; Veranth, J.M.; Reilly, C.A. Differential Activation of TRPA1 by Diesel Exhaust Particles: Relationships between Chemical Composition, Potency, and Lung Toxicity. *Chem. Res. Toxicol.* **2019**, *32*, 1040–1050. [CrossRef] [PubMed]
46. Deering-Rice, C.E.; Romero, E.G.; Shapiro, D.; Hughen, R.W.; Light, A.R.; Yost, G.S.; Veranth, J.M.; Reilly, C.A. Electrophilic components of diesel exhaust particles (DEP) activate transient receptor potential ankyrin-1 (TRPA1): A probable mechanism of acute pulmonary toxicity for DEP. *Chem. Res. Toxicol.* **2011**, *24*, 950–959. [CrossRef] [PubMed]
47. Shapiro, D.; Deering-Rice, C.E.; Romero, E.G.; Hughen, R.W.; Light, A.R.; Veranth, J.M.; Reilly, C.A. Activation of transient receptor potential ankyrin-1 (TRPA1) in lung cells by wood smoke particulate material. *Chem. Res. Toxicol.* **2013**, *26*, 750–758. [CrossRef]
48. Sun, L.; Zhang, J.; Niu, C.; Deering-Rice, C.E.; Hughen, R.W.; Lamb, J.G.; Rose, K.; Chase, K.M.; Almestica-Roberts, M.; Walter, M.; et al. CYP1B1-derived epoxides modulate the TRPA1 channel in chronic pain. *Acta Pharm. Sin. B* **2023**, *13*, 68–81. [CrossRef]
49. Balsamo, R.; Lanata, L.; Egan, C.G. Mucoactive drugs. *Eur. Respir. Rev.* **2010**, *19*, 127–133. [CrossRef]
50. Udobi, K.F.; Childs, E.; Touijer, K. Acute respiratory distress syndrome. *Am. Fam. Physician* **2003**, *67*, 315–322.
51. Seagrave, J.; Albrecht, H.H.; Hill, D.B.; Rogers, D.F.; Solomon, G. Effects of guaifenesin, N-acetylcysteine, and ambroxol on *MUC5AC* and mucociliary transport in primary differentiated human tracheal-bronchial cells. *Respir. Res.* **2012**, *13*, 98. [CrossRef]
52. Lin, R.; Peng, H.; Nguyen, L.P.; Dudekula, N.B.; Shardonofsky, F.; Knoll, B.J.; Parra, S.; Bond, R.A. Changes in beta 2-adrenoceptor and other signaling proteins produced by chronic administration of 'beta-blockers' in a murine asthma model. *Pulm. Pharmacol. Ther.* **2008**, *21*, 115–124. [CrossRef] [PubMed]
53. Nguyen, L.P.; Al-Sawalha, N.A.; Parra, S.; Pokkunuri, I.; Omoluabi, O.; Okulate, A.A.; Windham Li, E.; Hazen, M.; Gonzalez-Granado, J.M.; Daly, C.J.; et al. beta2-Adrenoceptor signaling in airway epithelial cells promotes eosinophilic inflammation, mucous metaplasia, and airway contractility. *Proc. Natl. Acad. Sci. USA* **2017**, *114*, E9163–E9171. [CrossRef]
54. Nguyen, L.P.; Lin, R.; Parra, S.; Omoluabi, O.; Hanania, N.A.; Tuvim, M.J.; Knoll, B.J.; Dickey, B.F.; Bond, R.A. Beta2-adrenoceptor signaling is required for the development of an asthma phenotype in a murine model. *Proc. Natl. Acad. Sci. USA* **2009**, *106*, 2435–2440. [CrossRef]
55. Nguyen, L.P.; Omoluabi, O.; Parra, S.; Frieske, J.M.; Clement, C.; Ammar-Aouchiche, Z.; Ho, S.B.; Ehre, C.; Kesimer, M.; Knoll, B.J.; et al. Chronic exposure to beta-blockers attenuates inflammation and mucin content in a murine asthma model. *Am. J. Respir. Cell Mol. Biol.* **2008**, *38*, 256–262. [CrossRef] [PubMed]
56. Nguyen, L.P.; Singh, B.; Okulate, A.A.; Alfaro, V.Y.; Tuvim, M.J.; Dickey, B.F.; Bond, R.A. Complementary anti-inflammatory effects of a beta-blocker and a corticosteroid in an asthma model. *Naunyn Schmiedebergs Arch. Pharmacol.* **2012**, *385*, 203–210. [CrossRef]
57. Thanawala, V.J.; Forkuo, G.S.; Al-Sawalha, N.; Azzegagh, Z.; Nguyen, L.P.; Eriksen, J.L.; Tuvim, M.J.; Lowder, T.W.; Dickey, B.F.; Knoll, B.J.; et al. beta2-Adrenoceptor agonists are required for development of the asthma phenotype in a murine model. *Am. J. Respir. Cell Mol. Biol.* **2013**, *48*, 220–229. [CrossRef]
58. Ha, E.V.; Rogers, D.F. Novel Therapies to Inhibit Mucus Synthesis and Secretion in Airway Hypersecretory Diseases. *Pharmacology* **2016**, *97*, 84–100. [CrossRef] [PubMed]
59. Bielory, L.; Lupoli, K. Herbal interventions in asthma and allergy. *J. Asthma* **1999**, *36*, 1–65. [CrossRef]
60. Zanasi, A.; Mazzolini, M.; Kantar, A. A reappraisal of the mucoactive activity and clinical efficacy of bromhexine. *Multidiscip. Respir. Med.* **2017**, *12*, 7. [CrossRef]

61. Kantar, A.; Klimek, L.; Cazan, D.; Sperl, A.; Sent, U.; Mesquita, M. An overview of efficacy and safety of ambroxol for the treatment of acute and chronic respiratory diseases with a special regard to children. *Multidiscip. Respir. Med.* **2020**, *15*, 511. [CrossRef]
62. Cazan, D.; Klimek, L.; Sperl, A.; Plomer, M.; Kolsch, S. Safety of ambroxol in the treatment of airway diseases in adult patients. *Expert Opin. Drug Saf.* **2018**, *17*, 1211–1224. [CrossRef]
63. Bromhexine. *Lancet* **1971**, *1*, 1058.
64. Gibbs, B.F. Differential modulation of IgE-dependent activation of human basophils by ambroxol and related secretolytic analogues. *Int. J. Immunopathol. Pharmacol.* **2009**, *22*, 919–927. [CrossRef]
65. Seifart, C.; Clostermann, U.; Seifart, U.; Muller, B.; Vogelmeier, C.; von Wichert, P.; Fehrenbach, H. Cell-specific modulation of surfactant proteins by ambroxol treatment. *Toxicol. Appl. Pharmacol.* **2005**, *203*, 27–35. [CrossRef]
66. Fois, G.; Hobi, N.; Felder, E.; Ziegler, A.; Miklavc, P.; Walther, P.; Radermacher, P.; Haller, T.; Dietl, P. A new role for an old drug: Ambroxol triggers lysosomal exocytosis via pH-dependent Ca^{2+} release from acidic Ca^{2+} stores. *Cell Calcium* **2015**, *58*, 628–637. [CrossRef]
67. Rayees, S.; Mabalirajan, U.; Bhat, W.W.; Rasool, S.; Rather, R.A.; Panda, L.; Satti, N.K.; Lattoo, S.K.; Ghosh, B.; Singh, G. Therapeutic effects of R8, a semi-synthetic analogue of Vasicine, on murine model of allergic airway inflammation via STAT6 inhibition. *Int. Immunopharmacol.* **2015**, *26*, 246–256. [CrossRef]
68. Ge, L.T.; Liu, Y.N.; Lin, X.X.; Shen, H.J.; Jia, Y.L.; Dong, X.W.; Sun, Y.; Xie, Q.M. Inhalation of ambroxol inhibits cigarette smoke-induced acute lung injury in a mouse model by inhibiting the Erk pathway. *Int. Immunopharmacol.* **2016**, *33*, 90–98. [CrossRef] [PubMed]
69. Sikder, M.A.; Lee, H.J.; Ryu, J.; Park, S.H.; Kim, J.O.; Hong, J.H.; Seok, J.H.; Lee, C.J. Apigenin and Wogonin Regulate Epidermal Growth Factor Receptor Signaling Pathway Involved in *MUC5AC* Mucin Gene Expression and Production from Cultured Airway Epithelial Cells. *Tuberc. Respir. Dis.* **2014**, *76*, 120–126. [CrossRef] [PubMed]
70. Green, D.; Ruparel, S.; Gao, X.; Ruparel, N.; Patil, M.; Akopian, A.; Hargreaves, K. Central activation of TRPV1 and TRPA1 by novel endogenous agonists contributes to mechanical allodynia and thermal hyperalgesia after burn injury. *Mol. Pain* **2016**, *12*, 1744806916661725. [CrossRef] [PubMed]
71. Santes-Palacios, R.; Marroquin-Perez, A.L.; Hernandez-Ojeda, S.L.; Camacho-Carranza, R.; Govezensky, T.; Espinosa-Aguirre, J.J. Human CYP1A1 inhibition by flavonoids. *Toxicol. In Vitro* **2020**, *62*, 104681. [CrossRef] [PubMed]
72. Zhai, S.; Dai, R.; Friedman, F.K.; Vestal, R.E. Comparative inhibition of human cytochromes P450 1A1 and 1A2 by flavonoids. *Drug Metab. Dispos.* **1998**, *26*, 989–992. [PubMed]
73. de Souza, A.R.; Traboulsi, H.; Wang, X.; Fritz, J.H.; Eidelman, D.H.; Baglole, C.J. The Aryl Hydrocarbon Receptor Attenuates Acute Cigarette Smoke-Induced Airway Neutrophilia Independent of the Dioxin Response Element. *Front. Immunol.* **2021**, *12*, 630427. [CrossRef] [PubMed]
74. Deering-Rice, C.E.; Johansen, M.E.; Roberts, J.K.; Thomas, K.C.; Romero, E.G.; Lee, J.; Yost, G.S.; Veranth, J.M.; Reilly, C.A. Transient receptor potential vanilloid-1 (TRPV1) is a mediator of lung toxicity for coal fly ash particulate material. *Mol. Pharmacol.* **2012**, *81*, 411–419. [CrossRef]
75. Pang, Z.; Chong, J.; Zhou, G.; de Lima Morais, D.A.; Chang, L.; Barrette, M.; Gauthier, C.; Jacques, P.E.; Li, S.; Xia, J. MetaboAnalyst 5.0: Narrowing the gap between raw spectra and functional insights. *Nucleic Acids Res.* **2021**, *49*, W388–W396. [CrossRef]
76. Pachitariu, M.; Stringer, C. Cellpose 2.0: How to train your own model. *Nat. Method.* **2022**, *19*, 1634–1641. [CrossRef]
77. Stringer, C.; Wang, T.; Michaelos, M.; Pachitariu, M. Cellpose: A generalist algorithm for cellular segmentation. *Nat. Method.* **2021**, *18*, 100–106. [CrossRef]
78. Waisman, A.; Norris, A.M.; Elias Costa, M.; Kopinke, D. Automatic and unbiased segmentation and quantification of myofibers in skeletal muscle. *Sci. Rep.* **2021**, *11*, 11793. [CrossRef] [PubMed]

pharmaceuticals

MDPI

Review

Hypericum perforatum L. and the Underlying Molecular Mechanisms for Its Choleretic, Cholagogue, and Regenerative Properties †

Ala Mohagheghzadeh [1], Parmis Badr [2], Abdolali Mohagheghzadeh [2,3] and Shiva Hemmati [1,4,5,*]

1 Department of Pharmaceutical Biotechnology, School of Pharmacy, Shiraz University of Medical Sciences, Shiraz 71468-64685, Iran; alamhz1376@gmail.com
2 Pharmaceutical Sciences Research Center, Shiraz University of Medical Sciences, Shiraz 71468-64685, Iran; badrparmis@gmail.com (P.B.); mohaghegh@sums.ac.ir (A.M.)
3 Department of Phytopharmaceuticals (Traditional Pharmacy), School of Pharmacy, Shiraz University of Medical Sciences, Shiraz 71468-64685, Iran
4 Biotechnology Research Center, Shiraz University of Medical Sciences, Shiraz 71468-64685, Iran
5 Department of Pharmaceutical Biology, Faculty of Pharmaceutical Sciences, UCSI University, Cheras, Kuala Lumpur 56000, Malaysia
* Correspondence: hemmatish@sums.ac.ir or shemmati7@gmail.com; Tel.: +98-7132424128

† Dedicated to the memory of Professor Wilhelm Alfermann (1942–2023).

Abstract: Any defects in bile formation, secretion, or flow may give rise to cholestasis, liver fibrosis, cirrhosis, and hepatocellular carcinoma. As the pathogenesis of hepatic disorders is multifactorial, targeting parallel pathways potentially increases the outcome of therapy. *Hypericum perforatum* has been famed for its anti-depressive effects. However, according to traditional Persian medicine, it helps with jaundice and acts as a choleretic medication. Here, we will discuss the underlying molecular mechanisms of *Hypericum* for its use in hepatobiliary disorders. Differentially expressed genes retrieved from microarray data analysis upon treatment with safe doses of *Hypericum* extract and intersection with the genes involved in cholestasis are identified. Target genes are located mainly at the endomembrane system with integrin-binding ability. Activation of α5β1 integrins, as osmosensors in the liver, activates a non-receptor tyrosine kinase, c-SRC, which leads to the insertion of bile acid transporters into the canalicular membrane to trigger choleresis. *Hypericum* upregulates CDK6 that controls cell proliferation, compensating for the bile acid damage to hepatocytes. It induces ICAM1 to stimulate liver regeneration and regulates nischarin, a hepatoprotective receptor. The extract targets the expression of conserved oligomeric Golgi (COG) and facilitates the movement of bile acids toward the canalicular membrane via Golgi-derived vesicles. In addition, *Hypericum* induces SCP2, an intracellular cholesterol transporter, to maintain cholesterol homeostasis. We have also provided a comprehensive view of the target genes affected by *Hypericum*'s main metabolites, such as hypericin, hyperforin, quercitrin, isoquercitrin, quercetin, kaempferol, rutin, and *p*-coumaric acid to enlighten a new scope in the management of chronic liver disorders. Altogether, standard trials using *Hypericum* as a neo-adjuvant or second-line therapy in ursodeoxycholic-acid-non-responder patients define the future trajectories of cholestasis treatment with this product.

Keywords: bile acid; bioactive compounds; cholesterol; *p*-coumaric acid; hypericin; hyperforin; medicinal plant; microbiota; natural products; ursodeoxycholic acid

Citation: Mohagheghzadeh, A.; Badr, P.; Mohagheghzadeh, A.; Hemmati, S. *Hypericum perforatum* L. and the Underlying Molecular Mechanisms for Its Choleretic, Cholagogue, and Regenerative Properties. *Pharmaceuticals* **2023**, *16*, 887. https://doi.org/10.3390/ph16060887

Academic Editors: Elena Y. Enioutina, Kathleen M. Job and Catherine Sherwin

Received: 22 May 2023
Revised: 9 June 2023
Accepted: 13 June 2023
Published: 15 June 2023

1. Introduction

Bile acids are biological surfactants synthesized from cholesterol in the liver. These steroidal molecules are involved in various cell-signaling pathways [1]. The bile acid-activated nuclear receptors, including farnesoid X receptor (FXR), pregnane X receptor (PXR), constitutive androstane receptor (CAR), and vitamin D receptor (VDR), have a vital role in the regulation of bile secretion and energy expenditure [2]. Bile is formed at the hepatocytes and travels through the bile canaliculi into the gallbladder [3]. Any defects in bile formation, secretion, or flow may lead to the accumulation of highly cytotoxic molecules in the hepatocytes and give rise to cholestasis. Chronic cholestasis will eventually bring about liver fibrosis, cirrhosis, and subsequent hepatocellular carcinoma (HCC) [4]. Besides idiopathic etiologies, drugs, ischemia, stenosis, pregnancy, viruses, bacteria, and fungi, the two typical cholangiopathies are primary biliary cholangitis (PBC) and primary sclerosing cholangitis (PSC). While both intra- and extrahepatic large bile ducts are affected by PSC, any damage to the intra-hepatic small bile duct leads to PBC [5,6].

Various treatments have been adopted in order to inhibit the progression of cholestasis. Alteration in the bile flow rate, bile synthesis, and bile detoxification are reported adaption mechanisms to resolve cholestasis. One of these treatments is to use an FXR ligand to reduce inflammation and hepatic bile acid production. There are fibroblast growth factor 19 mimetics that regulate bile acid synthesis [7]. Through competitive removal of toxic hydrophobic bile acid molecules, ursodeoxycholic acid (UDCA) prevents damage to hepatocytes and bile ducts. UDCA, with a dose of 13–15 mg/Kg/day, is a multifunctional medication in PBC management [8]. However, more than 40% of the patients do not respond to UDCA and are considered to experience severe hepatic complications within 10 years [9,10]. Hence, a precise and helpful outcome of UDCA, as the first-line treatment, in the various stages of PBC, is considered doubtful, and the efficacy of second-line treatments has been investigated in trials [11–14]. UDCA seems not to be promising in unfavorable consequences of intrahepatic cholestasis of pregnancy [15]. It also elevates the morbidity and mortality rate in cholestatic neonates and infants [16] and might be intolerable in some patients due to its side effects, such as diarrhea, nausea, and vomiting [17]. Required evidence on the helpful impact of UDCA for other hepatic afflictions such as PSC or metabolic liver disorders is insufficient [10]. While UDCA is not beneficial in PSC, obeticholic acid (OCA) is the only approved alternative for PBC patients who are UDCA-intolerant or non-responders [18]. To attenuate the extrahepatic manifestation of cholestasis, such as pruritis, cholestyramine, rifampicin, naltrexone, and sertraline, might be prescribed. Fibrates and statins are recommended to regulate dyslipidemia [19]. Antioxidants might be also proposed to protect the liver from the damage of bile acids [20–22]. Diverse immunomodulators have been tested for cholestatic liver disorders [9]. Glucocorticoid medications such as prednisolone and budesonide as anti-inflammatory agents, and fibrates that, besides triggering biliary secretion, show anti-inflammatory properties and mycophenolate mofetil are some of the immunomodulators that might be used as alternatives to UDCA [23]. However, long-term uses of immunosuppressants are not recommended due to side effects [23]. The utmost treatment is liver transplantation, restrained by the shortage of organ donor candidates with the hazard of post-transplantation complications [6]. These observations fueled the ongoing controversy on the complete efficacy of UDCA in hepatobiliary disorders, and adjuvants or second-line therapies are profoundly necessary.

Plants are known as a rich source of pharmaceutically valuable primary and secondary metabolites [24,25]. *Hypericum perforatum* L., as one of the most famous medicinal herbs in the world, is reported to ameliorate liver-related disorders, including hepatic steatosis, impaired hepatic lipid metabolism, and cholestasis [26]. This plant is known as St. John's wort (SJW) (*Hypericum* or Millepertuis), and is a member of the Hypericaceae (Clusiacaeae) family. It is a herbaceous perennial plant indigenous to Europe, Western Asia, and Northern Africa [27–29]. Its flowers are yellow to coppery, having four or five petals, many stamens, and a pistil. Bioactive compounds are stored as a red-colored liquid in golden petals [28]. Pedanios Dioskourides (a famous herbalist) was the first to introduce *Hypericum* as a medicinal plant in the first century. *Hypericum* flowers and aerial parts, including its leaf, are the main parts that are consumed [30,31]. Today, dried aerial parts of *Hypericum* are commercially available as tablets, capsules, tea, and tinctures for their therapeutic potential [28,31,32]. Low cost, good accessibility, high efficacy, low major side effects, high tolerability, and a lack of dependence in comparison with conventional anti-depressants are commonly reported reasons for self-treatment with *Hypericum* [33].

One of the main therapeutic approaches in treating cholestasis is increasing the bile flow (choleretic effect) and excreting excess bile by feces (cholagogue effect). *Hypericum* has been suggested for ileus or intestinal obstruction, and also biliary obstruction in Traditional Persian Medicine (TPM) [34]. According to TPM, *Hypericum* is a natural bile laxative with choleretic and cholagogue effects. Both seeds and leaves are cholagogue agents and increase bile secretion [34]. In addition, according to Turkish folk medicine, *Hypericum* can help with jaundice, hepatic, and biliary disorders [35]. Within this study, we aimed to describe the most important pharmacological effects and specialized metabolites of *H. perforatum*. Then, we will discuss the target genes associated with *Hypericum*'s total extract and bioactive compounds involved in its cholagogue, choleretic, and regenerative properties. We believe that a comprehensive view of the underlying molecular mechanisms of *Hypericum* is promising in targeting multiple pathways and lights a new scope in the management of liver chronic disorders such as cholestasis, fibrosis, and HCC.

2. Results and Discussion

2.1. *Hypericum Medical Attributes and Its Bioactive Compounds*

Hypericum has been used traditionally for the treatment of several disorders such as mental illness, insomnia, gastrointestinal tract diseases, skin wounds, eczema and burns. It is now one of the most greatly studied medicinal herbs in the world [36]. For example, in TPM, its vaginal formulation, as an emmenagogue, increases menstrual flow [34]. The urethral dosage form has a diuretic effect [37]. The alcoholic extract of the leaves relieves sciatica pain and gout [38]. Topical formulations have antimicrobial effects, useful for wound healing, particularly burn wounds. *Hypericum*'s aerial parts are widely used to treat mild to moderate depression, anxiety, irritability, neuralgia, sciatica, viral infections including HSV, vaginal problems such as vaginal atrophy and vaginal dryness, menopausal complications, and cystitis [30,39]. Many investigations have approved that *Hypericum* has anti-inflammatory [40], anti-tumor, anti-bacterial (Gram-positive bacteria), anti-oxidative, and neuroprotective effects in Parkinson's and Alzheimer's disease [41]. The SARS-CoV-2 virus resulted in a global pandemic called COVID-19, and various naturally derived compounds could target this pathogen [42,43]. This virus can be affected by the antiviral properties of *Hypericum* and its metabolites [44]. *Hypericum* is also utilized widely as a natural source of food flavor [45]. A growing interest has been observed in enriched or functional foods in the last few decades [46]. There is increased attention to *Hypericum*, as a mood enhancer, to be added to different foods, including cookies [47], functional beverages [48], and probiotic beverages [49]. Its antioxidant activity for long-term storage of food products has been also reported [50]. The most dominant pharmacological properties of *Hypericum* are summarized in Table 1.

Concerning its diverse medical attributes, *Hypericum* is abundant in bioactive metabolites such as flavonoids, phenylpropanes, xanthones, tannins, proanthocyanidins, phloroglucinols, naphthodianthrones, biflavonoids, flavonol aglycones, and several volatile oils. The potential medical benefits of *Hypericum* are mostly attributed to naphthodianthrones and phloroglucinols (Figure 1). The naphthodianthrones in *H. perforatum* are mainly hypericin, pseudohypericin, protohypericin, pseudoprotohypericin, cyclopseudohypericin, and emodinanthrone. This plant contains several phloroglucinols, including hyperforin, adhyperforin, and hydroperoxycadiforin [30,51]. Cell, tissue, and organ culturing is an important tool for the identification and isolation of secondary metabolites [52,53]. This strategy has been employed for the propagation of *Hypericum* as an industrially vital plant for the production of hypericin [54].

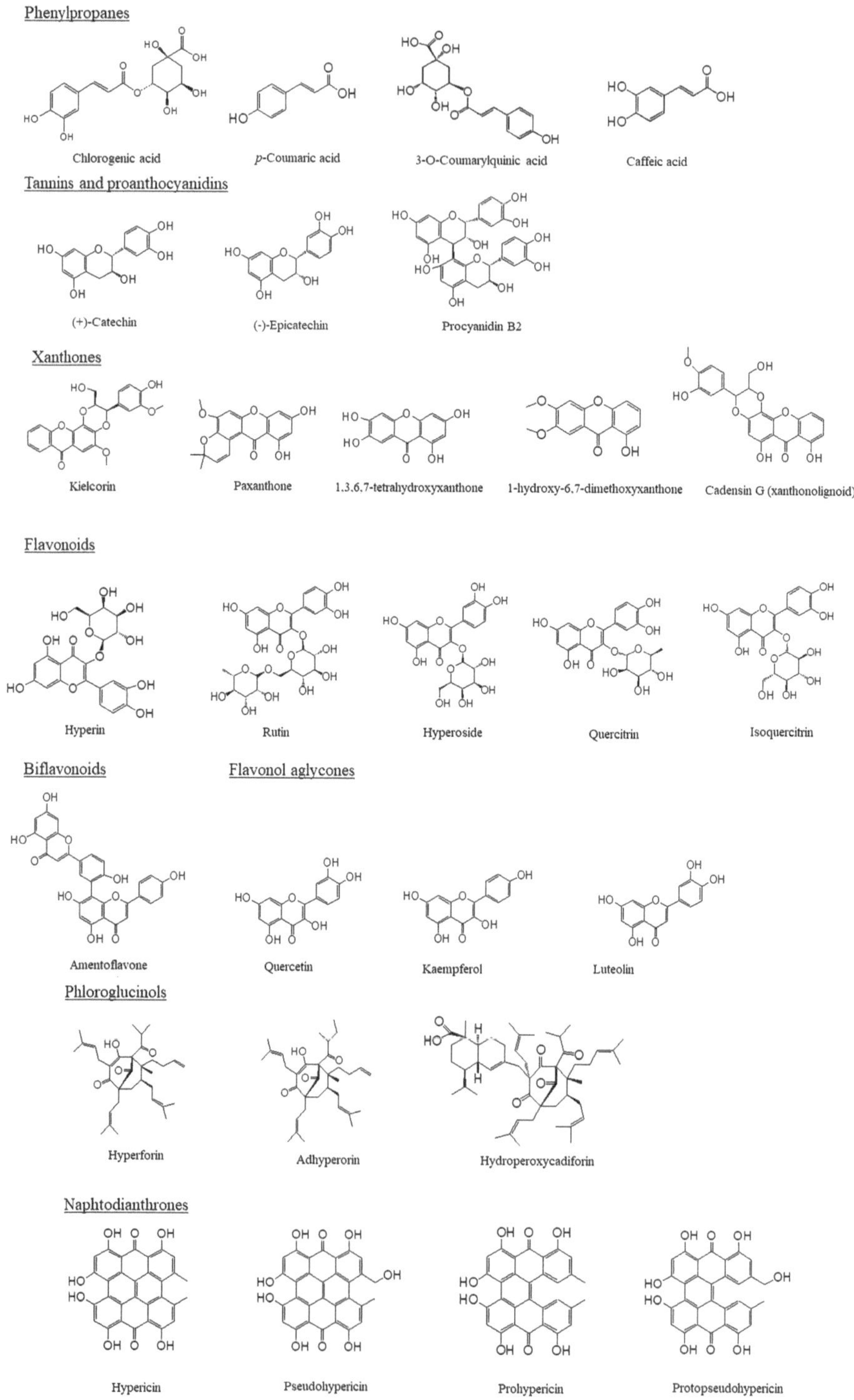

Figure 1. Chemical structures of the main specialized metabolites of *Hypericum perforatum*.

Table 1. Various pharmacological effects of *Hypericum perforatum* L., its mode of actions, and corresponding metabolites for each effect.

Effect	Mechanism	Metabolite	Model of Study
Antidepression	NT * metabolism ↓, Regulation of NT receptors sensitivity, NT synaptic reuptake ↓	Total extract [29]	*In vivo* animal model [29]
Antioxidative	Free radical scavenger	Total extract [55,56], Rutin, quercetin [57]	*In vivo* animal model [55,56] *In vitro* assay and ex vivo rat membrane model [57]
Anti-inflammatory	NF-κb ↓, GSH ↑, Ca influx ↓, IL-6 ↓, IL-12 ↓, TNF-α ↓	Total extract [56], Pseudohypericin, Quercetin, Amentoflavone, Chlorogenic acid [58], Hyperforin [59]	*In vivo* animal model [56] RAW 264.7 macrophage cell line [58] A549 cells & *in vivo* animal model [59]
Antitumor	Apoptosis ↑	Hyperforin, Hypericin [60]	*In vivo* animal model [60]
Hypolipidemic	FAS ↓, ACC ↓, PPAR-α ↑	Total extract [26,61]	*In vivo* animal model [26] 3T3L1 adipocyte [61]
Cholesterol ↓	HMG-CoA reductase ↓, Cholesterol excretion via secreted bile acids ↑	Total extract [62–64] Rutin [65]	*In vivo* animal model [62–65]
Triglycerides ↓	(LP1) ↓, (Dgat1) ↓	Total extract, Rutin [61]	3T3L1 adipocyte [61]
HDL ↑	(Apo-A1) ↑	Total extract [66]	*In vivo* animal model [66]
Hepatoprotective (hepatic steatosis ↓)	PPAR-γ ↑	Chlorogenic acid [67]	3T3L1 preadipocyte [67]
	AMPK ↑	Hypericin [61,68], Rutin [69]	L02 and HepG2 cells & *in vivo* animal models [61,68], HepG2 cells [69]
ALT ↓, AST ↓	Free radical scavenger, Neutrophil activation	Quercetin [70], Hyperoside [71]	*In vivo* animal model [70,71]

* ACC: Acetyl-CoA carboxylase; ALT: Alanine transaminase; Apo-A1: apolipoprotein-A1; AMPK: AMP-activated protein kinase; AST: Aspartate aminotransferase; Dgat1: Diacylglycerol *O*-acyltransferase 1; FAS: Fatty acid synthase; GSH: Glutathione; HDL: High-density lipoprotein; HMG-CoA reductase: 3-hydroxy-3-methylglutaryl coenzyme-A reductase; IL: Interleukin; LP1: Lipid transfer protein 1; NT: Neurotransmitter; NF-κb: Nuclear factor kappa B; PPAR: Peroxisome proliferator-activated receptors; TNF-α: Tumor necrosis factor α. Upward (↑) and downward arrows (↓) represent increase and decrease, respectively.

2.1.1. Mechanisms of Antidepressant Activity of *H. perforatum*

As the only approved herbal substitute for synthetic anti-depressants, *Hypericum* is now registered in many countries to treat mild to moderate depression with a daily dose of 500 mg, which is equivalent to 1–2 mg of hypericin [72]. Although neurotransmitter (NT) reuptake inhibitory effect and non-selective monoamine oxidase (MAO) inhibition seem to be the main pharmacological actions of *Hypericum*, the exact mode of its antidepressant activity is not well understood [73]. *Hypericum* modulates some genes, such as the corticotropin-releasing factor (CRF) involved in the hypothalamic–pituitary–adrenal axis, as the hyperactivity of this system is a sign of depression [73]. The anti-depressive effect of *Hypericum* is majorly attributed to hyperforin, hypericin, and its flavonoids [74]. Selective antagonization of CRF is observed by pseudohypericin [75]. Adhyperforin binds to serotonin and noradrenalin receptors resulting in the inhibition of NT reuptake [76]. Some *in vitro* investigations admit the MAO inhibitory effect of hypericin [77]. *In vitro* administration of hyperforin inhibits the uptake of several NTs at presynaptic terminals, including dopamine, noradrenaline, GABA, L-glutamate, and especially serotonin [78]. This observed effect is mainly due to the disruption of intracellular Na^+ concentrations as a result of transient receptor protein potential channel (TRPPC6) activation by hyperforin [79]. Hyperforin is also believed to impair the monoamine storage at vesicles and probably affects the solute carrier (SLC) gene family, including SLC 17, 18, and 32 [78]. Taken together, considering its few side effects, *Hypericum* can be a good "household alternative" to medications such as selective serotonin reuptake inhibitors (SSRIs) or tricyclic antidepressants (TCA) [30].

2.1.2. Hepatoprotective and Anti-Atherogenic Activity of *Hypericum*

Compared to a single chemical medication such as UDCA, *Hypericum* extract contains plentiful metabolites, interfering with various metabolic pathways to ameliorate cholestasis consequences. For example, in UDCA non-responsive PBC patients, biochemical indices are not improved [80]. However, according to *in vivo* animal models, *Hypericum* extract helps with hepatic biochemical markers such as ALT and AST [70]. Although UDCA reduces total cholesterol, it does not have a significant effect on triglyceride (TG), high-density lipoprotein (HDL), and low-density lipoprotein (LDL) [8]. *Hypericum* helps with hepatotoxicity, hepatitis, hepatocyte peroxidation, non-alcoholic fatty liver disease (NAFLD), hepatic lipid metabolism, and hepatic steatosis [26,68]. *Hypericum* extract lowers total cholesterol, raises HDL, and decreases TG content in *in vivo* animal models [81,82] (Table 1). Similarly, *in vivo* studies show that hyperforin can attenuate serum TG, cholesterol, and LDL levels [62]. Hyperoside, a pivotal flavonoid found in *Hypericum* species, regulates cholesterol metabolism and therefore attenuates NAFLD [83]. Since free radicals can damage cellular macromolecules, excessive production of free radicals in the liver may contribute to a variety of hepatic disorders [84]. *Hypericum* is best known for its anti-inflammatory and anti-oxidative activity, which gives a sense of hepatoprotection. *Hypericum*'s hepatoprotective activity can be attributed to the suppression of TNF-α and IL-6 cytokine contents in the liver [26,61]. These two pro-inflammatory cytokines are produced mainly by adipocytes, and their concentration adjusts the percentage and distribution of fat [85]. Similar to fibrates, *Hypericum* extract has been shown to increase the expression of PPAR-α in animal models promoting bile acid excretion [26]. There is a close connection between lysophosphatidylcholine (LysoPC) content as a hepatic inflammation biomarker and TGF-β/SMAD3 pro-inflammatory signaling pathway, which is associated with bile acid accumulation in the liver [86]. *Hypericum* is also said to regulate LysoPC content according to *in vivo* animal trials [26].

By modulating the peroxisome proliferator-activated receptor (PPAR-γ), *Hypericum* regulates the secretion and expression of adiponectin, which balances glucose and fatty acid metabolism [87]. *Hypericum* also improves glucose and lipid metabolism by inhibiting protein tyrosine phosphatase 1B catalytic activity in obese mice models [88]. The dysbiosis in gut bacteria is observed in cholestatic liver disorders due to the damage to bile-acid-sensitive species. Fecal microbiota transplantation and the use of probiotics are recommended as alternative treatments to UDCA for cholestasis [9]. It has been defined in animal models that *H. perforatum* modulates the gut microbiome and consequently normalizes serum lipid profile and reverses the hepatic steatosis symptoms [62]. Finally, to conclude a clear positioning statement, standard trials using *Hypericum* alone and in combination with UDCA as the neo-adjuvant or second-line therapy define the future trajectories of cholestasis treatment with this plant.

2.2. Analysis of Differentially Expressed Genes (DEGs) upon Treatment of HepG2 Cells with H. perforatum Crude Extract

A study by Ozturk et al. suggested that *Hypericum*, as a choleretic and cholagogue agent, exerts its hepatoprotective effects by increasing bile secretion and flow [35]. In addition, according to TPM, *Hypericum* has been used because of its choleretic and cholagogue activities. Bile-duct-ligated rodent models have been used as classic cholestatic *in vivo* models, which are replaced by genetically modified mice, and inducible models using toxicants [89]. Cell lines, such as human hepatoma HuH-7, known for high expression and localization of bile acid transporters and bile salt export pumps, are also appropriate models to investigate the underlying choleretic mechanisms [90]. However, due to feasible access and culture conditions, HepG2 cells are favorable models to study drugs that target hepatic functions [91]. To define the underlying mechanism of choleretic and cholagogue activities, DEGs in HepG2 cells treated with a safe amount of *H. perforatum* extract (2.5 μg/mL) or DMSO were analyzed (according to the available microarray data from VanderMolen et al. in the GEO database as described in the Section 3). Analysis of the box plot quartiles and their median reconfirms that the data distribution is valid and there is no outlier sample. A total of 73 DEGs were identified in GSE144235 considering a p-value < 0.05 and | log Fc (fold change) | > 0.2 as the cut-off criteria. As a result, 52 and 21 genes were up- and down-regulated, respectively, represented by volcano plots (Figure 2A) (Table S1).

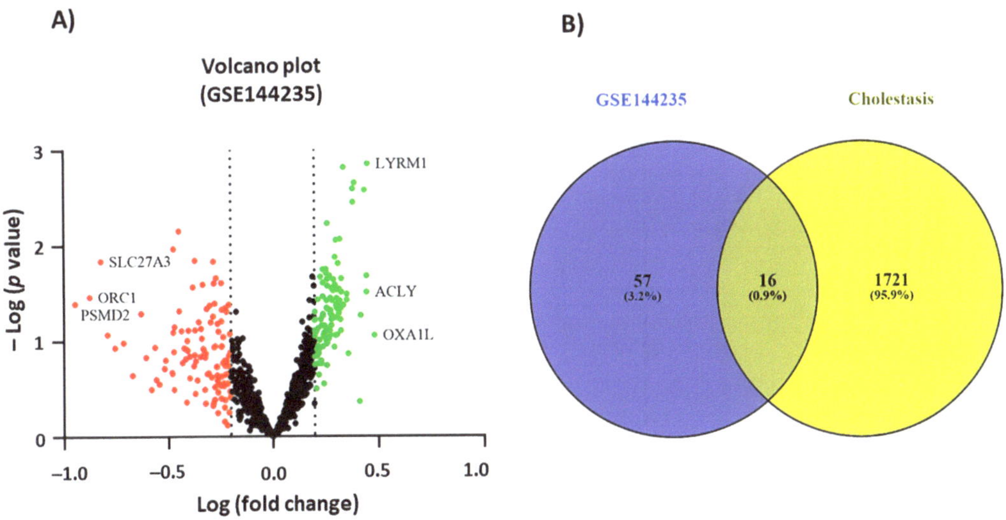

Figure 2. (**A**) Volcano plots related to differentially expressed genes (DEGs) of GSE144235. Differences in gene expressions of HepG2 cells treated with 2.5 μg/mL *Hypericum* extract compared to the DMSO-treated control. Each dot in the plot is a symbol of gene expression. A | log F_c (fold change) | > 0.2 (x-axis) and a p-value < 0.05 (y-axis) were set as statistical significant criteria. The red dots represent down-regulated genes and the green dots represent up-regulated genes. (**B**) A Venn diagram representing 73 DEGs upon treatment with *Hypericum* crude extract and 1737 genes related to cholestasis. The overlapped section is the symbol of mutually expressed genes in both conditions. There are 16 expressed genes related to cholestasis among 73 monitored DEGs.

2.3. Identification of Target Genes

A total of 1737 genes related to cholestasis were retrieved using the GeneCards database (Table S2). To define the potential choleretic and anti-cholestatic mechanisms of *Hypericum*, the intersection of 73 DEGs upon treatment with the safe dose of plant extract and 1737 genes related to cholestasis was determined and displayed using a Venn diagram (Figure 2B). A total of 16 common genes, including EZH2, SCP2, ILK, CDK6, EGF, SPP1, PLOD3, SKIV2L, CXCL2, NISCH, ICAM1, SRC, CAT, COG7, BAX, and COG4 were identified.

For additional investigation on the function and mechanism, all the sixteen retrieved genes were imported to DAIVID as a functional enrichment analysis tool. Gene Ontology (GO) enrichment results are listed in Table 2. The table includes MF, BP, and CC, which refer to molecular function, biological process, and cellular components, respectively, ranking by p-value. GO enrichment analysis revealed that the most significant biological pathways for enriched genes were involved in the regulation of MAP kinase activity, as well as lipid and metabolic processes. It seems that *Hypericum* regulates P38 mitogen-activated protein kinase

(MAPK). The MAPK signaling pathway regulates various hepatic functions, including bile acid synthesis, bile acid excretion, and bile-acid-induced apoptosis, and involves in the pathogenesis of hepatic steatosis. MAPK also regulates the insertion and retrieval of the bile salt export pump (BSEP) and the multidrug-resistance-associated protein 2 (MRP2) into the plasma membrane [92]. Hence, *Hypericum* as a choleretic agent prompts the insertion of these transports by regulating MAPK. Regarding cellular components and molecular function, DEGs were mainly at the endomembrane system with integrin binding ability. The top KEGG pathway analysis of mutual genes revealed that these genes are mainly related to lipid and atherosclerosis as well as EGFR tyrosine kinase inhibitor resistance.

Table 2. Gene ontology and KEGG enrichment results of differentially expressed genes upon treatment with *H. perforatum* extract overlapped with cholestasis-involved genes. MF, BP, and CC, refer to molecular function, biological process, and cellular components, respectively.

Category	Term	*p*-Value	Target Gene
MF	Integrin binding	6×10^{-7}	NISCH, SRC, SPP1, ILK, ICAM1
Bp	GO:0043406~positive regulation of MAP kinase activity	4×10^{-4}	SRC, EGF, ILK, EZH2
	GO:0033993~response to lipid	7×10^{-4}	SRC, CAT, SPP1, CXCL2, EZH2, ICAM1
	GO:0009893~positive regulation of metabolic process	4×10^{-3}	CDK6, SCP2, SRC, EGF, SPP1, BAX, ILK, EZH2, ICAM1
	GO:0014065~phosphatidylinositol 3-kinase signaling	4×10^{-3}	SRC, EGF, CAT
CC	Endomembrane system	2×10^{-3}	NISCH, COG7, SCP2, SRC, EGF, COG4, CAT, SPP1, BAX, PLOD3
KEGG pathway	Lipid and atherosclerosis	3×10^{-3}	SRC, BAX, CXCL2, ICAM1
	EGFR tyrosine kinase inhibitor resistance	5×10^{-3}	SRC, BAX, EGF

2.4. Protein–Protein Interaction (PPI) Network of DEGs

A PPI network of 16 overlapped DEGs after treatment with *H. perforatum* extract and cholestasis is observed in Figure 3. The interaction was ranked by a degree method through CytoHubba. *Hypericum* can upregulate Src, a non-receptor tyrosine kinase, as an essential member of the SRC family kinases. The SRC family kinases are of significant importance thanks to regulating many liver functions, such as bile flow and bile formation [93,94]. Anisoosmotic hepatocyte volume changes regulate the expression of SRC family kinases. Hepatocyte swelling caused by ambient hypo-osmolarity will lead to the rapid activation of the integrin system as osmo-sensors in the liver. Activation of β1 and α5β1 integrins activates the upstream c-Src, epidermal growth factor receptor (EGFR), mitogen-activated protein kinase (MAPK), focal adhesion kinase (FAK), and phosphatidylinositol kinase 3 (PI3 kinase). This will expedite the downstream activation of extracellular signal-regulated kinases (Erks) and p38 mitogen-activated protein kinase (p38 MAPK). The downstream activation of Erk and p38 will lead to the insertion of the bile salt export pump (BSEP) and multidrug-resistance-associated protein 2 (MRP2) as two important bile acid transporters into the canalicular membrane and triggers choleresis (Figures 4 and 5A) [94]. The other cholestasis-related genes affected by *Hypericum* are discussed further.

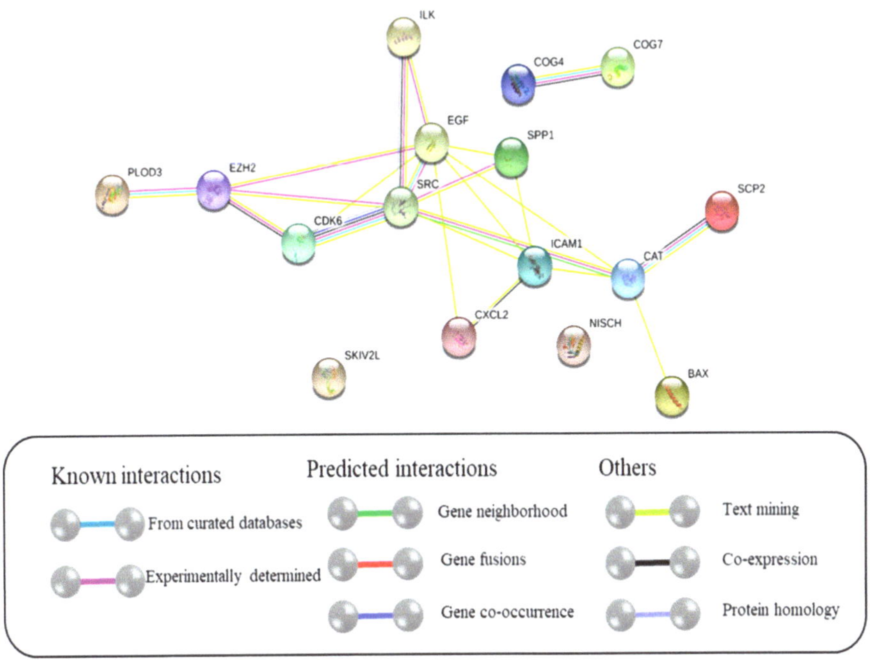

Figure 3. Protein–protein interaction (PPI) network of DEGs in treated groups with *Hypericum* extract in common with the genes involved in cholestasis.

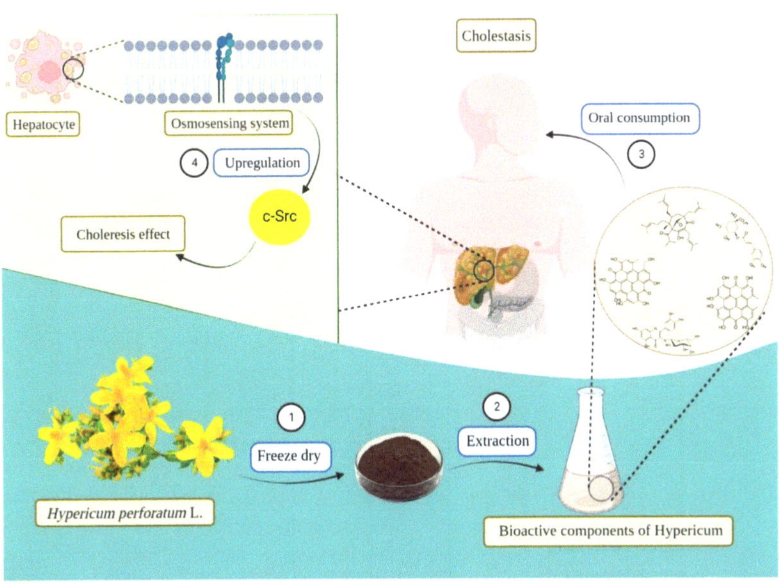

Figure 4. The role of c-Src in the choleretic effect of *Hypericum perforatum*. The up-regulation of c-Src by *Hypericum* extract eventually results in the insertion of the bile salt export pump and multidrug resistance protein 2 as two important bile acid transporters into the canalicular membrane and trigger choleresis.

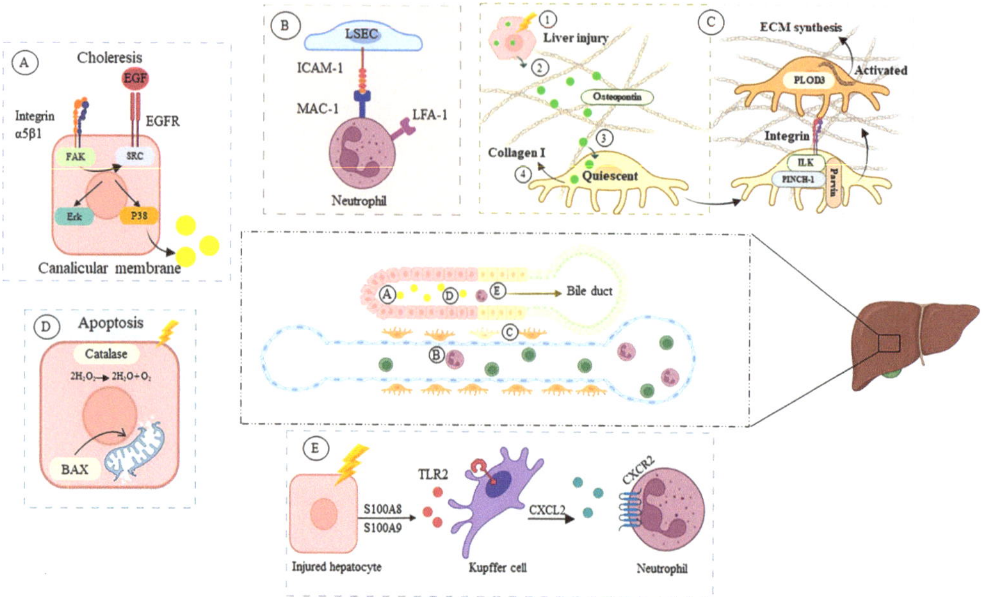

Figure 5. A summary of the function of cholestasis-related genes affected by *Hypericum* extract (**A**) EGFR activation by EGF or any EGFR ligands leads to activating SRC and eventually induces choleresis (**B**) ICAM-1 is an expressed binding molecule on neutrophils, which mediates the neutrophil recruitment to the inflammatory sites (**C**) OPN expression in the liver helps with liver regeneration, regulating hepatic infiltration of macrophages and neutrophils. When a ligand binds to integrin, the structure of integrin changes, and ILK binds to the tail of integrin, resulting in the activation of the ternary complex of ILK, PINCH, and PARVIN. As a result of activating this signaling pathway, HSCs become activated, motile, and synthesize more ECM components, including collagen type I, α-actin, and fibronectin. PLOD3 generates hydroxylysine-linked carbohydrates, which are important for collagen biosynthesis (**D**) Cholestasis can cause apoptosis and necrosis in hepatocytes and cholangiocytes. Following oxidative stress and increased accumulation of ROS, cholestasis induces BAX expression. BAX, as a pro-apoptotic member of the Bcl-2 family, activates caspases, and releases mitochondrial inter-membrane space (IMS). Catalase is increased in cholestasis, which is due to the increased demand for hepatocyte detoxification from excess production of H_2O_2 (**E**) TLR2/S100A8/S100A9 signaling pathway is introduced as hepatic CXCL2 regulator, which results in neutrophil recruitment.

- Epidermal growth factor (EGF)

The EGF gene encodes a polypeptide of 6 kDa that belongs to the epidermal growth factor superfamily. *Hypericum* upregulates EGF as a mitogenic factor that binds specifically to the epidermal growth factor receptor (EGFR), which activates several signaling pathways, including JAK/STAT, Ras/ERK, and PI3K/AKT [95]. EGFR signaling is characterized as a hepatoprotective factor and prevents cholestatic liver injury [96]. Studies have shown that ablation of the EGFR signaling pathway results in aggravated bile-acid-induced liver injury, collagen deposition in periportal areas, and upregulation of the bile acid biosynthesis enzyme. The STAT3 pathway regulates the EGFR signaling pathway, IL6, and IGF-1 and protects the liver from hepatocyte apoptosis and cholestatic injury. Due to EGFR's role in regulating compensatory cell proliferation mechanisms, EGFR ablation will result in defective liver regeneration. The EGFR signaling pathway is also used therapeutically to prevent liver injury and fibrosis [97]. Previous studies have shown that pretreatment of hepatocytes with bile acids, including deoxycholic acid (DCA), activates the EGFR signaling pathway. EGFR activation by DCA was transduced to the MAPK pathway via Ras and the PI3 kinase pathway, as expected when hepatocytes are treated with natural EGFR ligands. Consequently, bile acid's toxic potential is limited by itself (Figure 5A) [98].

- Intercellular Adhesion Molecule-1 (ICAM-1)

As a result of cholestasis and activation of the MAPK signaling pathway, early growth response factor 1 (Egr-1) is activated, which plays a crucial role in the progression of inflammation. In cholestasis, Egr-1 is the main inducer of ICAM-1 overexpression [99]. According to many studies, ICAM-1 expression in sinusoidal and perisinusoidal areas in cholestatic patients is higher than that in healthy controls [100]. ICAM-1 encodes a cell surface glycoprotein, named intercellular adhesion molecule 1 (ICAM-1) which binds to different types of integrins. The expression of ICAM-1 on HSCs and liver sinusoidal endothelial cells (LSEC) is critical for the attachment of leukocytes to the site of injury for the alleviation of cholestatic symptoms [100]. Excess bilirubin, bile salts, and overexpression of TNF-α in the cholestatic liver will lead to the activation of Kupffer cells [101]. Following this, hepatocytes, HSCs, and endothelial cells become involved due to TNF-α release. Neutrophils are recruited to inflamed liver sites by platelet-activating factor (PAF) and monocyte chemotactic protein-1 (MCP-1) secreted by activated HSCs. HSCs will also express ICAM-1 which helps with the neutrophil adhesion to the endothelial cells. ICAM-1 participates in many adhesion pathways, including MAC-1, and LFA-1 (expressed binding molecules on neutrophiles' surface) to mediate neutrophil recruitment into hepatic inflamed sites (Figure 5B) [102]. Several studies have evaluated the role of neutrophils as the largest population of circulating leukocytes in the pathogenesis of many liver diseases [103]. Liver sinusoids are regularly patrolled by neutrophils, with a few resident neutrophils. Neutrophil infiltration is a necessary step in confronting liver diseases; however, excess neutrophil infiltration and activation will lead to chronic inflammation and subsequent organ dysfunction. In fact, neutrophils have been introduced as a promising target for treating several liver diseases [104]. Hepatocyte mitogens, IL-6, and TNF are released by neutrophils when they bind ICAM-1, which is a liver regeneration stimulus [104].

- Integrin-linked kinase (ILK)

The extracellular matrix (ECM) plays an important role in hepatocyte differentiation, motility, and liver regeneration. The architecture of ECM also influences hepatocyte-specific gene expression. These developmental and differentiation signals transmit to the cell interior from ECM via integrins and signal-transducing molecules. There are some ECM–hepatocyte adhesion proteins, including integrin-linked kinase (ILK) and focal adhesion kinase (FAK), that facilitate the communication between ECM and cells [105]. As the name implies, ILK encodes the intracellular kinase linked with integrin. The ILK ternary complex consists of ILK, PINCH-1, and PARVIN, which transmit ECM signals via the binding of ligands (such as collagen type I) to integrins. When a ligand binds to integrin, the structure of the integrin changes and ILK binds to the tail of integrin, resulting in the activation of the ternary complex of ILK, PINCH, and PARVIN. As a result of activating this signaling pathway, hepatic stellate cells (HSCs) become activated, motile, and synthesize more ECM components, including collagen type I, α-actin, and fibronectin (Figure 5C) [106,107]. Many cellular processes, including hepatocyte differentiation, growth, migration, and survival depend on ILK expression and its interaction with the extracellular matrix [108]. Researchers have shown that knocking down ILK results in dedifferentiated hepatocytes that can be regenerated by adding hydrated complex matrix preparations (Matrigel®), indicating that ILK contributes to maintaining extracellular microarchitecture. It is convincing that ILK protects cells from anoikis because of its role in the ECM, and knocking it out leads to uncontrolled apoptosis [109].

- Secreted phosphoprotein 1 (SPP1)

SPP1, located on chromosome 4 in humans, encodes a highly negatively charged protein named osteopontin (OPN) [110]. Depending on the number of post-translationally modified residues, OPN has a molecular weight ranging from 41 to 75 kDa. OPN is a multi-functional protein that is associated with ECM maintenance and turnover. It is composed of three integrin-binding domains, two heparin-binding domains, and one CD44 binding domain. By binding to these domains, signaling pathways that are involved in cell proliferation, adhesion, motility, invasion, and fibrosis are triggered. In the liver, OPN plays a role as a cytokine-like protein that is involved in fibrinogenesis [111]. The highest levels of OPN expression in the liver can be found in cholangiocytes, followed by macrophages, hepatocytes, sinusoidal endothelial cells, HSCs, and natural killer cells (NKs). OPN is related to integrin and ERK signaling pathways. OPN expression in the liver helps with liver regeneration, regulating hepatic infiltration of macrophages and neutrophils, and activation of signaling pathways, including IL6 and STAT3 in Kupffer cells (Figure 5C) [111]. Hepatic inflammation is associated with OPN expression, which serves as a chemoattractant of macrophages and neutrophils. Additionally, overexpression of OPN during liver inflammation activates integrin molecules and CD44 signaling pathways for macrophage migration, dendritic cell maturation, and T cell activation and differentiation [112].

Several studies indicate that OPN expression in liver cells is associated with PPAR-α inhibition; therefore, there is a positive correlation between OPN serum levels and hepatic cholesterol and triglycerides [113]. In addition, OPN serum levels are correlated with subsequent liver fibrosis in chronic alcoholics. OPN expression increases the wound healing ability of HSCs, as well as collagen type I production and the PI3K-pAkt-NFB pathway activation. Normal biliary epithelial cells (BECs) express OPN, whereas liver injury induces OPN overexpression, suggesting a pathogenic role for OPN in cholangiopathies [114]. Based on a microarray analysis in intrahepatic cholangiocarcinoma (ICC) patients, the most expressed gene is SPP1, which has a positive correlation with tumor size [114]. According to studies, extracellular OPN is related to obesity and lipid synthesis. OPN knockdown reduces inflammation of adipose tissue and insulin resistance in high-fat diets, suggesting that OPN contributes to metabolic syndrome. OPN$^{-/-}$ mice demonstrate increased hepatic cholesterol after injection of recombinant OPN, but decreased levels of cytochrome P450 family-7 subfamily-A member-1 (CYP7A1), indicating that OPN regulates bile acids, which play a role in hepatic lipogenesis [111].

- Procollagen-Lysine,2-Oxoglutarate 5-Dioxygenase 3 (PLOD3)

PLOD3 encodes lysyl hydroxylase 3 (LH3), which belongs to the PLOD family (PLOD1-3) [115]. Due to its galactosyl- and glucosyl-galactosyl-transferase activities, LH3, also known as PLOD3, is the only isoenzyme that can also generate hydroxylysine-linked carbohydrates, which are important for collagen biosynthesis (Figure 5C) [116,117]. As a major component of the ECM, collagen promotes hepatic microenvironment hemostasis both biochemically and physically, making PLOD3 even more important. There are many studies demonstrating that a few weeks after a hepatic injury, the activity of lysyl hydroxylase increases, which is an indicator of the increased rate of collagen biosynthesis [118]. The abnormal expression of the PLOD family promotes tumor progression and metastasis in HCC patients, making PLODs potential treatment targets. Meanwhile, scientific studies have shown that PLODs' expression correlates with immune cell infiltration. Overall, PLODs are responsible for balancing the hepatic microenvironment, especially in HCC [116]. In a recent study, LH3 was found to recruit matrix metalloproteinase 9, which is involved in ECM remodeling and TGF-β activation [117]. Banushi et al. has shown that VIPAR, a trafficking protein, is responsible for regulating the interaction of LH3 and collagen-containing organelles from the trans-Golgi network (TGN). VIPAR deficiency causes arthrogryposis, renal dysfunction, and cholestasis syndrome (ARC), which involves functional defects throughout several organs, including the liver. A surprising feature of this syndrome is that some clinical phenotypes overlap with those found in patients with inherited LH3 deficiencies [117].

- Catalase (CAT)

The CAT gene encodes catalase, an essential enzyme located in the peroxisomes of almost all aerobic cells, which breakdowns the intracellular H_2O_2 into water and oxygen without generating free radicals. Studies have shown that oxidative stress contributes to the pathogenesis of cholestasis via cytokines, and it is believed that tissue injury in cholestatic patients is caused by lipid peroxidation [91,119]. A complex antioxidative system such as catalase is activated in the presence of free oxygen radicals, so it makes sense that mean catalase levels are reported to be significantly higher in hepatocytes of cholestatic patients than in controls. Catalase is involved in defining hepatic antioxidant capacity and is increased in many hepatic injuries, especially cholestasis, which is due to increased demand for hepatocyte detoxification from excess production of H_2O_2 [120]. There are approved mechanisms for the flavonoid-rich extract of *Hypericum* against H_2O_2-induced apoptosis in PC12 cells, including decreased H_2O_2 cytotoxicity, and reduced DNA laddering (Figure 5D) [121].

- Bcl-2-Associated X-protein (BAX)

The BAX gene encodes a 21 kDa pro-apoptotic protein, named Bcl-2-Associated X-protein (BAX), an important member of the Bcl-2 gene family, which regulates intrinsic apoptosis [122]. The intrinsic pathway of apoptosis is triggered by free radicals, toxins, and impaired DNA [123]. Cholestasis can cause hepatocyte and cholangiocyte apoptosis and necrosis. Following oxidative stress and increased accumulation of ROS, cholestasis induces BAX expression. BAX, as a pro-apoptotic factor, activates caspases and releases mitochondrial inter-membrane space (IMS). In general, cholestasis alters the expression of apoptosis-related proteins, including Bax and Bcl-2. An elevated BAX level and apoptotic body index are observed in the liver of cholestatic patients (Figure 5D) [123]. There is a proposed anti-apoptotic mechanism for hyperforin salt, including the down-regulation of BAX protein, which helps with the amelioration of solid tumors [124]. *Hypericum* ethanolic extract can regulate BAX expression, which can be considered one of the anti-cholestatic mechanisms of this precious herb. Upon increased toxin and ROS formation following cholestasis, brain damage is expected. There are studies evaluating the positive effect of neuroprotective treatments on cholestasis-induced brain injury [123]. *Hypericum*, as an anti-oxidant that exerts neuroprotective effects, may also have potential benefits on central nervous system injury second to cholestasis.

- Chemokine (C-X-C motif) ligand 2 (CXCL2)

Bile acids induce CXCL2 expression, which recruits neutrophils to inflamed sites during cholestasis [99,125]. CXCL2 is a secreted chemokine that belongs to the chemokine superfamily and plays an important role in immunoregulation and inflammatory processes [126]. The TLR2/S100A8/S100A9 signaling pathway is introduced as a hepatic CXCL2 regulator, which results in neutrophil recruitment (Figure 5E) [127]. Neutrophil production is regulated via granulocyte-colony-stimulating factor (G-CSF), and CXCL2 as a chemokine. In response to CXCL2 gradients and other stimuli, mature neutrophils migrate into inflamed sites [104]. Several studies have reported increased levels of CXCL2 and its receptor (CXCR2) after bile duct ligation (BDL) and subsequent liver injury. The activation of this pathway leads to the formation of chemokine gradients, neutrophil recruitment, and regulation of hepatocyte proliferation and death during liver damage [128]. There is a biological link between hepatic c-Jun NH2-terminal kinase (JNK), the AP1 signal transduction pathway, and CXCL2 [129]. This axis is regarded as being responsible for insulin resistance and hepatic steatosis. The JNK axis inhibits PPARα which is an important lipid and bile acid hemostasis regulator, affecting intracellular fatty acid transport. The JNK axis blockade activates PPARα in hepatocytes which modulate bile acid hemostasis. Several studies have introduced this axis as a therapeutic target for treating cholestasis and hepatic steatosis [130]. Studies have shown the beneficial effects of low-dose fenofibrate on the JNK-AP1-CXCL2 axis and subsequent PPARα activation, which ultimately ameliorates cholestatic liver [131]. Bile acid regulates bile metabolism by activating the JNK signaling pathway and therefore downregulating CYP7A1, which ultimately leads to bile acid over-production and cholestasis [131].

- Enhancer of zeste homolog 2 (EZH2)

EZH2, a histone methyltransferase (HMT) subunit of the polycomb repressive complex 2 (PRC2), is a key regulator of downstream gene expression. EZH2 has an essential role in silencing tumor-suppressive microRNAs and its overexpression is correlated with the development of solid tumors such as HCC. EZH2 overexpression inhibits insulin-like growth factor binding protein 4 (IGFBP4), which is normally expressed in the liver and functions as a tumor suppressor. In addition to being a diagnostic biomarker of HCC, EZH2 is also considered a good therapeutic target for this disease. EZH2 inhibitors reduce serum levels of inflammatory cytokines, including IL-6, IL-1β, and IFN-γ [132,133]. EZH2 regulates cellular cholesterol homeostasis via DNA methyltransferase 1 (DNMT1) recruitment and downregulation of ATP-binding cassette transporter A1 (ABCA1). ABCA1 exerts atheroprotection properties and is mainly expressed in macrophages and hepatocytes. EZH2-induced DNMT1 recruitment in macrophage-derived foam cells promotes CpG methylation of the ABCA1 gene, which ultimately impairs cholesterol efflux and leads to atherosclerosis [134].

- Sterol Carrier Protein 2 (SCP2)

SCP2 encodes two distinct isoforms, SCP2 and SCPx, which have a common 13 kDa carboxy terminus. It has been found that the amino acid sequence of SCP2/SCPx is conserved across different species, indicating that these two proteins serve important functions. The 58 kDa protein (SCPx) is localized to peroxisomes [135,136] and serves a catalytic role as a thiolase in cholesterol biosynthesis. Studies have shown that SCPx expression is sex-dependent; male murine models of puberty show an increase in hepatic levels of SCPx, while female murine models show a decrease. The fact that SCPx expression is specifically controlled by androgens during sexual maturation suggests that androgens play a significant role in controlling SCPx expression [137]. In diseases associated with impaired bile acid synthesis and cholesterol binding, the gene is highly expressed [138]. The liver plays a key role in regulating the cholesterol synthesis rate. Furthermore, it coordinates the removal of cholesterol from the body by either removing it directly into the bile or converting it into more water-soluble bile acids [139]. Free cholesterol (FC) or non-esterified cholesterol cannot move between cell membranes or within cellular compartments due to its hydrophobicity. Intracellular cholesterol transport is facilitated by intracellular lipid transporter proteins such as SCP2 (13 kDa) (Figure 6). The expression of this carrier is induced by *Hypericum* and is closely correlated with the rate of intracellular cholesterol metabolism in different tissues, especially the liver, which maintains cholesterol homeostasis. He et al. evaluated the effect of SCP2/SCPx deficiency on intestinal cholesterol absorption [138]. There is a close correlation between decreased levels of hepatic lipid transport proteins, including SCPx and SCP2 and Niemann–Pick type C (NPC) disease, which is characterized by accumulated hepatic cholesterol in lysosomes and Golgi [138]. As lysosomal cholesterol is the primary precursor of androgens, a deficiency of intracellular cholesterol transport from lysosomes in NPC patients is responsible for disrupting androgen production [140].

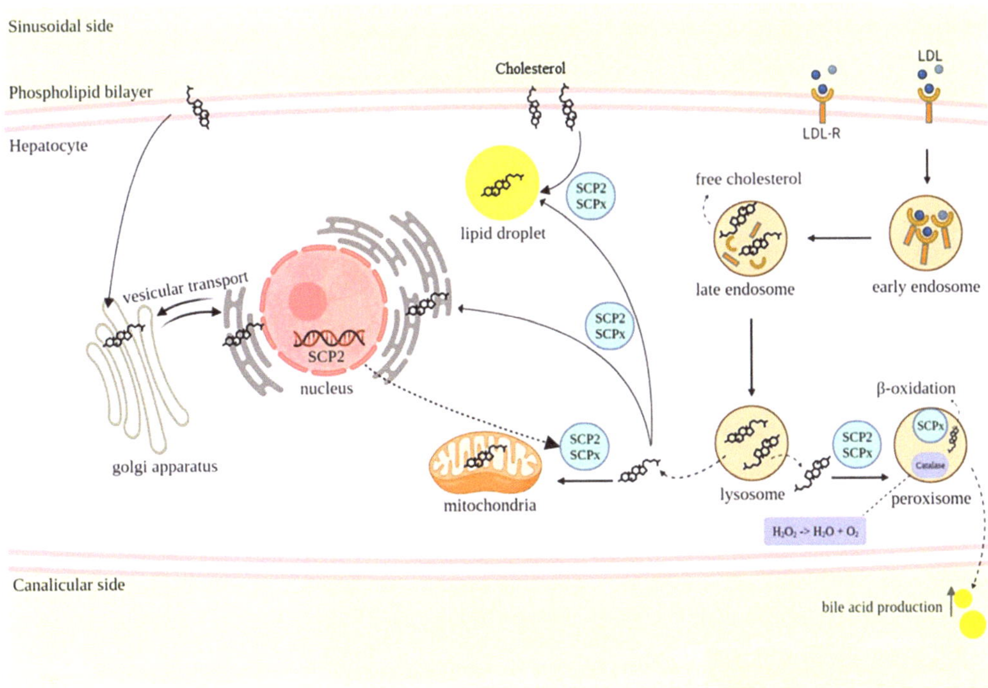

Figure 6. SCP2/SCPx function in cholestasis. LDL transport from the sinusoidal side to the hepatocyte via the LDL receptor (LDL-R). Due to the acidic pH of endosomes, LDL-R breaks into free cholesterol. The transportation of free cholesterol between different organelles, including mitochondria, plasma membrane, peroxisome, and lysosomes is facilitated by SCP2/SCPx. The entrance of free cholesterol into the lipid droplet from the sinusoidal side is also carried out via SCP2/SCPx. Apart from these, SCPx is a key factor in peroxisomal β-oxidation of fatty acids and bile acid production.

- Cyclin-dependent kinase 6 (CDK6)

CDK6 is a member of the CDK family that is generally responsible for regulating DNA replication. CDKs are characterized as essential signaling factors for hepatocyte proliferation in the late gestation period of fetal liver development [141]. CDK6 is a protein-coding gene that encodes a 37 kDa serine/threonine protein kinase. The encoded kinase is a mitogenic factor, in complex with D-type cyclins (D1, D2, and D3 cyclins), promoting G1 phase progression and G1/S transition, and is ubiquitously expressed. The CDK6-cyclin complex regulates retinoblastoma (Rb), a tumor suppressor protein, and therefore plays a key role in the early phases of several human cancers. Rb will release E2F, a transcription activator of necessary genes for DNA replication when the CDK-cyclin complex phosphorylates it. The Rb-E2F pathway exerts a key role in the regulation of cell proliferation and differentiation during the G1 phase of the cell cycle. Overexpression of CDK6 will lead to phosphorylation and activation of the Rb-E2F regulating pathway. Rb phosphorylation can be controlled by members of the INK family and the CIP/KIP family [142]. It has been observed that bile acids may cause DNA damage to hepatocytes in previous studies [143]. As a result, the upregulation of CDK6 by *H. perforatum* can be considered a hepatoprotective mechanism against cholestasis.

- Superkiller Viralicidic Activity 2-Like (SKIV2L)

The human super killer (SKI) complex works alongside RNA exosomes to mediate RNA surveillance. The human SKI complex is made up of four proteins: TPR encoded by tetratricopeptide repeat domain-containing protein 37 (TTC37), two WD40-containing subunits encoded by WDR61, and SKI2W which is encoded by super killer viralicidic activity 2 (SKIV2L) [144]. It is believed that pathogenic variants in SKIV2L and TTC37 often relate to a rare recessive genetic disorder known as trichohepatoenteric syndrome (THES). A third of THES cases are reported to be caused by SKIV2L gene mutations, and another third are caused by TTC37 gene mutations [145]. In a recent study, severe infantile liver disease has been associated with a novel homozygous frame-shift mutation (c.3391 delC) in SKIV2L [146]. The syndrome is characterized by intractable diarrhea, hepatic problems, facial and hair dysmorphisms, and intellectual disabilities in the first few months of life. These patients often suffer from cardiac abnormalities and immune dysregulations. Patients with SKIV2L mutations may benefit from growth hormone therapy [145]. Therefore, SKIV2L expression under *Hypericum* treatment could be involved in regulating bile flow and hepatic hemostasis.

- NISCH

The NISCH encodes imidazoline receptor antisera-selected (IRAS), also known as nischarin, which is a novel protein interacting with α5 cytoplasmic domain of integrins, and therefore affects cell migration and ECM microarchitecture [147]. It was claimed that nischarin may function as an imidazoline 1 receptor (I1R) in some cells [148]. However, this hypothesis was later challenged by Arnoux et al., who concluded that NISCH and I1R are not the same [149]. Liver fibrosis, as a life-threatening result of cholestasis, is progressed by releasing of pro-inflammatory cytokines, activation of HSCs, and Kupffer cells. Activation of I1R serves a hepatoprotective role in the fibrotic liver by interacting with the Nrf2 signaling pathway. Activation of the Nrf2 signaling pathway is associated with the inhibition of the TLR4/NF-*k*B pathway and TGF-β, as one of the most important cytokines related to fibrosis [150].

- Conserved oligomeric Golgi (COG 4,7)

COG encodes conserved oligomeric Golgi complex with eight subunits, and exerts its role in the maintenance of Golgi apparatus structure and function. COG4 is one of the subunits and is located in lobe A of this complex and COG7 is located in lobe B [151]. The Golgi apparatus is an important site for protein and lipid glycosylation [152]. There is a reported vesicular pathway of transportation of bile acid into the hepatocyte which mainly involves the Golgi apparatus. After the uptake of bile acids by hepatocyte sinusoidal plasma membrane, they bind to proteins. The complex formed (bile acid + protein) can be taken up by the Golgi apparatus and move towards the canalicular membrane via Golgi-derived vesicles [153]. It can be hypothesized that any defect in genes that are related to the Golgi apparatus maintenance and function, including COGs, can lead to impairment in bile flow and ultimately cholestasis.

2.5. Interacting Network of Hypericum Metabolites and Their Target Genes

As mentioned earlier, *Hypericum* contains several metabolites, with a broad-spectrum pharmacological attribute. In order to define the potential target genes of the named bioactive constituents, we used the STITCH database [154]. Bioactive compounds were uploaded to STITCH in order to achieve hub genes of each specialized metabolite. The organism was limited to "homo sapiens". Only targets with an interaction score >0.4 were selected for subsequent analysis. The intersection of target genes for each *Hypericum* metabolite and cholestasis-related genes (obtained from GeneCards) were determined [155]. Retrieved target genes for each metabolite are classified in Table S3 and those that are involved in cholestasis are displayed in Figure 7. A full description of the genes that are mainly involved in hepatobiliary disorders is discussed below.

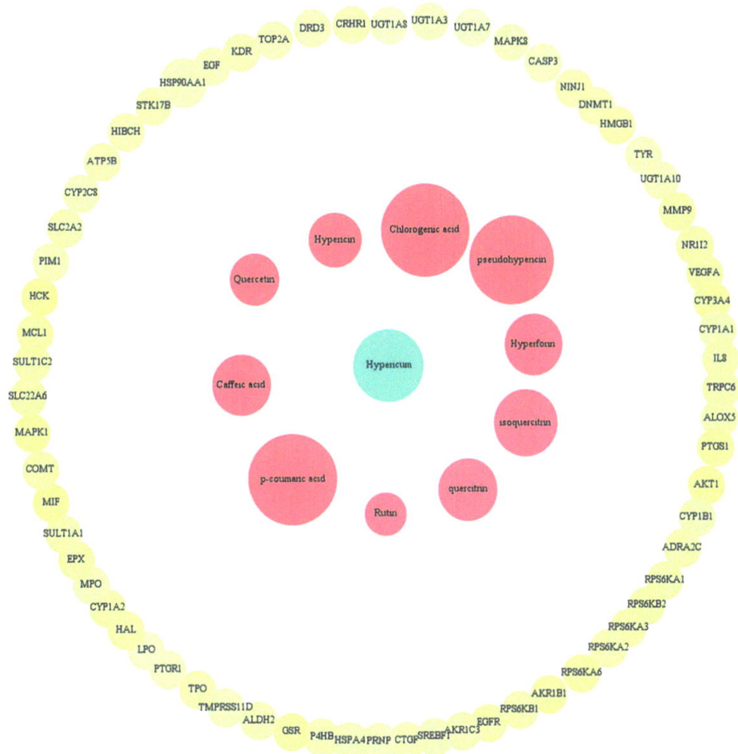

Figure 7. Potential target genes against cholestasis associated with each of the *Hypericum perforatum* L. bioactive metabolites. Hypericin, hyperforin, quercitrin, isoquercitrin, caffeic acid, *p*-coumaric acid, chlorogenic acid, rutin, quercetin, and pseudohypericin are located as central nodes.

Caffeic acid is capable of affecting MAPK1/8 expression, which is involved in liver toxicity during cholestasis [92]. Caffeic acid, hyperforin, and hypericin have the capacity to affect arachidonate 5-lipoxygenase (ALOX5) expression, which is believed to accelerate atherosclerosis by elevated leukotriene synthesis via leukocytes and therefore increased inflammation within arterial walls [156]. As observed in the interaction network (Figure 7), caffeic acid can also regulate the expression of organic anion transporter 1 (OAT1/SLC22A6) involved in the regulation of bile acid secretion and transportation. This is in agreement with experimental observations that demonstrate a decreased serum level of bile acid compared to the wild-type in OAT1 knockout mice [157].

Chlorogenic acid also alters MAPK8 regulation, according to the interacting network of *Hypericum* metabolites and target genes. Chlorogenic acid and kaempferol are capable of changing UGT1A3/7/8/10 expression, which encodes the enzyme UDP-glucuronosyltransferase (UGT). Any defect in UGT expression, as the bile acid detoxifier, is believed to be related to the accumulation of toxic molecules in the body, including bile acids [158]. Chlorogenic acid also regulates DNMT1 expression, which is involved in the impairment of cholesterol efflux as mentioned earlier. This metabolite regulates high-mobility group box 1 (HMGB1) expression, which is released after liver injury, activates HSCs, and ultimately induces liver fibrosis as a repair response [159].

As observed in Figure 7, the expression of CYP1A1 is inhibited by several metabolites, including hypericin, hyperforin, pseudohypericin, quercitrin, quercetin, and *p*-coumaric acid. This observation is in agreement with previous studies conducted on *Hypericum* extract [160]. Previous studies have shown that CYP1A1 is upregulated by bile acids, which may explain the carcinogenesis effect of cholestasis [161]. Generally, CYP1A (including CYP1A1/2) is found to regulate cholesterol biosynthesis pathways which provide new insights into the treatment of hypercholesterolemia. *p*-coumaric acid, a main metabolite of *Hypericum*, affects CYP1A2 expression and is suitable to regulate cholesterol homeostasis [162]. The expression of myeloperoxidase (MPO), an enzyme related to oxidative stress, inflammation, and liver fibrosis, is affected by *p*-coumaric acid [163]. Elevated MPO activity in hepatic neutrophils has shown correlations with hepatocyte damage and nonalcoholic steatohepatitis (NASH) [164].

The interacting network of metabolites and target genes shows that hypericin, hyperforin, and quercitrin affect CYP3A4 expression (Figure 7), which is in agreement with the previous studies stating that *H. perforatum* induces CYP3A4 [165]. CYP3A4, as the potential bile acid detoxifier, is recommended as one of the therapeutic mechanisms against cholestasis facilitating the consequent bile acid glucuronidation reaction by UGTs [166]. Other CYPs, such as CYP1B1 and CYP2C8, can be potential targets for the treatment of metabolic diseases [167]. CYP1B1 is targeted by quercitrin, isoquercitrin, rutin, quercetin, and kaempferol. The interaction network shows that quercetin, a common flavonol aglycone, affects CYP2C8 and CYP1B1 expression. In addition, quercetin affects anti-apoptotic Mcl-1, which exerts hepatoprotective effects following cholestasis-induced bile duct ligation. Overexpressing hepatic Mcl-1 is a suggested therapeutic mechanism against liver injury [168].

Vascular endothelial growth factor A (VEGFA) from hepatocytes is contributed to NAFLD with the mechanism of activating HSCs in the liver, so it can be counted as a good therapeutic target against NAFLD [169]. Antiangiogenic therapies have been evaluated as a good therapeutic choice for improving chronic liver disease-induced cholestasis [170]. Interestingly, hyperforin shows also antiangiogenic activity by inhibiting VEGFA [171]. According to the identified hub genes, both hyperforin and hypericin target VEGFA (Figure 7, Table S3). Matrix metalloproteinase 9 (MMP9), involved in hepatic tissue repair, remodeling, and cellular movement, is regulated by hyperforin, hypericin, quercetin, and luteolin. MMP9 can be secreted from Kupffer cells and HSCs, and induce the release of growth factors from ECM [172].

There is evidence that heat shock protein 90 (HSP90) is associated with liver injury, and HSP90 inhibitors serve as protectors of several organs. Administration of 17-DMAG, an HSP90 inhibitor, was related to the amelioration of cholestasis and the reduction of IL-1β and IL-18 expression [173]. Amongst *Hypericum* metabolites, hypericin affects HSP90 expression, which is worth further in-depth investigation (Figure 7).

3. Materials and Methods

In this article, the key points of pharmacological mechanisms of *Hypericum* choleretic and anti-cholestasis characteristics appear in two distinct sections as follows:

3.1. Hypericum Bioactive Components and Their Pharmacological Attributes with an Emphasis on Cholestasis Found in Literature

First, we searched medical attributes to *H. perforatum* known as "Houfariqun" with a phonetic spelling as/hu:fɑ:rɪɢu:n/in Makhzan-ol-advieh, a traditional Persian pharmacopeia collected by "Aqili al-Alavi" (1772 A.D.) to investigate its traditional medicinal properties. Then, different terms, including "*Hypericum perforatum*", "St. John's wort", "Cholestasis", "bile acid", "pharmacological mechanisms", and "bioactive components", were searched through engines such as "PubMed" and "Google Scholar" until September 2022.

3.2. Potential H. perforatum Target Genes against Cholestasis

H. perforatum expression microarray data sets were extracted using the GEO website (http://www.ncbi.nlm.nih.gov/geo/, accessed on 1 May 2023). The study type was restricted to expression profiling by an array. The GEO website contains three expression microarray datasets for *H. perforatum* L., including GSE56571, GSE21841, and GSE144235 [174–176]. Since sample numbers were limited for GSE56571 and GSE21841, we only selected GSE144235 [174]. To investigate the potential target genes related to cholestasis, we used GSE144235 with 228 samples containing 48 controls [174]. The transcriptional profile of GSE144235 was retrieved via Genometry L1000™ Expression Profiling using four human cell lines, including MCF7, Ishikawa, HepG2, and A549, to evaluate the toxicity of a dietary supplement containing *Hypericum*, ginger, kava kava, chaste tree, and ashwagandha [174]. We have performed an in-depth analysis on HepG2 cells that were treated with three different concentrations of *H. perforatum* extract (2.5, 25, 250 µg/mL) or DMSO as a vehicle for a 6-h time point. Notably, *Hypericum* extracts with a concentration of 25 and 250 µg/ml were defined to be cytotoxic according to VanderMolen et al. Therefore, we have intensively considered hepatocytes treated with 2.5 µg/ml *Hypericum* extract. The differentially expressed genes (DEGs) were identified and analyzed using GEO2R. Benjamini–Hochberg false discovery rate was used to adjust the *p*-value. $|\log \text{Fc}$ (fold change)$| > 0.2$ and a p-value < 0.05 were set as statistical significance criteria.

To acquire genes involved in cholestasis, we used "cholestasis" as the keyword to search in GeneCards as a human gene database [177]. Genes with "gifts > 30" were selected as potential genes involved in cholestasis. The intersections of DEGs upon treatment with *Hypericum* extract and potential genes that are involved in cholestasis were generated and defined using the Bioinformatics & Evolutionary Genomics online tool (https://bioinformatics.psb.ugent.be/webtools/Venn/), accessed on 1 May 2023, to display the Venn diagram. Overlapped DEGs were used to define hub genes. The DAVID online analysis tool, which is a database for annotation, visualization, and integrated discovery was used for gene ontology (GO) enrichment analysis [178].

To retrieve a protein–protein interaction (PPI) network by defining Homo sapiens as the target organism, we used "String", a search tool for the retrieval of interacting genes and proteins [179]. The protein interaction network of DEGs was constructed by Cytoscape software [180]. The Cytohubba plug-in was utilized in order to introduce potential hub genes [181]. Then, each gene was searched using different terms, including "cholestasis", "cholagogue", "bile acid", and "cholesterol". Finally, in order to predict potential target genes associated with each *Hypericum* metabolite, we used the STITCH database [154]. The main secondary metabolites of *Hypericum* as bioactive compounds were uploaded to STITCH using the SMILE format in order to achieve the target genes of each bioactive component. The organism was limited to "Homo sapiens". Only targets with an interaction score >0.4 were selected for subsequent analysis. The cholestasis-related genes obtained from GeneCards and the predicted genes of each *Hypericum* bioactive metabolite were intersected to define the target gene for each metabolite [155].

4. Conclusions

Effective therapeutics against hepatic disorders are worryingly limited and might eventually result in liver transplantation with a high mortality rate. Therefore, hepatic afflictions can be considered complex disorders which require multi-targeted drug discovery. One of the main therapeutic approaches in treating cholestasis is increasing the bile flow (choleretic effect) and excreting excess bile by feces (cholagogue effect). *Hypericum* helps with hepatitis, hepatocyte peroxidation, NAFLD, hepatic lipid metabolism, and hepatic steatosis. *Hypericum*'s hepatoprotective activity can be attributed to the suppression of TNF-α and IL-6 cytokine contents in the liver. *Hypericum* regulates LysoPC content as a hepatic inflammation biomarker and regulates the secretion and expression of adiponectin, which balances glucose and fatty acid metabolism. *Hypericum* extract lowers total cholesterol, raises HDL, and decreases triglyceride content. As degeneration and lytic necrosis are features of cholestatic hepatitis, *Hypericum* triggers the regulatory mechanism for liver regeneration. A total of 16 common genes, including EZH2, SCP2, ILK, CDK6, EGF, SPP1, PLOD3, SKIV2L, CXCL2, NISCH, ICAM1, SRC, CAT, COG7, BAX, and COG4, which are also involved in cholestasis, were identified under the treatment with the low dose of *Hypericum* extract. *Hypericum* targets the MAPK signaling pathway, which in turn regulates various hepatic functions, including bile acid synthesis, bile acid excretion, bile-acid-induced apoptosis, and hepatic steatosis. Target genes that are affected by *Hypericum* extract or its metabolites regulate cholesterol homeostasis to control hypercholesterolemia, detoxify bile acids, regulate hepatocyte differentiation, growth, migration, and survival, and increase the wound healing ability of HSCs toward liver regeneration through the modulation of collagen production. For example, hyperforin, one of the most important specialized metabolites of *Hypericum*, shows antiangiogenic activity by inhibiting VEGFA, which is suitable for controlling NAFLD. Quercetin, which affects the anti-apoptotic Mcl-1 protein, prevents liver injury following cholestasis. Taken together, merging the data retrieved through traditional medicine with the target genes that are affected by *Hypericum* improves the treatment approaches against cholestasis and related hepatic injuries such as hepatic carcinoma. Finally, standard trials using *Hypericum* alone and in combination with UDCA as adjuvant or second-line therapy should be designed to define the placement of this plant species in the treatment of cholestasis and its symptoms.

Supplementary Materials: The following supporting information can be downloaded at: https://www.mdpi.com/article/10.3390/ph16060887/s1: Table S1: Differentially expressed genes in HepG2 cells under the treatment with 2.5 µg/ml *Hypericum perforatum* extract; Table S2: The involved genes in cholestasis; Table S3: Predicted target genes affected by *Hypericum perforatum* metabolites.

Author Contributions: Conceptualization, P.B. and S.H.; methodology, A.M. (Ala Mohagheghzadeh) and S.H.; software, A.M. (Ala Mohagheghzadeh) and S.H.; validation, P.B., S.H. and A.M. (Abdolali Mohagheghzadeh); formal analysis, A.M. (Ala Mohagheghzadeh); investigation, A.M. (Ala Mohagheghzadeh); resources, A.M. (Abdolali Mohagheghzadeh) and S.H.; data curation, S.H.; writing—original draft preparation, A.M. (Ala Mohagheghzadeh); writing—review and editing, P.B., A.M. (Abdolali Mohagheghzadeh) and S.H.; visualization, P.B., A.M. (Abdolali Mohagheghzadeh) and S.H.; supervision, S.H.; project administration, S.H.; funding acquisition, S.H. All authors have read and agreed to the published version of the manuscript.

Funding: This research was funded by Shiraz University of Medical Sciences: 28411.

Institutional Review Board Statement: Not applicable.

Data Availability Statement: Data sharing not applicable.

Acknowledgments: Authors would like to thank Shiraz University of Medical Sciences for the project #28411.

Conflicts of Interest: The authors declare no conflict of interest.

References

1. Li, T.; Apte, U. Bile Acid Metabolism and Signaling in Cholestasis, Inflammation, and Cancer. *Adv. Pharmacol.* **2015**, *74*, 263–302. [PubMed]
2. Ding, L.; Yang, L.; Wang, Z.; Huang, W. Bile acid nuclear receptor FXR and digestive system diseases. *Acta Pharm. Sin. B* **2015**, *5*, 135–144. [CrossRef]
3. Cai, S.-Y.; Ouyang, X.; Chen, Y.; Soroka, C.J.; Wang, J.; Mennone, A.; Wang, Y.; Mehal, W.Z.; Jain, D.; Boyer, J.L. Bile acids initiate cholestatic liver injury by triggering a hepatocyte-specific inflammatory response. *JCI Insight.* **2017**, *2*, e90780. [CrossRef] [PubMed]
4. Wu, H.; Chen, C.; Ziani, S.; Nelson, L.J.; Ávila, M.A.; Nevzorova, Y.A.; Cubero, F.J. Fibrotic Events in the Progression of Cholestatic Liver Disease. *Cells* **2021**, *10*, 1107. [CrossRef] [PubMed]
5. Saffioti, F.; Gurusamy, K.S.; Eusebi, L.H.; Tsochatzis, E.; Davidson, B.R.; Thorburn, D. Pharmacological interventions for primary biliary cholangitis: An attempted network meta-analysis. *Cochrane Database Syst. Rev.* **2017**, *3*, Cd011648. [PubMed]
6. Rajapaksha, I.G.; Angus, P.W.; Herath, C.B. Current therapies and novel approaches for biliary diseases. *World J. Gastrointest. Pathophysiol.* **2019**, *10*, 1–10. [CrossRef]

7. Di Ciaula, A.; Bonfrate, L.; Baj, J.; Khalil, M.; Garruti, G.; Stellaard, F.; Wang, H.H.; Wang, D.Q.-H.; Portincasa, P. Recent Advances in the Digestive, Metabolic and Therapeutic Effects of Farnesoid X Receptor and Fibroblast Growth Factor 19: From Cholesterol to Bile Acid Signaling. *Nutrients* **2022**, *14*, 4950. [CrossRef]
8. Simental-Mendía, L.E.; Simental-Mendía, M.; Sánchez-García, A.; Banach, M.; Serban, M.-C.; Cicero, A.F.G.; Sahebkar, A. Impact of ursodeoxycholic acid on circulating lipid concentrations: A systematic review and meta-analysis of randomized placebo-controlled trials. *Lipids Health Dis.* **2019**, *18*, 88. [CrossRef]
9. Santiago, P.; Scheinberg, A.R.; Levy, C. Cholestatic liver diseases: New targets, new therapies. *Ther. Adv. Gastroenterol.* **2018**, *11*, 1756284818787400. [CrossRef]
10. de Vries, E.; Beuers, U. Management of cholestatic disease in 2017. *Liver Int.* **2017**, *37* (Suppl. S1), 123–129. [CrossRef]
11. Khakoo, N.S.; Sultan, S.; Reynolds, J.M.; Levy, C. Efficacy and Safety of Bezafibrate Alone or in Combination with Ursodeoxycholic Acid in Primary Biliary Cholangitis: Systematic Review and Meta-Analysis. *Dig. Dis. Sci.* **2023**, *68*, 1559–1573. [CrossRef] [PubMed]
12. Li, C.; Zheng, K.; Chen, Y.; He, C.; Liu, S.; Yang, Y.; Li, M.; Zeng, X.; Wang, L.; Zhang, F. A randomized, controlled trial on fenofibrate in primary biliary cholangitis patients with incomplete response to ursodeoxycholic acid. *Ther. Adv. Chronic Dis.* **2022**, *13*, 20406223221114198. [CrossRef] [PubMed]
13. Yang, C.; Guo, G.; Li, B.; Zheng, L.; Sun, R.; Wang, X.; Deng, J.; Jia, G.; Zhou, X.; Cui, L.; et al. Prediction and evaluation of high-risk patients with primary biliary cholangitis receiving ursodeoxycholic acid therapy: An early criterion. *Hepatol. Int.* **2023**, *17*, 237–248. [CrossRef] [PubMed]
14. Namisaki, T.; Fujinaga, Y.; Moriya, K.; Yoshiji, H. The association of histological progression with biochemical response to ursodeoxycholic acid in primary biliary cholangitis. *Hepatol. Res.* **2021**, *51*, 31–38. [CrossRef]
15. Chappell, L.C.; Bell, J.L.; Smith, A.; Linsell, L.; Juszczak, E.; Dixon, P.H.; Chambers, J.; Hunter, R.; Dorling, J.; Williamson, C.; et al. Ursodeoxycholic acid versus placebo in women with intrahepatic cholestasis of pregnancy (PITCHES): A randomised controlled trial. *Lancet* **2019**, *394*, 849–860. [CrossRef]
16. Kotb, M.A.; Mosallam, D.; Basanti, C.W.S.; El Sorogy, S.T.M.; Badr, A.M.; Abd El Baky, H.E.H.; Draz, I.H. Ursodeoxycholic acid use is associated with significant risk of morbidity and mortality in infants with cholestasis: A strobe compliant study. *Medicine* **2020**, *99*, e18730. [CrossRef]
17. Agrawal, R.; Majeed, M.; Attar, B.M.; Abu Omar, Y.; Mbachi, C.; Wang, Y.; Flores, E.; Shaqib, S.; Wang, Y.; Udechukwu, V.; et al. Effectiveness of bezafibrate and ursodeoxycholic acid in patients with primary biliary cholangitis: A meta-analysis of randomized controlled trials. *Ann. Gastroenterol.* **2019**, *32*, 489–497. [CrossRef]
18. Goldstein, J.; Levy, C. Novel and emerging therapies for cholestatic liver diseases. *Liver Int.* **2018**, *38*, 1520–1535. [CrossRef]
19. Lu, L. Guidelines for the Management of Cholestatic Liver Diseases (2021). *J. Clin. Transl. Hepatol.* **2022**, *10*, 757–769. [CrossRef]
20. Clichici, S.; David, L.; Moldovan, B.; Baldea, I.; Olteanu, D.; Filip, M.; Nagy, A.; Luca, V.; Crivii, C.; Mircea, P.; et al. Hepatoprotective effects of silymarin coated gold nanoparticles in experimental cholestasis. *Mater. Sci. Eng. C Mater Biol. Appl.* **2020**, *115*, 111117. [CrossRef]
21. Shen, K.; Feng, X.; Pan, H.; Zhang, F.; Xie, H.; Zheng, S. Baicalin Ameliorates Experimental Liver Cholestasis in Mice by Modulation of Oxidative Stress, Inflammation, and NRF2 Transcription Factor. *Oxidative Med. Cell. Longev.* **2017**, *2017*, 6169128. [CrossRef] [PubMed]
22. Li, S.; Tan, H.-Y.; Wang, N.; Zhang, Z.-J.; Lao, L.; Wong, C.-W.; Feng, Y. The Role of Oxidative Stress and Antioxidants in Liver Diseases. *Int. J. Mol. Sci.* **2015**, *16*, 26087–26124. [CrossRef] [PubMed]
23. Wang, L.; Zhang, F.C.; Zhang, X. Therapeutic advances for primary biliary cholangitis: The old and the new. *Eur. J. Gastroenterol. Hepatol.* **2016**, *28*, 615–621. [CrossRef] [PubMed]
24. Mohagheghzadeh, A.; Hemmati, S.; Mehregan, I.; Alfermann, A.W. *Linum persicum*: Lignans and placement in Linaceae. *Phytochem. Rev.* **2003**, *2*, 363–369. [CrossRef]
25. Rahmatabadi, S.S.; Sadeghian, I.; Ghasemi, Y.; Sakhteman, A.; Hemmati, S. Identification and characterization of a sterically robust phenylalanine ammonia-lyase among 481 natural isoforms through association of in silico and in vitro studies. *Enzym. Microb. Technol.* **2019**, *122*, 36–54. [CrossRef]
26. Pérez-Ramírez, I.F.; Gallegos-Corona, M.A.; González-Dávalos, M.L.; Mora, O.; Rocha-Guzmán, N.E.; Reynoso-Camacho, R. Mechanisms Associated with the Effect of *Hypericum perforatum* and *Smilax cordifolia* Aqueous Extracts on Hepatic Steatosis in Obese Rats: A Lipidomic Approach. *Eur. J. Lipid Sci. Technol.* **2019**, *121*, 1800403. [CrossRef]
27. Barnes, J.; Anderson, L.A.; Phillipson, J.D. St John's wort (*Hypericum perforatum* L.): A review of its chemistry, pharmacology and clinical properties. *J. Pharm. Pharmacol.* **2001**, *53*, 583–600. [CrossRef]
28. Greeson, J.M.; Sanford, B.; Monti, D.A. St. John's wort (*Hypericum perforatum*): A review of the current pharmacological, toxicological, and clinical literature. *Psychopharmacology* **2001**, *153*, 402–414. [CrossRef]
29. Ben-Eliezer, D.; Yechiam, E. *Hypericum perforatum* as a cognitive enhancer in rodents: A meta-analysis. *Sci. Rep.* **2016**, *6*, 35700. [CrossRef]
30. Romm, A.; Hardy, M.L.; Mills, S. ST. John's Wort. In *Botanical Medicine for Women's Health*; Romm, A., Hardy, M.L., Mills, S., Eds.; Churchill Livingstone: Saint Louis, MO, USA, 2010; pp. 544–546.
31. Booker, A.; Agapouda, A.; Frommenwiler, D.A.; Scotti, F.; Reich, E.; Heinrich, M. St John's wort (*Hypericum perforatum*) products—An assessment of their authenticity and quality. *Phytomedicine* **2018**, *40*, 158–164. [CrossRef]

32. Klemow, K.M.; Bartlow, A.; Crawford, J.; Kocher, N.; Shah, J.; Ritsick, M. *Medical Attributes of St. John's Wort (Hypericum Perforatum)*, 2nd ed.; CRC Press/Taylor & Francis: Boca Raton, FL, USA, 2011.
33. Russo, E.; Scicchitano, F.; Whalley, B.J.; Mazzitello, C.; Ciriaco, M.; Esposito, S.; Patanè, M.; Upton, R.; Pugliese, M.; Chimirri, S.; et al. *Hypericum perforatum*: Pharmacokinetic, Mechanism of Action, Tolerability, and Clinical Drug–Drug Interactions. *Phytother. Res.* **2014**, *28*, 643–655. [CrossRef]
34. Khorasani, M.A. Makhzan al Advieh (The Storehouse of Medicaments). In *Research Institute for Islamic and Complementary Medicine*; Iran University of Medical Sciences Bavardaran Press: Tehran, Iran, 2001; Volume 351. (In Persian)
35. Öztürk, Y.; Aydin, S.; Başer, K.H.C.; Kirimer, N.; Kurtar-Öztürk, N. Hepatoprotective activity of *Hypericum perforatum* L. alcoholic extract in rodents. *Phytother. Res.* **1992**, *6*, 44–46. [CrossRef]
36. Bokelmann, J.M. 67—St. John's Wort (*Hypericum perforatum*): Flowering Buds and Tops. In *Medicinal Herbs in Primary Care*; Bokelmann, J.M., Ed.; Elsevier: Philadelphia, PA, USA, 2021; pp. 569–577.
37. Zhang, R.; Ji, Y.; Zhang, X.; Kennelly, E.J.; Long, C. Ethnopharmacology of *Hypericum* species in China: A comprehensive review on ethnobotany, phytochemistry and pharmacology. *J. Ethnopharmacol.* **2020**, *254*, 112686. [CrossRef]
38. Galeotti, N. *Hypericum perforatum* (St John's wort) beyond depression: A therapeutic perspective for pain conditions. *J. Ethnopharmacol.* **2017**, *200*, 136–146. [CrossRef]
39. Wölfle, U.; Seelinger, G.; Schempp, C.M. Topical application of St. John's wort (*Hypericum perforatum*). *Planta Med.* **2014**, *80*, 109–120.
40. Hammer, K.D.; Birt, D.F. Evidence for Contributions of Interactions of Constituents to the Anti-Inflammatory Activity of *Hypericum perforatum*. *Crit. Rev. Food Sci. Nutr.* **2014**, *54*, 781–789. [CrossRef]
41. Shrivastava, M.; Dwivedi, L. Therapeutic potential of *Hypericum perforatum*: A review. *Int. J. Pharm. Sci. Res.* **2015**, *6*, 4982–4988.
42. Hemmati, S.; Behzadipour, Y.; Haddad, M. Decoding the proteome of severe acute respiratory syndrome coronavirus 2 (SARS-CoV-2) for cell-penetrating peptides involved in pathogenesis or applicable as drug delivery vectors. *Infect. Genet Evol.* **2020**, *85*, 104474. [CrossRef] [PubMed]
43. Behzadipour, Y.; Gholampour, M.; Pirhadi, S.; Seradj, H.; Khoshneviszadeh, M.; Hemmati, S. Viral 3CL(pro) as a Target for Antiviral Intervention Using Milk-Derived Bioactive Peptides. *Int. J. Pept. Res. Ther.* **2021**, *27*, 2703–2716. [CrossRef]
44. Mohamed, F.F.; Anhlan, D.; Schöfbänker, M.; Schreiber, A.; Classen, N.; Hensel, A.; Hempel, G.; Scholz, W.; Kühn, J.; Hrincius, E.R.; et al. *Hypericum perforatum* and Its Ingredients Hypericin and Pseudohypericin Demonstrate an Antiviral Activity against SARS-CoV-2. *Pharmaceuticals* **2022**, *15*, 530. [CrossRef] [PubMed]
45. Bilia, A.R.; Costa, M.D.C. Medicinal plants and their preparations in the European market: Why has the harmonization failed? The cases of St. John's wort, valerian, ginkgo, ginseng, and green tea. *Phytomedicine* **2021**, *81*, 153421. [CrossRef]
46. Colombo, F.; Restani, P.; Biella, S.; Di Lorenzo, C. Botanicals in Functional Foods and Food Supplements: Tradition, Efficacy and Regulatory Aspects. *Appl. Sci.* **2020**, *10*, 2387. [CrossRef]
47. Jakubczyk, A.; Kiersnowska, K.; Ömeroğlu, B.; Gawlik-Dziki, U.; Tutaj, K.; Rybczyńska-Tkaczyk, K.; Szydłowska-Tutaj, M.; Złotek, U.; Baraniak, B. The Influence of *Hypericum perforatum* L. Addition to Wheat Cookies on Their Antioxidant, Anti-Metabolic Syndrome, and Antimicrobial Properties. *Foods* **2021**, *10*, 1379. [CrossRef]
48. Ang, C.Y.W.; Hu, L.; Heinze, T.M.; Cui, Y.; Freeman, J.P.; Kozak, K.; Luo, W.; Liu, F.F.; Mattia, A.; DiNovi, M. Instability of St. John's Wort (*Hypericum perforatum* L.) and Degradation of Hyperforin in Aqueous Solutions and Functional Beverage. *J. Agric. Food Chem.* **2004**, *52*, 6156–6164. [CrossRef]
49. Tiwari, P.; Tiwari, P. Probiotic Novel Beverages and Their Applications. *Syst. Rev. Pharm.* **2011**, *2*, 41–47. [CrossRef]
50. Sánchez-Muniz, F.J.; Olivero-David, R.; Triki, M.; Salcedo, L.; González-Muñoz, M.J.; Cofrades, S.; Ruiz-Capillas, C.; Jiménez-Colmenero, F.; Benedi, J. Antioxidant activity of *Hypericum perforatum* L. extract in enriched n-3 PUFA pork meat systems during chilled storage. *Food Res. Int.* **2012**, *48*, 909–915. [CrossRef]
51. Carrubba, A.; Lazzara, S.; Giovino, A.; Ruberto, G.; Napoli, E. Content variability of bioactive secondary metabolites in *Hypericum perforatum* L. *Phytochem. Lett.* **2021**, *46*, 71–78. [CrossRef]
52. Hemmati, S.; Schneider, B.; Schmidt, T.J.; Federolf, K.; Alfermann, A.W.; Fuss, E. Justicidin B 7-hydroxylase, a cytochrome P450 monooxygenase from cell cultures of *Linum perenne* Himmelszelt involved in the biosynthesis of diphyllin. *Phytochemistry* **2007**, *68*, 2736–2743. [CrossRef] [PubMed]
53. Mohagheghzadeh, A.; Dehshahri, S.; Hemmati, S. Accumulation of Lignans by in vitro Cultures of Three *Linum* Species. *Z. Nat. C* **2009**, *64*, 73–76. [CrossRef] [PubMed]
54. Danova, K.; Motyka, V.; Trendafilova, A.; Dobrev, P.I.; Ivanova, V.; Aneva, I. Evolutionary Aspects of Hypericin Productivity and Endogenous Phytohormone Pools Evidenced in *Hypericum* Species In Vitro Culture Model. *Plants* **2022**, *11*, 2753. [CrossRef] [PubMed]
55. De Paola, R.; Muià, C.; Mazzon, E.; Genovese, T.; Crisafulli, C.; Menegazzi, M.; Caputi, A.P.; Suzuki, H.; Cuzzocrea, S. Effects of *Hypericum perforatum* Extract in a Rat Model of Ischemia and Reperfusion Injury. *Shock* **2005**, *24*, 255–263. [CrossRef]
56. Aydin, A.; Sakrak, O.; Yilmaz, T.U.; Kerem, M. The effects of Hypericum perforatum on hepatic ischemia-reperfusion injury in rats. *Bratisl. Lek. Listy* **2014**, *115*, 209–215. [CrossRef]
57. Saija, A.; Scalese, M.; Lanza, M.; Marzullo, D.; Bonina, F.; Castelli, F. Flavonoids as antioxidant agents: Importance of their interaction with biomembranes. *Free. Radic. Biol. Med.* **1995**, *19*, 481–486. [CrossRef]

58. Huang, N.; Rizshsky, L.; Hauck, C.; Nikolau, B.J.; Murphy, P.A.; Birt, D.F. Identification of anti-inflammatory constituents in *Hypericum perforatum* and *Hypericum gentianoides* extracts using RAW 264.7 mouse macrophages. *Phytochemistry* **2011**, *72*, 2015–2023. [CrossRef]
59. Koeberle, A.; Rossi, A.; Bauer, J.; Dehm, F.; Verotta, L.; Northoff, H.; Sautebin, L.; Werz, O. Hyperforin, an Anti-Inflammatory Constituent from St. John's Wort, Inhibits Microsomal Prostaglandin E2 Synthase-1 and Suppresses Prostaglandin E2 Formation in vivo. *Front. Pharmacol.* **2011**, *2*, 7. [CrossRef]
60. Menegazzi, M.; Masiello, P.; Novelli, M. Anti-Tumor Activity of *Hypericum perforatum* L. and Hyperforin through Modulation of Inflammatory Signaling, ROS Generation and Proton Dynamics. *Antioxidants* **2020**, *10*, 18. [CrossRef]
61. Tokgöz, H.B.; Altan, F. *Hypericum perforatum* L.: A medicinal plant with potential as a curative agent against obesity-associated complications. *Mol. Biol. Rep.* **2020**, *47*, 8679–8686. [CrossRef] [PubMed]
62. Chen, L.; Liu, Y.; Tang, Z.; Shi, X.; Song, Z.; Cao, F.; Wei, P.; Li, M.; Li, X.; Jiang, D.; et al. Improvements in estrogen deficiency-induced hypercholesterolemia by *Hypericum perforatum* L. extract are associated with gut microbiota and related metabolites in ovariectomized (OVX) rats. *Biomed. Pharmacother.* **2021**, *135*, 111131. [CrossRef] [PubMed]
63. Maleki, M.; Moghaddam, M.H.G.; Roghani, M. Effect of *Hypericum perforatum* aqueous extracts on serum lipids, aminotransferases, and lipid peroxidation in hyperlipidemic rats. *Res. Cardiovasc. Med.* **2016**, *5*, e31326. [CrossRef] [PubMed]
64. Zou, Y.; Lu, Y.; Wei, D. Hypocholesterolemic effects of a flavonoid-rich extract of *Hypericum perforatum* L. in rats fed a cholesterol-rich diet. *J. Agric. Food Chem.* **2005**, *53*, 2462–2466. [CrossRef] [PubMed]
65. Hsu, C.-L.; Wu, C.-H.; Huang, S.-L.; Yen, G.-C. Phenolic Compounds Rutin and *o*-Coumaric Acid Ameliorate Obesity Induced by High-Fat Diet in Rats. *J. Agric. Food Chem.* **2009**, *57*, 425–431. [CrossRef] [PubMed]
66. Asgary, S.; Parkhideh, S.; Mahzouni, P.; Solhpour, A.; Madani, H.; Kabiri, N. Effect of hydroalcoholic extract of *Hypericum perforatum* on selected traditional and novel biochemical factors of cardiovascular diseases and atherosclerotic lesions in hypercholesterolemic rabbits: A comparison between the extract and lovastatin. *J. Pharm. Bioallied Sci.* **2012**, *4*, 212–218. [CrossRef] [PubMed]
67. Peng, S.G.; Pang, Y.L.; Zhu, Q.; Kang, J.H.; Liu, M.X.; Wang, Z. Chlorogenic Acid Functions as a Novel Agonist of PPARγ2 during the Differentiation of Mouse 3T3-L1 Preadipocytes. *BioMed Res. Int.* **2018**, *2018*, 8594767. [CrossRef]
68. Liang, C.; Li, Y.; Bai, M.; Huang, Y.; Yang, H.; Liu, L.; Wang, S.; Yu, C.; Song, Z.; Bao, Y.; et al. Hypericin attenuates nonalcoholic fatty liver disease and abnormal lipid metabolism via the PKA-mediated AMPK signaling pathway in vitro and in vivo. *Pharmacol. Res.* **2020**, *153*, 104657. [CrossRef]
69. Wu, C.-H.; Lin, M.-C.; Wang, H.-C.; Yang, M.-Y.; Jou, M.-J.; Wang, C.-J. Rutin Inhibits Oleic Acid Induced Lipid Accumulation via Reducing Lipogenesis and Oxidative Stress in Hepatocarcinoma Cells. *J. Food Sci.* **2011**, *76*, T65–T72. [CrossRef]
70. Chen, X. Protective effects of quercetin on liver injury induced by ethanol. *Pharmacogn. Mag.* **2010**, *6*, 135–141. [CrossRef]
71. Shi, Y.; Qiu, X.; Dai, M.; Zhang, X.; Jin, G. Hyperoside Attenuates Hepatic Ischemia-Reperfusion Injury by Suppressing Oxidative Stress and Inhibiting Apoptosis in Rats. *Transplant. Proc.* **2019**, *51*, 2051–2059. [CrossRef]
72. Skalkos, D.; Gioti, E.; Stalikas, C.D.; Meyer, H.; Papazoglou, T.G.; Filippidis, G. Photophysical properties of *Hypericum perforatum* L. extracts—Novel photosensitizers for PDT. *J. Photochem. Photobiol. B Biol.* **2006**, *82*, 146–151. [CrossRef]
73. Velingkar, V.S.; Gupta, G.L.; Hegde, N.B. A current update on phytochemistry, pharmacology and herb–drug interactions of *Hypericum perforatum*. *Phytochem. Rev.* **2017**, *16*, 725–744. [CrossRef]
74. Oliveira, A.I.; Pinho, C.; Sarmento, B.; Dias, A.C.P. Neuroprotective Activity of *Hypericum perforatum* and Its Major Components. *Front. Plant Sci.* **2016**, *7*, 1004. [CrossRef] [PubMed]
75. Simmen, U.; Bobirnac, I.; Ullmer, C.; Lübbert, H.; Büter, K.B.; Schaffner, W.; Schoeffter, P. Antagonist effect of pseudohypericin at CRF1 receptors. *Eur. J. Pharmacol.* **2003**, *458*, 251–256. [CrossRef]
76. Tian, J.; Zhang, F.; Cheng, J.; Guo, S.; Liu, P.; Wang, H. Antidepressant-like activity of adhyperforin, a novel constituent of *Hypericum perforatum* L. *Sci. Rep.* **2014**, *4*, 5632. [CrossRef] [PubMed]
77. Herraiz, T.; Guillén, H. Monoamine Oxidase-A Inhibition and Associated Antioxidant Activity in Plant Extracts with Potential Antidepressant Actions. *BioMed Res. Int.* **2018**, *2018*, 4810394. [CrossRef] [PubMed]
78. Sell, T.S.; Belkacemi, T.; Flockerzi, V.; Beck, A. Protonophore properties of hyperforin are essential for its pharmacological activity. *Sci. Rep.* **2014**, *4*, 7500. [CrossRef] [PubMed]
79. Leuner, K.; Kazanski, V.; Muller, M.; Essin, K.; Henke, B.; Gollasch, M.; Harteneck, C.; Müller, W.E. Hyperforin—A key constituent of St. John's wort specifically activates TRPC6 channels. *Faseb J.* **2007**, *21*, 4101–4111. [CrossRef]
80. Örnolfsson, K.T.; Lund, S.H.; Olafsson, S.; Bergmann, O.M.; Björnsson, E.S. Biochemical response to ursodeoxycholic acid among PBC patients: A nationwide population-based study. *Scand. J. Gastroenterol.* **2019**, *54*, 609–616. [CrossRef] [PubMed]
81. Arokiyaraj, S.; Balamurugan, R.; Augustian, P. Antihyperglycemic effect of Hypericum perforatum ethyl acetate extract on streptozotocin–induced diabetic rats. *Asian Pac. J. Trop. Biomed.* **2011**, *1*, 386–390.
82. Ansari, I.; Roghani, M.; Moghaddam, M.; Ghanem, A.; Mehdizade, N. The Effect of Oral Administration of Hypericum Perforatum on Serum Glucose and Lipids, Hepatic Enzymes and Lipid Peroxidation in Streptozotocin-Induced Diabetic Rats. *Galen Med. J.* **2017**, *6*, 319–329.
83. Duan, J.; Chen, W.; Zhao, Y.; He, L.; Li, E.; Bai, Z.; Wang, Y.; Zhang, C. Flavonoids from *Hypericum patulum* enhance glucose consumption and attenuate lipid accumulation in HepG2 cells. *J. Food Biochem.* **2021**, *45*, e13898. [CrossRef] [PubMed]

84. Thuy, L.T.T.; Hai, H.; Kawada, N. Role of cytoglobin, a novel radical scavenger, in stellate cell activation and hepatic fibrosis. *Clin. Mol. Hepatol.* **2020**, *26*, 280–293. [CrossRef] [PubMed]
85. Popko, K.; Gorska, E.; Stelmaszczyk-Emmel, A.; Plywaczewski, R.; Stoklosa, A.; Gorecka, D.; Pyrzak, B.; Demkow, U. Proinflammatory cytokines IL-6 and TNF-α and the development of inflammation in obese subjects. *Eur. J. Med. Res.* **2010**, *15* (Suppl. S2), 120–122. [CrossRef]
86. Lehmann, R.; Franken, H.; Dammeier, S.; Rosenbaum, L.; Kantartzis, K.; Peter, A.; Zell, A.; Adam, P.; Li, J.; Xu, G.; et al. Circulating Lysophosphatidylcholines Are Markers of a Metabolically Benign Nonalcoholic Fatty Liver. *Diabetes Care* **2013**, *36*, 2331–2338. [CrossRef]
87. Mizuno, H.; Taketomi, A.; Nakabayashi, T. Potentially Beneficial Effects of St. John's Wort (*Hypericum perforatum*) in Patients with Metabolic Syndrome. *OBM Integr. Complement. Med.* **2018**, *3*, 021. [CrossRef]
88. Tian, J.Y.; Tao, R.Y.; Zhang, X.L.; Liu, Q.; He, Y.B.; Su, Y.L.; Ji, T.F.; Ye, F. Effect of *Hypericum perforatum* L. extract on insulin resistance and lipid metabolic disorder in high-fat-diet induced obese mice. *Phytother. Res.* **2015**, *29*, 86–92. [CrossRef] [PubMed]
89. Mariotti, V.; Cadamuro, M.; Spirli, C.; Fiorotto, R.; Strazzabosco, M.; Fabris, L. Animal models of cholestasis: An update on inflammatory cholangiopathies. *Biochim. Biophys. Acta (BBA)-Mol. Basis Dis.* **2019**, *1865*, 954–964. [CrossRef]
90. Saran, C.; Fu, D.; Ho, H.; Klein, A.; Fallon, J.K.; Honkakoski, P.; Brouwer, K.L.R. A novel differentiated HuH-7 cell model to examine bile acid metabolism, transport and cholestatic hepatotoxicity. *Sci. Rep.* **2022**, *12*, 14333. [CrossRef]
91. Sadeghian, I.; Khalvati, B.; Ghasemi, Y.; Hemmati, S. TAT-mediated intracellular delivery of carboxypeptidase G2 protects against methotrexate-induced cell death in HepG2 cells. *Toxicol. Appl. Pharmacol.* **2018**, *346*, 9–18. [CrossRef] [PubMed]
92. Anwer, M. Role of P38 MAPK in Bile Formation and Cholestasis. *Gastroenterol. Hepatol. Res.* **2018**, *3*, 22.
93. Reinehr, R.; Becker, S.; Wettstein, M.; Häussinger, D. Involvement of the Src family kinase yes in bile salt-induced apoptosis. *Gastroenterology* **2004**, *127*, 1540–1557. [CrossRef]
94. Reinehr, R.; Sommerfeld, A.; Häussinger, D. The Src family kinases: Distinct functions of c-Src, Yes, and Fyn in the liver. *Biomol. Concepts* **2013**, *4*, 129–142. [CrossRef] [PubMed]
95. Zerdes, I.; Matikas, A.; Bergh, J.; Rassidakis, G.Z.; Foukakis, T. Genetic, transcriptional and post-translational regulation of the programmed death protein ligand 1 in cancer: Biology and clinical correlations. *Oncogene* **2018**, *37*, 4639–4661. [CrossRef] [PubMed]
96. Santamaría, E.; Rodríguez-Ortigosa, C.M.; Uriarte, I.; Latasa, M.U.; Urtasun, R.; Alvarez-Sola, G.; Bárcena-Varela, M.; Colyn, L.; Arcelus, S.; Jiménez, M.; et al. The Epidermal Growth Factor Receptor Ligand Amphiregulin Protects from Cholestatic Liver Injury and Regulates Bile Acids Synthesis. *Hepatology* **2019**, *69*, 1632–1647. [CrossRef] [PubMed]
97. Svinka, J.; Pflügler, S.; Mair, M.; Marschall, H.-U.; Hengstler, J.G.; Stiedl, P.; Poli, V.; Casanova, E.; Timelthaler, G.; Sibilia, M.; et al. Epidermal growth factor signaling protects from cholestatic liver injury and fibrosis. *J. Mol. Med.* **2017**, *95*, 109–117. [CrossRef] [PubMed]
98. Centuori, S.M.; Gomes, C.J.; Trujillo, J.; Borg, J.; Brownlee, J.; Putnam, C.W.; Martinez, J.D. Deoxycholic acid mediates non-canonical EGFR-MAPK activation through the induction of calcium signaling in colon cancer cells. *Biochim. Biophys. Acta* **2016**, *1861*, 663–670. [CrossRef] [PubMed]
99. Ye, X.; Zhang, T.; Han, H. PPARα: A potential therapeutic target of cholestasis. *Front. Pharmacol.* **2022**, *13*, 916866. [CrossRef] [PubMed]
100. Sun, F.; Li, X.; Xu, C.; Li, P.; Wu, J.; Sui, J. Effect of compound Yindan decoction on alpha-naphthylisothiocyanate-Induced acute intrahepatic cholestasis in rats. *J. Tradit. Chin. Med.* **2019**, *39*, 315–323.
101. Cai, S.-Y.; Li, M.; Boyer, J.L. The Liver: Biology and Pathobiology. In *The Role of Bile Acid-Mediated Inflammation in Cholestatic Liver Injury*; Wiley: Oxford, UK, 2020; pp. 728–736.
102. Nakamura, K.; Kageyama, S.; Kupiec-Weglinski, J.W. The Evolving Role of Neutrophils in Liver Transplant Ischemia-Reperfusion Injury. *Curr. Transplant. Rep.* **2019**, *6*, 78–89. [CrossRef]
103. Bartneck, M.; Wang, J. Therapeutic Targeting of Neutrophil Granulocytes in Inflammatory Liver Disease. *Front. Immunol.* **2019**, *10*, 2257. [CrossRef]
104. Tang, J.; Yan, Z.; Feng, Q.; Yu, L.; Wang, H. The Roles of Neutrophils in the Pathogenesis of Liver Diseases. *Front. Immunol.* **2021**, *12*, 625472. [CrossRef]
105. Michalopoulos, G.K.; Bhushan, B. Liver regeneration: Biological and pathological mechanisms and implications. *Nat. Rev. Gastroenterol. Hepatol.* **2021**, *18*, 40–55. [CrossRef]
106. Górska, A.; Mazur, A.J. Integrin-linked kinase (ILK): The known vs. the unknown and perspectives. *Cell. Mol. Life Sci.* **2022**, *79*, 100. [CrossRef] [PubMed]
107. Shafiei, M.S.; Rockey, D.C. The function of integrin-linked kinase in normal and activated stellate cells: Implications for fibrogenesis in wound healing. *Lab. Investig.* **2012**, *92*, 305–316. [CrossRef]
108. Martucci, N.; Michalopoulos, G.K.; Mars, W.M. Integrin Linked Kinase (ILK) and its Role in Liver Pathobiology. *Gene Expr.* **2021**, *20*, 201–207. [CrossRef] [PubMed]
109. Almasabi, S.; Ahmed, A.U.; Boyd, R.; Williams, B.R.G. A Potential Role for Integrin-Linked Kinase in Colorectal Cancer Growth and Progression via Regulating Senescence and Immunity. *Front. Genet.* **2021**, *12*, 638558. [CrossRef] [PubMed]
110. Yim, A.; Smith, C.; Brown, A.M. Osteopontin/secreted phosphoprotein-1 harnesses glial-, immune-, and neuronal cell ligand-receptor interactions to sense and regulate acute and chronic neuroinflammation. *Immunol. Rev.* **2022**, *311*, 224–233. [CrossRef]

111. Bruha, R.; Vitek, L.; Smid, V. Osteopontin—A potential biomarker of advanced liver disease. *Ann. Hepatol.* **2020**, *19*, 344–352. [CrossRef]
112. Shirasaki, T.; Honda, M.; Yamashita, T.; Nio, K.; Shimakami, T.; Shimizu, R.; Nakasyo, S.; Murai, K.; Shirasaki, N.; Okada, H.; et al. The osteopontin-CD44 axis in hepatic cancer stem cells regulates IFN signaling and HCV replication. *Sci. Rep.* **2018**, *8*, 13143. [CrossRef]
113. Meng, F.-G.; Zhang, X.-N.; Liu, S.-X.; Wang, Y.-R.; Zeng, T. Roles of peroxisome proliferator-activated receptor α in the pathogenesis of ethanol-induced liver disease. *Chem. Interact.* **2020**, *327*, 109176. [CrossRef]
114. Song, Z.; Chen, W.; Athavale, D.; Ge, X.; Desert, R.; Das, S.; Han, H.; Nieto, N. Osteopontin Takes Center Stage in Chronic Liver Disease. *Hepatology* **2021**, *73*, 1594–1608. [CrossRef]
115. Vahidnezhad, H.; Youssefian, L.; Saeidian, A.H.; Touati, A.; Pajouhanfar, S.; Baghdadi, T.; Shadmehri, A.A.; Giunta, C.; Kraenzlin, M.; Syx, D.; et al. Mutations in PLOD3, encoding lysyl hydroxylase 3, cause a complex connective tissue disorder including recessive dystrophic epidermolysis bullosa-like blistering phenotype with abnormal anchoring fibrils and type VII collagen deficiency. *Matrix Biol.* **2019**, *81*, 91–106. [CrossRef]
116. Yang, B.; Zhao, Y.; Wang, L.; Zhao, Y.; Wei, L.; Chen, D.; Chen, Z. Identification of PLOD Family Genes as Novel Prognostic Biomarkers for Hepatocellular Carcinoma. *Front. Oncol.* **2020**, *10*, 1695. [CrossRef]
117. Banushi, B.; Forneris, F.; Straatman-Iwanowska, A.; Strange, A.; Lyne, A.-M.; Rogerson, C.; Burden, J.J.; Heywood, W.E.; Hanley, J.; Doykov, I.; et al. Regulation of post-Golgi LH3 trafficking is essential for collagen homeostasis. *Nat. Commun.* **2016**, *7*, 12111. [CrossRef] [PubMed]
118. Du, H.; Pang, M.; Hou, X.; Yuan, S.; Sun, L. PLOD2 in cancer research. *Biomed. Pharmacother.* **2017**, *90*, 670–676. [CrossRef] [PubMed]
119. Zhang, Y.; Lu, Y.; Ji, H.; Li, Y. Anti-inflammatory, anti-oxidative stress and novel therapeutic targets for cholestatic liver injury. *Biosci. Trends* **2019**, *13*, 23–31. [CrossRef] [PubMed]
120. Brzački, V.; Mladenović, B.; Dimić, D.; Jeremić, L.; Živanović, D.; Djukić, D.; Stojanović, N.M.; Sokolović, D.T. Comparison between the effects of selenomethionine and S-adenosylmethionine in preventing cholestasis-induced rat liver damage. *Amino Acids* **2019**, *51*, 795–803. [CrossRef]
121. Zou, Y.P.; Lu, Y.H.; Wei, D.Z. Protective effects of a flavonoid-rich extract of *Hypericum perforatum* L. against hydrogen peroxide-induced apoptosis in PC12 cells. *Phytother. Res.* **2010**, *24* (Suppl. S1), S6–S10. [CrossRef]
122. Hemmati, S.; Kazerooni, H.R. Polypharmacological Cell-Penetrating Peptides from Venomous Marine Animals Based on Immunomodulating, Antimicrobial, and Anticancer Properties. *Mar. Drugs* **2022**, *20*, 763. [CrossRef]
123. Nasehi, M.; Torabinejad, S.; Hashemi, M.; Vaseghi, S.; Zarrindast, M.R. Effect of cholestasis and NeuroAid treatment on the expression of Bax, Bcl-2, Pgc-1α and Tfam genes involved in apoptosis and mitochondrial biogenesis in the striatum of male rats. *Metab. Brain Dis.* **2020**, *35*, 183–192. [CrossRef]
124. Brankiewicz, A.; Trzos, S.; Mrożek, M.; Opydo, M.; Szostak, E.; Dziurka, M.; Tuleja, M.; Łoboda, A.; Pocheć, E. Cytotoxic and Antioxidant Activity of *Hypericum perforatum* L. Extracts against Human Melanoma Cells from Different Stages of Cancer Progression, Cultured under Normoxia and Hypoxia. *Molecules* **2023**, *28*, 1509. [CrossRef]
125. Cai, S.-Y.; Boyer, J.L. Studies on the mechanisms of bile acid initiated hepatic inflammation in cholestatic liver injury. *Inflamm. Cell Signal.* **2017**, *4*, e1561.
126. Subat, S.; Mogushi, K.; Yasen, M.; Kohda, T.; Ishikawa, Y.; Tanaka, H. Identification of genes and pathways, including the CXCL2 axis, altered by DNA methylation in hepatocellular carcinoma. *J. Cancer Res. Clin. Oncol.* **2019**, *145*, 675–684. [CrossRef]
127. Moles, A.; Murphy, L.; Wilson, C.L.; Chakraborty, J.B.; Fox, C.; Park, E.J.; Mann, J.; Oakley, F.; Howarth, R.; Brain, J.; et al. A TLR2/S100A9/CXCL-2 signaling network is necessary for neutrophil recruitment in acute and chronic liver injury in the mouse. *J. Hepatol.* **2014**, *60*, 782–791. [CrossRef] [PubMed]
128. Konishi, T.; Schuster, R.M.; Goetzman, H.S.; Caldwell, C.C.; Lentsch, A.B. Cell-specific regulatory effects of CXCR2 on cholestatic liver injury. *Am. J. Physiol. Gastrointest. Liver Physiol.* **2019**, *317*, G773–G783. [CrossRef]
129. Luo, Y.; Kang, J.; Luo, J.; Yan, Z.; Li, S.; Lu, Z.; Song, Y.; Zhang, X.; Yang, J.; Liu, A. Hepatocytic AP-1 and STAT3 contribute to chemotaxis in alphanaphthylisothiocyanate-induced cholestatic liver injury. *Toxicol. Lett.* **2023**, *373*, 184–193. [CrossRef] [PubMed]
130. Manieri, E.; Folgueira, C.; Rodríguez, M.E.; Leiva-Vega, L.; Esteban-Lafuente, L.; Chen, C.; Cubero, F.J.; Barrett, T.; Cavanagh-Kyros, J.; Seruggia, D.; et al. JNK-mediated disruption of bile acid homeostasis promotes intrahepatic cholangiocarcinoma. *Proc. Natl. Acad. Sci. USA* **2020**, *117*, 16492–16499. [CrossRef] [PubMed]
131. Dai, M.; Yang, J.; Luo, Y.; Xu, L.; Zhang, H.; Xu, G.; Liu, A. Therapeutic action against chronic cholestatic liver injury by low-dose fenofibrate involves anti-chemotaxis via JNK-AP1-CCL2/CXCL2 signaling. *Pharmacol. Rep.* **2020**, *72*, 935–944. [CrossRef]
132. Lee, Y.-Y.; Mok, M.T.; Kang, W.; Yang, W.; Tang, W.; Wu, F.; Xu, L.; Yan, M.; Yu, Z.; Lee, S.-D.; et al. Loss of tumor suppressor IGFBP4 drives epigenetic reprogramming in hepatic carcinogenesis. *Nucleic Acids Res.* **2018**, *46*, 8832–8847. [CrossRef]
133. Lee, S.; Woo, D.-C.; Kang, J.; Ra, M.; Kim, K.H.; Lee, S.R.; Choi, D.K.; Lee, H.; Hong, K.B.; Min, S.-H.; et al. The Role of the Histone Methyltransferase EZH2 in Liver Inflammation and Fibrosis in STAM NASH Mice. *Biology* **2020**, *9*, 93. [CrossRef]
134. Lv, Y.-C.; Tang, Y.-Y.; Zhang, P.; Wan, W.; Yao, F.; He, P.-P.; Xie, W.; Mo, Z.-C.; Shi, J.-F.; Wu, J.-F.; et al. Histone Methyltransferase Enhancer of Zeste Homolog 2-Mediated ABCA1 Promoter DNA Methylation Contributes to the Progression of Atherosclerosis. *PLoS ONE* **2016**, *11*, e0157265. [CrossRef]

135. Xu, C.; Li, H.; Tang, C.-K. Sterol carrier protein 2: A promising target in the pathogenesis of atherosclerosis. *Genes Dis.* **2023**, *10*, 457–467. [CrossRef]
136. Xu, C.; Li, H.; Tang, C.-K. Sterol carrier protein 2 in lipid metabolism and non-alcoholic fatty liver disease: Pathophysiology, molecular biology, and potential clinical implications. *Metabolism* **2022**, *131*, 155180. [CrossRef]
137. Vuolo, D.; Do Nascimento, C.C.; D'Almeida, V. Reproduction in Animal Models of Lysosomal Storage Diseases: A Scoping Review. *Front. Mol. Biosci.* **2021**, *8*, 773384. [CrossRef]
138. He, H.; Wang, J.; Yannie, P.J.; Kakiyama, G.; Korzun, W.J.; Ghosh, S. Sterol carrier protein-2 deficiency attenuates diet-induced dyslipidemia and atherosclerosis in mice. *J. Biol. Chem.* **2018**, *293*, 9223–9231. [CrossRef]
139. Wang, J.; Bie, J.; Ghosh, S. Intracellular cholesterol transport proteins enhance hydrolysis of HDL-CEs and facilitate elimination of cholesterol into bile. *J. Lipid Res.* **2016**, *57*, 1712–1719. [CrossRef]
140. Galano, M.; Venugopal, S.; Papadopoulos, V. Role of STAR and SCP2/SCPx in the Transport of Cholesterol and Other Lipids. *Int. J. Mol. Sci.* **2022**, *23*, 12115. [CrossRef] [PubMed]
141. Wu, H.; Reizel, Y.; Wang, Y.J.; Lapiro, J.L.; Kren, B.T.; Schug, J.; Rao, S.; Morgan, A.; Herman, A.; Shekels, L.L.; et al. A negative reciprocal regulatory axis between cyclin D1 and HNF4α modulates cell cycle progression and metabolism in the liver. *Proc. Natl. Acad. Sci. USA* **2020**, *117*, 17177–17186. [CrossRef]
142. Topacio, B.R.; Zatulovskiy, E.; Cristea, S.; Xie, S.; Tambo, C.S.; Rubin, S.M.; Sage, J.; Kõivomägi, M.; Skotheim, J.M. Cyclin D-Cdk4,6 Drives Cell-Cycle Progression via the Retinoblastoma Protein's C-Terminal Helix. *Mol. Cell* **2019**, *74*, 758–770.e4. [CrossRef]
143. Di Ciaula, A.; Wang, D.Q.-H.; Molina-Molina, E.; Baccetto, R.L.; Calamita, G.; Palmieri, V.O.; Portincasa, P. Bile Acids and Cancer: Direct and Environmental-Dependent Effects. *Ann. Hepatol.* **2017**, *16*, S87–S105. [CrossRef] [PubMed]
144. Gao, J.; Hu, X.; Hu, W.; Sun, X.; Chen, L. Novel TTC37 mutations in a patient with Trichohepatoenteric syndrome: A case report and literature review. *Transl. Pediatr.* **2022**, *11*, 1050–1057. [CrossRef]
145. Poulton, C.; Pathak, G.; Mina, K.; Lassmann, T.; Azmanov, D.; McCormack, E.; Broley, S.; Dreyer, L.; Gration, D.; Taylor, E.; et al. Tricho-hepatic-enteric syndrome (THES) without intractable diarrhoea. *Gene* **2019**, *699*, 110–114. [CrossRef] [PubMed]
146. Morgan, N.V.; Hartley, J.L.; Setchell, K.; Simpson, M.A.; Brown, R.; Tee, L.; Kirkham, S.; Pasha, S.; Trembath, R.C.; Maher, E.R.; et al. A combination of mutations in AKR1D1 and SKIV2L in a family with severe infantile liver disease. *Orphanet J. Rare Dis.* **2013**, *8*, 74. [CrossRef] [PubMed]
147. Okpechi, S.C.; Yousefi, H.; Nguyen, K.; Cheng, T.; Alahari, N.V.; Collins-Burow, B.; Burow, M.E.; Alahari, S.K. Role of Nischarin in the pathology of diseases: A special emphasis on breast cancer. *Oncogene* **2022**, *41*, 1079–1086. [CrossRef] [PubMed]
148. Sun, Z.; Chang, C.-H.; Ernsberger, P. Identification of IRAS/Nischarin as an I1-imidazoline receptor in PC12 rat pheochromocytoma cells. *J. Neurochem.* **2007**, *101*, 99–108. [CrossRef] [PubMed]
149. Arnoux, A.; Aubertin, G.; Da Silva, S.; Weiss, M.; Bousquet, P.; Monassier, L.; Niederhoffer, N. Nischarin Is Not the Functional I1 Imidazoline Receptor Involved in Blood Pressure Regulation. *J. Cardiovasc. Pharmacol.* **2022**, *79*, 229–234. [CrossRef] [PubMed]
150. Zhang, W.; Li, X.; Liu, Y.; Chen, H.; Gong, J. Activation of imidazoline I 1 receptor by moxonidine regulates the progression of liver fibrosis in the Nrf2-dependent pathway. *Biomed. Pharmacother.* **2017**, *90*, 821–834. [CrossRef]
151. Blackburn, J.B.; Kudlyk, T.; Pokrovskaya, I.; Lupashin, V.V. More than just sugars: Conserved oligomeric Golgi complex deficiency causes glycosylation-independent cellular defects. *Traffic* **2018**, *19*, 463–480. [CrossRef]
152. Zhang, X.; Wang, Y. Glycosylation Quality Control by the Golgi Structure. *J. Mol. Biol.* **2016**, *428*, 3183–3193. [CrossRef]
153. Nicastro, E.; D'Antiga, L. Genetic Cholestatic Disorders. In *Pediatric Hepatology and Liver Transplantation*; D'Antiga, L., Ed.; Springer: Cham, Switzerland; Bergamo, Italy, 2019; pp. 227–245. [CrossRef]
154. Kuhn, M.; von Mering, C.; Campillos, M.; Jensen, L.J.; Bork, P. STITCH: Interaction networks of chemicals and proteins. *Nucleic Acids Res.* **2008**, *36*, D684–D688. [CrossRef]
155. Noor, F.; Rehman, A.; Ashfaq, U.A.; Saleem, M.H.; Okla, M.K.; Al-Hashimi, A.; AbdElgawad, H.; Aslam, S. Integrating Network Pharmacology and Molecular Docking Approaches to Decipher the Multi-Target Pharmacological Mechanism of *Abrus precatorius* L. Acting on Diabetes. *Pharmaceuticals* **2022**, *15*, 414. [CrossRef]
156. Demetz, E.; Schroll, A.; Auer, K.; Heim, C.; Patsch, J.R.; Eller, P.; Theurl, M.; Theurl, I.; Theurl, M.; Seifert, M.; et al. The Arachidonic Acid Metabolome Serves as a Conserved Regulator of Cholesterol Metabolism. *Cell Metab.* **2014**, *20*, 787–798. [CrossRef]
157. Granados, J.C.; Nigam, A.K.; Bush, K.T.; Jamshidi, N.; Nigam, S.K. A key role for the transporter OAT1 in systemic lipid metabolism. *J. Biol. Chem.* **2021**, *296*, 100603. [CrossRef]
158. Lampou, V.K.; Poller, B.; Huth, F.; Fischer, A.; Kullak-Ublick, G.A.; Arand, M.; Schadt, H.S.; Camenisch, G. Novel insights into bile acid detoxification via CYP, UGT and SULT enzymes. *Toxicol. Vitr.* **2023**, *87*, 105533. [CrossRef]
159. Khambu, B.; Yan, S.; Huda, N.; Yin, X.-M. Role of High-Mobility Group Box-1 in Liver Pathogenesis. *Int. J. Mol. Sci.* **2019**, *20*, 5314. [CrossRef]
160. Schwarz, D.; Kisselev, P.; Schunck, W.H.; Roots, I. Inhibition of 17β-estradiol activation by CYP1A1: Genotype- and regioselective inhibition by St. John's Wort and several natural polyphenols. *Biochim. Biophys Acta* **2011**, *1814*, 168–174. [CrossRef]
161. Ibrahim, Z.S. Chenodeoxycholic acid increases the induction of CYP1A1 in HepG2 and H4IIE cells. *Exp. Ther. Med.* **2015**, *10*, 1976–1982. [CrossRef] [PubMed]

162. Lu, J.; Shang, X.; Yao, B.; Sun, D.; Liu, J.; Zhang, Y.; Wang, H.; Shi, J.; Chen, H.; Shi, T.; et al. The role of CYP1A1/2 in cholesterol ester accumulation provides a new perspective for the treatment of hypercholesterolemia. *Acta Pharm. Sin. B* **2022**, *13*, 648–661. [CrossRef] [PubMed]
163. Bal, S.S.; Leishangthem, G.D.; Sethi, R.S.; Singh, A. P-coumaric acid ameliorates fipronil induced liver injury in mice through attenuation of structural changes, oxidative stress and inflammation. *Pestic. Biochem. Physiol.* **2022**, *180*, 104997. [CrossRef]
164. Rensen, S.S.; Slaats, Y.; Nijhuis, J.; Jans, A.; Bieghs, V.; Driessen, A.; Malle, E.; Greve, J.W.; Buurman, W.A. Increased Hepatic Myeloperoxidase Activity in Obese Subjects with Nonalcoholic Steatohepatitis. *Am. J. Pathol.* **2009**, *175*, 1473–1482. [CrossRef]
165. Roby, C.A.; Anderson, G.D.; Kantor, E.; Dryer, D.A.; Burstein, A.H. St John's Wort: Effect on CYP3A4 activity. *Clin. Pharmacol. Ther.* **2000**, *67*, 451–457. [CrossRef] [PubMed]
166. Chen, J.; Zhao, K.N.; Chen, C. The role of CYP3A4 in the biotransformation of bile acids and therapeutic implication for cholestasis. *Ann. Transl. Med.* **2014**, *2*, 7.
167. Li, F.; Zhu, W.; Gonzalez, F.J. Potential role of CYP1B1 in the development and treatment of metabolic diseases. *Pharmacol. Ther.* **2017**, *178*, 18–30. [CrossRef] [PubMed]
168. Kahraman, A.; Mott, J.L.; Bronk, S.F.; Werneburg, N.W.; Barreyro, F.J.; Guicciardi, M.E.; Akazawa, Y.; Braley, K.; Craig, R.W.; Gores, G.J. Overexpression of Mcl-1 Attenuates Liver Injury and Fibrosis in the Bile Duct–Ligated Mouse. *Dig. Dis. Sci.* **2009**, *54*, 1908–1917. [CrossRef] [PubMed]
169. Shen, H.; Yu, H.; Li, Q.-Y.; Wei, Y.-T.; Fu, J.; Dong, H.; Cao, D.; Guo, L.-N.; Chen, L.; Yang, Y.; et al. Hepatocyte-derived VEGFA accelerates the progression of non-alcoholic fatty liver disease to hepatocellular carcinoma via activating hepatic stellate cells. *Acta Pharmacol. Sin.* **2022**, *43*, 2917–2928. [CrossRef] [PubMed]
170. Elpek, G.Ö. Angiogenesis and liver fibrosis. *World J. Hepatol.* **2015**, *7*, 377–391. [CrossRef] [PubMed]
171. Merhi, F.; Tang, R.; Legrand, O.; Nguyen-Khac, F.; Susin, S.A.; Bauvois, B. The antiangiogenic phloroglucinol hyperforin inhibits the secretion of proMMP-2, proMMP-9 and VEGF-A during apoptosis of primary acute myeloid leukemia cells. *J. Cancer Metastasis Treat.* **2021**, *7*, 42. [CrossRef]
172. Palladini, G.; Ferrigno, A.; Richelmi, P.; Perlini, S.; Vairetti, M. Role of matrix metalloproteinases in cholestasis and hepatic ischemia/reperfusion injury: A review. *World J. Gastroenterol.* **2015**, *21*, 12114–12124. [CrossRef]
173. Tong, C.; Li, J.; Lin, W.; Cen, W.; Zhang, W.; Zhu, Z.; Lu, B.; Yu, J. Inhibition of heat shock protein 90 alleviates cholestatic liver injury by decreasing IL-1β and IL-18 expression. *Exp. Ther. Med.* **2021**, *21*, 241. [CrossRef]
174. VanderMolen, K.M.; Naciff, J.M.; Kennedy, K.; Otto-Bruc, A.; Shan, Y.; Wang, X.; Daston, G.P.; Mahony, C. Incorporation of in vitro techniques for botanicals dietary supplement safety assessment—Towards evaluation of developmental and reproductive toxicity (DART). *Food Chem. Toxicol.* **2020**, *144*, 111539. [CrossRef]
175. Manna, S.K.; Golla, S.; Golla, J.P.; Tanaka, N.; Cai, Y.; Takahashi, S.; Krausz, K.W.; Matsubara, T.; Korboukh, I.; Gonzalez, F.J. St. John's Wort Attenuates Colorectal Carcinogenesis in Mice through Suppression of Inflammatory Signaling. *Cancer Prev. Res.* **2015**, *8*, 786–795. [CrossRef]
176. Hammer, K.D.; Yum, M.-Y.; Dixon, P.M.; Birt, D.F. Identification of JAK–STAT pathways as important for the anti-inflammatory activity of a Hypericum perforatum fraction and bioactive constituents in RAW 264.7 mouse macrophages. *Phytochemistry* **2010**, *71*, 716–725. [CrossRef] [PubMed]
177. Lancet, D. The GeneCards Suite. In *Practical Guide to Life Science Databases*; Springer: Singapore, 2022; pp. 27–56.
178. Dennis, G.; Sherman, B.T.; Hosack, D.A.; Yang, J.; Gao, W.; Lane, H.C.; Lempicki, R.A. DAVID: Database for Annotation, Visualization, and Integrated Discovery. *Genome Biol.* **2003**, *4*, R60. [CrossRef]
179. Szklarczyk, D.; Franceschini, A.; Wyder, S.; Forslund, K.; Heller, D.; Huerta-Cepas, J.; Simonovic, M.; Roth, A.; Santos, A.; Tsafou, K.P.; et al. STRING v10: Protein-Protein Interaction Networks, Integrated Over the Tree of Life. *Nucleic Acids Res.* **2015**, *43*, D447–D452. [CrossRef] [PubMed]
180. Doncheva, N.T.; Morris, J.H.; Gorodkin, J.; Jensen, L.J. Cytoscape StringApp: Network Analysis and Visualization of Proteomics Data. *J. Proteome Res.* **2019**, *18*, 623–632. [CrossRef]
181. Chin, C.-H.; Chen, S.-H.; Wu, H.-H.; Ho, C.-W.; Ko, M.-T.; Lin, C.-Y. cytoHubba: Identifying hub objects and sub-networks from complex interactome. *BMC Syst. Biol.* **2014**, *8*, S11. [CrossRef] [PubMed]

pharmaceuticals

MDPI

Review

Natural Products Targeting PI3K/AKT in Myocardial Ischemic Reperfusion Injury: A Scoping Review

Syarifah Aisyah Syed Abd Halim [1], Norhashima Abd Rashid [2], Choy Ker Woon [3,*] and Nahdia Afiifah Abdul Jalil [1,*]

1. Department of Anatomy, Faculty of Medicine, Universiti Kebangsaan Malaysia, Cheras 56000, Kuala Lumpur, Malaysia; syarifahaisyah@ukm.edu.my
2. Department of Biomedical Science, Faculty of Applied Science, Lincoln University College, Petaling Jaya 47301, Selangor, Malaysia; norhashima@lincoln.edu.my
3. Department of Anatomy, Faculty of Medicine, Universiti Teknologi MARA, Sungai Buloh 47000, Selangor, Malaysia

* Correspondence: choykerwoon@uitm.edu.my (C.K.W.); nahdia.afiifah@ukm.edu.my (N.A.A.J.)

Abstract: This scoping review aimed to summarize the effects of natural products targeting phosphoinositide-3-kinases/serine/threonine kinase (PI3K/AKT) in myocardial ischemia-reperfusion injury (MIRI). The review details various types of natural compounds such as gypenoside (GP), gypenoside XVII (GP-17), geniposide, berberine, dihydroquercetin (DHQ), and tilianin which identified to reduce MIRI in vitro and in vivo by regulating the PI3K/AKT signaling pathway. In this study, 14 research publications that met the inclusion criteria and exclusion criteria were shortlisted. Following the intervention, we discovered that natural products effectively improved cardiac functions through regulation of antioxidant status, down-regulation of Bax, and up-regulation of Bcl-2 and caspases cleavage. Furthermore, although comparing outcomes can be challenging due to the heterogeneity in the study model, the results we assembled here were consistent, giving us confidence in the intervention's efficacy. We also discussed if MIRI is associated with multiple pathological condition such as oxidative stress, ERS, mitochondrial injury, inflammation, and apoptosis. This brief review provides evidence to support the huge potential of natural products used in the treatment of MIRI due to their various biological activities and drug-like properties.

Keywords: medicinal plants; PI3K/AKT; myocardial ischemic reperfusion injury; phytochemicals; cardiovascular disease

Citation: Syed Abd Halim, S.A.; Abd Rashid, N.; Woon, C.K.; Abdul Jalil, N.A. Natural Products Targeting PI3K/AKT in Myocardial Ischemic Reperfusion Injury: A Scoping Review. *Pharmaceuticals* **2023**, *16*, 739. https://doi.org/10.3390/ph16050739

Academic Editors: Elena Y. Enioutina, Kathleen M. Job and Catherine Sherwin

Received: 8 March 2023
Revised: 11 April 2023
Accepted: 19 April 2023
Published: 12 May 2023

1. Introduction

Coronary heart disease is the third leading cause of global mortality which associated with 17.8 million of deaths yearly [1]. Coronary heart disease occurs most commonly in patients who present with an acute ST-segment elevation myocardial infarction (STEMI). Infarction deprives the heart from necessary oxygen and nutrients to pump blood effectively to the body system [2]. Therefore, rapid reperfusion is much needed to resuscitate the dying area, which involves angioplasty, primary percutaneous coronary intervention, and thrombolytic therapy. Ironically, the perfusion process can be harmful by intensifying the tissue injury known as myocardial ischemia-reperfusion injury (MIRI) [3]. Ischemia-reperfusion injury refers to the situation where the restoration of the blood flow to the particular tissues that were previously deprived of oxygen paradoxically worsens their function and leads to cellular death. Although the re-establishment of blood flow is necessary to save the ischemic tissue, the reperfusion process could lead to additional damage, endangering the survival and function of the organ. Ischemic-reperfusion injury is not only limited to the myocardium but also affects other organs such as the brain, kidney, gut, and skeletal muscle, depending on the impaired blood vessel [4–6]. The damage includes fulminant migration of inflammatory cells, oedema and apoptotic processes, an extension of the infarct area and a dysfunctional microcirculation [4,7].

Natural products (NP) derived from plants could be an alternative source of promising drugs to mitigate the harmful aftereffects of MIRI. NP offers various medicinal values and health benefits [8–12], including to the heart attributed to anti-apoptotic, antioxidant, and anti-inflammatory properties [13–17]. Furthermore, accumulating studies suggest bioactive compounds and extracts of NPs improved the viability of cardiomyocytes in post-MIRI, ameliorated endothelial function, and modulated the inflammatory and stress process [16,17]. Thus, numerous research focused on the bioactive compounds of NPs to reduce MIRI.

The phosphoinositide-3-kinases/serine/threonine kinase (PI3K/AKT) is an intracellular signaling pathway involved in the regulation of cellular metabolism, survival, and apoptosis [18]. Many studies supported the role of PI3K/AKT to inhibit apoptosis by improving cellular viability [13,14,19]. Phosphorylation of PI3K begins when ligands bind to the receptor tyrosine kinase. Consequently, phosphorylated PI3K generates a second messenger, phosphatidylinositol (3,4,5)-triphosphate, which in turn activates downstream signaling cascades by mediating through phosphorylation of AKT [20]. In cell survival/apoptosis, PI3K/AKT inhibits the activity of pro-apoptotic proteins by downregulating the expression of the Bcl-2 family, Bim protein via downstream PI3K/AKT/FOXO3a pathway, thus enhancing cell survival [17]. PI3K/AKT also regulates apoptosis via GSK3 by phosphorylating GSK3 isoforms on the N-terminal regulatory site [20].

Accordingly, the damages related to MIRI are reduced when the PI3K/AKT pathway is regulated, implying its significance in cardioprotection [13–15]. Activation of PI3K/Akt pathway reduced the apoptosis in the cardiomyocytes and mitochondrial oxidative damage, leading to better survival of the cardiac function [21].Therefore, the study aims to systematically review the existing literature regarding NPs that effectively hinder the MIRI in MIRI models via PI3K/AKT signaling pathway, which may provide insight for investigators and future research.

2. Results

2.1. Literature Search

A total of 178 studies were found from the database search. After removing the duplicates, 176 articles were shortlisted. After title-abstract screening, 123 articles were excluded because the articles were not relevant to the topic. The reasons for the irrelevance are non-MIRI models (diabetic cardiomyopathy, myocardial fibrosis, cardiotoxicity, and myocardial infarction, high glucose-induced injury in cardiomyocytes, inorganic mercury-induced cardiac injury), other signaling pathways such as PI3-kinase/glycogen synthase kinase 3β/β-catenin pathway, NFkB signaling, IGF-1R/Nrf2 signaling, and the PI3k/Akt signaling pathway were not measured. By full-text screening of the remaining article 53 articles, a total of 39 articles were eliminated based on the inclusion/exclusion criteria; study models used were not MIRI experiment models (n = 36), combination of herbs in the treatment (n = 2), and no availability of full text (n = 1). Thus, a total of 14 articles from January 2016 to January 2021 were selected in this scoping review. A flowchart depicting the search process and study selection is presented in Preferred Reporting Items for Systematic Reviews and Meta-Analyses (PRISMA) for Scoping Review (Figure 1). The characteristics of the selected studies were summarized in Table 1.

2.2. MIRI Models Used

Several experimental models were used in the selected review to mimic ischemic-reperfusion injury either using in vivo, in vitro, and ex vivo methods (Table 2). Four studies used in vivo methods only [15,22–24], five studies used in vitro methods [13,25–28], and another five studies used a combined experimental design [14,29–32]. A study by Yu et al. 2016 compared the effect of pretreatment of gypenoside in both in vivo and in vitro experiments. The results for both experiments showed gypenoside to have a strong capacity to reduce cell apoptotic rates modulated by upregulation of phosphorylated Akt. The results of protein expression of targeted molecules were comparable and similar between these experimental designs.

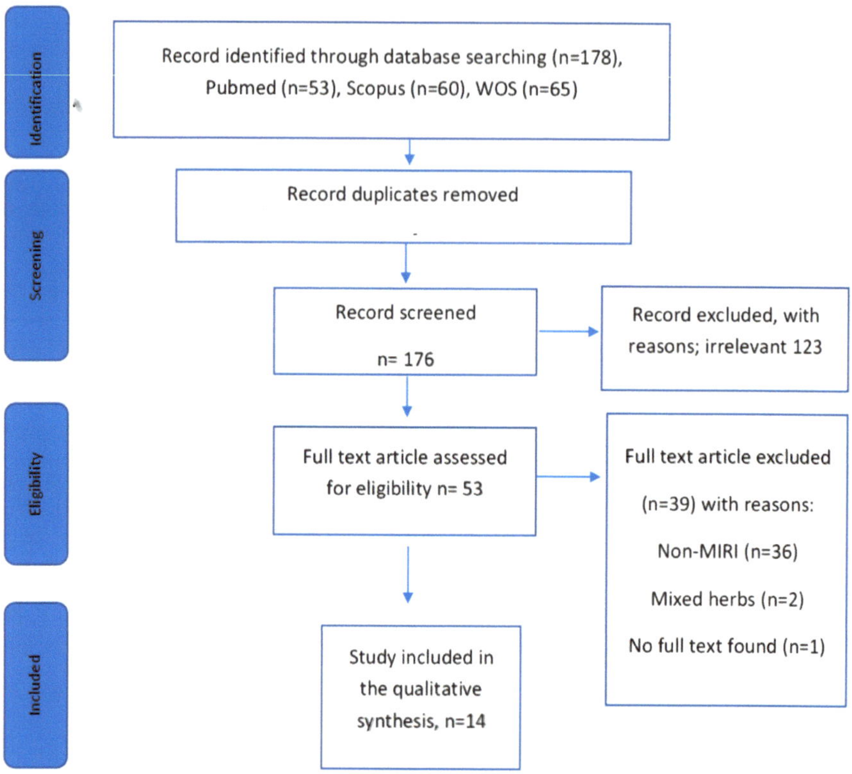

Figure 1. Flow diagram of the article selection.

Table 1. Study characteristics of the selected articles.

Study Characteristics		Count *n* (%)
Year of publication	2016	5 (35.7%)
	2017	3 (21.4%)
	2018	3 (21.4%)
	2019	3 (21.4%)
Country of publication	China	14 (100%)
Source of plant	Part of the plant, method of extraction and the solvents used were mentioned.	5 (35.7%)
	Processed plants were purchased.	5 (35.7%)
	Not mentioned source of plant	4 (28.6%)
MIRI model used	In vitro	5 (35.7%)
	In vivo	4 (28.6%)
	Mixed in vitro and ex vivo	2 (14.3%)
	Mixed in vitro and in vivo	2 (14.3%)
	In vivo, in vitro, ex vivo	1 (7.1%)

Table 2. MIRI models used and method to inflict MIRI.

MIRI Model Used	Brief Explanation of Method to Inflict MIRI	Duration of Ischemic/Reperfusion (I/R)
In vitro	Hypoxia-reperfusion (H/R) injury was elicited in H9c2 cardiomyocytes. To induce hypoxia, the cells were incubated in an anaerobic box with or without the media changed to non-glucose DMEM. To mimic reperfusion, the cells were moved to the regular incubator with or without the media being replaced with high-glucose media. Duration of ischemia and reperfusion varies according to the studies.	4 h of hypoxia, 24 h of reperfusion [29]
		6 h of hypoxia and 12 h of reoxygenation [14]
		H/R time: 4/2, 6/3, 12/4, 14/5, 16/6, 22/10 h [25]
		6 h of ischemia, 16 h of reperfusion [31]
		8 h of hypoxia followed by 4 h of reoxygenation [13]
		6 h of ischemia, followed by reoxygenation [26]
		10 h of ischemia, followed by 2 h of reperfusion [27]
		6 h of hypoxia, followed by 12 h of reoxygenation [28]
In vivo	Left anterior descending coronary arteries (LAD) of MIRI rat model were ligated temporarily to induce ischemia, followed by a period of reperfusion by releasing the ligation. Duration of ischemia and reperfusion varies according to the studies.	LAD were reversibly occluded for 45 min, followed by 3 h of reperfusion [29]
		LAD was occluded for 30 min followed by reperfusion for 4 h [15]
		45 min of ischemia followed by 4 h of reperfusion [22]
		Ischemia for 45 min, followed by 12 h of reperfusion [23]
		45 min ischemia, followed by 24 h of reperfusion [24]
		Ligation LAD for 30 min followed by 24 h of reperfusion [32].
	Cold ischemia was performed to induce ischemia followed by reperfusion.	Cold ischemia for 18 h, followed by 8 h of reperfusion [30]
Ex vivo	Langendorff perfusion of rat hearts was used to induce global ischemia and reperfusion.	Global ischemia for 40 min and reperfusion for 60 min [14].
		45 min of ischemia, 1 h reperfusion [31]
		Ischemic state was induced for 30 min by no-flow followed by 30 min of reperfusion [32].

In the in vivo method, the left anterior descending coronary arteries (LAD) of the animals were ligated to induce ischemia for some period. Subsequently, ligation was released to mimic reperfusion. Even though the research adopted a similar in vivo design, the timings for ischemia and reperfusion were different. For example, Yu et al., 2016, ligated and occluded LAD for 45 min followed by 3 h of reperfusion, Jiang et al., 2016, occluded the LAD for 30 min followed by 4 h of reperfusion, Zeng et al., 2018, introduced ischemia for 45 min, followed by 4 h of reperfusion, Zeng et al., 2018, and Zhao et al., 2018, ligated the LAD for 45 min mimicking ischemia, followed by 12 h of reperfusion and Wu et al., 2016, induced ischemia by ligation of LAD for 30 min, followed by 24 h of reperfusion.

Additionally, IR can also be induced with prolonged cold ischemia (18 h) and followed by 8 h of reperfusion in rat. For the in vitro model, hypoxic-reoxygenation (H/R) injury was established by culturing H9c2 cell in glucose-free DMEM medium placed in the anaerobic glove box or hypoxic chamber containing high percentage of nitrogen gas to mimic hypoxia. Then, the medium of the cells was changed with glucose containing medium and placed in the regular incubator with atmosphere of 95% air. Using similar H/R injury method in H9c2 cells, Wu et al., 2013, induced 8 h of hypoxia followed by 4 h of reoxygenation, Shen et al., 2018, induced 10 h of ischemia followed by 2 h of reperfusion, and Liao et al., 2016, induced 6 h of hypoxia and 12 h of reoxygenation.

In addition, MIRI can be induced ex vivo using Langendorff perfusion model. There were 3 studies using this model. A study by Mei-ping Wu et al., 2016, stopped the perfusion on the isolated heart for 30 min to induce ischemia and then reperfusion for another 30 min, Zun Peng Shu et al., 2019, found the perfusion on the isolated heart was stopped for 45 min to induce cardiac ischemia and then reperfusion occurred for another 60 min, while Yingli Yu et al., 2019, introduced global ischemia for 40 min and reperfusion for 60 min.

2.3. Source of Plant

Five studies mentioned the part of the plant, method of extraction, and the solvents used [13,22,23,26,28]. Bark of Cortex Dictamni was aqueously extracted and *Dracocephalum moldavica* was extracted in ethanol [13,23]. HPLC was performed to analyze the chemical constituents in TFDM. The dry powder of *Dracocephalum moldavica* was further extracted in aqueous ethanol and purified to obtain tilianin, which was then identified by HPLC [22]. Whereas the bark of Myrica rubra was extracted with methanol and the plant of Bauhinia championii was extracted with ethanol and further partitioned with ethyl acetate [26,28]. Another five studies purchased processed plant to be tested with the experimental design, whereas another four studies did not mention the source of the natural products [15,30–32] (Table 1). The details of plants selected in the articles, including the doses and duration used were presented in Table 3.

Table 3. Source of plants, dose, and duration of intervention.

Natural Product	Source	Dose and Duration	References
Gypenoside (GP)	*Gynostema pentaphyllum* (Thunb.) Makino	For in vivo Short term: GP 50, 100, 200 mg/kg 1 h before MIRI. Long term: GP 200 mg/kg 1 h before MIRI; 24 and 72 h post-MIRI. For in vitro GP 5μM, 10μM, 20μM incubated before OGD/R	[29]
Gypenoside XVII (GP-17)	Antioxidant phytoestrogen of the gypenoside group.	For in vitro GP-17 1.25, 2.5, 5, 10, 20, 40, 100 μM incubated 24 h before H/R injury. For ex vivo GP-17 5, 10, 20 μM were dissolved in Krebs–Henseleit (KH) buffer	[14]
Geniposide (glycoside)	An extract from *Gardenia jasminoides* J. Ellis	For in vitro Geniposide 2.5, 5, 10, 20, 40, 80, 160, 320 μM for 30 min before H/R	[25]
Berberine	An alkaloid derivative. The source of plant was not mentioned	For in vivo 10 mg/kg berberine OD for 30 days For in vitro 10 mg/mL berberine for 24 h	[30]
Berberine	The source of plant was not mentioned	For in vivo Berberine 25, 50, 100 mg/kg for 14 days	[15]
Dihydroquercetin (DHQ)	Belongs to the flavanonol subclass in the flavonoids. The source of plant was not mentioned	For in vitro DHQ 2.5, 5, 10, 20, 40, 80 μM incubated for 12 h before H/R	[31]
Aqueous extract of Cortex Dictamni (AECD)	A species of Dictamnus dasycarpus Turcz. This plant was aqueously extracted.	For in vitro AECD 0.39, 1.56, 6.25, 25, 100 μg/mL were pretreated with the cells for 24 h.	[13]
Tilianin (is a flavonoid antioxidant)	Tilianin is a powerful flavonoid from dried *Dracocephalum moldavica* L. (DML). Its dried powder was extracted in aqueous ethanol.	For in vivo Tilianin 2.5, 5, 10 mg/kg for 14 days	[22]
Total flavonoid extract from *Dracocephalum moldavica* L. (TFDM)	The plant was extracted in 40% ethanol andHPLC was preformed	For in vivo TFDM 3, 10, 30 mg/kg for 2 weeks	[23]
Schisandrin B. (Sch B)	Natural monomer extracted from *Schisandra chinensis* (Turcz.) Baill.	For in vivo Sch. B 60 mg/kg for 15 days	[24]
Higenamine	An alkaloid derivative. The source of plant was not mentioned	For in vivo Higenamine 10 mg/kg 2 h before surgery For in vitro Higenamine 30, 60, 120 μM For ex vivo Higenamine 100μM	[32]
Myrica rubra flavonoids (MRF)	The bark of Myrica rubra was extracted with methanol using reflux extraction. Myrica rubra flavonoid was then chemically identified at the Institute of Medicinal Plant Development.	For in vitro MRF 6.25μg/mL was incubated for 12 h before H/R injury	[26]
Total paeony glycoside (TPG)	TPG powder was obtained from Haoxuan Biological Technology Co., Ltd. (Xi'an, China).	For in vitro TPG 10, 40, 160 μg/mL post I/R injury	[27]
Bauhinia championii flavone	Dried Bauhinia championii (Benth.) Benth. was extracted with ethanol.	For in vitro BCF 3.125 μg/mL	[28]

2.4. *Effects of Natural Products in MIRI via PI3K/AKT Signaling Pathway*

2.4.1. Gypenoside

Gypenoside is the main component of *Gynostemma pentaphyllum* (Thunb.) Makino [33,34], and exist mainly as dammarane type-triterpene glycosides [35]. In an oxygen–glucose deprivation/reperfusion (OGD/R) cell and MIRI rat models, gypenoside treatment ameliorated impairments in cardiac morphology at a dose of 50 mg/kg, 100 mg/kg, and 200 mg/kg [29]. In the MIRI group, myocardial tissues showed up-regulation of Bax and cleaved caspase-3 and down-regulation of Bcl-2, which were reversed by gypenoside. The administration of gypenoside significantly reduced the apoptotic rates in both rat and cell models and effectively improved the cardiac function as determined by hemodynamic parameters, lactate dehydrogenase levels (LDH), and creatine kinase (CK). Western blotting showed that these effects of gypenoside against MIRI were achieved via inhibition of endoplasmic reticulum stress (ERS) and apoptotic pathway, which subsequently lead to PI3K/AKT pathway activation. Pre-treatment of gypenoside in rats increased the reduction in p-AKTs and p-GSK3β from ischemic-reperfusion (I/R) injury and reduced the ERS markers, namely GRP78, CHOP, cleaved-caspase 12, p-PERK, p-eIF2α, and ATF4 upregulated by I/R injury [29].

2.4.2. Gypenoside XVII

Gypenoside XVII (GP17) is an antioxidant phytoestrogen of the gypenosides group has a similar structure as estradiol [14,36]. GP17-treated-MIRI-H92c cells improved cell viability, reduced LDH release and caspase-3 activity. GP17 at a dose of 1.25–100 μM ameliorated cardiac contractility dysfunction, oxidative damage, and myocardial apoptosis, leading to mitochondrial injury. Mitochondrial injury was associated with mitochondrial permeability transition pore (mPTP) opening, ROS accumulation, and decreased calcium concentration. Mitochondrial apoptosis caused the accumulation of cytochrome-C in the cytosol and increased Bax expression, which was reversed by GP17, thereby suppressing MIRI-induced mitochondrial injury and apoptosis. PERK/eIF2a- and IRE1-related pathway was found to mediate ERS-cardiomyocytes apoptosis. GP17 relieved the ERS and apoptosis by reducing ERS response; GRP78, ERS sensors; PERK and IRE1 levels, as well as pro-apoptotic proteins; p-JNK, CHOP, Bad, Bax, and caspase-12. Preconditioning with PI3K inhibitor and P38/MAPK inhibitor greatly impaired the favorable effects of GP-17 on ERS, mitochondrial injury and apoptosis, suggesting the involvement of PI3K/AKT signaling pathway in the cardioprotective role of GP17 [14].

2.4.3. Geniposide

In a hypoxia/reoxygenation (H/R) of H9c2 cells, pre-treatment with geniposide, an extract from *Gardenia jasminoides* J. Ellis inhibited cardiomyocytes apoptosis, thus improving cell viability and decreased LDH levels [25]. Mitochondrial dysfunction induced by MIRI was reversed by geniposide at a dose of 2.5–320 μM via inhibition of oxidative stress, namely ROS/RNS and MDA, elevating the level T-SOD, improvement of mitochondrial morphology, attenuation of mitochondrial calcium overload, and blunting depolarization of the mitochondrial membrane. Geniposide enhanced the Bcl-2/Bax ratio and p-AKTserine473. In addition, geniposide attenuated the cleaved caspase-3 and cytochrome-c. The protective effects of geniposide were reversed by glucagon-like peptide-1 receptor antagonist exendin-(9-39) (GLP-1R) and the PI3K inhibitor LY294002, which further confirms that geniposide improved H/R-induced myocardial apoptosis by reversing mitochondrial dysfunction through GLP-1R and PI3K/AKT signaling activation [25].

2.4.4. Berberine

Berberine is an alkaloid derivative, isolated from Coptis chinensis Franch [37] and *Berberis vulgaris* L. [38]. In the MIRI mouse model, berberine improves blood lipid levels, blood pressure, and myocardial function (9). Berberine also reduced inflammatory responses via the nuclear factor (NF)-κB signaling pathway. Berberine increased the expression of PI3K/AKT in myocardial cells. Berberine reduced apoptotic protease-activating factor-1 (apaf-1), caspase-3 and caspase-9 expression while up-regulation of Bcl2-associated agonist of cell death, Bcl-2-like protein 1, and cellular tumor antigen p53. In conclusion, berberine suppressed the apoptosis of myocardial cells via the PI3K/AKT signaling pathway at a dose of 10 mg/kg which was administered to rats for 30 days [30]. In a separate study, 25 mg/kg, 50 mg/kg, and 100 mg/kg of berberine were administered to rats for 14 consecutive days. It was demonstrated to reduce ventricular arrhythmia (VA) score and improve histopathological changes of the myocardium. The underlying cardioprotective mechanism of berberine was caused by decreased p85 activity, a regulatory subunit of PI3K, leading to AKT activation. Suppression of PI3K/AKT signaling pathway is accompanied by a decrease in tumor necrosis factor-α (TNF-α), interleukin-6 (IL-6) and IL-1β levels resulting in a reduction in inflammatory cells infiltration. Berberine protected against MIRI through suppression of PI3K/AKT signaling and, subsequently, in the inflammatory response [15].

2.4.5. Dihydroquercetin

Dihydroquercetin (DHQ) is a flavonoid that is commonly found in *Allium cepa* L. and *Silybum marianum* (L.) Gaertn [39]. In H9c2 cells and rat hearts Langendorff perfusion model, DHQ pre-treatment significantly reduced the cardiac dysfunction via scavenging free radical, reduction in lipid peroxidation, and elevation of the antioxidant enzyme activity [31]. Two myocardial enzymes, namely AST and CK, were reduced following DHQ. Western blot revealed that DHQ downregulated CHOP, Caspase-12, and p-JNK. Moreover, DHQ delayed the occurrence of ERS via reduction in GRP78, p-PERK, and p-eif2α expression levels and by up-regulation of HO-1 expression and Nrf2 binding to antioxidant elements. The effects of DHQ were inhibited by PI3K/AKT inhibitor LY294002, which suggest that DHQ alleviated MIRI at a dose of 2.5, 5, 10, 20, 40, and 80 μM via activation of PI3K/AKT pathway, which subsequently reduced oxidative stress and apoptosis induced by ERS [31].

2.4.6. Cortex Dictamni

Cortex Dictamni (CD) is a species of *Dictamnus dasycarpus* Turcz [40,41]. Aqueous extract of Cortex Dictamni (AECD) on MIRI-induced-H92c cells demonstrated improvement of cell viability while reducing LDH and cardiac troponin I (cTn-I) release at a dose of 0.39, 1.56, 6.25, 25, and 100 μg/mL. AECD silenced both the initial and late phase of apoptosis via reduction in nucleus chromatin condensation, phosphatidylserine externalization, and fragmentation of DNA. AECD significantly controlled the oxidative stress via elimination of ROS and MDA while promoting SOD in MIRI. The nrf2-mediated antioxidant pathway was enhanced during AECD pre-treatment. The mitochondrial-dependent apoptosis process was also suppressed by AECD, evidenced by elevation of Bcl-2/Bax ratio, inhibition of cytochrome-c release, and caspase-3 and -9 activation. The anti-apoptotic effects of AECD in MIRI are mainly by activating the PI3K/AKT pathway and GSK-3β phosphorylation. LY294002 inhibited p-GSK-3β and suppressed the Nrf2 expression, which AECD reversed via PI3K/AKT mechanism [13].

2.4.7. *Dracocephalum moldavica*

Dracocephalum moldavica L. is a herbaceous plant that belongs to the Lamiaceae family [42]. Total flavonoid extract of *Dracocephalum moldavica* (TFDM) was found to decrease MIRI severity by decreasing CK-MB, LDH, MDA, and apoptotic cells index at aa dose of 3, 10, and 30 mg/kg. Furthermore, it was also able to reduce the infarction size, preserved cell membrane, and mitochondria. In addition, antioxidative and anti-apoptotic properties of TFDM were confirmed by increased SOD and Bcl-2/Bax ratio and decreased cleaved caspase-3, -7 and -9 levels. Additionally, TFDM elevated p-PI3K and p-AKT as well p-PI3K/PI3K and p-AKT/AKT ratio. Activation of PI3K/AKT signaling was facilitated by protein expression of p-GSK-3β and p-ERK1/2. The cardioprotective effect of TFDM was abolished upon administration of LY294002 and PD98059, which were the inhibitor of PI3K and ERK 1/2 phosphorylation, respectively [23].

2.4.8. Tilianin

Tilianin is a powerful flavonoid in dried *Dracocephalum moldavica* L.(DML) [43]. Tilianin at a dose of 2.5, 5, and 10 mg/kg was administered to rats for 14 days. It was found to improve MIRI via promoting cell survival, reducing apoptosis, and scavenging free radical activity. Tilianin reduced CK-MB, LDH, MDA and increased SOD levels. Tilianin inhibited myocardial apoptosis by increasing the Bcl-2/Bax ratio and lowering caspase-7 and -9 levels. X-linked inhibitor of apoptosis protein (XIAP) particularly binds to caspase-3, -7, and -9 and regulates their activities. Following tilianin treatment, Smac/Diablo and HtrA2/Omi protease activity were reduced in the treated-MIRI group, thus suppressing caspases proteolytic activity and improving XIAP degeneration, resulting in the diminished ischemic area with the betterment of myocardial function. Tilianin inhibited apoptosis in MIRI by activating PI3K/AKT signaling and suppressing the mitochondrial leakage of Smac/Diablo and HtrA2/Omi, XIAP degeneration, and caspase activity [22].

2.4.9. Schisandrin B

Schisandrin B (Sch B) is a natural medicinal monomer extracted from *Schisandra chinensis* (Turcz.) Baill. [44] Sch B reduced apoptotic nuclei number, Bax, and cleaved-caspase-3 while increased Bcl-2 at a dose of 60 mg/kg. Furthermore, the significant elevation of p-AKT expression showed that Sch exerted its protective role via PI3K/AKT signaling [24]. AKT activation preserved the mitochondrial integrity via blocking the opening of mPTP and phosphorylation GSK-3β [23,45].

2.4.10. Higenamine

Higenamine derives from plant-based protoberberines alkaloids [46]. Higenamine at a dose of 10 mg/kg increased the cardiomyocytes survival by decreasing the infarct size and apoptotic nuclei. In addition to that, the administration of higenamine at doses of 30, 60, 100, and 120 μM was able to attenuate early and late H_2O_2-induced cardiomyocyte apoptosis. The protective effect of higenamine was achieved via upregulation of cleaved-caspase-3 and -9 and protein expression of p-AKT. However, $ß_2$-adrenergic receptor (AR) antagonist and PI3K inhibitor eliminated these protective effects [32]. In summary, higenamine protected against MIRI through β2-AR/PI3K/AKT pathway.

2.4.11. *Myrica rubra*

Myrica rubra (Lour) Siebold and Zucc. belongs to the family Myricaceae. Hypoxic/reoxygenation of H9c2 cells revealed that *Myrica rubra* flavonoid (MRF), at a dose of 6.25 μg/mL, was able to attenuate intracellular ROS level, protected the cells against mitochondrial membrane potential depolarization, inhibited caspase-3 activity, and alleviated the ratio of apoptotic cells [26]. This protective function of MRF is contributed by the upregulation of Akt and GSK-3ß proteins phosphorylation [26].

2.4.12. Total Paeony Glycoside

Total paeony glycoside (TPG) is a major constituent of *Paeonia lactiflora* Pall. [47]. TPG reduced H9c2 cells apoptotic rate, downregulated the cleaved-caspase-3, PARP1, and Bax, and it upregulated Bcl-2 and pro-caspase-3 at doses of 10, 40, and 160 μg/mL. The anti-apoptotic mechanism of TPG was closely related to its ability to suppress oxidative stress. TPG significantly attenuated the protein expression of PI3K/AKT, which was inhibited by insulin growth factor (IGF-1). These findings suggested that the protective function of TPG was achieved by suppressing the PI3K/AKT mechanism [27].

2.4.13. *Bauhinia championii* Benth

Bauhinia championii Benth. or *Phanera championii* Benth. belongs to the genus Bauhinia [48]. *Bauhinia championii* flavone (BCF), at a dose of 3.125 μg/mL, markedly attenuated apoptotic rate, caspase-3, Bax, and cytochrome-C. BCF also significantly increased the protein expression of p-PI3K and p-AKT. In addition, BCF significantly decreased the level of ROS-generating mitochondria, attenuated mitochondrial transmembrane potential ($\Delta\Psi m$) dissipation, reduced the mPTP opening and increased ATP production. However, co-administration of LY294002 eliminated the protective effect of BCF [28]. Figure 2 shows the chemical structure of the natural products compound that were able to attenuate MIRI through PI3K/AKT signaling pathway.

2.5. Techniques to Detect PI3K/Akt Activation and Its Related Mechanism

The studies reported in this review utilized Western blotting analysis for detection of PI3K and Akt. Western blot is not only able to detect the protein expression but also able to quantitate protein phosphorylation, which is the fundamental mechanism to study cell signaling [49]. Analysis of phosphorylation demonstrated the status of the signaling. Most studies in this review measured Akt, PI3K and its phosphorylated proteins. However, some researches only quantified Akt and p-Akt [13,15,24–26,29,32]. Akt is the primary protein effector downstream of the PI3K signaling pathway. Some research also measured GSK-3ß, the downstream effector of Akt which participated in mediating apoptosis [13,23,26,29]

Activation of PI3K/Akt signaling involved in the protection against MIRI-induced apoptosis. In order to evaluate the cardioprotective effect played by PI3K/Akt signaling on cell survival, its effects in the apoptotic-related mechanism were observed. There were many assays with various techniques used to measure various aspect of apoptosis. Some studies used flow cytometric quantitation of cell death using Annexin-V/propidium staining to detect early and late apoptotic events. Annexin has greater specificity to bind to the phosphotidylserine (PS), which is the membrane phospholipid. As apoptosis failed to maintain the phospholipid in the cell membrane, PS appear on the outer leaflet of the cell membrane which will be stained with Annexin V. Cells stained positive with Annexin V and negative for PI was suggestive for early apoptotic event, whereas Annexin V positive and PI negative population indicate late apoptotic event [32]. Another study performed terminal deoxynucleotidyl transferase-mediated dUTP-biotin nick end-labeling (TUNEL) assay for detection of apoptotic cells that exhibited the DNA fragmentation. Most of the studies measured the molecular players related to apoptosis/apoptotic cascade such as bcl-2 family protein and caspases activity. Although mitochondria played a key role in apoptosis, only five of the researches measured the parameters related to mitochondrial apoptosis such as mitochondrial membrane potential, mPTP opening, and release of cytochrome-c from mitochondria to cytosol [13,14,25,28,31]. The cardioprotective effect of NP against MIRI on cell survival was measured by regulation of PI3K/AKT signaling and its effects in the apoptotic-related mechanism (Table 4).

2.6. PI3K Inhibitor

The antagonizing effect of PI3K/Akt inhibitors against NP were important to be verified to confirm the PI3K/Akt signaling pathway involvement. Protective effects of NPs in this review were abolished upon administration of PI3K inhibitors such as LY 294002, LY 204002, and wortmannin. There were two studies that did not use PI3K inhibitor [15,27] (Table 4). PI3K inhibitor caused the rapid induction in cell death. Therefore, the incubation of cell line with PI3K/Akt inhibitors inhibited the effect of NPs on cellular apoptotic rate, reversed the expression of pro- and anti-apoptotic molecules, and eliminated the anti-apoptotic effect of NPs.

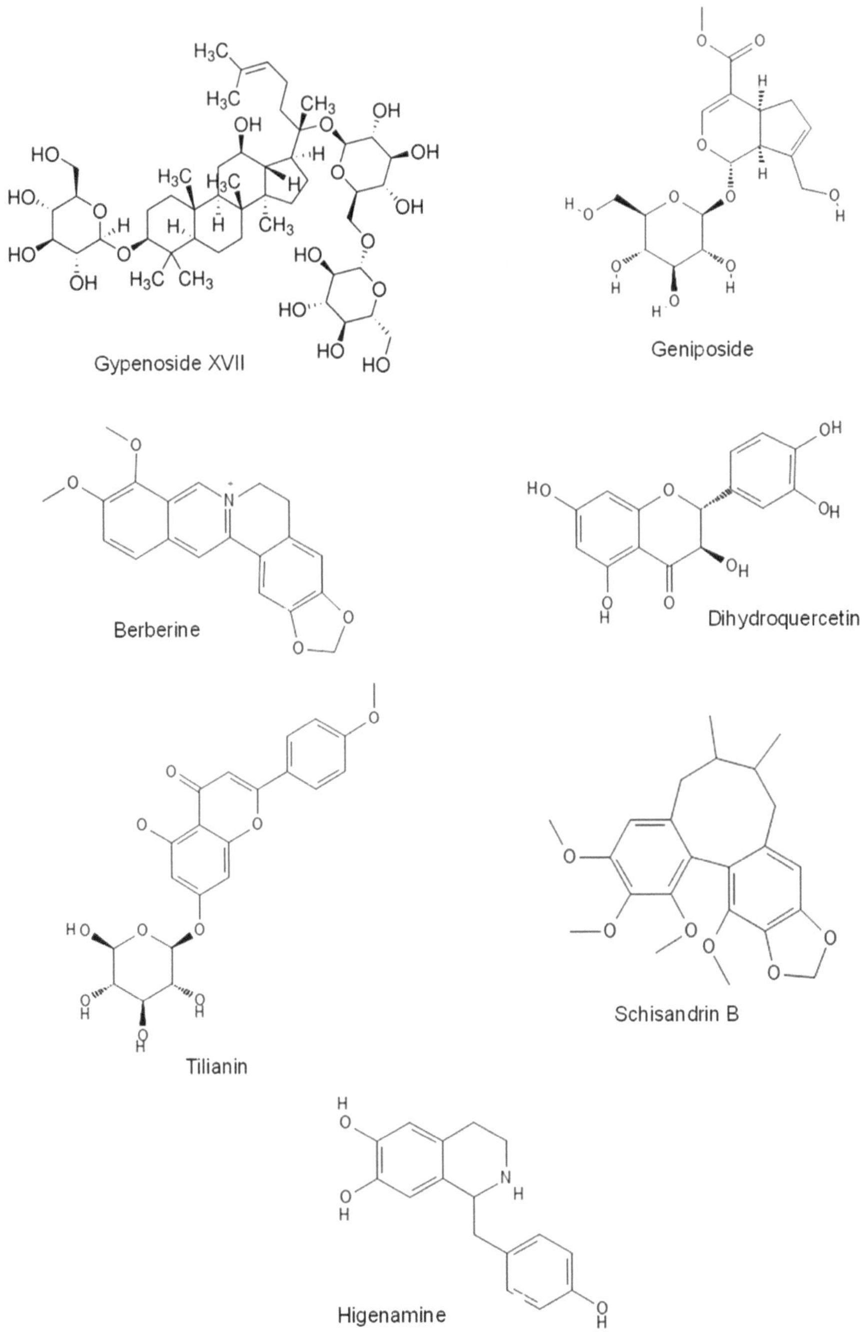

Figure 2. Chemical structures of natural products compound which attenuate MIRI through PI3K/AKT signaling.

Table 4. Summary of regulation of PI3K/Akt by NPs to alleviate MIRI and its possible mechanism.

Natural Products	Regulation of PI3K/Akt Signaling	Administration of PI3K Inhibitor	Parameters Used to Measure Cardioprotective Mechanism of NPs on Cell Survival					References
			Apoptosis	Mitochondrial Injury/ Cytochrome C/Caspase-3,9	Bcl-2/Bax	Endoplasmic Reticulum Stress Marker	Oxidative Stress/Antioxidant	
Gypenoside (GP)	↑p-Akt/Akt, p-GSK3β/GSK3β	√	√ (TUNEL)	×	√	√	×	[29]
Gypenoside XVII (GP-17)	↑p-PI3K/PI3K, p-Akt/Akt ratios	√	√ (Annexin V/PI)	√	√	√	√	[14]
Geniposide (glycoside)	↑p-Akt/Akt	√	√ (Annexin-V/PI)	√	√	×	√	[25]
Berberine	↑expression of PI3K, Akt, p-Akt	√	√	√	√	×	×	[30]
Berberine	↓p-Akt/Akt ratio ↓p-p85/p85	×	×	×	×	×	×	[15]
Dihydroquercetin (DHQ)	↑p-PI3K/PI3K and p-AKT/AKT ratios	√	×	√	√	√	√	[31]
Aqueous extract of Cortex Dictamni (AECD)	↑p-Akt, p-GSK-3β	√	√ (TUNEL, Annexin/PI)	√	√	×	√	[13]
Tilianin (is a flavonoid antioxidant)	↑p-Akt, p-PI3K, p-Akt/Akt, p-PI3K/PI3K	√	√ (TUNEL)	√	√	×	√	[22]
Total flavonoid extract from *Dracocephalum moldavica* L. (TFDM)	↑protein expression of p-PI3K, p-Akt ↑p-PI3K/PI3K, p-Akt/Akt ratios ↑p-GSK-3β, p-ERK 1/2	√	√ (TUNEL)	√	√	×	√	[23]
Schisandrin B. (Sch B)	↑p-Akt	√	√ (TUNEL)	√	√	×	×	[24]
Higenamine	↑p-Akt, p-Akt/Akt ratio	√	√	√	×	×	×	[32]
Myrica rubra flavonoids (MRF)	↑p-Akt/Akt, p-GSK-3β/GSK-3β	√	√ (Annexin V/PI)	√	√	×	√	[26]
Total paeony glycoside (TPG)	↓p-PI3K, p-Akt	×	√ (Annexin V-FITC/PI)	√	√	×	√	[27]
Bauhinia championii flavone	↑p-Akt/Akt, p-PI3K	√	√ (Annexin V-FITC/PI)	√	√	×	√	[28]

3. Discussion

This scoping review suggests the evidence of the NP-based therapies that provide cardioprotection in MIRI targeting the PI3K/AKT mechanism. This became a novel therapeutic strategy in the treatment of MIRI. There are increasing numbers of NP-derived drugs used in medicine due to their various biological activities and drug-like properties. One of the major metabolites in the plant is a flavonoid. Previous studies showed that a high intake of dietary flavonoids and their subclasses were associated with lower mortality of cardiovascular disease [50]. The NPs also enriched with other secondary metabolite compounds such as alkaloid and saponin, which display cardioprotective function [14,30].

MIRI is associated with multiple pathological condition such as oxidative stress, ERS, mitochondrial injury, inflammatory process, and apoptosis. Therefore, the role of PI3K/Akt signaling pathway post MIRI is very crucial, as it improves the cell survival and viability by limiting the apoptotic event. Generally, the apoptotic signaling pathway can either be stimulated by intrinsic or extrinsic pathways [51]. Bcl-2 and Bax proteins are integral regulatory factors in all apoptotic pathways [51,52]. The intrinsic pathway mainly involves mitochondrial injury and caspase-9 activation, whereas the extrinsic pathway is mediated by the death receptor Bcl-2/Bax [51,52]. Another pathway is regulated through the activation of caspase-12 [53]. Caspase-9 activates caspases-3 and -7, causing the conformation and biochemical processes related to apoptosis [51]. Apoptotic cascade includes mitochondria dysfunction, disturbed ATP supply, loss of mitochondrial membrane potential, the opening of mPTP, and release of cytochrome-C [54,55]. Therefore, inhibition of apoptosis and oxidative stress by targeting Bcl-2/Bax, cytochrome-C, caspase-3, -7, -9, mitochondrial ROS attenuated the progression of MIRI.

ERS is a type of oxidative stress which induces cell dysfunction in MIRI via regulation of the PI3K/AKT pathway [56]. Oxygen deficit and ROS accumulation during MIRI can trigger unfolded protein response (UPR) [56,57], through three ER transmembrane sensors: PERK, Activating Transcription Factor 6 (ATF6), and Inositol requiring 1 (IRE1). Uncontrolled ERS dissociates GRP78 from ER transmembrane sensors [58]. Inhibition of caspase-12 prevents subsequent caspase-9 and -3 activation and eventually suppressing apoptosis, and promoting cell survival [14,58]. Failure to control ERS might lead to apoptosis via increased GRP78, CHOP pathway, and caspase-12 activation, therefore dysregulating the PI3K/AKT signaling leading to MIRI.

Nrf2 is a redox-sensitive transcription factor that plays vital role to combat oxidative stress [59]. Nrf2 coordinates transcriptional activation of antioxidant genes including HO-1, NQO1 and SOD to eliminate ROS in reperfused cardiomyocytes [60,61]. Modulation of PI3K/AKT signaling pathway is important to increase SOD, CAT, and GSH enzymes activity and reduce MDA value in MIRI cardiomyocytes [62,63]. Previous studies demonstrated that attenuating the inflammation is critical for protection against MIRI [64] via PI3K/AKT pathway. The inhibition of PI3K/AKT pathway reduced IL-6, IL-1β, and TNFα in serum and histopathological analysis [15]. The PI3K/AKT pathway is believed to regulate the adaptive immune response and innate immune cells and suppress the inflammation associated with MIRI [65].

PI3K/AKT pathway is a key signaling cascade that mitigates MIRI. Most of NPs in Figure 1 conferred cardioprotection against MIRI via activation of PI3K/AKT pathway [13,14,22–24,26,28–32] except berberine [15] and TPG (41), which suppressed PI3K/AKT pathway. Further phosphorylation of downstream effectors of AKT, GSK-3β, involved cell survival in mitigating MIRI [13,23,26,29,66] by inhibiting mPTP opening, protecting the cell against mitochondrial-mediated cell death, and limiting infarct size [23]. β2-AR agonist activated PI3K/AKT cascade to promote myocyte survival [32]. The phosphorylation of PI3K/AKT pathway to mitigate MIRI was markedly reversed by a specific PI3K inhibitor, eliminating the unwanted effects on cytochrome-C release, caspase-9/3 activity, Bcl-2/Bax ratio, mPTP opening, ERS, p53 level, and XIAP expression. These findings conclude the key role of the PI3K/AKT pathway to suppress MIRI by attenuating ERS, oxidative stress, inflammation, and apoptosis [29–31]. The mechanism underlying NPs alleviates MIRI through activation of PI3K/Akt pathway is summarized in Figure 3.

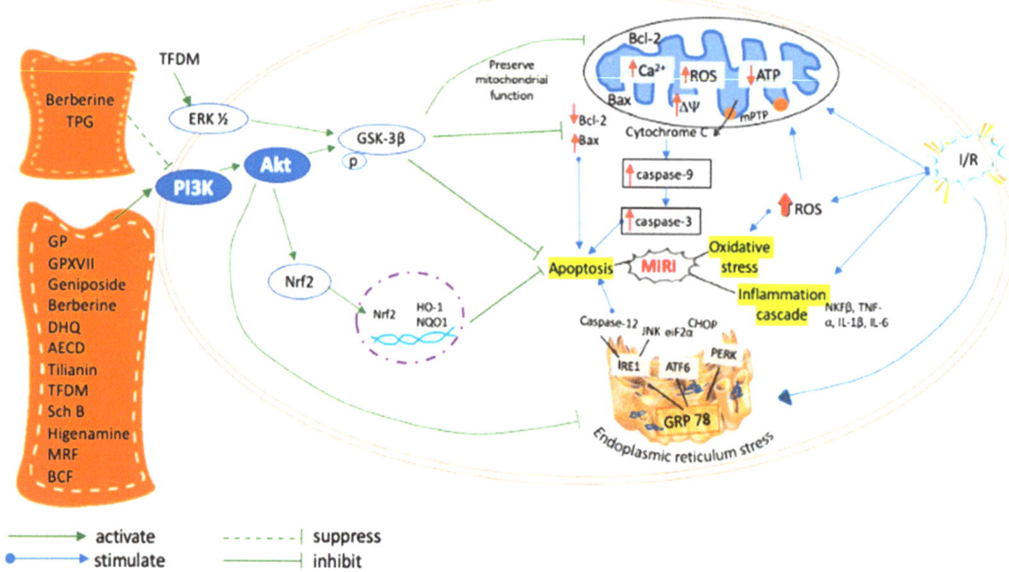

Figure 3. Mechanism of action of NPs alleviates MIRI in cardiomyocytes through PI3K/Akt signaling pathway.

4. Materials and Methods

A systematic search was conducted to identify the NP that alleviate MIRI targeting on PI3K/AKT pathway using PRISMA framework for scoping review [67]. Peer-reviewed and English full-text articles were gathered from January 2016 to January 2021 using PubMed, Scopus, and Web of Science (WOS) databases. The search terms used together with the Boolean operators AND and OR were as follows: "natural product" OR "herb* medicine" OR "plant-derived" OR "natural medicine" OR "plant extract" OR "plant ground" AND "myocardial injury" OR "myocardial infarction" OR "myocardial damage" OR "myocardial isch*" OR "myocardial inflammation" OR "myocardial dysfunction" AND "PI3K/AKT". The inclusion criteria of this study were (1) targeting on PI3K/AKT signaling, (2) availability of English full text, and (3) experiment using MIRI model (Table 5). The exclusion criteria were (1) a combination of herbs in the treatment and (2) not plant-derived. All titles and abstracts from the search results were screened and critiqued independently by all authors. Following the inclusion and exclusion criteria, the articles were shortlisted for eligibility upon reaching a consensus by all authors.

Table 5. Eligibility criteria for article selection.

Eligibility Criteria	Criteria
For title selection	1. Title in English 2. Year of publication from January 2016 to January 2021 3. Title reflects on MIRI

Table 5. *Cont.*

Eligibility Criteria	Criteria
For abstract selection	1. Abstract reflects that the article is an original article. 2. Abstract provides evidence of a robust study design. 3. Abstract highlights at least one measurable outcome that reflects PI3K/Akt signaling pathway. 4. Abstract clearly mentions the usage of MIRI model. The abstract reflects the use of natural product as intervention.
For full text of article selection	1. The article is available as a full-text article. 2.The article provides well-designed research methodology and/or intervention. 3. The article measures the outcome that related to PI3K/Akt. 4. The article uses natural product as an intervention. 5. The natural product used as intervention was not a combination of multiple natural products. The article explicitly explains the usage of MIRI model.

5. Limitations

The findings from this scoping review were restricted by several factors. First, our search strategy was focused solely on targeting one signaling pathway, namely the PI3K/Akt pathway, while MIRI is a complex injury that involves various other pathways such as TGFβ1/Smads signaling pathway [68], Parkin-mediated mitophagy [69], protein kinase A pathway [70], and activation of endogenous pro survival pathways such as protein kinase G [71]. Therefore, targeting one mechanism at a time may not be sufficient to produce a strong and robust effect in clinical situations where many uncontrolled variables usually coexist. Second, the therapeutic use of natural products was only limited to pre-clinical studies with no clinical trials included. Although all animal models in the papers presented were rodents, there was a difference in the genus. Additionally, we used a small sample size, which may have limited the generalizability of our findings. Third, several of the included studies provided experimental values in graphic form and, thus, the authors were unable to compare the findings in one study to another study that measured the same parameter. Fourth, translation into clinical situations is unfeasible because myocardial infarction is unpredictable, and most of the NPs-based drugs were designed as a pretreatment in MIRI models. Finally, only English articles with accessibility of full text were included. However, given the limitations faced in conducting this scoping review, it is unlikely that any missed data would possibly amend the conclusion drawn based on this review due to a clear focus on pre-clinical studies and because the electronic database search was performed to include citations and anywhere the keywords appeared in the article.

6. Conclusions

We summarized that NPs enriched with various bioactive compounds are beneficial to mitigate the pathological effects in post-MIRI. Recent studies suggest that these harmful effects can be alleviated by targeting the PI3K/AKT pathway, which might reduce apoptosis, inflammation, and oxidative stress. Further research is warranted to validate the safety and efficacy of NPs-based drugs in MIRI.

Author Contributions: All authors contributed to the writing; N.A.A.J., N.A.R., C.K.W. and S.A.S.A.H. conceived, designed, wrote, and revised the manuscript. All authors have read and agreed to the published version of the manuscript.

Funding: This research received no external funding.

Institutional Review Board Statement: Not applicable.

Informed Consent Statement: Not applicable.

Data Availability Statement: Data is contained within the article.

Acknowledgments: The authors also thank the Faculty of Medicine, Universiti Kebangsaan Malaysia and Faculty of Medicine, Universiti Teknologi MARA for the funding support for article processing fee.

Conflicts of Interest: The authors declare no conflict of interest.

References

1. Brown, J.C.; Gerhardt, T.E.; Kwon, E. *Risk Factors for Coronary Artery Disease*; StatPearls Publishing: Treasure Island, FL, USA, 2022.
2. Li, X.; Liu, M.; Sun, R.; Zeng, Y.; Chen, S.; Zhang, P. Protective Approaches against Myocardial Ischemia Reperfusion Injury. *Exp. Ther. Med.* **2016**, *12*, 3823–3829. [CrossRef]
3. Garcia-Dorado, D.; Rodríguez-Sinovas, A.; Ruiz-Meana, M.; Inserte, J. Protection Against Myocardial Ischemia-Reperfusion Injury in Clinical Practice. *Rev. Española Cardiol. (Engl. Ed.)* **2014**, *67*, 394–404. [CrossRef]
4. Dohmen, C.; Bosche, B.; Graf, R.; Reithmeier, T.; Ernestus, R.I.; Brinker, G.; Sobesky, J.; Heiss, W.D. Identification and Clinical Impact of Impaired Cerebrovascular Autoregulation in Patients With Malignant Middle Cerebral Artery Infarction. *Stroke* **2007**, *38*, 56–61. [CrossRef] [PubMed]
5. Malek, M.; Nematbakhsh, M. Renal Ischemia/Reperfusion Injury; from Pathophysiology to Treatment. *J. Ren. Inj. Prev.* **2015**, *4*, 20. [CrossRef]
6. Cowled, P.; Fitridge, R. Pathophysiology of Reperfusion Injury. In *Mechanisms of Vascular Disease: A Reference Book for Vascular Specialists*; University of Adelaide Press: Adelaide, Australia, 2011; pp. 331–350. [CrossRef]
7. Heusch, G. The Coronary Circulation as a Target of Cardioprotection. *Circ. Res.* **2016**, *118*, 1643–1658. [CrossRef]
8. Abd Rashid, N.; Mohammed, S.N.F.; Syed Abd Halim, S.A.; Abd Ghafar, N.; Abdul Jalil, N.A. Therapeutic Potential of Honey and Propolis on Ocular Disease. *Pharmaceuticals* **2022**, *15*, 1419. [CrossRef] [PubMed]
9. Adib Ridzuan, N.; Teoh, S.; Abdul Rashid, N.; Othman, F.; Baharum, S.; Hussan, F. *Polygonum Minus* Ethanolic Extracts Attenuate Cisplatin—Induced Oxidative Stress in the Cerebral Cortex of Rats via Its Antioxidant Properties. *Asian Pac. J. Trop. Biomed.* **2019**, *9*, 196–203. [CrossRef]
10. Abd Rashid, N.; Hussan, F.; Hamid, A.; Adib Ridzuan, N.R.; Teoh, S.L.; Budin, S.B. Preventive Effects of Polygonum Minus Essential Oil on Cisplatin-Induced Hepatotoxicity in Sprague Dawley Rats. *Sains Malays.* **2019**, *48*, 1975–1988. [CrossRef]
11. Abd Rashid, N.; Abd Halim, S.A.S.; Teoh, S.L.; Budin, S.B.; Hussan, F.; Adib Ridzuan, N.R.; Abdul Jalil, N.A. The Role of Natural Antioxidants in Cisplatin-Induced Hepatotoxicity. *Biomed. Pharmacother.* **2021**, *144*, 112328. [CrossRef]
12. Rashid, N.A.; Hussan, F.; Hamid, A.; Ridzuan, N.R.A.; Halim, S.A.S.A.; Jalil, N.A.A.; Najib, N.H.M.; Teoh, S.L.; Budin, S.B. Polygonum Minus Essential Oil Modulates Cisplatin-Induced Hepatotoxicity through Inflammatory and Apoptotic Pathways. *EXCLI J.* **2020**, *19*, 1246–1265. [CrossRef]
13. Li, L.; Zhou, Y.; Li, Y.; Wang, L.; Sun, L.; Zhou, L.; Arai, H.; Qi, Y.; Xu, Y. Aqueous Extract of Cortex Dictamni Protects H9c2 Cardiomyocytes from Hypoxia/Reoxygenation-Induced Oxidative Stress and Apoptosis by PI3K/Akt Signaling Pathway. *Biomed. Pharmacother.* **2017**, *89*, 233–244. [CrossRef]
14. Yu, Y.; Wang, M.; Chen, R.; Sun, X.; Sun, G.; Sun, X. Gypenoside XVII Protects against Myocardial Ischemia and Reperfusion Injury by Inhibiting ER Stress–Induced Mitochondrial Injury. *J. Ginseng Res.* **2019**, *45*, 642–653. [CrossRef]
15. Zhu, Q.W.; Li, Y.G. Berberine Attenuates Myocardial Ischemia Reperfusion Injury by Suppressing the Activation of PI3K/AKT Signaling. *Exp. Ther. Med.* **2016**, *11*, 978–984. [CrossRef]
16. Guo, X.; Cao, W.; Yao, J.; Yuan, Y.; Hong, Y.; Wang, X.; Xing, J. Cardioprotective Effects of Tilianin in Rat Myocardial Ischemia-Reperfusion Injury. *Mol. Med. Rep.* **2015**, *11*, 2227–2233. [CrossRef] [PubMed]
17. Sun, Y.-H.; Bu, R.; Wang, Y.-W.; Hu, Y.-C.; Wang, X.-M.; Dong, X.; Zu, W.; Niu, Y.; Zhao, P.-W.; Sun, P.; et al. Validation of Efficacy and Mechanism of Sanwei-Tanxiang Powder in Improving Myocardial Ischemia Reperfusion Injuries. *Sci. Rep.* **2021**, *11*, 664. [CrossRef] [PubMed]
18. Xie, Y.; Shi, X.; Sheng, K.; Han, G.; Li, W.; Zhao, Q.; Jiang, B.; Feng, J.; Li, J.; Gu, Y. PI3K/Akt Signaling Transduction Pathway, Erythropoiesis and Glycolysis in Hypoxia (Review). *Mol. Med. Rep.* **2019**, *19*, 783–791. [CrossRef] [PubMed]
19. Zhao, G.X.; Pan, H.; Ouyang, D.Y.; He, X.H. The Critical Molecular Interconnections in Regulating Apoptosis and Autophagy. *Ann. Med.* **2015**, *47*, 305–315. [CrossRef]
20. Franke, T.F.; Hornik, C.P.; Segev, L.; Shostak, G.A.; Sugimoto, C. PI3K/Akt and Apoptosis: Size Matters. *Oncogene* **2003**, *22*, 8983–8998. [CrossRef]
21. Yu, D.; Xiong, J.; Gao, Y.; Li, J.; Zhu, D.; Shen, X.; Sun, L.; Wang, X. Resveratrol Activates PI3K/AKT to Reduce Myocardial Cell Apoptosis and Mitochondrial Oxidative Damage Caused by Myocardial Ischemia/Reperfusion Injury. *Acta Histochem.* **2021**, *123*, 151739. [CrossRef]
22. Zeng, C.; Jiang, W.; Zheng, R.; He, C.; Li, J.; Xing, J. Cardioprotection of Tilianin Ameliorates Myocardial Ischemia-Reperfusion Injury: Role of the Apoptotic Signaling Pathway. *PLoS ONE* **2018**, *13*, e0193845. [CrossRef]
23. Zeng, C.; Jiang, W.; Yang, X.; He, C.; Wang, W.; Xing, J. Pretreatment with Total Flavonoid Extract from *Dracocephalum moldavica*, L. Attenuates Ischemia Reperfusion-Induced Apoptosis. *Sci. Rep.* **2018**, *8*, 17491. [CrossRef]

24. Zhao, X.; Xiang, Y.; Cai, C.; Zhou, A.; Zhu, N.; Zeng, C. Schisandrin B Protects against Myocardial Ischemia/Reperfusion Injury via the PI3K/Akt Pathway in Rats. *Mol. Med. Rep.* **2018**, *17*, 556–561. [CrossRef]
25. Jiang, Y.-Q.; Chang, G.; Wang, Y.; Zhang, D.-Y.; Cao, L.; Liu, J. Geniposide Prevents Hypoxia/Reoxygenation-Induced Apoptosis in H9c2 Cells: Improvement of Mitochondrial Dysfunction and Activation of GLP-1R and the PI3K/AKT Signaling Pathway. *Cell. Physiol. Biochem.* **2016**, *39*, 407–421. [CrossRef]
26. Wang, M.; Liu, Y.; Pan, R.L.; Wang, R.Y.; Ding, S.L.; Dong, W.R.; Sun, G.B.; Ye, J.X.; Sun, X.B. Protective Effects of Myrica Rubra Flavonoids against Hypoxia/Reoxygenation-Induced Cardiomyocyte Injury via the Regulation of the PI3K/Akt/GSK3β Pathway. *Int. J. Mol. Med.* **2019**, *43*, 2133–2143. [CrossRef]
27. Shen, P.; Chen, J.; Pan, M. The Protective Effects of Total Paeony Glycoside on Ischemia/Reperfusion Injury in H9C2 Cells via Inhibition of the PI3K/Akt Signaling Pathway. *Mol. Med. Rep.* **2018**, *18*, 3332–3340. [CrossRef]
28. Liao, P.; Sun, G.; Zhang, C.; Wang, M.; Sun, Y.; Zhou, Y.; Sun, X.; Jian, J. Bauhinia Championii Flavone Attenuates Hypoxia-Reoxygenation Induced Apoptosis in H9c2 Cardiomyocytes by Improving Mitochondrial Dysfunction. *Molecules* **2016**, *21*, 1469. [CrossRef]
29. Yu, H.; Zhang, H.; Zhao, W.; Guo, L.; Li, X.; Li, Y.; Zhang, X.; Sun, Y. Gypenoside Protects against Myocardial Ischemia-Reperfusion Injury by Inhibiting Cardiomyocytes Apoptosis via Inhibition of CHOP Pathway and Activation of PI3K/Akt Pathway In Vivo and In Vitro. *Cell. Physiol. Biochem.* **2016**, *39*, 123–136. [CrossRef] [PubMed]
30. Wang, L.; Ma, H.; Xue, Y.; Shi, H.; Ma, T.; Cui, X. Berberine Inhibits the Ischemia-Reperfusion Injury Induced Inflammatory Response and Apoptosis of Myocardial Cells through the Phosphoinositide 3-Kinase/RAC-α Serine/Threonine-Protein Kinase and Nuclear Factor-KB Signaling Pathways. *Exp. Ther. Med.* **2018**, *15*, 1225–1232. [CrossRef] [PubMed]
31. Shu, Z.; Yang, Y.; Yang, L.; Jiang, H.; Yu, X.; Wang, Y. Cardioprotective Effects of Dihydroquercetin against Ischemia Reperfusion Injury by Inhibiting Oxidative Stress and Endoplasmic Reticulum Stress-Induced Apoptosis: Via the PI3K/Akt Pathway. *Food Funct.* **2019**, *10*, 213–215. [CrossRef]
32. Wu, M.P.; Zhang, Y.S.; Zhou, Q.M.; Xiong, J.; Dong, Y.R.; Yan, C. Higenamine Protects Ischemia/Reperfusion Induced Cardiac Injury and Myocyte Apoptosis through Activation of B2-AR/PI3K/AKT Signaling Pathway. *Pharmacol. Res.* **2016**, *104*, 115–123. [CrossRef] [PubMed]
33. Qin, R.; Zhang, J.; Li, C.; Zhang, X.; Xiong, A.; Huang, F.; Yin, Z.; Li, K.; Qin, W.; Chen, M.; et al. Protective Effects of Gypenosides against Fatty Liver Disease Induced by High Fat and Cholesterol Diet and Alcohol in Rats. *Arch. Pharm. Res.* **2012**, *35*, 1241–1250. [CrossRef]
34. Zhang, G.-L.; Deng, J.-P.; Wang, B.-H.; Zhao, Z.-W.; Li, J.; Gao, L.; Liu, B.-L.; Xong, J.-R.; Guo, X.-D.; Yan, Z.-Q.; et al. Gypenosides Improve Cognitive Impairment Induced by Chronic Cerebral Hypoperfusion in Rats by Suppressing Oxidative Stress and Astrocytic Activation. *Behav. Pharmacol.* **2011**, *22*, 633–644. [CrossRef]
35. Zhuang, Q.; Cheng, J.; Xia, J.; Ning, M.; Wu, S.; Shen, S.; Shi, Y.; Huang, D.; Dong, Z.; Wan, X. Gypenosides Prevent and Dissolve Cholesterol Gallstones by Modulating the Homeostasis of Cholesterol and Bile Acids. *Front. Med.* **2022**, *9*, 818144. [CrossRef] [PubMed]
36. Yang, K.; Zhang, H.; Luo, Y.; Zhang, J.; Wang, M.; Liao, P.; Cao, L.; Guo, P.; Sun, G.; Sun, X. Gypenoside XVII Prevents Atherosclerosis by Attenuating Endothelial Apoptosis and Oxidative Stress: Insight into the ERα-Mediated PI3K/Akt Pathway. *Int. J. Mol. Sci.* **2017**, *18*, 77. [CrossRef]
37. Tie, G.; Yan, J.; Yang, Y.; Park, B.D.; Messina, J.A.; Raffai, R.L.; Nowicki, P.T.; Messina, L.M. Oxidized Low-Density Lipoprotein Induces Apoptosis in Endothelial Progenitor Cells by Inactivating the Phosphoinositide 3-Kinase/Akt Pathway. *J. Vasc. Res.* **2010**, *47*, 519–530. [CrossRef]
38. Cui, G.; Qin, X.; Zhang, Y.; Gong, Z.; Ge, B.; Zang, Y.Q. Berberine Differentially Modulates the Activities of ERK, P38 MAPK, and JNK to Suppress Th17 and Th1 T Cell Differentiation in Type 1 Diabetic Mice. *J. Biol. Chem.* **2009**, *284*, 28420–28429. [CrossRef] [PubMed]
39. Sunil, C.; Xu, B. An Insight into the Health-Promoting Effects of Taxifolin (Dihydroquercetin). *Phytochemistry* **2019**, *166*, 112066. [CrossRef] [PubMed]
40. Yu, S.M.; Ko, F.N.; Su, M.J.; Wu, T.S.; Wang, M.L.; Huang, T.F.; Teng, C.M. Vasorelaxing Effect in Rat Thoracic Aorta Caused by Fraxinellone and Dictamine Isolated from the Chinese Herb Dictamnus Dasycarpus Turcz: Comparison with Cromakalim and Ca2+ Channel Blockers. *Naunyn. Schmiedebergs Arch. Pharmacol.* **1992**, *345*, 349–355. [CrossRef]
41. Chen, R.; Su, W.; Li, P.; Huo, L.; Lu, R.; Peng, M. Free Radical-Scavenging and Antioxidant Activity of Skin of Dictamnus Dasycarpus. *Asian J. Chem.* **2013**, *25*, 1753–1754. [CrossRef]
42. Dastmalchi, K.; Damien Dorman, H.J.; Laakso, I.; Hiltunen, R. Chemical Composition and Antioxidative Activity of Moldavian Balm (*Dracocephalum moldavica* L.) Extracts. *LWT—Food Sci. Technol.* **2007**, *40*, 1655–1663. [CrossRef]
43. García-Díaz, J.A.; Navarrete-Vázquez, G.; García-Jiménez, S.; Hidalgo-Figueroa, S.; Almanza-Pérez, J.C.; Alarcón-Aguilar, F.J.; Gómez-Zamudio, J.; Cruz, M.; Ibarra-Barajas, M.; Estrada-Soto, S. Antidiabetic, Antihyperlipidemic and Anti-Inflammatory Effects of Tilianin in Streptozotocin-Nicotinamide Diabetic Rats. *Biomed. Pharmacother.* **2016**, *83*, 667–675. [CrossRef]
44. Panossian, A.; Wikman, G. Pharmacology of Schisandra Chinensis Bail.: An Overview of Russian Research and Uses in Medicine. *J. Ethnopharmacol.* **2008**, *118*, 183–212. [CrossRef] [PubMed]

45. Chiu, P.Y.; Leung, H.Y.; Siu, A.H.L.; Poon, M.K.T.; Ko, K.M. Schisandrin B Decreases the Sensitivity of Mitochondria to Calcium Ion-Induced Permeability Transition and Protects against Ischemia-Reperfusion Injury in Rat Hearts. *Acta Pharmacol. Sin.* **2007**, *28*, 1559–1565. [CrossRef] [PubMed]
46. Kosuge, T.; Yokota, M. Studies on Cardiac Principle of Aconite Root. *Chem. Pharm. Bull.* **1976**, *24*, 176–178. [CrossRef] [PubMed]
47. Tan, Y.-Q.; Chen, H.-W.; Li, J.; Wu, Q.-J. Efficacy, Chemical Constituents, and Pharmacological Actions of Radix Paeoniae Rubra and Radix Paeoniae Alba. *Front. Pharmacol.* **2020**, *11*, 1054. [CrossRef] [PubMed]
48. Zhang, Y.; Yan, G.; Sun, C.; Li, H.; Fu, Y.; Xu, W. Apoptosis Effects of Dihydrokaempferol Isolated from Bauhinia Championii on Synoviocytes. *Evid.-Based Complement. Altern. Med.* **2018**, *2018*, 9806160. [CrossRef]
49. Bass, J.; Wilkinson, D.; Rankin, D.; Phillips, B.; Szewczyk, N.; Smith, K.; Atherton, P. An Overview of Technical Considerations for Western Blotting Applications to Physiological Research. *Scand. J. Med. Sci. Sports* **2017**, *27*, 4–25. [CrossRef]
50. Bondonno, N.P.; Dalgaard, F.; Kyrø, C.; Murray, K.; Bondonno, C.P.; Lewis, J.R.; Croft, K.D.; Gislason, G.; Scalbert, A.; Cassidy, A.; et al. Flavonoid Intake Is Associated with Lower Mortality in the Danish Diet Cancer and Health Cohort. *Nat. Commun.* **2019**, *10*, 3651. [CrossRef]
51. D'Arcy, M.S. Cell Death: A Review of the Major Forms of Apoptosis, Necrosis and Autophagy. *Cell Biol. Int.* **2019**, *43*, 582–592. [CrossRef] [PubMed]
52. Tzifi, F.; Economopoulou, C.; Gourgiotis, D.; Ardavanis, A.; Papageorgiou, S.; Scorilas, A. The Role of BCL2 Family of Apoptosis Regulator Proteins in Acute and Chronic Leukemias. *Adv. Hematol.* **2012**, *2012*, 524308. [CrossRef]
53. Wu, N.; Zhang, X.; Jia, P.; Jia, D. Hypercholesterolemia Aggravates Myocardial Ischemia Reperfusion Injury via Activating Endoplasmic Reticulum Stress-Mediated Apoptosis. *Exp. Mol. Pathol.* **2015**, *99*, 449–454. [CrossRef]
54. Ahn, H.J.; Kim, K.I.; Kim, G.; Moon, E.; Yang, S.S.; Lee, J.S. Atmospheric-Pressure Plasma Jet Induces Apoptosis Involving Mitochondria via Generation of Free Radicals. *PLoS ONE* **2011**, *6*, e28154. [CrossRef]
55. Du, J.K.; Cong, B.H.; Yu, Q.; Wang, H.; Wang, L.; Wang, C.N.; Tang, X.L.; Lu, J.Q.; Zhu, X.Y.; Ni, X. Upregulation of MicroRNA-22 Contributes to Myocardial Ischemia-Reperfusion Injury by Interfering with the Mitochondrial Function. *Free Radic. Biol. Med.* **2016**, *96*, 406–417. [CrossRef]
56. Yuan, Y.; Guo, Q.; Ye, Z.; Pingping, X.; Wang, N.; Song, Z. Ischemic Postconditioning Protects Brain from Ischemia/Reperfusion Injury by Attenuating Endoplasmic Reticulum Stress-Induced Apoptosis through PI3K-Akt Pathway. *Brain Res.* **2011**, *1367*, 85–93. [CrossRef] [PubMed]
57. Yu, L.; Lu, M.; Wang, P.; Chen, X. Trichostatin A Ameliorates Myocardial Ischemia/Reperfusion Injury Through Inhibition of Endoplasmic Reticulum Stress-Induced Apoptosis. *Arch. Med. Res.* **2012**, *43*, 190–196. [CrossRef] [PubMed]
58. Choy, K.W.; Murugan, D.; Mustafa, M.R. Natural Products Targeting ER Stress Pathway for the Treatment of Cardiovascular Diseases. *Pharmacol. Res.* **2018**, *132*, 119–129. [CrossRef] [PubMed]
59. Xu, B.; Zhang, J.; Strom, J.; Lee, S.; Chen, Q.M. Myocardial Ischemic Reperfusion Induces de Novo Nrf2 Protein Translation. *Biochim. Biophys. Acta—Mol. Basis Dis.* **2014**, *1842*, 1638–1647. [CrossRef] [PubMed]
60. Surh, Y.J.; Kundu, J.K.; Na, H.K. Nrf2 as a Master Redox Switch in Turning on the Cellular Signaling Involved in the Induction of Cytoprotective Genes by Some Chemopreventive Phytochemicals. *Planta Med.* **2008**, *74*, 1526–1539. [CrossRef]
61. Eggler, A.L.; Gay, K.A.; Mesecar, A.D. Molecular Mechanisms of Natural Products in Chemoprevention: Induction of Cytoprotective Enzymes by Nrf2. *Mol. Nutr. Food Res.* **2008**, *52*, S84–S94. [CrossRef]
62. Ighodaro, O.M.; Akinloye, O.A. First Line Defence Antioxidants-Superoxide Dismutase (SOD), Catalase (CAT) and Glutathione Peroxidase (GPX): Their Fundamental Role in the Entire Antioxidant Defence Grid. *Alex. J. Med.* **2018**, *54*, 287–293. [CrossRef]
63. Ho, E.; Karimi Galougahi, K.; Liu, C.C.; Bhindi, R.; Figtree, G.A. Biological Markers of Oxidative Stress: Applications to Cardiovascular Research and Practice. *Redox Biol.* **2013**, *1*, 483–491. [CrossRef]
64. Liu, Z.Z.; Kong, J.B.; Li, F.Z.; Ma, L.L.; Liu, S.Q.; Wang, L.X. Ischemic Postconditioning Decreases Matrix Metalloproteinase-2 Expression during Ischemiareperfusion of Myocardium in a Rabbit Model: A Preliminary Report. *Exp. Clin. Cardiol.* **2013**, *18*, 99.
65. Shrimali, D.; Shanmugam, M.K.; Kumar, A.P.; Zhang, J.; Tan, B.K.H.; Ahn, K.S.; Sethi, G. Targeted Abrogation of Diverse Signal Transduction Cascades by Emodin for the Treatment of Inflammatory Disorders and Cancer. *Cancer Lett.* **2013**, *341*, 139–149. [CrossRef] [PubMed]
66. Haupt, M.; Zechmeister, B.; Bosche, B.; Lieschke, S.; Zheng, X.; Zhang, L.; Venkataramani, V.; Jin, F.; Hein, K.; Weber, M.S.; et al. Lithium Enhances Post-Stroke Blood-Brain Barrier Integrity, Activates the MAPK/ERK1/2 Pathway and Alters Immune Cell Migration in Mice. *Neuropharmacology* **2020**, *181*, 108357. [CrossRef]
67. Tricco, A.C.; Lillie, E.; Zarin, W.; O'Brien, K.K.; Colquhoun, H.; Levac, D.; Moher, D.; Peters, M.D.J.; Horsley, T.; Weeks, L.; et al. PRISMA Extension for Scoping Reviews (PRISMA-ScR): Checklist and Explanation. *Ann. Intern. Med.* **2018**, *169*, 467–473. [CrossRef]
68. Zheng, Q.N.; Wei, X.H.; Pan, C.S.; Li, Q.; Liu, Y.Y.; Fan, J.Y.; Han, J.Y. QiShenYiQi Pills® Ameliorates Ischemia/Reperfusion-Induced Myocardial Fibrosis Involving RP S19-Mediated TGFβ1/Smads Signaling Pathway. *Pharmacol. Res.* **2019**, *146*, 104272. [CrossRef] [PubMed]
69. Yang, H.X.; Wang, P.; Wang, N.N.; Li, S.D.; Yang, M. hui Tongxinluo Ameliorates Myocardial Ischemia-Reperfusion Injury Mainly via Activating Parkin-Mediated Mitophagy and Downregulating Ubiquitin-Proteasome System. *Chin. J. Integr. Med.* **2021**, *27*, 542–550. [CrossRef]

70. Li, X.D.; Yang, Y.J.; Geng, Y.J.; Jin, C.; Hu, F.A.; Zhao, J.L.; Zhang, H.T.; Cheng, Y.T.; Qian, H.Y.; Wang, L.L.; et al. Tongxinluo Reduces Myocardial No-Reflow and Ischemia-Reperfusion Injury by Stimulating the Phosphorylation of ENOS via the PKA Pathway. *Am. J. Physiol. Heart Circ. Physiol.* **2010**, *299*, H1255–H1261. [CrossRef] [PubMed]
71. Davidson, S.M.; Ferdinandy, P.; Andreadou, I.; Bøtker, H.E.; Heusch, G.; Ibáñez, B.; Ovize, M.; Schulz, R.; Yellon, D.M.; Hausenloy, D.J.; et al. Multitarget Strategies to Reduce Myocardial Ischemia/Reperfusion Injury: JACC Review Topic of the Week. *J. Am. Coll. Cardiol.* **2019**, *73*, 89–99. [CrossRef] [PubMed]

pharmaceuticals MDPI

Review

Natural Ingredients to Improve Immunity

Amin Gasmi [1], Mariia Shanaida [2], Oleksandra Oleshchuk [2], Yuliya Semenova [3], Pavan Kumar Mujawdiya [4], Yana Ivankiv [2], Olena Pokryshko [2], Sadaf Noor [5], Salva Piscopo [1,6], Stepan Adamiv [7] and Geir Bjørklund [8,*]

1 Société Francophone de Nutrithérapie et de Nutrigénétique Appliquée, 69100 Villeurbanne, France
2 I. Horbachevsky Ternopil National Medical University, 46001 Ternopil, Ukraine
3 School of Medicine, Nazarbayev University, 5/1 Kerey and Zhanibek Khandar Str., Astana 010000, Kazakhstan
4 Inochi Care Private Limited, New Delhi 110017, India
5 Institute of Molecular Biology and Biotechnology, Bahauddin Zakariya University Multan, Multan 60000, Pakistan
6 Department of Nutritional Research and Development, Nutri-Logics SA, 9990 Luxembourg, Luxembourg
7 Department of General Dentistry, Odessa National Medical University, 65000 Odessa, Ukraine
8 Council for Nutritional and Environmental Medicine, 8610 Mo i Rana, Norway
* Correspondence: bjorklund@conem.org

Abstract: The immune system protects the body from infectious agents such as bacteria, viruses, or fungi. Once encountered with pathogens or antigens, the innate and adaptive arms of the immune system trigger a strong immune response to eliminate them from the system and protect the body. Thus, well-balanced immunity is pivotal for maintaining human health, as an insufficient level of immune defense leads to infections and tumors. In contrast, the excessive functioning of the immune system causes the development of autoimmune diseases and allergies. Strong immunity requires adequate nutrition, dietary interventions, and sufficient intake of certain vitamins (vitamin C, vitamin D, and folic acid) and minerals (magnesium, zinc, and selenium). Therefore, nutritional and micronutrient deficiencies lead to compromised immunity. Several natural ingredients have shown potent immunomodulatory properties. The immune-enhancing properties of many plants and fungi are due to containing bioactive phytoconstituents such as polyphenols, terpenoids, β-glucans, vitamins, etc. Probiotics and prebiotics can be used as innovative tools to reduce intestinal inflammation and downregulate hypersensitivity reactions. Plant sources of melatonin, a multifunctional molecule with proven anti-inflammatory and immunomodulatory properties, have been discovered relatively recently. The bioactive compounds augment the immune response by directly increasing the cytotoxic activity of natural killer cells, macrophages, and neutrophils. Many phytoconstituents prevent cell damage due to their powerful antimicrobial, antioxidant, and anti-inflammatory properties. The present review attempts to understand the molecular mechanisms underlying the immune-enhancing properties of some bioactive compounds from plants, fungi, animals, microorganisms, and other natural sources.

Keywords: natural bioactive compounds; medicinal plants; vitamins; minerals; melatonin; propolis; probiotics; prebiotics; dosages; immunomodulators; antioxidants

Citation: Gasmi, A.; Shanaida, M.; Oleshchuk, O.; Semenova, Y.; Mujawdiya, P.K.; Ivankiv, Y.; Pokryshko, O.; Noor, S.; Piscopo, S.; Adamiv, S.; et al. Natural Ingredients to Improve Immunity. *Pharmaceuticals* **2023**, *16*, 528. https://doi.org/10.3390/ph16040528

Academic Editor: Elena Y. Enioutina

Received: 26 February 2023
Revised: 28 March 2023
Accepted: 30 March 2023
Published: 1 April 2023

1. Introduction

Humans are constantly exposed to various external influences, such as environmental pollutants or harmful pathogens, that affect homeostasis [1]. In recent decades, the rapid growth of the frequency of various infectious diseases, inflammatory conditions, allergies, cancers, and autoimmune disorders has brought much suffering to human beings. At the beginning of the 21st century, Parkin and Cohen [2] summarized that an insufficient level of immune defense leads primarily to the occurrence of severe infections or/and tumors, while the excessive functioning of the immune system causes the development of allergic or/and autoimmune diseases. Thus, well-balanced immunity is pivotal for maintaining human health [3]. Therefore, the importance of using natural substances with immunomodulating properties to prevent or augment the treatment of the abovementioned conditions is becoming quite obvious [4].

The immune system comprises a wide range of immune cells, various cytokines, and signaling pathways that protect the skin, intestinal tract, and respiratory tract from foreign invaders such as bacteria, viruses, and fungi. The host immune system has two arms: the innate immune system and the adaptive immune system [2]. While innate immunity lacks immunological memory, it is a hallmark of adaptive immunity [5].

Medicinal plants, beekeeping products, probiotics and prebiotics, melatonin, and other natural compounds with immunomodulating properties could explore new therapeutic ways to enhance immunity against various diseases [6–9]. Many vitamins and minerals are also very effective in supporting the proper functioning of immunity [7]. The high cost of synthetic drugs, their anticipated toxicity, and various adverse effects are undesirable for patients. In contrast, herbal substances as health promoters have gained increasing attention in both scientific circles and among consumers [10]. Some medicinal plants can exhibit immunomodulatory effects such as phagocytosis promotion and macrophage activation, modulation of cytokine secretion, immunoglobulin production, and lymphocyte proliferation [10]. In addition to the significant growth of interest in so-called superfoods (berries, nuts, green tea, sea products, and honey, among many others) in the era of the coronavirus pandemic [11], COVID-19 has prompted a search for new effective natural remedies for immunomodulation to prevent this disease. Natural phytotherapeutics were regarded as effective immune boosters in the case of COVID-19 disease [12]. Despite the progressive successes in developing various vaccines against COVID-19, the importance of natural substances as immune-enhancing agents cannot be underestimated [7]. Recently, herbal medicines have been considered the drugs of choice to enhance immunity in pre- and post-COVID-19 patients [13].

Plant-based natural ingredients promote health and help fight infections by boosting host immunity. Some phytoconstituents increase the proportion of beneficial gut bacteria, which are crucial for maintaining immunity. Recently, Rondanelli et al. described the pivotal role of vitamins (C, D), zinc, and *Echinacea* preparations in self-care for the prevention or treatment of common colds [14]. The natural ingredients of garlic (*Allium sativum*) boost immunity by increasing the functions of innate immune system cells such as lymphocytes, $\gamma\delta$-T cells, and natural killer (NK) cells, which kill invading pathogens [15]. β-Glucans are a category of naturally derived ingredients (from some plants, fungi, and bacteria) that modulate innate and adaptive immune responses. However, the immune response generated by β-glucans varies based on the structure [16]. The appropriate intake of some polyphenols, vitamins, and minerals helps boost immune functions and fight infections, including COVID-19 [17]. The immune-boosting properties of flavonoids help fight cancer, inflammation, and viral infections [18,19].

It should be noted that a balanced immune response also requires the suppression of unnecessary and harmful immune reactions. As it is known, dendritic cells (DCs) directly link the innate and adaptive immune systems, and their abnormal activation leads to chronic inflammation, rejection of transplants, and autoimmunity. It was revealed that quercetin, as a representative of flavonoids, can act as an immunosuppressant by inhibiting the activation of DCs [20]. Nowadays, scientists have concluded that using nanoformulations helps successfully solve the problem of poor aqueous solubility and low bioavailability of some natural constituents such as curcumin, quercetin, gingerol, etc. [21–23]. Nanodelivery of drugs makes it possible to provide targeted delivery of bioactive components and helps significantly reduce their dosage.

Micronutrients, such as vitamin C, also improve immune functions by augmenting chemotaxis and phagocytosis and generating free radicals by immune cells [24]. Similarly, vitamin D increases the Th2 cell response and suppresses Th1 cell activation [25]. Overall, deficiencies in certain vitamins and minerals can lead to the weakening of the immune system [26]. It should be also mentioned that propolis, a famous beekeeping product, is widely used for managing upper respiratory tract infections, which occur when the level of immunity decreases [8,27]. It is also worth adding that research in recent years has revealed that appropriate administration of the hormone melatonin plays a significant role in improving immunity [28,29].

This review attempts to describe the modern approaches to the immune-boosting roles of a variety of natural ingredients from different sources and their use in managing infections or other diseases related to the dysfunction of the immune system.

2. Medicinal Plants as Immunomodulators

Several botanical families comprise many plants with proven immunomodulating properties, including *Asteraceae, Rutaceae, Araliaceae, Zingiberaceae, Alliaceae, Lamiaceae*, etc. [30–33]. For example, the immune-stimulating properties of *Echinacea*, ginger, and fresh citrus juice have been well-known worldwide for several decades [1,32,34,35]. In recent years, an increasing number of herbs with immunostimulating properties have been researched and discovered for official medicine based on the study of plant species from different parts of the globe. Herbal preparations are regarded as effective and inexpensive natural immunomodulators [1,36–38]. Williamson summarized that the molecular pharmacology of herbal drugs is a tremendous challenge, as phytoextracts are multicomponent substances with multileveled modes of action compared to synthetic pharmaceuticals [39].

Thomford et al. [40] noted that modern approaches to medicine in the 21st century, as a rule, require the isolation and purification of one or two active compounds from medicinal plants. However, the isolation of an active compound could lead to the loss of its pharmacological activity [40]. For instance, the effectiveness of multi-component herbal prescriptions in traditional Chinese medicine is highly appreciated by modern health care practitioners. It should be noted that individually, many of the ingredients in these combinations do not possess therapeutic activities because of the simultaneous and synergistic action of several bioactive compounds [40]. The modern technologies such as metabolomics, genomics, proteomics, transcriptomics, and computational strategies open the way for choosing better drug candidates with immunomodulatory effects extracted from medicinal plants [41].

According to Boozari and Hosseinzadeh, the consumption of herbal substances prepared from *Echinacea* spp., *Zingiber officinale, Camellia sinensis, Hypericum perforatum, Allium sativum, Glycyrrhiza glabra*, and *Nigella sativa* can significantly improve the immune response in the fight against the novel coronavirus COVID-19 [42]. It was found that phytoconstituents from such ayurvedic medicinal plants as Ashwagandha (*Withania somnifera*), Tulsi (*Ocimum sanctum*), and Giloy (*Tinospora cordifolia*) were effective COVID-19 virus proteases [30,43]. Coriander (*Coriandrum sativum*) was regarded as the most commonly used ingredient in homemade remedies in Sri Lanka during the COVID-19 pandemic [44]. Herbal preparations are regarded as effective and inexpensive natural immunomodulators [1]. Recent findings of Al Kury et al. [45] demonstrate that an extract from the aerial part of *Xanthium spinosum* (*Asteraceae* family) has significant anticancer and immunomodulatory effects.

Many polyphenols, terpenoids, sulfur-containing compounds, polysaccharides, and some alkaloids possess the ability to enhance immunity [33,46,47]. Venter et al. [48] concluded that unsaturated omega-3 fatty acids from plants sources also play an important role in the maintenance of immunity in the context of autoimmune and allergic diseases.

However, the lack of reliable standardization of bioactive ingredients and rigorous tests for efficacy constitute a significant obstacle regarding the poor progress in research studying the immunomodulatory effects of herbal remedies [1,36]. Recently, Sun et al. [49] concluded that increased solubility, bioavailability, and efficacy of herbal formulations with immunomodulatory effects can be achieved using nano-engineered delivery systems. Chaudhary et al. [21] found that the synthesis of new antimicrobial drugs using 'green nanoparticles' from plant extracts has attracted a lot of attention from scientists in recent years.

2.1. Coneflower (Echinacea ssp.)

Coneflower (*Echinacea)* is a genus of herbaceous plants (*Asteraceae* family) originating from North America. Three species (*E. purpurea*, *E. pallida*, and *E. angustifolia*) have been used by Native Americans for the treatment of respiratory infections and inflammatory conditions, including bronchitis and inflammation of the mouth [1]. Phytopreparations from the coneflower rhizome with roots or herbs are also widely used in the 21st century in the pharmaceutical industry. They are the best-selling herbal drugs in the USA and Europe as effective natural immunomodulators [50].

The quality of *E. purpureae herba* and *radix* may be determined by the content of cichoric acid, which is regarded as their main bioactive compound, while dominating echinacoside is characteristic of the *E. angustifoliae* and *E. pallidae radices* [1]. In addition to these phytoconstituents, several other bioactive chemicals have been identified in *Echinacea* species. Thus, their N-alkylamides also possess significant immunomopharmacological effects [51]. Primary metabolites such as polysaccharide arabinogalactan from *E. purpurea* could also enhance macrophage activation [52]. It was suggested that treatment with standardized *Echinacea* extracts at 2.4 g/day over 120 days is beneficial for prophylactic use and a dose of 4.0 g/day during acute stages of colds [14]. The extract from the fresh aerial part of *E. purpurea* (10–250 µg/mL) could effectively modulate the human Jurkat T-cell cytokine response through interleukin-2 and interferon-gamma cytokine secretions [53].

In vitro studies of the ethanolic extract prepared from *E. purpurea* showed its significant effect on inhibiting highly pathogenic SARS-CoV-2 [54]. Vimalanathan et al. [55] showed the broad antiviral actions of *E. purpurea* against SARS-CoV-2. Recently, Kolev et al. [56] demonstrated in randomized clinical studies the ability of *E. purpurea* hydroethanolic extract to prevent respiratory tract viral infections during the COVID-19 pandemic in the long term.

2.2. Artemisia afra/annua

Artemisia (*Asteraceae* family) is a widely known genus of immense medicinal value. It comprises almost 500 species of plants. The famous antimalarial drug artemisinin was isolated from the Chinese species sweet wormwood (*A. annua*). The significant interest in this compound has increased in the past three years, due to the COVID-19 pandemic, as it also possesses antiviral effect [57].

Several volatile secondary phytoconstituents from *Artemisia* species are part of traditional medicinal systems worldwide. In the South African region, *A. afra* is one of the most common and widely used herbs to manage diabetes, malaria, and cough [58]. *A. afra* also possesses powerful antimicrobial properties due to the presence of bioactive terpenoids. The essential oils of *A. afra* showed antimicrobial properties against 41 bacterial strains, indicating broad antimicrobial activity, which favors its use as a preservative in the food and cosmetic industries [59]. Three compounds of *A. afra*, scopoletin, betulinic acid, and acacetin, have shown potent antimicrobial activity against a wide range of gram-negative and gram-positive bacterial species and *Candida albicans* [60]. Appalasamy et al. reported the antimicrobial properties of *A. annua*. However, the compounds in *A. annua* were not found to be effective against *Candida albicans* [61]. The extract of *A. annua* also showed dose-dependent inhibition of tumor necrosis factor-alfa (TNF-α) in activated neutrophils. At 25, 10, and 5 µg/mL concentrations, *A. annua* inhibited TNF-α secretion by 89%, 54%, and 38%, respectively. It also inhibited the secretion of prostaglandin E2 by activated neutrophils [62]. It is pertinent to mention that some studies have reported hepatotoxic effects of *A. annua*, where consumption of *A. annua* herbal tea was associated with acute cholestatic hepatitis. Therefore, the authors recommend its discontinuation for use in malaria due to its ineffectiveness and toxic effects on the liver [63]. A 2012 report by the European Food Safety Authority classified several *Artemisia* species in a category that "*contain naturally occurring substances of possible concern for human health when used in food and food supplements.*" Moreover, the Medicine Control Council of South Africa has also banned the use of *A. afra* for the treatment of malaria due to its lack of efficacy [64].

2.3. Ginseng (Panax ginseng)

Numerous studies have demonstrated that ginseng (*Panax ginseng*) as well as several other species from the *Araliaceae* family can modulate the immune system, thereby preventing many health disorders and treating immunity-related diseases [48]. Many isolated ginsenosides (including Re, Rf, and Rg2) possess noticeable positive effects on innate and adaptive immunity [65].

Interestingly, the immune-stimulating properties of ginseng are modulated by the fermentation process. For instance, the fermentation of an ethanol extract of red ginseng by *Lactobacillus plantarum* M-2 enhanced the immunological benefits of red ginseng. In the mouse model, intraperitoneal injection of 500 μg fermented red ginseng (FRG-E) was more effective in reducing lung metastasis than nonfermented red ginseng (NFRG-E) (81.1% v/s 66.9%). Moreover, FRG-E improved immunity in healthy subjects by increasing the levels of IgA and IgG. Surprisingly, NRFG-E reduced IgA and IgG levels in subjects compared with the baseline values (5.14 mg/mL v/s −14.5 mg/mL at one week), indicating improved immunological activity of FRG-E compared with NFRG-E [66].

A study conducted in patients with non-small cell lung cancer demonstrated that ginseng polysaccharides (GPS) alter the immune response of T helper cells (Th1 and Th2) compared to DCs alone. Both the GPS + DC and DC groups showed higher levels of Th1 cytokines (INF-γ and IL-2) and reduced levels of Th2 cytokines (IL-4 and IL-5), leading to a higher ratio of Th1/Th2 cytokines. Importantly, patients in the GPS + DC group showed higher immune functions than those in the DC alone group, indicating the potent immunomodulatory effects of GPS [67].

A randomized, placebo-controlled, parallel, double-blind study on 72 healthy subjects demonstrated that ginseng polysaccharide Y-75 (6 g/day) significantly increased immune functions compared to the control group. Intake of Y-75 enhanced NK cell activity by 35.2% and 40.2% from baseline values after 8 and 14 weeks of treatment, respectively. Similarly, the phagocytic activity of peripheral blood cells increased significantly by 25.2% and 39.4%. Moreover, serum TNF-α levels showed 38.2% and 44.5% increases at 8- and 14-weeks posttreatment, respectively. Importantly, Y-75 was found to be safe and efficacious in improving immune functions [68]. Sun et al. demonstrated that oral administration of 200 and 400 mg/day ginseng polysaccharides in cyclophosphamide-induced immunocompromised mice significantly improved immunity by increasing NK cell cytotoxic activity and increasing the secretion of perforin and granzyme [69].

2.4. Spices

A lot of different spices are widely used in cooking. As it turned out, some of them have a significant effect on the functioning of the immune system. Many spices that are commonly known as medicinal plants possess immune-enhancing properties. Thus, the rhizome of ginger (*Zingiber officinale*) contains dozens of compounds with antioxidant activities that could be used to treat various inflammations as well as modulate metabolic biomarkers. Karimi et al. [70] demonstrated that four capsules of ginger extract (750 mg) were used daily for six weeks by obese women with breast neoplasms to reduce systemic inflammation and metabolic syndrome. Yücel et al. [23] described gingerols' anti-inflammatory and immunomodulatory potential and their nanoformulations. The presence of a significant amount of eugenol in the essential oil as well as polyphenols (including apigenin, quercetin, and ferulic acid) in the aerial parts of 'Holy basil' or 'Tulsi' (*Ocimum sanctum*) from the *Lamiaceae* family could be the substantial reason for its excellent anti-inflammatory and immunostimulating activity [71]. The main biocompounds of garlic (*Allium sativum*) belong to γ-glutamyl cysteine derivatives, allyl methyl cysteine, and diallyl thiosulfinate compound families [72]. Allicin orally applied at doses of 3–9 mg/kg/day reduced parasitemia in mice infected with *Plasmodium malaria* and prolonged their survival by improving host immune responses [73]. The cumin (*Nigella* ssp.) seeds contain thymoquinone, β-elemen, dihydrofarnesol, and other bioactive terpenoids [74] that exhibit significant antioxidant and anti-inflammatory effects. Clinical trials revealed that *Nigella* seed oil has substantial potential to alleviate inflammation in the case of rheumatoid arthritis [74].

Figure 1 presents the most important medicinal plants and spices with immunomodulatory effects.

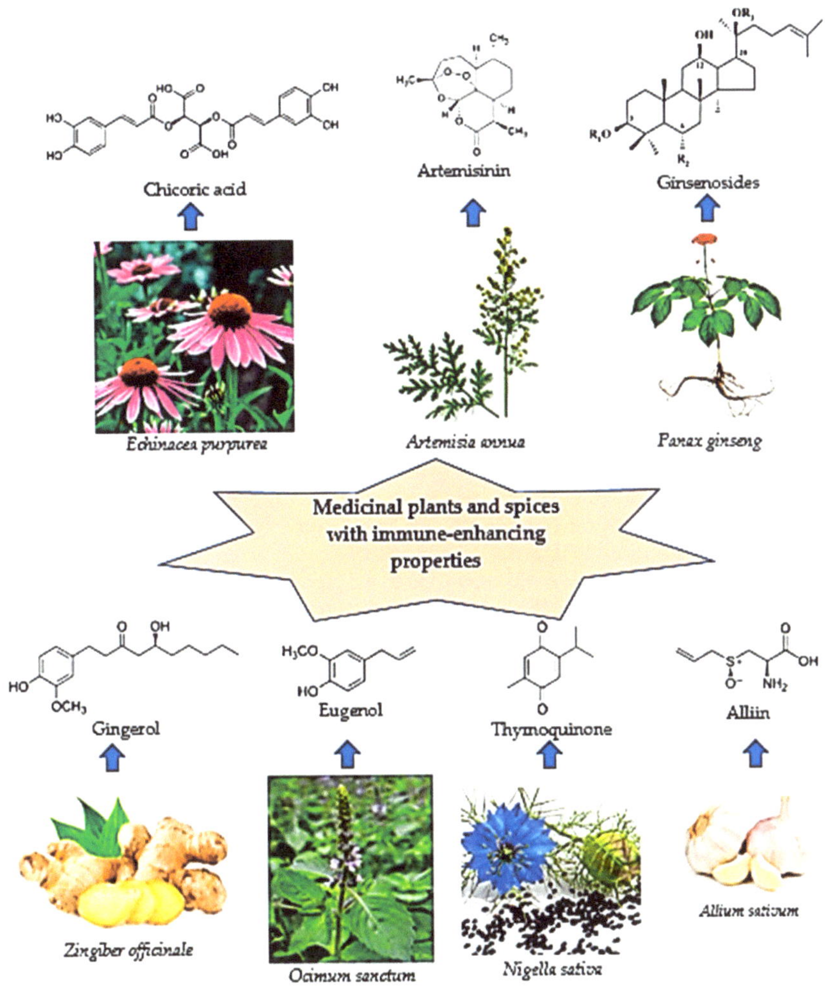

Figure 1. The most important medicinal plants and spices with immunomodulatory activity.

Thus, a lot of herbs are quite effective and inexpensive natural sources of phytoconstituents with immune-enhancing properties. Some polyphenols, terpenoids, sulfur-containing compounds, polysaccharides, etc., from medicinal plants and spices possess significant potential to improve immunity.

3. Selected Natural Compounds with Immunomodulating Properties

Quercetin, curcumin, luteolin, and other polyphenols demonstrate prominent immunostimulatory actions on macrophages as well as the ability to increase the proliferation of T cells and B cells [75]. Polyphenols can also reduce inflammation by suppressing proinflammatory cytokines and causing immunomodulatory effects against autoimmune diseases and allergic reactions [76]. According to Mollazadeh et al. [77], the positive effects of curcumin on human immunity could be related to its ability to increase IL-10-mediated effects.

Among other well-known components with an immunomodulatory effect, it should be mentioned propolis as a beekeeping product, melatonin as a representative of the class of neurohormones, or some polysaccharides of plants and mushrooms. Xylitol, as a non-digestible carbohydrate of natural origin, beyond its significant role in maintaining dental health, also modulates the immune response of the body [78,79]. It contributes to a reduced respiratory tract infection risk [79].

Below are the results of scientific research on the immunomodulatory potential of some biologically active components that have different resource origins.

3.1. Quercetin

Quercetin is a flavonoid with the chemical name 3,3′,4′,5,7-pentahydroxyflavone. Quercetin is not synthesized in the human body, and it is found in several plant species. Its anti-inflammatory, antioxidant, antiviral, and antibacterial properties are well reported in the literature [75,80].

In a randomized, double-blind, placebo-controlled clinical trial conducted in 50 women with rheumatoid arthritis, the intervention of quercetin (500 mg/day) for eight weeks significantly improved disease symptoms by reducing pain, disease activity, and plasma levels of hs-TNFα compared with the placebo group. Although quercetin supplementation affected the erythrocyte sedimentation rate, the difference was insignificant [81]. In a meta-analysis, quercetin supplementation significantly reduced CRP levels, total cholesterol, and low-density lipoprotein in patients suffering from metabolic disorders. However, no effect on IL-6, TNF-α, or high-density lipoprotein was observed [82]. However, a randomized, crossover study in 20 athletes showed that intake of four quercetin-based chews 15 min before a 2 h run did not reduce post-exercise inflammation or immune changes caused by increased levels of various cytokines, such as GM-CSF, IL-2, IL-6, IL-8, CRP, TNF-α, and IL-1β. The four quercetin-based chews provided to runners were made using 1000 mg quercetin, 1000 mg vitamin C, 400 mg each of isoquercetin, eicosapentaenoic acid, and docosahexaenoic acid, 120 mg epigallocatechin 3-gallate, and 40 mg niacinamide. Although quercetin levels significantly increased in the quercetin-based chews group, no statistically significant difference was observed in the postexercise inflammation levels compared to the placebo group [83].

Heinz et al. conducted a double-blinded, placebo-controlled, randomized trial to evaluate the impact of long-term supplementation of quercetin on the innate immune system. Supplementation of quercetin (500 mg/day and 1000 mg/day) to adult female subjects for 12 weeks had no significant impact on plasma IL-6 and TNF-α levels, and no significant impact on NK-cell activity and granulocyte phagocytosis was observed compared to the placebo group, indicating no direct impact on innate immunity and inflammation [84]. Figure 2 presents an overview of the immunomodulatory properties of quercetin and preparations from ginseng.

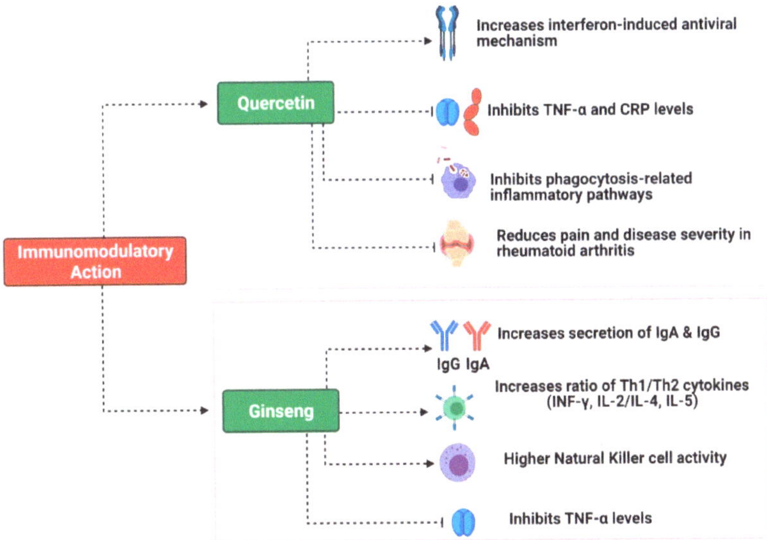

Figure 2. Immunomodulatory activities of quercetin and ginseng.

3.2. Propolis

Propolis is a highly viscous and resinous natural product produced by honeybees and possesses substantial pharmacological and biological properties [8]. Propolis is recommended for managing upper respiratory tract infections, flu, colds, wound healing, fighting bacterial, viral, and fungal infections, and treating acne or burns [27]. The antioxidant properties of propolis primarily contribute to its medicinal properties. A meta-analysis and systemic review of six studies with 406 participants concluded that propolis use significantly lowered serum TNF-α and CRP levels in study participants [85]. A double-blind, placebo-controlled clinical trial in 50 type 2 diabetes mellitus patients showed that the treated group receiving Iranian propolis (1000 mg/day) for 90 days showed a significant reduction in serum levels of CRP, TNF-α, glycosylated hemoglobin, and insulin [86]. A randomized, double-blind trial conducted in 60 elderly subjects (average age: 72.8 years) living at higher latitudes (2260 m above sea level) demonstrated that propolis intake (0.8 g; 24 months) significantly reduced serum IL-1β and IL-6 levels, but serum TNF-α levels were not statistically significant. However, the propolis-treated group showed significantly higher levels of TGF-β1 [87].

Similarly, in an 18-week randomized controlled study involving 33 type 2 diabetes mellitus patients, supplementation with 900 mg/day of Brazilian green propolis significantly reduced serum TNF-α levels but significantly increased serum IL-1β and IL-6 levels. Moreover, serum antioxidant capacity and total polyphenol concentrations were significantly higher in the propolis-treated group, while serum carbonyls and lactate dehydrogenase activity were significantly lower [88]. Diabetic foot is a major diabetes-associated complication. The use of propolis has been proposed to heal diabetic foot ulcers due to its anti-inflammatory, antioxidant, and wound-healing properties. A randomized trial conducted on 31 diabetic foot ulcer patients showed that propolis spray (3%) applied to wounds for eight weeks reduced the wound area by 4 cm^2 and facilitated wound healing via increased tissue deposition at the wound site.

Moreover, propolis reduced TNF-α but increased IL-10 and the glutathione/glutathione disulfide ratio. Therefore, propolis may be used as an adjuvant therapy in managing diabetic foot due to its anti-inflammatory and antioxidant potential [89]. A meta-analysis of six studies comprising 406 participants demonstrated that propolis intake significantly reduced serum levels of CRP and TNF-α [85]. In a double-blind, randomized, placebo-controlled clinical trial conducted on 31 dengue hemorrhagic fever patients in Indonesia, patients were given two capsules of 200 mg of Propoelix™ three times a day for seven days. The PropoelixTM-treated group showed faster recovery, as evidenced by increased platelets compared to the placebo group. Moreover, the treated group had a significantly lower TNF-α level on day seven than the placebo group. Overall, the treated group had lower hospitalization stays and better recovery [90].

3.3. Glucans

β-Glucan is a dietary fiber and a long-chain polymer of D-glucose, where D-glucose moieties are joined through glycosidic linkages. β-Glucans are a common constituent of the cell walls of several bacteria, algae, and fungi (*Saccharomyces cerevisiae, Aspergillus, Ganoderma applanatum,* and *Inonotus obliquus*), as well as cereals and grains (barley, wheat, oats, and rye) [29,60]. It was found that β-glucan contains various types of glycosidic linkages, β-(1,3)/β-(1,4)/β-(1,6), which vary depending on the source [91]. β-Glucans are a dietary source of soluble fermentable prebiotic fibers that provide a substrate for host microbiota within the large intestine, producing short-chain fatty acids and increasing fecal bulk.

It has been reported that β-glucan improves host immunity by activating the complement system and increasing the cytotoxic activity of macrophages and NK cells. Moreover, the interactions of β-glucan with several cell surface receptors, such as complement receptor 3, dectin-1, and lactosylceramide selected scavenger receptors, also trigger immune functions [92].

In animal models, beta 1,3/1,6 glucan from the mushroom reishi (*Ganoderma lucidum*) improved immunity by inducing the expression of IgA or IgG in serum and small intestinal fluid. Moreover, it also increased the expression of the poly-Ig receptor in the small intestine and promoted NK cell activity [93]. Water-insoluble β-(1→3)-D-glucan extracted from *G. lucidum* displayed potent anti-inflammatory properties in lipopolysaccharide (LPS)-induced Raw 264.7 cells by downregulating iNOS and TNF-α mRNA expression and inhibiting IκBα and JNK1/2 phosphorylation. At the molecular level, the anti-inflammatory activity of β-(1→3)-D-glucan was due to the inhibition of the NF-κB and JNK MAPK pathways, with TLR2 receptors playing a central role [94].

It has been demonstrated that the chemical structure of glucans (α or β) alters the bioactivity of glucans. For instance, β-(1→6), β-(1→3), (1→6), and α-(1→3) glucans were purified from a polysaccharide-enriched extract from *Lentinula edodes* (shiitake mushrooms). However, only the β-(1→6) and β-(1→3), (1→6) fractions displayed antioxidant properties against DPPH free radicals and lowered IL-1β and IL-6 secretion in LPS-stimulated THP-1/M cells, indicating the crucial role played by chemical structure in the biological activity of glucans [95]. In a similar observation, Murphy et al. reported that the extraction process of β-glucans from the same source also creates a difference in immunomodulatory properties. In this study, the "in-house" extract of the edible mushroom (IHL) *Lentinula edodes* was compared with commercially available (Carbosynth-Lentinan, CL) lentinan extract. The CL extract is rich in α-glucans and contains lower concentrations of β-glucans. In human alveolar epithelial A549 cells, both IHL and CL extracts reduced NF-κB activation at lower doses, but the IHL extract was more effective in lowering NF-κB activation. However, the CL extract was more potent in inhibiting the release of proinflammatory cytokines, such as IL-2, TNF-α, IL-22, IL-8, and IL-6, than the IHL extract. These findings demonstrate that β-glucans from the same source can have different immunomodulatory and pulmonary protective properties, which may have implications for treating disorders caused by a cytokine storm in COVID-19 [96].

Gaullier et al. conducted a double-blind, crossover, placebo-controlled study in healthy Caucasian adults to understand the bioactivity of (1–6,1–3)-beta-glucan (lentinan) from *Lentinula edodes*. In this study, adults were either given lentinex (2.5 mg/day) or a placebo for six weeks. After a four-week washout period, alternate supplementation was given for an additional six weeks. The results demonstrated that both groups showed a higher number of NK cells and circulating B cells. However, no difference in the levels of antibodies, cytokines, and complement proteins was observed. Lentinex supplementation was safe and well tolerated by the study participants [97]. Gordon et al. reported that a combination of lentinan and didanosine increased the number of CD4 cells and neutrophil activity in some HIV patients [98].

Cordyceps is a well-known Chinese fungus and possesses powerful immune-boosting properties. An extract from *Cordyceps* mycelium at a dose of 1.68 g/day for eight weeks significantly enhanced the cytotoxic activity of NK-cell activity (38.8 ± 17.6% increase) in healthy human subjects (n = 40) compared to the control group (n = 39) [99]. In another study, the aqueous and alkaline extracts of *Cordyceps militaris* mushrooms containing β-D-Glcp (1→3)-linked polysaccharides were studied for their immunomodulatory properties. The aqueous extracts stimulated the expression of various cytokines (TNF-α, IL-1β, COX-2) in THP-1 macrophages, while the alkaline extract did not elicit any immune response. However, alkaline did show potent anti-inflammatory activity in LPS-stimulated cells by inhibiting proinflammatory genes. Furthermore, the purified β-(1→3)-D-glucan from *C. militaris* was the most potent anti-inflammatory agent under in vivo conditions and reduced the migration of total leucocytes but did not affect neutrophil migration [100]. A clinical study conducted in healthy male adults (n = 39) demonstrated that capsules of *C. militaris* (dose: 1.5 g/day, 4 weeks) significantly enhanced cell-mediated immunity. The treated group displayed higher NK cell activity and lymphocyte proliferation index and induced the secretion of IFN-Y GREEK by Th1 cells compared to the placebo group. Therefore, *C. militaris* effectively enhanced cell-mediated immunity in adults without causing side effects [101].

Lehne et al. reported that oral supplementation with 400 mg/day soluble branched yeast β-1,3-D-glucan derived from the *S. cerevisiae* cell wall for four days significantly increased the salivary concentrations of IgA (65·8 ± 29·4 v/s 105·4 ± 73·9 ug/mL). The 400 mg/day dose was well tolerated, and no adverse events were reported [102]. In a double-blind placebo-controlled trial, oyster mushrooms (*Pleurotus cornucopiae*) containing a β-glucan concentration of 24 mg/meal for eight weeks increased the serum levels of IFN-Y and IL-12, whereas IL-10 and IL-13 did not change considerably. Moreover, the treated group showed increased activity of NK cells. It may help fight infection and cancer due to its immune-boosting properties [103]. Figure 3 presents an overview of the immunomodulatory properties of propolis and β-glucans.

3.4. Melatonin

Melatonin is a multifunctional molecule known as an anti-inflammatory agent, immunoregulator, and antioxidant that might be beneficial and broadly applicable to treat a variety of proinflammatory diseases by inhibiting the immune response and reducing the production of proinflammatory cytokines [104]. It is a hormone that is an indole derivative of serotonin [28,105].

For a long time, melatonin was considered an animal neurohormone, and only at the end of the 20th century were discovered various plant sources of phytomelatonin [106]. The richest sources of melatonin are the seeds of *Coffea arabica* (6800 ng/g) and black pepper (1093 ng/g) [106]. It has been found also in cherries, grapes, pistachio, olives, walnuts, tomatoes, maize, rice, and some medicinal plants (*Curcuma longa*, *Tanacetum parthenium*, *Hypericum perforatum*, etc.).

Previous studies have shown that melatonin, a potent scavenger of reactive oxygen species and a potent inhibitor of myeloperoxidases, inhibits nuclear factor kappa B (NF-κB) signaling pathways, which play an important role in reducing the expression of inflammatory genes, including the signal transducer and activator of transcription expressed in T cells and GATA-binding protein 3, an apoptosis-associated speck-like protein containing the recruitment domain of caspase and caspase-1 [107]. Reviews highlight the important role of melatonin as a potential adjuvant in the treatment of COVID-19 due to its ability to influence mechanisms that alter immune regulation; melatonin has been included as a preventive and therapeutic option against COVID-19 along with vitamin D, vitamin C, zinc, and selenium [108]. These nutrients show synergistic effects and play a central role in maintaining the function and integrity of the immune system, so even a minor deficiency can impair metabolism and immune responses [105,109].

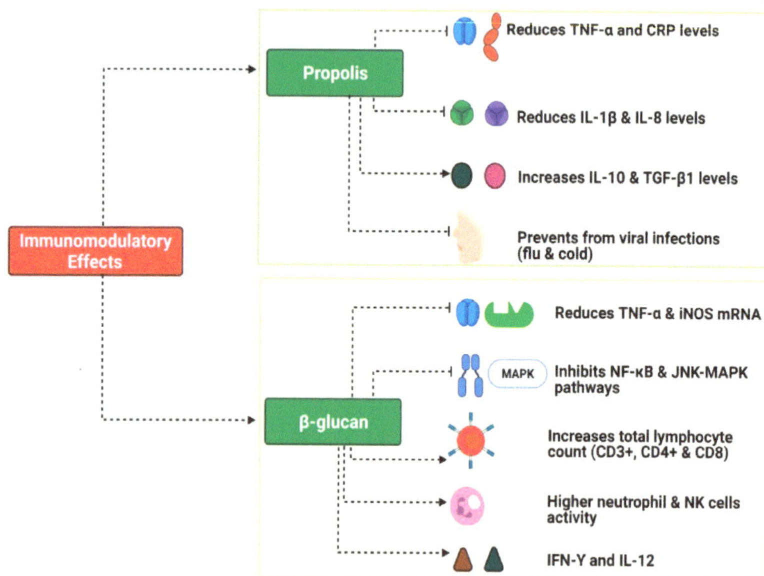

Figure 3. Immunomodulatory activities of propolis and β-glucans.

Melatonin has a regulatory effect on the immune system and directly enhances the immune response by increasing the proliferation and maturation of cells (T and B lymphocytes, granulocytes, and monocytes), enhancing antigen presentation in macrophages. The additional use of melatonin is associated with a significant decrease in the levels of the proinflammatory cytokines TNF-α, IL-1β, and IL-6 [110]. Considering the high effectiveness of oral melatonin as an adjuvant therapy added to standard treatment, the safety, and availability of the drug, it is suggested to conduct additional studies with larger sample sizes and longer observation periods on the use of melatonin for the prevention of complications and the treatment of COVID-19 patients of varying degrees of severity.

Therefore, a lot of in vitro, in vivo, and clinical studies convincingly demonstrate the significant immunomodulatory activities of quercetin and other polyphenols, as well as melatonin, β-glucans, and propolis, which have different resource origins and various mechanisms of immunomodulatory effects.

4. Micronutrients: Vitamins and Minerals

Many micronutrients play a crucial role in augmenting immune function and acting as immune boosters [111]. Some dietary micronutrients have been recognized as key components of the world-famous Mediterranean diet [112]. Each stage of an adequate immune response requires many specific elements, including zinc, selenium, magnesium, and vitamins, which play vital, often synergistic roles. As is known, many vitamins can be obtained from natural sources. For instance, a lot of fresh fruits and vegetables contain high amounts of vitamin C. However, some vitamins have a synthetic origin nowadays.

The daily demand for the consumption of micronutrients for proper functioning may be higher than the recommended dietary allowances [113]. As it was revealed recently, micronutrients are important immunomodulatory tools for COVID-19 management [75].

4.1. Vitamin C

Vitamin C, or ascorbic acid, is well known for its anti-inflammatory properties. It can increase the synthesis of cortisol and vasopressors and absorb free radicals affecting the functioning of leukocytes through the extracellular traps of neutrophils, thus strengthening the arsenal against various pathogens, including viruses and bacteria. However, there is still considerable controversy regarding vitamin C supplementation in various meta-analyses and multiple reviews due to the varied methodologies of the studies and the evaluation of the clinical efficacy of vitamin C use [114]. For example, vitamin C from fresh fruits and vegetables reduces cellular oxidative stress, improves immune functions by enhancing innate and adaptive immune responses, and acts as a cofactor for several enzymatic reactions. Moreover, the accumulation of vitamin C in neutrophils enhances chemotaxis and phagocytosis activity, leading to the killing of bacterial cells. It also promotes the clearance of spent neutrophils from the infection site and prevents tissue damage [24]. The preventive role of vitamin C in the common cold is well documented. Studies have shown that vitamin C supplements (1–2 g/day) reduce the severity of the common cold in children and adults.

Vitamin C concentrations are depleted during viral infections, and vitamin C deficiency is associated with postherpetic neuralgia. In 67 participants suffering from shingles, the intravenous administration of vitamin C (Pascorbin® 7.5 g/50 mL) for two weeks in combination with standard therapy reduced herpes zoster-associated pain and other complaints, indicating the beneficial effects of vitamin C during viral infections [115]. In a randomized clinical trial conducted in 200 patients, supplementation with vitamin C and vitamin E in combination with triple therapy of antibiotics (lansoprazole + amoxicillin + clarithromycin) for 14 days increased the clearance rate of *Helicobacter pylori* by increasing antibiotic effectiveness and augmenting immune functions [116].

Network meta-analysis compared different doses of vitamin C (<6 g/day), high doses of vitamin C (<12, ≥6 g/day), very high doses of vitamin C (≥12 g/day), glucocorticoids (<400 mg/day of hydrocortisone), vitamin B1, and combinations of these drugs with placebo or usual treatment, and discovered that there were no significant differences in early mortality in adults with sepsis or septic shock between treatment and placebo/usual treatment or between treatments and found no evidence that vitamin C affects organ dysfunction or duration of stay in the intensive care unit [117].

4.2. Vitamin D

As it is known, vitamin D can be synthesized in the human skin in the sun and also enter the body thorugh the process of nutrition. The main natural sources of vitamin D are fish oil, cod fish liver, egg yolk, butter, and some fungi [118]. 1,25-Dihydroxyvitamin D, the active form of vitamin D, exerts anti-inflammatory effects through the presence of immune cells, including B and T cells, DCs, and macrophages expressing the vitamin D receptor and 1α-hydroxylase. It was found a significant association between vitamin D deficiency and increased incidence or exacerbation of infectious diseases and inflammatory autoimmune diseases. However, the impact of vitamin D on the treatment and prevention of infectious diseases and the relationship between inflammatory diseases and vitamin D are still controversial [119].

There is increasing evidence that vitamin D is physiologically important for the human host's defense against bacterial and viral infections through vitamin D innate immune signaling mechanisms, including the production of cytokines, antimicrobial proteins, and pattern recognition receptors, and that vitamin D supplementation can combat viral infections, including those caused by SARS-CoV-2, which is supported by increasing clinical evidence of the beneficial effects of vitamin D supplementation in cases of vitamin D deficiency, which is common in most countries in North America and Europe and is particularly common in nursing homes, which are severely affected by the COVID-19 pandemic [120].

Based on recent studies, it is reasonable to avoid vitamin D deficiency in the population to maximize innate and adaptive immunity and prevent adverse cardiovascular outcomes during the COVID-19 pandemic by supplementing with vitamin D at doses recommended by the Endocrine Society to maintain 25-hydroxyvitamin D concentrations in blood serum at a level of at least 30 ng/mL, which can help reduce the risk of SARS-CoV-2 infection and its severe consequences, including mortality [121]. In a study involving 100 participants (50 with COVID-19 and 50 healthy subjects), it was noted that patients with COVID-19 had significantly lower serum 25-hydroxyvitamin D levels than healthy controls [23.10 ± 10.89 vs. 32.06 ± 17.22, $p = 0.0024$]. Additionally, the total numbers of lymphocytes, TCD4+, TCD8+, and NK cells were significantly decreased in patients with COVID-19 ($p < 0.0001$), and IL-12, IFN-γ, and TNF-α were significantly increased in patients with COVID-19 compared to controls. In contrast, IFN-α was reduced in the COVID-19 group; these data suggest a possible relationship between vitamin D concentration, immune system function, and risk of infection with COVID-19 [122].

During the recent COVID-19 outbreak, individuals suffering from vitamin D and selenium deficiency developed acute respiratory tract infections. Vitamin D enhances immunity by stimulating the production of antimicrobial peptides. Furthermore, vitamin D also prevents cytokine storms by reducing the secretion of inflammatory cytokines by immune cells. Selenium, on the other hand, boosts the cytotoxic effects of immune cells [111]. Interestingly, vitamin D receptors and other related enzymes are expressed by both innate and adaptive systems, probably explaining the immunomodulatory properties of vitamin D. Therefore, vitamin D deficiency is often linked with allergies, infections, and autoimmune disorders [123].

A randomized, active-control, double-blind study in HIV patients showed that high-dose vitamin D supplementation (120,000 IU/month) reduced T-cell activation/exhaustion and monocyte activation, preventing abnormal immune activation and immune response in HIV patients, a leading cause of comorbidities in HIV patients [104]. In a clinical trial, sarcopenia patients aged $\geq$65 were given 20 g of whey protein, 3 g of leucine, and 800 IU of vitamin D twice daily for 13 weeks. After the intervention period, IL-6 and IL-1Ra levels increased, but IL-8 levels were reduced. The study concluded that vitamin D and whey protein supplementation may reduce the immune response in sarcopenia patients [124].

Interestingly, vitamin D prevents autoimmunity by preventing the activation of T-regulatory cells. A double-blind, placebo-controlled study in 60 subjects showed that high-dose vitamin D for 12 weeks (140,000 IU/month) significantly increased the numbers of T_{reg} cells without changing the numbers of other immune cells such as monocytes, T and B cells, NK cells, and dendritic cells. The high dose of vitamin D was found to be safe and did not cause any side effects [125].

4.3. Folic Acid

Folic acid is also known as vitamin B9. The important natural sources of this vitamin are peanuts (246 μg/100 g), sunflower seeds (238 μg/100 g), asparagus (149 μg/100 g), lettuce (136 μg/100 g), etc. The nutritional recommendations of the National Institutes of Health (USA) describe that the tolerable upper intake of folic acid levels for adults are regarded as 1000 μg/day [126].

A cellular experiment was designed to evaluate the role of folic acid in the proinflammatory and antiviral molecular pathways of B-lymphocytes infected with a modified live vaccine. It was established that folic acid could modulate the response of B-lymphocytes to improve the molecular pathways of their antiviral and innate immune proinflammatory responses [127]. A study that identified key genes and effective compounds through the analysis of effective compounds and drug targets against COVID-19 showed that folic acid acts on SARS-CoV-2 N through molecular docking and antagonizes the inhibitory effect of the protein on the RNA interference pathway, which is the perspective of the therapeutic use of FC supplements [128]. Importantly, these results were confirmed by the more severe clinical course of COVID-19 and the worse outcomes associated with micronutrient deficiencies, especially low levels of folic acid [129]. However, isolated clinical folic acid deficiency cases are extremely rare; most of the symptoms coincide with cobalamin deficiency; the proliferative effects of folic acid may increase the risk of cancer [130]; it is suggested to follow practical advice on micronutrient provision and monitoring during nutritional support [131]. To conclude, knowledge of the main mechanisms of the interaction between the virus and the host has expanded the use of folic acid supplementation and the opportunities for developing new medications.

4.4. *Magnesium*

Magnesium is an essential micronutrient required for various physiological processes, and there is increasing evidence that it is needed to support the normal functioning of the body's immune system. The main natural dietary sources of magnesium are bananas, nuts, black beans, whole grains, flaxseed, green vegetables, and pumpkin seeds [132]. Hypomagnesemia can lead to various chronic inflammatory diseases [76].

Several studies have shown that magnesium may have a protective role against COVID-19 by reducing lung inflammation [133]. According to the results of this study, magnesium levels were lower in patients with more severe symptoms of COVID-19, and the median magnesium level in patients with severe symptoms of COVID-19 was 38.33 mg/L. In contrast, the median magnesium level in the group with mild symptoms was 39.46 mg/L, giving a p value of 0.002 between the two groups. This study shows that higher magnesium levels may protect against severe symptoms of COVID-19 [134]. Mechanisms include its calcium channel-blocking effects, which lead to inhibition of interleukin-6, CRP, nuclear factor Kβ, and other potentially disruptive factors. In addition, magnesium deficiency is associated with increased IL-6, a proinflammatory cytokine and a likely target for the treatment of COVID-19 [135].

Magnesium contributes to the regulation of the immune response by affecting the cells of the innate and adaptive immune systems. The low magnesium content increases the reactivity to various immune reactions and participates in the pathophysiology of many common chronic diseases; it increases the level of cytokines and the oxidation of granulocytes, stimulates phagocytes, activates endothelial cells, and thus, promotes inflammation [136].

Importantly, altered magnesium homeostasis may contribute to long-term COVID syndrome and exacerbate it after the acute phase; increasing reports describe persistent and long-lasting effects after acute COVID-19 affecting the lungs, heart, brain, and gastrointestinal system, as well as neurological manifestations of magnesium deficiency such as insomnia, anxiety, depression, dizziness, and headache. Hence, assessing and correcting magnesium levels is essential for facilitating recovery [137].

There are many formulations of magnesium, including inorganic (oxide, sulfate, and chloride) and organic (citrate, malate, and taurate) compounds. The doses of administered Mg2+ varied widely among studies (from 100 to 1000 mg/day) [138]. As it was observed by Fiorentini et al. [138], toxic hypermagnesemia occurred if oral magnesium doses were higher than 2500 mg/day. Generally, magnesium was regarded as a safe and cost-effective mineral that could help restore the damaged homeostatic equilibrium of the human body [137].

4.5. *Zinc*

The irreplaceable trace element zinc is of crucial importance for many physiological processes; it plays a significant role in maintaining immune homeostasis by affecting the functional capacity of the cells of the innate and adaptive immune systems and has a regulatory effect on the production of cytokines and antibodies and the activity of the complement system, so the deficiency of this element can contribute to the violation of immune function and thus have a significant impact on health [139]. The richest source of zinc is found in foods obtained from animals, such as seafood, meat, and milk products [140].

Some cereal-based products and vegetables were also regarded as appropriate natural sources of zinc. A meta-analysis and systematic review conducted by Jafari et al. aimed to investigate the effect of zinc supplementation on immune factors in a total of 35 randomized controlled trials with 1995 participants. It was observed a significant decrease in circulating serum CRP (weighted mean difference (WMD): −32.4; 95% confidence interval (CI): from −44.45 to −19.62, $p < 0.001$), high sensitivity C reactive protein concentrations (WMD: −0.95; 95% CI: from −1.01 to −0.89, $p < 0.001$), neutrophil levels (standard mean difference (SMD): −0.46; 95% CI: −0.90 to −0.01, $p = 0.043$), and CD4 levels (WMD: 1.79; 95% CI: 0.57 to 3, $p = 0.004$) after zinc supplementation [141].

A previous study showed that the expression of angiotensin-converting enzyme 2 (ACE2) regulates the signaling of reactive oxygen species and NF-κB in a human lung cell line; zinc supplementation enhances the inhibitory effect and not only destroys the balance of the immune response but also affects the expression of ACE2 receptors, which are necessary for penetration into target cells for ACE2-associated diseases such as COVID-19 and should be considered for treatment. Moreover, zinc has the potential to restore depleted immune cell function or improve normal immune cell function and may also act synergistically when used concurrently with standard antiviral therapy [142].

A meta-analysis of trace element zinc levels in COVID-19 patients and controls, according to severity and nonseverity, as well as nonsurvivors and survivors, using a random-effects model from 11 studies, showed that the overall SMD in zinc levels between patients with COVID-19 and controls was −0.83 (−1.19 to 0.46, $p < 0.05$), indicating that patients with COVID-19 had significantly lower zinc levels. In addition, the difference in zinc levels between severe and nonsevere patients, or survivors and nonsurvivors, was assessed, and severe COVID-19 patients had significantly lower zinc levels than nonsevere COVID-19 patients (SMD: −0.47, 95% CI: −0.75 to −0.18, $p < 0.05$). However, zinc levels in nonsurvivors were not significantly different from those in survivors with COVID-19 (SMD: −1.46, 95% CI: −3.98 to 1.06, $p < 0.05$) [143].

A randomized clinical trial showed that zinc supplementation during severe pneumonia did not improve recovery from respiratory disorders and only showed marginal improvement in the severity of symptoms. The study outcomes do not support using zinc as an adjunct therapy for treating severe pneumonia in zinc-replete children [144]. A randomized controlled trial in children ($n = 512$) aged 6–23 months demonstrated that zinc supplementation (7 mg/day) combined with a multiple micronutrient powder for nine months did not affect cytokine secretion or the number of T cells. However, zinc supplementation altered the numbers of lymphocytes and eosinophils [145]. Daily ingestion of zinc supplements (40 mg/day in adults) was generally considered safe [146].

It was considered zinc as a preventive and adjunctive therapy against COVID-19 for groups at risk of zinc deficiency. In addition, existing zinc deficiency exacerbates inflammatory disease, whereas prophylactic zinc supplementation reduces the severity of the disease or even prevents its development. Research evidence highlights the important role of zinc in immune function, but there are also conflicting results showing that high doses of zinc cause immune dysfunction and related health problems. Regular assessment of zinc status should be performed, and such knowledge should help link existing zinc deficiency to the development and severity of certain diseases [147].

4.6. Selenium

Selenium is a trace element that is found in the body in minimal concentrations but can play an important role in the functioning of the immune system, protecting the body from infections, especially those of viral origin. It takes part in the enzymatic functions of catalyzing glutathione peroxidase, deiodinase, and thioredoxin reductase, serves as an antioxidant, and protects cell membranes and organelles from peroxide destruction [148]. Selenium may be a potential agent for preventing viral infections, including coronavirus, according to the mechanism of enhancing the proliferation of NK cells. T-lymphocytes also have a positive effect in combination with vitamins D and E [149]. Considering that increased oxidative stress and excessive production of inflammatory cytokines are critical components of coronavirus disease, selenium reduces the level of viral infection, reduces oxidative stress and inflammation, strengthens the immune system, and is necessary for critically ill patients. Moreover, selenium deficiency is often associated with the severity and mortality of the disease, providing new insight into the relationship between selenium deficiency and the severity of COVID-19 [150].

The study has shown that selenium deficiency reduced the expression of some antioxidant selenoproteins, thereby additionally inducing the accumulation of reactive oxygen species and oxidative stress, reducing the activity of glutathione peroxidase ($p < 0.05$), thioredoxin reductase, and catalase, as well as the inhibitory capacity for hydroxyl radicals, and increasing ($p < 0.05$) the content of malondialdehyde and nitrogen oxide. Its deficiency increased ($p < 0.05$) NF-κB transcription factor expression and regulated inflammatory cytokines. Se deficiency increased ($p < 0.05$) the expression of IL-6, IL-8, IL-12, IL-17, and cyclooxygenase-2 and decreased ($p < 0.05$) the expression of IL-10, IL-13, and TGF-β, which indicates the regulation of selenoproteins of oxidative stress and inflammation [151].

Research by Fath et al. focused on selenium supplementation, which reduces the ability of SARS-CoV-2 to infect human cells by increasing T cells, especially CD4+ T cells, the percentage of NK cells, and subsequently NK cell cytotoxicity [152]. The main sources of organic selenium are beef/sheep liver, red meats, poultry, eggs, seafood, dairy products, some fungi, brazil nuts, broccoli, and whole grain foods [111]. WHO recommends that the daily intake of selenium by adults should be 40–70 μg/day, depending on body condition and gender (weight, pregnancy in women, etc.) [111]. It should be noted that selenium in doses above 400 μg/day demonstrates harmful actions [149]. Recently, Vahidi et al. [153], during a study of the anticancer properties of selenium, concluded that its nano-formulations could be developed for targeted delivery to tumors and that they would significantly decrease the dosage of selenium to minimize the possible adverse effects.

Considering the research results, selenium supplementation seems promising, so blood levels should be carefully monitored. While taking selenium supplements, it is important to follow the appropriate dosage to minimize potential toxic side effects.

It could be concluded that certain vitamins and minerals play a pivotal role in boosting immune function. A very important aspect of their applications in the last 3 years is that micronutrients are important immunomodulators for COVID-19 management.

5. Probiotics, Prebiotics, Synbiotics, and Immunity

Probiotics are described as live bacteria that, when consumed adequately, confer a health benefit on the host [154]. The first records of ingestion of live bacteria by humans were over 2000 years old. Prebiotics have been defined as nondigestible food ingredients that beneficially affect the host by selectively stimulating the growth and/or activity of one or a limited number of bacterial species already resident in the colon and thus attempt to improve host health [155]. Various molecules can be prebiotics, but most are dietary fibers. They serve as substrates for probiotic commensal bacteria that release short-chain fatty acids in the intestinal tract along with some other metabolites. A synbiotic contains both prebiotics and probiotics, which can stimulate and increase the survival of autochthonous microbiota and probiotic bacteria, particularly lactobacilli and bifidobacteria.

The best-studied and best-characterized probiotics belong to the lactic acid bacteria group, which mainly includes the genera *Lactobacillus*, *Bifidobacterium*, *Leuconostoc*, *Lactococcus*, *Pediococcus*, and *Streptococcus* [156]. *Lactobacillus* strains can enhance the humoral immune response to infections [157] and vaccination [158].

Probiotics impact intestinal microbiota balance, making it benign and promoting the absorption of active substances, improving human physiological functions. Thus, severe dysbiosis due to reducing the concentration of *Lactobacillus* spp., *Bacteroides* spp., etc., in patients with rheumatoid arthritis led to an overgrowth of pathogenic microorganisms [159]. Probiotics promote the digestion and absorption of nutrients and maintain gut microbiota homeostasis. As beneficial natural inhabitants of the human microbiome, probiotics play an important role in producing various nutrients, preventing infectious diseases caused by intestinal pathogens, and modulating the immune response [160]. Probiotics are chosen as alternatives because they act as natural immune enhancers [161]. The mechanisms by which probiotic strains modulate the immune response are not completely known. Probiotics affect innate immunity by preventing bacterial adherence and translocation and improving the mechanisms of pathogen destruction. Prevention of the initial step of tissue colonization by pathogens may improve the treatment of some infectious diseases. For example, *Saccharomyces boulardii* significantly reduces some adverse effects of *Helicobacter pylori* eradication therapy by preventing adherence of this pathogen to the mucous membrane of the stomach [162].

Probiotic strains can produce bacteriocins, contributing to the antimicrobial activity of the gut microbiome [163]. Species from the genus *Lactobacillus* release various bacteriocins that inhibit taxonomically related gram-positive bacteria. Some are active against a much wider range of gram-positive and gram-negative bacteria, yeasts, and molds. Adhesion and invasion of an intestinal epithelial cell line (Intestine 407) by adherent invasive *E. coli* isolated from patients with Crohn's disease (CD) were substantially diminished by co- or pre-incubation with the probiotic strain *E. coli* Nissle 1917 [164]. *E. coli* Nissle is known to secrete microcins to antagonize its competitors [165]. These findings have shown that probiotics avert epithelial injury induced by pathogenic bacteria, contribute to an improved mucosal barrier, and limit enteric pathogen access.

Probiotic bacteria can stimulate enterocytes to produce cytoprotective substances, such as heat shock proteins and antimicrobial peptides, e.g., defensin and mucin. The induction of defensins by probiotics might be an interesting new therapeutic strategy to strengthen innate defense mechanisms. *E. coli* Nissle 1917, *L. fermentum*, *L. acidophilus* PZ 1138, *Pediococcus pentosaceus*, and other probiotics activate the human-beta defensin 2 promoter, inducing the intestinal barrier defense system without provoking inflammation in patients, while the induction of human-beta defensin 2 expression by the pathogenic strains *Salmonella* ssp. and *H. pylori* provokes inflammation [166]. It was investigated and found that flagellin is the major stimulatory factor of *E. coli* Nissle 1917 [164].

Probiotics can downregulate the expression of proinflammatory cytokines and ameliorate intestinal inflammatory diseases. They can suppress the nuclear NF-κB signaling pathway [167], possibly related to alterations in mitogen-activated protein kinases and pattern recognition receptor pathways. Probiotics can also inhibit the binding of LPS to the CD14 receptor, reducing the overall activation of NF-κβ and produce proinflammatory cytokines [168]. Kim et al. showed that conjugated linoleic acids produced by probiotics interact with IkB kinase and heat shock protein 90 to activate the NF-kB signaling pathway in human gastric epithelial cells infected with *H. pylori* [169]. Lv et al. have shown that probiotics generally cannot eliminate *H. pylori*, although they decrease the density of colonization, thereby maintaining lower levels of *H. pylori* in the stomach [170].

Regarding the adaptive immune response, numerous studies have shown that probiotic impacts seem to be variable. Many probiotic strains seem capable of stimulating IgA production by B cells. In children with viral gastroenteritis caused by rotavirus, probiotics such as *L. rhamnosus* have been shown to stimulate rotavirus-specific IgA antibody responses. A stronger significant inverse correlation was observed between small intestinal HRV IgA titres and mean fecal scores in Vac + Pro piglets compared with vaccinated probiotic-colonized piglets [171]. Thus, reinfections can be partly prevented by probiotic intestinal cell-mediated responses. *Pediococcus acidilactici* K15, as well as LAB, was found to be the most effective in inducing IgAs, which are mainly induced via IL-10, as well as IL-6, secreted by K15-stimulated dendritic cells. In a clinical trial, an increase in salivary sIgA concentration by K15 ingestion was confirmed [172]. The health benefits ascribed to one strain of probiotic may not be obligatory when applied to another strain [173]. Díaz-Ropero et al. showed that the consumption of *L. fermentum* CECT5716 enhanced the production of Th1 cytokines by spleen cells and increased the IgA concentration in feces. Therefore, this probiotic has an immunostimulatory effect. However, the consumption of *L. salivarius*

CECT 5713 induced IL-10 production by spleen cells, demonstrating the anti-inflammatory effect [174].

The potential of probiotics to boost health benefits has been reported, as they can regulate allergic reactions, alleviate inflammatory bowel disease, reduce tumor growth in some cancer models, prevent colon cancer, control the levels of blood cholesterol, and protect hosts from bacterial and viral infections [175]. The prominent probiotic *Escherichia coli* NISSLE 1917 is used in the treatment of intestinal diseases such as diarrhea and inflammatory bowel disease because it has high adhesive properties and demonstrates immunomodulation and anti-inflammation abilities [176]. The effects of *Bifidobacterium infantis* supplementation in an inflammatory bowel disease mouse model demonstrated relief of intestinal epithelial injury and increased production of cytokines, such as transforming TGF-β1, IL-10, and IL-35, which play an immunosuppressive role in maintaining the body's immune tolerance [177]. The research of Xiao Joe et al. using principal component analysis and cluster analysis heatmaps showed that the novel candidate probiotic mixture is effective against the nervous necrosis virus as a consequence of stimulation of innate and adaptive immunity [178]. Probiotics from the *Bifidobacterium* and *Lactobacillus* genera have exhibited feasible antiviral activities against rotavirus [179] and enterovirus [180]. Randomized controlled trials found that supplementation with probiotics or prebiotics as adjuvant therapy for COVID-19 might positively affect the outcome of COVID-19, and improvements in fatigue, anosmia, breathlessness, nausea, vomiting, and other gastrointestinal symptoms were reported [181,182]. The administration of probiotics in the diet of patients with gastrointestinal symptoms related to COVID-19 and those with mild-to-moderate systemic symptoms can be an alternative for preventing cytokine storms [182].

Prebiotics can induce a microbiota-independent effect by directly acting on gut-associated epithelial and innate immune cells through Toll-like receptors. Studies in the animal model showed that the prebiotics inulin/oligofructose primarily activated immune cells in Peyer's patches, including IL-10 production and NK cell cytotoxicity. They modulated the concentration of secretory IgA in the ileum and caecum [183]. Intestinal DCs are located within gut-associated lymphoid tissue and express pattern recognition receptors such as TLR-2 and TLR-4. Prebiotics or their fermentation byproducts can bind to these receptors and trigger the maturation process involving upregulation or downregulation of membrane CD83, CD86, HLA-DR, and DC-SIGN molecules and induce the secretion of cytokines. The activation of DCs through particular pattern recognition and immunity receptors defines the polarization of effector T cells to either the T-helper 1 (Th1), Th2, Th17, or Treg phenotype [184]. Some authors showed that butyrate, acetate, and soybean oligosaccharides could enhance the activity of NK cells in comparison with the control group [185,186]. The symbiotic combination of enriched inulin with probiotics such as *Lactobacillus rhamnosus* GG and *Bifidobacterium lactis* Bb12 enhanced NK cell activity in the blood [185]. Studies in poultry flocks indicated that the probiotic strain *Enterococcus faecium* combined with prebiotics inulin and fructooligosaccharides might inhibit pathogen proliferation, insomuch as significantly extending the lag time for pathogenic *E. coli* O1/O18 and *Salmonella enterica* serotype *Enteritidis* strains [187].

The global nutraceutical market, including the probiotics market, is one of the fastest-growing segments of the food industry. Widespread use of probiotic products due to growing reports about the health demands to estimate their bioavailability, safety, and side effects. The European Food Safety Authority has developed guidelines for the safety assessment of probiotics as a food additive (FEEDAP, 2014). Currently, probiotic products have been commercially regulated in three forms: functional foods (fermented foods), dietary supplements, and drugs (pharmaceuticals) [188]. Probiotics are a priori nonpathogenic; therefore, they are never supposed to cause or potentiate any disease in humans. The safety of medicinal probiotics is still being discussed. The safety of probiotics was confirmed as apparent due to the absence of toxicity by randomized trials in different target populations, conditions, and age groups in a specific clinical scenario [189–193].

Probiotics are categorized in accordance with the site of action (the oral, upper respiratory, or gastrointestinal tract). As it is known, the dosage form must be in adequate amounts to confer a health benefit. The dose of a drug is indirectly proportional to its bioavailability. The viability of probiotic bacteria is a requirement to meet the definition of a probiotic. It is questionable when probiotics are exposed to harsh environments during processing (i.e., dehydration), storage, and delivery to their site of action. Their efficacy is dependent upon delivering an adequate dose throughout the product's shelf life. The World Health Organization (WHO) and the Food and Agriculture Organization (FAO) reported that the viability of probiotics in food products should be counted at least at 106 colony-forming units /g alive microbial cells [194–197]. According to the majority of human clinical studies, probiotic dosages typically range between 107 and 1011 colony-forming units /day. The appropriate dose, duration, and composition of a synbiotic needed to confer a health benefit are likely to be specific to outcome and baseline host target site microbiota, as well as coexisting environmental factors such as medication, habitual diet, and host genetic factors [198].

Despite the tremendously beneficial effects of probiotics and prebiotics on health, the WHO and FAO reported [199] that they might have some side effects, and safety issues may arise due to the use of living microbial cells [200]. The topic of probiotic safety is still being discussed [201,202]. Evidence from clinical trials is mixed and controversial [194]. The long-term colonizing probiotics have potential risks, such as that the probiotic could displace a microbe performing an important function; negatively impact the structure and function of the surrounding microbiota; and if the normal gut barrier is breached, the probiotic could access the systemic circulation, resulting in invasive infection [203]. Suez J. and colleagues [204] found that resident gut bacteria in a subset of individuals resist the mucosal presence of probiotic strains, limiting their modulatory effect on the microbiome. Evidence of probiotic gut mucosal colonization efficacy remains sparse. The elicited cytokine production via probiotic supplementation might cause inordinate immunological effects. Theoretically, probiotic administration might lead to auto-immune disease development or certain inflammations [205]. Building a strong safety profile for probiotic strains will solidify their use in individuals that can benefit the most from microbial modulation.

As could be seen from the results of the experimental and clinical studies described above, a lot of probiotics, prebiotics, and synbiotics are very useful for improving immune function. When probiotics are mainly alive, useful bacteria, prebiotics are regarded as dietary polysaccharides or oligosaccharides of plants. A symbiotic relationship contains both of these groups and can increase the survival of autochthonous microbiota and probiotic bacteria (mainly lactobacilli and bifidobacteria).

6. Conclusions

The body's immune system fights against a huge number of pathogens and antigens and plays a central role in our survival. Therefore, enhancing the immune system's ability is highly beneficial in preventing many health disorders. Some medicinal plants and different natural ingredients have been effectively used to augment immunity and prevent infections since ancient times. In today's era, there have been a lot of experimental and clinical studies demonstrating that some natural ingredients from plants, fungi, animals, and microorganisms can directly modulate multiple signaling pathways, alter gene expression, and change the secretion of pro- and anti-inflammatory cytokines. Moreover, these bioactive natural ingredients increase the activity of numerous immune cells, including neutrophils, basophils, mast cells, macrophages, NK cells, and lymphocytes, thereby increasing immune functions.

The present review is an attempt to explore the health-promoting effects of certain natural ingredients from medicinal plants and different dietary sources. Some of these natural ingredients have been used by humankind since time immemorial. Nowadays, a lot of preclinical and clinical studies have also found that many of these traditional sources as well as some comparatively recently discovered health-promoting agents (vitamins, minerals, polyphenols, terpenoids, polysaccharides, melatonin, pre- and probiotics) are efficacious in boosting immunity and safe to consume. However, there is a lack of clinical trials for some of the natural ingredients covered in the present review. Hence, future research must be directed toward finding their efficacy, an appropriate dose range, and dosage forms, as well as mechanisms of action, for further promoting their use as immunity-enhancing agents.

Author Contributions: Conceptualization, A.G. and G.B.; methodology, M.S.; software, O.O.; validation, Y.S., P.K.M. and Y.I.; formal analysis, O.P.; investigation, S.N.; resources, S.P.; data curation, S.A.; writing—original draft preparation, A.G.; writing—review and editing, G.B.; visualization, M.S.; supervision, O.O.; project administration, Y.S.; funding acquisition, G.B. and M.S. All authors have read and agreed to the published version of the manuscript.

Funding: This research received no external funding.

Institutional Review Board Statement: Not applicable.

Informed Consent Statement: Not applicable.

Data Availability Statement: Data sharing not applicable.

Conflicts of Interest: The authors declare no conflict of interest.

References

1. Catanzaro, M.; Corsini, E.; Rosini, M.; Racchi, M.; Lanni, C. Immunomodulators Inspired by Nature: A Review on Curcumin and Echinacea. *Molecules* **2018**, *23*, 2778. [CrossRef] [PubMed]
2. Parkin, J.; Cohen, B. An overview of the immune system. *Lancet* **2001**, *357*, 1777–1789. [CrossRef] [PubMed]
3. Raducanu, A.E.; Tihauan, B.M.; Marinas, I.C.; Ciuperca, O.T.; Tebrencu, C.E.; Ionescu, E.; Onisei, T. The Biological Effects of Novel Nutraceuticals with Curcuminoids and Other Plant-Derived Immunomodulators and Pre-Probiotics. *Pharmaceutics* **2021**, *13*, 666. [CrossRef]
4. Tieu, S.; Charchoglyan, A.; Wagter-Lesperance, L.; Karimi, K.; Bridle, B.; Karrow, N.; Mallard, B. Immunoceuticals: Harnessing Their Immunomodulatory Potential to Promote Health and Wellness. *Nutrients* **2022**, *14*, 4075. [CrossRef] [PubMed]
5. Marshall, J.S.; Warrington, R.; Watson, W.; Kim, H.L. An introduction to immunology and immunopathology. *Allergy Asthma Clin. Immunol.* **2018**, *14* (Suppl. S2), 49. [CrossRef]
6. Sultan, M.; Buttxs, M.; Qayyum, M.; Suleria, H. Immunity: Plants as Effective Mediators. *Crit. Rev. Food Sci. Nutr.* **2014**, *54*, 1298–1308. [CrossRef]
7. Vishwakarma, S.; Panigrahi, C.; Barua, S.; Sahoo, M.; Mandliya, S. Food nutrients as inherent sources of immunomodulation during COVID-19 pandemic. *Lebensm.-Wiss. Und-Technol.* **2022**, *158*, 113154. [CrossRef]
8. Wieczorek, P.P.; Hudz, N.; Yezerska, O.; Horcinova-Sedlackova, V.; Shanaida, M.; Korytniuk, O.; Jasicka-Misiak, I. Chemical Variability and Pharmacological Potential of Propolis as a Source for the Development of New Pharmaceutical Products. *Molecules* **2022**, *27*, 1600. [CrossRef]
9. Ilina, T.; Kashpur, N.; Granica, S.; Bazylko, A.; Shinkovenko, I.; Kovalyova, A.; Goryacha, O.; Koshovyi, O. Phytochemical Profiles and In Vitro Immunomodulatory Activity of Ethanolic Extracts from *Galium aparine* L. *Plants* **2019**, *8*, 541. [CrossRef]
10. Mahima; Rahal, A.; Deb, R.; Latheef, S.K.; Abdul Samad, H.; Tiwari, R.; Verma, A.K.; Kumar, A.; Dhama, K. Immunomodulatory and therapeutic potentials of herbal, traditional/indigenous and ethnoveterinary medicines. *Pak. J. Biol. Sci.* **2012**, *15*, 754–774.
11. Hassoun, A.; Harastani, R.; Jagtap, S.; Trollman, H.; Garcia-Garcia, G.; Awad, N.; Zannou, O.; Galanakis, C.; Gökşen, G.; Nayik, G.; et al. Truths and myths about superfoods in the era of the COVID-19 pandemic. *Crit. Rev. Food Sci. Nutr.* **2022**, 1–18. [CrossRef] [PubMed]
12. Khanna, K.; Kohli, S.K.; Kaur, R.; Bhardwaj, A.; Bhardwaj, V.; Ohri, P.; Sharma, A.; Ahmad, A.; Bhardwaj, R.; Ahmad, P. Herbal immune-boosters: Substantial warriors of pandemic COVID-19 battle. *Phytomedicine* **2021**, *85*, 153361. [CrossRef] [PubMed]
13. Prajapati, S.K.; Malaiya, A.; Mishra, G.; Jain, D.; Kesharwani, P.; Mody, N.; Ahmadi, A.; Paliwal, R.; Jain, A. An exhaustive comprehension of the role of herbal medicines in Pre- and Post-COVID manifestations. *J. Ethnopharmacol.* **2022**, *296*, 115420. [CrossRef]
14. Rondanelli, M.; Miccono, A.; Lamburghini, S.; Avanzato, I.; Riva, A.; Allegrini, P.; Faliva, M.; Peroni, G.; Nichetti, M.; Perna, S. Self-Care for Common Colds: The Pivotal Role of Vitamin D, Vitamin C, Zinc, and *Echinacea* in Three Main Immune Interactive Clusters (Physical Barriers, Innate and Adaptive Immunity) Involved during an Episode of Common Colds—Practical Advice on Dosages and on the Time to Take These Nutrients/Botanicals in order to Prevent or Treat Common Colds. *Evid.-Based Complement. Altern. Med.* **2018**, *2018*, 5813095.
15. Nantz, M.; Rowe, C.; Muller, C.; Creasy, R.; Stanilka, J.; Percival, S. Supplementation with aged garlic extract improves both NK and γδ-T cell function and reduces the severity of cold and flu symptoms: A randomized, double-blind, placebo-controlled nutrition intervention. *Clin. Nutr.* **2012**, *31*, 337–344. [CrossRef]

16. de Oliveira, C.A.F.; Vetvicka, V.; Zanuzzo, F.S. Beta-Glucan successfully stimulated the immune system in different jawed vertebrate species. *Comp. Immunol. Microbiol. Infect. Dis.* **2019**, *62*, 1–6. [CrossRef] [PubMed]
17. Arshad, M.S.; Khan, U.; Sadiq, A.; Khalid, W.; Hussain, M.; Yasmeen, A.; Asghar, Z.; Rehana, H. Coronavirus disease (COVID-19) and immunity booster green foods: A mini review. *Food Sci. Nutr.* **2020**, *8*, 3971–3976. [CrossRef] [PubMed]
18. Burkard, M.; Leischner, C.; Lauer, U.M.; Busch, C.; Venturelli, S.; Frank, J. Dietary flavonoids and modulation of natural killer cells: Implications in malignant and viral diseases. *J. Nutr. Biochem.* **2017**, *46*, 1–12. [CrossRef]
19. Gasmi, A.; Mujawdiya, P.K.; Noor, S.; Lysiuk, R.; Darmohray, R.; Piscopo, S.; Lenchyk, L.; Antonyak, H.; Dehtiarova, K.; Shanaida, M.; et al. Polyphenols in Metabolic Diseases. *Molecules* **2022**, *27*, 6280. [CrossRef]
20. Huang, R.Y.; Yu, Y.L.; Cheng, W.C.; OuYang, C.N.; Fu, E.; Chu, C.L. Immunosuppressive effect of quercetin on dendritic cell activation and function. *J. Immunol.* **2010**, *184*, 6815–6821. [CrossRef]
21. Chaudhary, P.; Sharma, R.; Rawat, S.; Janmeda, P. Antipyretic Medicinal Plants, Phytocompounds, and Green Nanoparticles: An Updated Review. *Curr. Pharm. Biotechnol.* **2023**, *24*, 23–49. [PubMed]
22. Quispe, C.; Cruz-Martins, N.; Manca, M.L.; Manconi, M.; Sytar, O.; Hudz, N.; Shanaida, M.; Kumar, M.; Taheri, Y.; Martorell, M.; et al. Nano-Derived Therapeutic Formulations with Curcumin in Inflammation-Related Diseases. *Oxid Med. Cell Longev.* **2021**, *2021*, 3149223. [CrossRef] [PubMed]
23. Yücel, Ç.; Şeker Karatoprak, G.; Bahadir, O.; Akkol, E.; Barak, T.H.; Sobarzo-SÁNchez, E.; Aschner, M.; Shirooie, S. Immunomodulatory and anti-inflammatory therapeutic potential of gingerols and their nanoformulations. *Front. Pharmacol.* **2022**, *13*. [CrossRef]
24. Carr, A.C.; Maggini, S. Vitamin C and Immune Function. *Nutrients* **2017**, *9*, 1211. [CrossRef] [PubMed]
25. Ota, K.; Dambaeva, S.; Kim, M.W.; Han, A.R.; Fukui, A.; Gilman-Sachs, A.; Beaman, K.; Kwak-Kim, J. 1,25-Dihydroxy-vitamin D3 regulates NK-cell cytotoxicity, cytokine secretion, and degranulation in women with recurrent pregnancy losses. *Eur. J. Immunol.* **2015**, *45*, 3188–3199. [CrossRef]
26. Mitra, S.; Paul, S.; Roy, S.; Sutradhar, H.; Emran, T.; Nainu, F.; Khandaker, M.; Almalki, M.; Wilairatana, P.; Mubarak, M. Exploring the Immune-Boosting Functions of Vitamins and Minerals as Nutritional Food Bioactive Compounds: A Comprehensive Review. *Molecules* **2022**, *27*, 555. [CrossRef]
27. Wagh, V.D. Propolis: A wonder bees product and its pharmacological potentials. *Adv. Pharmacol. Sci.* **2013**, *2013*, 308249. [CrossRef]
28. Oleshchuk, O.; Ivankiv, Y.; Falfushynska, H.; Mudra, A.; Lisnychuk, N. Hepatoprotective Effect of Melatonin in Toxic Liver Injury in Rats. *Medicina* **2019**, *55*, 304. [CrossRef]
29. Ivankiv, Y.; Oleshchuk, O. Immunomodulatory effect of melatonin supplementation in experimental diabetes. *Pharmacia* **2020**, *67*, 223–228. [CrossRef]
30. Yates, C.R.; Bruno, E.J.; Yates, M.E.D. Tinospora Cordifolia: A review of its immunomodulatory properties. *J. Diet. Suppl.* **2022**, *19*, 271–285. [CrossRef]
31. Ahmed, H.; Babakir-Mina, M. Investigation of rosemary herbal extracts (Rosmarinus officinalis) and their potential effects on immunity. *Phytother. Res.* **2020**, *34*, 1829–1837. [CrossRef] [PubMed]
32. Miles, E.; Calder, P. Effects of Citrus Fruit Juices and Their Bioactive Components on Inflammation and Immunity: A Narrative Review. *Front. Immunol.* **2021**, *12*, 712608. [CrossRef]
33. Shanaida, M.; Pryshlyak, A.; Golembiovska, O. Determination of triterpenoids in some Lamiaceae species. *Res. J. Pharm. Technol.* **2018**, *7*, 3113–3118. [CrossRef]
34. Al-Ataby, I.A.; Talib, W.H. Daily Consumption of Lemon and Ginger Herbal Infusion Caused Tumor Regression and Activation of the Immune System in a Mouse Model of Breast Cancer. *Front. Nutr.* **2022**, *9*, 829101. [CrossRef]
35. Aryaeian, N.; Shahram, F.; Mahmoudi, M.; Tavakoli, H.; Yousefi, B.; Arablou, T. The effect of ginger supplementation on some immunity and inflammation intermediate genes expression in patients with active Rheumatoid Arthritis. *Gene* **2019**, *698*, 179–185. [CrossRef] [PubMed]
36. Bałan, B.; Sokolnicka, I.; Skopińska-Różewska, E.; Skopiński, P. The modulatory influence of some *Echinacea*-based remedies on antibody production and cellular immunity in mice. *Cent.-Eur. J. Immunol.* **2016**, *41*, 12–18. [CrossRef] [PubMed]
37. Ilina, T.; Skowronska, W.; Kashpur, N.; Granica, S.; Bazylko, A.; Kovalyova, A.; Goryacha, O.; Koshovyi, O. Immunomodulatory Activity and Phytochemical Profile of Infusions from Cleavers Herb. *Molecules* **2020**, *25*, 3721. [CrossRef] [PubMed]
38. Mykhailenko, O.; Lesyk, R.; Finiuk, N.; Rostyslav, S.; Tetyana, Y.; Anna, O.; Valentina, V.; Volodymyr, M.; Georgiyants, V. In vitro anticancer activity screening of Iridaceae plant extracts. *J. Appl. Pharm. Sci.* **2020**, *10*, 59–63.
39. Williamson, E.M. Synergy and other interactions in phytomedicines. *Phytomedicine* **2001**, *8*, 401–409. [CrossRef]
40. Thomford, N.E.; Senthebane, D.A.; Rowe, A.; Munro, D.; Seele, P.; Maroyi, A.; Dzobo, K. Natural Products for Drug Discovery in the 21st Century: Innovations for Novel Drug Discovery. *Int. J. Mol. Sci.* **2018**, *19*, 1578. [CrossRef]
41. Harvey, A.L.; Edrada-Ebel, R.; Quinn, R.J. The re-emergence of natural products for drug discovery in the genomics era. *Nat. Rev. Drug. Discov.* **2015**, *14*, 111–129. [CrossRef] [PubMed]
42. Boozari, M.; Hosseinzadeh, H. Natural products for COVID-19 prevention and treatment regarding to previous coronavirus infections and novel studies. *Phytother. Res.* **2020**, *35*, 864–876. [CrossRef] [PubMed]

43. Shree, P.; Mishra, P.; Selvaraj, C.; Singh, S.K.; Chaube, R.; Garg, N.; Tripathi, Y.B. Targeting COVID-19 (SARS-CoV-2) main protease through active phytochemicals of ayurvedic medicinal plants—Withania somnifera (Ashwagandha), Tinospora cordifolia (Giloy) and Ocimum sanctum (Tulsi)—A molecular docking study. *J. Biomol. Struct. Dyn.* **2022**, *40*, 190–203. [CrossRef] [PubMed]
44. Francis, T.; Sooriyaarachchi, P.; Jayawardena, R. Usage of nutritional supplements to improve immunity during the COVID-19 pandemic: An online survey. *Clin. Nutr. Open Sci.* **2022**, *43*, 6–19. [CrossRef]
45. Al Kury, L.T.; Taha, Z.; Mahmod, A.I.; Talib, W.H. Xanthium spinosum L. Extracts Inhibit Breast Cancer in Mice by Apoptosis Induction and Immune System Modulation. *Pharmaceuticals* **2022**, *15*, 1504. [CrossRef]
46. Drenkhan, R.; Kaldmäe, H.; Silm, M.; Adamson, K.; Bleive, U.; Aluvee, A.; Erik, M.; Raal, A. Comparative Analyses of Bioactive Compounds in Inonotus obliquus Conks Growing on Alnus and Betula. *Biomolecules* **2022**, *12*, 1178. [CrossRef]
47. Rios, J.L. Effects of triterpenes on the immune system. *J. Ethnopharmacol.* **2010**, *128*, 1–14. [CrossRef]
48. Venter, C.; Eyerich, S.; Sarin, T.; Klatt, K.C. Nutrition and the Immune System: A Complicated Tango. *Nutrients* **2020**, *12*, 818. [CrossRef]
49. Mangla, B.; Javed, S.; Sultan, M.H.; Kumar, P.; Kohli, K.; Najmi, A.; Alhazmi, H.A.; Al Bratty, M.; Ahsan, W. Sulforaphane: A review of its therapeutic potentials, advances in its nanodelivery, recent patents, and clinical trials. *Phytother. Res.* **2021**, *35*, 5440–5458. [CrossRef]
50. Barrett, B. Medicinal properties of *Echinacea*: A critical review. *Phytomedicine* **2003**, *10*, 66–86. [CrossRef]
51. Chicca, A.; Raduner, S.; Pellati, F.; Strompen, T.; Altmann, K.H.; Schoop, R.; Gertsch, J. Synergistic immunomopharmacological effects of N-alkylamides in *Echinacea purpurea* herbal extracts. *Int. Immunopharmacol.* **2009**, *9*, 850–858. [CrossRef]
52. Luettig, B.; Steinmuller, C.; Gifford, G.E.; Wagner, H.; Lohmann-Matthes, M.L. Macrophage activation by the polysaccharide arabinogalactan isolated from plant cell cultures of *Echinacea purpurea*. *J. Natl. Cancer Inst.* **1989**, *81*, 669–675. [CrossRef]
53. Fonseca, F.; Papanicolaou, G.; Lin, H.; Lau, C.; Kennelly, E.; Cassileth, B.; Cunningham-Rundles, S. *Echinacea purpurea* (L.) Moench modulates human T-cell cytokine response. *Int. Immunopharmacol.* **2014**, *19*, 94–102. [CrossRef]
54. Signer, J.; Jonsdottir, H.R.; Albrich, W.C.; Strasser, M.; Zust, R.; Ryter, S.; Ackermann-Gaumann, R.; Lenz, N.; Siegrist, D.; Suter, A.; et al. Author Correction: In vitro virucidal activity of Echinaforce®, an *Echinacea purpurea* preparation, against coronaviruses, including common cold coronavirus 229E and SARS-CoV-2. *Virol. J.* **2020**, *17*, 172. [CrossRef]
55. Vimalanathan, S.; Shehata, M.; Sadasivam, K.; Delbue, S.; Dolci, M.; Pariani, E.; D'Alessandro, S.; Pleschka, S. Broad Antiviral Effects of *Echinacea purpurea* against SARS-CoV-2 Variants of Concern and Potential Mechanism of Action. *Microorganisms* **2022**, *10*, 2145. [CrossRef] [PubMed]
56. Kolev, E.; Mircheva, L.; Edwards, M.R.; Johnston, S.L.; Kalinov, K.; Stange, R.; Gancitano, G.; Berghe, W.V.; Kreft, S. *Echinacea Purpurea* For the Long-Term Prevention of Viral Respiratory Tract Infections During COVID-19 Pandemic: A Randomized, Open, Controlled, Exploratory Clinical Study. *Front. Pharmacol.* **2022**, *13*, 856410. [CrossRef]
57. Fuzimoto, A.D. An overview of the anti-SARS-CoV-2 properties of *Artemisia annua*, its antiviral action, protein-associated mechanisms, and repurposing for COVID-19 treatment. *J. Integr. Med.* **2021**, *19*, 375–388. [CrossRef] [PubMed]
58. Liu, N.Q.; van der Kooy, F.; Verpoorte, R. Artemisia afra: A potential flagship for African medicinal plants? *S. Afr. J. Bot.* **2009**, *75*, 185–195. [CrossRef]
59. Ncube, T.; Muyima, N. Comparative evaluation of the antimicrobial activities of essential oils of Artemisia afra, Pteronia incana and Rosmarinus officinalis on selected Bacteria and yeast strains. *Lett. Appl. Microbiol.* **1999**, *28*, 291–296.
60. More, G.; Lall, N.; Hussein, A.; Tshikalange, T.E. Antimicrobial Constituents of Artemisia afra Jacq. ex Willd. against Periodontal Pathogens. *Evid.-Based Complement. Altern. Med.* **2012**, *2012*, 252758. [CrossRef]
61. Appalasamy, S.; Lo, K.Y.; Ch'ng, S.J.; Nornadia, K.; Othman, A.S.; Chan, L.K. Antimicrobial activity of artemisinin and precursor derived from in vitro plantlets of *Artemisia annua* L. *Biomed. Res. Int.* **2014**, *2014*, 215872. [CrossRef]
62. Hunt, S.; Yoshida, M.; Davis, C.E.; Greenhill, N.S.; Davis, P.F. An extract of the medicinal plant *Artemisia annua* modulates production of inflammatory markers in activated neutrophils. *J. Inflamm. Res.* **2015**, *8*, 9–14. [CrossRef] [PubMed]
63. Ruperti Repilado, F.J.; Haefliger, S.; Rehm, S.; Zweier, M.; Rentsch, K.; Blum, J.; Jetter, A.; Heim, M.; Leuppi-Taegtmeyer, A.; Terracciano, L.; et al. Danger of Herbal Tea: A Case of Acute Cholestatic Hepatitis Due to *Artemisia annua* Tea. *Front. Med.* **2019**, *6*, 221. [CrossRef] [PubMed]
64. du Toit, A.; van der Kooy, F. Artemisia afra, a controversial herbal remedy or a treasure trove of new drugs? *J. Ethnopharmacol.* **2019**, *244*, 112127. [CrossRef] [PubMed]
65. Ratan, Z.A.; Youn, S.H.; Kwak, Y.S.; Han, C.K.; Haidere, M.F.; Kim, J.K.; Min, H.; Jung, Y.J.; Hosseinzadeh, H.; Hyun, S.H.; et al. Adaptogenic effects of Panax ginseng on modulation of immune functions. *J. Ginseng. Res.* **2021**, *45*, 32–40. [CrossRef] [PubMed]
66. Kim, B.G.; Shin, K.S.; Yoon, T.J.; Yu, K.W.; Ra, K.S.; Kim, J.M.; Kim, S.Y.; Suh, H.J. Fermentation of Korean red ginseng by Lactobacillus plantarum M-2 and its immunological activities. *Appl. Biochem. Biotechnol.* **2011**, *165*, 1107–1119. [CrossRef]
67. Ma, J.; Liu, H.; Wang, X. Effect of ginseng polysaccharides and dendritic cells on the balance of Th1/Th2 T helper cells in patients with non-small cell lung cancer. *J. Tradit. Chin. Med.* **2014**, *34*, 641–645. [CrossRef] [PubMed]
68. Cho, Y.J.; Son, H.J.; Kim, K.S. A 14-week randomized, placebo-controlled, double-blind clinical trial to evaluate the efficacy and safety of ginseng polysaccharide (Y-75). *J. Transl. Med.* **2014**, *12*, 283. [CrossRef]
69. Sun, Y.; Guo, M.; Feng, Y.; Zheng, H.; Lei, P.; Ma, X.; Han, X.; Guan, H.; Hou, D. Effect of ginseng polysaccharides on NK cell cytotoxicity in immunosuppressed mice. *Exp. Ther. Med.* **2016**, *12*, 3773–3777. [CrossRef]

70. Karimi, N.; Dabidi Roshan, V.; Bayatiyani, Z. Individually and Combined Water-Based Exercise with Ginger Supplement, on Systemic Inflammation and Metabolic Syndrome Indices, Among the Obese Women with Breast Neoplasms. *Iran. J. Cancer Prev.* **2015**, *8*, e3856. [CrossRef]
71. Khatoon, S.; Kalam, N.; Balasubramaniam, V.R.; Shaikh, M.F.; Ansari, M.T. Chemotherapeutic Role of Polyphenols Present in Ocimum sanctum. *Anticancer Agents Med. Chem.* **2022**, *22*, 3325–3342. [PubMed]
72. Arreola, R.; Quintero-Fabian, S.; Lopez-Roa, R.I.; Flores-Gutierrez, E.O.; Reyes-Grajeda, J.P.; Carrera-Quintanar, L.; Ortuno-Sahagun, D. Immunomodulation and anti-inflammatory effects of garlic compounds. *J. Immunol. Res* **2015**, *2015*, 401630. [CrossRef] [PubMed]
73. Feng, Y.; Zhu, X.; Wang, Q.; Jiang, Y.; Shang, H.; Cui, L.; Cao, Y. Allicin enhances host pro-inflammatory immune responses and protects against acute murine malaria infection. *Malar. J.* **2012**, *11*, 268. [CrossRef] [PubMed]
74. Poles, J.; Karhu, E.; McGill, M.; McDaniel, H.R.; Lewis, J.E. The effects of twenty-four nutrients and phytonutrients on immune system function and inflammation: A narrative review. *J. Clin. Transl. Res.* **2021**, *7*, 333–376. [PubMed]
75. Gasmi, A.; Mujawdiya, P.K.; Lysiuk, R.; Shanaida, M.; Peana, M.; Gasmi Benahmed, A.; Beley, N.; Kovalska, N.; Bjorklund, G. Quercetin in the Prevention and Treatment of Coronavirus Infections: A Focus on SARS-CoV-2. *Pharmaceuticals* **2022**, *15*, 1049. [CrossRef]
76. Shakoor, H.; Feehan, J.; Apostolopoulos, V.; Platat, C.; Al Dhaheri, A.S.; Ali, H.I.; Ismail, L.C.; Bosevski, M.; Stojanovska, L. Immunomodulatory Effects of Dietary Polyphenols. *Nutrients* **2021**, *13*, 728. [CrossRef]
77. Mollazadeh, H.; Cicero, A.F.G.; Blesso, C.N.; Pirro, M.; Majeed, M.; Sahebkar, A. Immune modulation by curcumin: The role of interleukin-10. *Crit. Rev. Food Sci. Nutr.* **2019**, *59*, 89–101. [CrossRef]
78. Gasmi Benahmed, A.; Gasmi, A.; Arshad, M.; Shanaida, M.; Lysiuk, R.; Peana, M.; Pshyk-Titko, I.; Adamiv, S.; Shanaida, Y.; Bjorklund, G. Health benefits of xylitol. *Appl. Microbiol. Biotechnol.* **2020**, *104*, 7225–7237. [CrossRef]
79. Salli, K.; Lehtinen, M.J.; Tiihonen, K.; Ouwehand, A.C. Xylitol's Health Benefits beyond Dental Health: A Comprehensive Review. *Nutrients* **2019**, *11*, 1813. [CrossRef]
80. Anand David, A.V.; Arulmoli, R.; Parasuraman, S. Overviews of Biological Importance of Quercetin: A Bioactive Flavonoid. *Pharmacogn. Rev.* **2016**, *10*, 84–89. [PubMed]
81. Javadi, F.; Ahmadzadeh, A.; Eghtesadi, S.; Aryaeian, N.; Zabihiyeganeh, M.; Rahimi Foroushani, A.; Jazayeri, S. The Effect of Quercetin on Inflammatory Factors and Clinical Symptoms in Women with Rheumatoid Arthritis: A Double-Blind, Randomized Controlled Trial. *J. Am. Coll. Nutr.* **2017**, *36*, 9–15. [CrossRef] [PubMed]
82. Tabrizi, R.; Tamtaji, O.; Mirhosseini, N.; Lankarani, K.; Akbari, M.; Heydari, S.; Dadgostar, E.; Asemi, Z. The effects of quercetin supplementation on lipid profiles and inflammatory markers among patients with metabolic syndrome and related disorders: A systematic review and meta-analysis of randomized controlled trials. *Crit. Rev. Food Sci. Nutr.* **2019**, *60*, 1855–1868. [CrossRef] [PubMed]
83. Konrad, M.; Nieman, D.C.; Henson, D.A.; Kennerly, K.M.; Jin, F.; Wallner-Liebmann, S.J. The acute effect of ingesting a quercetin-based supplement on exercise-induced inflammation and immune changes in runners. *Int. J. Sport Nutr. Exerc. Metab.* **2011**, *21*, 338–346. [CrossRef] [PubMed]
84. Heinz, S.; Henson, D.; Nieman, D.; Austin, M.; Jin, F. A 12-week supplementation with quercetin does not affect natural killer cell activity, granulocyte oxidative burst activity or granulocyte phagocytosis in female human subjects. *Br. J. Nutr.* **2010**, *104*, 849–857. [CrossRef] [PubMed]
85. Jalali, M.; Ranjbar, T.; Mosallanezhad, Z.; Mahmoodi, M.; Moosavian, S.P.; Ferns, G.A.; Jalali, R.; Sohrabi, Z. Effect of Propolis Intake on Serum C-Reactive Protein (CRP) and Tumor Necrosis Factor-alpha (TNF-alpha) Levels in Adults: A Systematic Review and Meta-Analysis of Clinical Trials. *Complement. Ther. Med.* **2020**, *50*, 102380. [CrossRef]
86. Zakerkish, M.; Jenabi, M.; Zaeemzadeh, N.; Hemmati, A.A.; Neisi, N. The Effect of Iranian Propolis on Glucose Metabolism, Lipid Profile, Insulin Resistance, Renal Function and Inflammatory Biomarkers in Patients with Type 2 Diabetes Mellitus: A Randomized Double-Blind Clinical Trial. *Sci. Rep.* **2019**, *9*, 7289. [CrossRef]
87. Zhu, A.; Wu, Z.; Zhong, X.; Ni, J.; Li, Y.; Meng, J.; Du, C.; Zhao, X.; Nakanishi, H.; Wu, S. Brazilian Green Propolis Prevents Cognitive Decline into Mild Cognitive Impairment in Elderly People Living at High Altitude. *J. Alzheimer's Dis.* **2018**, *63*, 551–560. [CrossRef]
88. Zhao, L.; Pu, L.; Wei, J.; Li, J.; Wu, J.; Zhonghao, X.; Gao, W.; Guo, C. Brazilian Green Propolis Improves Antioxidant Function in Patients with Type 2 Diabetes Mellitus. *Int. J. Environ. Res. Public Health* **2016**, *13*, 498. [CrossRef]
89. Mujica, V.; Orrego, R.; Fuentealba, R.; Leiva, E.; Zuniga, J. Propolis as an Adjuvant in the Healing of Human Diabetic Foot Wounds Receiving Care in the Diagnostic and Treatment Centre from the Regional Hospital of Talca. *J. Diabetes Res.* **2019**, *2019*, 2507578. [CrossRef]
90. Lardo, S.; Bagus, S.; Yongkie, I.; Djoko, W. The effect of a unique propolis compound (PropoelixTM) on clinical outcomes in patients with dengue hemorrhagic fever. *Infect. Drug Resist.* **2014**, *7*, 323–329. [CrossRef]
91. Maheshwari, G.; Sowrirajan, S.; Joseph, B. Extraction and Isolation of beta-Glucan from Grain Sources-A Review. *J. Food Sci.* **2017**, *82*, 1535–1545. [CrossRef] [PubMed]
92. Akramiene, D.; Kondrotas, A.; Didziapetriene, J.; Kevelaitis, E. Effects of beta-glucans on the immune system. *Medicina* **2007**, *43*, 597–606. [CrossRef] [PubMed]

93. Wu, Y.-S.; Ho, S.-Y.; Nan, F.-H.; Chen, S.-N. Ganoderma lucidum beta 1,3/1,6 glucan as an immunomodulator in inflammation induced by a high-cholesterol diet. *BMC Complement. Altern. Med.* **2016**, *16*, 500. [CrossRef]
94. Wang, J.; Yuan, Y.; Yue, T. Immunostimulatory activities of beta-d-glucan from Ganoderma Lucidum. *Carbohydr. Polym.* **2014**, *102*, 47–54. [CrossRef] [PubMed]
95. Morales, D.; Rutckeviski, R.; Villalva, M.; Abreu, H.; Soler-Rivas, C.; Santoyo, S.; Iacomini, M.; Smiderle, F.R. Isolation and comparison of alpha- and beta-D-glucans from shiitake mushrooms (Lentinula edodes) with different biological activities. *Carbohydr. Polym.* **2020**, *229*, 115521. [CrossRef] [PubMed]
96. Murphy, E.J.; Masterson, C.; Rezoagli, E.; O'Toole, D.; Major, I.; Stack, G.D.; Lynch, M.; Laffey, J.G.; Rowan, N.J. beta-Glucan extracts from the same edible shiitake mushroom Lentinus edodes produce differential in-vitro immunomodulatory and pulmonary cytoprotective effects—Implications for coronavirus disease (COVID-19) immunotherapies. *Sci. Total Environ.* **2020**, *732*, 139330. [CrossRef]
97. Gaullier, J.M.; Sleboda, J.; Ofjord, E.S.; Ulvestad, E.; Nurminiemi, M.; Moe, C.; Tor, A.; Gudmundsen, O. Supplementation with a soluble beta-glucan exported from Shiitake medicinal mushroom, Lentinus edodes (Berk.) singer mycelium: A crossover, placebo-controlled study in healthy elderly. *Int. J. Med. Mushrooms* **2011**, *13*, 319–326. [CrossRef]
98. Gordon, M.; Guralnik, M.; Kaneko, Y.; Mimura, T.; Goodgame, J.; DeMarzo, C.; Pierce, D.; Baker, M.; Lang, W. A phase II controlled study of a combination of the immune modulator, lentinan, with didanosine (ddI) in HIV patients with CD4 cells of 200–500/mm^3. *J. Med.* **1995**, *26*, 193–207.
99. Jung, S.J.; Jung, E.S.; Choi, E.K.; Sin, H.S.; Ha, K.C.; Chae, S.W. Immunomodulatory effects of a mycelium extract of Cordyceps (Paecilomyces hepiali; CBG-CS-2): A randomized and double-blind clinical trial. *BMC Complement. Altern. Med.* **2019**, *19*, 77. [CrossRef]
100. Smiderle, F.; Baggio, C.; Borato, D.; Santana-Filho, A.; Sassaki, G.; Iacomini, M.; Van Griensven, L. Anti-Inflammatory Properties of the Medicinal Mushroom Cordyceps militaris Might Be Related to Its Linear (1→3)-β-D-Glucan. *PLoS ONE* **2014**, *9*, e110266. [CrossRef]
101. Kang, H.J.; Baik, H.W.; Kim, S.J.; Lee, S.G.; Ahn, H.Y.; Park, J.S.; Park, S.J.; Jang, E.J.; Park, S.W.; Choi, J.Y.; et al. Cordyceps militaris Enhances Cell-Mediated Immunity in Healthy Korean Men. *J. Med. Food.* **2015**, *18*, 1164–1172. [CrossRef] [PubMed]
102. Lehne, G.; Haneberg, B.; Gaustad, P.; Johansen, P.; Preus, H.; Abrahamsen, T. Oral administration of a new soluble branched β-1,3-D-glucan is well tolerated and can lead to increased salivary concentrations of immunoglobulin A in healthy volunteers. *Clin. Exp. Immunol.* **2006**, *143*, 65–69. [CrossRef] [PubMed]
103. Tanaka, A.; Nishimura, M.; Sato, Y.; Sato, H.; Nishihira, J. Enhancement of the Th1-phenotype immune system by the intake of Oyster mushroom (Tamogitake) extract in a double-blind, placebo-controlled study. *J. Tradit. Complement. Med.* **2016**, *6*, 424–430. [CrossRef] [PubMed]
104. Farnoosh, G.; Akbariqomi, M.; Badri, T.; Bagheri, M.; Izadi, M.; Saeedi-Boroujeni, A.; Rezaei, E.; Ghaleh, H.; Aghamollaei, H.; Fasihi-Ramandi, M.; et al. Efficacy of a Low Dose of Melatonin as an Adjunctive Therapy in Hospitalized Patients with COVID-19: A Randomized, Double-blind Clinical Trial. *Arch. Med. Res.* **2020**, *53*, 79–85. [CrossRef] [PubMed]
105. Bocheva, G.; Slominski, R.M.; Janjetovic, Z.; Kim, T.K.; Bohm, M.; Steinbrink, K.; Reiter, R.J.; Kleszczynski, K.; Slominski, A.T. Protective Role of Melatonin and Its Metabolites in Skin Aging. *Int. J. Mol. Sci.* **2022**, *23*, 1238. [CrossRef]
106. Talib, W.H.; Alsayed, A.R.; Abuawad, A.; Daoud, S.; Mahmod, A.I. Melatonin in Cancer Treatment: Current Knowledge and Future Opportunities. *Molecules* **2021**, *26*, 2506. [CrossRef]
107. Faridzadeh, A.; Tabashiri, A.; Heidarian Miri, H.; Mahmoudi, M. The role of melatonin as an adjuvant in the treatment of COVID-19: A systematic review. *Heliyon* **2022**, *8*, e10906. [CrossRef]
108. Giovane, R.A.; Di Giovanni-Kinsley, S.; Keeton, E. Micronutrients for potential therapeutic use against COVID-19; a review. *Clin. Nutr. ESPEN* **2021**, *46*, 9–13. [CrossRef]
109. Borges, L.; Gennari-Felipe, M.; Dias, B.B.; Hatanaka, E. Melatonin, Zinc, and Vitamin C: Potential Adjuvant Treatment for COVID-19 Patients. *Front. Nutr.* **2021**, *8*, 821824. [CrossRef]
110. Zhang, R.; Wang, X.; Ni, L.; Di, X.; Ma, B.; Niu, S.; Liu, C.; Reiter, R. COVID-19: Melatonin as a potential adjuvant treatment. *Life Sci.* **2020**, *250*, 117583. [CrossRef]
111. Bjorklund, G.; Shanaida, M.; Lysiuk, R.; Antonyak, H.; Klishch, I.; Shanaida, V.; Peana, M. Selenium: An Antioxidant with a Critical Role in Anti-Aging. *Molecules* **2022**, *27*, 6613. [CrossRef]
112. Castiglione, D.; Platania, A.; Conti, A.; Falla, M.; D'Urso, M.; Marranzano, M. Dietary Micronutrient and Mineral Intake in the Mediterranean Healthy Eating, Ageing, and Lifestyle (MEAL) Study. *Antioxidants* **2018**, *7*, 79. [CrossRef] [PubMed]
113. Gombart, A.F.; Pierre, A.; Maggini, S. A Review of Micronutrients and the Immune System-Working in Harmony to Reduce the Risk of Infection. *Nutrients* **2020**, *12*, 236. [CrossRef] [PubMed]
114. Rawat, D.; Roy, A.; Maitra, S.; Gulati, A.; Khanna, P.; Baidya, D.K. Vitamin C and COVID-19 treatment: A systematic review and meta-analysis of randomized controlled trials. *Diabetes Metab. Syndr.* **2021**, *15*, 102324. [CrossRef] [PubMed]
115. Schencking, M.; Vollbracht, C.; Weiss, G.; Lebert, J.; Biller, A.; Goyvaerts, B.; Kraft, K. Intravenous vitamin C in the treatment of shingles: Results of a multicenter prospective cohort study. *Med. Sci. Monit.* **2012**, *18*, CR215–CR224. [CrossRef]
116. Sezikli, M.; Cetinkaya, Z.A.; Guzelbulut, F.; Yesil, A.; Cosgun, S.; Kurdas, O.O. Supplementing vitamins C and E to standard triple therapy for the eradication of Helicobacter pylori. *J. Clin. Pharm. Ther.* **2012**, *37*, 282–285. [CrossRef] [PubMed]

117. Fujii, T.; Salanti, G.; Belletti, A.; Bellomo, R.; Carr, A.; Furukawa, T.A.; Luethi, N.; Luo, Y.; Putzu, A.; Sartini, C.; et al. Effect of adjunctive vitamin C, glucocorticoids, and vitamin B1 on longer-term mortality in adults with sepsis or septic shock: A systematic review and a component network meta-analysis. *Intensive Care Med.* **2022**, *48*, 16–24. [CrossRef] [PubMed]
118. Chang, S.W.; Lee, H.C. Vitamin D and health—The missing vitamin in humans. *Pediatr. Neonatol.* **2019**, *60*, 237–244. [CrossRef]
119. Ao, T.; Kikuta, J.; Ishii, M. The Effects of Vitamin D on Immune System and Inflammatory Diseases. *Biomolecules* **2021**, *11*, 1624. [CrossRef]
120. Griffin, T.P.; Wall, D.; Blake, L.; Griffin, D.G.; Robinson, S.M.; Bell, M.; Mulkerrin, E.C.; O'Shea, P.M. Vitamin D Status of Adults in the Community, in Outpatient Clinics, in Hospital, and in Nursing Homes in the West of Ireland. *J. Gerontol. Ser. A Biol. Sci. Med. Sci.* **2020**, *75*, 2418–2425. [CrossRef]
121. Bae, M.; Kim, H. Mini-Review on the Roles of Vitamin C, Vitamin D, and Selenium in the Immune System against COVID-19. *Molecules* **2020**, *25*, 5346. [CrossRef] [PubMed]
122. Soltani-Zangbar, M.S.; Mahmoodpoor, A.; Dolati, S.; Shamekh, A.; Valizadeh, S.; Yousefi, M.; Sanaie, S. Serum levels of vitamin D and immune system function in patients with COVID-19 admitted to intensive care unit. *Gene Rep.* **2022**, *26*, 101509. [CrossRef]
123. Mailhot, G.; White, J.H. Vitamin D and Immunity in Infants and Children. *Nutrients* **2020**, *12*, 1233. [CrossRef] [PubMed]
124. Eckard, A.R.; O'Riordan, M.A.; Rosebush, J.C.; Lee, S.T.; Habib, J.G.; Ruff, J.H.; Labbato, D.; Daniels, J.E.; Uribe-Leitz, M.; Tangpricha, V.; et al. Vitamin D supplementation decreases immune activation and exhaustion in HIV-1-infected youth. *Antivir. Ther.* **2018**, *23*, 315–324. [CrossRef] [PubMed]
125. Liberman, K.; Njemini, R.; Luiking, Y.; Forti, L.N.; Verlaan, S.; Bauer, J.M.; Memelink, R.; Brandt, K.; Donini, L.M.; Maggio, M.; et al. Thirteen weeks of supplementation of vitamin D and leucine-enriched whey protein nutritional supplement attenuates chronic low-grade inflammation in sarcopenic older adults: The PROVIDE study. *Aging Clin. Exp. Res.* **2019**, *31*, 845–854. [CrossRef]
126. Folate, Folate—Fact Sheet for Health Professionals. U.S. Department of Health & Human Services: US National Institutes of Health. 2022. Available online: https://ods.od.nih.gov/factsheets/folate-HealthProfessional/ (accessed on 30 November 2022).
127. Prietl, B.; Treiber, G.; Mader, J.; Hoeller, E.; Wolf, M.; Pilz, S.; Graninger, W.; Obermayer-Pietsch, B.; Pieber, T. High-dose cholecalciferol supplementation significantly increases peripheral CD4+ Tregs in healthy adults without negatively affecting the frequency of other immune cells. *Eur. J. Nutr.* **2013**, *53*, 751–759. [CrossRef] [PubMed]
128. Uribe-Diaz, S.; Nazeer, N.; Jaime, J.; Vargas-Bermudez, D.S.; Yitbarek, A.; Ahmed, M.; Rodriguez-Lecompte, J.C. Folic acid enhances proinflammatory and antiviral molecular pathways in chicken B-lymphocytes infected with a mild infectious bursal disease virus. *Br. Poult. Sci.* **2022**, *63*, 1–13. [CrossRef]
129. Chen, Y.M.; Wei, J.L.; Qin, R.S.; Hou, J.P.; Zang, G.C.; Zhang, G.Y.; Chen, T.T. Folic acid: A potential inhibitor against SARS-CoV-2 nucleocapsid protein. *Pharm. Biol.* **2022**, *60*, 862–878. [CrossRef]
130. Voelkle, M.; Gregoriano, C.; Neyer, P.; Koch, D.; Kutz, A.; Bernasconi, L.; Conen, A.; Mueller, B.; Schuetz, P. Prevalence of Micronutrient Deficiencies in Patients Hospitalized with COVID-19: An Observational Cohort Study. *Nutrients* **2022**, *14*, 1862. [CrossRef]
131. Berger, M.M.; Shenkin, A.; Schweinlin, A.; Amrein, K.; Augsburger, M.; Biesalski, H.K.; Bischoff, S.C.; Casaer, M.P.; Gundogan, K.; Lepp, H.L.; et al. ESPEN micronutrient guideline. *Clin. Nutr.* **2022**, *41*, 1357–1424. [CrossRef]
132. Razzaque, M. Magnesium: Are We Consuming Enough? *Nutrients* **2018**, *10*, 1863. [CrossRef] [PubMed]
133. Mathew, A.; Panonnummal, R. 'Magnesium'-the master cation-as a drug—Possibilities and evidences. *BioMetals* **2021**, *34*, 955–986. [CrossRef] [PubMed]
134. Eskander, M.; Razzaque, M. Can Maintaining Optimal Magnesium Balance Reduce the Disease Severity of COVID-19 Patients? *Front. Endocrinol.* **2022**, *13*, 843152. [CrossRef] [PubMed]
135. Wallace, T.C. Combating COVID-19 and Building Immune Resilience: A Potential Role for Magnesium Nutrition? *J. Am. Coll. Nutr.* **2020**, *39*, 685–693. [CrossRef] [PubMed]
136. Maier, J.A.; Castiglioni, S.; Locatelli, L.; Zocchi, M.; Mazur, A. Magnesium and inflammation: Advances and perspectives. *Semin. Cell Dev. Biol.* **2021**, *115*, 37–44. [CrossRef]
137. Trapani, V.; Rosanoff, A.; Baniasadi, S.; Barbagallo, M.; Castiglioni, S.; Guerrero-Romero, F.; Iotti, S.; Mazur, A.; Micke, O.; Pourdowlat, G.; et al. The relevance of magnesium homeostasis in COVID-19. *Eur. J. Nutr.* **2022**, *61*, 625–636. [CrossRef]
138. Fiorentini, D.; Cappadone, C.; Farruggia, G.; Prata, C. Magnesium: Biochemistry, Nutrition, Detection, and Social Impact of Diseases Linked to Its Deficiency. *Nutrients* **2021**, *13*, 1136. [CrossRef]
139. Weyh, C.; Kruger, K.; Peeling, P.; Castell, L. The Role of Minerals in the Optimal Functioning of the Immune System. *Nutrients* **2022**, *14*, 644. [CrossRef]
140. Rangan, A.M.; Samman, S. Zinc intake and its dietary sources: Results of the 2007 Australian National Children's Nutrition and Physical Activity Survey. *Nutrients* **2012**, *4*, 611–624. [CrossRef]
141. Jafari, A.; Noormohammadi, Z.; Askari, M.; Daneshzad, E. Zinc supplementation and immune factors in adults: A systematic review and meta-analysis of randomized clinical trials. *Crit. Rev. Food Sci. Nutr.* **2022**, *62*, 3023–3041. [CrossRef]
142. Kumar, A.; Kubota, Y.; Chernov, M.; Kasuya, H. Potential role of zinc supplementation in prophylaxis and treatment of COVID-19. *Med. Hypotheses* **2020**, *144*, 109848. [CrossRef]
143. Li, Y.; Luo, W.; Liang, B. Circulating trace elements status in COVID-19 disease: A meta-analysis. *Front. Nutr.* **2022**, *9*, 982032. [CrossRef] [PubMed]

144. Howie, S.; Bottomley, C.; Chimah, O.; Ideh, R.C.; Ebruke, B.; Okomo, U.; Onyeama, C.; Donkor, S.; Rodrigues, O.; Tapgun, M.; et al. Zinc as an adjunct therapy in the management of severe pneumonia among Gambian children: Randomized controlled trial. *J. Glob. Health* **2018**, *8*, 010418. [CrossRef] [PubMed]
145. Kewcharoenwong, C.; Schuster, G.U.; Wessells, K.R.; Hinnouho, G.M.; Barffour, M.A.; Kounnavong, S.; Brown, K.H.; Hess, S.Y.; Samer, W.; Tussakhon, I.; et al. Daily Preventive Zinc Supplementation Decreases Lymphocyte and Eosinophil Concentrations in Rural Laotian Children from Communities with a High Prevalence of Zinc Deficiency: Results of a Randomized Controlled Trial. *J. Nutr.* **2020**, *150*, 2204–2213. [CrossRef] [PubMed]
146. Saper, R.B.; Rash, R. Zinc: An essential micronutrient. *Am. Fam. Physician* **2009**, *79*, 768–772.
147. Wessels, I.; Fischer, H.J.; Rink, L. Dietary and Physiological Effects of Zinc on the Immune System. *Annu. Rev. Nutr.* **2021**, *41*, 133–175. [CrossRef]
148. Razaghi, A.; Poorebrahim, M.; Sarhan, D.; Bjornstedt, M. Selenium stimulates the antitumour immunity: Insights to future research. *Eur. J. Cancer* **2021**, *155*, 256–267. [CrossRef]
149. Kieliszek, M.; Lipinski, B. Selenium supplementation in the prevention of coronavirus infections (COVID-19). *Med. Hypotheses* **2020**, *143*, 109878. [CrossRef]
150. Khatiwada, S.; Subedi, A. A Mechanistic Link Between Selenium and Coronavirus Disease 2019 (COVID-19). *Curr. Nutr. Rep.* **2021**, *10*, 125–136. [CrossRef]
151. Li, S.; Zhao, Q.; Zhang, K.; Sun, W.; Jia, X.; Yang, Y.; Yin, J.; Tang, C.; Zhang, J. Se deficiency induces renal pathological changes by regulating selenoprotein expression, disrupting redox balance, and activating inflammation. *Metallomics* **2020**, *12*, 1576–1584. [CrossRef]
152. Fath, M.K.; Naderi, M.; Hamzavi, H.; Ganji, M.; Shabani, S.; Ghahroodi, F.N.; Khalesi, B.; Pourzardosht, N.; Hashemi, Z.S.; Khalili, S. Molecular mechanisms and therapeutic effects of different vitamins and minerals in COVID-19 patients. *J. Trace. Elem. Med. Biol.* **2022**, *73*, 127044. [CrossRef] [PubMed]
153. Vahidi, H.; Barabadi, H.; Muthupandian, S. Emerging Selenium Nanoparticles to Combat Cancer: A Systematic Review. *J. Clust. Sci.* **2020**, *31*, 301–309. [CrossRef]
154. Guarner, F.; Schaafsma, G.J. Probiotics. *Int. J. Food Microbiol.* **1998**, *39*, 237–238. [CrossRef] [PubMed]
155. Schrezenmeir, J.; de Vrese, M. Probiotics, prebiotics, and synbiotics–approaching a definition. *Am. J. Clin. Nutr.* **2001**, *73* (Suppl. S2), 361S–364S. [CrossRef]
156. Batista, V.; Da Silva, T.; de Jesus, L.; Coelho Rocha, N.; Lima, F.; Tavares, L.; Azevedo, V.; Mancha-Agresti, P.; Drumond, M. Probiotics, Prebiotics, Synbiotics, and Paraprobiotics as a Therapeutic Alternative for Intestinal Mucositis. *Front. Microbiol.* **2020**, *11*, 544490. [CrossRef]
157. Lubiech, K.; Twaruzek, M. Lactobacillus Bacteria in Breast Milk. *Nutrients* **2020**, *12*, 3783. [CrossRef]
158. Kazemifard, N.; Dehkohneh, A.; Baradaran Ghavami, S. Probiotics and probiotic-based vaccines: A novel approach for improving vaccine efficacy. *Front. Med.* **2022**, *9*, 940454. [CrossRef]
159. Kuchmak, O.B.; Klymnyuk, S.I.; Romanyuk, L.B.; Pokryshko, O.V. The Use of Probiotics in Patients with Rheumatoid Arthritis. *Lik. Sprava* **2014**, *12*, 63–65.
160. Yeşilyurt, N.; Yılmaz, B.; Ağagündüz, D.; Capasso, R. Involvement of Probiotics and Postbiotics in the Immune System Modulation. *Biologics* **2021**, *1*, 89–110. [CrossRef]
161. Lakshmi, B.; Viswanath, B.; Sai Gopal, D.V.R. Probiotics as Antiviral Agents in Shrimp Aquaculture. *J. Pathog.* **2013**, *2013*, 424123. [CrossRef]
162. Naghibzadeh, N.; Salmani, F.; Nomiri, S.; Tavakoli, T. Investigating the effect of quadruple therapy with Saccharomyces boulardii or Lactobacillus reuteri strain (DSMZ 17648) supplements on eradication of Helicobacter pylori and treatments adverse effects: A double-blind placebo-controlled randomized clinical trial. *BMC Gastroenterol.* **2022**, *22*, 107.
163. Kanmani, P.; Satish Kumar, R.; Yuvaraj, N.; Paari, K.A.; Pattukumar, V.; Arul, V. Probiotics and its functionally valuable products-a review. *Crit. Rev. Food Sci. Nutr.* **2013**, *53*, 641–658. [CrossRef] [PubMed]
164. Schlee, M.; Wehkamp, J.; Altenhoefer, A.; Oelschlaeger, T.; Stange, E.; Fellermann, K. Induction of Human -Defensin 2 by the Probiotic Escherichia coli Nissle 1917 Is Mediated through Flagellin. *Infect. Immun.* **2007**, *75*, 2399–2407. [CrossRef] [PubMed]
165. Hare, P.; Englander, H.; Mok, W. Probiotic Escherichia coli Nissle 1917 Inhibits Bacterial Persisters that Survive Fluoroquinolone Treatment. *J. Appl. Microbiol.* **2022**, *132*, 4020–4032. [CrossRef] [PubMed]
166. Schlee, M.; Harder, J.; Koten, B.; Stange, E.F.; Wehkamp, J.; Fellermann, K. Probiotic lactobacilli and VSL#3 induce enterocyte beta-defensin 2. *Clin. Exp. Immunol.* **2008**, *151*, 528–535.
167. Gupta, T.; Kaur, H.; Kapila, S.; Kapila, R. Lactobacillus fermentum (MTCC-5898) alleviates Escherichia coli-induced inflammatory responses in intestinal epithelial cells by modulating immune genes and NF-kappaB signalling. *J. Appl. Microbiol.* **2021**, *131*, 3008–3017. [CrossRef]
168. Yousefi, B.; Eslami, M.; Ghasemian, A.; Kokhaei, P.; Salek Farrokhi, A.; Darabi, N. Probiotics importance and their immunomodulatory properties. *J. Cell. Physiol.* **2018**, *234*, 8008–8018. [CrossRef]
169. Kim, J.M.; Kim, J.S.; Kim, Y.J.; Oh, Y.K.; Kim, I.Y.; Chee, Y.J.; Han, J.S.; Jung, H.C. Conjugated linoleic acids produced by Lactobacillus dissociates IKK-gamma and Hsp90 complex in Helicobacter pylori-infected gastric epithelial cells. *Lab. Investig.* **2008**, *88*, 541–552. [CrossRef]

170. Lv, Z.; Wang, B.; Zhou, X.; Wang, F.; Xie, Y.; Zheng, H.; Lv, N. Efficacy and safety of probiotics as adjuvant agents for Helicobacter pylori infection: A meta-analysis. *Exp. Ther. Med.* **2015**, *9*, 707–716. [CrossRef]
171. Kandasamy, S.; Chattha, K.S.; Vlasova, A.N.; Rajashekara, G.; Saif, L.J. Lactobacilli and Bifidobacteria enhance mucosal B cell responses and differentially modulate systemic antibody responses to an oral human rotavirus vaccine in a neonatal gnotobiotic pig disease model. *Gut Microbes* **2014**, *5*, 639–651. [CrossRef]
172. Kawashima, T.; Ikari, N.; Kouchi, T.; Kowatari, Y.; Kubota, Y.; Shimojo, N.; Tsuji, N.M. The molecular mechanism for activating IgA production by Pediococcus acidilactici K15 and the clinical impact in a randomized trial. *Sci. Rep.* **2018**, *8*, 5065. [CrossRef] [PubMed]
173. Chapman, C.; Gibson, G.R.; Rowland, I. In vitro evaluation of single- and multi-strain probiotics: Inter-species inhibition between probiotic strains, and inhibition of pathogens. *Anaerobe* **2012**, *18*, 405–413. [CrossRef] [PubMed]
174. Diaz-Ropero, M.P.; Martin, R.; Sierra, S.; Lara-Villoslada, F.; Rodriguez, J.M.; Xaus, J.; Olivares, M. Two Lactobacillus strains, isolated from breast milk, differently modulate the immune response. *J. Appl. Microbiol.* **2007**, *102*, 337–343. [CrossRef]
175. You, S.; Ma, Y.; Yan, B.; Pei, W.; Wu, Q.; Ding, C.; Huang, C. The promotion mechanism of prebiotics for probiotics: A review. *Front. Nutr.* **2022**, *9*, 1000517. [CrossRef] [PubMed]
176. Zhao, Z.; Xu, S.; Zhang, W.; Wu, D.; Yang, G. Probiotic Escherichia coli NISSLE 1917 for inflammatory bowel disease applications. *Food Funct.* **2022**, *13*, 5914–5924. [CrossRef]
177. Zhou, L.; Liu, D.; Xie, Y.; Yao, X.; Li, Y. Bifidobacterium infantis Induces Protective Colonic PD-L1 and Foxp3 Regulatory T Cells in an Acute Murine Experimental Model of Inflammatory Bowel Disease. *Gut Liver* **2019**, *13*, 430–439. [CrossRef]
178. Xiao Joe, J.T.; Shi Sung, H.T.; Wu, J.L.; Lai, Y.S.; Lu, M.W. Dietary Administration of Novel Multistrain Probiotics from Healthy Grouper Intestines Promotes the Intestinal Immune Response against NNV Infection. *Life* **2021**, *11*, 1053. [CrossRef]
179. Olaya, G.N.; Rubiano, J.; Velez, F.; Duarte, K.; Salas Cárdenas, S.; Fernandez, M. In vitro antiviral activity of Lactobacillus casei and Bifidobacterium adolescentis against rotavirus infection monitored by NSP4 protein production. *J. Appl. Microbiol.* **2016**, *120*, 1041–1051. [CrossRef]
180. Ang, L.Y.; Too, H.K.; Tan, E.L.; Chow, T.V.; Shek, L.P.; Tham, E.H.; Alonso, S. Erratum to: Antiviral activity of Lactobacillus reuteri Protectis against Coxsackievirus A and Enterovirus 71 infection in human skeletal muscle and colon cell lines. *Virol. J.* **2016**, *13*, 186. [CrossRef]
181. Loniewski, I.; Skonieczna-Zydecka, K.; Solek-Pastuszka, J.; Marlicz, W. Probiotics in the Management of Mental and Gastrointestinal Post-COVID Symptomes. *J. Clin. Med.* **2022**, *11*, 5155. [CrossRef]
182. Xavier-Santos, D.; Padilha, M.; Fabiano, G.; Vinderola, G.; Cruz, A.; Sivieri, K.; Antunes, A. Evidences and perspectives of the use of probiotics, prebiotics, synbiotics, and postbiotics as adjuvants for prevention and treatment of COVID-19: A bibliometric analysis and systematic review. *Trends Food Sci. Technol.* **2022**, *120*, 174–192. [CrossRef] [PubMed]
183. Watzl, B.; Girrbach, S.; Roller, M. Inulin, oligofructose and immunomodulation. *Br. J. Nutr.* **2005**, *93* (Suppl. S1), S49–S55. [CrossRef]
184. Pujari, R.; Banerjee, G. Impact of prebiotics on immune response: From the bench to the clinic. *Immunol. Cell Biol.* **2021**, *99*, 255–273. [CrossRef] [PubMed]
185. Seifert, S.; Watzl, B. Inulin and oligofructose: Review of experimental data on immune modulation. *J. Nutr.* **2007**, *137* (Suppl. S11), 2563S–2567S. [CrossRef] [PubMed]
186. Poggi, A.; Benelli, R.; Vene, R.; Costa, D.; Ferrari, N.; Tosetti, F.; Zocchi, M.R. Human Gut-Associated Natural Killer Cells in Health and Disease. *Front. Immunol.* **2019**, *10*, 961. [CrossRef]
187. Fuhrmann, L.; Vahjen, W.; Zentek, J.; Gunther, R.; Saliu, E.M. The Impact of Pre- and Probiotic Product Combinations on Ex vivo Growth of Avian Pathogenic Escherichia coli and Salmonella Enteritidis. *Microorganisms* **2022**, *10*, 121. [CrossRef]
188. Zuntar, I.; Petric, Z.; Bursac Kovacevic, D.; Putnik, P. Safety of Probiotics: Functional Fruit Beverages and Nutraceuticals. *Foods* **2020**, *9*, 947. [CrossRef]
189. Dronkers, T.M.G.; Ouwehand, A.C.; Rijkers, G.T. Data on global analysis of clinical trials with probiotics. *Data Brief* **2020**, *32*, 106269. [CrossRef]
190. Dudek-Wicher, R.; Junka, A.; Paleczny, J.; Bartoszewicz, M. Clinical Trials of Probiotic Strains in Selected Disease Entities. *Int. J. Microbiol.* **2020**, *2020*, 8854119. [CrossRef]
191. Mirashrafi, S.; Hejazi Taghanaki, S.Z.; Sarlak, F.; Moravejolahkami, A.R.; Hojjati Kermani, M.A.; Haratian, M. Effect of Probiotics Supplementation on Disease Progression, Depression, General Health and Anthropometric Measurements in Relapsing-Remitting Multiple Sclerosis Patients: A Systematic Review and Meta-analysis of Clinical Trials. *Int. J. Clin. Pract.* **2021**, *75*, e14724. [CrossRef]
192. Boggio Marzet, C.; Burgos, F.; Del Compare, M.; Gerold, I.; Tabacco, O.; Vinderola, G. Approach to probiotics in pediatrics: The role of Lactobacillus rhamnosus GG. *Arch. Argent. Pediatr.* **2022**, *120*, e1–e7.
193. Ceccherini, C.; Daniotti, S.; Bearzi, C.; Re, I. Evaluating the Efficacy of Probiotics in IBS Treatment Using a Systematic Review of Clinical Trials and Multi-Criteria Decision Analysis. *Nutrients* **2022**, *14*, 2689. [CrossRef]
194. Zmora, N.; Zilberman-Schapira, G.; Suez, J.; Mor, U.; Dori-Bachash, M.; Bashiardes, S.; Kotler, E.; Zur, M.; Regev-Lehavi, D.; Ben Zeev, R.; et al. Personalized Gut Mucosal Colonization Resistance to Empiric Probiotics Is Associated with Unique Host and Microbiome Features. *Cell* **2018**, *174*, 1388–1405.e21. [CrossRef]

195. Mikawlrawng, K.; Kumar, S.; Bhatnagar, K. Drug Interactions, Safety and Efficacy of Probiotics. *Asian J. Med. Health* **2016**, *1*, 1–8. [CrossRef]
196. Shah, N.P. Probiotic bacteria: Selective enumeration and survival in dairy foods. *J. Dairy Sci.* **2000**, *83*, 894–907. [CrossRef]
197. Bansal, S.; Mangal, M.; Sharma, S.K.; Gupta, R.K. Non-dairy Based Probiotics: A Healthy Treat for Intestine. *Crit. Rev. Food Sci. Nutr.* **2016**, *56*, 1856–1867. [CrossRef]
198. Swanson, K.; Gibson, G.; Hutkins, R.; Reimer, R.; Reid, G.; Verbeke, K.; Scott, K.; Holscher, H.; Azad, M.; Delzenne, N.; et al. The International Scientific Association for Probiotics and Prebiotics (ISAPP) consensus statement on the definition and scope of synbiotics. *Nat. Rev. Gastroenterol. Hepatol.* **2020**, *17*, 687–701. [CrossRef]
199. FAO; WHO. *Report of a Joint FAO/WHO Working Group on Drafting Guidelines for the Evaluation of Probiotics in Food: London, Ontario, Canada, April 30–May 1, 2002*; World Health Organization: Roma, Italy, 2006; pp. 34–50. Available online: http://www.who.int/foodsafety/publications/fs_management/probiotics2/en/ (accessed on 28 March 2023).
200. Markowiak, P.; Slizewska, K. Effects of Probiotics, Prebiotics, and Synbiotics on Human Health. *Nutrients* **2017**, *9*, 1021. [CrossRef]
201. van den Nieuwboer, M.; Claassen, E. Dealing with the remaining controversies of probiotic safety. *Benef. Microbes* **2019**, *10*, 605–616. [CrossRef]
202. Yoha, K.S.; Nida, S.; Dutta, S.; Moses, J.A.; Anandharamakrishnan, C. Targeted Delivery of Probiotics: Perspectives on Research and Commercialization. *Probiotics Antimicrob Proteins* **2022**, *14*, 15–48. [CrossRef]
203. Merenstein, D.; Pot, B.; Leyer, G.; Ouwehand, A.C.; Preidis, G.A.; Elkins, C.A.; Hill, C.; Lewis, Z.T.; Shane, A.L.; Zmora, N.; et al. Emerging issues in probiotic safety: 2023 perspectives. *Gut Microbes* **2023**, *15*, 2185034. [CrossRef]
204. Suez, J.; Zmora, N.; Elinav, E. Probiotics in the next-generation sequencing era. *Gut Microbes* **2019**, *11*, 77–93. [CrossRef]
205. Kothari, D.; Patel, S.; Kim, S.-K. Probiotic supplements might not be universally-effective and safe: A review. *Biomed. Pharmacother.* **2019**, *111*, 537–547. [CrossRef]

MDPI AG
Grosspeteranlage 5
4052 Basel
Switzerland
Tel.: +41 61 683 77 34

Pharmaceuticals Editorial Office
E-mail: pharmaceuticals@mdpi.com
www.mdpi.com/journal/pharmaceuticals

www.ingramcontent.com/pod-product-compliance
Lightning Source LLC
Chambersburg PA
CBHW041431210926
51850CB00013B/3402